Core Techniques in Flap Reconstructive Microsurgery

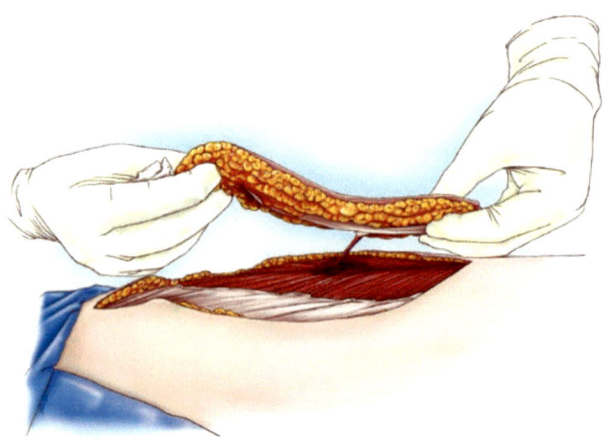

Dariush Nikkhah • Jeremy Rawlins
Georgios Pafitanis
Editors

Core Techniques in Flap Reconstructive Microsurgery

A Stepwise Guide

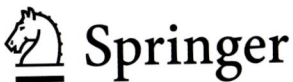

Editors
Dariush Nikkhah
Department of Plastic, Reconstructive and
Aesthetic Surgery
Royal Free Hospital & University College
London (UCL) Division of Surgical Sciences
London, UK

Jeremy Rawlins
Department of Plastic Surgery
Royal Perth Hospital
Perth, WA, Australia

Georgios Pafitanis
London Reconstructive Microsurgery Unit
(LRMU), Department of Plastic Surgery,
Emergency Care and Trauma Division (ECAT)
The Royal London Hospital, Barts Health NHS
Trust & University College Hospital London
(UCLH)
London, UK

ISBN 978-3-031-07677-0   ISBN 978-3-031-07678-7 (eBook)
https://doi.org/10.1007/978-3-031-07678-7

© Springer Nature Switzerland AG 2023

This work is subject to copyright. All rights are reserved by the Publisher, whether the whole or part of the material is concerned, specifically the rights of translation, reprinting, reuse of illustrations, recitation, broadcasting, reproduction on microfilms or in any other physical way, and transmission or information storage and retrieval, electronic adaptation, computer software, or by similar or dissimilar methodology now known or hereafter developed.

The use of general descriptive names, registered names, trademarks, service marks, etc. in this publication does not imply, even in the absence of a specific statement, that such names are exempt from the relevant protective laws and regulations and therefore free for general use.

The publisher, the authors, and the editors are safe to assume that the advice and information in this book are believed to be true and accurate at the date of publication. Neither the publisher nor the authors or the editors give a warranty, expressed or implied, with respect to the material contained herein or for any errors or omissions that may have been made. The publisher remains neutral with regard to jurisdictional claims in published maps and institutional affiliations.

This Springer imprint is published by the registered company Springer Nature Switzerland AG
The registered company address is: Gewerbestrasse 11, 6330 Cham, Switzerland

This book is dedicated to my patients and to the great mentors I have had in my training. I must also thank my dearest wife, Mahdis, who supported me through the editing of this book since 2018 and my wonderful children Rose and Alborz. I must thank my father and mother, who have given me all the opportunities throughout my life.
This book is also dedicated to the brave people of Iran and for my dream to return to a free Homeland.
'Women, Life, Freedom'

Dariush Nikkhah

Foreword

Reconstructive microsurgery has been developed for decades. However, there are still occasional failures and complications especially when a junior plastic surgeon starts to practice microsurgery. To minimise pitfalls, a book with concise description of the core free flaps step-by-step procedures would be beneficial for any plastic surgeon with special interest in reconstructive microsurgery.

It would act as a useful guide before surgery and act as a rapid reading reference for the procedure's crucial steps in conjunction with the copious reading from a long and detailed chapter of a formal textbook. With the accumulation of large experience from world masters, this book provides a shortcut to the core skillset and theoretical knowledge required for the competent and confident beginners in reconstructive microsurgery. It can also serve as an aide-memoire for surgeons in training or even for senior surgeons that do not perform specific flaps routinely in their daily practice or they may not be familiar with the challenges entailing a particular flap.

Georgios Pafitanis ('Gio') has been working with us as a microsurgery fellow, and he is very keen to make each flap perfect. Dariush Nikkhah demonstrated his deep insights in microsurgery during his visit to our department. Their efforts in providing this step-by-step guidebook to reconstructive microsurgery literature are an attempt to simplify and empirically dissect flap raising to provide an easy, but also an insightful, reminder to the key characteristics, the critical anatomy and nomenclature and the challenges that each core flap entails.

Our vast experience, at China Medical University Hospital, with major trauma and oncological reconstruction and the large number of patients requiring microsurgery, such as replantation, peripheral nerve repair and free tissue transfer reconstruction, allowed us to formulate a training pathway for young surgeons with safe and robust framework for the patient. The loss of a free flap or function is a disaster. The direction to improve the function and appearance instead of just achieving survival is a major motivation to publish this book. I hope it is very helpful for both surgeons and patients, also hope that this book can be expanded to more topics for reconstruction of acute and chronic problems in the future.

Hung-Chi Chen

Plastic Surgery
China Medical University
Taichung City, Taiwan

International Medical Service Center
China Medical University Hospital
Taichung City, Taiwan

Preface

Thou shalt make a Plan (Sir Harold Gillies) [1]

Microsurgery is a powerful tool that enables the Plastic Surgeon to reconstruct any defect with free tissue transplantation. In the early days there was no understanding of the blood supply of the body and surgeons like Gillies popularised tube pedicle flaps. It was not until McGregor and Jackson popularised the pedicled groin flap based on an axial blood supply that pushed the field of flap surgery forward [2]. This culminated in the first free tissue transplant performed in the west by Taylor and his subsequent landmark work on the Angiosomes of the human body [3]. These disruptions led to great innovations in the field that has led us to this book.

My experience in reconstructive microsurgery started at the Queen Victoria Hospital, East Grinstead, one of the modern powerhouses of plastic surgery where the first great toe transplant was performed in 1968 by Cobbett [4]. This hospital was the centre of Burns and Plastic surgery during the second world war and was purposefully built outside the capital. The epicentre of what is complex trauma is now in central London at the Major Trauma Centres.

Royal Perth where I did my fellowship offered a unique experience in the full spectrum of reconstructive microsurgery, extremity, head and neck, breast reconstruction, trauma and perineal reconstruction. The free tissue transplants I performed under the guidance of surgeons in that unit form the basis of much of my philosophy as a Consultant Plastic Surgeon in London. Replace like with like, take care of the donor site, preserve recipient vessels if you can and do not sacrifice major vessels. Another important point is that plastic surgeons are often the surgeons' surgeon and in many scenarios solve surgical problems for other specialities.

This book is a guidebook to the junior microsurgeon and provides a succinct, stepwise guide to workhorse flaps for the plastic surgeon in training and those who want to refresh their memories on more obscure flaps. Some of the cases have videos demonstrating pertinent steps in flap elevation or long-term outcomes. Each flap also has a discussion of the key papers and selected texts from the literature discussing the origins, pitfalls and technical refinements of those flaps. We have also managed to draw experts from a truly international stage, the UK, Australia, USA, South Korea, Japan, China, Europe to name a few.

In my career I have tried to refine and improve techniques in flap elevation; simplicity is the key to a successful operation. Complexity can invite failure unless meticulous planning for the case is undertaken. In this book the microsurgeon can be carried through steps with clinical illustrations. The book covers everything from microsurgical anastomosis, management of flap complications to stepwise description of fasciocutaneous and muscle flaps. I do hope over the course of my career this book will have many editions and be a useful guide to the Plastic Surgeon.

References

1. Gillies SH, Millard DR. The principles and art of plastic surgery. Boston, MA; Toronto, ON: Little, Brown & Co; 1957.
2. McGregor IA, Jackson IT. The groin flap. Br J Plast Surg. 1972;25(1):3–16.

3. Taylor GI, Palmer JH. The vascular territories (angiosomes) of the body: experimental study and clinical applications. Br J Plast Surg. 1987;40(2):113–41.
4. Cobbett JR. Free digital transfer: report of a case of transfer of a great toe to replace an amputated thumb. J Bone Joint Surg (Br). 1969;51:677–9.

London, UK   Dariush Nikkhah

Acknowledgements

The editors and the publisher especially acknowledge the collaboration of the following authors: Doctor Yelena Akelina for Chap. 1, Doctor Sandra Shurrey for Chap. 2, Doctor Petr Vondra for Chap. 29, and also thank Doctor Georgios Pafitanis for Chaps. 1–4, 15, 17, 23, 31 and 35, as well as Doctor Dariush Nikkhah for Chap. 22. Without their unwavering commitment, this work would not have been possible.

Contents

Part I Introduction to Reconstructive Microsurgery

1 **Microsurgery Essentials: Preconditions, Instrumentation, and Setup** 3
Alberto Ballestín and Sandra Shurey

2 **Basic and Advanced Microvascular Anastomotic Techniques** 11
Alberto Ballestín and Yelena Akelina

3 **Decision-Making in Flap Surgery: Reconstructive Ladder Versus Elevator** 19
Mohammed Farid, Thessa Friebel, and Dariush Nikkhah

4 **Assessment of Flap Perfusion: Microvascular Flowmetry** 25
Joshua Luck

5 **Re-exploration, Complications and Flap Salvage** 39
Paul Caine, Johann A. Jeevaratnam, Adam Misky, and Dariush Nikkhah

6 **The Use of Ultrasound Technology in Planning Perforator Flaps
and Lymphatic Surgery** 47
Giuseppe Visconti, Alessandro Bianchi, Akitatsu Hayashi,
and Marzia Salgarello

7 **Novel Microscopic Technologies in Reconstructive
Microsurgery/Microvascular Surgery** 55
Michalis Hadjiandreou and Georgios Pafitanis

8 **Robotic Microvascular and Free Flap Surgery: Overview of Current Robotic
Applications and Introduction of a Dedicated Robot for Microsurgery** 77
Joost A. G. N. Wolfs, Rutger M. Schols, and Tom J. M. van Mulken

9 **Technical Tips in Microvascular Surgery** 87
Marios Nicolaides and Georgios Pafitanis

Part II Core Flaps

10 **Temporal Artery Flaps** 99
Oliver J. Smith, Greg O'Toole, and Walid Sabbagh

11 **Supraorbital and Supratrochlear Artery Flaps - Forehead
Flap and Modifications** 105
Daniel B. Saleh and Alex Dearden

12 **Cervicofacial Flap** 117
Luke Geoghegan, Dariush Nikkhah, and Tiew Chong Teo

13 **Bowel Flaps - Jejunum Flap** 123
Georgios Pafitanis, Shin-Heng Chen, and Hung-Chi Chen

14	**Thoracodorsal Artery Flap: Latissimus Dorsi Flap**	133
	Mohammed Farid, Dariush Nikkhah, and Jeremy Rawlins	
15	**Thoracodorsal Artery Perforator Flap**	153
	Youn Hwan Kim and Lan Sook Chang	
16	**The Scapular Axis Flaps: An Expendable Direct Cutaneous Perforator with Many Options**	165
	Daniel Saleh and John Henton	
17	**Thoracoacromial Artery Flap: Pectoralis Major Muscle Flap**	171
	Jonathan A. Dunne, Ian C. C. King, Dariush Nikkhah, and Jeremy Rawlins	
18	**Transverse Cervical Artery Flap - Supraclavicular Flap**	181
	Pedro Ciudad, Juste Kaciulyte, Georgios Pafitanis, and Hung-Chi Chen	
19	**Inferior Epigastric Artery Flap: Deep Inferior Epigastric Artery Perforator Flap**	189
	Alexandra O'Neill, Dariush Nikkhah, Ahmed M. Yassin, and Bernard Luczak	
20	**Inferior and Superior Epigastric Artery Flaps: The Rectus Abdominis Muscle Flap**	205
	Matthew Wordsworth, Dariush Nikkhah, Alex Woollard, and Norbert Kang	
21	**Superficial Inferior Epigastric Artery and Superficial Circumflex Iliac Artery Perforator Combined Flaps**	213
	Hidehiko Yoshimatsu, Yuma Fuse, Ryo Karakawa, and Akitatsu Hayashi	
22	**Superior Gluteal Artery Perforator Flap**	219
	Mohammed Farid and Mohamed Shibu	
23	**Inferior Gluteal Artery Perforator Flap**	227
	Maleeha Mughal and Paul Roblin	
24	**The Lumbar Artery Perforator Flap: A True Alternative in Autologous Breast Reconstruction**	231
	Filip B. J. L. Stillaert, Phillip Blondeel, and Koenraad Van Landuyt	
25	**Right Gastroepiploic Artery: Omental Flap**	243
	Vladimir Anikin and Katherine de Rome	
26	**Dorsal Metacarpal Artery Flaps**	249
	Prateush Singh, Andreas Georgiou, Julia Ruston, and Dariush Nikkhah	
27	**Digital Artery Flaps: Homodigital and Heterodigital Island Flaps**	259
	Sirke Rinkoff, Julia Ruston, and Dariush Nikkhah	
28	**Radial Forearm Flap**	271
	Shahriar Raj Zaman, Qadir Khan, Jeremy M. Rawlins, Allan Ponniah, and Dariush Nikkhah	
29	**Posterior Interosseous Artery Flap**	281
	Douglas Copson, Dariush Nikkhah, and Mark Pickford	
30	**Venous Flaps**	289
	Christopher Deutsch and Jamil Moledina	
31	**Free Thenar Flap**	297
	Dimitris Reissis, Petr Vondra, and Zheng Yumao	

Contents

32 Medial and Lateral Arm Fasciocutaneous Flaps 305
Katerina Kyprianou, Georgios Pafitanis, Dajiang Song, and Youmao Zhen

33 The Groin Flap: The Workhorse Flap for Upper Limb Reconstruction 313
Hari Venkatramani, David Zargaran, Dariush Nikkhah, Julia Ruston,
and S. Raja Sabapathy

**34 Superficial Circumflex Iliac Artery Perforator Flap: A Thin
and Versatile Option for Limb and Head and Neck Reconstruction** 325
Juan Enrique Berner, Dariush Nikkhah, and Tiew Chong Teo

**35 Lateral Circumflex Femoral Artery—Anterolateral Thigh Flap:
Anterolateral Thigh Flap** 333
Robert Miller, Dariush Nikkhah, Edmund Fitzgerald O'Connor,
and Jeremy Rawlins

**36 Transverse Upper Gracilis (TUG) Flap: A Reliable Alternative
for Breast Reconstruction** 343
Juan Enrique Berner and Adam Blackburn

37 Medial Circumflex Femoral Artery: Gracilis Muscle Flap 353
Robert Miller, Dariush Nikkhah, and Graeme Glass

38 Profunda Artery Perforator Flap 365
Tomoyuki Yano

39 Medial Femoral Condyle Flap 373
Anthony L. Logli and Alexander Y. Shin

40 Medial Sural Artery Perforator Flap 385
Dimitris Reissis, Dariush Nikkhah, Bernard Luczak, and Georgios Orfaniotis

41 Peroneal Artery Flaps: The Free Fibula Flap 397
Amitabh Thacoor, Daniel Butler, Dariush Nikkhah, and Jeremy Rawlins

42 Posterior Tibial and Peroneal Perforators Flaps 409
Ahmed M. Yassin, Muholan Kanapathy, and Georgios Pafitanis

43 Second Toe Free Flap 419
Dariush Nikkhah, Juan Enrique Berner, Petr Vondra, Bran Sivakumar,
and Mark Pickford

44 Great Toe Flaps 429
Dariush Nikkhah and Norbert Kang

45 The Medial Plantar Flap 443
Alexander E. J. Trevatt, Miguel A. Johnson, and Tiew C. Teo

Part III Common Recipient Vessels

46 Chest Wall Recipient Vessels Access 455
Pennylouise Hever, Dariush Nikkhah, Alexandra Molina, and Martin Jones

47 Head and Neck Recipient Vessels Access 465
Alexandra O'Neill, Juan Enrique Berner, and Georgios Pafitanis

48 Upper Limb Recipient Vessels Access 473
Zhi Yang Ng, Calum Honeyman, Amir Sadr, and Dariush Nikkhah

49 Lower Limb Recipient Vessels Access 481
Yezen Sheena, Georgios Pafitanis, Dariush Nikkhah,
Edmund Fitzgerald O'Connor, and Jeremy Rawlins

50 Lymphatic Supermicrosurgery 489
Takumi Yamamoto and Nana Yamamoto

Part IV   Appendix

51 Cadaveric Anatomy: Microvascular Flaps Dissection 499
Georgios Pafitanis, Dajiang Song, and Youmao Zheng

List of Videos

Video 5.1 Hyperaemia in the immediate post-operative period following great toe to hand transfer

Video 5.2 Demonstration of a congested gracilis flap in a lower limb flap reconstruction

Video 14.1 This video narrated by Dr Dariush Nikkhah demonstrates the elevation of a Free LD flap for extremity reconstruction

Video 19.1 Narrated video demonstrating tips and tricks on DIEP flap elevation, recipient vessel preparation, microsurgery (arterial anastomosis and Venous anastomosis with Vein coupler) and inset. Case performed and narrated by Dariush Nikkhah

Video 22.1 SGAP flap elevation, demonstrating good capillary refill and pulsating perforator. Flap is rotated into perineum

Video 22.2 SGAP flap de epitheliasation before transfer as a propeller flap to obliterate dead space in perineum

Video 29.1 Identification of ECU/EDM septum by flexion and extension of the little finger during PIA flap harvest

Video 29.2 Large SCC of the right thumb necessitating amputation and coverage with a reverse PIA flap

Video 34.1 SCIP flap raising technique demonstration (Part 1)

Video 34.2 SCIP flap raising technique demonstration (part 2)

Video 35.1 A demonstration of the de-roofing technique in ALT flap harvest

Video 35.2 Post operative outcome for upper limb defect reconstruction with an ALT flap

Video 35.3 This video narrated by Dr Dariush Nikkhah demonstrated an overview of the ALT flap raise

Video 37.1 This video demonstrates the post-operative outcome from a free functional gracilis muscle transfer for elbow reanimation after a brachial plexus injury

Video 41.1 Demonstration of an osteotomy of a fibula flap whilst protecting the underlying pedicle with a malleable retractor

Video 41.2 Narrated video by Dr Dariush Nikkhah demonstrating steps in raising a osteocutaneous free fibula flap to reconstruct the mandible in a patient with a large odontogenic myxoma

Video 43.1 This narrated video by Dr. Dariush Nikkhah, Juan Berner and TC Teo demonstrates a second toe to hand transfer for thumb reconstruction

Video 44.1 Demonstration of dexterity after the great toe transfer by passing a coin between the reconstructed thumb and opposing digits

Video 44.2 Demonstration of circumduction of the great toe transfer

Video 49.1 Preoperative markings in planning a free flap reconstruction of the right lateral ankle. The surgeon is planning extension along the fasciotomy lines to access the anterior tibial vessels

Part I
Introduction to Reconstructive Microsurgery

Microsurgery Essentials: Preconditions, Instrumentation, and Setup

Alberto Ballestín and Sandra Shurey

1.1 Introduction

Reconstructive microsurgery is the surgical technique that uses the optical magnification of a microscope, the precision of specific instruments, and the accuracy of small sutures (8/0 to 13/0) to achieve fine dissections and free tissue transfers by performing vascular and nerve anastomoses of small diameter. Although nowadays microsurgery is a fundamental part of reconstructive surgery, it has a relatively short but intense history.

The development of reconstructive microsurgery was primarily influenced by advances in vascular surgery. The main vascular anastomosis techniques were not described until the beginning of the twentieth century until the experimental work of Carrel and Guthrie [1]. Later, in 1921, the microscope was introduced for the first time in surgery by the otolaryngologist Nylen [2]. Then, the progressive improvement of microscopes, together with the synthesis of anticoagulants and antibiotics, laid the necessary foundations for surgeons Julius H. Jacobson and Ernesto L. Suárez to perform the first vascular anastomoses in vessels of 1 mm diameter in the 1960s [3]. Subsequently, first successes were obtained in replantation of severed body parts during the following years [4]. During that period, Harry J. Buncke and other pioneers carried out innovative studies on replantation and tissue transplants in animals, developing many of the basic principles of this discipline [5]. After years of research, the first free tissue transfer was performed on a patient in 1972 [6]. Since then, a multitude of designs and techniques have been described for performing free tissue transfers and microsurgical repairs which are used in countless procedures: replantation, transplantation, neurosurgery, limb reconstruction, head and neck surgery, breast reconstruction, peripheral nerve surgery, lymphedema, etc.

Microsurgery has ostensibly improved the treatment of patients affected by a wide range of tissue defects. In this book chapter, we first describe the necessary materials for microsurgery, such as specific instruments, optical magnification, and sutures. Then, we detail the microsuture techniques, the main formal training programs, and some different microsurgical setups.

1.2 Surgical Magnification: Loupes and Microscopes

Microscopy is an integral part of reconstructive surgery but also of many other surgical disciplines nowadays. Otolaryngology was the first discipline to incorporate the microscope into its surgeries [2], ophthalmology added illumination [7], and neurosurgery allowed the use of infrared and other wavelength cameras to use contrast-enhancing techniques for specific anatomical structure visualization [8]. The technical evolution of surgical microscopy over decades has been impressive and very useful for surgeons. The microscopic magnification of the surgical field improves visual acuity and enhances precise treatments. Small anatomical details are appreciated allowing the performance of fine dissections and microsuture techniques in a precise and easier way nowadays.

In reconstructive surgery, a surgeon's first introduction to magnification is usually with the use of surgical loupes. Magnifying loupes are tremendously useful for dissections that do not require great magnification capacity but require working in large or distant surgical approaches. However, when high magnification is required to perform microsurgery, the use of a microscope is essential, as loupes typically have 2.5–5× magnification, while microscopes provide 2–40× magnification. In addition, the ergonomic improvements of microscopes, the variation of the magnification and its high-

---

A. Ballestín (✉)
Tumor Microenvironment Laboratory, Institut Curie, Paris, France

S. Shurey
MicroShure Ltd, Brixham, England, UK

© Springer Nature Switzerland AG 2023
D. Nikkhah et al. (eds.), *Core Techniques in Flap Reconstructive Microsurgery*, https://doi.org/10.1007/978-3-031-07678-7_1

quality visualization, allow the performance of procedures with high precision that are not possible to perform with surgical loupes. However, surgical loupes are portable, easy to use, and cost-effective compared to surgical microscopes [9].

1.2.1 Surgical Loupes

Surgical loupes are very useful when high magnification is not required but an improvement in technical precision is needed. Three different optical systems can be used for its manufacture: simple, compound (Galilean), and prismatic [10].

- Simple loupes consist of a single meniscus lens; they are not currently marketed by almost any company since the other two systems are better.
- Compound (Galilean) loupe systems are the most common; they are made up of two magnifying lenses separated from each other. Compared to the simple system, the Galilean system offers greater magnification, greater depth of view, and longer working distances.
- Prismatic loupes consist of a more complex optical system that provide higher magnification and typically longer working distances than simple and compound loupes. However, its weight is greater, as well as its cost.

Regarding the placement of the loupes on the glasses, there are two types of designs: through-the-lens (TTL) and flip-up loupes (Fig. 1.1). They are different; the choice of surgical loupes should be based on personal preferences prioritizing surgical-specific needs. Both designs have advantages and disadvantages when compared.

- TTL: It is a custom design of loupes, which are mounted through the lens of the glasses depending on the user's specific interpupillary distance. The loupes are positioned at a steep declination angle to the eyeglass lenses to allow the user to achieve an ergonomic posture during surgery.
- Flip-up loupes: It is a foldable design of loupes that have the optics attached to a hinge mechanism. This system allows magnifying lenses to be moved out or in to work with or without magnification. They are cheaper than TTL, and usually interpupillary variation is possible; therefore they can be used by surgeons with different interpupillary distances. However, TTL loupes offer a wider field of view than flip-up loupes, because lenses are closer to the user's eyes, which means that users can see a larger area of surgical field than with the same magnification with flip-up loupes.

Loupes are usually available with a fixed magnification between 2.5× and 5×, although there are some allowing more magnification. However, for all optical systems, the higher the magnification of the loupes, the greater their weight, the smaller the field of view, and the narrower the depth of focus becomes.

It is also possible to use a light source with surgical loupes. Usually the light source is connected by cable to a battery that can be carried in surgeon's pocket, but there are also rechargeable or battery-powered models that have the batteries in the temple of the glasses.

Loupes offer flexibility, portability, and lower cost compared to microscopes. However, they offer lower magnification power and do not have coaxial illumination, and surgeon's ergonomics are much poorer. The working distance of surgical loupes is fixed; therefore, surgeon must find a correct position to obtain a focused view. This can lead to improper body positions causing neck and back fatigue and even leading to musculoskeletal injuries.

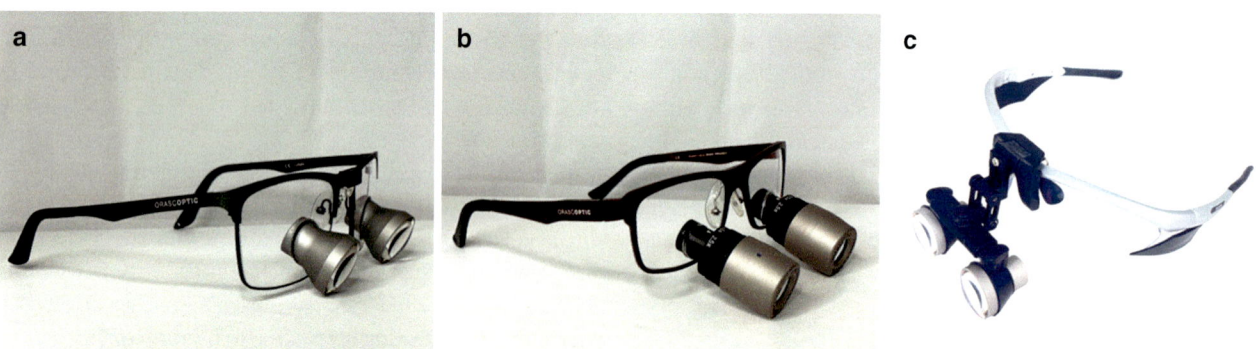

Fig. 1.1 Different types of surgical loupes. (**a**) Through-the-lens Galilean loupes (2.5×). (**b**) Through-the-lens variable magnification loupes (2.5×–3.5×–4.5×). (**c**) Flip-up Galilean loupes (2.5×). (*Images courtesy of Optimedic*)

1.2.2 Surgical Microscope

Surgical microscopes allow for stereoscopic vision and therefore for in-depth orientation. This, in turn, allows safe and precise use of instruments and improves ergonomics, since it can be operated while maintaining an upright position, preventing fatigue and postural alterations that could lead to muscle strain or injury.

To use surgical instruments on the patient using a microscope, a certain distance is required between the surgical approach and the main lens of the microscope. This space is called the working distance. In reconstructive microsurgery, the working distance is generally between 200 and 400 mm and must be adapted in each situation regarding the surgeon to maintain a correct working posture.

The magnification factor of a microscope is variable and allows varying between 1.5× and 30× magnifications. Microscopes permit modifying the magnification/zoom during surgery, maintaining the focal length while having a relaxed posture for the surgeon.

Microscopes also allow variation of the working distance, allowing to evaluate different anatomical planes with good focus and high image quality. Thus, it makes the surgeon work in a comfortable way.

Today the surgical microscope (Fig. 1.2) is indispensable in reconstructive surgery. Its main parts are:

- Binocular tubes. They are mobile to adapt the interpupillary distance of the surgeon. It is also possible to regulate the diopters; for this, it is recommended that each eye binocular is individually focused to achieve maximum visual acuity.

- To facilitate ergonomics, usually 180° tiltable binocular tubes are used; also it can be turned about its optical axis. The widefield eyepieces usually have 10× or 12.5× providing magnification. Usually there are two binoculars, allowing face-to-face surgery by two surgeons. The mounting of three or four binoculars is also possible in some microscopes if further assistance was needed.
- Variation system. Progressive zoom allows going from low to high magnification during surgery.
- Lens of the main objective. It largely defines the image quality, and its positioning usually sets the focal length ranging from 100 to 400 mm.

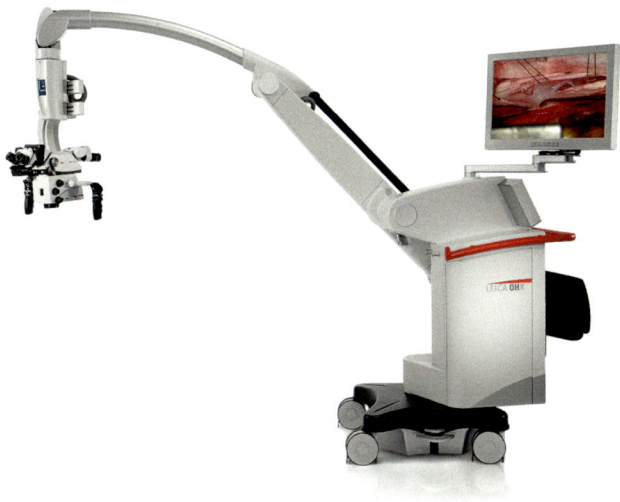

Fig. 1.2 Surgical microscope. (*Courtesy of Leica*)

- Coaxial field lighting, which usually is halogen or xenon light.
- Camera to record procedures and take images to follow up surgeries.
- Some models have an infrared camera that allows, through the use of contrasts such as ICG (Indocyanine Green), to evaluate the lymphatic system or to perform intraoperative angiography.
- Pedal. It allows movement in XY without manipulating the stand with the hands; it also allows ordering the taking of images or video, as well as launching programs for evaluation with an infrared camera.

1.2.3 Heads-Up 3D Microscopy and Exoscopes

New 3D heads-up microscopes (Fig. 1.3) have made it possible to improve the comfort of the microsurgeon since they allow to operate sitting or standing with the head up, without compromising the quality of the image or the technical accuracy [11].

Although its use has been anecdotal, exoscopes provide a high-definition image of the field from a digital camera system projected onto a 2D or 3D high-resolution monitor [12, 13].

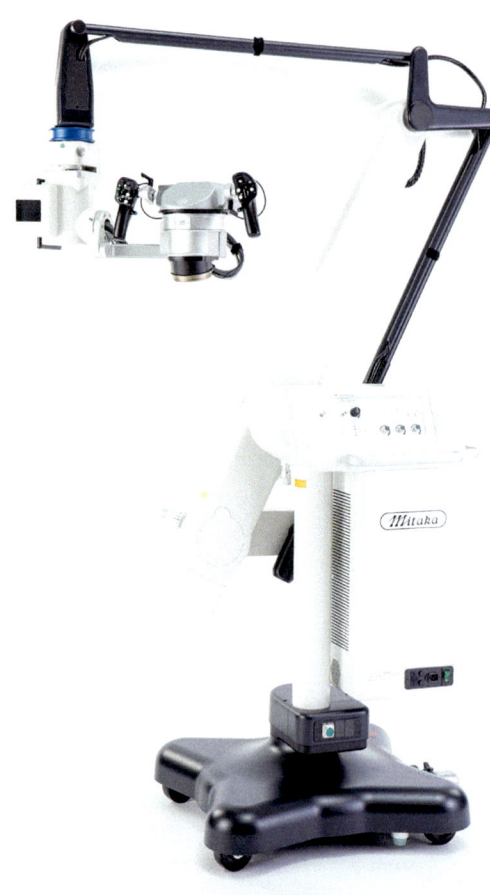

Fig. 1.3 3D heads-up microscopes. (*Courtesy of Mitaka*)

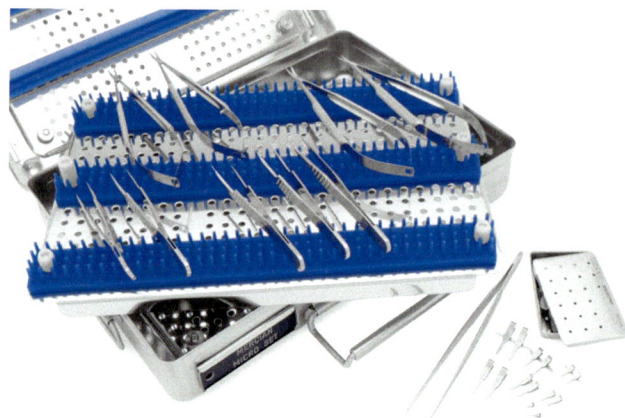

Fig. 1.4 Microsurgery instrument set. (*Courtesy of Mercian*)

1.3 Microsurgical Equipment, Instruments, and Sutures

Specific and high-quality instruments are key to the performance and precision of microsurgical techniques. Each instrument should have a satin finish to avoid glare under the microscope and should be long enough to rest properly in the surgeon's hands. Some instruments are spring-loaded; on these instruments the closing tension should be gentle enough to avoid fatigue.

A set of microsurgical instruments (Fig. 1.4) should contain microneedle holder, straight and curved Dumont forceps, vasodilator forceps, microscissors, clamps, microvascular clamp applicator, and sutures.

Needle holders usually have spring-loaded handles that can have a round or flat grip. The fine tips can be curved, angled, or straight. The tip should be fine enough to hold the needle without distorting its curve during use. Needle holders with lock ratchets should not be used because the release of the lock makes impossible to control the movement; therefore, it can be a problem when working with high magnification since precision is reduced. Angled microsurgical forceps can also be used as needle holders to handle very small sutures as they are less bulky and allow fine handling.

Microsurgical forceps no. 3 and 5 are essential in any microsurgical instrument set. Their tips should evenly coincide over a length of 2 mm so that the 10/0 and 11/0 nylon thread can be easily collected without damaging it. These microforceps can be straight, angled, or curved.

Vasodilator forceps are modified forceps, and at the tip they are rounded and polished, so they can be inserted into the end of a cut vessel, and through their gentle opening, counterpressure is provided while suturing. Furthermore, vasodilation prior to the anastomosis performance can facilitate the procedure.

Microscissors should have a spring handle, and curved or straight blades can be short or long depending on personal preference. The tips should be rounded so that the tissues adjacent to the vessels can be dissected without damaging them.

The adventitia scissors are similar, but with straight and sharp blades; they are used to remove the adventitia from the vessels and/or remove the sutures made.

Microvascular clamps are used to block blood flow; depending on the diameter of the vessel, a different clamp must be chosen. Caution must be exercised during use; blood on the clamp joint can render them ineffective.

Clamp applicator forceps are specifically designed for the proper handling of microvascular clamps.

Microsurgical sutures must be inert and antithrombogenic. That is why nonabsorbable synthetic monofilaments are commonly used. Nylon has these characteristics, its *strength* and handling during knotting are adequate, and it is usually black, which makes it clearly visible under the microscope. Polypropylene monofilament and polyester monofilament are also inert sutures that retain their strength well in the tissue, and the material is softer than nylon; however, their light color makes them more difficult to see under the microscope, and special care is necessary when handling them to not to damage them.

All these materials are available in different sizes: 8/0 (0.4 metric), 9/0 (0.3 metric), 10/0 (0.2 metric), and 11/0 (0.1 metric). The 11/0 sutures have an average diameter of 18 µm, those of 10/0 of 25 µm, those of 9/0 of 35 µm, and those of 8/0 of 45 µm. Nowadays, 12/0 and 13/0 sutures are also available for supramicrosurgery.

Regarding the needle, the monofilament material is usually inserted into a 3/8 circle needle end. Different characteristics are important to take into account when selecting the best needle for each situation: needle length (size of the needle in mm), needle profile (curved and usually 3/8, but half circle needles are occasionally used), needle diameter (measured in microns and dependent on the needs, until very recently, 130 µm needles were the finest available, but diameters as fine as 30 µm are now manufactured), and cross section (the vast majority of needles used in microsurgery have an atraumatic tip and a round body).

1.4 Microsurgical Training

Microsurgical techniques have historically been learned through observation and practice in the operating room and also through courses developed in multiple laboratories around the world. Microsurgery has a steep learning curve; therefore, following a proper training program and deliberate repetitive practice are essential to obtain the necessary skills.

1.4.1 Formal Microsurgery Training Curriculum

Educational programs for microsurgery include the use of surgical microscopes, the handling of specific microsurgical instruments, and practice with small sutures. Basic techniques of suturing and anastomosis are also taught. Increasing restrictions on the use of live animals for surgical training courses have led to the development of synthetic, inert organic, and virtual simulation for learning surgical skills.

Most of the courses begin with basic suturing exercises either on surgical gloves, gauzes, or microsuture cards [14]. Many programs continue with different silicone elastomer tubes to simulate blood vessels, but there are also some laboratories that work with cryopreserved arteries [15].

For the practice of microdissection and vascular anastomoses, various inert organic models are used. The main organic models are the chicken wing [16] and the chicken thigh [17] that allow the practice in vessels of optimal size for teaching microsurgery and supermicrosurgical techniques. Furthermore, these models can be used to practice flaps, such as the chicken thigh adductor profundus free muscle flap [18].

The highest fidelity simulator for clinical microsurgery is the rat, which remains as an indispensable live animal model for many training courses worldwide. It allows interaction with bleeding, spasm, thrombosis, and a real anatomy [19]. Despite the new simulation models for supermicrosurgery [20], the rat continues to be the best preparation model for achieving high standards of competency. Different submillimetric vessels in the rat have been described for performing supermicrosurgical anastomoses [21], vascularized lymph node transfers [22], and lymphovenous anastomoses [23].

In addition, and despite the anatomical variations, the pig has proven to be a great translational model for teaching free and perforator flaps [24–27]. But the cost and the requirements to work with this animal restrict its use to specific surgical training centers with a highly specialized team of veterinarians.

Due to the great disparity of training programs, the International Society for Experimental Microsurgery (ISEM) published some recommendations [28]. In addition, the International Microsurgery Simulation Society (IMSS) reached an international consensus of experts in which the minimum standards for a basic microsurgery course and the minimum thresholds for training were established [29] and suggested the use of microsurgical anastomosis global rating scales [30] to assess learning.

Recently, the pandemic situation of Covid-19 significantly affected medical education and made face-to-face microsurgical teaching adapt to the new times [31]; also mass online forums emerged to help learning in times of social isolation [32, 33]. We are perhaps facing nowadays a paradigm shift that will lead to new evolutions in the learning of reconstructive microsurgery.

1.4.2 Home Microsurgical Training Setup

Following a well-established curricular program and receiving training from experts is the best form of learning microsurgery. Then, to strengthen knowledge and refine skills, repetitive individual practice is needed. However, the lack of time and access to microscopy and instruments are impediments in this regard. The ideal situation would be to have several periodical weeks of practice in a microsurgery laboratory, although this optimal form of training is not always possible. One way to complement the formal training would be to establish a home setup for microsurgery training and then to follow online teaching contents made by experts for the correct review and practice of microsurgical techniques [34].

The most expensive required materials are the microscope and instruments. However, nowadays a cheap tabletop microscope with an ×5–40 magnification can be purchased online [35]; it is important that focal distance allows practice. Basic suture practice can even be performed using a smartphone [36] although magnification, working distance, and quality vary greatly with respect to clinical practice.

Training can be performed with a basic set of instruments (needle holder, straight and angled forceps, and microsurgical scissors), vascular clamps, and microsutures. All these materials can be found online at cheap prices, although without the quality standards required for clinical practice. Furthermore, simulation methods described previously can be used (surgical gloves, gauzes, silastic tubes, chicken thighs and wings) which are inexpensive and easily available. This training method will not replace formal courses but is a useful complement for continued practice.

References

1. Carrel A. La technique opératoire des anastomoses vasculaires et de la transplantation des visceres. Lyon: Association Typographique; 1902.
2. Nylen CO. The microscope in aural surgery, its first use and later development. Acta Otolaryngol Suppl. 1954;116:226–40.
3. Jacobson JH, Suarez EL. Microsurgery in anastomosis of small vessels. Surg Forum. 1960;11:243–5.
4. Malt RA, McKhann C. Replantation of severed arms. JAMA. 1964;189:716–22.
5. Buncke HJ, Buncke GM, Kind GM. The early history of microsurgery. Plast Reconstr Surg. 1996;98(6):1122–3.
6. McLean DH, Buncke HJ Jr. Autotransplant of omentum to a large scalp defect, with microsurgical revascularization. Plast Reconstr Surg. 1972;49(3):268–74.
7. Troutman RC. The operating microscope in ophthalmic surgery. Trans Am Ophthalmol Soc. 1965;63:335–48.
8. La Rocca G, Della Pepa GM, Menna G, Altieri R, Ius T, Rapisarda A, et al. State of the art of fluorescence guided techniques in neurosurgery. J Neurosurg Sci. 2019;63(6):619–24.
9. Stanbury SJ, Elfar J. The use of surgical loupes in microsurgery. J Hand Surg [Am]. 2011;36(1):154–6.
10. Baker JM, Meals RA. A practical guide to surgical loupes. J Hand Surg [Am]. 1997;22(6):967–74.
11. Mendez BM, Chiodo MV, Vandevender D, Patel PA. Heads-up 3D microscopy: an ergonomic and educational approach to microsurgery. Plast Reconstr Surg Glob Open. 2016;4(5):e717.
12. De Virgilio A, Costantino A, Ebm C, Conti V, Mondello T, Di Bari M, et al. High definition three-dimensional exoscope (VITOM 3D) for microsurgery training: a preliminary experience. Eur Arch Otorhinolaryngol. 2020;277(9):2589–95.
13. Pafitanis G, Hadjiandreou M, Alamri A, Uff C, Walsh D, Myers S. The exoscope versus operating microscope in microvascular surgery: a simulation non-inferiority trial. Arch Plast Surg. 2020;47(3):242–9.
14. Uson J, Calles MC. Design of a new suture practice card for microsurgical training. Microsurgery. 2002;22(8):324–8.
15. Lausada NR, Escudero E, Lamonega R, Dreizzen E, Raimondi JC. Use of cryopreserved rat arteries for microsurgical training. Microsurgery. 2005;25(6):500–1.
16. Olabe J. Microsurgical training on an in vitro chicken wing infusion model. Surg Neurol. 2009;72(6):695–9.
17. Chen WF, Eid A, Yamamoto T, Keith J, Nimmons GL, Lawrence WT. A novel supermicrosurgery training model: the chicken thigh. J Plast Reconstr Aesthet Surg. 2014;67(7):973–8.
18. Pafitanis G, Serrar Y, Raveendran M, Ghanem A, Myers S. The chicken thigh adductor profundus free muscle flap: a novel validated non-living microsurgery simulation training model. Arch Plast Surg. 2017;44(4):293–300.
19. Shurey S, Akelina Y, Legagneux J, Malzone G, Jiga L, Ghanem AM. The rat model in microsurgery education: classical exercises and new horizons. Arch Plast Surg. 2014;41(3):201–8.
20. Pafitanis G, Narushima M, Yamamoto T, Raveendran M, Veljanoski D, Ghanem AM, et al. Evolution of an evidence-based supermicrosurgery simulation training curriculum: a systematic review. J Plast Reconstr Aesthet Surg. 2018;71(7):976–88.
21. Zheng Y, Corvi JJ, Nicolas CF, Akelina Y. Supermicrosurgery simulation training program for submillimeter anastomoses in the rat epigastric artery and vein. Microsurgery. 2019;39(8):773–4.
22. Najjar M, Lopez MM Jr, Ballestin A, Munabi N, Naides AI, Noland RD, et al. Reestablishment of lymphatic drainage after vascularized lymph node transfer in a rat model. Plast Reconstr Surg. 2018;142(4):503e–8e.
23. Yamamoto T, Yamamoto N, Yamashita M, Furuya M, Hayashi A, Koshima I. Establishment of supermicrosurgical lymphaticovenular anastomosis model in rat. Microsurgery. 2017;37(1):57–60.
24. Bodin F, Diana M, Koutsomanis A, Robert E, Marescaux J, Bruant-Rodier C. Porcine model for free-flap breast reconstruction training. J Plast Reconstr Aesthet Surg. 2015;68(10):1402–9.
25. Gonzalez-Garcia JA, Chiesa-Estomba CM, Alvarez L, Altuna X, Garcia-Iza L, Thomas I, et al. Porcine experimental model for perforator flap raising in reconstructive microsurgery. J Surg Res. 2018;227:81–7.
26. Gonzalez-Garcia JA, Chiesa-Estomba CM, Larruscain E, Alvarez L, Sistiaga JA. Porcine experimental model for gracilis free flap transfer to the head and neck area with novel donor site description. J Plast Reconstr Aesthet Surg. 2020;73(1):111–7.
27. Nistor A, Ionac M, Spano A, Georgescu A, Hoinoiu B, Jiga LP. Mastering the approach of internal mammary vessels: a new training model in pigs. Plast Reconstr Surg. 2013;131(5):859e–61e.
28. Tolba RH, Czigany Z, Osorio Lujan S, Oltean M, Axelsson M, Akelina Y, et al. Defining standards in experimental microsurgical training: recommendations of the European Society for Surgical Research (ESSR) and the International Society for Experimental Microsurgery (ISEM). Eur Surg Res. 2017;58(5–6):246–62.
29. Ghanem A, Kearns M, Ballestin A, Froschauer S, Akelina Y, Shurey S, et al. International microsurgery simulation society (IMSS) consensus statement on the minimum standards for a basic microsurgery course, requirements for a microsurgical anastomosis global rating scale and minimum thresholds for training. Injury. 2020;51(Suppl 4):S126–S30.
30. Ghanem AM, Al Omran Y, Shatta B, Kim E, Myers S. Anastomosis Lapse Index (ALI): a validated end product assessment tool for simulation microsurgery training. J Reconstr Microsurg. 2016;32(3):233–41.
31. Oltean M, Nistor A, Hellstrom M, Axelsson M, Yagi S, Kobayashi E, et al. Microsurgery training during COVID-19 pandemic: practical recommendations from the International Society for Experimental

Microsurgery and International Microsurgery Simulation Society. Microsurgery. 2021;41(4):398–400.
32. Santamaria E, Nahas-Combina L, Altamirano-Arcos C, Vargas-Flores E. Master Series microsurgery for residents: results from a comprehensive survey of a multitudinous online course during COVID-19 pandemic. J Reconstr Microsurg. 2021;37:602.
33. Kwon SH, Goh R, Wang ZT, Ting-Hsuan Tang E, Chu CF, Chen YC, et al. Tips for making a successful online microsurgery educational platform: the experience of international microsurgery club. Plast Reconstr Surg. 2019;143(1):221e–33e.
34. Shurey S. MicroShure microsurgery. YouTube. 2020. https://www.youtube.com/channel/UCytdJXQfxRijsyJRRPai1jg.
35. Loh CY, Tiong VT, Loh AY, Athanassopoulos T. Microsurgery training--a home do-it-yourself model. Microsurgery. 2014;34(5):417–8.
36. Kim DM, Kang JW, Kim JK, Youn I, Park JW. Microsurgery training using a smartphone. Microsurgery. 2015;35(6):500–1.

Basic and Advanced Microvascular Anastomotic Techniques

2

Alberto Ballestín and Yelena Akelina

2.1 Introduction

Reconstructive microsurgery is a surgical technique that has been practiced since the 1960s, when Jacobson and Suárez performed vascular anastomoses in 1 mm vessels with the use of a surgical microscope, specific instruments, and microsutures [1]. However, the first vascular anastomosis techniques were previously described on large-caliber vessels by Carrel and Guthrie at the beginning of the twentieth century [2]. Due to those technical advances that changed surgery forever, Carrel was awarded the Nobel Prize in Physiology or Medicine in 1912 "in recognition of his work on vascular sutures and the transplantation of blood vessels and organs."

The development of surgical microscopes, the refinement of instruments, and the manufacture of microsutures made possible to describe several microsurgical anastomosis techniques. Success on small vessel and nerve anastomoses have allowed the surgical replantation of severed parts and the performance of a wide variety of free tissue transfers in patients. Therefore, innumerable surgical approaches have changed for reconstructing patients suffering from high-intensity trauma or burn injuries or after receiving resective cancer surgeries. This chapter describes, step-by-step, each of the main microvascular anastomosis techniques as well as indicates essential handling tips for a proper dissection of the tissues involved in these surgeries.

A. Ballestín (✉)
Tumor Microenvironment Laboratory, UMR3347 CNRS/U1021 INSERM, Institut Curie, Paris, France

Y. Akelina
Microsurgery Research and Training Laboratory, Columbia University, New York, NY, USA

2.2 Tissue Handling

Microvascular anastomoses are common techniques in reconstructive surgery; they are the essence of free tissue transfers. Fundamental to its successful performance are the execution of careful tissue dissections, the understanding of anatomical differences between arteries and veins, and the appropriate vessel pedicle preparation.

Gentle tissue dissections are required prior to perform anastomoses. Accordingly, smooth harmonic movements should be performed, applying a very small amount of forces while dissecting, most of which are below the surgeons' tactile sensory threshold.

Respect innate anatomy of vessel pedicle is a prerequisite to accomplish success. Blood vessels must be handled with great care, parallel dissection of perivascular tissues is recommended to avoid damaging, but if necessary, vessels can be gently manipulated by holding the tunica adventitia, its outermost layer.

Arteries and veins have three layers (tunica intima, tunica media, and tunica adventitia) that are formed and have different characteristics among them. Veins have an anatomy that makes the free edges to be anastomosed more collapsible and easy to damage. This is due to the fact that they have less collagen fibers compared to arteries. Thus, it is necessary to be especially delicate when manipulating veins to avoid damage, as well as working with irrigation to visualize the vascular lumen during the microsurgical procedure.

Vascular damage during dissection would lead to specific injuries at the tunica intima, media, and/or adventitia. It would cause vessel spasm that would make it difficult to perform the anastomotic technique. And furthermore, it would stimulate platelet aggregation and, consequently, the development of thrombus that would lead to failure.

© Springer Nature Switzerland AG 2023
D. Nikkhah et al. (eds.), *Core Techniques in Flap Reconstructive Microsurgery*, https://doi.org/10.1007/978-3-031-07678-7_2

The main cause of spasm is improper vessel handling and dissection. In addition, the loss of temperature in the surgical field may lead to spasm too. This can be favored by a low external temperature or by the lack of proper tempered irrigation. Therefore, adequate warm moistening of the vessels is required to prevent vascular drying and smooth fiber contraction. If spasm occurs despite taking these precautions, vasodilators can be applied locally.

Regarding thrombosis and besides vessel injury, other factors can also contribute to its development which usually occurs in the first 24 h after surgery. Poor microsurgical technique, torsion of the vascular pedicle when performing flap insetting, or a prolonged ischemic time [3] will favor the development of thrombus and the failure of surgery [4].

Once the blood vessels to be anastomosed are clamped and exposed under the microscope, local irrigation with heparinized serum is necessary to avoid having any blood inside the lumen as well as to keep vessels in a hydrated and correct elasticity state.

Next, adventitiectomy of vessel ends must be performed to prevent adventitia from entering in the lumen. Adventitia may disturb correct laminar blood flow after anastomosis and even act as a thrombogenic attractant that will lead to anastomotic failure.

Finally, to facilitate the microsurgical anastomosis technique, blunt-tipped vasodilator forceps can be used to widen vessel lumen and help in size matching of the vessel ends to be anastomosed. It has to be a delicate maneuver, since over-dilation can damage vascular endothelium.

2.3 Microvascular End-to-End Anastomotic Techniques

2.3.1 End-to-End Anastomosis Using Biangulation Technique

1. Perform blunt dissection to expose the vessels to be anastomosed.
2. Isolate arteries from veins.
3. Ligate small vessel branches if needed, or use a bipolar cautery.
4. Once vessels are exposed and cut, use heparinized saline solution to wash out both vessel lumens and their edges.
5. Place a double clamp to approach both vessel ends and locate a contrast background to enhance visualization (Fig. 2.1a).
6. Prepare vessel edges by trimming adventitia using fine forceps and microsurgical scissors (Fig. 2.1b).
7. Dilate vessel ends using a polished blunt-tipped vessel dilator.
8. Place two interrupted stay sutures at 180° (12 o'clock and 6 o'clock positions). If using a clamp with frame, fix the ends of each stay suture to the frame (Fig. 2.1c).
9. Place three more interrupted sutures starting at 3 o'clock, then 1 o'clock, and 4 o'clock positions. Middle stitch may be left longer for vessel handling to avoid catching the back wall while suturing (Fig. 2.2a).
10. Flip the double clamp 180° to expose the posterior wall, check the lumen by irrigating heparinized saline solution, and complete the anastomosis in the same manner as anterior wall (Fig. 2.2b).

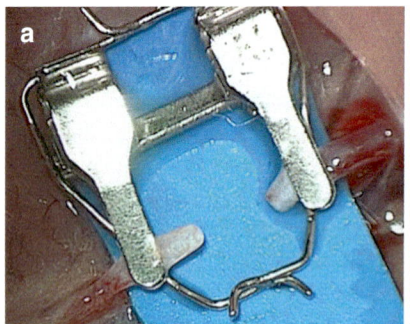
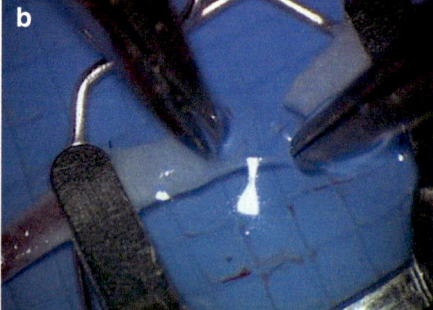
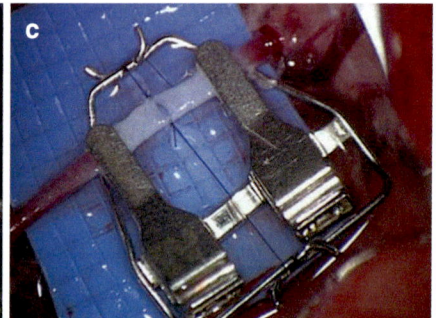

Fig. 2.1 First steps of an end-to-end arterial microsurgical anastomosis using biangulation technique. (**a**) Microscopic view of an artery after clamping and washing out using heparinized serum saline. (**b**) Excess of adventitia removal. (**c**) Placement of two stay sutures 180° apart one from each other

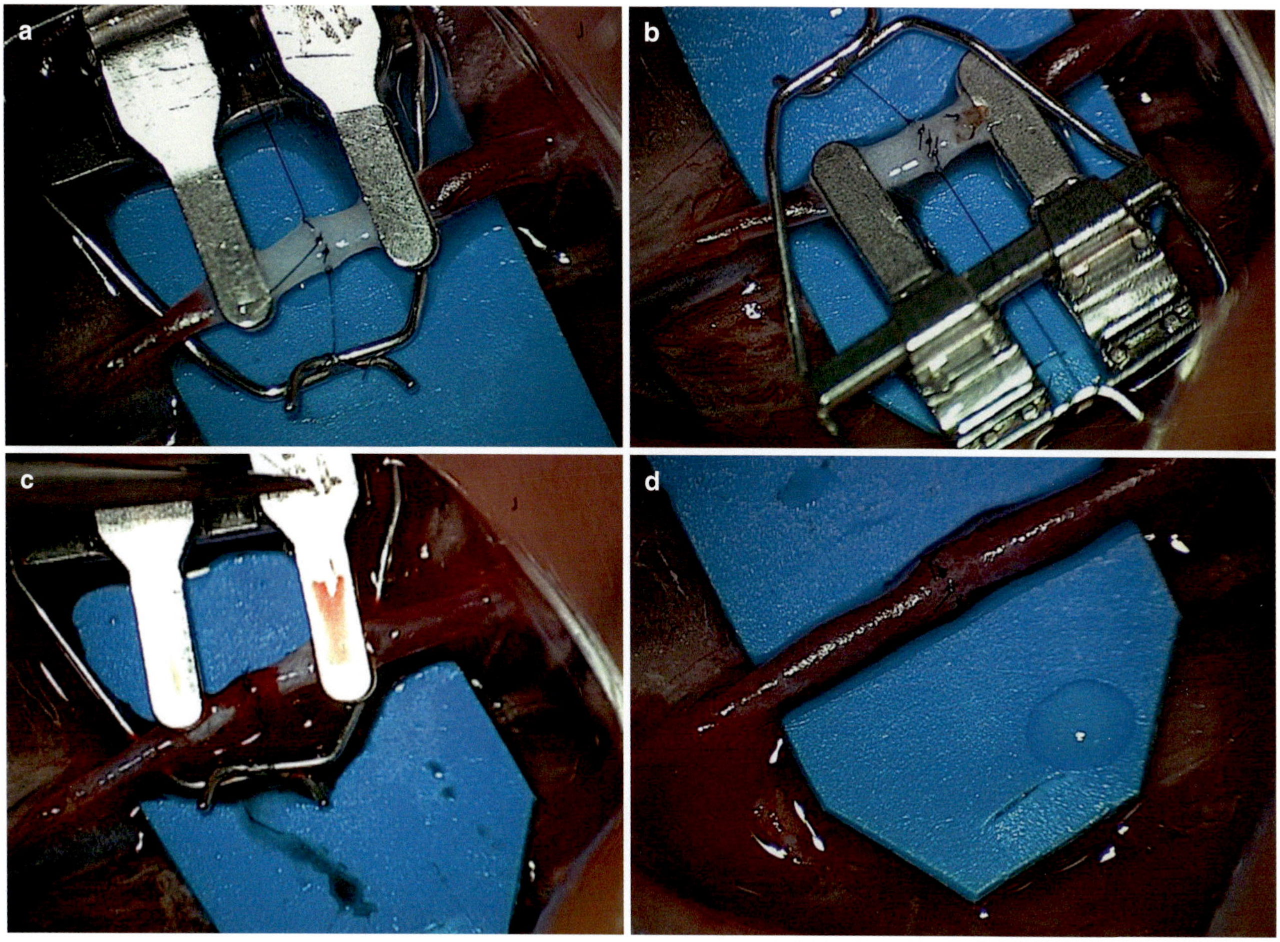

Fig. 2.2 End-to-end arterial microsurgical anastomosis using biangulation technique. (**a**) Placement of microsurgical stitches on the anterior wall. (**b**) Placement of microsurgical stitches on the posterior wall after having turned the microvascular clamp 180°. (**c**) Microvascular clamp removal. (**d**) Patent end-to-end arterial anastomosis

11. After completion, release the stay sutures and remove the clamp (Fig. 2.2c).
12. Place some adipose tissue and a surgical gauze over the anastomosis site for a few minutes for hemostasis [5] before evaluating patency.
13. Check vessel after completing the anastomosis (Fig. 2.2d).
14. If bleeding occurs, repair the anastomosis with additional stitches using the partial occlusion techniques [6] to avoid thrombus development (Fig. 2.3).

2.3.2 End-to-End Anastomosis Using One-Way-Up Technique

1. Prepare the vessel as previously described for end-to-end biangulation anastomosis technique.
2. Place and secure the first stay suture at 12 o'clock position.

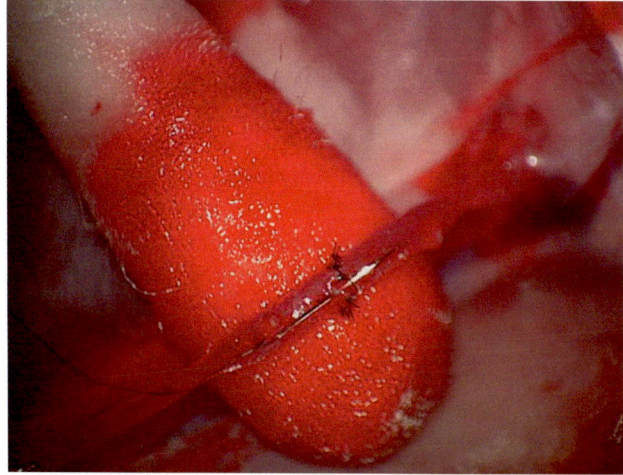

Fig. 2.3 Partial occlusion technique to perform anastomosis repair without clamps [6] to avoid thrombus development

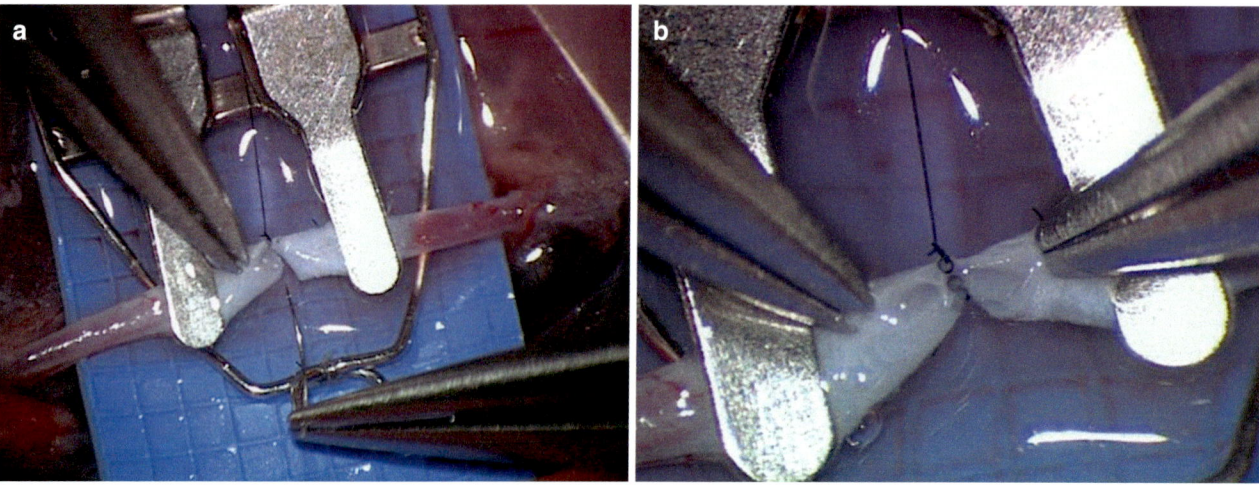

Fig. 2.4 End-to-end anastomosis using one-way-up technique. (**a**) Backhand technique for placing posterior wall stitches, first pass outside in in the left side. (**b**) Microscopic view of the anterior wall after the placement of the first two stitches of an anastomosis using one-way-up technique

3. For the all posterior wall stitches, make the first pass outside in using a backhand technique and the second pass inside out with the forehand technique for having the knot outside of the lumen (Fig. 2.4a, b).
4. Fix the 6 o'clock stay stitch once midpoint of the anastomosis is reached.
5. Proceed closing the anterior wall in the normal, single pass forehand manner.
6. Upon completion of the vessel sutures, release the stay suture and the vessel clamp.

2.4 Microvascular End-to-Side Anastomotic Technique

The most common technique in vascular microsurgery is the end-to-end anastomosis, which is performed between vessels of the same or similar caliber. When end-to-end cannot be done because it is necessary to preserve the blood flow of a vessel, or when there are size discrepancies greater than 2:1 between the vessels to be anastomosed, end-to-side anastomosis is performed [7].

Size discrepancy is a common issue in reconstructive microsurgery, because vessel caliber change can cause turbulent blood flow and, therefore, predisposes to platelet aggregation. Small size discrepancies can be resolved by mechanical expansion with vasodilator forceps. Other option if the size of the donor vessel is small is to enlarge lumen diameter by cutting the end of the vessel obliquely. However, in the event of large discrepancies, other techniques such as sleeve anastomosis could be considered [8].

Clinically, end-to-side anastomoses are commonly performed in tissue revascularizations and organ transplants and during free tissue transfers. The end-to-side technique consists of three steps: preparation of the donor vessel, preparation of the recipient vessel, and the microsuture technique.

2.4.1 Preparing Donor Vessel (Vessel End)

1. Perform careful blunt dissection of the vessel under high magnification. If needed, ligate or coagulate small vessel branches.
2. Place a single clamp on the proximal end of the vessel and ligate distally.
3. Transect the vessel close to the ligature and flush with heparinized saline.
4. Trim the excess of adventitia at the vessel edge and dilate its lumen by using vessel dilators.

2.4.2 Preparing Recipient Vessel (Vessel Side)

1. Place two single clamps on both the proximal and distal end of the recipient vessel.
2. Position the donor vessel next to the recipient vessel to help visualize the space required for the size of the arteriotomy or venotomy (depending on the type of vessel being used).
3. Before creating the side cut, remove completely adventitia over an area twice as large as the arteriotomy or venotomy size.
4. Plan the lateral arteriotomy/venotomy in an area that will help to avoid tension during the anastomosis. To avoid tension more dissection may be performed or mobilizing the tissues involved may be needed. Do not place the lateral arteriotomy/venotomy directly over any marginal branch.

5. Gently lift the vessel wall with straight forceps or by using a microsuture stitch to pull the vessel. Make a small "v-shaped" cut underneath the forceps or suture (Fig. 2.5a). To do so, position your scissors longitudinally along the vessel at a 45° angle, and make a small nick in the vessel. Flush through the newly made cut with heparinized saline. And then, dilate the cut opening using a vessel dilator to a size that is approximately 20% larger than the diameter of the donor vessel that is going to be anastomosed to the recipient vessel.

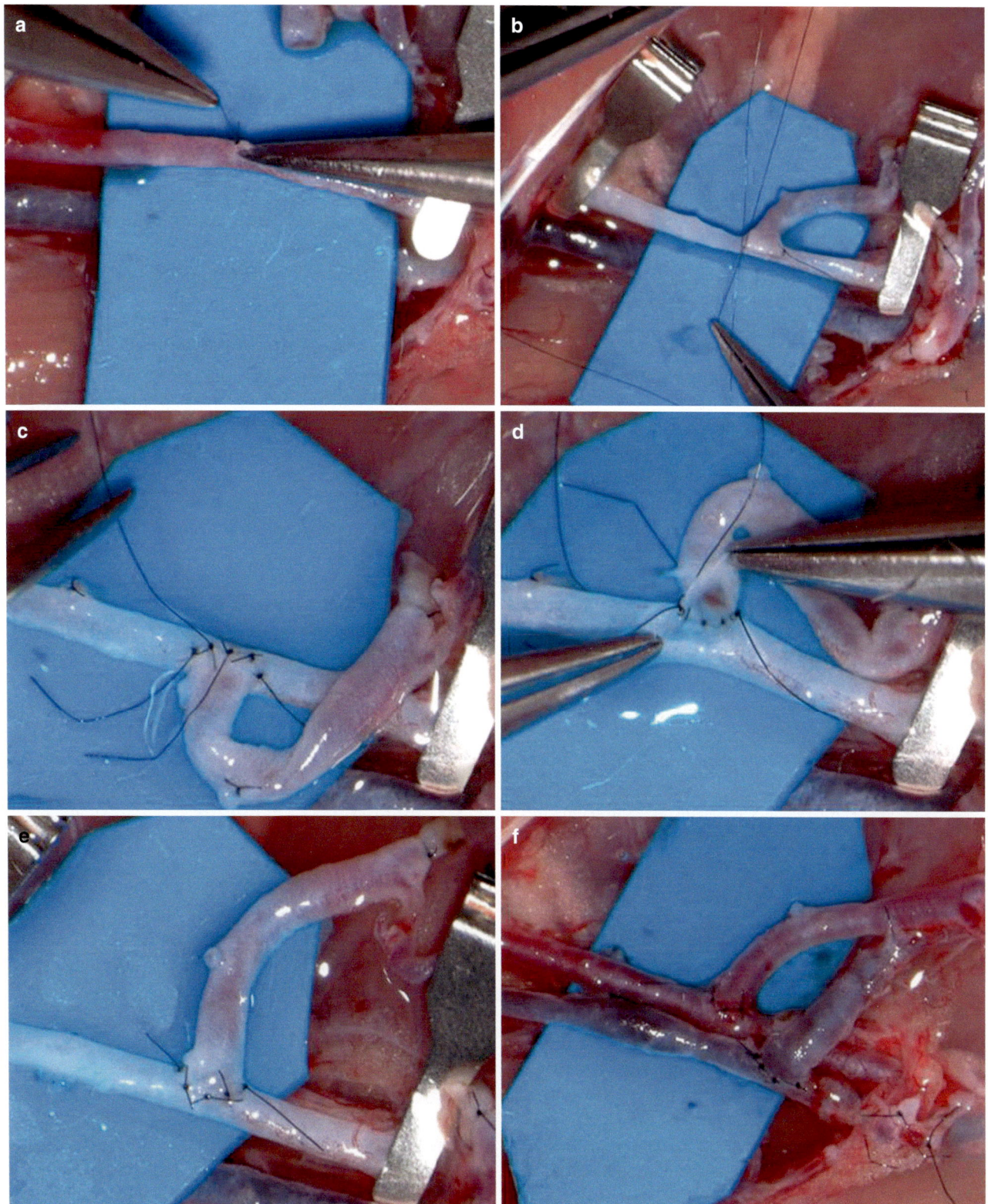

Fig. 2.5 End-to-side anastomosis. (**a**) Cut of an oval-shaped opening that is similar in size to the vessel to be approximated. (**b**) Placement of two stitches at 180° to connect the donor and recipient vessels together. (**c**) Back-wall sutures of the end-to-side anastomosis. (**d**) Inspection of the vessel lumen after posterior wall suture. (**e**) Front wall sutures of the end-to-side anastomosis. (**f**) Patent end-to-side anastomoses

2.4.3 Microsuture Technique for End-to-Side Anastomosis

1. Connect the end of the donor vessel with the side of the recipient vessel with the first stitch that should be placed closest to the proximal end of the donor vessel at the longitudinal aspect of the elliptical arteriotomy/venotomy (9 o'clock position). The second stitch should be placed 180° opposite the first stitch (3 o'clock position). Make sure the stitches are made "outside in, inside out" to let the knot outside the anastomosis lumen (Fig. 2.5b).
2. After this, complete circumferential stitches on the wall that is opposite the surgeon; complete the back wall first (Fig. 2.5c). This will help prevent inadvertent back-wall stitches throughout the procedure. Make sure the middle stitch is placed straight and the two others radially. Pay attention to the spacing between the stitches. Be sure to make small bites when throwing stitches (between 1 and 2 needle widths from the suture line).

    Note: In case the vessel cannot be mobilized, or it is very difficult to interrupt suturing of the back wall, interrupted stitches can be placed "outside in, inside out" in a similar way to the one-way-up technique, or even a continuous hemisuture can be made on the back wall.
3. After completing the back wall, irrigate with heparin solution to remove any blood residue remaining in the lumen and to inspect for back-walling stitches (Fig. 2.5d).
4. Perform suturing of the front wall (Fig. 2.5e). In order to avoid the back-wall stitches, we suggest keeping the middle stitch open while also placing two radial stitches. Then, close both radial stitches before closing the middle stitch. Again, place all stitches in the same "outside in, inside out" manner.
5. Once the procedure is completed, examine the anastomosis for gaps before clamps are removed. The order of clamp release should follow the lowest blood pressure to highest blood pressure.
6. Finally, check for patency to ensure re-establishment of blood flow through the anastomosis (Fig. 2.5f).

2.5 Interpositional Venous Grafting

Interpositional vein grafts have become a standard procedure for bridging segmental vascular defects in reconstructive microsurgery [9].

In the past, in replantation surgery, the bones and soft tissues were shortened to achieve direct anastomosis. Nowadays, vein grafts are essential to face defects in which vascular tissue has been lost due to trauma, after debridement or resection surgery. But grafts can also be considered when there is a significant size discrepancy between the recipient vessels and the flap pedicle [10]. In addition vein grafting can also be used to help in difficult anastomoses with short vessel stumps, to avoid bifurcations, or to place the anastomoses away from infected, radiated, atherosclerotic, or otherwise altered vessels [11].

Interpositional microvascular vein grafting consists of three steps: preparation of the artery, preparation of vein graft, and the microsuture technique.

2.5.1 Preparation of the Artery

1. Clamp and wash out the artery with heparinized saline.
2. Trim the adventitia from the edge and insert the vasodilator forceps into the arterial ends to slightly enlarge the lumen.
3. Using the small ruler, measure the length of the gap between the edges of the artery to determine the exact length of the graft needed to cover that defect (Fig. 2.6a).

2.5.2 Preparation of Vein Graft

1. Place marking stiches in the vein adventitia so that you can align the graft in the proper orientation of the valves and blood flow. This means that the graft will need to be reversed when inserted into the artery such that the distal end of the vein is sutured to the proximal end of the artery. Leave one marking stitch longer to facilitate keeping track of the proximal end.
2. Ligate both ends of the vein, ensuring you have at least 1 mm more length than the artery defect on each end.
3. Excise the distal end of the vein first, irrigate with heparinized saline, and trim the adventitia before excising the other end, as it is easier to flush and trim with one end still attached. Then, excise the proximal end of the vein and bring it to the arterial defect to start suturing (Fig. 2.6b).

2.5.3 Microsuture Technique for Interpositional Vein Graft Technique

1. Place the first stay suture at 12 o'clock through the proximal end of the artery to the distal end of the vein. Then place the second stay suture at the 12 o'clock in the distal end of the artery to the proximal end of the vein, using the marking stitches to ensure proper alignment with no twisting of the vein.

    Note: When working with medium- or large-sized vessels, there are greater gaps, so it may be needed to use a double clamp to approximate the artery and vein first on the proximal anastomosis and then on the distal.
2. Then place the third and fourth stay sutures at 6 o'clock on both sides. Leave some length on each stay suture for easier manipulation of the vessels.

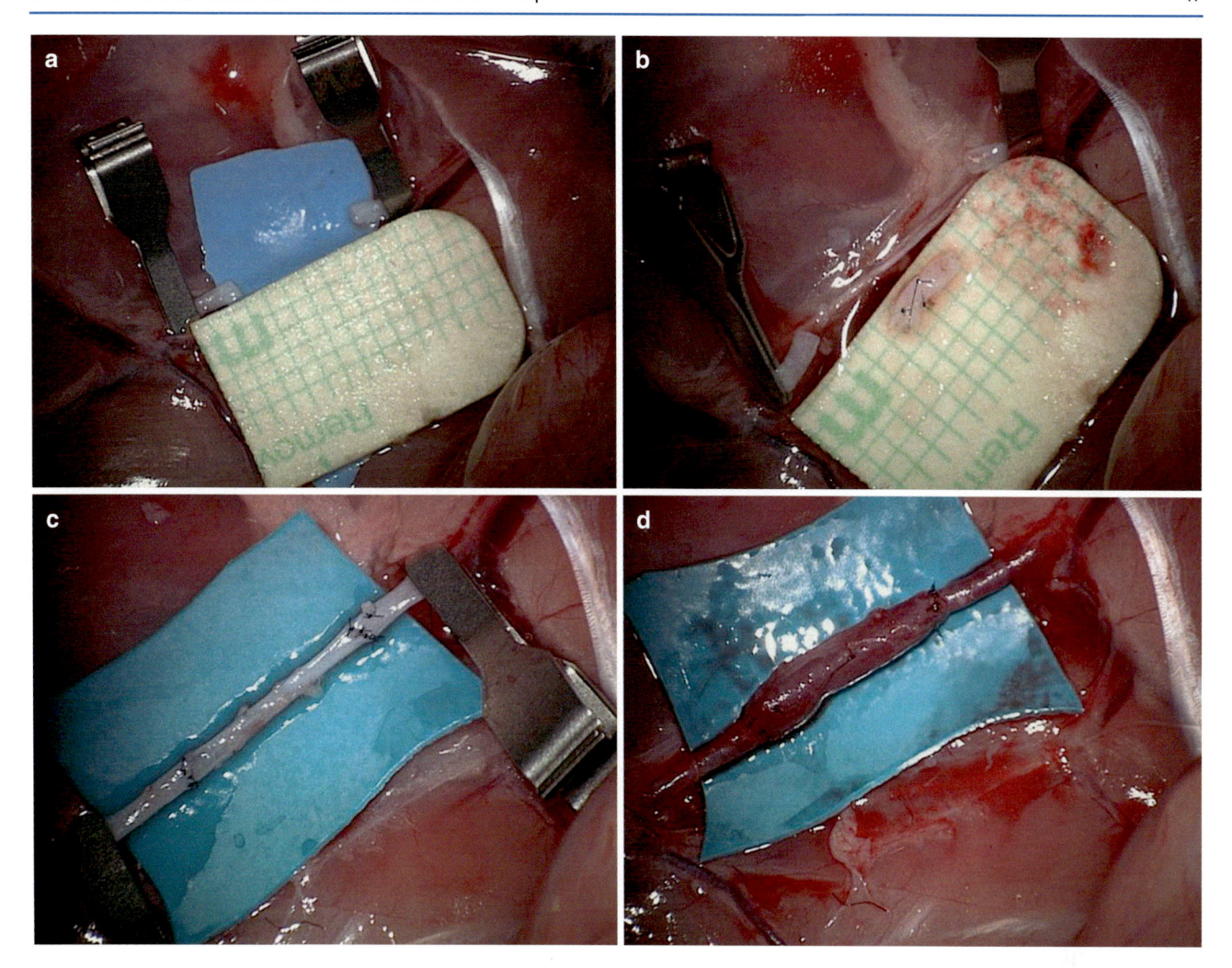

Fig. 2.6 Interpositional vein graft. (**a**) Artery defect requiring a vein graft. (**b**) Vein graft positioned in the field. Its size is larger than the existing arterial defect, although it may not seem like it because after its harvesting the vessel is naturally retracted. (**c**) Anastomosed vein graft. (**d**) Patent microvascular vein graft

   Note: In case of a large-sized discrepancy, oblique cuts can be made to spatulate the edges of the artery and reduce the diameter differences.
3. Complete the anterior walls on both anastomoses with three middle evenly spaced stitches.
   Note: Make sure that the marking stitches are aligned to ensure that there is no twisting of the vein.
4. Flip microvascular clamps to complete suturing of posterior walls.
5. Upon completion of both anastomoses, examine the suture lines for any gaps and place extra sutures if needed (Fig. 2.6c).
6. Release the distal clamp first and let the retrograde flow open the lumen to show any defects. Then open the proximal clamp (Fig. 2.6d).
7. Finally, check the patency distally from the distal anastomosis.

2.6 Supermicrosurgery and Future Perspectives

Supermicrosurgery is the part of microsurgery that includes the dissection and anastomosis of vessels smaller than 0.8 mm [12]. Thanks to the use of 11/0, 12/0, and 13/0 sutures, this technique allows anastomosing of very small arterial, venous, and lymphatic vessels that were previously inaccessible.

It is a technique that enabled to refine multiple soft tissue reconstruction techniques such as finger-tip replantation, toe tip transfers for fingertip loss, and free perforator-to-perforator flaps. Furthermore, it has had a paramount impact in the surgical treatment of lymphedema, allowing to perform vascularized lymph node transfers [13, 14] and lymphaticovenular [15] and lymphatico-lymphatic anastomoses [16].

Microsurgery will continue to evolve. Technical refinements in microscopy, designs of specific instruments, innovations in contrast media, and the development of new specific robots for microsurgery to enhance precision and eliminate tremor [17] may be some of the next steps forward in this field.

References

1. Jacobson JH, Suarez EL. Microsurgery in anastomosis os small vessels. Surg Forum. 1960;11:243–5.
2. Carrel A. La technique opératoire des anastomoses vasculaires et de la transplantation des visceres. Lyon: Association Typographique; 1902.
3. Ballestin A, Casado JG, Abellan E, Vela FJ, Alvarez V, Uson A, et al. Ischemia-reperfusion injury in a rat microvascular skin free flap model: a histological, genetic, and blood flow study. PLoS One. 2018;13(12):e0209624.
4. Shaughness G, Blackburn C, Ballestin A, Akelina Y, Ascherman JA. Predicting thrombosis formation in 1-mm-diameter arterial anastomoses with transit-time ultrasound technology. Plast Reconstr Surg. 2017;139(6):1400–5.
5. Akelina Y, Danilo P. Endogenous adipose tissue as a hemostatic: use in microsurgery. Microsurgery. 2008;28(3):192–6.
6. Harb A, Levi M, Akelina Y, Kadiyala R, Ascherman JA. A novel technique to perform microvascular anastomosis revisions without clamps. J Reconstr Microsurg Open. 2018;3(2):e58–61.
7. Djohan RS, Gage E, Bernard SL. Microsurgical techniques. In: Siemionow M, Eisenmann-Klein M, editors. Plastic and reconstructive surgery. New York, NY: Springer; 2010. p. 89–100.
8. Lopez-Monjardin H, de la Pena-Salcedo JA. Techniques for management of size discrepancies in microvascular anastomosis. Microsurgery. 2000;20(4):162–6.
9. Cooley BC. History of vein grafting. Microsurgery. 1998;18(4):234–6.
10. Miller MJ, Schusterman MA, Reece GP, Kroll SS. Interposition vein grafting in head and neck reconstructive microsurgery. J Reconstr Microsurg. 1993;9(3):245–51; discussion 51–2.
11. Biemer E. Role of vein grafts in reconstructive microsurgery. Microsurgery. 1998;18(4):237–41.
12. Koshima I, Yamamoto T, Narushima M, Mihara M, Iida T. Perforator flaps and supermicrosurgery. Clin Plast Surg. 2010;37(4):683–9, vii–iii.
13. Najjar M, Lopez MM Jr, Ballestin A, Munabi N, Naides AI, Noland RD, et al. Reestablishment of lymphatic drainage after vascularized lymph node transfer in a rat model. Plast Reconstr Surg. 2018;142(4):503e–8e.
14. Patel KM, Lin CY, Cheng MH. A prospective evaluation of lymphedema-specific quality-of-life outcomes following vascularized lymph node transfer. Ann Surg Oncol. 2015;22(7):2424–30.
15. Koshima I, Inagawa K, Urushibara K, Moriguchi T. Supermicrosurgical lymphaticovenular anastomosis for the treatment of lymphedema in the upper extremities. J Reconstr Microsurg. 2000;16(6):437–42.
16. Yamamoto T, Yoshimatsu H, Koshima I. Navigation lymphatic supermicrosurgery for iatrogenic lymphorrhea: supermicrosurgical lymphaticolymphatic anastomosis and lymphaticovenular anastomosis under indocyanine green lymphography navigation. J Plast Reconstr Aesthet Surg. 2014;67(11):1573–9.
17. van Mulken TJM, Schols RM, Scharmga AMJ, Winkens B, Cau R, Schoenmakers FBF, et al. First-in-human robotic supermicrosurgery using a dedicated microsurgical robot for treating breast cancer-related lymphedema: a randomized pilot trial. Nat Commun. 2020;11(1):757.

Decision-Making in Flap Surgery: Reconstructive Ladder Versus Elevator

Mohammed Farid, Thessa Friebel, and Dariush Nikkhah

3.1 Introduction: The History of Reconstructive Plastic Surgery

The earliest descriptions for the use of random pattern flaps in facial reconstruction by Susruta are dated to 600 BC [1]. The second pioneer was Tagliacozzi who demonstrated the use of distant tubed pedicle flaps from the biceps region to reconstruct the nose in 1497. During World War I, the sheer volume of injuries which Gillies faced led to the evolution of local and distant pedicled flaps in reconstruction of soft tissue defects, first described in 1917 [2].

The development of microsurgery techniques and reconstructive surgery principles during the late nineteeth and early twentieth centuries was profound. Murphy performed the first end-to-end vascular anastomosis on animals and femoral artery repair for a gunshot wound in 1896 [3, 4] (Fig. 3.1). Shortly after, Carrel introduced the concept of "triangulation" into vascular anastomosis in 1902 [5]. Six decades later, in 1960, the first microvascular anastomosis was performed under the microscope by Jacobson and Suarez [6]. A Nobel Laureate winner, Joseph Murray, was a plastic surgeon who performed the first successful organ

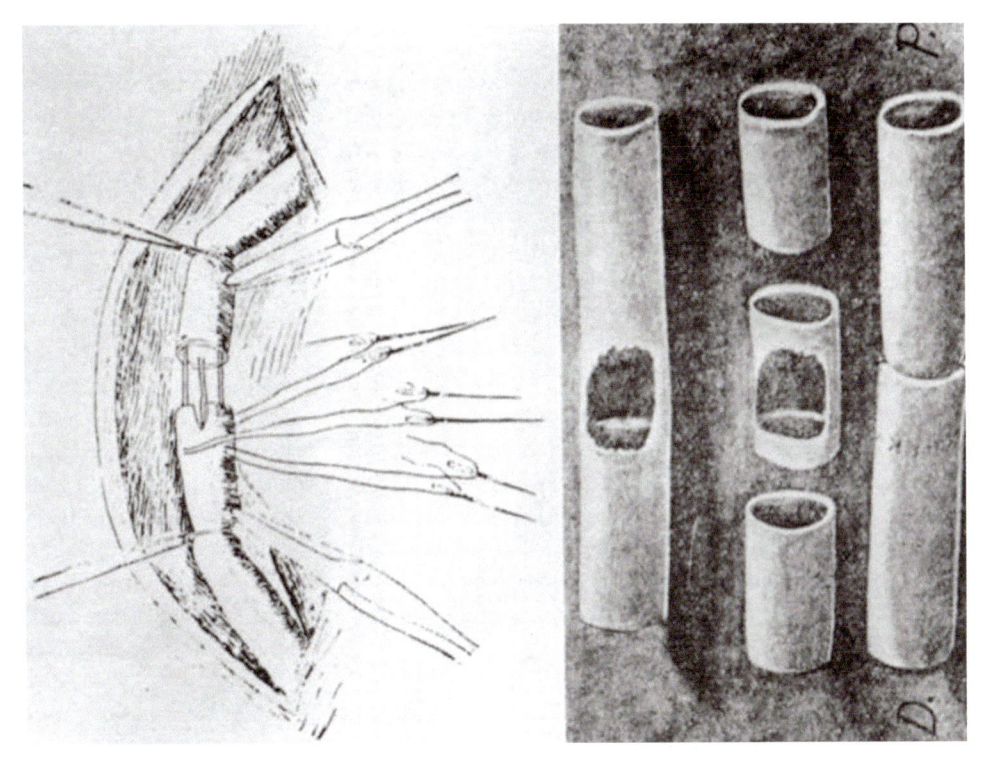

Fig. 3.1 Murphy's illustration in performing the first end-to-end vascular anastomosis

M. Farid (✉)
Royal Stoke University Hospital, Stoke-on-Trent, UK

T. Friebel
James Cook University Hospital, Middlesbrough, UK

D. Nikkhah
Royal Free Hospital, London, UK
e-mail: d.nikkhah@nhs.net

© Springer Nature Switzerland AG 2023
D. Nikkhah et al. (eds.), *Core Techniques in Flap Reconstructive Microsurgery*, https://doi.org/10.1007/978-3-031-07678-7_3

Table 3.1 Reconstructive surgery milestones and pioneers

Year	Pioneer	Milestone/technique
600 BC	Susruta	Random pattern local flaps in facial reconstruction
1497	Taglocozzi	Random pattern pedicled flaps in nasal reconstruction
1896	Murphy	First arterial end-to-end anastomosis
1917	Gillies	Local and distant pedicled flaps
1958	Seidenburg	First free jejunal anastomosis for oesophageal reconstruction
1959	Murray	First successful organ transplant
1968	Cobbett	Toe to thumb transfer
1972	Buncke	Free omental flap for scalp reconstruction
1972	Jackson	First pedicled groin flap (based on a named vessel)
1973	Taylor	First free fasciocutaneous groin flap
1987	Taylor	Angiosome Concept
1994	Pribaz	Flap Prelamination
2005	Lantieri	First face transplant

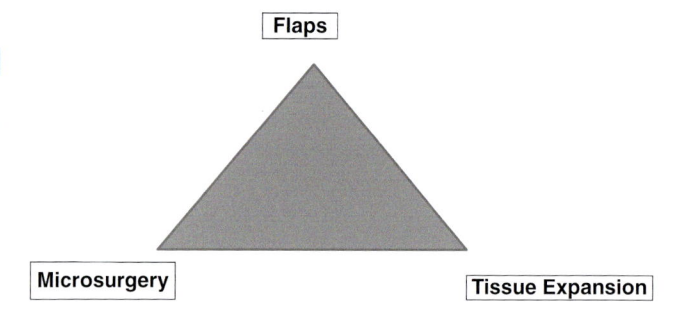

Fig. 3.2 The reconstructive triangle

(kidney) transplant in 1959 [7]. During the same period, Seidenberg in 1958 performed a free jejunal anastomosis to reconstruct the oesophagus in a dog [8]. This was followed by the first successful toe to thumb transfer in 1968 by Cobbett [9]. The work by Buncke was revolutionary whereby he performed a free omental flap to cover a scalp defect in 1972 [10]. In the same year, the work of McGregor and Jackson in describing the groin pedicled flap based on a named vessel was an important turning point in reconstructive surgery [11]. A year later, the first free fasciocutaneous flap (groin) to the foot was successfully transferred by Daniel and Taylor [12]. Further work by Taylor describing the angiosome concept in mapping the human body vasculature had opened the gates to the birth of a new era in reconstructive free flap and perforator microsurgery in 1987 [13]. The focus on microsurgery until this point was to achieve milestone achievements in reconstructive principles. While reconstructive microsurgery continued to evolve, the concept of *the reconstructive ladder* was introduced by Mathes and Nahai in 1982 [14]. An important milestone in reconstructive microsurgery is the introduction of prefabrication and prelamination principles. Prefabrication was first described by Shen in 1982 and then popularised by Pribaz who also integrated prelamination concept in 1994 [15, 16]. These concepts of reconstruction achieved a pinnacle in composite tissue allotransplantation with the first successful cases performed in France (Table 3.1) [17–19].

3.2 The Reconstructive Ladder vs. Elevator

Integrating Gillies principles in terms of "thou shalt make a plan" has been instinctively applied in our advanced reconstructive thinking nowadays [20]. The plan suggested by the rungs of the reconstructive ladder provided a step-by-step framework to determine the best reconstructive option from simple (healing by secondary intention) to more complex (free flap). A more safe and reliable outcome with less morbidity is achieved with the simplest option for wound closure based on the ladder. It still forms a stepping-stone in our thinking towards soft tissue defects. Nonetheless, the evolution of microsurgery during the 1980s onwards projected itself to introduce different dimensions into the reconstructive ladder [21].

The limitations of the stepwise approach by the ladder pushed towards a new term *reconstructive elevator* coined by Gottlieb in 1993 [22]. This advanced towards the freedom to ascend up the ladder based on the complexity of reconstruction. The emphasis was on form and function indicating that the simplest option may not be the best choice. It encouraged a problem-solving strategy integrating available reconstructive options and patient and wound factors to newly advanced technologies. This approach allowed creativity in reconstructive thinking and the ability to make choices based on desired form and function rather than only an option to cover a defect. The ideals of soft tissue cover no longer followed a linear approach and therefore utilised various methods/ways in reconstructive surgery [23]. However, other factors like surgeon operative skills and their ability to perform complex reconstruction may rule out particular options for coverage based on the elevator principle [24]. In 1997, Nahai introduced the concept of the *reconstructive triangle*, consisting of integrated flaps, microsurgery and tissue expansion (Fig. 3.2) [25]. This was an attempt to address the potential pitfalls in the *reconstructive ladder* and allow a degree of flexibility when thinking about options for reconstruction. It also acknowledged the importance of donor site morbidity when making such choices.

3.3 The Reconstructive Toolbox

There have been many advances and innovations in the field of reconstructive surgery. New techniques and options for reconstruction evolved over the past two decades. These are considered as a first-line option or adjuncts in management of defects. A list of such methods to be integrated to the reconstructive algorithm includes:

- Fat transfer
- Implants/expanders
- Dermal matrices
- Fillers
- Allotransplantation
- Tissue engineering
- Stem cells

Starting with fat transfer, this has been used as an adjunct or even the only option in breast reconstruction and in facial, hand or scar rejuvenation [26, 27]. Implants had no place in the *reconstructive ladder or elevator* but are commonly used in reconstruction (e.g. chin augmentation) [28]. Implants are deemed a primary form of reconstruction in breast surgery based on patient or surgeon choice [29]. The use of dermal matrices whether biological or synthetic has gained popularity in complex soft tissue reconstruction (e.g. chest wall, abdominal) and as a temporising measure prior to definite repair [30, 31]. Fillers either temporary or permanent are used in facial rejuvenation for medical (e.g. HIV lipodystrophy) or aesthetic (e.g. lip, rhinoplasty) reasons [32, 33]. Composite tissue allotransplantation particularly for hand proved to be a successful tool in the reconstructive algorithm [34]. Nonetheless, only a small number of cases worldwide have been performed due to a myriad of reasons including ethical, immunological, financial and the complexity of such operations [35]. Tissue engineering determined new alternatives to autograft or allograft reconstruction and is gaining a new popularity [36]. This has already been in use clinically for complex defects including chest wall reconstruction [37]. At its infancy, stem cell technology seems to be the forthcoming paradigm to introduce new methods to reconstruction [38].

The new adjuncts can be considered as a *reconstructive toolbox* to be utilised as deemed appropriate (Fig. 3.3). This can be as a sole form of reconstruction or integrated to the *reconstructive elevator* methods.

3.4 Defect Reconstruction: Function, Form and Aesthetic

The modern era in reconstruction should ideally aim to address achieving excellent form, function and aesthetics of any defect. A detailed analysis of the defect is crucial as an initial step to determine all components (skin, subcutaneous

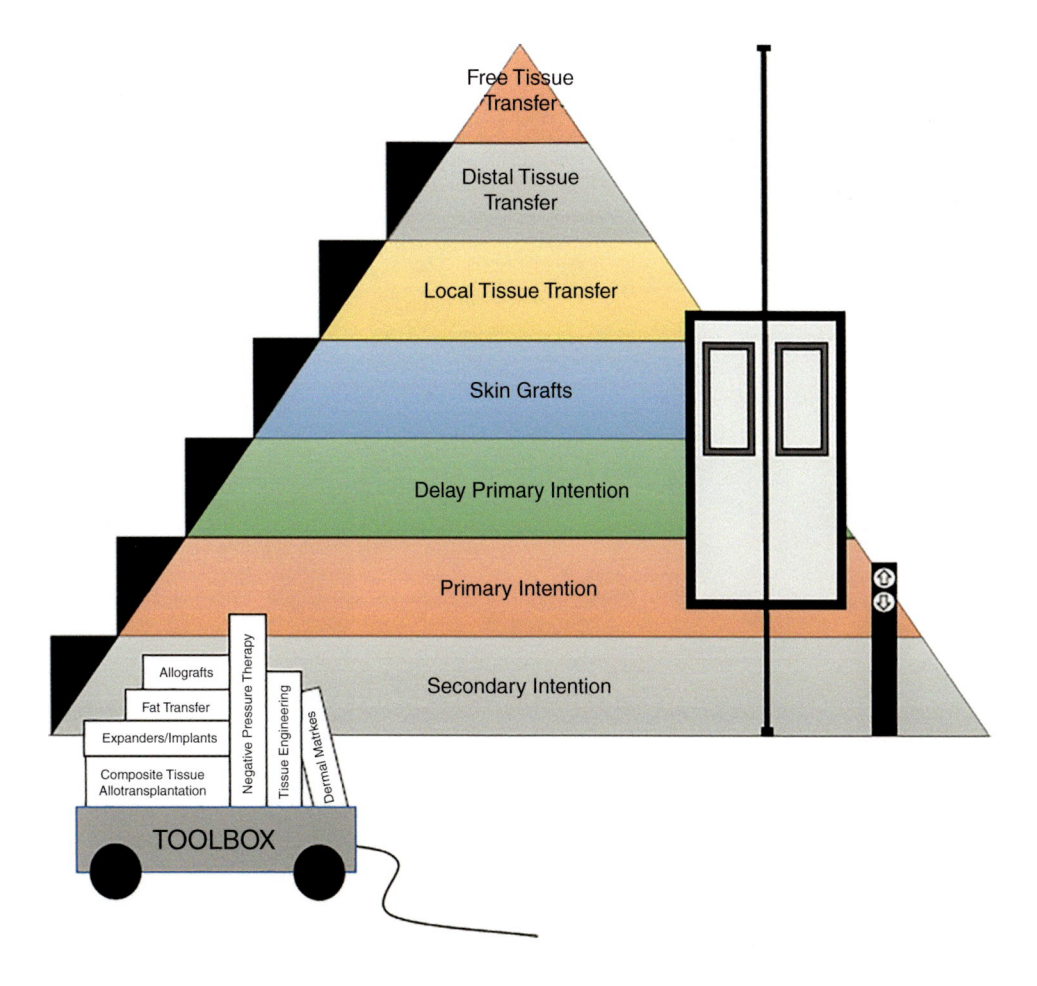

Fig. 3.3 The reconstructive toolbox—adjuncts to the elevator

fat, muscle, bone, tendons and ligaments) to be reconstructed. The principle of "like for like" is to be applied in reconstructive surgery when choosing an ideal option. This is particularly a key step following traumatic or oncological resection of tissue defects. Working within a multidisciplinary setting and putting patients' choices first is rather paramount in making good choices for reconstruction. Patients may opt for a less than optimal choice for reconstruction which should be respected. The transition of form and function to integrate aesthetics happened over the past decade. The diverse and advanced field of reconstructive microsurgery in offering free flaps has led to having more than one option for a particular defect. We advocate the application of an option in reconstruction taking into account patient choice, defect and donor site in achieving the best outcome. The flexibility in such choices would also be limited by the surgeon's own experience in applying all the available tools for reconstruction.

3.5 Clinical Scenarios

Case 1: (Surgeons Dariush Nikkhah and Jeremy Rawlins) This case demonstrates a 46-year-old man who developed necrotising fasciitis of the right flank and upper thigh. He subsequently underwent multiple skin graft procedures but developed a chronic wound at the right ischial region. He underwent local fasciocutaneous flaps and negative pressure therapy dressing which all subsequently failed. Due to the poor local tissues, a decision was made to perform a free ALT (anterolateral thigh) flap from the contralateral thigh. A preoperative CT angiogram demonstrated suitable recipient vessels at the lateral circumflex femoral artery (LCFA). The ALT flap was anastomosed to the LCFA. The patient had an unremarkable post-operative outcome. This case demonstrates the concept of the reconstructive elevator with the use of a free flap being the most suitable option (Figs. 3.4, 3.5, 3.6, and 3.7).

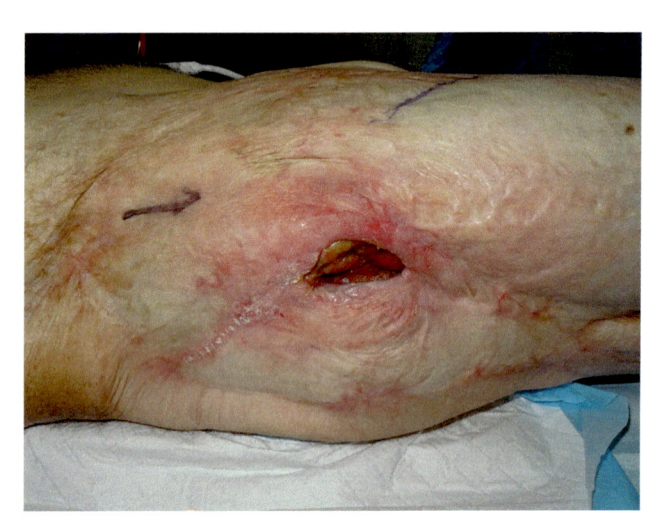

Fig. 3.4 Right ischial chronic wound

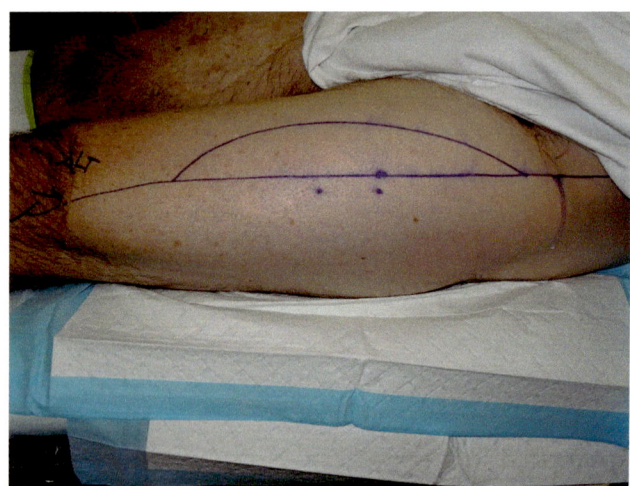

Fig. 3.5 Marking of contralateral ALT free flap

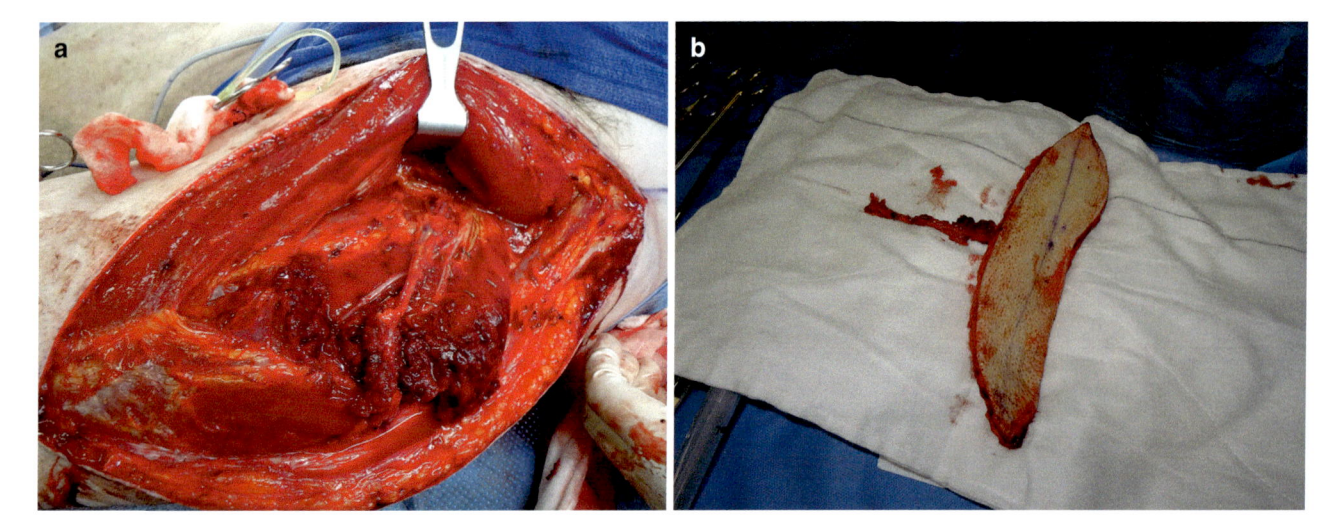

Fig. 3.6 (**a**) Elevation of contralateral ALT flap demonstrating long intramuscular course (**b**) ALT flap with long pedicle ready for transfer

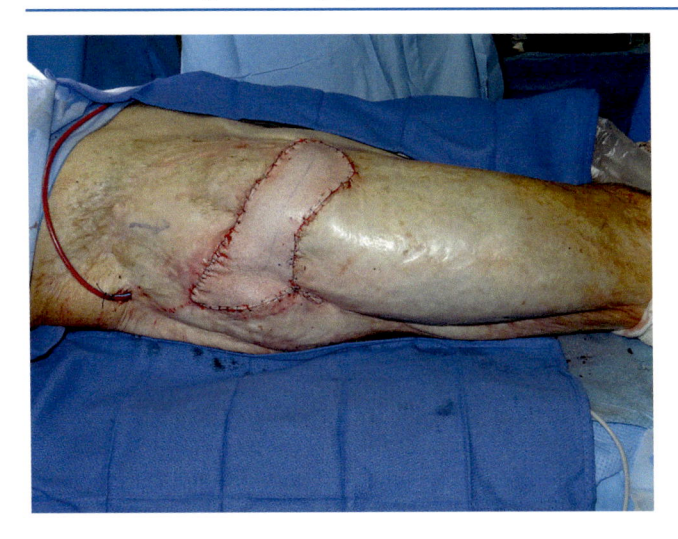

Fig. 3.7 Right ischial chronic wound reconstruction with free ALT flap (contralateral)

3.6 Selected Readings

- Agrawal N, Zavlin D, Louis M, Reece E. Stem cells and plastic surgery. Semin Plast Surg. 2019;33:162–6.

- *Adipose-derived stem cells and cultured epithelial autografts are the most relevant clinical examples in plastic surgery and the stem cell technology. The future induction of pluripotent stem cells leads to breakthrough in regenerative medicine. The limitations of current signalling pathway, inhibition of differentiations into carcinomas and new advancing technologies are key to clinical application in medicine.*

- Iske J, Nian Y, Maenosono R, Maurer M, Sauer I, Tullius S. Composite tissue allotransplantation: opportunities and challenges. Cell Mol Immunol. 2019;16:343–9.

- *Vascularised composite tissue allotransplantation offers unique opportunities for severely injured patients. The current protocols of immunosuppression are effective in preventing acute rejection. A more balanced approach of benefits vs. risks of long-term immunosuppression is to be considered. The future is to determine a tolerance regime to allow immunological acceptance of donor tissue without the need for immunosuppression.*

- Jessop Z, Al-Sabah A, Gardiner M, Combellack E, Hawkins K, Whitaker I. 3D bioprinting for reconstructive surgery: principles, applications and challenges. J Plast Reconstr Aesthet Surg. 2017;70(9):1155–70.

- *The three-dimensional (3D) biomanufacturing of human tissue would ultimately replace autologous tissue transfer and further remove the need for immunosuppression. Overcoming the challenges in bioprinting whether biological, technological or regulatory would translate into clinical practice in reconstructive surgery.*

- Taylor I, Corlett R, Dhar S, Ashton M. The anatomical (angiosome) and clinical territories of cutaneous perforating arteries: development of the concept and designing safe flaps. Plast Reconstr Surg. 2011;127(4):1447–59.

- *This paper illustrates the concept of cutaneous (angiosomes) creating a network of vessels covering the entire body. A detailed description of the anatomical and clinical territory of a perforator is described on the bases of choke connections. It highlighted the important work on perforasome theory by Saint-Cyr. Clinical examples related to DIEP flap integrated these concepts to provide safe flap planning and patient selection.*

- Guo L, Pribaz J. Chapter 11: Prefabrication and prelamination. In: Wei F-C, Mardini S, editors. Flaps and reconstructive surgery; 2009. p. 103–16.

- *Flap prefabrication is a two-stage process involving a vascular pedicle being introduced into tissue for a desired reconstruction which is followed by a transfer of neovascularised tissue into the defect. Flap prelamination refers to a two-stage process whereby one or more tissues are engrafted into a reliable vascular bed to create a multilayered composite flap which is subsequently transferred on its original vascular supply en bloc to the site of reconstruction. A clear understanding of the difference between the two techniques is helpful in choosing the appropriate technique to deal with a specific clinical problem and also for scientific communication.*

References

1. Wallace A. History of plastic surgery: the early development of pedicle flaps. J R Soc Med. 1978;71:834–8.
2. Marck KW, Palyvoda R, Bamji A, et al. The tubed pedicle flap centennial: its concept, origin, rise and fall. Eur J Plast Surg. 2017;40:473–8.
3. Murphy JB. Resection of arteries and veins injured in continuity end-to-end sutured experimental and clinical research. Med Rec. 1897;51:73.
4. Friedman SG. The end-to-end anastomosis of John B. Murphy. J Vasc Surg. 2015;62(2):515–7.
5. Carrel A, Morel B. Anastomose bout about de la jugulaireet de la 5. carotide primitive. Lyon Méd. 1902;99:114–6.
6. Tamai S. History of microsurgery – from the beginning until the end of the 1970s. Microsurgery. 1993;14(1):6–13.
7. Starzl T. The birth of clinical organ transplantation. J Am Coll Surg. 2001;192(4):431–46.
8. Seidenberg B, Rosenak S, Hurwitt E. Immediate reconstruction of the cervical esophagus by a revascularized isolated jejunal segment. Ann Surg. 1959;149(2):162–71.
9. Whitworthm I, Pickford M. The first toe-to-hand transfer: a thirty-year follow-up. J Hand Surg. 2001;25(6):608–10.

10. McLean DH, Buncke HJ Jr. Autotransplant of omentum to a large scalp defect, with microsurgical revascularization. Plast Reconstr Surg. 1972;49(3):268–74.
11. McGregor I, Jackson I. The groin flap. Br J Plast Surg. 1972;25:3–16.
12. Daniel RK, Taylor GI. Distant transfer of an island flap by microvascular anastomoses: a clinical technique. Plast Reconstr Surg. 1973;52:111–7.
13. Taylor I, Palmer J. The vascular territories (angiosomes) of the body: experimental study and clinical applications. Br J Plast Surg. 1987;40(2):113–41.
14. Mathes SJ, Nahai F. Clinical applications for muscle and musculocutaneous flaps. St. Louis, MO: C.V. Mosby; 1982.
15. Shen ZY. Microvascular transplantation of prefabricated free thigh flap (letter). Plast Reconstr Surg. 1982;69:568.
16. Maitz PK, Pribaz JJ, Duffy FJ, Hergrueter CA. The value of the delay phenomenon in flap prefabrication: an experimental study in rabbits. Br J Plast Surg. 1994;47:149–54.
17. Dubernard JM, Owen E, Herzberg G, et al. Human hand allograft: report on first 6 months. Lancet. 1999;353:1315–20.
18. Dubernard JM, et al. Outcomes 18 months after the first human partial face transplantation. N Engl J Med. 2007.
19. Siemionow M, Kulahci Y. Facial transplantation. Semin Plast Surg. 2007;21(4):259–68.
20. Gillies HD, Millard DR. Principles and art of plastic surgery. Boston, MA: Little Brown; 1957.
21. Wei FC, Mardini S. Free-style free flaps. Plast Reconstr Surg. 2004;114(4):910–6.
22. Gottlieb LJ, Krieger LM. From the reconstructive ladder to the reconstructive elevator. Plast Reconstr Surg. 1994;93(7):1503–4.
23. Lineaweaver WC. Microsurgery and the reconstructive ladder. Microsurgery. 2005;25:185–6.
24. Wong CJ, Niranjan N. Reconstructive stages as an alternative to the reconstructive ladder. Plast Reconstr Surg. 2008;121:362e–3e.
25. Mathes SJ, Nahai F. Reconstructive surgery: principles, anatomy & technique, vol. 2. New York, NY; St. Louis, MO: Churchill Livingstone; Quality Medical; 1997.
26. Abu-Ghname A, Perdanasari A, Reece E. Principles and applications of fat grafting in plastic surgery. Semin Plast Surg. 2019;33(3):147–54.
27. Manconi A, De Lorenzi F, Chahuan B, Valeria Berrino V, Berrino P, Zucca-Matthes G, Petit J, Rietjens M. Total breast reconstruction with fat grafting after internal expansion and expander removal. Ann Plast Surg. 2017;78(4):392–6.
28. Nahai F. Surgery of the chin. Facial Plast Surg. 2012;28(1):34–9.
29. Apte A, Walsh M, Balaji P, Khor B, Chandrasekharan S, Chakravorty A. Single stage immediate breast reconstruction with acellular dermal matrix and implant: defining the risks and outcomes of post-mastectomy radiotherapy. Surgeon. 2020;18(4):202–7.
30. Ge P, Imai T, Aboulian A, Van Natta T. The use of human acellular dermal matrix for chest wall reconstruction. Ann Thorac Surg. 2010;90(6):1799–804.
31. Maxwell D, Hart A, Keifer O, Halani S, Losken A. A comparison of acellular dermal matrices in abdominal wall reconstruction. Ann Plast Surg. 2019;82(4):435–40.
32. Jagdeo J, Ho D, Lo A, Carruthers A. A systematic review of filler agents for aesthetic treatment of HIV facial lipoatrophy (FLA). J Am Acad Dermatol. 2015;73(6):1040–54.e14.
33. Lee J, Lorenc Z. Synthetic fillers for facial rejuvenation. Clin Plast Surg. 2016;43(3):497–503.
34. Jones JW, Gruber SA, Barker JH, Breidenbach WC. Successful hand transplantation: one-year follow-up. Louisville Hand Transplant Team. N Engl J Med. 2000;343:468–73.
35. Petit F, Minns A, Dubernard J-M, Hettiaratchy S, Lee W. Composite tissue allotransplantation and reconstructive surgery: first clinical applications. Ann Surg. 2003;237(1):19–25.
36. Al-Himdani S, Jessop Z, Al-Sabah A, Combellack E, Ibrahim A, Doak S, Hart A, Archer C, Thornton C, Whitaker I. Tissue-engineered solutions in plastic and reconstructive surgery: principles and practice. Front Surg. 2017;23(4):4.
37. Moradiellos J, Amor S, Córdoba M, Rocco G, Vidal M, Varela A. Functional chest wall reconstruction with a biomechanical three-dimensionally printed implant. Ann Thorac Surg. 2017;103(4):e389–91.
38. Strong A, Neumeister M, Levi B. Stem cells and tissue engineering: regeneration of the skin and its contents. Clin Plast Surg. 2017;44(3):635–50.

Assessment of Flap Perfusion: Microvascular Flowmetry

Joshua Luck

4.1 Introduction

4.1.1 Rationale for Microvascular Flowmetry

Since the advent of microsurgical free tissue transfer in the 1950s, various surgical and technical advancements have markedly improved flap survival rates. Although success rates of over 95% are now widely achievable [1], flap failure remains a rare but disastrous outcome.

At present, intraoperative evaluation of flap perfusion relies on a subjective assessment of tissue colour, capillary refill and bleeding quality; this assessment is even more challenging for flaps without a cutaneous component. Anastomotic patency can be further interrogated with the Acland test; however this is only able to subjectively differentiate between 'some flow' and 'no flow' at a single time point [2]. Although partial or total flap failure may be prevented by on-table revision, the threshold doing so is poorly defined and varies according to surgeon experience [3]. In addition, although insufficient flap edge circulation can lead to various adverse outcomes (including wound dehiscence and fat necrosis), accurately identifying subtle features that indicate suboptimal tissue perfusion at the time of flap inset is often difficult.

Post-operatively, early recognition of flap compromise is directly linked to salvage rates [4, 5]. Given that flap ischaemia becomes irreversible after only a few hours [6], prompt re-exploration of the failing flap is essential to avoid 'no-reflow' outcomes. However, clinical assessment is subjective, labour-intensive and prone to error [4]. When used alone, clinical monitoring leads to variable salvage rates, ranging from 30% to 80% [7, 8].

4.1.2 How Can Microvascular Flowmetry Help the Reconstructive Microsurgeon?

Flowmeter measurements are routinely used in cardiac surgery to qualitatively and quantitatively assess graft patency. Although there is currently limited evidence for microvascular free flap flowmetry [2], these technologies may have a role in determining the need for on-table flap revision and as adjunct tools in post-operative flap monitoring.

Microvascular flowmeters may be used intraoperatively to objectively and reliably evaluate anastomotic patency and flap perfusion. When used in conjunction with traditional clinical assessment, flowmetry tools provide objective data to aid surgical decision-making. For example, they may provide reassurance about the viability of larger flaps [9] or indicate the need for immediate anastomotic revision [10]. There is emerging evidence that their use leads to shorter surgical procedures [11, 12], altered flap design (by including additional perforators [13, 14], excising poorly perfused areas [15, 16] or converting to a different flap [17]) and improved flap survival rates [3].

Clinical surveillance throughout the post-operative period remains the gold standard monitoring technique. However, subjective assessments of colour, turgor, capillary refill, temperature and pinprick bleeding may be augmented by the use of flowmeter devices. Subtle clinical changes may be missed by inexperienced medical or nursing personnel—here, objective monitoring adjuncts can improve salvage rates by promoting earlier take back. Clinical monitoring is especially challenging in buried flaps and in anatomical areas with difficult access, such as the head and neck. Although this can be partially mitigated by including a distal skin paddle [18, 19] or exteriorised segment [20, 21], significant caution must be exercised when evaluating the status of these monitoring or sentinel flaps. Here, there is a clinical need for surgical technologies that can provide direct, objective and real-time information about the perfusion of the primary flap.

J. Luck (✉)
Department of Plastic & Reconstructive Surgery, Stoke Mandeville Hospital, Aylesbury, UK
e-mail: joshua.luck1@nhs.net

4.2 Intraoperative Flowmetry

4.2.1 Fluorescence Angiography

4.2.1.1 What Is It?

Fluorescence angiography (FA) is real-time, semiquantitative imaging modality used to assess microvascular flow. It has a well-established role in ophthalmic, cardiothoracic and neurosurgical settings. Although the technique was developed with fluorescein dye, modern flowmetry devices preferentially use indocyanine green (ICG) as it has a shorter half-life, quicker onset of action and superior side effect profile [22]. In ICG angiography (ICGA), a near-infrared light source (750–800 nm) is used to excite intravenously administered ICG, while a digital camera positioned over the flap captures fluorescence within the downstream microvasculature. Bolus doses of 3–5 mL are injected before a cinegraphic image is captured after 15–20 s [10]. Perforators and small vessels appear as 'fluorescent blushes' against a black background, whereas ischaemic areas remain dark (Fig. 4.1). Multiple injections—up to a maximum dose of 5 mg/kg [24]—may be administered within the same surgical procedure [25].

4.2.1.2 How Is It Used?

In autologous breast reconstruction, ICGA may help to select a dominant perforator [15, 26, 27], identify inadequately perfused areas of the free flap [14, 28–30] and ensure viability of the mastectomy skin flaps [22]. Although ICGA is able to provide a dynamic, topographic representation of dermal blood flow, various commercially available systems have been developed to perform more complex semiquantitative analyses (see Table 4.1). The most widely used ICGA device is the SPY Elite system which, in conjunction with the corresponding SPY-Q software, can provide objective measures of microvascular flow. For example, the intrinsic transit time (ITT)—namely, the time taken for the dye to pass from the arterial to the venous anastomosis—has been shown to strongly predict flap failure. Over 90% of flaps with an ITT of greater than 50 s require post-operative re-exploration or fail [31], and a number of authors recommend on-table revision above this threshold [3].

4.2.1.3 Technical Considerations and Limitations

ICGA is necessarily invasive, requiring the administration of a water-soluble, biliary-excreted dye. Although serious allergic reactions are rare [32], ICG is contraindicated in patients

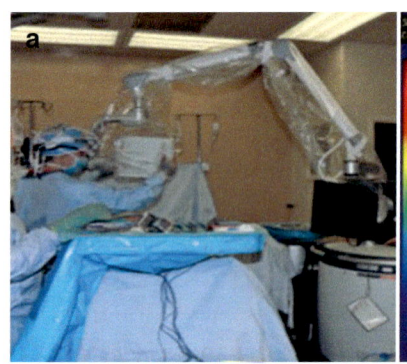

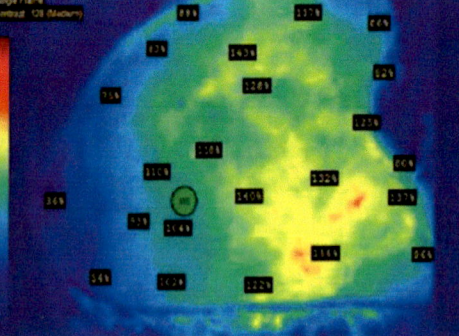

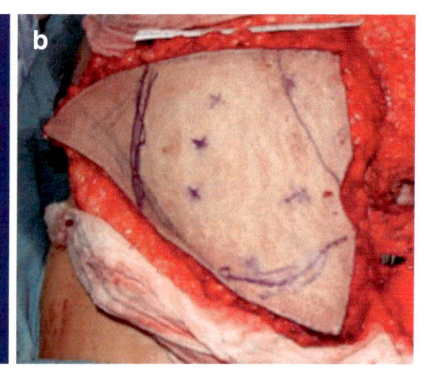

Fig. 4.1 Intraoperative ICG angiography using the SPY Elite system (reproduced from Hanasano [23] with permission). An articulating arm allows the surgeon to position the cinegraphic camera over the operative field. Images (**a**) and (**b**) correspond to the same right-sided transverse rectus abdominis flap. In (**a**), the user has assigned a value of 100% to the area of maximal perfusion; the SPY-Q software then provides relative perfusion values for the rest of the flap. In (**b**), the surgeon has marked several perforators centrally and areas of poor perfusion peripherally

Table 4.1 Commercially available ICGA detection systems

	SPY Elite	FLARE	PDE-Neo	Fluobeam 800
Manufacturer	Novadaq (Stryker), Canada	Curadel LLC, USA	Hamamatsu Photonics, Japan	Fluoptics, France
Software	SPY-Q	XIP	N/A	N/A
Data	Quantitative	Quantitative	Qualitative	Qualitative

FLARE fluorescence-assisted resection and exploration, *PDE* photodynamic eye

who are pregnant, as well as individuals with liver disease or a known iodine allergy. Importantly, ICGA can only assess perfusion up to a depth of 1 cm; hence it is unlikely to supersede computed tomographic (CT) or magnetic resonance (MR) angiography in pre-operative flap planning (especially in clinical cases where a thick pannus may be preferred, such as with a DIEP). In addition, ICGA is limited in its ability to reliably detect venous occlusion [2]; however, when there are concerns about venous congestion, some authors suggest re-imaging at 5–20 min to confirm dye clearance [23]. Furthermore, it is important that clinicians remain aware of the various systemic factors (including volume status, blood pressure and temperature) that influence superficial dermal perfusion.

Although a range of commercially available ICGA systems are available, the most commonly used system is the SPY Elite device. The initial investment required is significant [22] and each use may cost up to 1200 USD [33]. Given that the hardware is difficult to transport between theatre suites and hospitals, to what extent this adversely impacts upon the cost-effectiveness of ICGA has yet to be determined. Finally, there is a surgical learning curve for the SPY-Q system, and there remains a lack of consensus as to how to interpret the various quantitative output measures it provides [3]. For example, there are no widely accepted thresholds indicative of inadequate tissue perfusion using either relative or absolute perfusion indices.

4.2.2 Transit Time Volume Flowmetry

4.2.2.1 What Is It?
Transit time volume flowmetry (TTVF) is a non-Doppler-based ultrasound technology that is commonly used to assess intraoperative coronary graft patency. The probe consists of two transducer crystals that sit at 45° to the long axis of the vessel with a reflector positioned halfway between them on the contralateral vessel wall. Both transducers emit an ultrasound beam which is reflected onto the other transducer. The ultrasound signal takes longer to pass upstream than downstream and this delay is proportional to blood flow [34]. Hence the transit time reflects blood flow across an anastomosis, represented as flow curves with quantitative mean flow and pulsatility index values (Fig. 4.2). Unlike Doppler-based ultrasound approaches, TTVF measurements are independent of vessel diameter and wall thickness [35]. Furthermore, TTVF readings are not influenced by heart rate, flow velocity or serum haemoglobin levels [36].

4.2.2.2 How Is It Used?
TTVF offers an intraoperative measurement of flow volume across a pedicle, providing the surgeon with useful information about the quality of the arterial anastomosis and reliability of the venous outflow. If TTVF demonstrates low, no or retrograde flow (or an unacceptably high pulsatility index), this should prompt the surgeon to revise the anastomosis. Similarly, TTVF has been shown to be useful in identifying venae comitans with the highest flow rates—importantly, this does not always correlate with vessel calibre [34]. Supporting evidence from the lymphaticovenous anastomosis (LVA) literature has shown that TTVF can be used to establish quantitative thresholds for minimum flow rates in target vessels in lieu of traditional judgements about their calibre or degree of sclerosis.

4.2.2.3 Technical Considerations and Limitations
Unlike ICGA, TTVF focusses specifically on pedicle flow—it therefore does not provide any direct assessment of end-organ perfusion. In a direct comparison between ICGA and TTVF for coronary grafts, TTVF was shown to be significantly less able to detect clinically relevant graft failures. Furthermore, TTVF may only be used to augment intraoperative decision-making; however, acceptable threshold flow rates for each workhorse flap have yet to be established. In an experimental pig model, flow rates less than 4 ml/min were found to be unreliable [35], although to what extent such low flow rates would be clinically relevant is unclear. Finally, some authors have reported technical issues in setting up the TTVF probe apparatus [3].

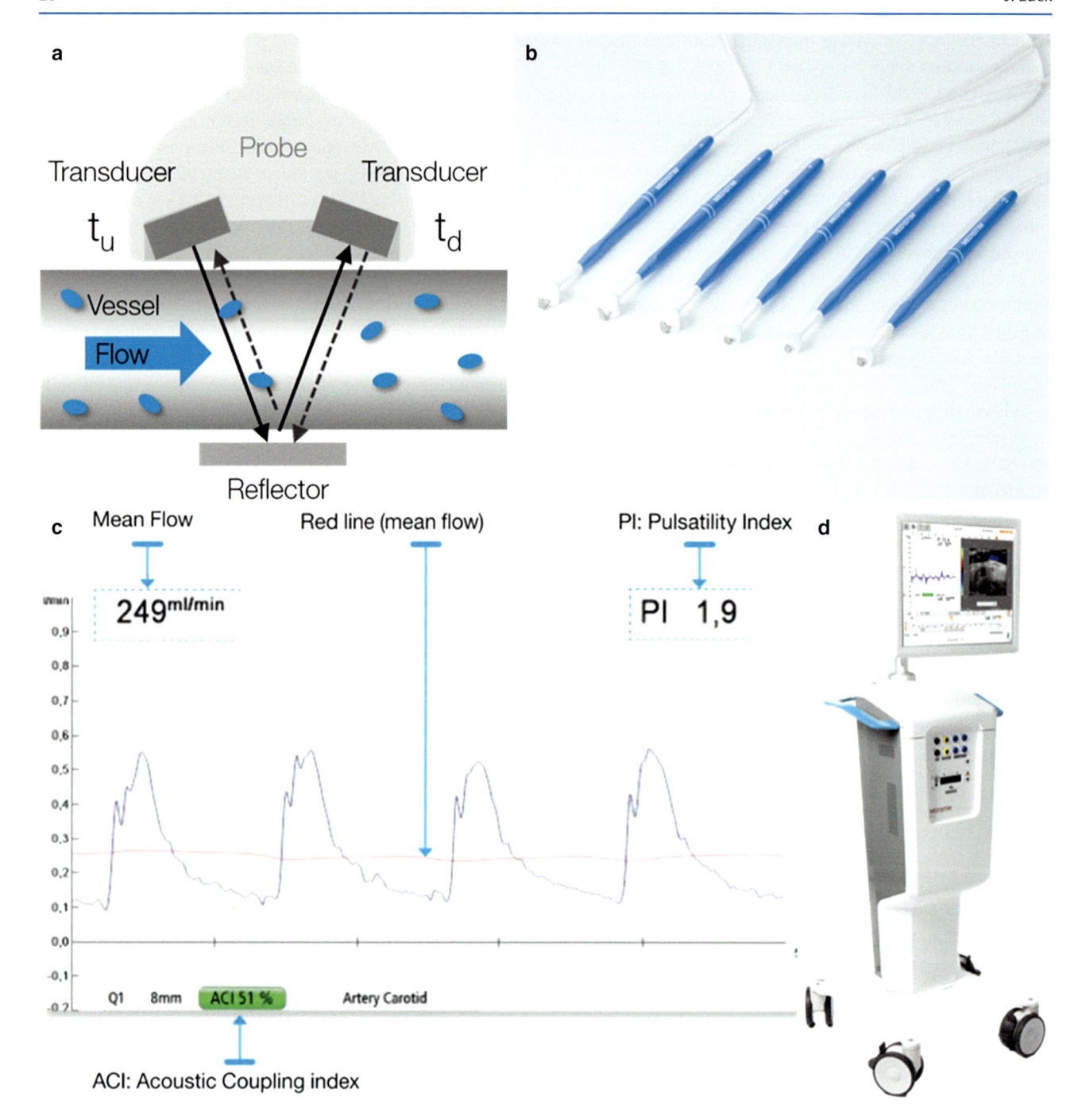

Fig. 4.2 Transit time volume flowmetry using the Medistim system (reproduced with permission from Medistim). (**a**) Each probe contains two transducers that fire ultrasound pulses in opposite directions. The time taken for the ultrasound beam to pass upstream (t_u) is slightly longer than downstream (t_d), and this delay is proportional to blood flow. (**b**) Medistim QuickFit™ vascular probes. (**c**) Quantitative mean flow values should be interpreted in the context of vessel size and blood pressure. The pulsatility index is calculated by dividing the difference between the maximum and minimum flow by the mean flow: a high pulsatility index (caused by turbulence or vasospasm) may suggest that the measurements are unreliable or may indicate the need for anastomotic revision. Before using the Medistim system, a baseline acoustic coupling index is recorded: to ensure that the measurements taken intraoperatively are reliable, this should remain >30%. (**d**) Medistim MiraQ™ vascular system

4.3 Post-operative Flowmetry

4.3.1 Non-invasive

4.3.1.1 Laser Doppler

What Is It?

Laser Doppler flowmetry (LDF) provides a continuous and non-invasive measurement of blood flow within a small (1 mm^3) volume of tissue located 0.5–8 mm beneath a surface probe [1]. The probe is held in place using either adhesive material or sutures, and it is connected to a 5 mW diode laser via a fibreoptic cable [37]. The target tissue is illuminated with coherent laser light, and the frequency shift of backscattered light reflects the average velocity of erythrocytes. It provides a real-time reflection of tissue perfusion expressed as a relative velocity (Fig. 4.3). Although measurements are typically given in mL/min/100 g tissue, they are often considered as arbitrary units [38, 39] and may be normalised to flow values before flap elevation [40]. Although tissue penetration is affected by skin pigmentation and probe geometry, LDF is particularly useful in muscle flaps and darker skin where clinical evaluation is more challenging [41].

How Is It Used?

Importantly, relative perfusion values vary between tissues and patients. As a result, it is the trend that is informative, as opposed to any absolute values. When arterial inflow is lost, flow values typically steeply decline towards zero [42]. This means that LDF may be used intraoperatively during flap inset when the pedicle may be compromised by kinking, stretching or excessive pressure [43]. In the post-operative surveillance period, a decline in normalised flow values should prompt close clinical review and possibly re-exploration [40, 43]. Some authors use a decrease in perfusion value of over 50% for >20 min as their threshold for clinical review [41] although there are no widely accepted standards across the literature [44]. With conventional LDF, venous obstruction is more subtle—here, there is a slower decline in flow values as blood is still able to enter the flap until the capacitance of the system is exceeded [42, 45]. To address this issue, more modern LDF devices (such as the Oxygen to See (O2C, LEA Medizintechnik, Germany) system) combine conventional LDF with white light spectrophotometry to better differentiate between arterial and venous insufficiency [46]. Similarly, some LDF probes have integrated surface temperature sensors to provide additional information about flap perfusion.

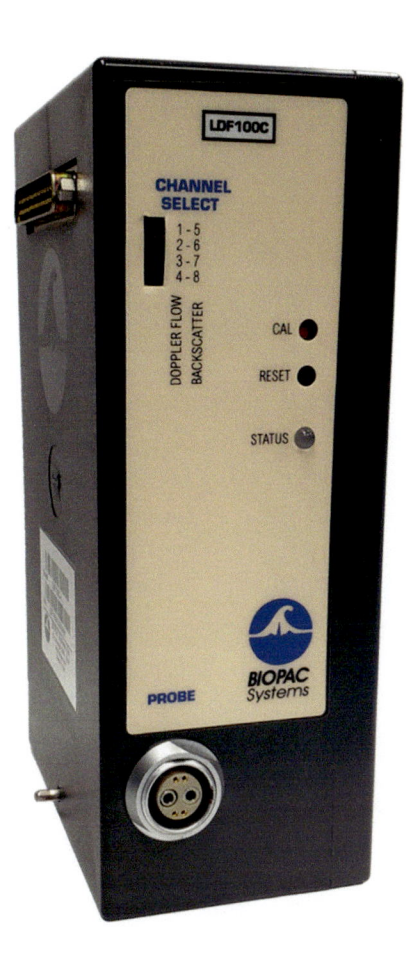

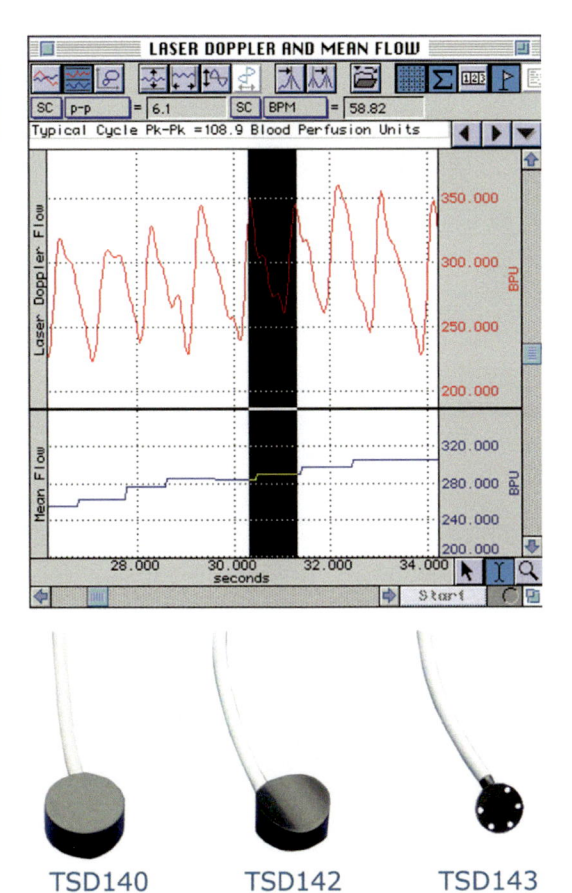

Fig. 4.3 Laser Doppler flowmetry system (reproduced with permission from BIOPAC). Various different fibreoptic surface probes (pictured) and invasive needle probes (not pictured) are compatible with the BIOPAC laser Doppler flowmetry system. Flow values are usually treated as arbitrary units, and it is the trend in relative perfusion (rather than any absolute value) that is informative

Technical Considerations and Limitations

Although LDF is highly sensitive and relatively easy to use [2], flow values may be falsely elevated by movement or vibration artefacts [39], and positive flow values have been observed even in 'no flow' conditions [47]. Furthermore, LDF calculations are influenced by erythrocyte density—hence laser Doppler techniques may be inaccurate in the context of anaemia or haemodilution, both of which are not uncommon following free tissue transfer. From a practical perspective, it can be difficult to maintain probe contact on moist or bloody surfaces, and probe dislodgement may produce falsely low readings [38]. On some devices, the last recorded value may still be displayed with an 'out of range' alert. As a result, inexperienced medical or nursing personnel could miss this warning and be falsely reassured [48]. It is also worth highlighting that the probe is only able to monitor a small tissue area and hence the anastomoses indirectly. Finally, as with any new technology, there are expensive start-up costs [43] that require rigorous cost-benefit evaluation in each clinical setting.

4.3.1.2 Near-Infrared Spectroscopy

What Is It?

Near-infrared spectroscopy (NIRS) uses the selective light absorption characteristics of haemoglobin to provide continuous, non-invasive monitoring of tissue perfusion [49]. A probe attached to the flap surface emits calibrated near-infrared wavelengths that penetrate up to 20 mm [50] (Fig. 4.4). Backscattered light is then collected by a receiver photodiode, and the ratio of oxyhaemoglobin to deoxyhaemoglobin is used to calculate tissue oxygen saturation (StO2) levels [4]. In principle, NIRS is not significantly different from traditional white/visible light spectroscopy; however, the absorption of visible light is 100 times greater than near-infrared wavelengths, meaning that NIRS is particularly useful in thick flaps [51]. Unlike other modalities (such as LDF), NIRS is not significantly influenced by movement artefact or temporary probe detachment [50], making it a practical adjunct in ward-based settings. Furthermore, StO2 is not affected by common confounding physiological (e.g. blood

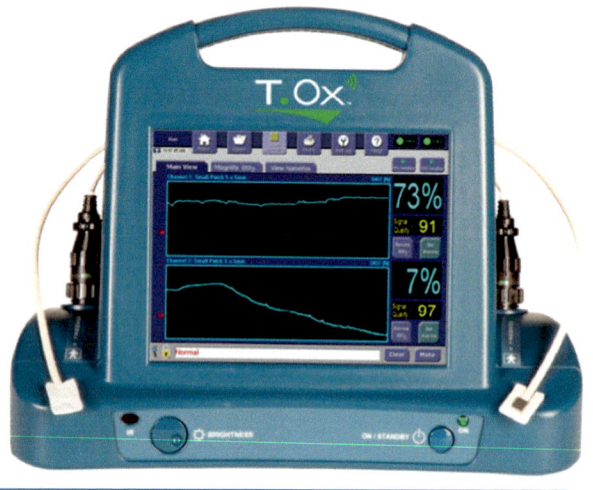

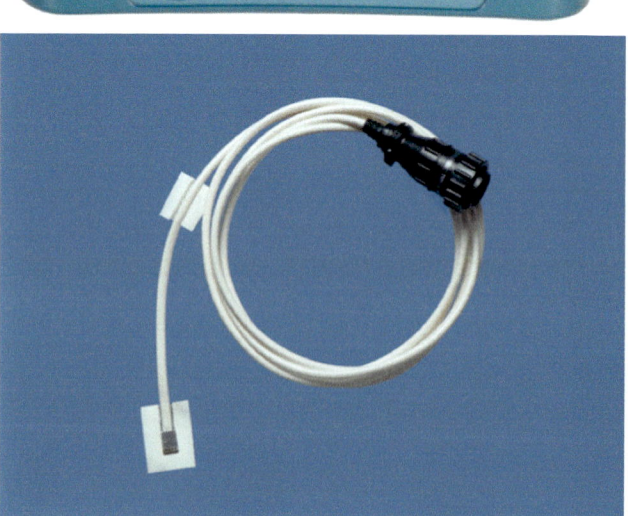

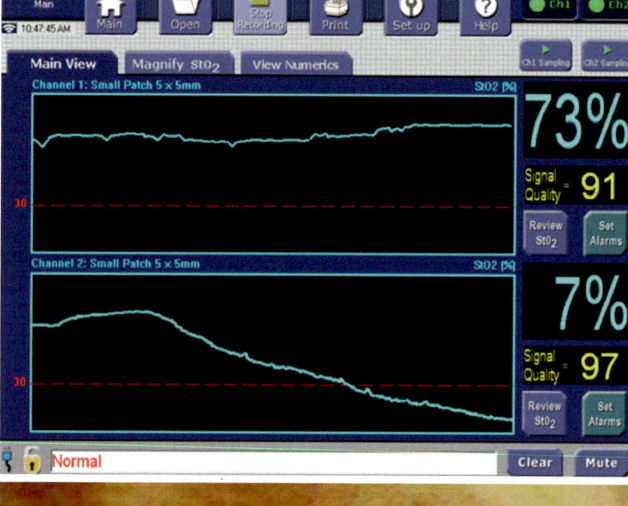

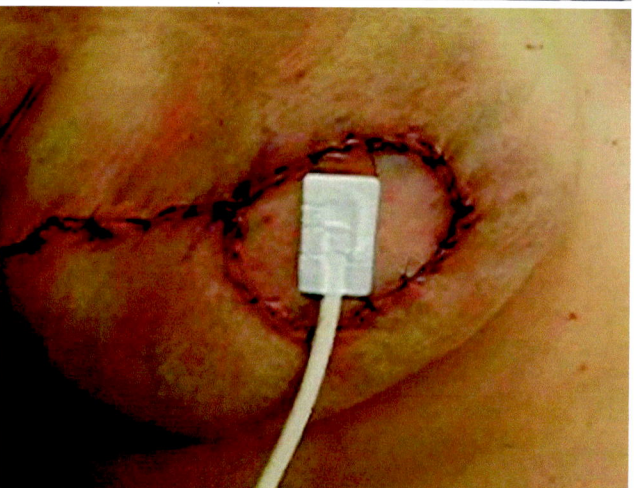

Fig. 4.4 Near-infrared spectroscopy T.Ox™ system (reproduced with permission from ViOptix). A probe attached to the flap surface emits calibrated near-infrared wavelengths and measures backscattered light. The ratio of oxyhaemoglobin to haemoglobin is then used to provide a continuous trace of tissue oxygen saturation

Table 4.2 Commercially available NIRS systems (adapted from Kagaya et al. [51])

	O2C	T.Ox Tissue Oximeter	T-Stat VLS	TOS-OR
Measurement depth	2–8 mm[a]	3–6 mm	2 mm	8–16 mm
Update interval	2 s	4 s	1 s	1 s
Measurement item(s)	StO2	StO2	StO2	StO2
	rHb		THB	HbI
	Flow velocity			
Device cost (USD)	Device: 27,000	Device: 40,000	Device: 32,500	Not currently in production
	Probe: 2240	Probe: 1600	Probe: 660–760	
Manufacturer	LEA Medizintechnik GmbH, Germany	ViOptix, USA	Spectros, USA	Fujita, Japan

USD US dollars, *StO2* tissue oxygen saturation, *Hb* haemoglobin, *rHb* relative amount of haemoglobin, *THI* tissue haemoglobin index, *HbI* haemoglobin index, *THB* total haemoglobin concentration
[a] Different depth probes available

pressure and supplemental oxygen) and flap (e.g. perforator number and size) variables [52].

How Is It Used?

Various proprietary NIRS systems are commercially available (see Table 4.2)—all of these measure StO2, and the majority provide additional information about tissue haemoglobin (Hb) which helps to differentiate between arterial and venous compromise. In general, arterial insufficiency is indicated by a reduction in both StO2 and Hb levels, whereas venous congestion is usually characterised by a transient increase in StO2 followed by a steady decline with rising Hb values. Although there is no widely accepted consensus as to the thresholds that prompt surgical re-exploration, StO2 levels below 30% (or falling by >15% per hour) should raise concerns about the status of the flap [51, 53]. To help in the interpretation of the NIRS data recorded, some authors advocate the use of a second probe on native, healthy tissue (e.g. the contralateral breast) to provide patient-specific reference values [54].

Technical Considerations and Limitations

While NIRS is able to act as an early warning system for impending flap failure, it is of limited use in the first 8–12 h post-operatively when a physiological decrease in StO2 is expected [49, 51, 55]. Commercially available NIRS monitors differ with respect to their hardware capabilities and proprietary algorithms, meaning that experience with one device may not be readily transferable to another system [49]. Traditionally, NIRS monitors need to be affixed to a cutaneous paddle, although there is emerging evidence that NIRS may be used with buried muscle or visceral organ flaps [55, 56]. Finally, while NIRS is associated with high upfront costs [50, 57] some studies have demonstrated that the routine use of NIRS is cost-effective overall [58].

4.3.1.3 Dynamic Infrared Thermography

What Is It?

Conventional surface temperature monitoring is often used as an adjunct in post-operative free flap monitoring. The primary mechanism of cutaneous heat loss is via infrared (IR) radiation; hence a heat-sensing camera may be used to generate a colour-coded representation of blood flow. In static IR thermography, 'hot' and 'cold' regions are shown on a single image; however, the information gained from a single image is relatively limited and may be subject to interference from complex vascular patterns [59]. As a result, dynamic IR thermography (DIRT) techniques have been developed to monitor the response of a flap to thermal stress—typically a transient cold challenge. To achieve physiological cooling, a conductive metal plate is applied to the area for 30 s [59], or a high-speed portable fan is used to accelerate the evaporation of topically applied isopropyl alcohol spray [60]. The rate and pattern of homeostatic temperature changes is then monitored to provide a visual and non-invasive representation of tissue perfusion (see Fig. 4.5).

How Is It Used?

DIRT may be used both intraoperatively and post-operatively. Several authors have described the use of DIRT in perforator selection [61–63], corroborated by handheld acoustic Doppler. Following completion of the anastomosis, DIRT may then be used to identify on-table issues with the pedicle [64]. Using this technique, it is possible to differentiate between arterial and venous insufficiency: if the entire flap fails to rewarm, this suggests an inflow problem; conversely, venous congestion manifests as adequate rewarming but without characteristic 'hot spots' [10]. Importantly, these features can reliably be identified using IR thermography before macroscopic changes are visible [63]. DIRT may also be used to interrogate flap perfusion post-operatively [65]— here, smartphone-compatible, portable thermographic cameras (such as the Forward Looking Infrared One (FLIR ONE®) device (FLIR Systems, Wilsonville, OR)) may be of particular benefit.

Technical Considerations and Limitations

Early IR thermographic cameras were limited in their ability to detect subtle (<0.1 °C) temperature changes. Since then, improvements in IR technologies mean that DIRT can be

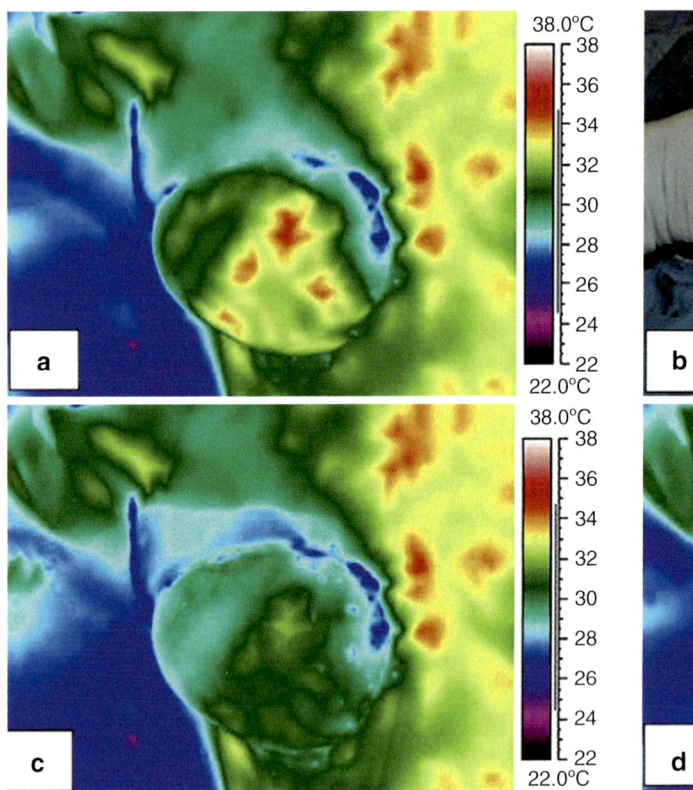

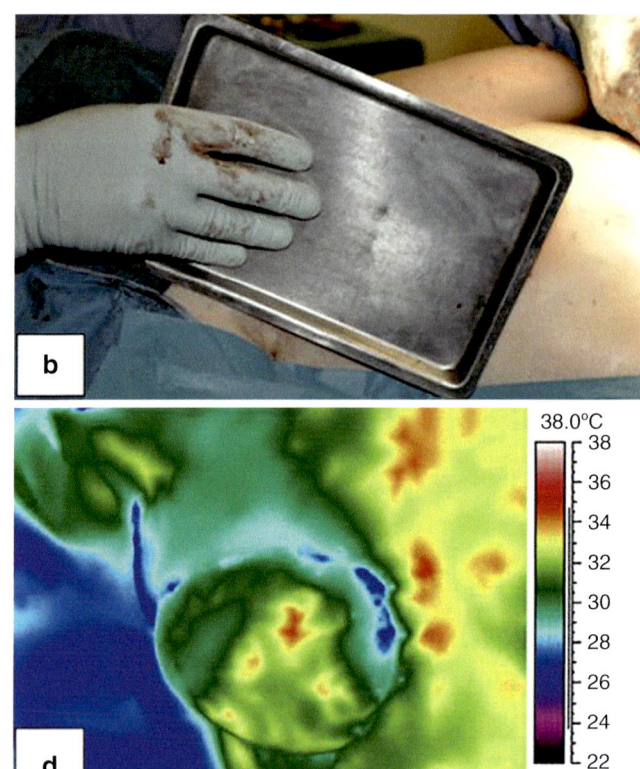

Fig. 4.5 Post-operative dynamic IR thermography images confirming DIEP flap viability in breast reconstruction (reproduced from de Weerd et al. [59] with permission). The thermogram in (**a**) shows the DIEP in situ before gentle cooling with a metal plate (**b**). The effect of cooling is demonstrated in (**c**) before reperfusion is confirmed by rapid return of thermal hot spots (**d**)

used to simply and non-invasively evaluate free flap perfusion. However, DIRT is not able to continuously monitor blood flow and, as the observer is required to make their own assessment of the topographic map displayed, it lacks true objectivity [60]. It is also important that clinicians are aware of this impact of external factors on flap temperature [66]; for example, room temperature, clothing and humidity can generate skin temperature fluctuations of up to 8 °C [67]. Dedicated thermal cameras are less likely to be misled by background thermal interference (such as 'heat hollows' or cutaneous veins [68]), although these are typically more expensive and less portable than their smartphone counterparts.

4.3.2 Invasive

4.3.2.1 Implantable Doppler

What Is It?
The Cook-Swartz implantable Doppler probe was first developed in 1988 [69]. It consists of a 1 mm³ piezoelectric crystal wrapped in a silastic sleeve. This sleeve is wrapped around the vascular pedicle and held in place using sutures [70], microclips [71], fibrin sealant [72] or an elongated soft silicone cuff [73]. When positioned correctly, the pulsed 20 MHz ultrasonic probe reflects flow as a qualitative 'all-or-nothing' phenomenon. A thin wire exiting through the wound connects the probe to a portable monitor via an intermediary extension cable that is sutured to the patient by a series of retention tabs [74]. The wire is then safely removed at between Day 5 and 10 [7] by applying gentle (50 g) tension.

How Is It Used?
The implantable Doppler provides continuous monitoring of blood flow across the pedicle. The probe may be placed on either the artery or vein and, as yet, there is no universal consensus as to which approach is superior [75]. In principle, arterial placement leads to a higher false negative rate as the probe is less able to detect early venous thrombosis [76]. In contrast, venous monitoring is able to promptly identify both inflow and outflow issues [56]. However, venous probes are more easily dislodged and poorly discriminate between true

thrombosis and technical malfunction [76]. Given that implantable Dopplers are especially useful in buried flaps when clinical correlation is challenging, these false positives can lead to unnecessary re-exploration. To some extent, the development of a wireless implantable Doppler system may mitigate against the risk of inadvertent probe dislodgment [77]. In addition, the Cook-Swartz Doppler may be useful during flap inset when it provides valuable information about on-table pedicle compromise [1].

Technical Considerations and Limitations
By design, the implantable Doppler is only able to measure blood flow across the pedicle and provides only limited information about tissue perfusion [1]. It is necessarily invasive and requires the permanent placement of a foreign body, theoretically increasing the risk of anastomotic rupture or thrombosis [56]. This may be particularly problematic in anatomical areas with challenging geometry, such as the head and neck [76], or when multiple probes are used [74]. In addition, its introduction into routine clinical practice involves a surgical learning curve, and, to some extent, the widely variable false positive and false negative rates seen across the literature may reflect operator experience [7]. Finally, as with all flowmetry technologies, rigorous financial evaluation is needed to justify its additional upfront costs in each clinical setting [76].

4.4 Future Directions

4.4.1 Characteristics of an Ideal Flowmetry Device

The ideal monitoring device should be non-invasive and provide real-time, objective measurements of tissue perfusion both intraoperatively and post-operatively [78]. It should

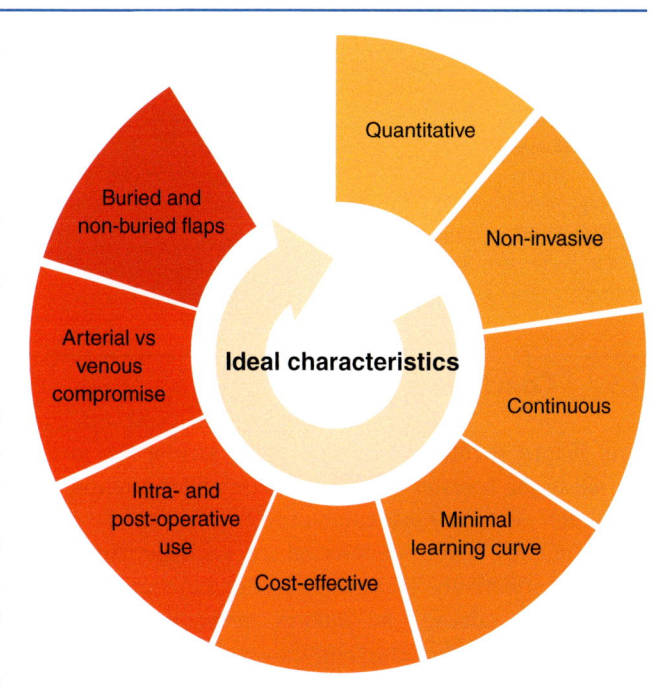

Fig. 4.6 Characteristics of an ideal flowmetry device (created with BioRender)

respond to subtle changes in blood flow and be able to distinguish arterial from venous compromise [37]. It should be applicable to all types of flaps, including those without a cutaneous paddle, and provide quantitative data that can be interpreted by even inexperienced personnel [1]. It should not put either the flap or patient at risk, and it should be cost-effective at scale (Fig. 4.6). Crucially, any flowmetry device must be sufficiently sensitive and specific to meaningfully improve clinical outcomes [4]. For example, post-operative monitoring devices should significantly increase flap salvage rates without an unnecessarily high number of false positive take backs [7]. The key features of each monitoring device discussed in this chapter are outlined in Table 4.3.

Table 4.3 Monitoring characteristics of different flowmetry techniques

Flowmetry technique	Invasive	Timing	Data	Frequency	Pedicle assessment	Buried flaps?
Fluorescence angiography	Yes	Intra-op[a]	Semiquantitative	Single use	A[b]	No
Transit time volume flowmetry	Yes	Intra-op	Quantitative	Single use	A and V	Yes
Laser Doppler	No	Intra- and post-op	Quantitative	Continuous	A and V	Yes
Near-infrared spectroscopy	No	Post-op	Quantitative	Continuous	A and V	Yes[c]
Dynamic infrared thermography	No	Intra- and post-op	Semiquantitative	Intermittent	A and V	No
Implantable Doppler	Yes	Intra- and post-op	Qualitative	Continuous	A and V	Yes

A arterial, *V* venous
[a] Can be used post-operatively
[b] May be able to indirectly demonstrate venous insufficiency
[c] Emerging evidence in buried flaps

Table 4.4 Additional microvascular flowmetry techniques in clinical studies

Non-invasive	Invasive
Colour Doppler	Microdialysis
Pulse oximetry	Contrast-enhanced ultrasound
Photoplethysmography	Nuclear medicine (PET)
Spatial frequency domain imaging	
White/visible light spectroscopy	
Sidestream dark field imaging	

4.5 Conclusions

This chapter reviews the role of microvascular flowmetry in free tissue transfer with a focus on understanding the key features of the most commonly encountered flowmetry techniques. It aims to describe how each modality may be most effectively used with an appreciation of each technique's relative advantages and disadvantages. However, many other emerging flowmetry techniques not discussed here have been trialled in clinical settings (Table 4.4).

Although clinical assessment remains the gold standard method of evaluating free flap perfusion, we anticipate that flowmetry devices will enter widespread clinical use as important intraoperative and post-operative adjunct technologies. At present, there is an unmet clinical need for objective, quantitative tools that are able to accurately predict and monitor free flap outcomes. When appraising the effectiveness of any flap monitoring tool in your own practice, we recommend that you consider the following framework set out by Lineaweaver [79]:

1. False positive rate
2. Sensitivity to true vascular complications
3. Clinical outcomes, including flap failure and flap salvage rates

4.6 Selected Readings

- Chae MP, Rozen WM, Whitaker IS, Chubb D, Grinsell D, Ashton MW, et al. Current Evidence for postoperative monitoring of microvascular free flaps: a systematic review. Ann Plast Surg. 2015;74:621–32.
- *Comprehensive review of post-operative flowmetry technologies with an emphasis on clinically relevant outcomes. In particular, it highlights which monitoring tools lead to improvements in flap salvage without unacceptably high false positive rates.*
- Hanasano MM. Chapter 4 - Emerging technology in reconstructive surgery. In: Wei F-C, Mardini S, editors. Flaps and reconstructive surgery. 2nd ed. Amsterdam: Elsevier; 2016. p. e11.
- *Detailed narrative review of how ICG angiography can be used intraoperatively to improve outcomes in both free tissue transfer and lymphatic surgery. However, no other microvascular flowmetry technologies are discussed.*
- Lohman RF, Ozturk CN, Ozturk C, Jayaprakash V, Djohan R. An analysis of current techniques used for intraoperative flap evaluation. Ann Plast Surg. 2015;75:679–85.
- *Quantitative systematic appraisal of the sensitivity and specificity of intraoperative ICG angiography, dynamic IR thermography and photospectrometry with an attempt to correlate flowmetry data with clinically relevant outcomes (e.g. revision, re-exploration and flap loss).*
- Newton E, Butskiy O, Shadgan B, Prisman E, Anderson DW. Outcomes of free flap reconstructions with near-infrared spectroscopy (NIRS) monitoring: a systematic review. Microsurgery. 2020;40:268–75.
- *PRISMA-compliant systematic review demonstrating the benefit of additional NIRS monitoring post-operatively. Based upon ten articles included in the final analysis, the detection of vascular compromise with NIRS preceded clinical changes, leading to higher salvage rates and reduced partial flap loss.*
- Pafitanis G, Raveendran M, Myers S, Ghanem AM. Flowmetry evolution in microvascular surgery: a systematic review. J Plast Reconstr Aesthet Surg. 2017;70:1242–51.
- *Systematic review of the preclinical and clinical microvascular flowmetry literature with an appraisal of the quality of evidence provided by each study. The article concludes with a discussion of how flowmetry monitoring changes surgical decision-making in both intraoperative and post-operative settings.*
- Smit JM, Zeebregts CJ, Acosta R, Werker PMN. Advancements in free flap monitoring in the last decade: a critical review. Plast Reconstr Surg. 2010;125(1):177–85.
- *Narrative review of commonly encountered flowmetry technologies with an overview of the scientific rationale underpinning each approach. It also assesses to what extent each technique conforms to the criteria for an ideal monitoring device.*
- Smit JM, Negenborn VL, Jansen SM, Jaspers MEH, de Vries R, Heymans MW, et al. Intraoperative evaluation of perfusion in free flap surgery: a systematic review and meta-analysis. Microsurgery. 2018;38:804–18.
- *Well-executed PRISMA-compliant systematic review and meta-analysis of intraoperative flowmeter devices, demonstrating that the use of fluorescence angiography and laser Doppler improves flap survival outcome; insufficient evidence to support the use of oxygen saturation monitoring, dynamic IR thermography, microdialysis and ultrasound-based approaches.*

References

1. Smit JM, Zeebregts CJ, Acosta R, Werker PMN. Advancements in free flap monitoring in the last decade: a critical review. Plast Reconstr Surg. 2010;125(1):177–85.
2. Pafitanis G, Raveendran M, Myers S, Ghanem AM. Flowmetry evolution in microvascular surgery: a systematic review. J Plast Reconstr Aesthet Surg. 2017;70:1242–51.
3. Smit JM, Negenborn VL, Jansen SM, Jaspers MEH, de Vries R, Heymans MW, et al. Intraoperative evaluation of perfusion in free flap surgery: a systematic review and meta-analysis. Microsurgery. 2018;38:804–18.
4. Newton E, Butskiy O, Shadgan B, Prisman E, Anderson DW. Outcomes of free flap reconstructions with near-infrared spectroscopy (NIRS) monitoring: a systematic review. Microsurgery. 2020;40:268–75.
5. Siemionow M, Arslan E. Ischemia/reperfusion injury: a review in relation to free tissue transfers. Microsurgery. 2004;24(6):468–75.
6. Chen K-T, Mardini S, Chuang DC-C, Lin C-H, Cheng M-H, Lin Y-T, et al. Timing of presentation of the first signs of vascular compromise dictates the salvage outcome of free flap transfers. Plast Reconstr Surg. 2007;120(1):187–95.
7. Chae MP, Rozen WM, Whitaker IS, Chubb D, Grinsell D, Ashton MW, et al. Current evidence for postoperative monitoring of microvascular free flaps: a systematic review. Ann Plast Surg. 2015;74:621–32.
8. Chubb D, Rozen WM, Whitaker IS, Acosta R, Grinsell D, Ashton MW. The efficacy of clinical assessment in the postoperative monitoring of free flaps: a review of 1140 consecutive cases. Plast Reconstr Surg. 2010;125(4):1157–66.
9. Holm C, Mayr M, Höfter E, Raab N, Ninkovic M. Interindividual variability of the SIEA Angiosome: effects on operative strategies in breast reconstruction. Plast Reconstr Surg. 2008;122(6):1612–20.
10. Lohman RF, Ozturk CN, Ozturk C, Jayaprakash V, Djohan R. An analysis of current techniques used for intraoperative flap evaluation. Ann Plast Surg. 2015;75:679–85.
11. Bigdeli AK, Gazyakan E, Schmidt VJ, Hernekamp FJ, Harhaus L, Henzler T, et al. Indocyanine green fluorescence for free-flap perfusion imaging revisited: advanced decision making by virtual perfusion reality in visionsense fusion imaging angiography. Surg Innov. 2016;23(3):249–60.
12. Mothes H, Dönicke T, Friedel R, Simon M, Markgraf E, Bach O. Indocyanine-green fluorescence video angiography used clinically to evaluate tissue perfusion in microsurgery. J Trauma. 2004;57(5):1018–24.
13. Beier JP, Horch RE, Arkudas A, Dragu A, Schmitz M, Kneser U. Decision-making in DIEP and ms-TRAM flaps: the potential role for a combined laser Doppler spectrophotometry system. J Plast Reconstr Aesthet Surg. 2013;66(1):73–9.
14. Newman MI, Samson MC. The application of laser-assisted indocyanine green fluorescent dye angiography in microsurgical breast reconstruction. J Reconstr Microsurg. 2009;25(1):21–6.
15. Pestana IA, Coan B, Erdmann D, Marcus J, Levin LS, Zenn MR. Early experience with fluorescent angiography in free-tissue transfer reconstruction. Plast Reconstr Surg. 2009;123(4):1239–44.
16. Yamaguchi S, De Lorenzi F, Petit JY, Rietjens M, Garusi C, Giraldo A, et al. The "perfusion map" of the unipedicled TRAM flap to reduce postoperative partial necrosis. Ann Plast Surg. 2004;53(3):205–9.
17. Pestana IA, Zenn MR. Correlation between abdominal perforator vessels identified with preoperative CT angiography and intraoperative fluorescent angiography in the microsurgical breast reconstruction patient. Ann Plast Surg. 2014;72(6):S144–9.
18. Tan NC, Shih H-S, Chen C-C, Chen Y-C, Lin P-Y, Kuo Y-R. Distal skin paddle as a monitor for buried anterolateral thigh flap in pharyngoesophageal reconstruction. Oral Oncol. 2012;48(3):249–52.
19. Revenaugh PC, Waters HH, Scharpf J, Knott PD, Fritz MA. Suprastomal cutaneous monitoring paddle for free flap reconstruction of laryngopharyngectomy defects. JAMA Facial Plast Surg. 2013;15(4):287–91.
20. Dionyssopoulos A, Odobescu A, Foroughi Y, Harris P, Karagergou E, Guertin L, et al. Monitoring buried jejunum free flaps with a sentinel: a retrospective study of 20 cases. Laryngoscope. 2012;122(3):519–22.
21. Kashimura T, Nakazawa H, Shimoda K, Soejima K. False-negative monitoring flap in free jejunal transfer. J Reconstr Microsurg. 2013;29(2):137–40.
22. Griffiths M, Chae MP, Rozen WM. Indocyanine green-based fluorescent angiography in breast reconstruction. Gland Surg. 2016;5(2):133–49.
23. Hanasano MM. Chapter 4 - Emerging technology in reconstructive surgery. In: Wei F-C, Mardini S, editors. Flaps and reconstructive surgery. 2nd ed. Amsterdam: Elsevier; 2016. p. e11.
24. Raabe A, Beck J, Gerlach R, Zimmermann M, Seifert V. Near-infrared indocyanine green video angiography: a new method for intraoperative assessment of vascular flow. Neurosurgery. 2003;52(1):132–9.
25. Liu DZ, Mathes DW, Zenn MR, Neligan PC. The application of indocyanine green fluorescence angiography in plastic surgery. J Reconstr Microsurg. 2011;27(6):355–64.
26. Azuma R, Morimoto Y, Masumoto K, Nambu M, Takikawa M, Yanagibayashi S, et al. Detection of skin perforators by indocyanine green fluorescence nearly infrared angiography. Plast Reconstr Surg. 2008;122(4):1062–7.
27. Alander JT, Kaartinen I, Laakso A, Pätilä T, Spillmann T, Tuchin VV, et al. A review of indocyanine green fluorescent imaging in surgery. Int J Biomed Imag. 2012;2012:940585.
28. Yeoh MS, Kim DD, Ghali GE. Fluorescence angiography in the assessment of flap perfusion and vitality. Oral Maxillofac Surg. 2013;25:61–6.
29. Duggal CS, Madni T, Losken A. An outcome analysis of intraoperative angiography for postmastectomy breast reconstruction. Aesthet Surg J. 2014;34(1):61–5.
30. Francisco BS, Kerr-Valentic MA, Agarwal JP. Laser-assisted indocyanine green angiography and DIEP breast reconstruction. Plast Reconstr Surg. 2010;125(3):116e–8e.
31. Holm C, Dornseifer U, Sturtz G, Basso G, Schuster T, Ninkovic M. The intrinsic transit time of free microvascular flaps: clinical and prognostic implications. Microsurgery. 2010;30(2):91–6.
32. Hope-Ross M, Yannuzzi LA, Gragoudas ES, Guyer DR, Slakter JS, Sorenson JA, et al. Adverse reactions due to indocyanine green. Ophthalmology. 1994;101(3):529–33.
33. Beckler AD, Ezzat WH, Seth R, Nabili V, Blackwell KE. Assessment of fibula flap skin perfusion in patients undergoing oromandibular reconstruction: comparison of clinical findings, fluorescein, and indocyanine green angiography. JAMA Facial Plast Surg. 2015;17(6):422–6.
34. Selber JC, Garvey PB, Clemens MW, Chang EI, Zhang H, Hanasono MM. A prospective study of transit-time flow volume measurement for intraoperative evaluation and optimization of free flaps. Plast Reconstr Surg. 2013;131(2):270–81.
35. Bonde CT, Holstein-Rathlou N-H, Elberg JJ. Validation of a 1-mm transit time flow probe and the potential for use in microsurgery. J Reconstr Microsurg. 2006;22(7):519–24.
36. Hirotani T, Kameda T, Shirota S, Nakao Y. An evaluation of the intraoperative transit time measurements of coronary bypass flow. Eur J Cardio-Thorac Surg. 2001;19(6):848–52.

37. Abdel-Galil K, Mitchell D. Postoperative monitoring of microsurgical free tissue transfers for head and neck reconstruction: a systematic review of current techniques-Part I. Non-invasive techniques. Br J Oral Maxillofac Surg. 2009;47(5):351–5.
38. Heller L, Levin LS, Klitzman B. Laser Doppler flowmeter monitoring of free-tissue transfers: blood flow in normal and complicated cases. Plast Reconstr Surg. 2001;107(7):1739–45.
39. Clinton MS, Sepka RS, Bristol D, Pederson WC, Barwick WJ, Serafin D, et al. Establishment of normal ranges of laser Doppler blood flow in autologous tissue transplants. Plast Reconstr Surg. 1991;87(2):299–309.
40. Yoshino K, Nara S, Endo M, Kamata N. Intraoral free flap monitoring with a laser Doppler flowmeter. Microsurgery. 1996;17(6):337–40.
41. Rimler J, Nguyen A, Evans GRD. Chapter 29 - Postoperative care. In: Wei F-C, Mardini S, editors. Flaps and reconstructive surgery. 2nd ed. Amsterdam: Elsevier; 2016. p. 348.
42. Yuen JC, Feng Z. Distinguishing laser Doppler flowmetric responses between arterial and venous obstructions in flaps. J Reconstr Microsurg. 2000;16(8):629–35.
43. Hallock GG. Acoustic doppler sonography, color duplex ultrasound, and laser doppler flowmetry as tools for successful autologous breast reconstruction. Clin Plast Surg. 2011;38:203–11.
44. Chao AH, Meyerson J, Povoski SP, Kocak E. A review of devices used in the monitoring of microvascular free tissue transfers. Exp Rev Med Dev. 2013;10:649–60.
45. Yuen JC, Feng Z. Monitoring free flaps using the laser Doppler flowmeter: five-year experience. Plast Reconstr Surg. 2000;105(1):55–61.
46. Hölzle F, Loeffelbein DJ, Nolte D, Wolff K-D. Free flap monitoring using simultaneous non-invasive laser Doppler flowmetry and tissue spectrophotometry. J Cranio-Maxillo-Facial Surg. 2006;34(1):25–33.
47. Marks NJ, Trachy RE, Cummings CW. Dynamic variations in blood flow as measured by laser Doppler velocimetry: a study in rat skin flaps. Plast Reconstr Surg. 1984;73(5):804–10.
48. Hallock GG. A "True" false-negative misadventure in free flap monitoring using laser Doppler flowmetry. Plast Reconstr Surg. 2002;110:1609–11.
49. Colwell AS, Craft RO. Near-infrared spectroscopy in autologous breast reconstruction. Clin Plast Surg. 2011;38:301–7.
50. Repez A, Oroszy D, Arnez ZM. Continuous postoperative monitoring of cutaneous free flaps using near infrared spectroscopy. J Plast Reconstr Aesthet Surg. 2008;61(1):71–7.
51. Kagaya Y, Miyamoto S. A systematic review of near-infrared spectroscopy in flap monitoring: current basic and clinical evidence and prospects. J Plast Reconstr Aesthet Surg. 2018;71:246–57.
52. Ozturk CN, Ozturk C, Ledinh W, Bozkurt M, Schwarz G, O'Rourke C, et al. Variables affecting postoperative tissue perfusion monitoring in free flap breast reconstruction. Microsurgery. 2015;35(2):123–8.
53. Keller A. Noninvasive tissue oximetry for flap monitoring: an initial study. J Reconstr Microsurg. 2007;23(4):189–97.
54. Vranken NPA, Weerwind PW, van Onna MA, Bouman EAC, van der Hulst RRWJ. Non-invasive tissue oximetry following unilateral DIEP-flap reconstruction: a pilot evaluation. J Plast Reconstr Aesthet Surg. 2017;12:59–65.
55. Cai Z, Zhang J, Zhang J, Zhao F, Yu G, Li Y, et al. Evaluation of near infrared spectroscopy in monitoring postoperative regional tissue oxygen saturation for fibular flaps. J Plast Reconstr Aesthet Surg. 2008;61(3):289–96.
56. Berthelot M, Ashcroft J, Boshier P, Hunter J, Henry FP, Lo B, et al. Use of near-infrared spectroscopy and implantable doppler for postoperative monitoring of free tissue transfer for breast reconstruction: a systematic review and meta-analysis. Plast Reconstr Surg Glob Open. 2019;7:e2437v, 1–8.
57. Koolen PGL, Vargas CR, Ho OA, Ibrahim AMS, Ricci JA, Tobias AM, et al. Does increased experience with tissue oximetry monitoring in microsurgical breast reconstruction lead to decreased flap loss? The learning effect. Plast Reconstr Surg. 2016;137(4):1093–101.
58. Pelletier A, Tseng C, Agarwal S, Park J, Song D. Cost analysis of near-infrared spectroscopy tissue oximetry for monitoring autologous free tissue breast reconstruction. J Reconstr Microsurg. 2011;27(8):487–94.
59. De Weerd L, Mercer JB, Weum S. Dynamic infrared thermography. Clin Plast Surg. 2011;38:277–92.
60. Hallock GG. Dynamic infrared thermography and smartphone thermal imaging as an adjunct for preoperative, intraoperative, and postoperative perforator free flap monitoring. Plast Aesthet Res. 2019;6:29.
61. Pereira N, Valenzuela D, Mangelsdorff G, Kufeke M, Roa R. Detection of perforators for free flap planning using smartphone thermal imaging: a concordance study with computed tomographic angiography in 120 perforators. Plast Reconstr Surg. 2018;141(3):787–92.
62. Nahabedian MY. Overview of perforator imaging and flap perfusion technologies. Clin Plast Surg. 2011;38:165–74.
63. John HE, Niumsawatt V, Rozen WM, Whitaker IS. Clinical applications of dynamic infrared thermography in plastic surgery: a systematic review. Gland Surg. 2016;5(2):122–32.
64. Tenorio X, Mahajan AL, Wettstein R, Harder Y, Pawlovski M, Pittet B. Early detection of flap failure using a new thermographic device. J Surg Res. 2009;151(1):15–21.
65. de Weerd L, Miland AO, Mercer JB. Perfusion dynamics of free DIEP and SIEA flaps during the first postoperative week monitored with dynamic infrared thermography. Ann Plast Surg. 2009;62(1):42–7.
66. Just M, Chalopin C, Unger M, Halama D, Neumuth T, Dietz A, et al. Monitoring of microvascular free flaps following oropharyngeal reconstruction using infrared thermography: first clinical experiences. Eur Arch Otorhinolaryngol. 2016;273(9):2659–67.
67. Hennessy O, Potter SM. Use of infrared thermography for the assessment of free flap perforators in autologous breast reconstruction: a systematic review, vol. 23. J Plast Reconstr Aesthet Surg; 2020. p. 60–70.
68. Tenorio X, Mahajan AL, Elias B, van Riempst JS, Wettstein R, Harder Y, et al. Locating perforator vessels by dynamic infrared imaging and flow Doppler with no thermal cold challenge. Ann Plast Surg. 2011;67(2):143–6.
69. Swartz WM, Jones NF, Cherup L, Klein A. Direct monitoring of microvascular anastomoses with the 20-MHz ultrasonic Doppler probe: an experimental and clinical study. Plast Reconstr Surg. 1988;81(2):149–61.
70. Oliver DW, Whitaker IS, Giele H, Critchley P, Cassell O. The Cook-Swartz venous Doppler probe for the post-operative monitoring of free tissue transfers in the United Kingdom: a preliminary report. Br J Plast Surg. 2005;58(3):366–70.
71. Whitaker IS, Smit JM, Acosta R. A simple method of implantable Doppler cuff attachment: experience in 150 DIEP breast reconstructions. J Plast Reconstr Aesthet Surg. 2008;61:1251–2.
72. Bill TJ, Foresman PA, Rodeheaver GT, Drake DB. Fibrin sealant: a novel method of fixation for an implantable ultrasonic microDoppler probe. J Reconstr Microsurg. 2001;17(4):257–62.
73. Rozen WM, Ang GG, McDonald AH, Sivarajah G, Rahdon R, Acosta R, et al. Sutured attachment of the implantable Doppler probe cuff for large or complex pedicles in free tissue transfer. J Reconstr Microsurg. 2011;27(2):99–102.
74. Abdel-Galil K, Mitchell D. Postoperative monitoring of microsurgical free-tissue transfers for head and neck reconstruction: a sys-

tematic review of current techniques-Part II. Invasive techniques. Br J Oral Maxillofac Surg. 2009;47(6):438–42.
75. Klifto KM, Milek D, Gurno CF, Seal SM, Hultman CS, Rosson GD, et al. Comparison of arterial and venous implantable Doppler postoperative monitoring of free flaps: systematic review and meta-analysis of diagnostic test accuracy. Microsurgery. 2020;40:501–11.
76. Chang TY, Lee YC, Lin YC, Wong STS, Hsueh YY, Kuo YL, et al. Implantable Doppler probes for postoperatively monitoring free flaps: efficacy. A systematic review and meta-analysis. Plast Reconstr Surg Glob Open. 2016;4(11):1–10.
77. Unadkat JV, Rothfuss M, Mickle MH, Sejdic E, Gimbel ML. The development of a wireless implantable blood flow monitor. Plast Reconstr Surg. 2015;136(1):199–203.
78. Creech B, Miller S. Evaluation of circulation in skin flaps. In: Grabb W, Myers M, editors. Skin flaps. Boston, MA: Little Brown; 1975. p. 21–38.
79. Lineaweaver W. Techniques of monitoring buried fasciocutaneous free flaps. Plast Reconstr Surg. 2009;124:1729–31.

Re-exploration, Complications and Flap Salvage

5

Paul Caine, Johann A. Jeevaratnam, Adam Misky, and Dariush Nikkhah

5.1 Introduction

Success rates of up to 95–99% have been reported for free flap surgery (FFS), with variation existing depending on whether the surgery is for breast, head and neck and lower limb reconstruction [1]. Elective DIEP flap failure rates have been quoted as low as 0.29%, while failure rates are reported as high as 6% in head and neck reconstruction and up to 9% in lower limb reconstruction [2, 3].

Despite often favourable outcomes, all surgeons who regularly undertake these procedures will at some point be faced with failing/failed flaps, which may not necessarily be attributed to poor technique. It is important to recognise evolving problems early and act accordingly to prevent flap loss and potential significant morbidity.

Adverse outcomes in FFS can present on a spectrum of severity and be categorised into complete flap loss, partial flap loss, failure to achieve desired outcome despite flap survival, donor site morbidity, medical complications and disappointed patients [1].

Beyond meticulous microsurgical technique, a number of other factors should be considered in aiming for a successful outcome. We discuss preoperative, perioperative and postoperative optimisation and management, together with an algorithm for surgical re-exploration and free flap salvage, and other associated complications.

5.2 Preoperative Assessment

This should serve to identify both potential technical challenges, relating to donor or recipient sites, and the fitness of the patient as a whole.

When selecting the appropriate donor site, one must consider volume and suitability of tissue, the functional and aesthetic result of the defect, available length of pedicle (and potential need for vein grafting) and vessel calibre, together with potential preoperative imaging. In terms of recipient site, key factors include the location of recipient vessels, potential for considerable size mismatch between vessels, previous irradiation, extent of zone of injury, need for adjuvant therapy and again the benefit of preoperative imaging [4]. This is of particular relevance in the head and neck, when often faced with an irradiated field, depleted recipient vessels and the need for interposition grafts to access the contralateral recipient site, all of which may contribute to high rates of failure [2]. Note, the correlation between free flap failure rates and use of vein grafts is controversial, with some reporting high success rates (>93%) when the need for a vein graft is identified in the preoperative planning phase [5]. Post-operative medical complications in FFS have been linked to high preoperative risk stratification tools such as the ASA (American Society of Anesthesiologists) and Charlson Comorbidity Index. However, the presence of pre-existing comorbidity does not increase the risk of surgical complications in patients undergoing FFS, and advanced age alone is also not a risk factor for surgical complications [4].

Where possible the patient should be optimised with regard to the following factors;

Supplementary Information The online version contains supplementary material available at [https://doi.org/10.1007/978-3-031-07678-7_5].

P. Caine (✉) · A. Misky · D. Nikkhah
The Royal Free Hospital NHS Foundation Trust, London, UK
e-mail: paul.caine@doctors.org.uk; p.caine@nhs.net; adam.misky@nhs.net; d.nikkhah@nhs.net

J. A. Jeevaratnam
Guy's & St Thomas' NHS Foundation Trust, London, UK
e-mail: jeevaj@doctors.org.uk

Hypertension has been linked with anastomotic failure, while diabetes, although known to increase the risk of wound complications, has not been shown to affect flap survival in large clinical series. Obesity (BMI > 30) has been shown to be significantly related to total/partial flap loss and the development of complications in free flap breast surgery, with a systematic review by Shin et al. showing obesity to play a significant role in the development of complications in breast free flaps when compared to non-breast free flaps [6].

The development of post-operative alcohol withdrawal symptoms has been specifically shown to be associated with flap complications. The literature has suggested that patients should cease smoking at least 1 week prior to undergoing free flap surgery, as an association has been demonstrated with smoking and flap-related wound complications, such as flap necrosis, haematoma and fat necrosis [7].

5.3 Perioperative Management

Patient physiology undergoes a multitude of changes during various stages of free tissue transfer: at induction, tissue resection, flap harvest, reperfusion of the flap and emergence from anaesthesia. Inadvertent hypothermia (core temperature <36.5 °C) in the immediate preoperative period can result in coagulopathy and later wound healing problems. Prewarming patients 1 h prior to the induction of anaesthesia and the maintenance of an ambient theatre temperature of 24 °C has been shown to counteract the drop in core temperature resulting from induction of anaesthesia. Studies have suggested that preoperative fasting of patients results in very minor insensible fluid loss, and preoperative fluid loading is therefore not necessary in those with normal circulation. Prophylaxis against venous thromboembolism is required in patients undergoing FFS, by way of graduated compression stockings (started on admission), intermittent pneumatic compression (started prior to induction of anaesthesia) and daily administration of low molecular weight heparin.

A hyperdynamic circulation (high cardiac output, peripheral vasodilation and large pulse pressure) is ideal in maintaining microcirculatory perfusion in FFS [8]. Goal-directed fluid therapy using oesophageal Doppler monitoring is the gold standard, as hypervolaemic haemodilution has been associated with medical complications in the post-operative period [4]. Aggressive fluid resuscitation has been shown to be an independent positive predictor for post-operative complications and length of hospital stay [9]. Studies have suggested that intraoperative fluid administration should not exceed 6 mL/kg/h and that a normovolaemic haemodilution with a haematocrit of 30–40% is preferable [10].

The perioperative and post-operative use of vasopressors in FFS has been widely debated. Many surgeons are concerned that these agents may compromise the blood supply to the flap, though they may at times be necessary to counteract vasodilatation resulting from anaesthetic agents. Though contrary to existing belief, studies looking at the use of intraoperative vasopressors have shown that they do not affect flap outcome [10]. A large study by Nelson et al. looking at complications in >1000 breast free flaps showed that vasopressors did not significantly impact thrombotic events or increase risk of free flap loss [11], with similar findings mirrored in the head and neck literature [12–14]. Evidence suggests that the maintenance of blood pressure through the use of vasopressors may be a preferable technique to fluid overload [13]. If vasopressors are to be used, evidence suggests that dobutamine is preferable and can even promote flap perfusion [10].

5.4 Post-operative Monitoring

Change in the status of the flap, which may or may not indicate a failing flap, must be identified early and managed aggressively to ensure the success of potential salvage procedures. Most flaps that are successfully salvaged are identified within the first 24 h post-operatively. Monitoring is therefore an essential component of post-operative care. There is no world-wide consensus regarding the nature or timing of monitoring; indeed there is evidence of significant variation in monitoring protocols between individual centres [15].

Clinical observation is the prime method of monitoring a free flap, by assessment of temperature, turgor, colour, capillary refill time (CRT) and Doppler signal. Ideally the distal course of the pedicle should be marked perioperatively, to avoid both difficulty in locating it and confusion with the recipient vessel on hand-held Doppler examination (Fig. 5.1). If necessary, other potential manoeuvres include dermal scratch or pin prick, which are of particular use in patients with darker skin tone, in whom identification of congestion can be difficult until the late stages. While a number of alternative monitoring methods exist, such as implantable Doppler probes and spectroscopy, these have not shown increased usefulness, particularly when taking cost and invasiveness into account [16].

Pedicle thrombosis is the most common cause for flap compromise, with 80% of pedicle thrombosis occurring within 48 h of surgery [4]. Venous thrombosis often occurs in the first 24 h and is twice as common as arterial thrombosis, which often occurs in the second 24 h [4]. Note, late venous thrombosis, after Day 3, which is rare, should be managed as per acute thrombosis [17]. After thrombosis, haematoma is the next most likely cause of compromise.

We suggest free flap monitoring according to the British Association of Plastic, Reconstructive and Aesthetic Surgeons (BAPRAS) guidelines for the first 48 h (Table 5.1)

5 Re-exploration, Complications and Flap Salvage

[18] and clinical assessment four times a day thereafter [19]. Clearly some of the recommendations documented in Table 5.1 are not possible with muscle flaps, which are discussed separately. It is important to audit the local centre's data regularly and adjust local monitoring guidelines accordingly, to ensure the highest possible rate of flap survival.

When faced with a pale flap, one should assume arterial insufficiency, which may be due to hypotension, vasospasm, thrombosis or external compression. It is however important to bear in mind that a pale flap, in a Caucasian patient, may well be healthy, with development of a pink/hyperaemic hue a potential sign of venous compromise. Often, fasciocutaneous flaps are hyperaemic in the immediate post-operative period but settle with time (Video 5.1). It is therefore good clinical practice for the surgeon to assess the flap on table, in recovery and on the ward, together with staff responsible for subsequent flap monitoring.

Clinical assessment of a pale flap may identify a prolonged CRT, decreased temperature, increased pallor and loss of tissue turgor. An audible Doppler signal and evidence of bleeding on scratch/prick may be absent, though one should be mindful of transmitted signal from the recipient vessel and the potential for signal from the pedicle, proximal to a thrombosed segment.

Venous insufficiency is more common than arterial, likely due to the low-flow system being more likely to succumb to stasis; however it is more likely to be detected [20]. It should be suspected with any evidence of congestion, which may be

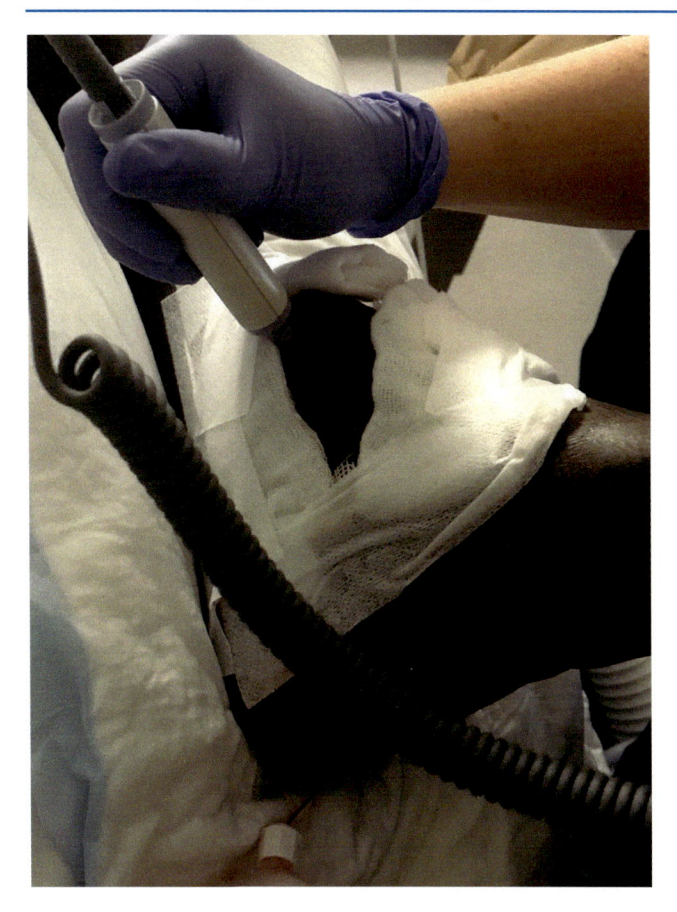

Fig. 5.1 Hand-held Doppler examination of an anterolateral thigh free flap

Table 5.1 British Association of Plastic, Reconstructive and Aesthetic Surgeons flap monitoring guidelines [18]

Recommendation	Action	Rationale
Monitor flap every 30 min for 24 h Hourly thereafter	Document flap observations on the chart regularly to identify changes quickly.	Flap problems are the most common in the first 72 h after surgery (50% in 4 h, 80% in first 24 h, 95% in first 72 h). Venous compromise with flap congestion is three times more common in these early stages.
Flap temperature	Check with the back of your hand or finger and compare with skin on shoulder. Keep patient warm and cover flap with warm gamgee. Strips for comparing flap temperature with surrounding skin are available	A cold flap (>2 °C different) can indicate venous or arterial problems.
Flap Turgor	Press gently on flap to assess turgor.	A 'full', swollen, tense flap with increased turgor indicates a flap with venous compromise and / or a haematoma. An 'empty', flat flap with decreased turgor may indicate arterial compromise.
Flap Colour	View flap in good light to assess colour.	A purple, cyanotic, bluish or dusky flap is present with venous compromise. A pale, mottled flap indicates a flap with arterial compromise.
Flap Capillary Refill	Press on flap gently with your finger or a shaped instrument (e.g. the handle of a pair of scissors) for 5 s. Release the pressure and time the return of the pink colour.	Capillary refill should take about 2 s. In venous congestion it is brisk (<2 s). In arterial compromise it is sluggish (>2 s).
Flap Doppler signal	A mark may be made on the flap at the site of the dominant perforator or pedicle. The Doppler probe should be applied in this area. Alternatively implantable devices are available.	A triphasic pulsatile signal can be heard if the artery is working and a lower pitched more constant sound can be heard if the venous outflow is patent.

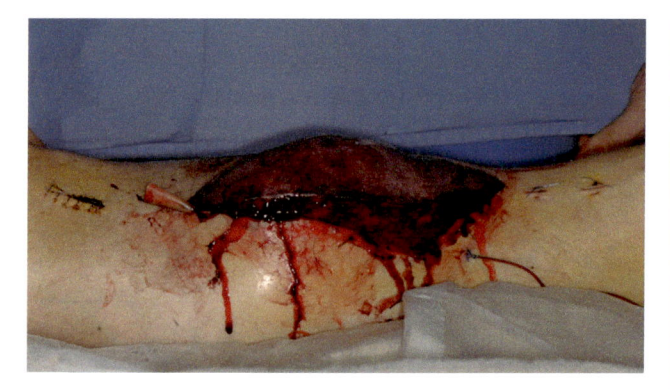

Fig. 5.2 An anterolateral thigh free flap at 48 h post-operatively, which has been congested for 12 h

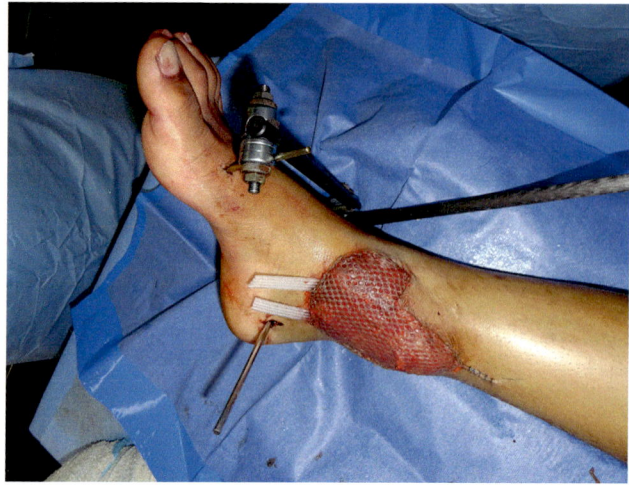

Fig. 5.3 Healthy free gracilis muscle flap with adherent overlying skin graft

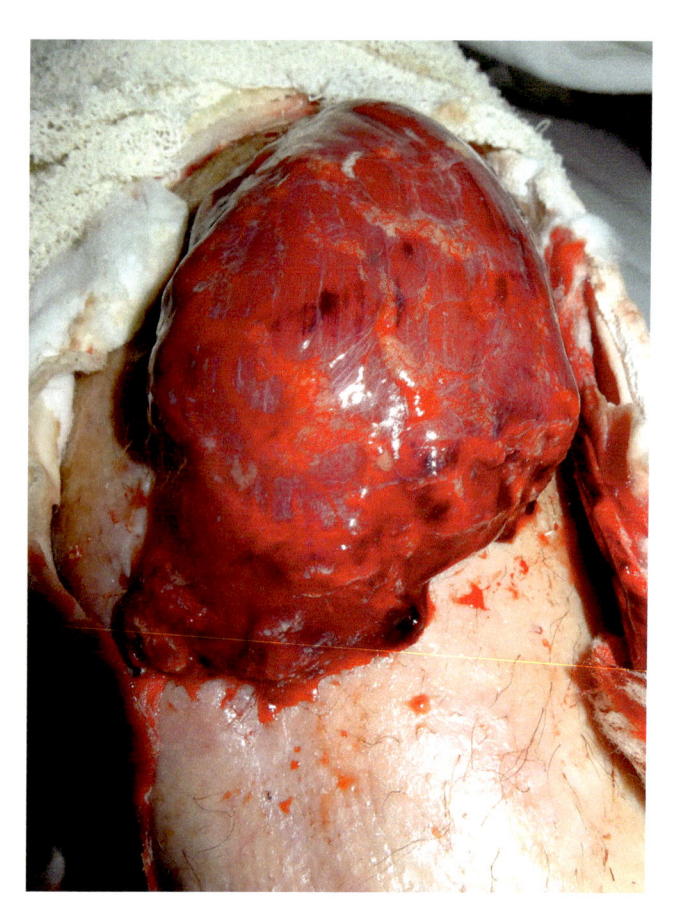

Fig. 5.4 A congested, swollen, free gracilis muscle flap with venous bleeding. Video 5.2 demonstrates a congested gracilis flap

due to venous thrombosis, compromise of the pedicle by kinking or external compression, from adjacent tissues or haematoma. It may manifest in the early stages with a purplish hue, which becomes progressively darker, a brisk CRT and increasing tissue turgor and temperature. Excessive bleeding from the flap edges, potentially leading to haematoma, may alert the clinician to venous compromise of the flap (Fig. 5.2).

If any doubt exists, the patient should be taken back to theatre urgently for re-exploration, as delayed return to theatre has been shown to be associated with a significantly increased rate of flap failure [20]. Delayed flap compromise due to any cause, which occurs after discharge home, is unlikely to be salvageable [21].

5.4.1 Muscle Flap Monitoring

Some differences exist when considering the monitoring of muscle flaps, due to potentially less obvious clinical signs and as they are more susceptible to ischaemic damage. Different compositions of flap tolerate different ischaemia times, due to differing basal metabolic rates. Biochemical changes have been reported in normothermic muscle tissue (at around 34 °C) after 2 h and 15 min [22], due to a higher metabolic rate than skin flaps, which are thought to tolerate a secondary ischaemia time of 7.2 h [23] and bone flaps up to 25 h [24]. Given the difficulty in clinical assessment of muscle-only flaps and time taken from decision to explore, to exploration, one should adopt a lower threshold of concern than with other flap types [25].

Muscle flaps should be salmon pink and contractile, with any overlying graft found to be adherent (Fig. 5.3). Conventional clinical monitoring should be undertaken but is less reliable than in fasciocutaneous flaps. Any change in contractility, colour or turgor should act as a warning of an underlying problem (Fig. 5.4). Anecdotally, some centres delay grafting of muscle flaps, to facilitate monitoring. Inclusion of a skin paddle may be considered, which will aid monitoring, expedite return to theatre and result in a higher salvage rate than their skin paddle-free counterparts [26]. Without a skin paddle, other, equally effective monitoring needs to be used.

A variety of alternative flap monitoring methods have been developed, with differing levels of efficacy, complexity and invasiveness, including implantable Doppler scanners, microdialysis and radionucleotide scanning. There is currently still no consensus as to which method should be the accepted standard [27]. More recently removable Dopplers have been incorporated in end-to-end anastomotic couplers, with no significant difference exhibited in free flap outcomes when compared to the longer-standing Cook-Swartz Doppler [28].

The non-invasive technique of hourly laser Doppler imaging with a commercially available camera, in addition to conventional clinical monitoring of the muscle flap, has been shown to detect vascular incompetence up to 17 h before clinical monitoring [29].

5.5 Flap Salvage

While preparing the patient for theatre, the following factors should be optimised:

- *Patient factors*
  - Normothermia
  - Haemodynamic stability (ideally without the use of vasopressors)

- *Flap factors*
  - Remove tight dressings.
  - Release tight sutures to ease tension on the flap while also decompressing any potential tense collection.
  - Position to avoid postural dependency of the flap.

These manoeuvres may buy time, but do not reduce the urgency for return to theatre.

5.5.1 Algorithm for Re-exploration of Flap

Intraoperatively, the following potential contributing factors must be assessed and addressed in a sequential systematic fashion, as per Chen [30].

5.5.1.1 Pedicle
Under the operating microscope, the entire course and position of the pedicle should be assessed, with great care and copious amounts of warm wash, to ensure there is no kinking or twisting. The position/inset of the flap should be checked, for tension or undue pressure on the pedicle. If concern exists, revision anastomoses with vein grafts should be considered to ensure the pedicle is without tension and with a favourable course.

5.5.1.2 Anastomoses
Working from proximal to distal (inflow to outflow), anastomoses should be examined for both patency and presence of thrombus. Patency may be assessed with the Acland flow test or by trimming a branch distal to the anastomosis to assess bleeding. To avoid undue trauma, the Acland flow test should not be performed repeatedly, while in irradiated vessels it should be carried out with extreme caution. If patent, the anastomoses should not be taken down; however, if any concern exists, a few sutures can be removed to examine the lumen. If localised thrombus is noted, the anastomosis should be taken down and thrombectomy performed, either by milking of the thrombus from the vessel and fishing out with vessel dilators or, if more extensive, by excision of the affected segment. Patency of the vascular circuit may be assessed by feeling for any resistance when flushing with heparinised saline.

There should be a low threshold for the use of vein grafts, to enable tension-free anastomoses between healthy vessels. If the thrombus is extensive and cannot be removed by simple measures and the affected segment cannot be excised, then thrombolytics should be considered, as discussed later. Vasospasm should be managed with vasodilators, such as lidocaine, verapamil or papaverine. Constricted segments may require adventitial excision. Supercharging, which is augmentation of either venous or arterial drainage by an additional distant (not intra-flap) anastomosis, should be borne in mind when attempting flap salvage.

5.5.1.3 Flap Inset
Once the pedicle and anastomoses have been evaluated and addressed, the flap should be re-inset, avoiding a tight inset, which may compress the pedicle. If too tight, a partial or delayed inset, with staples followed by secondary closure, should be considered.

5.5.1.4 Pharmacological Salvage
Thrombolytic drugs should be considered in the salvage of failing free flaps, though as yet no consensus has been reached regarding optimal agent and strategy [31]. Indications include intra-flap thrombus and cases of no-reflow. This is characterised by failure of tissue perfusion despite adequate arterial input and venous drainage, when systemic causes such as low arterial pressure and hypothermia-induced vasospasm have been ruled out [1]. At a cellular level, this is characterised by vascular endothelial cell swelling, intravascular aggregation of platelets and fluid leakage into the interstitial space. Pharmacological salvage should be considered, even in cases when venous thrombosis has been identified late, such as in cases of flap congestion of up to 12 h (Fig. 5.2) [32].

We advocate the use of tissue plasminogen activator (TPA), also known as alteplase, as a primary thrombolytic agent, as it is relatively clot selective and not antigenic and has minimal systemic side effects. It can be administered via an arterial side branch or through the original arterial anastomosis, with either a few sutures removed or completely taken down. A paediatric cannula is placed and an 8-0 suture placed around it to prevent leakage. The artery proximal to the site of infiltration should be clamped and the draining veins of the flap disconnected, to prevent systemic administration of the thrombolytic agent [32].

Our preferred recipe is for dilution of a 1 mg/mL preparation of TPA with 4 mL normal saline, to provide 5 mL with a concentration of 0.2 mg/mL. This 5 mL is infiltrated and alternated with 5 mL of heparinised saline, at a strength of 100 units/mL (5000 units heparin in 50 mL normal saline), infused over 5 min, and the cycle repeated [32]. In theory this cycle may be repeated ad infinitum; however there must come a point when there is no venous return, despite patient inflow and outflow and numerous cycles of thrombolysis, that the flap should be considered unsalvageable, likely due to the no-reflow phenomenon.

Prior to re-anastomosis of the successfully salvaged flap, the venous effluent should be allowed to drain for at least 10 min, once again to reduce the risk of systemic administration. At the time of clamp release, 5000 IU of heparin should be administered systemically (Figs. 5.5 and 5.6).

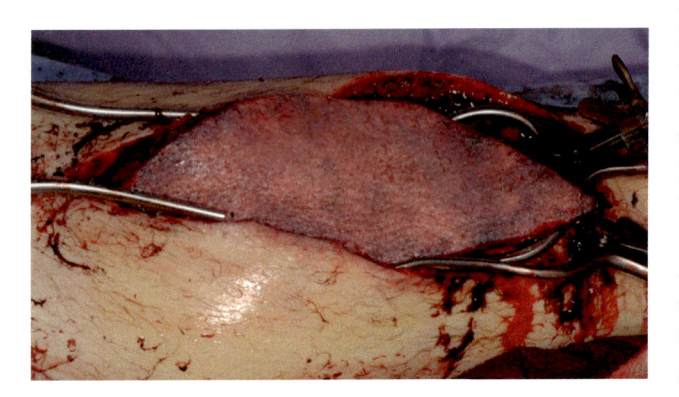

Fig. 5.5 Appearance of anterolateral thigh free flap immediately following successful administration of alteplase, prior to inset

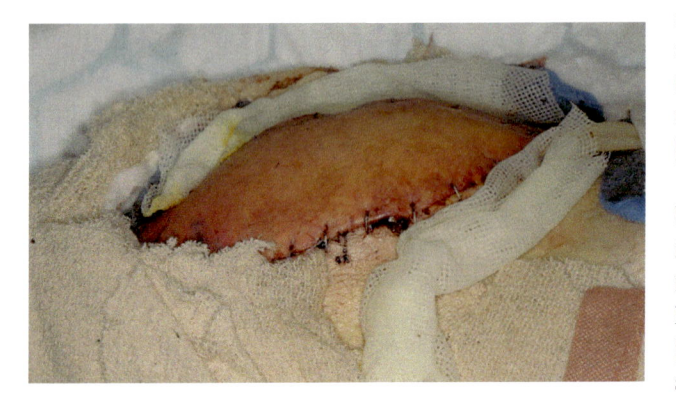

Fig. 5.6 Anterolateral thigh free flap, following successful pharmacological salvage, after 12 h of venous congestion

5.5.1.5 Hirudotherapy

Leeching, both live and chemical, is not a first-line therapy in free flap surgery, but is commonly used following digital replantation [33]. It may also be considered in cases of limited partial (distal) flap compromise or if flap salvage is medically or technically not possible. *Hirudo medicinalis* medicinal leeches may be applied in a cyclical manner, with appropriate antibiotic prophylaxis. Chemical leeching can be undertaken by way of multiple dermal punctures and the application of topical heparin. With both of these interventions, one must be mindful of the high likelihood for requiring blood transfusion [34].

5.5.1.6 Human Factors

Flap salvage procedures are stressful and the importance of having breaks and recruiting help from colleagues should not be underestimated. Taking a step back and approaching the situation with a fresh perspective, whether your own or a colleague's, is incredibly valuable.

5.6 Donor Site Morbidity

The success of FFS is, by most surgeons, based on flap survival, with minimal emphasis placed on donor site morbidity. As free survival rates improve, one cannot forget and must actively strive to reduce donor site morbidity. Problems with donor sites can be both troublesome for patients and hinder post-operative recovery. Potential donor site complications may be illustrated by looking at the radial forearm free flap (RFFF) and anterolateral thigh flap (ALT), both of which can be particularly problematic.

RFFF donor site complications are numerous. Most commonly, poor wound healing (>30%), including graft failure and unstable scar, results in long-term cosmetic and functional morbidity, such as reduced range of movement and grip strength post-operatively [35, 36]. Paraesthesia in the radial nerve distribution has also been documented. In cases of osteocutaneous RFFF, fractures of the radius are possible post-operatively [36]. Various techniques to reduce donor site morbidity and improve functional outcome have been suggested, such as full-thickness grafts in preference to split thickness skin grafts, suprafascial elevation of the flap and use of an ulnar-based transposition flap for donor site closure [35].

ALT donor sites have been reported, by Townley et al., to be complicated by reduced sensibility around the donor scar in 59% of patients, found to be correlated with the width of flap [37]. Muscle 'bulging' was reported by 12% of patients; however there were no clinical findings of discrete herniation [37]. Debate exists as to whether quadriceps function is affected post-ALT harvest, though even in cases of intramuscular perforator dissection, Townley et al. found no alteration in quadriceps function [37]. Other donor site complications

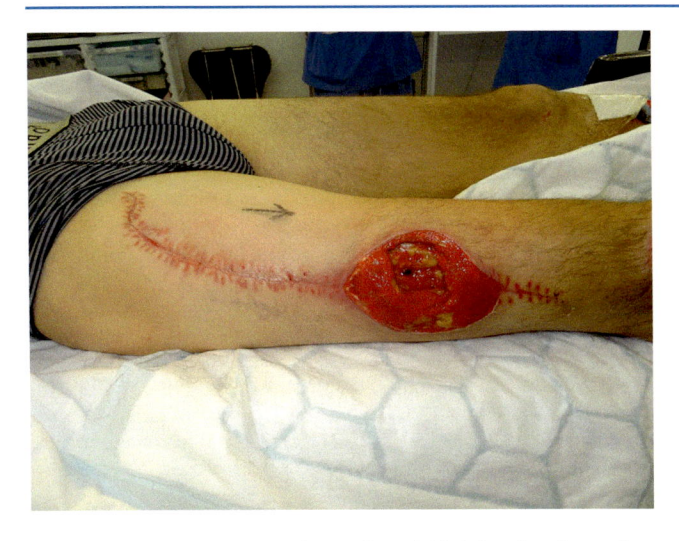

Fig. 5.7 Wound dehiscence of anterolateral thigh free flap donor site

from ALT free flap harvest may include pain, seroma, haematoma, wound infection, wound dehiscence and rarely compartment syndrome (Fig. 5.7). Avoidance of epidural use and avoiding the closure of donor site fascia could mitigate against potential compartment syndrome [35].

Potential donor site morbidity, particularly functional, should not be underestimated or disregarded. Every effort should be made to reduce any associated morbidity.

5.7 Summary

Any microsurgeon will inevitably be faced with the challenging scenario of a failing free flap. Every effort should be made to avoid this, through diligent preoperative and perioperative planning, though this will serve to reduce, rather than completely prevent, flap compromise. Careful post-operative monitoring should be undertaken to identify the failing flap early, at which point aggressive measures should be undertaken to attempt to salvage the flap. One should have an algorithm to ensure potential contributing factors are sought out and addressed in a systematic fashion. Above all, do not forget the patient, to which the flap is attached, and consider them foremost in all decision-making.

5.8 Selected Readings

- Bui DT, Cordeiro PG, Hu QY, Disa JJ, Pusic A, Mehrara BJ. Free flap reexploration: indications, treatment, and outcomes in 1193 free flaps. Plast Reconstr Surg. 2007;119(7):2092–100.

  A retrospective review of 1193 free flaps over a 9-year period, with a 98.8% success rate. Venous thrombosis could largely be salvaged (71% salvaged), while arterial thrombosis led to a worse outcome (40% salvaged). Time to re-exploration was found to be significantly correlated with rate of salvage.

- Gardiner MD, Nanchahal J. Strategies to ensure success of microvascular free tissue transfer. J Plast Reconstr Aesthet Surg. 2010;63(9):e665–73.

  A literature review examining the current evidence pertaining to preoperative optimisation of perioperative management of patients undergoing free tissue transfer.

- Winterton RI, Pinder RM, Morritt AN, Knight SL, Batchelor AG, Liddington MI, Kay SP. Long term study into surgical re-exploration of the 'free flap in difficulty'. J Plast Reconstr Aesthet Surg. 2010;63(7):1080–6.

  A prospective study of 2569 free flaps over a 23-year period. 13% of flaps were re-explored, of which 83% were successfully salvaged. They highlight two key areas to achieve favourable outcomes: firstly, a model of monitoring based primarily upon clinical examination, by experienced individuals, at its core and, secondly, nursing in a specialised post-operative environment, with the ability to return patients to theatre in an expeditious manner.

- Chen WF, Kung YP, Kang YC, Eid A, Tsao CK. Protocolisation and 'end' point of free-flap salvage. J Plast Reconstr Aesthet Surg. 2012;65(9):1272–5.

  A correspondence article summarising the standardised approach, and established endpoint, to flap salvage at Chang Gung Memorial Hospital.

- Griffin JR, Thornton JF. Microsurgery: free tissue transfer and replantation. SRPS. 2015;10(5):1–39.

  Includes a thorough overview of the mechanisms and pathophysiology relevant to free tissue transfer.

- Zoccali G, Molina A, Farhadi J. Is long-term post-operative monitoring of microsurgical flaps still necessary? J Plast Reconstr Aesthet Surg. 2017;70(8):996–1000.

  A literature review and case series, examining the correlation between time of complication onset and probability of flap salvage. As the first 48 hours are key, monitoring during this period is crucial; however beyond this time monitoring was not felt to affect the rate of flap salvage.

- Brouwers K, Kruit AS, Hummelink S, Ulrich DJO. Management of free flap salvage using thrombolytic drugs: a systematic review. J Plast Reconstr Aesthet Surg. 2020;73(10):1806–14.

  A systematic review examining the current evidence (a total of 27 studies and case reports) for pharmacological thrombolysis as a method of free flap salvage. Though deemed a useful adjunct, the level of evidence is low, and no consensus has been reached regarding their optimal use or of the benefit of one specific thrombolytic agent over another.

References

1. Koul AR, Patil RK, Nahar S. Unfavourable results in free tissue transfer. Indian J Plast Surg. 2013;46(2):247–55.
2. Davison SP, Clemens MW, Kochuba AL. Anatomy of free flap failures: dissection of a series. Mod Plast Surg. 2013;3(3):89–95.
3. Culliford AT IV, Spector J, Blank A, Karp NS, Kasabian A, Levine JP. The fate of lower extremities with failed free flaps: a single institution's experience over 25 years. Ann Plast Surg. 2007;59(1):18–21.
4. Gardiner MD, Nanchahal J. Strategies to ensure success of microvascular free tissue transfer. J Plast Reconstr Aesthet Surg. 2010;63(9):e665–73.
5. Classen DA. The indications and reliability of vein graft use in free flap transfer. Can J Plast Surg. 2004;12(1):27–9.
6. Shin JY, Roh SG, Lee NH, Yang KM. Is obesity a predisposing factor for free flap failure and complications? Comparison between breast and nonbreast reconstruction: systematic review and meta-analysis. Medicine (Baltimore). 2016;95(26):e4072.
7. Hwang K, Son JS, Ryu WK. Smoking and flap survival. Plast Surg. 2018;26(4):280–5.
8. Nimalan N, Branford OA, Stocks G. Anaesthesia for free flap breast reconstruction. BJA Educ. 2016;16(5):162–6.
9. Patel RS, McCluskey SA, Goldstein DP, Minkovich L, Irish JC, Brown DH, Gullane PJ, Lipa JE, Gilbert RW. Clinicopathologic and therapeutic risk factors for perioperative complications and prolonged hospital stay in free flap reconstruction of the head and neck. Head Neck. 2010;32(10):1345–53.
10. Vincent A, Sawhney R, Ducic Y. Perioperative care of free flap patients. Semin Plast Surg. 2019;33(1):5–12.
11. Nelson JA, Fischer JP, Grover R, Nelson P, Au A, Serletti JM, Wu LC. Intraoperative vasopressors and thrombotic complications in free flap breast reconstruction. J Plast Surg Hand Surg. 2017;51(5):336–41.
12. Kinzinger MR, Bewley AF. Perioperative care of head and neck free flap patients. Curr Opin Otolaryngol Head Neck Surg. 2017;25(5):405–10.
13. Rossmiller SR, Cannady SB, Ghanem TA, Wax MK. Transfusion criteria in free flap surgery. Otolaryngol Head Neck Surg. 2010;42(3):359–64.
14. Khouri RK, Cooley BC, Kunselman AR, Landis JR, Yeramian P, Ingram D, Natarajan N, Benes CO, Wallemark C. A prospective study of microvascular free-flap surgery and outcome. Plast Reconstr Surg. 1998;102(3):711–21.
15. Jallali N, Ridha H, Butler P. Postoperative monitoring of free flaps in UK plastic surgery units. Microsurgery. 2005;25:469–72.
16. Cervenka B, Bewley AF. Free flap monitoring: a review of the recent literature. Curr Opin Otolaryngol Head Neck Surg. 2015;23(5):393–8.
17. Nelson JA, Kim EM, Eftekhari K, Low DW, Kovach SJ, Wu LC, Serletti JM. Late venous thrombosis in free flap breast reconstruction: strategies for salvage after this real entity. Plast Reconstr Surg. 2012;129(1):8e–15e.
18. British Association of Plastic Reconstructive and Aesthetic Surgeons and Association of Breast Surgery. Oncoplastic Breast Reconstruction Guidelines for Best Practice. 2012. http://www.bapras.org.uk/docs/default-source/commissioning-and-policy/final-oncoplastic-guidelines%2D%2D-healthcare-professionals.pdf?sfvrsn=0. Accessed 21 Jan 2021.
19. Zoccali G, Molina A, Farhadi J. Is long-term post-operative monitoring of microsurgical flaps still necessary? J Plast Reconstr Aesthet Surg. 2017;70(8):996–1000.
20. Bui DT, Cordeiro PG, Hu QY, Disa JJ, Pusic A, Mehrara BJ. Free flap reexploration: indications, treatment, and outcomes in 1193 free flaps. Plast Reconstr Surg. 2007;119(7):2092–100.
21. Largo RD, Selber JC, Garvey PB, Chang EI, Hanasono MM, Yu P, Butler CE, Baumann DP. Outcome analysis of free flap salvage in outpatients presenting with microvascular compromise. Plast Reconstr Surg. 2018;141(1):20e–7e.
22. Eckert P, Schnackerz K. Ischemic tolerance of human skeletal muscle. Ann Plast Surg. 1991;26(1):77–84.
23. Kerrigan CL, Zelt RG, Daniel RK. Secondary critical ischemia time of experimental skin flaps. Plast Reconstr Surg. 1984;74(4):522–6.
24. Berggren A, Weiland AJ, Dorfman H. The effect of prolonged ischemia time on osteocyte and osteoblast survival in composite bone grafts revascularized by microvascular anastomoses. Plast Reconstr Surg. 1982;69(2):290–8.
25. Griffin JR, Thornton JF. Microsurgery: free tissue transfer and replantation. SRPS. 2015;10(5):1–39.
26. Stranix JT, Jacoby A, Lee ZH, Anzai L, Saadeh PB, Thanik V, Levine JP. Skin paddles improve muscle flap salvage rates after microvascular compromise in lower extremity reconstruction. Ann Plast Surg. 2018;81(1):68–70.
27. Top H, Sarikaya A, Aygit A, Benlier E, Kiyak M. Review of monitoring free muscle flap transfers in reconstructive surgery: role of 99mTc sestamibi scintigraphy. Nucl Med Commun. 2006;27(1):91–8.
28. Um GT, Chang J, Louie O, Colohan SM, Said HK, Neligan PC, Mathes DW. Implantable Cook-Swartz Doppler probe versus Synovis Flow Coupler for the post-operative monitoring of free flap breast reconstruction. J Plast Reconstr Aesthet Surg. 2014;67(7):960–6.
29. Tschumi C, Seyed Jafari SM, Rothenberger J, Van de Ville D, Keel M, Krause F, Shafighi M. Post-operative monitoring of free muscle transfers by Laser Doppler Imaging: a prospective study. Microsurgery. 2015;35(7):528–35.
30. Chen WF, Kung YP, Kang YC, Eid A, Tsao CK. Protocolisation and 'end' point of free-flap salvage. J Plast Reconstr Aesthet Surg. 2012;65(9):1272–5.
31. Brouwers K, Kruit AS, Hummelink S, Ulrich DJO. Management of free flap salvage using thrombolytic drugs: a systematic review. J Plast Reconstr Aesthet Surg. 2020;73(10):1806–14.
32. Nikkhah D, Tudor-Green B, Sapountzis S, Gilleard O, Sidhnu A, Blackburn A. Resurrection of an ALT flap with recombinant tissue plasminogen activator and heparin. Eur J Plast Surg. 2016;39:221–4.
33. Pickrell BB, Daly MC, Freniere B, Higgins JP, Safa B, Eberlin KR. Leech therapy following digital replantation and revascularization. J Hand Surg [Am]. 2020;45(7):638–43.
34. Herlin C, Bertheuil N, Bekara F, Boissiere F, Sinna R, Chaput B. Leech therapy in flap salvage: systematic review and practical recommendations. Ann Chir Plast Esthet. 2017;62(2):e1–e13.
35. Harris BN, Bewley AF. Minimizing free flap donor-site morbidity. Curr Opin Otolaryngol Head Neck Surg. 2016;24(5):447–52.
36. Timmons MJ, Missotten FE, Poole MD, Davies DM. Complications of radial forearm flap donor sites. Br J Plast Surg. 1986;39(2):176–8.
37. Townley WA, Royston EC, Karmiris N, Crick A, Dunn RL. Critical assessment of the anterolateral thigh flap donor site. J Plast Reconstr Aesthet Surg. 2011;64(12):1621–6.

The Use of Ultrasound Technology in Planning Perforator Flaps and Lymphatic Surgery

Giuseppe Visconti, Alessandro Bianchi, Akitatsu Hayashi, and Marzia Salgarello

6.1 Introduction

Since the introduction of perforator flaps in 1989 [1], reconstructive microsurgery was revolutionized because more customized reconstructions could be performed, minimizing morbidity in many cases. Moreover, the rigidity of the reconstructive ladder was converted to a more flexible approach, and the concept of the flap of choice, applied since then to traditional pedicled and free flaps, was progressively converted to the flap chosen [2].

Anatomically speaking, one of the main differences between traditional and perforator flaps is in the knowledge of microvascular anatomy. In fact, the microvascular anatomy of traditional flaps has been well defined. Position and dimension of microvascular structures is quite constant and few anatomical variants are present. On the other side, perforator flaps microvascular anatomy is peculiar for each donor site of each patient, unless the main pedicle on which the flap is based; moreover, it is also true that in some anatomical areas (i.e., thigh and lateral thoracic area), perforators located in watershed area could originate from different source vessels.

For all these reasons and not only, preoperative knowledge of microvascular anatomy can help the surgeon to know the exact microvascular anatomy before surgery, thus allowing to plan precisely the surgery before and make it safer, faster, and efficient. Moreover, advances in ultrasound technology can expand knowledge to very tiny details which makes this technology very helpful also in preoperative evaluation of thin, superthin, and pure skin perforator flaps as well as for lymphatic supermicrosurgery. Exploration time and sometimes frustration in understanding perforator anatomy intraoperatively will leave space to efficiency and creativity, because the microvascular anatomy is known. To achieve this confidence, it is important that the operating surgeon performs ultrasound evaluation by herself/himself without delegating it.

6.2 Background

In the late 1980s, the anatomical work by Taylor and Palmer led to the introduction of the angiosome concept and to the description of an average of 374 major perforators through the human body [3]. Later, the clinical work by Koshima and Soeda opened the perforator era in microsurgery [1].

Although the perforator flap concept has been frequently counterposed to that of conventional flaps, nowadays it is clear that perforator flap represents the natural evolution of conventional flaps [3]. In fact, conventional flaps are an unselective harvest of soft tissues on the main source pedicle to guarantee the perfusion of the tissue(s) of interest, whereas perforator flaps represent a selective tissue harvest based on its peripheral microvasculature (i.e., perforator) which supply skin and adipose tissue up to the main source pedicle, without sacrificing unneeded tissues (i.e., muscle, fascia, nerves, lymphatics).

Perforator flap era has been influenced by the definition of "reliable perforators" that are considered those with a caliber greater than 0.7 mm and with a visible pulsation. This definition is very likely related to the technical consideration that perforator of smaller dimension cannot be skeletonized safely, being more prone to spasm and to unwanted injury during dissection [2, 3].

The recent advent of supermicrosurgery brings the perforator concept to a further level of technical sophistication, and nowadays it is possible to harvest single tissue component (i.e., skin only) or thin flaps (i.e., skin and portion of

---

G. Visconti (✉) · A. Bianchi · M. Salgarello
Department of Plastic and Reconstructive Surgery, Università Cattolica del "Sacro Cuore" – Fondazione Policlinico Universitario "Agostino Gemelli" IRCSS, Rome, Italy
e-mail: giuseppe.visconti@policlinicogemelli.it

A. Hayashi
Department of Breast Center, Kameda Medical Center, Chiba, Japan

superficial adipose tissue) based on peripheral arborization of the perforator vessel as well as choosing smaller perforator (also called capillary perforators) in selected cases [4–7]. Technical ability to manipulate such tiny structures leads also to the development of a new microsurgical field, lymphatic supermicrosurgery [8].

One of the main difficulties in perforator flap surgery and even more in supermicrosurgery is the knowledge of microvascular anatomy. There is such a great variability in perforator location, size, course, and even sometimes presence of perforator. In the same person, microvascular anatomy is not specific for every donor site. For example, anterolateral thigh perforators of the right thigh are completely different from the left thigh.

Knowledge of perforator microanatomy has evolved in the last 30 years, starting with intraoperative exploration only which has been progressively abandoned by most.

The most frequent approach is to evaluate preoperatively the location of perforator by using the portable handheld Doppler [9, 10]. This method has been introduced in the 1970s and nowadays it still represents the method of choice for many microsurgeons. Although the main advantage of portable handheld Doppler is the easiness of use, high portability (pocket-size), and cheapness, this device has been proven to be poor in sensitivity and specificity [11, 12]. The most frequently used devices are unidirectional; thus they only give an audible signal of any type of vascular flow (Fig. 6.1). The intensity and the ability of finding audible signals are related to the angularity of the probe. This means that not only true perforators may be audible but also indirect and linking vessels within the subcutaneous tissue. Moreover, in some anatomical location and especially in thin patients, signals coming from deeper vascular structures may interfere with the examination (i.e., groin area).

Lastly, in the best scenario, the "true" perforators are luckily located; there is no knowledge on their caliber, flow, and supra- and subfascial course. Moreover, in perforator watershed area, it is not possible to know to which source vessel the perforator is coming from.

So far, nevertheless the portable handheld Doppler may give some preoperative information; its inaccuracy and low reliability still ask for an intraoperative exploration to confirm the presence of the perforators. All the other steps of dissection, including choosing the dominant perforator, are delegated to the intraoperative exploration.

Ultrasound technology has tremendously evolved, and nowadays we have the possibility to use high performance machines which can give us very detailed and precise information of the soft tissue anatomy and its microvascular network, including perforators (Fig. 6.2).

It is interesting to note that almost any medical specialty has incorporated in its daily practice the use of ultrasound

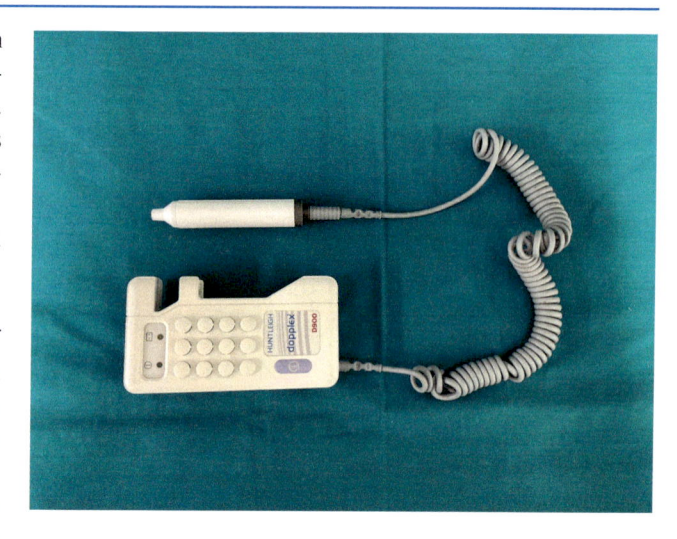

Fig. 6.1 Picture of handheld portable unidirectional Doppler

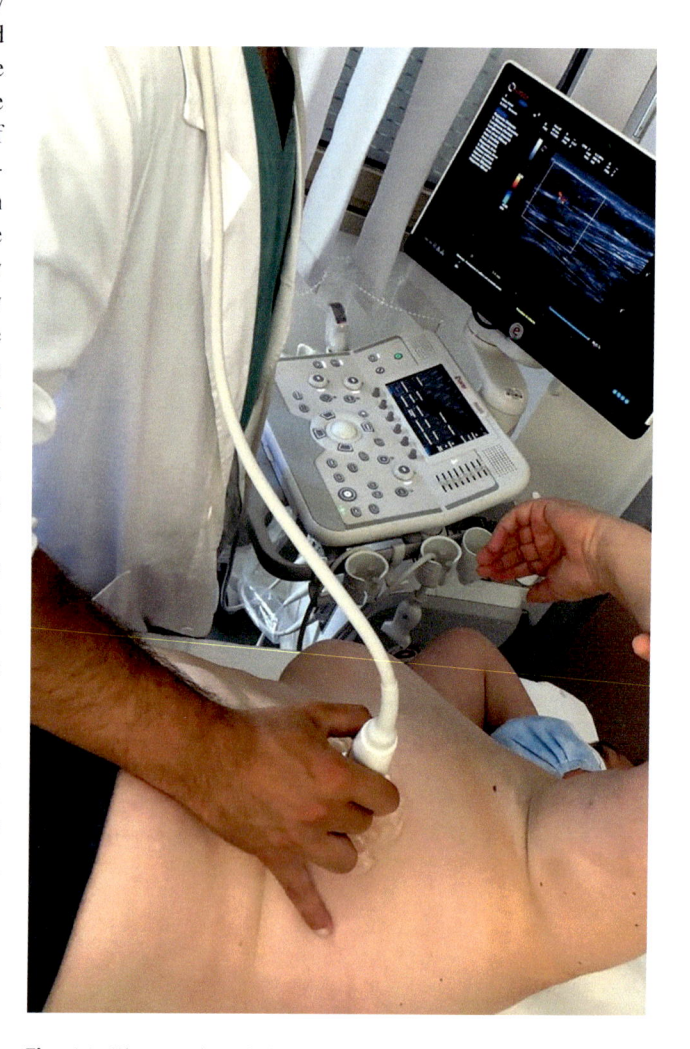

Fig. 6.2 Picture taken during a preoperative planning of immediate partial breast reconstruction using perforator flap of the lateral thoracic area. In the picture, a 1.1 mm LICAP (lateral intercostal artery perforator) was found using high-frequency ultrasound

technology for diagnosis and treatment purposes. To do so, specific training is needed to understand the technology and its potential and to correctly use it daily.

Plastic surgery remains one of the few specialties in which the use of ultrasound is still not common and when needed is delegated to radiologist. However, in our specialty we can benefit a lot from ultrasound, from general plastic surgery patient check and follow-up (postoperative scan of any surgical site when in doubt of seroma, fluid accumulation, hematoma) up to very sophisticated preoperative planning in microsurgery.

Even though many plastic surgeons may believe that in case the ultrasound examination is needed it is better to delegate it to radiologists to save time for other specific works, this attitude is not far-sighted. In fact, once the ultrasound skills are acquired, basic postoperative checkups may take few minutes to be performed. This will enhance a lot patients' compliance, adherence, and esteem.

When used in preoperative planning for sophisticated microsurgical procedures such as perforator flap and lymphatic surgery, ultrasound examination allows to save intraoperative time needed for exploration leaving energy for creativity and other important aspect of the surgery. In lymphatic surgery, ultrasound is the quintessence to perform LVA in an effective and efficient way.

6.3 Color-Coded Duplex Sonography (CCDS)

CCDS using high-resolution ultrasound allows to have detailed information on microvascular and soft tissue anatomy of any donor site [12–16]. In the field of plastic surgery, linear probes from 4 to 19 MHz are the most indicated. High-frequency ultrasound (>15 MHz) allows to expand knowledge on more superficial plane, thus allowing a further analysis of the perforator vessels and superficial microanatomy.

The anatomical details can be studied using B-mode, and information on microvascular network are better studied using color Doppler and power Doppler (Figs. 6.3, 6.4, and 6.5).

In literature, different studies have demonstrated a high sensitivity of color-coded ultrasound in preoperative perforator evaluation [12–16].

Compared to other imaging technology, such as multidetector CT (MDCT) scan angiography and magnetic resonance angiography (MRA) [17], US allows a live evaluation of the perforators which gives the possibility to mark their location precisely on the skin. Moreover, high-frequency probes allow a resolution up to 100 μm with the possibility to visualize microvessels up to 0.2 mm in caliber, which goes beyond the ability of other imaging modalities (Fig. 6.2).

Moreover, a dynamic evaluation of flow and velocity can be performed along with measuring its caliber, which helps

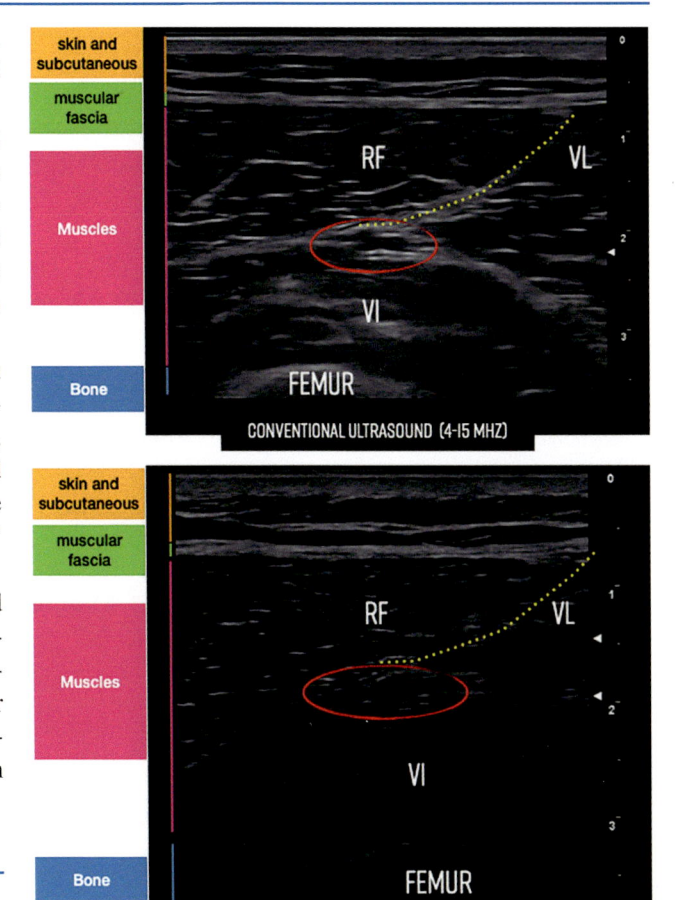

Fig. 6.3 Comparison of B-mode ultrasound scan of anterolateral thigh area taken with conventional (above) and high-frequency (below) ultrasound using same depth and focus point of the same spot. The anterolateral thigh (ALT) is a very common donor site for perforator flaps. The gross differences between conventional and high-frequency ultrasound are clear: the first gives clearer detail of deeper structures compared to the second. The intramuscular septum between rectus femoris (RF) muscle and vastus lateralis (VL) muscle is highlighted by yellow spots. Down to the septum, into the virtual space below RF and above vastus intermedius (VI) muscle, it is visible the descending branch of the lateral circumflex femoral artery (DB-LCFA)

in selecting the perforator preoperatively. The precise subfascial course of the perforator is available (septal/intramuscular/mixed course) up to the source vessel, thus precisely delineating the dissection route that will be performed intraoperatively (Fig. 6.4).

When planning local perforator flaps, the exact axis of a perforator within the subcutaneous tissue can be delineated, which helps to precisely include the perforator tree within flap design [18].

In LVA surgery, high-frequency ultrasound is useful in preoperative evaluation of recipient venules, whereas it gives limited information on lymphatic channels compared to ultrahigh-frequency [19].

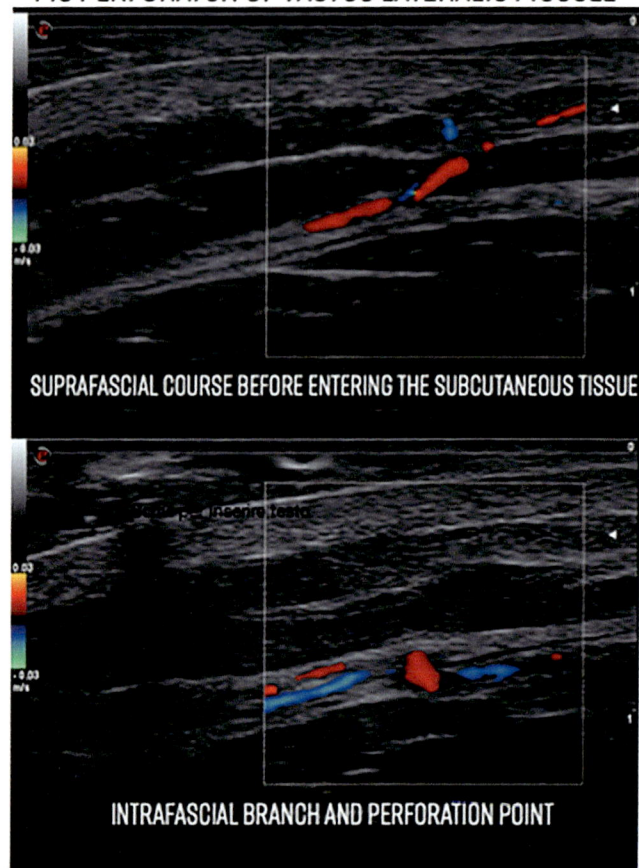

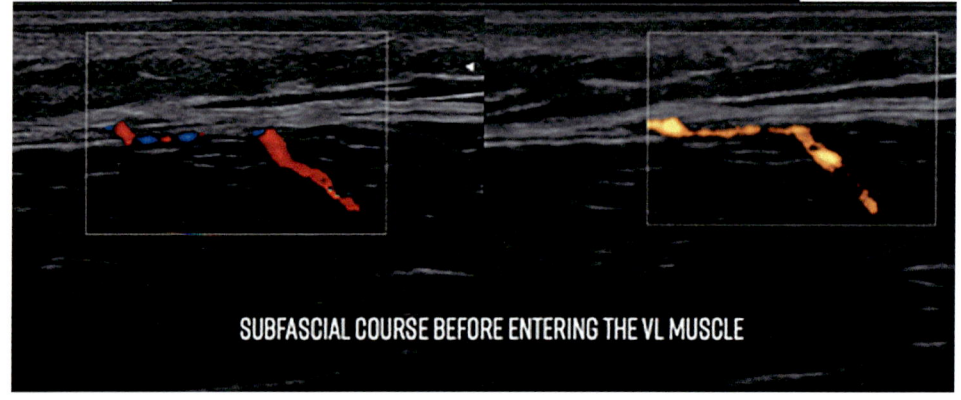

Fig. 6.4 DB-LCFA perforator course. (Above) Perforator visualization using the color flow mapping (CFM) just after piercing the muscular fascia. It is evident that the perforator has a strict suprafascial course for half centimeter and then enters the subcutaneous tissue. (Center) At the point when the perforator pierces the muscular fascia. It is visible an intrafascial branch. (Below, left) Perforator intramuscular course through VL muscle. At CFM, the perforator course from the muscular fascia perforator point to the intramuscular branch is not clear. (Above, right) To improve the sensibility of the signal, it is possible to switch to power Doppler mode which clearly highlights a strict subfascial course of the perforator for 0.5 cm before piercing the fascia. Compared to CFM, we do not have the flow direction information. Figure gives an idea of the most common information that can be acquired from a preoperative planning of an ALT flap. The perforator caliber, position, and course are already very clear before starting surgery

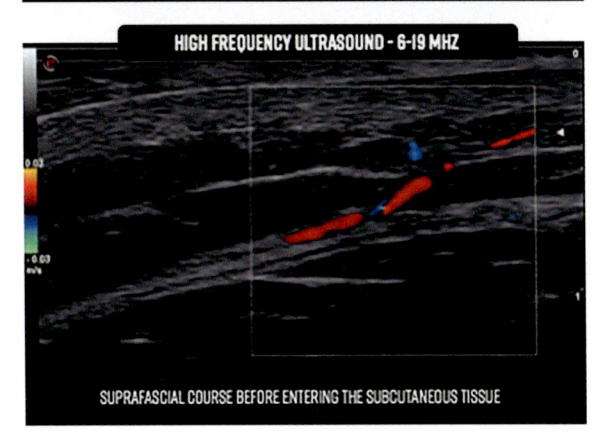

Fig. 6.5 The same perforator of Fig. 6.4 was scanned with ultrahigh-frequency ultrasound (UHFUS) linear probe (70 MHz). This technology allows to obtain very superficial details. The scale on the right is in millimeter compared to the scale of the high frequency which is in centimeter. (Above) With UHFUS, it is possible to identify the exact perforator dermis entry point as well as intradermal plexus. This information is particularly useful when planning thin and pure skin perforator flaps. This is a type 2 perforator, and the image above shows the left branch, barely appreciable with the high-frequency ultrasound (below)

6.4 Ultrahigh-Frequency Ultrasound (UHFUS)

The latest evolution in ultrasound technology has been the introduction of ultrahigh-frequency probes (48 and 70 MHz) available for use in humans. These frequencies allow a resolution up to 30 μm (70 MHz) and 50 μm (48 MHz) which enables clear and detailed visualization of very tiny structures and details, not possible before. The main disadvantages of such frequency is the depth analysis related to the low penetration. Accurate analysis down to 1 cm from the skin is possible with 70 MHz probes and down to 2 cm with the 48 MHz probes.

For these features, UHFUS should be seen as an upgrade of HF-US for some specific application in plastic surgery, especially for perforator and lymphatic imaging [20–28].

For perforator flaps, we usually proceed first with CCDS to delineate all features of the perforator. In case we are planning a thin, superthin, or pure skin perforator (PSP) flap, we further evaluate the identified perforators using the UHFUS. In fact, UHFUS allows to expand the knowledge of subcutaneous tissue anatomy and its microvascular network. We recently proposed a practical classification for harvesting thin, superthin, and PSP flaps based on UHFUS information [21].

Perforators are classified as *type 1 perforators*, when the perforator shows a direct course from the muscular fascia to dermis. Its caliber is preserved up to the superficial fascia (Camper's fascia), where it can branch or proceed directly to the dermis. One to three dermis entry points are identifiable and the intradermal plexus (for the arterial and venous component) is visible.

The microanatomical features of type 1 perforators make them very favorable when a superthin or PSP is planned. In fact, for superthin flaps, the main important step during the surgery is the identification of the proper superficial fascia (Camper's fascia). Once this plane is identified, the dissection proceeds along this plane up to the perforator, without needing explorative approach and/or microdissection. There is no fear to jeopardize flap vascularity by ligation of further microvessels that are encountered during elevation, because the chosen perforator has no branches below this level. For PSP, the dissection is similar with the difference that the elevation is made just below the dermis, as when a full-thickness skin graft is raised.

Conversely, *type 2 perforators* start to arborize in different collaterals within the subcutaneous tissue, after piercing the Scarpa's fascia. The perforator cannot be easily followed within the subcutaneous tissue with 48 and 70 MHz probes. Compared to type 1 perforator, it is not possible to detect a direct perforator course from muscular fascia to the dermis in type 2 perforators.

Type 2 perforators are thus chosen when a thin flap is planned (elevated on the Scarpa's fascia plane). If those perforators are chosen for superthin or PSP flap elevation, microdissection of all the tiny subcutaneous collaterals is needed not to jeopardize flap vascularity.

This classification does not apply for conventional supra- or subfascial perforator flap elevation, because in both cases, the perforator vascular tree is included in the flap.

In our experience, there are two main advantages of proposed UHFUS perforator classification:

- *Safer, faster elevation of PSP and superthin flap.* The precise knowledge of the perforator subcutaneous anatomy allows the surgeon to concentrate more on correctly finding the plane of elevation, which is sometimes hard, and to proceed with a precise superthin elevation.
- *Choose the perforators on which the flap is based.* In fact, we can choose the best perforator for our needs within the same donor site or choose the donor site based on perfora-

Fig. 6.6 Ultrahigh-frequency ultrasound scan of lower limb lymphedema using a 48 MHz linear probe. ICG lymphography did not show clear linear patterns. UHFUS allowed to identify an incision point with two lymphatic channels (yellow arrows) and a favorable recipient venule with a branch (blue arrows)

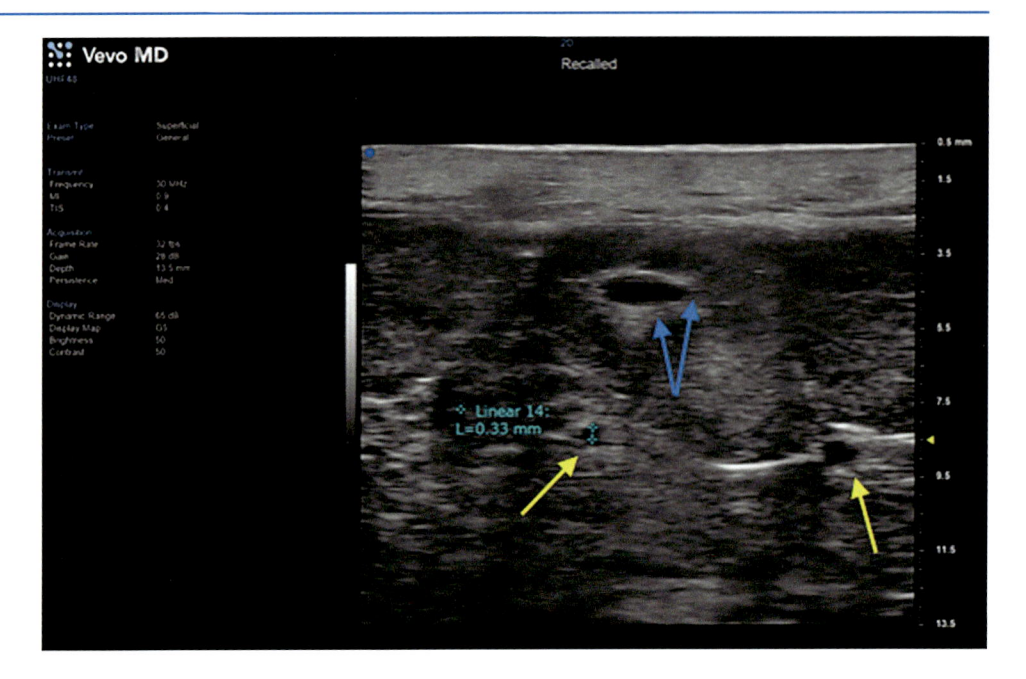

tor features. To give an example, ALT donor site is the most used for soft tissue reconstruction. It is not uncommon to find two to three sizeable and appropriate perforators on which we can harvest our flap. With the information given by US, we can choose the simplest, the least-invasive, and most appropriate perforator for our needs in case of thin flaps (type 1 or type 2).

UHFUS has also application in capillary perforator flap planning and in supermicrosurgical field [20].

In LVA surgery, UHFUS is the quintessence of preoperative planning [20, 23–28] that can be resumed in these points:

- Identification of functional lymphatic channels in dermal backflow areas (Fig. 6.6)
- Evaluation of lymphatic channels seen as linear pattern at the indocyanine green lymphography (ICG-L)
- Intraoperative selection of lymphatic channels
- Entire preoperative study in iodine-allergy patients that cannot undergo ICG-L
- Differentiation between functional and less-functional lymphatic channels as the UHFUS provides details comparable to those of histology
- Functional and static evaluation of favorable recipient venules
- Planning alternative methods in incisions devoid of venules

6.5 Conclusions

Ultrasound technology is largely available in all hospitals and small clinics as this technology represents the stethoscope for many specialties. Plastic surgeons should acquire sonographic skills to incorporate this tool in their practice, either this includes microsurgery or not.

CCDS allows to preoperatively study perforator anatomy, comprehensively. Information on size, hemodynamics, and anatomical course of a perforator allows to preoperatively plan the surgery, allowing to avoid time wasted for intraoperative exploration and frustration related to unknown microanatomy. This energy can be saved for improving creativity and to focus on other reconstructive needs. The patient will benefit from a safer, faster, and less destructive surgery.

UHFUS is advisable when planning superthin and PSP flaps. It represents the quintessence in LVA surgery.

Lastly, it is our opinion that ultrasonographic examination should be performed by the operating surgeon and not delegated to other colleagues or other specialists. It is only in this way that the operating surgeon can really feel to have preoperative knowledge of the microanatomy. This may have infinite potentials for further development of microsurgery.

Disclosure Giuseppe Visconti and Akitatsu Hayashi are Medical Advisors for Fujifilm Japan. Alessandro Bianchi and Marzia Salgarello have no interest in any of the products, devices, or drugs mentioned in this manuscript.

Conflict of Interest None.

Funding None.

References

1. Koshima I, Soeda S. Inferior epigastric artery skin flaps without rectus abdominis muscle. Br J Plast Surg. 1989;42(6):645–8.
2. Kim JT, Kim SW. Perforator flap versus conventional flap. J Korean Med Sci. 2015;30(5):514–22.
3. Taylor GI, Palmer JH. The vascular territories (angiosomes) of the body: experimental study and clinical applications. Br J Plast Surg. 1987;40:113–41.
4. Tashiro K, Yamashita S, Araki J, Narushima M, Iida T, Koshima I. Preoperative color Doppler ultrasonographic examination in the planning of thoracodorsal artery perforator flap with capillary perforators. J Plast Reconstr Aesthet Surg. 2016;69(3):346–50.
5. Narushima M, Yamasoba T, Iida T, Matsumoto Y, Yamamoto T, Yoshimatsu H, Timothy S, Pafitanis G, Yamashita S, Koshima I. Pure skin perforator flaps: the anatomical vascularity of the superthin flap. Plast Reconstr Surg. 2018;142(3):351e–60e.
6. Visconti G, Salgarello M. Free-style capillary perforator-based island flaps for reconstruction of skin cancer defects of the face, body, and extremities. Ann Plast Surg. 2018;81(2):192–7.
7. Yamamoto T. Onco-reconstructive supermicrosurgery. Eur J Surg Oncol. 2019;45(7):1146–51.
8. Koshima I, Inagawa K, Urushibara K, Moriguchi T. Supermicrosurgical lymphaticovenular anastomosis for the treatment of lymphedema in the upper extremities. J Reconstr Microsurg. 2000;16(6):437–42.
9. Aoyagi F, Fujino T, Ohshiro T. Detection of small vessels for microsurgery by a Doppler flowmeter. Plast Reconstr Surg. 1975;55(3):372–3.
10. Karkowski J, Buncke HJ. A simplified technique for free transfer of groin flaps, by use of a Doppler probe. Plast Reconstr Surg. 1975;55(6):682–6.
11. Stekelenburg CM, Sonneveld PMDG, Bouman MB, van der Wal MBA, Knol DL, de Vet HCW, van Zuijlen PPM. The hand held Doppler device for the detection of perforators in reconstructive surgery: what you hear is not always what you get. Burns. 2014;40:1702–6.
12. Thomas B, Warszawski J, Falkner F, Nagel SS, Schmidt VJ, Kneser U, Bigdeli AK. A comparative study of preoperative color-coded Duplex ultrasonography versus handheld audible Dopplers in ALT flap planning. Microsurgery. 2020;40(5):561–7.
13. Kehrer A, Sachanadani NS, da Silva NPB, Lonic D, Heidekrueger P, Taeger CD, Klein S, Jung EM, Prantl L, Hong JP. Step-by-step guide to ultrasound-based design of alt flaps by the microsurgeon - basic and advanced applications and device settings. J Plast Reconstr Aesthet Surg. 2020;73(6):1081–90.
14. Cho MJ, Kwon JG, Pak CJ, Suh HP, Hong JP. The role of duplex ultrasound in microsurgical reconstruction: review and technical considerations. J Reconstr Microsurg. 2020;36(7):514–21.
15. Feng S, Min P, Grassetti L, Lazzeri D, Sadigh P, Nicoli F, Torresetti M, Gao W, di Benedetto G, Zhang W, Zhang YX. A Prospective head-to-head comparison of color doppler ultrasound and computed tomographic angiography in the preoperative planning of lower extremity perforator flaps. Plast Reconstr Surg. 2016;137(1):335–47.
16. Cina A, Salgarello M, Barone-Adesi L, Rinaldi P, Bonomo L. Planning breast reconstruction with deep inferior epigastric artery perforating vessels: multidetector CT angiography versus color Doppler US. Radiology. 2010;255(3):979–87.
17. Cina A, Barone-Adesi L, Rinaldi P, Cipriani A, Salgarello M, Masetti R, Bonomo L. Planning deep inferior epigastric perforator flaps for breast reconstruction: a comparison between multidetector computed tomography and magnetic resonance angiography. Eur Radiol. 2013;23(8):2333–43.
18. Almadori G, De Corso E, Visconti G, Almadori A, Di Cintio G, Mele DA, Settimi S, Paludetti G, Salgarello M. Impact of internal mammary artery perforator propeller flap in neck resurfacing and fistula closure after salvage larynx cancer surgery: our experience. Head Neck. 2019;41(11):3788–97.
19. Hayashi A, Yamamoto T, Yoshimatsu H, Hayashi N, Furuya M, Harima M, Narushima M, Koshima I. Ultrasound visualization of the lymphatic vessels in the lower leg. Microsurgery. 2016;36(5):397–401.
20. Visconti G, Hayashi A, Yoshimatsu H, Bianchi A, Salgarello M. Ultra-high frequency ultrasound in planning capillary perforator flaps: preliminary experience☆. J Plast Reconstr Aesthet Surg. 2018;71(8):1146–52.
21. Visconti G, Bianchi A, Hayashi A, Cina A, Maccauro G, Almadori G, Salgarello M. Thin and superthin perforator flap elevation based on preoperative planning with ultrahigh-frequency ultrasound. Arch Plast Surg. 2020;47(4):365–70.
22. Yoshimatsu H, Hayashi A, Yamamoto T, Visconti G, Karakawa R, Fuse Y, Iida T. Visualization of the "intradermal plexus" using ultrasonography in the dermis flap: a step beyond perforator flaps. Plast Reconstr Surg Glob Open. 2019;7(11):e2411.
23. Visconti G, Yamamoto T, Hayashi N, Hayashi A. Ultrasound-assisted lymphaticovenular anastomosis for the treatment of peripheral lymphedema. Plast Reconstr Surg. 2017;139(6):1380e–1e.
24. Hayashi A, Giacalone G, Yamamoto T, Belva F, Visconti G, Hayashi N, Handa M, Yoshimatsu H, Salgarello M. Ultra high-frequency ultrasonographic imaging with 70 MHz scanner for visualization of the lymphatic vessels. Plast Reconstr Surg Glob Open. 2019;7(1):e2086.
25. Visconti G, Hayashi A, Tartaglione G, Yamamoto T, Bianchi A, Salgarello M. Preoperative planning of lymphaticovenular anastomosis in patients with iodine allergy: a multicentric experience. J Plast Reconstr Aesthet Surg. 2020;73(4):783–808.
26. Bianchi A, Visconti G, Hayashi A, Santoro A, Longo V, Salgarello M. Ultra-high frequency ultrasound imaging of lymphatic channels correlates with their histological features: a step forward in lymphatic surgery. J Plast Reconstr Aesthet Surg. 2020;73(9):1622–9.
27. Hayashi A, Visconti G, Yamamoto T, Giacalone G, Hayashi N, Handa M, Yoshimatsu H, Salgarello M. Intraoperative imaging of lymphatic vessel using ultra high-frequency ultrasound. J Plast Reconstr Aesthet Surg. 2018;71(5):778–80.
28. Visconti G, Bianchi A, Hayashi A, Salgarello M. Ultra-high frequency ultrasound preoperative planning of the rerouting method for lymphaticovenular anastomosis in incisions devoid of vein. Microsurgery. 2020;40:717. https://doi.org/10.1002/micr.30600. Epub ahead of print. PMID: 32369213.

Novel Microscopic Technologies in Reconstructive Microsurgery/Microvascular Surgery

Michalis Hadjiandreou and Georgios Pafitanis

Abbreviations

3D	Three-dimensional
ALT	Anterolateral thigh
AR	Augmented reality
CGAP	Cranial gluteal artery perforator
CVAs	Cerebrovascular accidents
DIEP	Deep inferior epigastric perforator
DOF	Depth of field
ENT	Ear, nose and throat
ETE	End-to-end
FOV	Field of view
HMM	Head-mounted microscope
HR	High resolution
HSI	Hyperspectral imaging
ICG	Indocyanine green
IMV	Internal mammary vein
iOCT	Integrated optical coherence tomography
LSCI	Laser speckle contrast imaging
MBARS	Microscope-based augmented reality system
MBVRS	Microscope-based virtual reality system
MIOCT	Microscope-integrated optical coherence tomography
MSI	Multispectral imaging
NIRF	Near-infrared fluorescence
OCT	Optical coherence tomography
OM	Operating microscope
OMiHSI	Operating microscope-integrated hyperspectral imaging
OM-NIRF	Operating microscope-near infrared fluoroscopy
PAL	Photoacoustic lymphangiography
PAM	Photoacoustic microscopy
PRDOCT	Phase-resolved Doppler optical coherence tomography
PU	Perfusion units
RM	Reconstructive microsurgery
VR	Virtual reality

7.1 Introduction

7.1.1 The Evolution of Operating Microscopy

Operating microscopy has gone through remarkable development over the last centuries. Technical advancements in the eighteenth and nineteenth centuries focused on improving the resolution of the monocular microscope. Amongst those, the placement of several low-powered lenses in a row with a certain distance between them by Joseph Jackson Lister and the proposal for a formula to calculate the numerical aperture by Ernst Abbe led to the enhancement of microscopy resolution [1].

Although the compound microscope had been invented in 1590 by two Dutch opticians, Zacharias and Hans Janssen, its several limitations including size and weight did not allow it to enter the operating theatre. Its limitations coupled with advancements in ophthalmology led to the development of binocular vision that was introduced by spectacle mounted magnifying systems. Head-worn magnification dominated the field of microscopy and preceded the operating microscope (OM) [2]. Devices were categorised into single-lens magnifiers (Figs. 7.1 and 7.2), prismatic magnifiers (Figs. 7.3 and 7.4) and telescopic systems [3]. In their simplest form, single-lens magnifiers were magnifying spectacles with convex lenses suspended at the end of the nose. Prismatic magnifiers were binocular magnifiers that used prism oculars and

---

M. Hadjiandreou (✉)
Centre for Plastic Surgery and Burns, St John's Hospital, Livingston, Scotland, UK

UCL Division of Surgery and Interventional Science, Royal Free Hospital, London, UK

G. Pafitanis
London Reconstructive Microsurgery Unit (LRMU), Emergency Care and Trauma Division (ECAT), The Royal London Hospital, Barts Health NHS Trust, London, UK

lenses and were first introduced in 1912 by the Carl Zeiss Company, offering a magnification in the range of 0.75–3.0×. It is of particular interest that the limitation of magnification and inflexibility in working distance paved the way for telescopic systems. The open Galilean loupes were the first device to offer this, followed by the first closed Galilean system that achieved focus of 15 cm and magnification of 3×. Finally, in 1952, the introduction of the *Keeler Galilean telescopic system* (Fig. 7.5) opened the door to modern microsurgery by providing a wide range of magnification (1.75–9×), working distance (34–16.5 cm) and the ability to adjust the interpupillary distance [3].

The need for stability in focusing and surgeon's discomfort with addition of a light source shifted the need to more stable devices such as monocular and, subsequently, binocular microscopes with tripod support and light attachment [3]. In 1921, the first monocular microscope was used intraoperatively by Carl Olof Nylén. The lack of depth perception led to the development of a *binocular Zeiss microscope* on a tripod with external light source in 1922 (Fig. 7.6). The operating microscope was widely adopted in the field of ENT surgery [1, 4]. However, several issues required improvements including image vibration at high magnification, fixed magnification insufficient illumination and single surgeon surgical field view.

In 1938, P. Tullio and P. Calicetti constructed a heavy tripod with counterweights that stabilised the image and allowed the optical unit to hang freely above the surgical table. Prisms were also mounted between the oculars to allow assistant to view the surgical field [5]. In 1952, Hans Littmann invented and introduced magnification change without changing focal length, in the form of *Zeiss-Opton* (Fig. 7.7) (working distance 200 mm, magnifications of 4, 6, 10, 16, 25, 40 or 63 as a rotary Galilean system) [4, 5]. In 1953, Littmann adopted improvements in manoeuvrability

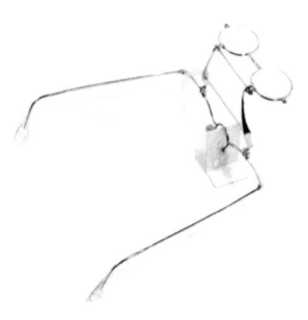

Fig. 7.1 Biconvex lenses on extended arm (single-lens magnifier)

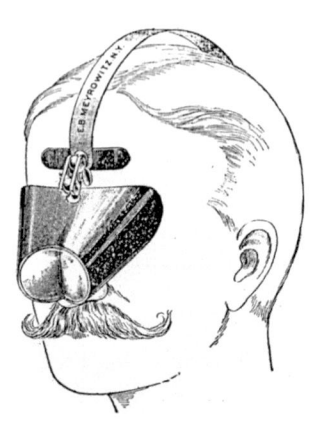

Fig. 7.2 Berger loupe (single-lens magnifier)

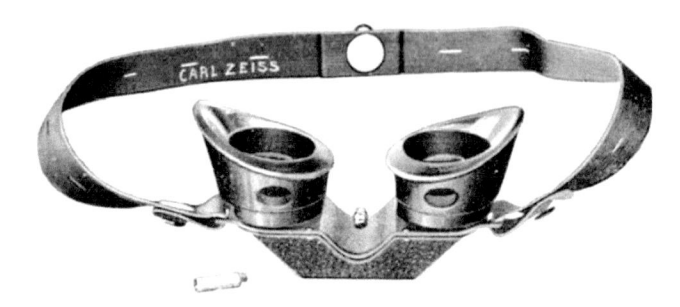

Fig. 7.3 Zeiss Prism binocular loupe (prismatic magnifier)

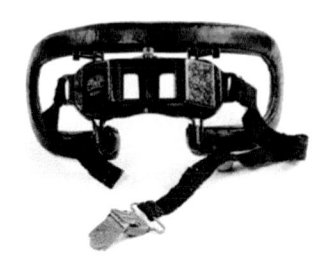

Fig. 7.4 Zeiss Prism binocular loupe on face frame (prismatic magnifier)

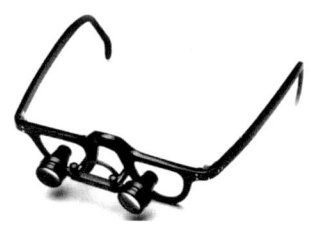

Fig. 7.5 Keeler Galilean telescopic system

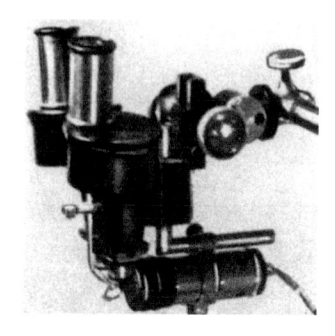

Fig. 7.6 The binocular Zeiss microscope modified by Holmgren

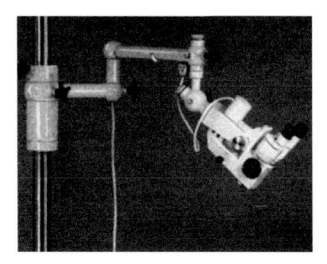

Fig. 7.7 Zeiss Opton microscope by Hans Littman

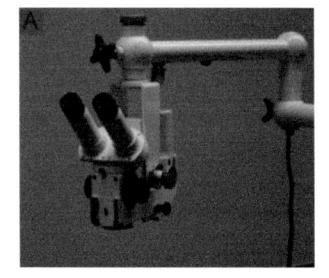

Fig. 7.8 The Zeiss OPMI 1

by Horst L. Wullstein and introduced the *Zeiss OPMI 1*, a milestone in the evolution of microscopy (Fig. 7.8), which offered more stability, easier operation and superior coaxial lighting than other microscopes available at the time (10–40.5 cm working distance and magnifications 2.5 and 50). Finally, in 1956, the OM had some significant innovations such as knee-controlled focusing lever and foot-controlled *x–y* coordinate system. These two developments allowed surgeons to operate in a hands-free manner and established the position of the OM in modern surgical practice [5].

7.1.2 Operating Microscopy in Reconstructive Microsurgery

The OM has numerous applications in the field of reconstructive microsurgery (RM). From finger replantation to lymphatic reconstruction, the OM offers unique capabilities to the reconstructive microsurgeon such as powerful magnification and unparalleled illumination. Numerous studies have highlighted the superiority of the OM compared to other means of magnification in the reconstructive outcome and safety of flap design [6–9].

Current limitations of the OM such as manoeuvrability, large volume, high cost and absence of three-dimensional (3D) vision remain the challenges that need to be addressed via technological advancements, namely, robotics and imaging modalities. This chapter will focus on presenting novel microscopic technologies for reconstructive microsurgery in three parts: (1) current novel microscopic technologies, (2) clinical applications of these technologies in the reconstructive field and (3) future directions of operative microscopy.

7.2 Novel Microscopic Technologies

7.2.1 Visualisation Technologies

7.2.1.1 HD Displays and 3D Visualisation

Visualisation is one of the most important technical characteristics of the modern OM. Stereopsis is a key feature of the binocular microscope that has enhanced visualisation by providing depth perception under magnification. This offered the microsurgeon a 3D impression of the surgical field. The depth information is clinically relevant in aiding diagnosis via recognition of anatomical location and morphology of tissue structures [4].

FusionOptics™ technology is a sophisticated optical approach technology that enhances stereo visualisation for surgical microscopes by providing simultaneous high depth of field (DOF) and high resolution (HR). This is achieved by one light path received by observer with higher resolution and lower DOF and, simultaneously, the other light path received by observer with lower resolution and higher DOF [10]. The human brain combines the images into a HR, high DOF optical spatial image.

High-definition (HD) display and 3D visualisation have transformed microsurgical practice and training and show potential in improving ergonomics. In 2010, *TrueVision Systems* developed a 'heads-up 3D microscopy' system which transmits the image on a HD 3D monitor to improve position of the microsurgeon. Mendez et al. evaluated the feasibility of using heads-up 3D microscopy to perform rat femoral artery anastomoses comparing the technique to traditional microscopy (Fig. 7.9). 3D visualisation was found to be equally safe to traditional technique with 100% patency rate and no significant difference in operative time. In addition, the 3D system was assessed by the majority of participants as equivalent or superior in-depth perception, image resolution and FOV. It is worth noting that all the participants found the 3D system to be a more valuable educational and interactive experience [11]. High-definition displays can show overlaid radiological or other images that can provide surgical guidance and intraoperative planning. A feasibility study by Belykh et al. presented the capabilities of the robotic visualisation platform, *ZEISS KINEVO 900*, including 3D display through polarising glasses for microvascular anastomoses on rat carotid arteries [12]. Further details on *KINEVO 900* can be found in Sect. 7.2.3.2 (Fig. 7.10).

7.2.1.2 Immersive Microscopy

Augmented Reality

Augmented reality (AR) overlays digital information on real-world objects to enhance user experience or capabilities [13]. AR has gained momentum in the field of RM due to its potential benefits and technical advancements of the OM. A recent systematic review by Vles et al. identified AR applications in preoperative planning for osteotomies in different plastic surgery procedures and perforator vessel identification; however, there was no utilisation of a microscope-based AR system (MBARS) in these applications [14]. Similarly, a systematic review by Al Omran et al. focusing on AR in RM identified five studies that incorporated three types of AR: head-mounted devices, hand-held devices and spatial augmentation reality. None of the studies identified involved the use of microscope-based AR system [15]. Despite the fact that MBARS is not popular within RM, it has been used in the field of neurosurgery. The MBARS allows overlaying 3D projections of preoperative surgical images into the bilateral eyepieces of the binocular optics with surgical field alignment [16].

There are a number of technical considerations prior to utilisation of MBARS. These can be categorised into calibration of optical system, tracking, registration and display. Table 7.1 summarises the technical interventions and their aim. Although not studied in RM directly, a MBARS has the potential to be used with near-infrared guided indocyanine green (NIR-ICG) technique in identification of lymphatic vessels for lymphaticovenous anastomosis (LVA) [17, 18]. Watson et al. demonstrated how real-time overlay of bright-field and NIR fluorescence images can be achieved. The objective lens receives both NIR and bright-field images of the specimen simultaneously. The augmentation module separates the NIR image from the bright-field image, and the NIR image is processed to generate a synthetic image. The synthetic image is then redirected to a single ocular piece. Equivalently, two cameras can capture the NIR image, and after processing, this is superimposed on the FOV, and the integrated image is projected to both ocular pieces [19]. Figure 7.11 shows a schematic of the MBARS reproduced from Watson et al. [19].

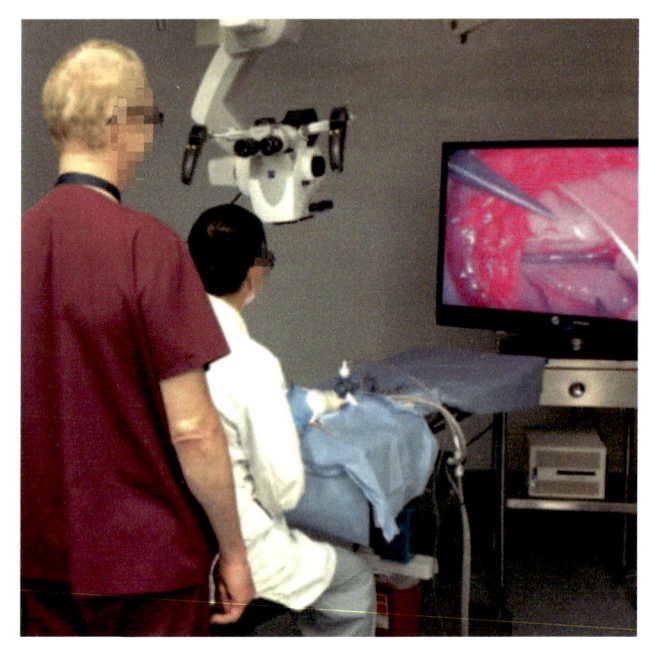

Fig. 7.9 (Left) 3D dimensional microscopy using 3D goggles. (Reproduced from Mendez et al. [11])

Table 7.1 Summary and aim of MBARS technical interventions (adapted from Ma L et al. [4])

MBARS technical interventions	Summary of intervention	Aim
Calibration (of optical system)	Determination of all camera parameters including optical errors	Production of projection matrix generating pixel position in the injected image of any 3D point relative to the frame of reference of microscope
Tracking	Pose estimation of objects in real time	Accuracy
Registration	Relating 2 or more data sets to each other to match their content	Essential as system very sensitive to misalignment of virtual image and real environment
Display	Image injection into microscope oculars and monitors	Accurate superposition of real and virtual image

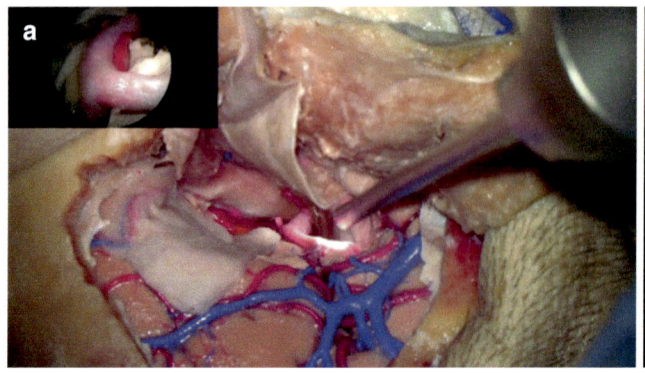

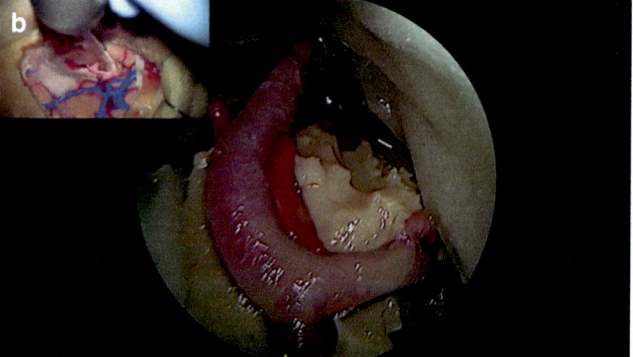

Fig. 7.10 (a, b) (Right) Overlaid image (picture-in-picture) feature of the robotic visualisation platform ZEISS KINEVO 900. (Reproduced from Belykh et al. [12])

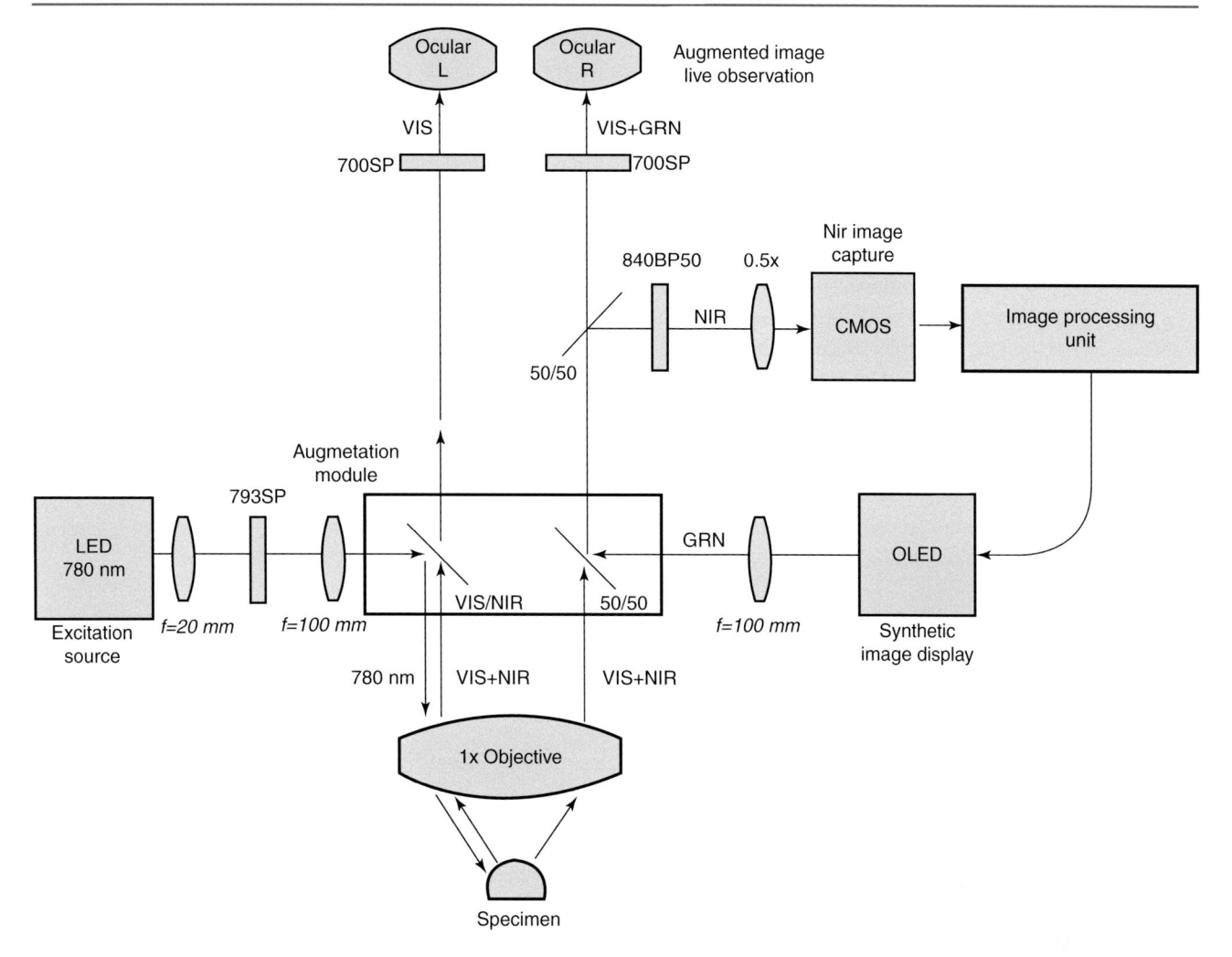

Fig. 7.11 MBARS illustration with augmented image projected to right eyepiece. (Reproduced from Watson et al. [19])

There are several obstacles in the design of AR before it is safely incorporated in routine RM practice: registration error from compounded sources, system latency resulting in visual asynchrony, obstruction of area of interest by virtual component and time consumption for registration and verification. Depth in AR refers to the understanding of spatial relationships between perspective, object in view and overlaid information. Incorrect depth interpretation is the most common perceptual problem in AR applications and can potentially have serious clinical implications [20]. The future of AR applications includes refinement and improvement of AR systems to allow seamless integration in the challenging microsurgical environment.

Virtual Reality

Virtual reality (VR) is a simulated, immersive experience that presents digital information in a 3D environment [21]. A review by Kim et al. identified VR applications in plastic surgery planning and training; however, none of the studies presented a microscopy-based VR system (MBVRS) used for RM purposes such as planning, intraoperative navigation or training [22].

7.2.2 Optical Imaging Modalities

7.2.2.1 Near-Infrared Fluorescence Imaging

Near-infrared fluorescence (NIRF) imaging modality is one of the most promising imaging techniques for image-guided surgery. Contrast agents with fluorescent characteristics (i.e. fluorophores including indocyanine green (ICG)) in the near-infrared spectrum (700–900 nm) can be visualised using dedicated NIR camera systems. A systematic review by Cornelissen et al. presents the multiple applications of NIRF imaging in plastic and reconstructive surgery including assessment of tissue perfusion in free flap surgery, perioperative assessment of mastectomy skin flap perfusion, bone perfusion and abdominal wall perfusion in abdominal wall reconstruction, planning of LVA and assessment of perfusion after revascularisation of upper limb extremity ischaemia [23].

Various NIRF systems are described in literature including hand-held, non-hand-held and operating microscope (OM)-NIRF system integration [24–31]. There are multiple advantages of OM-NIRF system integration including improved ergonomics, surgeon's hand freedom and uninterrupted surgical workflow. In its simplest form, an OM-NIRF system incorporates an excitation light source, one short-pass filter for light excitation, one long-pass filter for fluorescence signal and camera for fluorescence capture. The process involves the short-pass filter placed in front of light source and the long-pass filter placed in the observation optical path. The fluorescence signal emitted combined with excitation light is filtered by the long-pass filter with combined signal reaching the camera (CCD), surgeon or observer via beam splitters [4, 32]. Figure 7.12 shows a schematic representation of the process.

Holm et al. reported the first human preliminary study on OM-NIRF that allowed for intraoperative imaging of microsurgical anastomoses. The authors utilised an *OPMI Pentero IR 800* (Carl Zeiss, Oberkochen Germany) (Table 7.1) with integrated indocyanine green technology into the optical path and suggested a considerable potential impact of the microscopic technique on early flap failure [33]. Sugawara et al. evaluated the blood flow after vascular anastomosis in breast reconstruction to the anterograde IMV and the retrograde IMV using a NIRF system installed on a *M525 OH4 surgical microscope (Leica Microsystems, Wetzlar, Germany)* (Table 7.2) [37]. Multiple clinical studies utilised the *SPY Elite imaging system (Stryker Corporation, United States)* (Table 7.2), which consists of an imaging head (camera and laser light source), a mobile cart and an articulated arm. Although the system employs the fluorescence properties of ICG, it is not a microscope as the surgeon sees the images on a monitor and not under microscopic vision [30, 31, 38–40] (Fig. 7.13). Table 7.2 summarises the technical specifications of the three NIRF technologies.

Fig. 7.12 Schematic representation of OM-NIRF integration system. (Reproduced from Stummer et al. [32])

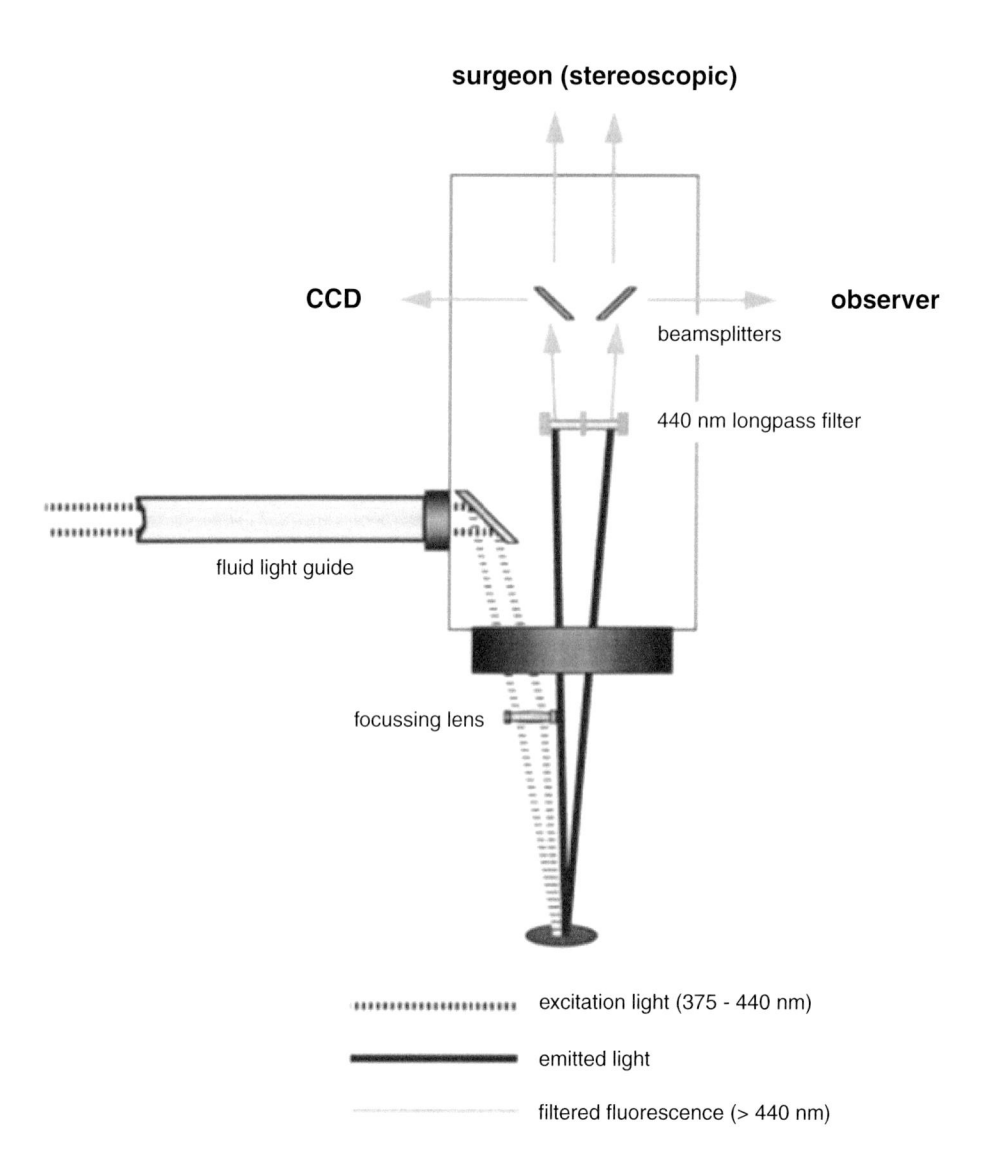

7 Novel Microscopic Technologies in Reconstructive Microsurgery/Microvascular Surgery

Table 7.2 Technical characteristics of commonly used NIR OMs in reconstructive microsurgery [34–36]

	Technical specifications of NIR OMs		
Name	OPMI Pentero IR 800	M525 OH4 Surgical Microscope	SPY elite imaging system
Design			
Components	Microscope, articulated arm, imaging console	Microscope, articulated arm, imaging console	Imaging unit, imaging console, articulated arm
Magnification range	Up to 39×	1.2–12.8× with 10× eyepiece	N/A
Working distance	200–500 mm	207–470 mm	N/A
Imaging agent	ICG (IR 800)	ICG (FL800) and 5-ALA (FL400) oncological fluorescence	ICG
Mode of Imaging	HD, NIR fluorescence imaging	HD, NIR fluorescence imaging	NIR fluorescence imaging

N/A not applicable

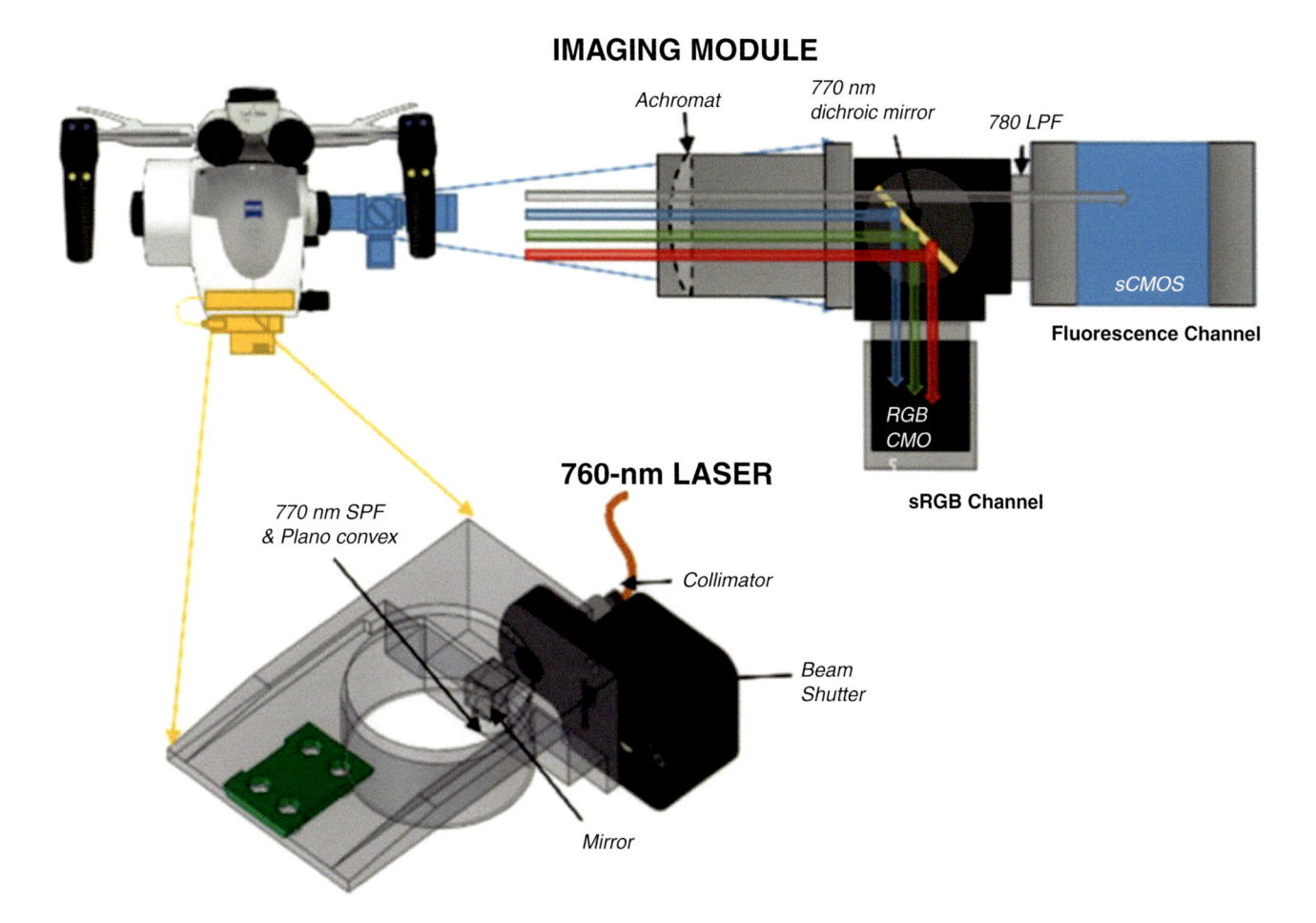

Fig. 7.13 Example of detection (blue) and illumination (yellow) modules for attachment on Zeiss OPMI Pentero head without affecting the standard operation of the OM. (Reproduced from Elliott et al. [41])

7.2.2.2 Optical Coherence Tomography

Optical coherence tomography (OCT) is a non-invasive optical imaging technology that can offer micrometre-scale-resolution 2D and 3D high-resolution images of biological samples such as submillimetre vessels and nerves [42, 43]. It has been widely used in the diagnosis and management of ocular pathology including various ophthalmological procedures [44–46], brain tumour imaging [47] and ENT [48, 49]. OCT operates on the principle of optical backscatter detection of NIR light from biological tissue with interferometry employed to measure time delays [43].

Intraoperative OCT has three main types of devices: hand-held OCT, needle-based probes and microscope-integrated OCT (MiOCT). MiOCT is a key technological advancement of OCT as surgeons can receive intraoperative, cost-effective, nonionising real-time feedback (relative to MRI or CT) with minimal surgical workflow interaction [4, 50]. In 2005, Geerling et al. presented a feasibility study on integrating the OCT technology with the OM for intraoperative 2D visualisation of the anterior segment of the eye [51]. A dichroic mirror was used to fold the OCT beam integrating its optical zoom with the optical zoom of the OM. Hence, the OCT lateral resolution and FOV were dependent on the microscope's optical zoom which could result in OCT performance compromise. This design was adopted and commercialised in the *Haag-Streit Surgical iOCT* (Fig. 7.14) [50]. Further MiOCT designs resulted in a number of improvements such as decoupling of the OCT resolution and lateral FOV from the OM zoom level [50], minimising the number of optical elements shared between the two modalities and use of spherical mirror relays to improve the optical transmission. These technological improvements were adopted in MiOCT commercial designs for human ocular surgery (Fig. 7.14) [50, 52–54].

MiOCT utilisation in RM is limited. Boppart et al. performed one of the earliest studies of OCT utilisation in microvascular anastomosis of in vitro rabbit (Fig. 7.14) and human arteries and nerves. It was reported that the imaging capabilities of OCT technology have the potential for intraoperative monitoring to improve patient outcomes (Fig. 7.15) [43]. Similarly, Huang et al. performed a proof-of-concept study utilising phase-resolved OCT (PRDOCT), albeit not MiOCT, to assist surgeons in avoiding microvascular anastomosis technical errors and evaluating the surgical outcome in terms of flow, lumen patency and thrombus formation in microvascular anastomosis. An in vivo rat popliteal artery anastomosis (diameter 0.4 mm) model was used (Figs. 7.16 and 7.17). It was demonstrated that PRDOCT can guide microvascular anastomosis reducing the risk of technical error and evaluating the surgical outcome [42]. In a further study by Huang et al., PRDOCT was used to generate high-resolution 3D structure views and flow information of 22 mouse femoral artery anastomoses and 17 mouse venous anastomoses. Flow status, vessel inner lumen and early thrombus detection were analysed based on PRDOCT imaging results. It was concluded that PRDOCT is an effective evaluation tool for microvascular anastomosis with 92% sensitivity and 90% specificity for arterial anastomoses [56]. In a step further, Zhu et al. utilised OCT technology for in vivo real-time imaging of

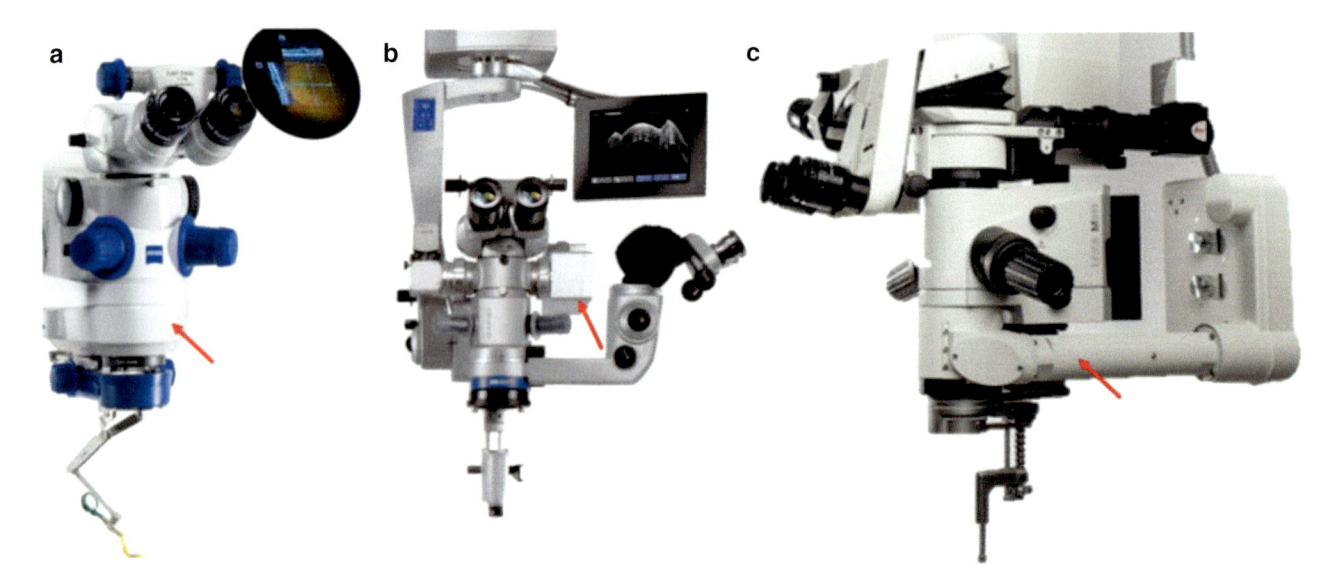

Fig. 7.14 Commercial MiOCT systems for human ocular procedures. (**a**) Zeiss RESCAN 700 B permanently integrated OCT system (red arrow) coupled directly prior to the microscope objective [52]. (**b**) Haag-Streit Surgical iOCT Modular OCT system (red arrow) attached to the camera port of microscope [53]. (**c**) Leica Microsystems Bioptigen EnFocus Modular OCT system (red arrow) attached prior to microscope objective [54]. (Reproduced from Carrasco-Zevallos et al. review [50])

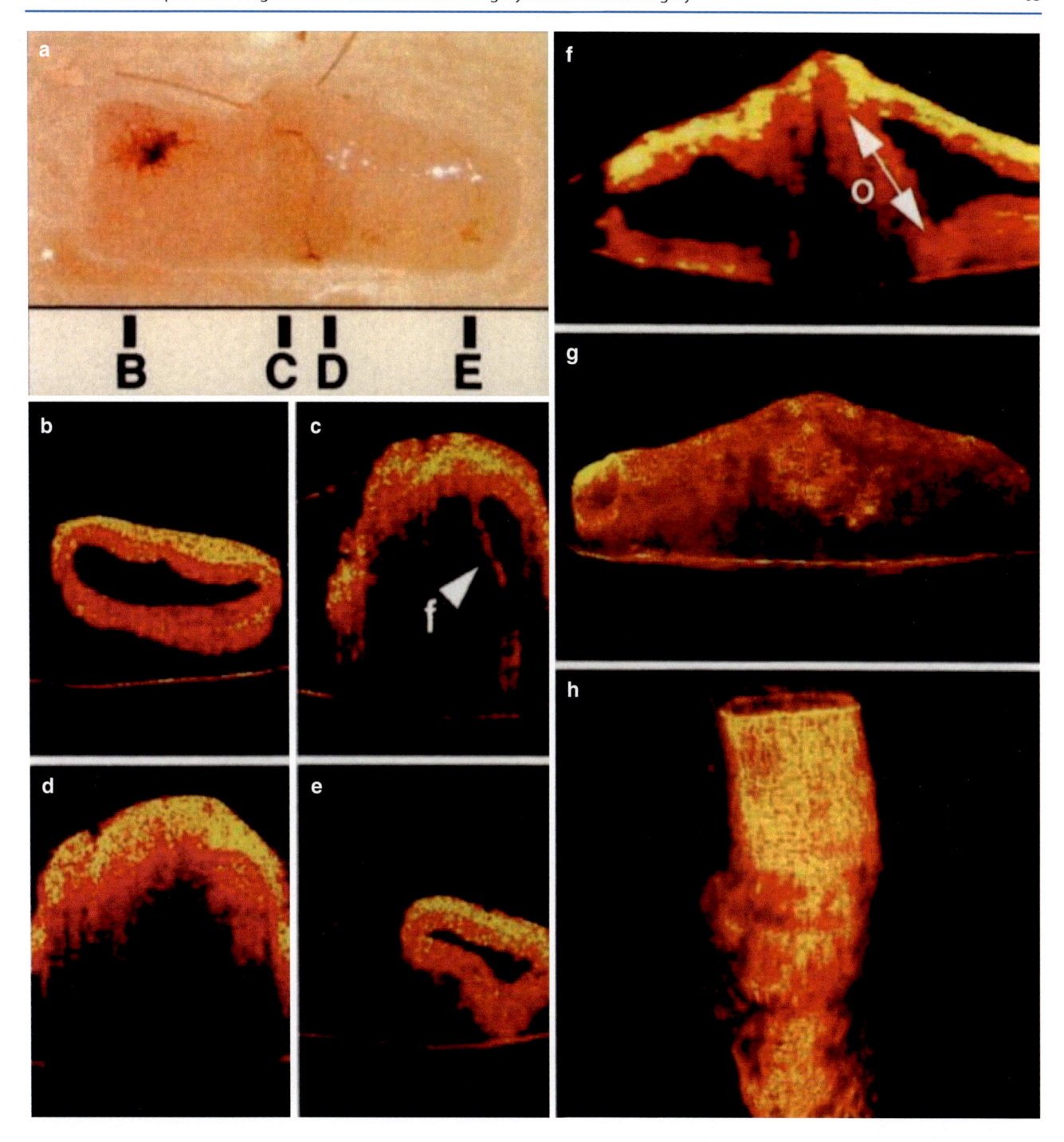

Fig. 7.15 3D OCT imaging of a rabbit artery anastomosis. (**a**) Digital image of 1-mm-diameter artery. (**b–e**) Planes for cross-sectional OCT images. (**b, e**) Lumen is patent. (**c**) Lumen partially obstructed with (arrowhead *f*) depicting thrombosis. (**d**) Fully obstructed portion of the anastomotic site. (**f**) Longitudinal section of the artery showing obstruction (double-headed arrow *o*). (**g, h**) 3D projection of rabbit artery. (Reproduced from Boppart et al. [43])

anastomoses for supermicrosurgical research. Forty mice underwent end-to-end (ETE) femoral artery anastomosis and in vivo monitoring by the OCT system at various time points. OCT was found to be a valid method to evaluate vessel patency, haemodynamics and structural changes of the anastomosed artery [57].

7.2.2.3 Hyperspectral Imaging

Hyperspectral imaging (HSI) is an emerging optical imaging technique. It uses wavelengths of visible light that detect chromophores for oxygenated and deoxygenated haemoglobin generating a datacube consisting of one spectral and two spatial dimensions (Fig. 7.17c) [55, 58]. The number of

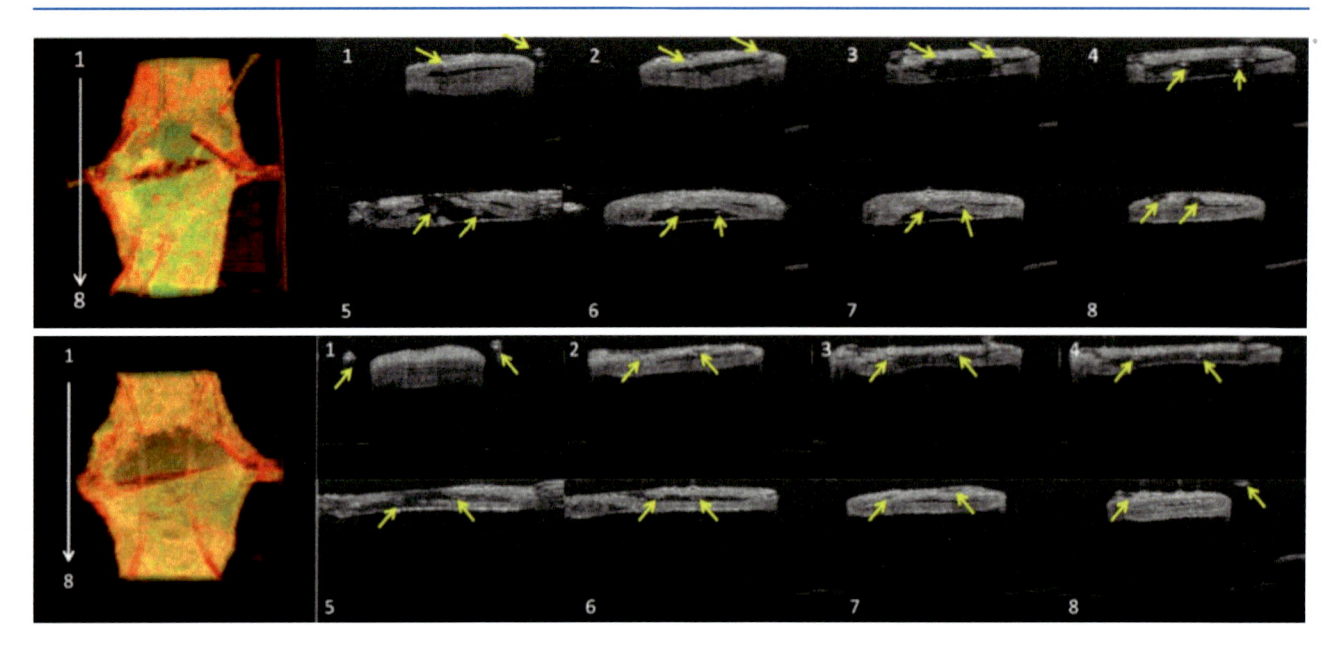

Fig. 7.16 (Top) OCT images showing vessel wall and incorrect suture placement for sutures 3 and 4. (Bottom) OCT showing vessel wall and correct suture placement for sutures 3 and 4. (Reproduced from Huang et al. [42])

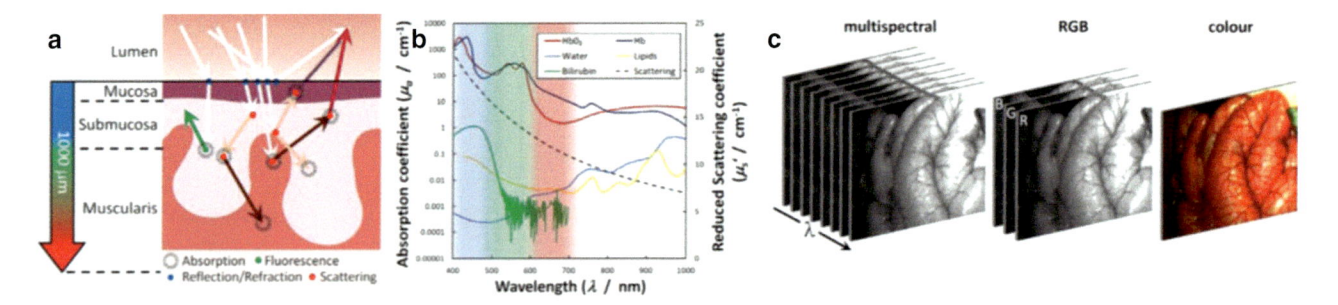

Fig. 7.17 (**a**) Propagation of light in bowel tissue. Light is being reflected, scattered or absorbed. (**b**) Optical properties of major absorbers such as oxygenated haemoglobin (HbO₂), deoxygenated haemoglobin (Hb), lipids, water and bilirubin. (**c**) Multispectral (MSI) Datacube bands acquired by the imaging system defines whether the system is termed multispectral (MSI; <10 s) or hyperspectral (HIS; <100 s). HSI offers multiple advantageous intraoperative characteristics: non-contact, non-invasive, nonionising, contrast agent-free and reproducible. HSI has the capacity to extend visual capabilities of surgeons delivering near real-time biomarker information and tissue pathophysiology through spectral characteristics. Thus, it has the potential of helping in disease diagnosis and surgical guidance [59].

HSI consists of four types of acquisition mode: point scanning, spectral scanning, line-scanning and snapshot [55]. Table 7.3 summarises the four types of acquisition mode.

HSI has not been extensively utilised in RM. Chin et al. demonstrated that HSI technology has the capacity to predictively assess the vascular evolution of wounds, allowing for early intervention [60]. The authors used the *OxyVu™-2 (HyperMed™, Inc. Greenwich, Connecticut)* device to gen-

of a segment of porcine bowel tissue. The same information in red, green and blue bands are collected by colour cameras to produce a colour image. (Reproduced from Clancy et al. [55])

Table 7.3 Details of the four types of HIS acquisition mode (adapted from Ma L et al. [4])

Acquisition mode	Details of acquisition mode
Point scanning	Point-by-point scanning, slow and not commonly used
Line-scanning	Scanning object along one spatial axis, complete spectrum for each pixel acquired in a row of pixels, requires relative motion between camera and patient
Spectral scanning	Capturing one greyscale image of the whole FOV at each step, better spatial and spectral resolution than snapshot
Snapshot	Spatial and spectral information captured simultaneously, fast video-rate acquisition speed

erate tissue oxygenation maps of the subpapillary plexus. No intraoperative microscope was used in this study. Similarly, in a more recent animal study, Chin et al. hypothesised that skin oxygenation changes seen at an early stage after flap surgery may non-invasively predict the long-term survival of the tissue in murine models [61]. The authors used the *OxyVu™-2 (HyperMed™, Imaging, Inc., Memphis, Tenn.)* device with no OM use. The same device has been used in a recent non-inferiority animal study by Jones et al. where an experimental animal model of ischaemic necrosis was used to compare the accuracy of ICG angiography and MSI in assessing tissue perfusion [62]. MSI did not appear to be inferior to ICG in detecting compromised tissue viability. Considering the advantages of the spectral technique, the study emphasised the exciting potential for widespread use of the technique in cosmetic and reconstructive procedures [62].

Currently, there are no reports or studies of operative microscope-integrated hyperspectral imaging (OMiHSI) utilisation in RM; however, other specialities have utilised OMiHSI [63].

7.2.2.4 Photoacoustic Microscopy

Photoacoustics is a physical phenomenon that describes the generation of acoustic waves from an object absorbing pulsed or intensity-modulated optical irradiation. Photoacoustic microscopy (PAM) operates by short-pulsed or intensity-modulated continuous-wave laser beam target irradiation inducing ultrasonic waves as a result of the transient thermoelastic expansion. In this way, excited photoacoustic signals are detected and can reveal the physiologically specific absorption signatures of endogenous chromophores [64].

PAM is an emerging imaging technique with multiple advantages over other established imaging techniques: label-free optical absorption information, non-invasiveness and high contrast and resolution [65]. PAM has been utilised in animal studies for characterisation of cerebral haemodynamics and oxygen metabolism in CVAs [66] and ocular imaging [67]; however, there has been limited utilisation for reconstructive microsurgical purposes. Hu et al. presented the utilisation of PAM as optical-resolution photoacoustic microscopy (OR-PAM) for characterisation of the microvasculature including microvascular-related physiological and pathophysiological research such as tumour-vascular interaction and haemodynamic monitoring [64]. Figure 7.18 demonstrates a schematic representation of OR-PAM [64]. Another application of PAM in the field of RM was presented recently by Suzuki et al. via a case series where LVAs were observed by photoacoustic lymphangiography (PAL) to assess the patency of LVAs (Fig. 7.19) [68].

7.2.2.5 Laser Speckle Contrast Imaging

Laser speckle contrast imaging (LSCI) is a full-field, non-invasive perfusion technique that does not require any contrast agents and enables perfusion measurements within seconds. It is based on the phenomenon of backscattering of light from a scattering medium that results in a speckle pattern. The phenomenon occurs due to irregularities in a surface causing a distance difference between the surface and the image plane. If the distance difference between two

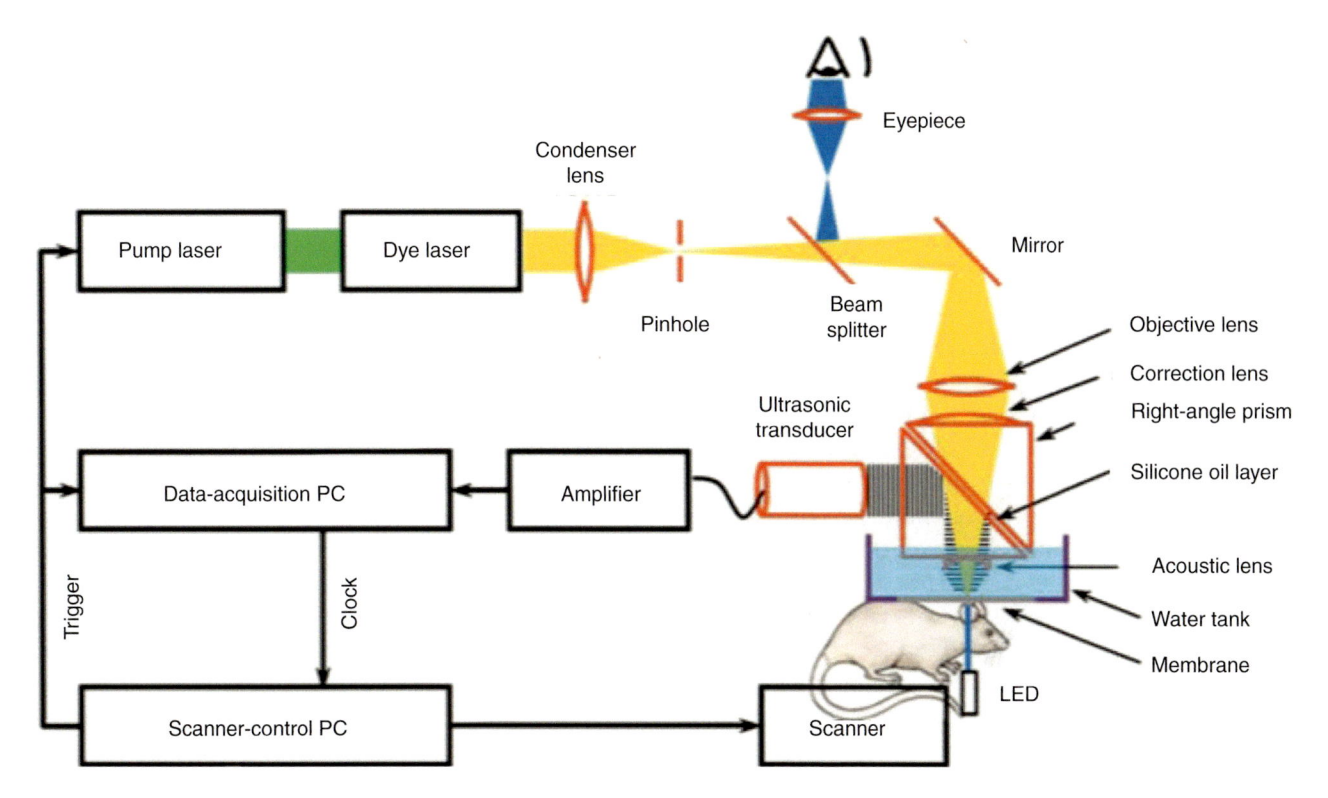

Fig. 7.18 Schematic representation of the OR-PAM. (Reproduced from Hu et al. [64])

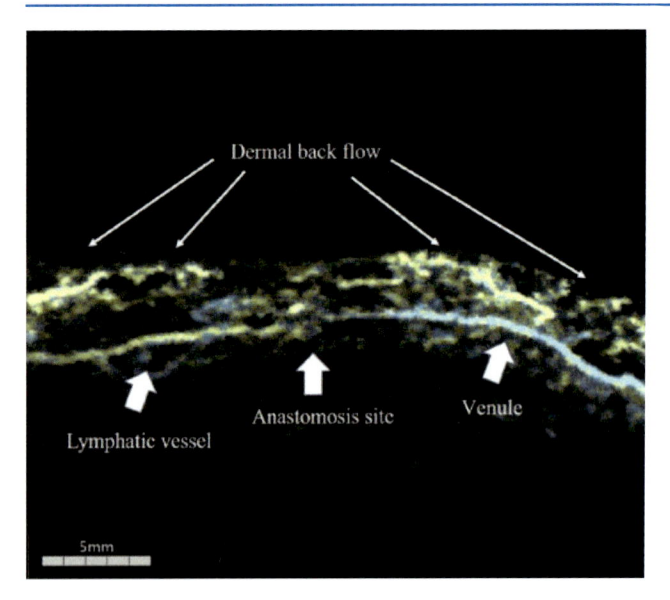

Fig. 7.19 Cross-sectional view of LVA. Dermal backflow is indicated in yellow (superiorly), the lymphatic vessel is indicated in yellow, and the venule is indicated in blue [68]

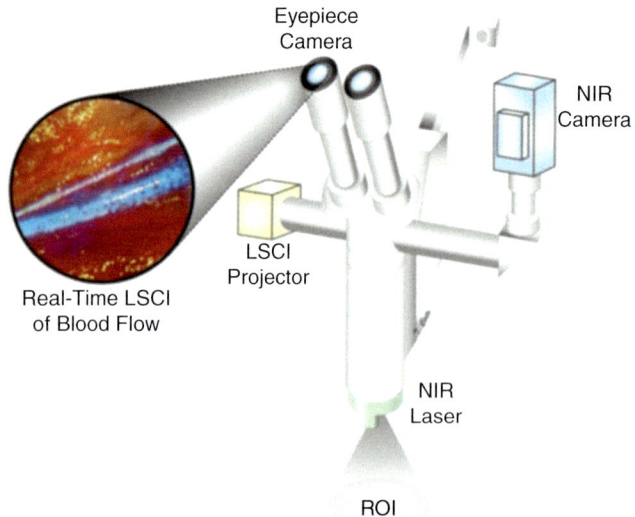

Fig. 7.20 Schematic representation of the SurgeON™ system with a NIR laser source (green), a NIR camera (blue) and LSCI projector (yellow). The NIR laser source irradiates the target images which are then captured by the NIR camera. The camera is connected to a computer which acquires laser speckle data, and the blood flow video feed is sent to the LSCI projector to be seen by operator via the eyepieces. (Reproduced from Mangraviti et al. [70])

irregularities corresponds to a multiple of the wavelength of light, there is constructive interference (or amplification). On the contrary, if the distance corresponds to half a wavelength, there is destructive interference (or cancellation). This results in a pattern of light and dark areas on a surface called a speckle pattern [69].

In a recent report of preclinical studies, Mangraviti et al. utilised LSCI technique in combination with the OM (Carl Zeiss OPMI) to develop a direct laser-speckle-video-imaging system, the SurgeON™ for cerebral blood flow assessment [70]. The system complements the OM with real-time LSCI and operates by displaying an on-demand video feed of blood flow information directly in the OM eyepiece. Figure 7.20 shows the schematic representation of the system and the imaging specifications suitable for neurosurgery [70].

The non-invasiveness and speed of the technique has been acknowledged by reconstructive microsurgeons for intraoperative and postoperative visualisation of surgical flap perfusion. In 1981, Fercher and Briers introduced the technique of single-exposure speckle photography to remove the need for scanning and offer a full-field technique. The technique was successfully demonstrated for retinal blood flow [71]. Subsequently, Briers and Webster introduced the digital version of the technique, laser speckle contrast analysis (LASCA) (Fig. 7.21) [72]. Nguyen et al. utilised LSCI (PeriCam PSI NR System, Perimed AB, Stockholm, Sweden) to examine blood perfusion of random pattern porcine model skin flaps after stretching and/or rotating. LSCI demonstrated two important findings: (1) blood perfusion is highly dependent on the length of the flap, and (2) rotation of the flap by up to 45° has no significant impact on blood perfusion. It is worth highlighting that investigators did not use a microscope-integrated LSCI system and commented on the inability of LSCI to quantify blood flow [73]. Similarly, Sheikh et al. investigated perfusion in full-thickness pig eyelid flaps measuring microvascular perfusion with the same LSCI system utilised by Nguyen et al. [74]. Du et al. utilised laser speckle imaging in an animal study of the role of haemodynamic alterations in flap delay and found that LSCI is a feasible method for predicting flap viability in rat models [75]. Karakawa et al. used LSCI successfully in a case of Tamai zone I fingertip replantation [76]. In a series of publications, Zötterman et al. evaluated LSCI as a method of perioperative planning in reconstructive surgery. LSCI was hypothesised that it can be utilised perioperatively to show negative perfusion trends to predict flap necrosis [77]. A cranial gluteal artery perforator (CGAP) porcine flap model was used, and it was concluded that a threshold perfusion of <25 PU at 30 min was a predictor for tissue morbidity 72 h after surgery (Fig. 7.22) [77]. In a further prospective case series study, Zötterman et al. used LSCI to investigate perfusion in deep inferior epigastric surgery perforator (DIEP) flap surgery and assess whether the technique assisted in prediction of postoperative complications. It was concluded that LSCI is a promising tool for measurement of flap perfusion and assessment of risk of postoperative ischaemic complications (Fig. 7.23) [78].

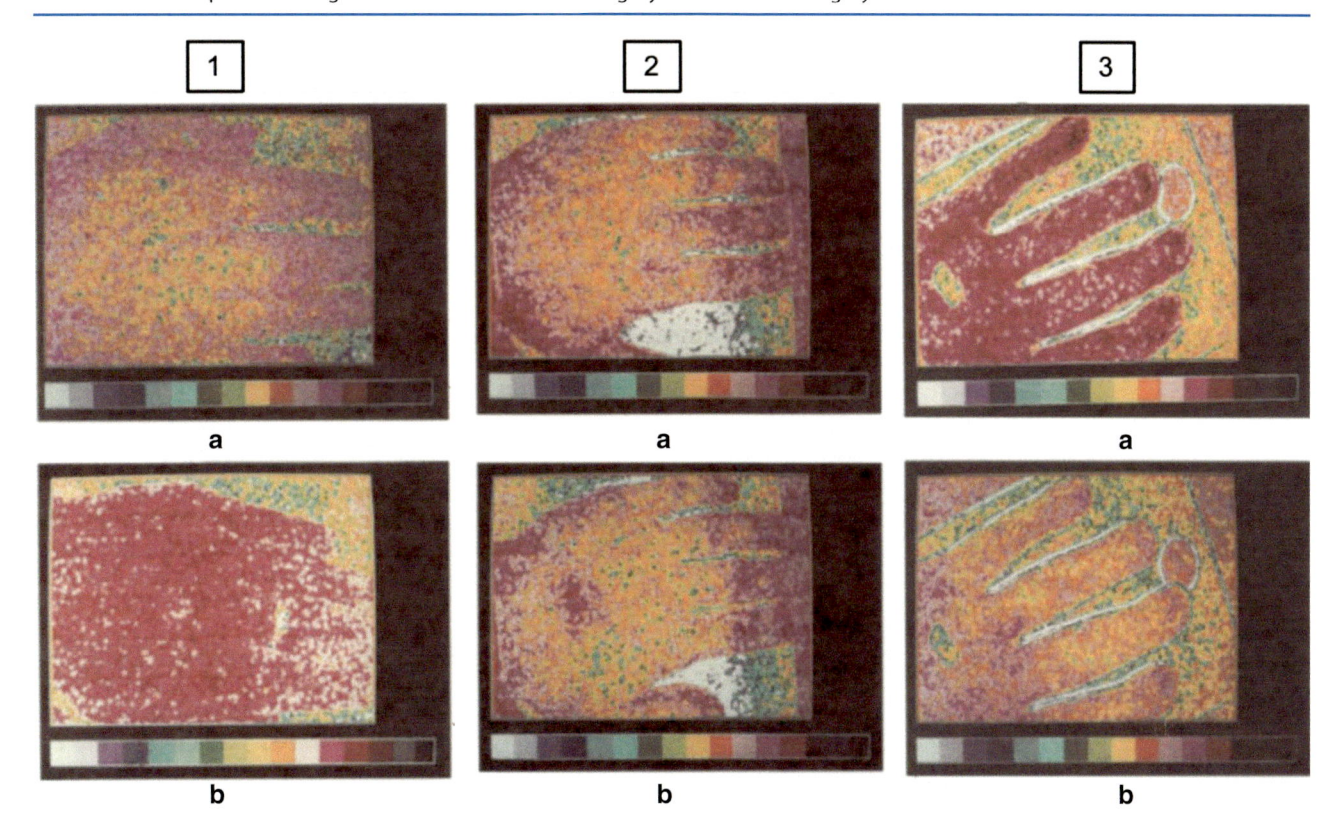

Fig. 7.21 LASCA hand images at different phases: (**1a**) hand in cold water, (**1b**) hand in hot water (contrast scale: contrast decreasing and velocity increasing from left to right), (**2a**) hand under normal conditions, (**2b**) hand area rubbed (small red area showing increased perfusion), (**3a**) hand under normal conditions, (**3b**) hand when blood pressure cuff is applied (reduced blood flow). (Adapted from Briers and Webster [72])

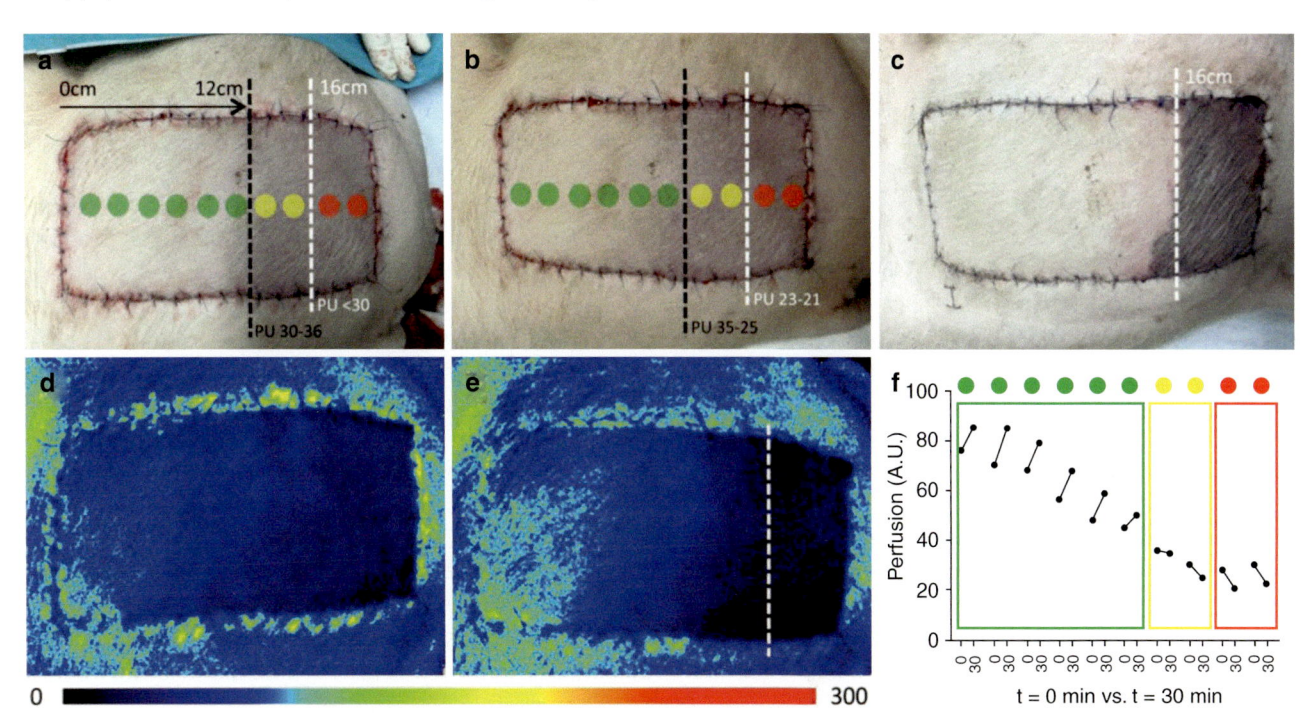

Fig. 7.22 Visual appearance (**a–c**) and perfusion (**d–f**) in a CGAP flap at time = 0 (**a, d**) and time = 30 min (**b, e**) after raising the flap. The dashed black line represents the proximal border where compromised circulation is predicted by clinical assessment. The dashed white line represents the proximal border of actual ischaemic necrosis at time = 72 h. Coloured dots represent the areas where perfusion was measured. (**f**) shows the change in perfusion from $t = 0$ to $t = 30$ min in the flap areas measured. (Reproduced from Zötterman J et al. [77])

Fig. 7.23 (**a**) Schematic representation of DIEP flap divided in Hartrampf zones I–IV. Perforator is labelled on zone I superior aspect. (**b**) LSCI perfusion image with zones I and II being highly perfused and hence more preferable for reconstruction. (Reproduced from Zötterman J et al. [78])

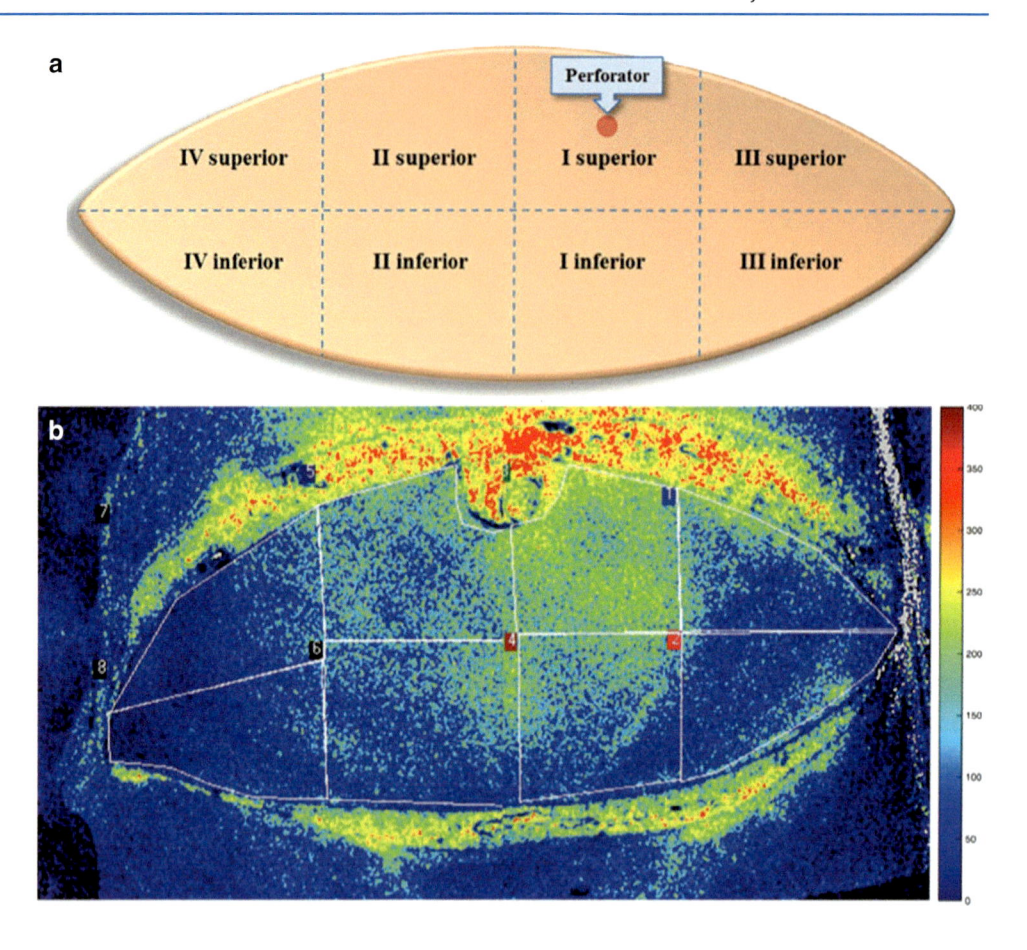

7.3 Heads-Up Operative Microscopes

7.3.1 The Exoscope

Advances in digital imaging and screen technology have led to the development of the exoscope as an alternative to the OM. The exoscope provides an array of theoretical advantages such as high-definition optics, 3D vision, high-quality illumination at depth, improved surgeon ergonomics and ease of use. Exoscopic devices currently available include the VITOM 2D and 3D (Karl Storz), ORBEYE (Sony Olympus) and Modus V (Synaptive Medical Inc.). Table 7.4 summarises the key characteristics of the available exoscopic devices [79–82].

Cheng et al. initially presented a 3D stereoscopic monitor system to improve the microsurgery environment during two head and neck cancer reconstruction cases. Although the microvascular anastomoses were successful, they proved time-consuming [83]. Piatkowski et al. performed a microvascular free flap for autologous breast reconstruction utilising the VITOM® 3D. Despite the fact that anastomoses were performed successfully, authors reported on the comfort and resolution while using higher magnifications not being adequate for routine microsurgical practice [84]. Ichikawa et al. highlighted the potential advantages of using the 3D exoscope for microvascular anastomosis in two cases of head and neck reconstruction with a free anterolateral thigh flap (ALT) transfer [85]. Pafitanis et al. performed a simulation non-inferiority trial utilising the Modus V exoscope and concluded patency non-inferiority in the microvascular anastomoses performed under exoscope compared to OM; nevertheless, duration of anastomoses under exoscope proved more time-consuming as previously shown in other studies [79]. In a recent case-control pilot study, Ahmad et al. utilised the ORBEYE exoscope for 49 consecutive microsurgical cases. Interestingly, authors reported that there was no difference in operative time, ischaemia time or microsurgical

Table 7.4 Summary of key characteristics of available exoscopic devices (reproduced from Pafitanis et al. [79])

Systems	VITOM® 2D and 3D, Karl Storz. 2011[24,25]	Computar MLH-10, CBC 2012[27]	ORBEYE, 3D-4K video Exoscope, Sony Olympus. 2017[28,29]	Modus V™ Synaptive Medical Inc. 2017
Demonstration				
Illumination	Xenon	SPD-300-W LED	×2 fibre optic LED	Quad (×4) LED
Magnification (optical zoom)	<2×	5–20×	<6×	<12.5×
Image quality	HD or 4K UHD	HD	4K	4K UHD
Field of view	50–150 mm	n/a	7.5–171 mm	6.5–207.9 mm
Portability	Portable base—manual setup	Portable	Mobile base with wheels	Mobile base with castor wheel brakes
Stereopsis – 3D capability	Yes	No	Yes	Pending released (2019)
Depth of field	35–100 mm	n/a	n/a	X2 of OM
Cost	$ (250K USD)	n/a	$$ (450K USD)	$$$ (500-750K USD)

LED light emission diode, *HD* high definition, *UHD* ultra high definition, *3D* three dimensional, *USD* United States dollars

complications between the exoscope and conventional microscopy groups, and participants reported favourable ergonomics, excellent image quality and ease of equipment manipulation [80].

7.3.2 Hybrid Visualisation Systems

The hybrid visualisation system, KINEVO® 900 (Carl Zeiss), can be utilised as an optical OM or exoscope with digital visualisation on an external 55″ 3D4k monitor plus an internal 24″ 3DHD system monitor. Technical specifications of the robotic, hybrid visualisation system are summarised in Table 7.5 [86, 87].

The use of KINEVO® 900 system is still at its early stages with studies being at a proof-of-concept stage. For example, Belykh et al. reported on the feasibility and effectiveness of performing microvascular bypass using the system above. The authors concluded on the feasibility to perform a microvascular anastomosis under the 3D hybrid system and, nevertheless, reported being unsuccessful when using the 2D imaging modality, thus emphasising the importance of appropriate depth perception [88]. Roethe et al. investigate the impact of the hybrid exoscope on surgical performance and team workflow in preclinical and clinical neurosurgical settings with results supporting clinical integration and improved surgeon ergonomics [86].

Table 7.5 Technical specifications of the digital and robotic visualisation system; KINEVO® 900 [86, 87]

Technical specifications of the KINEVO® 900	
Working distance	200–625 mm
Focal length	170 mm
Maximum magnification in exoscope mode	11
XY robotic movement	6 axes
3D4k stereo video cameras	2× 3-chip 4 K, 2160 p
Surgeon-controlled robotics	Wireless 10-button plus joystick food control panel

To the authors' knowledge, there are currently no studies published that utilise KINEVO® 900 in RM.

7.3.3 Head-Mounted Microscope

Head-mounted microscope (HMM) has been developed in an attempt to improve surgeon's ergonomics. The Leica HM500 is an ergonomic headset with a magnification capability of 2–9× and working distance of 300–700 mm (from eyepiece lens to object). The HMM also offers an automatic or manual focus function. In a preliminary study, Chen et al. utilised the Leica HM500 to perform five microlaryngoscopic operations. The study demonstrated a decrease in surgical fatigue and improved ergonomics in laryngoscopic microsurgery [89]. To the authors' knowledge, there is no published evidence of Leica HM500 utilisation in RM.

7.4 Clinical Applications of Microscopic Technologies in RM (Table 7.6)

Table 7.6 Clinical applications of microscopic technologies in RM

Novel microscopic technology	Study	Year	Type of study	Clinical application	Results	Comments
Visualisation						
Heads-up 3D microscopy	Mendez et al. [11]	2016	Feasibility study (heads-up 3D vs. traditional)	Femoral artery anastomoses on 8 rats	Anastomosis time = no difference. Heads-up 3D ≥ traditional for ergonomics, FOV, technical feasibility	TrueVision Systems
3D HMD	Kim et al. [90]	2019	Feasibility study	Rat axillary lymph node dissection	Eye fatigue not significantly different between eyepiece and 3D HMD, posture discomfort lower with 3D HMD than eyepiece	
KINEVO 900	No published studies on the utilisation of the technology in RM					
AR	Nishimoto et al. [17]	2016	Feasibility study, case report	LVA—IR image overlaid on real operation field	Feasibility of AR system with see-through glasses achieved	Eyeglasses type display: Moverio BT-200/AV
	Watson et al. [19]	2010	Feasibility study	AR microscopy: real-time overlay of bright-field and NIR fluorescence image	Image-guided surgery in anaesthetised rats using augmented microscopy	
VR	No published studies on the utilisation of this technology in RM					
Optical imaging (OM)-NIRF	Holm et al. [33]	2009	Preliminary study	Assessment of anastomotic patency in reconstructive microsurgery (OM: OPMI PENTERO IR 800)	22% (11/50) of anastomoses had a form of blood flow alteration	OM-NIRF is an excellent method for identifying significant anastomotic problems
	Sugawara et al. [37]	2015	Case series	Dynamic blood flow to the retrograde limb of the IMV in BR (OM: Leica M525 OH4)	Thrombosis prone to occur in the second recipient vein in 27.5% of cases	
	Valerio et al. [30]	2015	Retrospective case series	Evaluation of perfusion of vascularised osseous flaps (OM: SPY Elite System)	100% flap survival	1 complication: delayed partial skin flap loss
	Ludolph et al. [31]	2016	Prospective case series	DIEP/ms-TRAM flaps (OM: SPY Elite System)	100% flap survival rate. Laser-assisted ICG angiography is a useful tool for intraoperative evaluation of flap perfusion	No partial flap losses
	Munabi et al. [38]	2014	Case series	Intraoperative perfusion mapping to predict mastectomy flap necrosis in BR (OM: SPY Elite System)	8 cases (13%) of full-thickness skin necrosis identified. Data suggestive that laser-assisted ICG angiography predicts postoperative outcomes with high accuracy	
	Komorowska et al. [39]	2010	Prospective case series	Predicting tissue complications in BR (OM: SPY Elite System)	100% identification of postoperative complication rate	
	Newman et al. [40]	2009	Prospective case series	Intraoperative decision-making in BR	Flap survival rate 100%	
MiOCT	Boppart et al. [43]	1998	Preclinical	3D OCT in the assessment of the microsurgical anastomoses of vessels and nerves	OCT permits rapid feedback for assessment of microsurgical procedures	
	Huang et al. [42]	2013	Proof-of-concept	Microvascular anastomosis	Real-time OCT can assist in decision-making process intraoperatively and avoid postoperative complications	
	Zhu et al. [57]	2014	Preclinical	Supermicrosurgery—LVA	2/40 anastomoses with back-wall suturing were identified by OCT	

(continued)

Table 7.6 (continued)

Novel microscopic technology	Study	Year	Type of study	Clinical application	Results	Comments
HSI	Chin et al. [61]	2017	Preclinical	Prediction of flap survival	Early changes in deoxygenated haemoglobin may predict the region and extent of flap necrosis	
	Jones et al. [62]	2020	Non-inferiority	Prediction of flap survival	MSI does not appear to be inferior to ICG in detecting compromised tissue viability	
PAM	Suzuki et al. [68]	2021	Case report	LVA anastomosis patency	Photoacoustic lymphangiography cannot be used to visualise the lymphatic vessels that are not contrasted by ICG	
LSCI	Nguyen et al. [91]	2016	Preclinical	Blood perfusion after manipulating random pattern porcine model skin flaps	Length of flap and degree of stretch influence perfusion. Rotation of skin flap appears not to have a significantly detrimental effect on perfusion	
	Sheikh et al. [74]	2018	Preclinical	Eyelid perfusion after dissection	Dissection of eyelid results in slight decrease in blood flow	
	Karakawa et al. [76]	2018	Case report	Fingertip replantation	Successful Tamai zone I fingertip replantation	Postoperative advantages for monitoring
	Zötterman et al. [77]	2019	Preclinical	Prediction of flap necrosis	Perfusion of <25 PU at $t = 30$ min was predictor for tissue morbidity 72 h after surgery	LSCI is a promising technique for perioperative monitoring in RM
	Zötterman et al. [78]	2020	Prospective Case series	(1) Perfusion distribution in relation to the selected perforator in DIEP flap. (2) predicting postoperative complications	Microvascular perfusion in the skin of the DIEP is highest in Hartrampf zone I. Flap areas with perfusion values of less than 30 PU are correlated with postoperative flap necrosis	
Heads-up OM						
Exoscope	Cheng et al. [83]	2012	Case report	3D stereoscopic system in microvascular anastomosis	Microvascular anastomoses successful although time-consuming	OM: Opmi Universal S3
	Piatkowski et al. [84]	2018	Case report	DIEP flap for autologous BR using VITOM 3D	Exoscope can be used to perform free flap surgery; needs improvement on zoom capability and low depth of field	OM: VITOM 3D
	Ichikawa et al. [85]	2019	Case report	H&N reconstruction with free ALT flap transfer	100% flap survival	OM: VITOM 3D
	Pafitanis et al. [79]	2020	Preclinical, non-inferiority	Exoscope vs. OM in microvascular anastomosis	Exoscope non-inferior to OM in microvascular anastomoses	OM: MODUS V
	Ahmad et al. [80]	2020	Case-control pilot study	Exoscope vs. OM in microsurgical cases	No difference in OT. No difference in IT. No difference in microsurgical complications. Favourable ergonomics, excellent image quality, and ease of use	OM: ORBEYE
Hybrid visualisation system (KINEVO 900)	No published studies on the utilisation of this technology in RM					
HMM	Kim et al. [90] developed a HMD previously described in the visualisation class of this table					

RM reconstructive microsurgery, *HMD* head-mounted display, *IMV* internal mammary vein, *BR* breast reconstruction, *ICG* indocyanine green, *MSI* multispectral imaging, *AR* augmented reality, *VR* virtual reality, *OM-NIRF* operating microscope-near-infrared fluoroscopy, *MiOCT* microscope-integrated optical coherence tomography, *HSI* hyperspectral imaging, *PAM* photoacoustic microscopy, *LSCI* laser speckle contrast imaging, *PU* perfusion units, *t* time, *min* minutes, *DIEP* deep inferior epigastric perforator, *HMM* head-mounted microscope, *H&N* head and neck, *ALT* antero-lateral thigh

7.5 Future Directions of Operating Microscopy

Modern OMs have developed dramatically compared to early OM models with multiple attractive features: advanced optics, longer working distances, high-resolution 3D visualisation, AR capabilities, integrated imaging technology options and robotic features. Despite the multiple developments and surgical potential, there are still challenges that need to be overcome before OM's smooth and seamless integration in the surgical workflow takes place. These challenges include volume, weight and manoeuvrability of OMs, the risk that high-power illumination poses on tissue damage [92], high cost and steep learning curve for trainees.

As RM develops further into supermicrosurgery territories, intraoperative OM-integrated optical imaging technologies such as iOCT and robotic features would be of great value. Furthermore, immersive microscopy via the convergence of confocal microscopy and VR could allow reconstructive microsurgeons to 'walk through' the defect and plan the surgical procedure accordingly [93]. AR could potentially allow the displaying of the procedure in real time which could be of value in microsurgery training and remote operation.

7.6 Conclusion

Novel microscopic technologies in RM are at an infancy stage with immense potential in terms of intraoperative surgical capabilities. It is anticipated by the author that the OM would further develop into a smaller, mobile structure that would transform microsurgical practice and benefit the patient.

7.7 Selected Readings

- Ma L, Fei B. Comprehensive review of surgical microscopes: technology development and medical applications. J Biomed Opt. 2021;26(1):010901.

  Importance to reader—This is a comprehensive review that presents the technological advances and clinical application developments in surgical microscopy over the last century. The reader can appreciate the way new imaging modalities and visualisation advances integrate with surgical microscopes.

- Zötterman J. Laser speckle contrast imaging in reconstructive surgery. 2020.

  Importance to reader—This thesis presents laser speckle contrast imaging as a novel, fast and non-invasive imaging modality for tissue monitoring in reconstructive microsurgery. The reader can appreciate the methodology required to progress from animal studies to the operating theatre and critically appraise the evidence of a highly promising technology.

- Pafitanis G, Hadjiandreou M, Alamri A, Uff C, Walsh D, Myers S. The exoscope versus operating microscope in microvascular surgery: a simulation non-inferiority trial. Arch Plast Surg. 2020;47(3):242.

  Importance to reader—Objective preclinical evidence of exoscope non-inferiority against the operating microscope. This study compares a novel surgical visualisation device against the gold-standard OM and offers the reader with a characterisation of the experts' learning curve in a standard microsurgical task.

References

1. Schultheiss D, Denil J. History of the microscope and development of microsurgery: a revolution for reproductive tract surgery. Andrologia. 2002;34(4):234–41.
2. Kriss TC, Kriss VM. History of the operating microscope: from magnifying glass to microneurosurgery. Neurosurgery. 1998;42(4):899–907.
3. Keeler R. The evolution of the ophthalmic surgical microscope. Hist Ophthal Intern. 2015;1:35.
4. Ma L, Fei B. Comprehensive review of surgical microscopes: technology development and medical applications. J Biomed Opt. 2021;26(1):010901.
5. Uluç K, Kujoth GC, Başkaya MK. Operating microscopes: past, present, and future. Neurosurg Focus. 2009;27(3):E4.
6. Bernstein DT, Hamilton KL, Foy C, Petersen NJ, Netscher DT. Comparison of magnification in primary digital nerve repair: literature review, survey of practice trends, and assessment of 90 cadaveric repairs. J Hand Surg. 2013;38(11):2144–50.
7. Meyer V. The place of the microscope in hand surgery. Thousand Oaks, CA: SAGE Publications; 1987.
8. Ross DA, Ariyan S, Restifo R, Sasaki CT. Use of the operating microscope and loupes for head and neck free microvascular tissue transfer: a retrospective comparison. Arch Otolaryngol Head Neck Surg. 2003;129(2):189–93.
9. Yamamoto T, Yamamoto N, Azuma S, Yoshimatsu H, Seki Y, Narushima M, et al. Near-infrared illumination system-integrated microscope for supermicrosurgical lymphaticovenular anastomosis. Microsurgery. 2014;34(1):23–7.
10. Microsystems. L. Key factors to consider when selecting a stereo microscope. https://www.leica-microsystems.com/science-lab/factors-to-consider-when-selecting-a-stereo-microscope/.
11. Mendez BM, Chiodo MV, Vandevender D, Patel PA. Heads-up 3D microscopy: an ergonomic and educational approach to microsurgery. Plast Reconstruct Surg Glob Open. 2016;4(5):e717.
12. Belykh EG, Zhao X, Cavallo C, Bohl MA, Yagmurlu K, Aklinski JL, et al. Laboratory evaluation of a robotic operative microscope-visualization platform for neurosurgery. Cureus. 2018;10(7):e3072.
13. Berryman DR. Augmented reality: a review. Med Ref Serv Q. 2012;31(2):212–8.
14. Vles MD, Terng NCO, Zijlstra K, Mureau MAM, Corten EML. Virtual and augmented reality for preoperative planning in plastic surgical procedures: a systematic review. J Plast Reconstr Aesthet Surg. 2020;73:1951.

15. Al Omran Y, Abdall-Razak A, Sohrabi C, Borg T-M, Nadama H, Ghassemi N, et al. Use of augmented reality in reconstructive microsurgery: a systematic review and development of the augmented reality microsurgery score. J Reconstr Microsurg. 2020;36(4):261–70.
16. Meola A, Cutolo F, Carbone M, Cagnazzo F, Ferrari M, Ferrari V. Augmented reality in neurosurgery: a systematic review. Neurosurg Rev. 2017;40(4):537–48.
17. Nishimoto S, Tonooka M, Fujita K, Sotsuka Y, Fujiwara T, Kawai K, et al. An augmented reality system in lymphatico-venous anastomosis surgery. J Surg Case Rep. 2016;2016(5):rjw047.
18. Bigdeli AK, Gazyakan E, Schmidt VJ, Hernekamp FJ, Harhaus L, Henzler T, et al. Indocyanine green fluorescence for free-flap perfusion imaging revisited: advanced decision making by virtual perfusion reality in visionsense fusion imaging angiography. Surg Innov. 2016;23(3):249–60.
19. Watson JR, Gainer CF, Martirosyan N, Skoch J, Lemole GM Jr, Anton R, et al. Augmented microscopy: real-time overlay of bright-field and near-infrared fluorescence images. J Biomed Opt. 2015;20(10):106002.
20. Kruijff E, Swan JE, Feiner S. Perceptual issues in augmented reality revisited. Washington, DC: IEEE; 2010.
21. Pensieri C, Pennacchini M. Virtual reality in medicine. Handbook on 3D3C platforms. New York, NY: Springer; 2016. p. 353–401.
22. Kim Y, Kim H, Kim YO. Virtual reality and augmented reality in plastic surgery: a review. Arch Plast Surg. 2017;44(3):179.
23. Cornelissen AJM, van Mulken TJM, Graupner C, Qiu SS, Keuter XHA, van der Hulst RRWJ, et al. Near-infrared fluorescence image-guidance in plastic surgery: a systematic review. Eur J Plast Surg. 2018;41(3):269–78.
24. Xu H, Zhang Z, Xia Y, Steinberger Z, Min P, Li H, et al. Preliminary exploration: when angiosome meets prefabricated flaps. J Reconstr Microsurg. 2016;32(9):683–7.
25. Narushima M, Yamamoto T, Ogata F, Yoshimatsu H, Mihara M, Koshima I. Indocyanine green lymphography findings in limb lymphedema. J Reconstr Microsurg. 2016;32(1):72–9.
26. Yamamoto T, Narushima M, Yoshimatsu H, Yamamoto N, Kikuchi K, Todokoro T, et al. Dynamic indocyanine green (ICG) lymphography for breast cancer-related arm lymphedema. Ann Plast Surg. 2014;73(6):706–9.
27. Vargas CR, Nguyen JT, Ashitate Y, Silvestre J, Venugopal V, Neacsu F, et al. Near-infrared imaging for the assessment of anastomotic patency, thrombosis, and reperfusion in microsurgery: a pilot study in a porcine model. Microsurgery. 2015;35(4):309–14.
28. Wormer BA, Huntington CR, Ross SW, Colavita PD, Lincourt AE, Prasad T, et al. A prospective randomized double-blinded controlled trial evaluating indocyanine green fluorescence angiography on reducing wound complications in complex abdominal wall reconstruction. J Surg Res. 2016;202(2):461–72.
29. Nasser A, Fourman MS, Gersch RP, Phillips BT, Hsi HK, Khan SU, et al. Utilizing indocyanine green dye angiography to detect simulated flap venous congestion in a novel experimental rat model. J Reconstr Microsurg. 2015;31(8):590–6.
30. Valerio I, Green Iii JM, Sacks JM, Thomas S, Sabino J, Acarturk TO. Vascularized osseous flaps and assessing their bipartate perfusion pattern via intraoperative fluorescence angiography. J Reconstr Microsurg. 2015;31(01):045–53.
31. Ludolph I, Arkudas A, Schmitz M, Boos AM, Taeger CD, Rother U, et al. Cracking the perfusion code?: laser-assisted Indocyanine Green angiography and combined laser Doppler spectrophotometry for intraoperative evaluation of tissue perfusion in autologous breast reconstruction with DIEP or ms-TRAM flaps. J Plast Reconstr Aesthet Surg. 2016;69(10):1382–8.
32. Stummer W, Stepp H, Möller G, Ehrhardt A, Leonhard M, Reulen HJ. Technical principles for protoporphyrin-IX-fluorescence guided microsurgical resection of malignant glioma tissue. Acta Neurochir. 1998;140(10):995–1000.
33. Holm C, Mayr M, Höfter E, Dornseifer U, Ninkovic M. Assessment of the patency of microvascular anastomoses using microscope-integrated near-infrared angiography: a preliminary study. Microsurgery. 2009;29(7):509–14.
34. Zeiss. INFRARED 800 from ZEISS. https://www.zeiss.com/meditec/int/product-portfolio/intraoperative-fluorescence-modules/infrared-800.html#technical-data.
35. Microsystems L. High-performance surgical microscope Leica M525 OH4 2021. https://www.leica-microsystems.com/products/surgical-microscopes/p/leica-m525-oh4/.
36. Stryker. SPY Elite Fluorescence imaging system. 2021. https://www.stryker.com/us/en/endoscopy/products/spy-elite.html.
37. Sugawara J, Satake T, Muto M, Kou S, Yasumura K, Maegawa J. Dynamic blood flow to the retrograde limb of the internal mammary vein in breast reconstruction with free flap. Microsurgery. 2015;35(8):622–6.
38. Munabi NCO, Olorunnipa OB, Goltsman D, Rohde CH, Ascherman JA. The ability of intra-operative perfusion mapping with laser-assisted indocyanine green angiography to predict mastectomy flap necrosis in breast reconstruction: a prospective trial. J Plast Reconstr Aesthet Surg. 2014;67(4):449–55.
39. Komorowska-Timek E, Gurtner GC. Intraoperative perfusion mapping with laser-assisted indocyanine green imaging can predict and prevent complications in immediate breast reconstruction. Plast Reconstr Surg. 2010;125(4):1065–73.
40. Newman MI, Samson MC. The application of laser-assisted indocyanine green fluorescent dye angiography in microsurgical breast reconstruction. J Reconstr Microsurg. 2009;25(1):21–6.
41. Elliott JT, Dsouza AV, Marra K, Pogue BW, Roberts DW, Paulsen KD. Microdose fluorescence imaging of ABY-029 on an operating microscope adapted by custom illumination and imaging modules. Biomed Opt Express. 2016;7(9):3280–8.
42. Huang Y, Ibrahim Z, Lee WPA, Brandacher G, Kang JU. Real-time 3D Fourier-domain optical coherence tomography guided microvascular anastomosis. Bellingham, WA: International Society for Optics and Photonics; 2013.
43. Boppart SA, Bouma BE, Pitris C, Tearney GJ, Southern JF, Brezinski ME, et al. Intraoperative assessment of microsurgery with three-dimensional optical coherence tomography. Radiology. 1998;208(1):81–6.
44. Eguchi H, Kusaka S, Arimura-Koike E, Tachibana K, Tsujioka D, Fukuda M, et al. Intraoperative optical coherence tomography (RESCAN® 700) for detecting iris incarceration and iridocorneal adhesion during keratoplasty. Int Ophthalmol. 2017;37(3):761–5.
45. Ray R, Barañano DE, Fortun JA, Schwent BJ, Cribbs BE, Bergstrom CS, et al. Intraoperative microscope-mounted spectral domain optical coherence tomography for evaluation of retinal anatomy during macular surgery. Ophthalmology. 2011;118(11):2212–7.
46. Lu CD, Waheed NK, Witkin A, Baumal CR, Liu JJ, Potsaid B, et al. Microscope-integrated intraoperative ultrahigh-speed swept-source optical coherence tomography for widefield retinal and anterior segment imaging. Ophthal Surg Lasers Imag Ret. 2018;49(2):94–102.
47. Assayag O, Grieve K, Devaux B, Harms F, Pallud J, Chretien F, et al. Imaging of non-tumorous and tumorous human brain tissues with full-field optical coherence tomography. NeuroImage Clin. 2013;2:549–57.
48. Cho NH, Jang JH, Jung W, Kim J. In vivo imaging of middle-ear and inner-ear microstructures of a mouse guided by SD-OCT combined with a surgical microscope. Opt Express. 2014;22(8):8985–95.
49. Vokes DE, Jackson R, Guo S, Perez JA, Su J, Ridgway JM, et al. Optical coherence tomography—enhanced microlaryngoscopy: preliminary report of a noncontact optical coherence tomography system integrated with a surgical microscope. Ann Otol Rhinol Laryngol. 2008;117(7):538–47.
50. Carrasco-Zevallos OM, Viehland C, Keller B, Draelos M, Kuo AN, Toth CA, et al. Review of intraoperative optical coherence

tomography: technology and applications. Biomed Opt Express. 2017;8(3):1607–37.
51. Geerling G, Müller M, Winter C, Hoerauf H, Oelckers S, Laqua H, et al. Intraoperative 2-dimensional optical coherence tomography as a new tool for anterior segment surgery. Arch Ophthalmol. 2005;123(2):253–7.
52. Zeiss. RESCAN 700 with integrated intraoperative OCT. https://www.zeiss.com/meditec/us/products/ophthalmology-optometry/glaucoma/therapy/surgical-microscopes/opmi-lumera-700.html#highlights.
53. Surgical H-S. Haag-Streit surgical iOCT. https://www.haag-streit.com/john-weiss/products/haag-streit-surgical/microscope-range/ioct/.
54. Leica. EnFocus intraoperative OCT imaging system. https://www.leica-microsystems.com/products/surgical-microscopes/p/enfocus/.
55. Clancy NT, Jones G, Maier-Hein L, Elson DS, Stoyanov D. Surgical spectral imaging. Med Image Anal. 2020;63:101699.
56. Huang Y, Tong D, Zhu S, Wu L, Mao Q, Ibrahim Z, et al. Evaluation of microvascular anastomosis using real-time ultra-high resolution Fourier domain Doppler optical coherence tomography. Plast Reconstr Surg. 2015;135(4):711e.
57. Zhu S, Tong D, Huang Y, Wu L, Ibrahim Z, Mao Q, et al. Abstract P14: in vivo real-time ultra-fast 3D fourier domain optical coherence tomography imaging of anastomoses for super-microsurgical research. Plast Reconstr Surg. 2014;133(3S):196–7.
58. Hardy JD, Hammel HT, Murgatroyd D. Spectral transmittance and reflectance of excised human skin. J Appl Physiol. 1956;9(2):257–64.
59. Lu G, Fei B. Medical hyperspectral imaging: a review. J Biomed Opt. 2014;19(1):010901.
60. Chin MS, Freniere BB, Lo Y-C, Saleeby JH, Baker SP, Strom HM, et al. Hyperspectral imaging for early detection of oxygenation and perfusion changes in irradiated skin. J Biomed Opt. 2012;17(2):026010.
61. Chin MS, Chappell AG, Giatsidis G, Perry DJ, Lujan-Hernandez J, Haddad A, et al. Hyperspectral imaging provides early prediction of random axial flap necrosis in a preclinical model. Plast Reconstr Surg. 2017;139(6):1285e–90e.
62. Jones GE, Yoo A, King VA, Sowa M, Pinson DM. Snapshot multispectral imaging is not inferior to SPY laser fluorescence imaging when predicting murine flap necrosis. Plast Reconstr Surg. 2020;145(1):85e–93e.
63. Pichette J, Laurence A, Angulo L, Lesage F, Bouthillier A, Nguyen DK, et al. Intraoperative video-rate hemodynamic response assessment in human cortex using snapshot hyperspectral optical imaging. Neurophotonics. 2016;3(4):045003.
64. Hu S, Wang LV. Photoacoustic imaging and characterization of the microvasculature. J Biomed Opt. 2010;15(1):011101.
65. Han S, Lee C, Kim S, Jeon M, Kim J, Kim C. In vivo virtual intraoperative surgical photoacoustic microscopy. Appl Phys Lett. 2013;103(20):203702.
66. Deng Z, Wang Z, Yang X, Luo Q, Gong H. In vivo imaging of hemodynamics and oxygen metabolism in acute focal cerebral ischemic rats with laser speckle imaging and functional photoacoustic microscopy. J Biomed Opt. 2012;17(8):081415.
67. de La Zerda A, Paulus YM, Teed R, Bodapati S, Dollberg Y, Khuri-Yakub BT, et al. Photoacoustic ocular imaging. Opt Lett. 2010;35(3):270–2.
68. Suzuki Y, Kajita H, Kono H, Okabe K, Sakuma H, Imanishi N, et al. The direct observation of lymphaticovenular anastomosis patency with photoacoustic lymphangiography. Plast Reconstruct Surg Glob Open. 2021;9(1):e3348.
69. Zötterman J. Laser speckle contrast imaging in reconstructive surgery. 2020.
70. Mangraviti A, Volpin F, Cha J, Cunningham SI, Raje K, Brooke MJ, et al. Intraoperative laser speckle contrast imaging for real-time visualization of cerebral blood flow in cerebrovascular surgery: results from pre-clinical studies. Sci Rep. 2020;10(1):1–13.
71. Fercher AF, Briers JD. Flow visualization by means of single-exposure speckle photography. Opt Commun. 1981;37(5):326–30.
72. Briers JD, Webster S. Laser speckle contrast analysis (LASCA): a nonscanning, full-field technique for monitoring capillary blood flow. J Biomed Opt. 1996;1(2):174–9.
73. Nguyen CD, Sheikh R, Dahlstrand U, Lindstedt S, Malmsjö M. Investigation of blood perfusion by laser speckle contrast imaging in stretched and rotated skin flaps in a porcine model. J Plast Reconstr Aesthet Surg. 2018;71(4):611–3.
74. Sheikh R, Memarzadeh K, Torbrand C, Blohmé J, Lindstedt S, Malmsjö M. Blood perfusion in a full-thickness eyelid flap, investigated by laser Doppler velocimetry, laser speckle contrast imaging, and thermography. Eplasty. 2018;18:e9.
75. Du Z, Zan T, Li H, Li Q. A study of blood flow dynamics in flap delay using the full-field laser perfusion imager. Microvasc Res. 2011;82(3):284–90.
76. Karakawa R, Yano T, Yoshimatsu H, Harima M, Kanayama K, Iida T, et al. Use of laser speckle contrast imaging for successful fingertip replantation. Plast Reconstruct Surg Glob Open. 2018;6(9):e1924.
77. Zötterman J, Tesselaar E, Farnebo S. The use of laser speckle contrast imaging to predict flap necrosis: an experimental study in a porcine flap model. J Plast Reconstr Aesthet Surg. 2019;72(5):771–7.
78. Zötterman J, Opsomer D, Farnebo S, Blondeel P, Monstrey S, Tesselaar E. Intraoperative laser speckle contrast imaging in DIEP breast reconstruction: a prospective case series study. Plast Reconstruct Surg Glob Open. 2020;8(1):e2529.
79. Pafitanis G, Hadjiandreou M, Alamri A, Uff C, Walsh D, Myers S. The Exoscope versus operating microscope in microvascular surgery: a simulation non-inferiority trial. Arch Plast Surg. 2020;47(3):242.
80. Ahmad FI, Mericli AF, DeFazio MV, Chang EI, Hanasono MM, Pederson WC, et al. Application of the ORBEYE three-dimensional exoscope for microsurgical procedures. Microsurgery. 2020;40(4):468–72.
81. Kadaba V, Shafi F, Ahluwalia HS. The VITOM® exoscope in oculoplastic surgery: the 5 year Coventry experience. Eye. 2021;35:1–4.
82. De Virgilio A, Iocca O, Di Maio P, Mercante G, Mondello T, Yiu P, et al. Free flap microvascular anastomosis in head and neck reconstruction using a 4K three-dimensional exoscope system (VITOM 3D). Int J Oral Maxillofac Surg. 2020;49(9):1169–73.
83. Cheng HT, Ma H, Tsai CH, Hsu WL, Wang TH. A three-dimensional stereoscopic monitor system in microscopic vascular anastomosis. Microsurgery. 2012;32(7):571–4.
84. Piatkowski AA, Keuter XHA, Schols RM, van der Hulst RRWJ. Potential of performing a microvascular free flap reconstruction using solely a 3D exoscope instead of a conventional microscope. J Plast Reconstr Aesthet Surg. 2018;71(11):1664–78.
85. Ichikawa Y, Senda D, Shingyochi Y, Mizuno H. Potential advantages of using three-dimensional exoscope for microvascular anastomosis in free flap transfer. Plast Reconstr Surg. 2019;144(4):726e–7e.
86. Roethe AL, Landgraf P, Schröder T, Misch M, Vajkoczy P, Picht T. Monitor-based exoscopic 3D4k neurosurgical interventions: a two-phase prospective-randomized clinical evaluation of a novel hybrid device. Acta Neurochir. 2020;162:2949–61.
87. Zeiss C. KINEVO 900 from ZEISS. 2019.
88. Belykh E, George L, Zhao X, Carotenuto A, Moreira LB, Yağmurlu K, et al. Microvascular anastomosis under 3D exoscope or endoscope magnification: a proof-of-concept study. Surg Neurol Int. 2018;9:115.
89. Chen T, Dailey SH, Naze SA, Jiang JJ. The head-mounted microscope. Laryngoscope. 2012;122(4):781–4.

90. Kim C-H, Ryu S-Y, Yoon J-Y, Lee H-K, Choi N-G, Park I-H, et al. See-through type 3D head-mounted display–based surgical microscope system for microsurgery: a feasibility study. JMIR Mhealth Uhealth. 2019;7(3):e11251.
91. Nguyen DC, Shahzad F, Snyder-Warwick A, Patel KB, Woo AS. Transcaruncular approach for treatment of medial wall and large orbital blowout fractures. Craniomaxillofac Trauma Reconstr. 2016;9(1):46–54.
92. Lopez J, Soni A, Calva D, Susarla SM, Jallo GI, Redett R. Iatrogenic surgical microscope skin burns: a systematic review of the literature and case report. Burns. 2016;42(4):e74–80.
93. Bioimaging Research Hub in the School of Biosciences CU. IN FOCUS: immersive microscopy – 3D visualisation and manipulation of microscopic samples through virtual reality. 2019.

Robotic Microvascular and Free Flap Surgery: Overview of Current Robotic Applications and Introduction of a Dedicated Robot for Microsurgery

Joost A. G. N. Wolfs, Rutger M. Schols, and Tom J. M. van Mulken

8.1 Introduction

Microvascular free flap surgery is performed in several specialties, such as plastic and reconstructive surgery, head and neck surgery, neurosurgery, and traumatology. The majority of free tissue transplants are used for breast, lower extremity, and transoral reconstructions following cancer treatment or trauma.

Performing the microsurgical vascular anastomosis is considered technically demanding. It requires great surgical skills as well as a significant level of experience. Due to the difficulty of the procedure and small surgical field, robotic assistance offers potential advantages. Robotic platforms are able to filter the physiological tremor of the surgeons' hand, improve movement of instruments in smaller spaces, and allow for motion scaling. Furthermore, enhanced dexterity of a robotic platform can reduce human-related fatigue. Altogether this increases the surgical precision [1, 2].

Robot-assisted microsurgery is used in both pedicled and free flap surgery. This chapter provides an overview of robotics in microvascular and free flap surgery. Different robotic systems are presented, and their applications in different steps of free flap surgery are elaborated, based on current (pre)clinical research. Future perspectives of robotic microvascular and free flap surgery are discussed.

8.2 Robotic Systems

A systematic literature search in the MEDLINE database and consequent selection of eligible papers using Covidence.org software were performed by two independent researchers (JW and RS). A third researcher was consulted in case no consensus was reached (TM). Thirty-five eligible articles were selected on robotic assistance in microvascular and free flap surgery from which a few robotic surgical systems have emerged. An overview of the robotic systems and their applications are shown in Table 8.1.

8.2.1 RAMS

The Robot-Assisted Microsurgery (RAMS) workstation (Jet Propulsion Laboratory NASA, CA, USA) concerns a robotic arm, which functions as an operating as well as an assisting instrument (Fig. 8.1). The RAMS was used as an operating assistant in microvascular anastomosis in an animal study in 2001 [3]. Advantages of the system comprise its precise functioning and its ability to replace an assisting person to some extent. It provides seven degrees of freedom including open-

Table 8.1 Robotic systems and their reported applications

Robotic surgical system	Specialty	Robotic procedure	Characteristics
RAMS	Plastic and reconstructive surgery	Microvascular anastomosis (preclinical)	NA
AESOP	Plastic and reconstructive surgery	Pedicle harvest	NA
ZEUS	Plastic and reconstructive surgery	Microvascular anastomosis	1, 2
DaVinci	Plastic and reconstructive surgery	Flap harvest	1, 2
	Head and neck surgery	Microvascular anastomosis	
	Neurosurgery Traumatology	Flap inset	
MUSA	Plastic and reconstructive surgery	Microvascular anastomosis (preclinical) Supermicrosurgery (lymphatic surgery)	1, 2, 3, 4

Characteristics: motion scaling (1), tremor filtration (2), dedicated microsurgical instruments (3), and usage in conjunction with high magnification microscope (4)

Joost A. G. N. Wolfs · R. M. Schols · T. J. M. van Mulken (✉)
Department of Plastic Surgery, Maastricht University Medical Center, Maastricht, the Netherlands

© Springer Nature Switzerland AG 2023
D. Nikkhah et al. (eds.), *Core Techniques in Flap Reconstructive Microsurgery*, https://doi.org/10.1007/978-3-031-07678-7_8

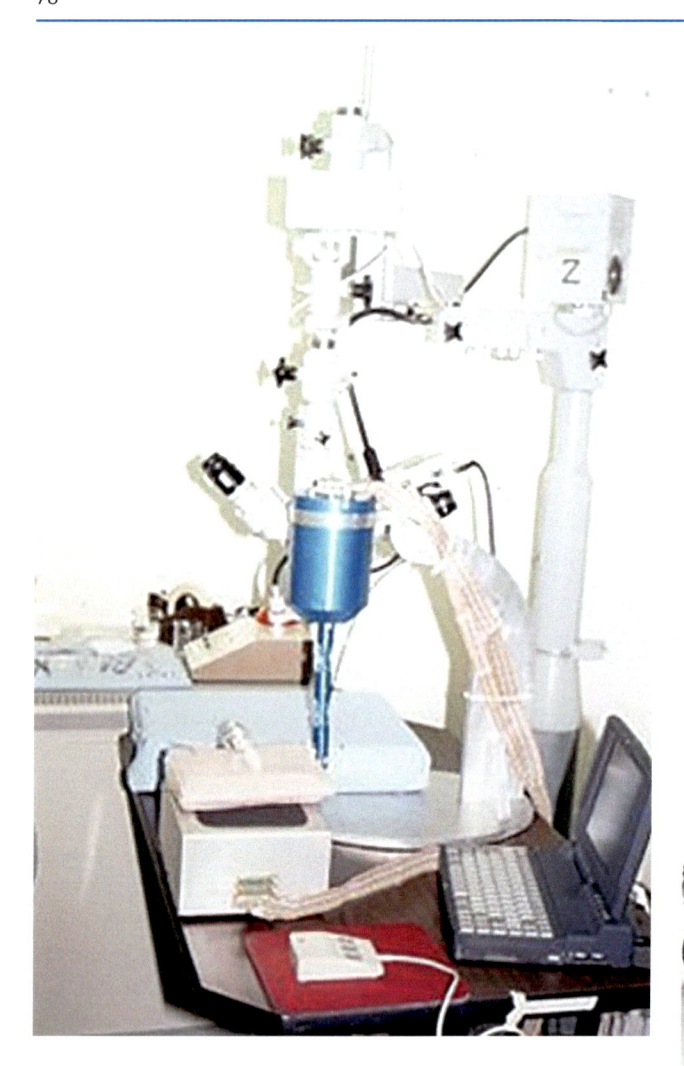

Fig. 8.1 RAMS Robot JPL. (Image courtesy of NASA/JPL-Caltech)

ing and closing of the forceps. Deficiencies of the system were startup time, the spatial conflict within the operative field, and the poor rotation of the robotic tip. Therefore, usage of this robotic platform in humans was not yet suitable. Hereafter, the RAMS is not further described in free flap surgery.

8.2.2 AESOP

The Automated Endoscopic System for Optimal Positioning (AESOP) voice-activated robotic arm (Computer Motion Inc, CA, USA) was reported as a surgeon's "third arm" in free flap surgery in 2006 [4]. The robotic system carried a high-definition video camera, and its motion was activated by the surgeon's voice, allowing precise visualization on a high-definition monitor (Fig. 8.2). Possible advantages of the AESOP system included improved accessibility in complex pedicle locations with the harvest of long pedicles in autologous breast reconstructions and both the surgeon's hands being free to operate. Subsequently, the use of this platform is not described in free flap surgery.

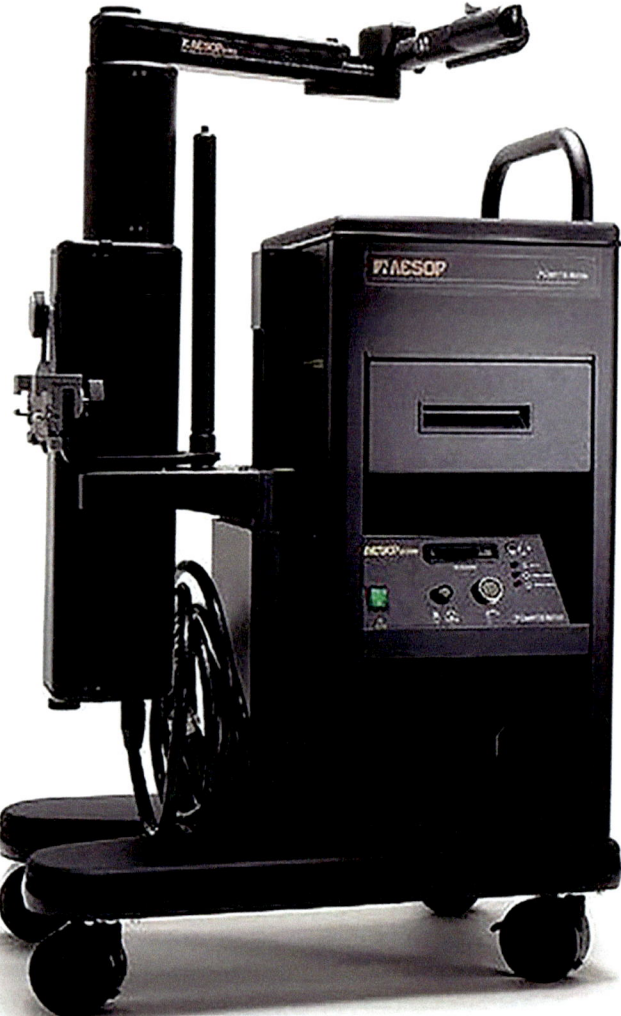

Fig. 8.2 AESOP system (Computer Motion Inc, CA, USA). (Reprinted by permission from Springer Nature: Springer, World Journal of Surgery, 30 Years of Robotic Surgery, Leal Ghezzi, T, Campos Corleta, O, Copyright 2016)

8.2.3 ZEUS

The ZEUS Robotic Surgical System (Computer Motion Inc, CA, USA) was the next generation of the AESOP technology as two arms were added to the video camera arm (Fig. 8.3). This system had certain advantages over the conventional human assistant, such as precise movement, lack of hand tremor, enhanced micro visualization, and improved ergonomics. The major advantage was the ability of the robot to scale down the surgeon's movements to a microscopic level. A limitation of the system was the surgeon's loss of tactile feedback and proprioception [5]. The use of the ZEUS system was discontinued following merger with its rival company Intuitive Surgical. Shortly after, the merged company developed the Da Vinci Surgical System.

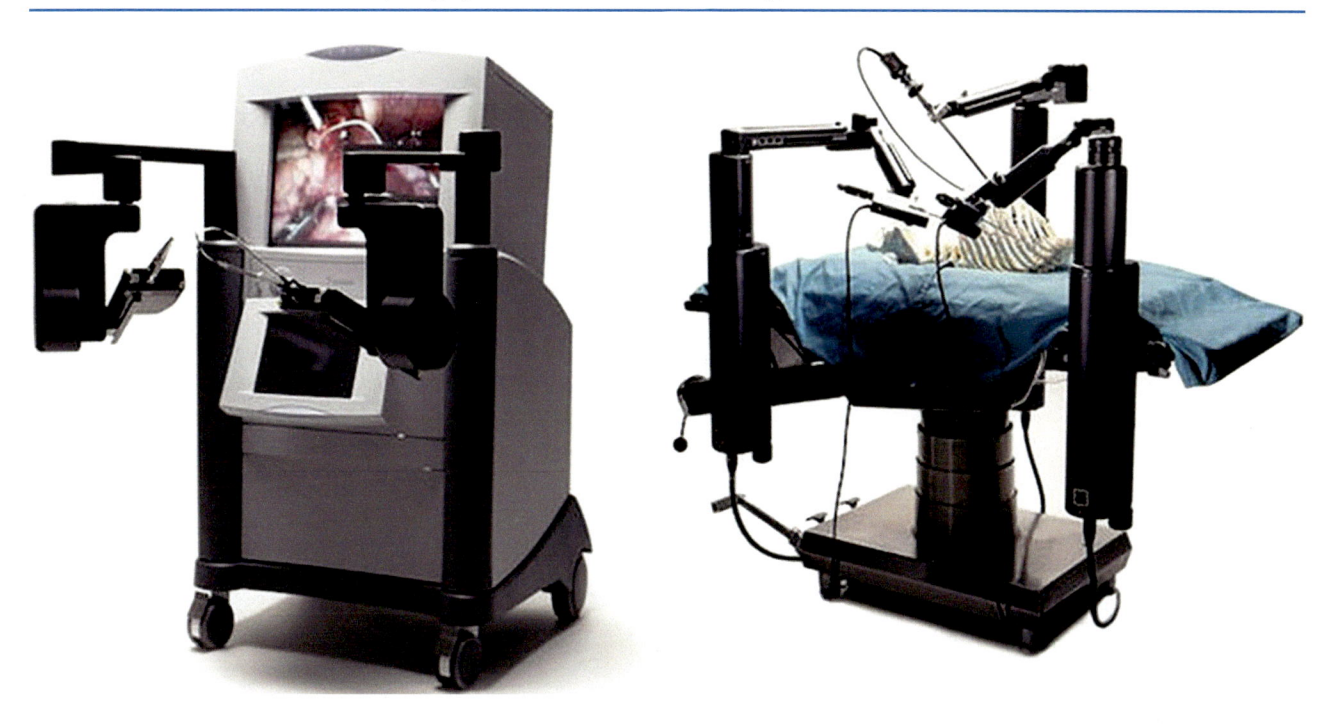

Fig. 8.3 ZEUS Robotic Surgical System (Computer Motion Inc, USA). (Reprinted by permission from Springer Nature: Springer, World Journal of Surgery, 30 Years of Robotic Surgery, Leal Ghezzi, T, Campos Corleta, O, Copyright 2016)

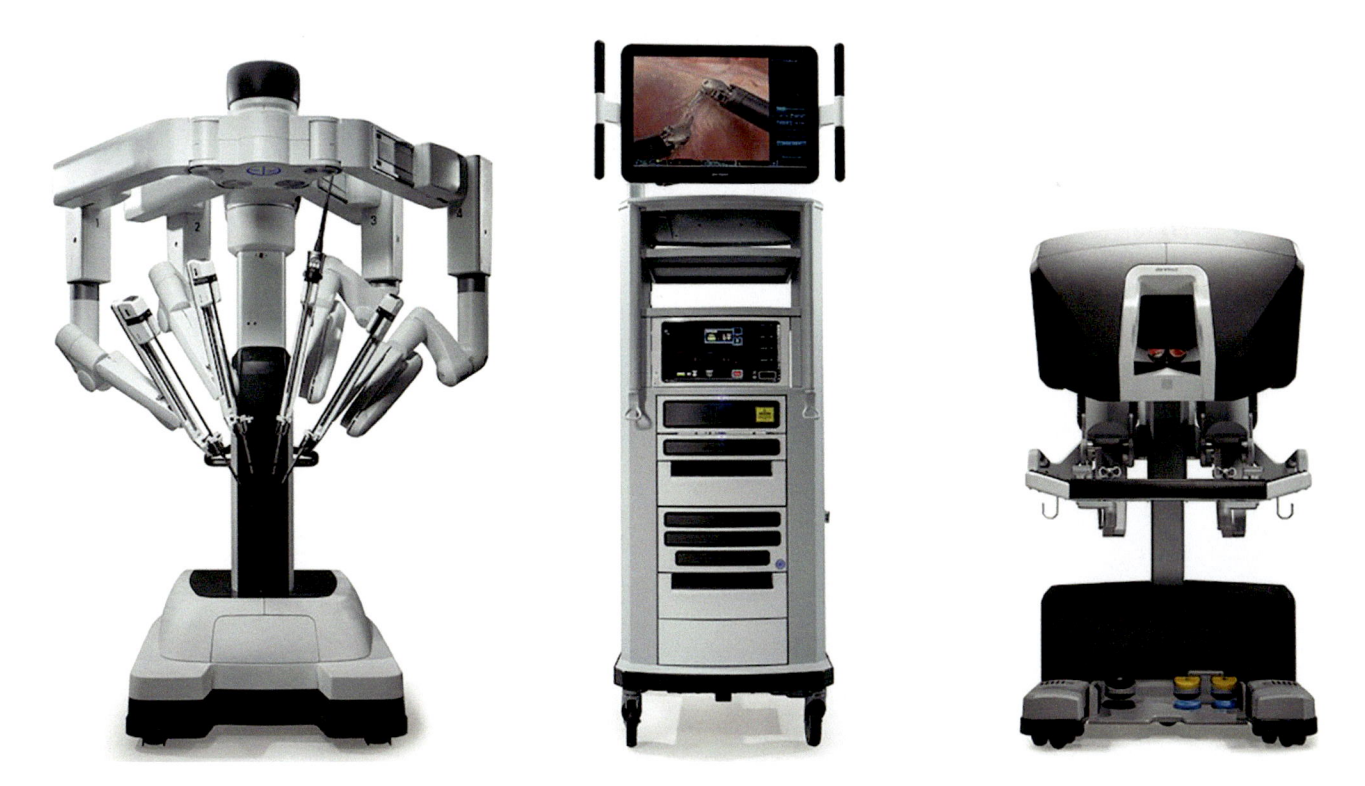

Fig. 8.4 Da Vinci Surgical System (Intuitive Surgical, Sunnyvale, CA, USA). (Reprinted by permission from Springer Nature: Springer, Surgical Endoscopy, Review of emerging surgical robotic technology, Peters, B.S. et al., Copyright 2018)

8.2.4 DaVinci

The Da Vinci Surgical System (Intuitive Surgical, Sunnyvale, CA, USA), consisting of a console for the operating surgeon and robotic arms, is the best known and most commonly used platform (Fig. 8.4) [6–20]. With tremor filtration, scalable movements, 3D visualization, and six degrees of motion freedom, the Da Vinci system contains proven benefits in endoscopic procedures in several surgical specialties [21–23]. Consequently, the system shows potential advantages in microsurgical free flap surgery regarding anatomical accessibility enabling endoscopic harvesting of flaps. However, the system is not particularly designed for use in microvascular anastomoses. In Maastricht University Medical Center (Maastricht, the Netherlands), the DaVinci system was first used in 2006 to perform a microvascular anastomosis in reconstructive microsurgery [24]. As the robotic system is not specifically created for the use in microvascular anastomoses, significant limitations of the system with respect to microsurgical procedures were found, such as limited optics and magnification, large and robust instruments, and a complex operation setup.

8.2.5 MUSA

The MUSA microsurgical robot (Microsure, Eindhoven, the Netherlands) is the first robotic platform that is specifically designed for microsurgery. The development of this novel robotic platform was initiated following the aforementioned experience with the DaVinci system leading to an intensive collaboration between microsurgeons of Maastricht University Medical Center and technical engineers of Eindhoven University of Technology (the Netherlands) [25, 26]. The MUSA robot incorporates two robotic arms that can be loaded with genuine microsurgical or supermicrosurgical instruments by using sterile 3D-printed adapters (Fig. 8.5).

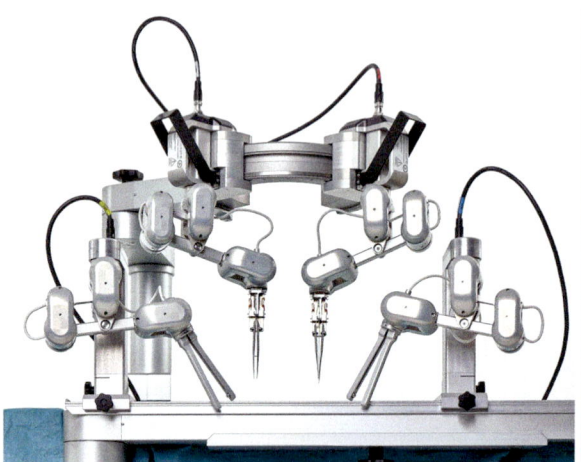

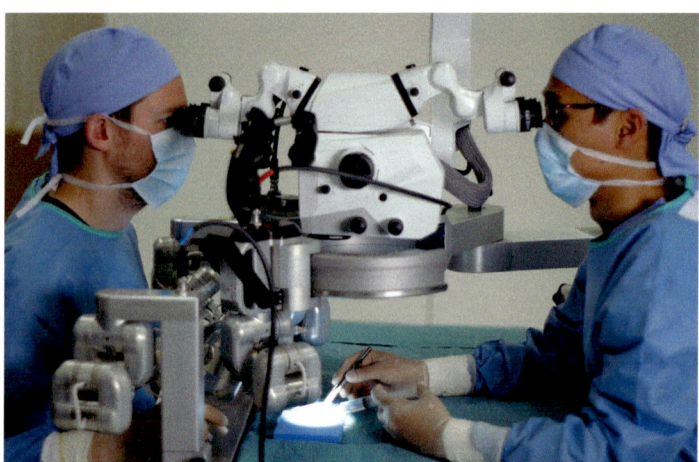

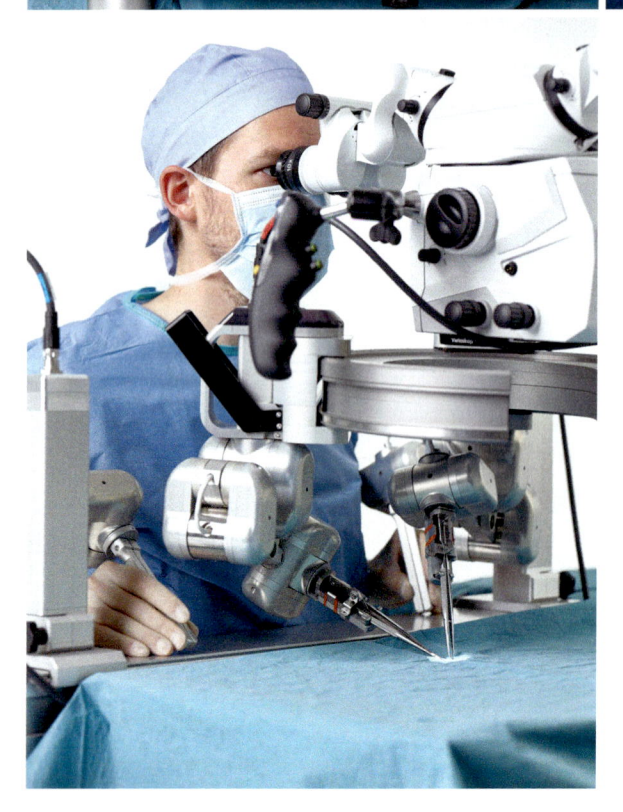

Figs. 8.5 and 8.6 The MUSA dedicated microsurgical robotic platform (Microsure, Eindhoven, the Netherlands)

The operating microsurgeon controls two master manipulators that are activated by a foot pedal (Fig. 8.6a, b). The robotic arms are attached to a suspension ring that is placed above the operating field and assist the microsurgeon by tremor filtration and motion scaling. Consequently, hand-eye coordination is improved and the precision of the surgeon is enhanced. The system can be used in combination with genuine surgical microscopes or camera systems. The size and weight of the system are small leaving the setup and workflow of a microvascular operation intact and making hybrid operations possible (quickly alternating conventional surgery and robot assistance).

8.3 Current Applications of Robotics in Microvascular and Free Flap Surgery

Robotic assistance with use of the Da Vinci Surgical System is originally known for its benefits in endoscopic procedures providing small incision surgery and reducing donor site morbidities. Compared with conventional surgery, the robot-assisted surgery contains 3D vision and wristed instruments which allow for increased accessibility and movement during endoscopic procedures. For robot-assisted microsurgery, additional advantages are motion scaling and tremor filtration. The MUSA is designed for these matters using slave arms that have the possibility to hold dedicated microsurgical instruments, downsize motions, and filter the physiological tremor to gain more precision during microsurgery.

8.3.1 Robotic Flap Harvesting

8.3.1.1 Deep Inferior Epigastric Perforator Flap
Several authors have described robot-assisted harvesting of a deep inferior epigastric perforator (DIEP) flap using the Da Vinci Surgical System. The use of this platform resulted in an improved precision of the DIEP flap harvest and decrease of the donor site morbidity by minimizing the incision length of the anterior rectus sheath [10]. Postoperatively, donor site pain was diminished, and hospital stay was shorter compared with a conventional DIEP flap procedure. However, the risk for posterior rectus sheath or bowel injury and the longer operation time can't be unnoticed.

When comparing the robot-assisted DIEP flap harvest in a transabdominal pre-peritoneal (TAPP) fashion with a totally extraperitoneal (TEP) approach, the duration of robotic harvest and pedicle dissection was not significantly different. Both approaches were considered feasible; however, the TEP procedure was less invasive by preserving the posterior rectus sheath, thereby decreasing the risk of complications such as bowel injury and pneumoperitoneum [15].

Selber et al. applied robot-assisted surgery on harvesting the flap pedicle. A long pedicle of 10–15 cm through a small fascial incision of 1–3 cm could be harvested, which is in fact a step forward in minimal-invasive autologous breast reconstruction [27].

8.3.1.2 Rectus Abdominis Muscle Flap
Robot assistance with the DaVinci system is also described in harvesting the rectus abdominis muscle for use as a free flap to cover defects on the extremity [18, 28]. One author harvested several rectus abdominis muscles in a porcine model where other authors described the robot-assisted harvest of this flap in patients [18, 28, 29]. A steep learning curve in robot-assisted harvesting was seen as adequate muscle flaps could be dissected. Furthermore, a decreased surgical-site morbidity was found without hernias, bulges, or conversions to the open technique.

8.3.1.3 Internal Mammary Vessels
The AESOP surgical system was used by Boyd et al. to explore an alternative approach of harvesting the internal mammary vessels in 20 breast reconstruction patients, including a muscle-sparing transverse rectus abdominis musculocutaneous (TRAM) flap, superior gluteal artery (SGA) flap, superficial inferior epigastric artery (SIEA) flap, and superior gluteal arterial perforator (SGAP) flap [4]. With this approach, the pedicle could be brought out through the second intercostal space without cartilage resection. This procedure could have been an advantage in skin-sparing mastectomies; however, in two patients flap loss was documented following venous congestion. The authors reported that the tunnel through the intercostal space was too narrow with constriction of the pedicle as a result. With these flap losses and six take-backs for hematoma evacuations, the complication rate was very high, suggesting this alternative approach had to be adjusted. This could also be the reason for the AESOP system not being described in further research regarding free flap surgery.

8.3.1.4 Miscellaneous
Robotic assistance for latissimus dorsi flap harvesting is described by different authors enabling an endoscopic approach using the DaVinci system [30–34]. This technique is actually associated with a lower complication rate at the expense of a longer operative time compared with conventional surgery [34]. In primary nipple sparing mastectomy and immediate breast reconstruction with robot-assisted harvesting of a latissimus dorsi flap, only one small and inconspicuous axillary wound was needed for reconstruction using the DaVinci system [33]. The prolonged surgical time and complexity of combining the mastectomy and robot-assisted reconstruction were considered as disadvantages. Additionally, the DaVinci system was used to perform endoscopic harvest of free omental flaps [17].

8.3.2 Robotic Microvascular Anastomosis

The RAMS, ZEUS, DaVinci, and MUSA systems have all been used to perform microvascular anastomoses. These anastomoses are performed in different surgical specialties and at different acceptor sites.

8.3.2.1 Preclinical Studies

Various authors have reported robotic assistance during microvascular anastomoses in animal models [6, 7, 12, 20, 35]. The DaVinci was used for dissection, fitting of a vascular clamp, section of the artery, and suturing of the anastomosis [20]. Additionally, the system was applied for the anastomosis for ureteral reconstruction using a long peritoneal flap [6]. The studies proved its feasibility as viable flaps with patent anastomoses were reported [12]. The time to perform the robot-assisted anastomoses was analyzed concluding relatively short learning curves. Besides the DaVinci system, robotic microvascular anastomoses on abdominal arteries and femoral arteries were successfully carried out with use of the MUSA robot in a rat model [36, 37]. All but one anastomosis were patent and again a steep learning curve was seen.

8.3.2.2 Clinical Studies

Several clinical free flaps have been described using robot-assisted microvascular anastomosis. For example, the DaVinci system was used to perform the microvascular anastomoses in oropharyngeal reconstruction using a free radial forearm flap (FRFF) and anterolateral thigh (ALT) flap [13, 19, 38–40]. These microvascular anastomoses were carried out without hand-sewn revisions or surgical complications such as flap failures, take-backs, or fistulas. All of these microvascular anastomoses were considered feasible and safe. When comparing conventional free flap reconstruction with robot-assisted reconstruction with a FRFF, smaller donor blood vessels could be selected when using the DaVinci system [13, 39]. Besides the aforementioned advantages, limitations of the DaVinci system were also reported. The longer operating time, large and robust instruments, limited optics and magnification, increased costs, and a complex operation setup were considered the disadvantages after performing the first microvascular anastomosis using this platform [24].

8.3.3 Robotic Flap Inset

Robot-assisted flap inset using the DaVinci system has been described during transoral free flap reconstructions. Robotic assistance with this platform was used for inset of FRFF, ALT flaps, and FAMM flaps [19, 38, 40]. The oropharynx is not easily accessible which leads to less visual cues when performing the inset of flaps. Robot-assisted surgery leads to more precision and, consequently, more chance of preservation of the mandible and lip without complications, such as flap failures or fistulas. The lack of visual cues to determine whether sufficient tension has been applied for tying knots for the anastomoses or flap inset raises the debate for incorporation of haptic feedback in robotic surgery.

8.3.4 Robotic Supermicrosurgery

Advancements in reconstructive microsurgery have evolved into supermicrosurgery completing anastomoses between 0.3 and 0.8 mm in diameter. Supermicrosurgery is limited by the dexterity and the precision of the surgeon's hand taking the physiological tremor into account. The MUSA robot has been designed for high surgical precision, safety, and user-friendliness. The system is compatible with standard (super) microsurgical instruments and microscopes. To date, the MUSA is used to perform lymphaticovenous anastomoses (LVA) connecting vessels of approximately 0.3 mm in patients suffering from lymphedema in the arm after breast cancer treatment (Fig. 8.7a) [41]. Comparing robot-assisted with conventional LVA procedure, no significant difference was found on postoperative outcome in terms of improvement in quality of life, arm circumference, and discontinuation of conservative treatment. Therefore, the MUSA was found to be feasible for supermicrosurgical anastomosis, which concerns anastomoses significantly smaller than standard free flap surgery.

Currently other indications of robot-assisted microsurgery using the MUSA such as perforator-to-perforator flaps and conventional free flaps are evaluated in clinical studies (Fig. 8.7b).

8.3.5 Robotic Microsurgical Training

In robot-assisted as well as conventional microsurgery, training is required to adequately perform microsurgical procedures. Microsurgical training is evaluated with use of different surgical systems. Comparing the conventional micro anastomosis with the robot-assisted procedure using the ZEUS system, both fully trained surgeons and residents showed longer anastomosis times and more errors of management during the robot-assisted procedure [5].

A steep learning curve in performing microvascular anastomoses with the DaVinci system was observed [42]. Robotic microsurgery videos were evaluated to validate the Structured Assessment of Robotic Microsurgical Skills (SARMS) as an assessment instrument [43]. Proficiency in robotic microsurgical skills could be achieved over a relatively limited number of practice sessions. A plateau following the steep learning curve was seen after performing 22 trials which is relatively short [41, 42, 44]. A side note is that the assessment instrument (SARMS) is specifically designed for the

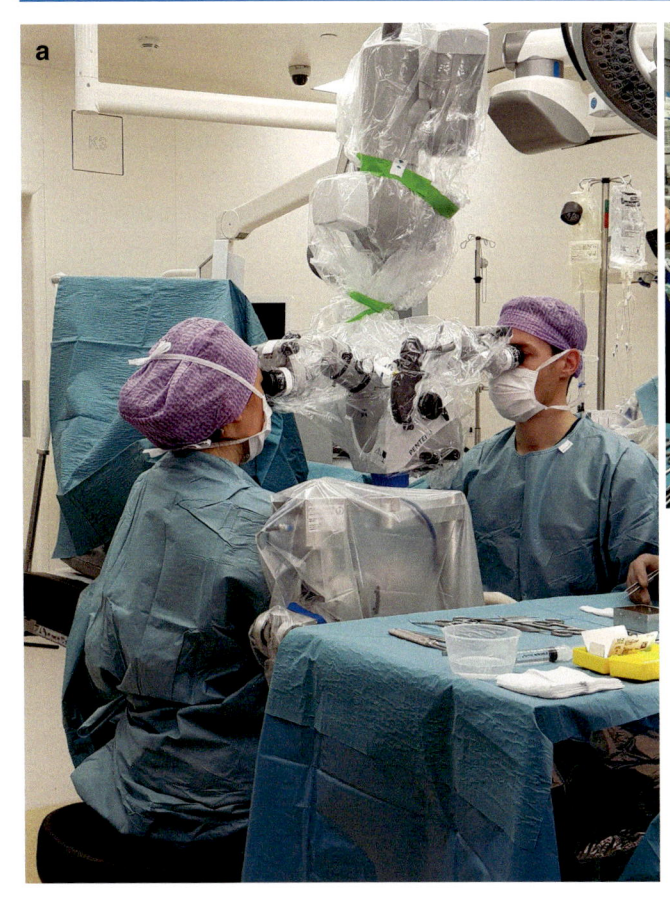

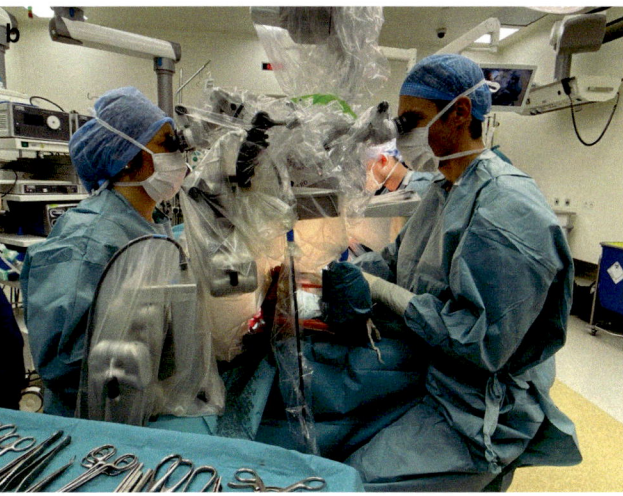

Fig. 8.7 Clinical application of the MUSA robot. (**a**) Lymphaticovenous anastomoses and (**b**) free flap anastomosis for lower extremity reconstruction

DaVinci system, as "camera movement" is part of the scoring items. Therefore, comparison to conventional microsurgery is not possible using this instrument.

To ensure user-friendly and quick-to-learn robotic microsurgery, the intention in developing the MUSA system was to minimize the number of new skills that must be learned and to maximize transfer of skills from the conventional method to the robot-assisted method. As a result, after evaluation of the Structured Assessment of Microsurgical Skills (SAMS), a comparable steep learning curve using the MUSA robot was seen for microsurgical training of surgeons and residents [37, 41]. Training in robot-assisted microsurgery seems easy to facilitate for inexperienced surgeons.

8.4 Future Perspectives

Robot assistance has great potential in the field of microvascular and free flap surgery. To date, a few robotic platforms have been described for this type of surgery. The DaVinci system was used in the majority of the studies. Robotic assistance has been applied for harvesting, microvascular anastomosis, and inset of free flaps. A reduction in postoperative pain and shorter length of hospital stay after robotic free flap surgery in comparison with conventional surgery was described keeping the risks of bowel injury during endoscopic pedicle harvest in mind. A steep learning curve in performing robot-assisted free flap surgery was reported by several authors. Nevertheless, the best outcome after robot-assisted free flap surgery was found in experienced robotic surgeons. The main disadvantages reported are the setup time, operating time, costs, lack of haptic feedback, limited optics and magnification, and large and robust instruments. Nowadays, robot assistance is even possible in supermicrosurgery using a newly developed dedicated microsurgical robot, the MUSA.

Clinically available robotic systems and novel robotic platforms (i.e., still under development) should be further improved. Current systems lack haptic feedback which might be considered as a limitation compared with conventional surgery. However, in (super)microsurgery forces are too low to rely on which also applies for conventional surgery. Hence, introduction of haptic feedback could be an advantage as the incorporation in (super)microsurgery would allow the surgeon to feel the small forces that occur. This advancement might improve tissue handling and surgical precision and, as a result, improve patient outcome. Another way to compensate the lack of haptic feedback is to provide intraoperative image guidance and add visual cues to improve surgical efficacy. Optimal visualization is paramount during microsurgery. The evolution of camera systems will enable high magnification with 3D vision, replacing the current setting of the microscope in the operation field. These camera systems can be incorporated into robotic platforms or can be used as external camera systems, such as exoscopes and heads-up microscopes [45]. In addition to these new camera systems, novel imaging techniques are promising areas in the continued refinement of microsurgery, such as HR stereotactic operation, spectral imaging, and real-time navigation systems. Near-infrared fluorescence (NIRF) imaging could contribute to critical decision-making by facilitating real-time intraoperative anatomical navigation [46].

The DaVinci system consists of a console in the operation room keeping the surgeon away from the surgical table. In tele-surgery, the surgeon carries out the procedure while located in a separate geographical location as the patient which may become common practice in future microsurgery. A reliable connection without any lag is mandatory to perform surgery safely.

Last but not least, a new trend that refers to intelligent robotic systems and the ability of self-learning is cognitive surgical robots which are supported by big data analytics. Nowadays, assessment of microsurgical skills has been conducted by subjective observations of other trained surgeons. The advantage of using robotic platforms for microsurgery is that every movement and force can be registered. This data can be used for the objective assessment using standardized evaluation methods and, therefore, creating objective microsurgical training programs. The improved surgical data science could also be used to enable semi-automated surgery, conducted by cognitive robots including artificial intelligence to help improve surgical performance.

Robot assistance in microvascular and free flap surgery is relatively underdeveloped compared to other surgical fields. This is partially due to the fact that most operation robots are not designed for microsurgery and therefore lack the delicate instruments and precision that is needed for free flaps and microsurgical operations. The evolution of endoscopic harvest and inset of flaps using current general robotic systems and the availability of new dedicated microsurgical robots such as the MUSA is propelling innovation and adoption of robotic technology in our field.

8.5 Selected Readings

- Dobbs TD, Cundy O, Samarendra H, Khan K, Whitaker IS. A systematic review of the role of robotics in plastic and reconstructive surgery-from inception to the future. Front Surg. 2017;4:66.

  A systematic literature search to identify all applications of robot assistance in plastic and reconstructive surgery. The feasibility of robotic plastic surgery has been demonstrated in several specific indications. As technology, knowledge, and skills in this area improve, these techniques have the potential to contribute positively to patient and provider experience and outcomes.

- Ibrahim AE, Sarhane KA, Selber JC. New Frontiers in robotic-assisted microsurgical reconstruction. Clin Plast Surg. 2017;44(2):415–23.

  The different clinical applications of robotic microsurgery are presented, highlighting its advantages over conventional microsurgery and outlining the main limitations that might prevent its widespread use.

- Tan YPA, Liverneaux P, Wong JKF. Current limitations of surgical robotics in reconstructive plastic microsurgery. Front Surg. 2018;5:22.

  Tan et al. performed a systematic review to evaluate current state of surgical robotics within the field of reconstructive microsurgery and their limitations. Despite the theoretical potential of surgical robots, current commercially available robotic systems are suboptimal for plastic or reconstructive microsurgery.

- van Mulken TJM, Boymans C, Schols RM, et al. Preclinical experience using a new robotic system created for microsurgery. Plast Reconstr Surg. 2018;142(5):1367–76.

  A preclinical study concluded that it is feasible to complete anastomotic microsurgery on silicone vessels using the newly developed Microsure robotic system.

- Selber JC. The robotic DIEP flap. Plast Reconstr Surg. 2020;145(2):340–3.

  Selber describes the robotic DIEP flap procedure. The robotic deep inferior epigastric artery perforator flap permits the longest possible pedicle harvest through the smallest possible fascial incision and, for this reason, may be the next stage in the evolution of minimally invasive, autologous breast reconstruction.

- van Mulken TJM, Scharmga AMJ, Schols RM, et al. The journey of creating the first dedicated platform for robot-assisted (super)microsurgery in reconstructive surgery. Eur J Plast Surg. 2020;43(1):1–6.

  This publication elaborates on the journey of creating the first dedicated microsurgical robot, currently known as the MUSA robot.

- van Mulken TJM, Schols RM, Scharmga AMJ, et al. First-in-human robotic supermicrosurgery using a dedicated microsurgical robot for treating breast cancer-related lymphedema: a randomized pilot trial. Nat Commun. 2020;11(1):757.

  This paper reports the first-in-human study of robot-assisted supermicrosurgery using a dedicated microsurgical robotic platform. A prospective randomized pilot study was conducted comparing robot-assisted and manual supermicrosurgical lymphaticovenous anastomosis (LVA) in treating breast cancer-related lymphedema.

- Murphy DC, Saleh DB. Artificial Intelligence in plastic surgery: what is it? Where are we now? What is on the horizon? Ann R Coll Surg Engl. 2020;102(8):577–80.

   Review article on artificial intelligence (e.g., machine learning, big data, etc.) in plastic surgery. Surgeons must collaborate with computer scientists to ensure that AI algorithms inform clinically relevant health objectives and are interpretable. Ethical concerns are also discussed.

References

1. Dobbs TD, Cundy O, Samarendra H, Khan K, Whitaker IS. A systematic review of the role of robotics in plastic and reconstructive surgery-from inception to the future. Front Surg. 2017;4:66.
2. Tan YPA, Liverneaux P, Wong JKF. Current limitations of surgical robotics in reconstructive plastic microsurgery. Front Surg. 2018;5:22.
3. Krapohl BD, Reichert B, Machens HG, Mailander P, Siemionow M, Zins JE. Computer-guided microsurgery: surgical evaluation of a telerobotic arm. Microsurgery. 2001;21(1):22–9.
4. Boyd B, Umansky J, Samson M, Boyd D, Stahl K. Robotic harvest of internal mammary vessels in breast reconstruction. J Reconstr Microsurg. 2006;22(4):261–6.
5. Karamanoukian RL, Finley DS, Evans GR, Karamanoukian HL. Feasibility of robotic-assisted microvascular anastomoses in plastic surgery. J Reconstr Microsurg. 2006;22(6):429–31.
6. Brandao LF, Laydner H, Akca O, et al. Robot-assisted ureteral reconstruction using a tubularized peritoneal flap: a novel technique in a chronic porcine model. World J Urol. 2017;35(1):89–96.
7. Clarke NS, Price J, Boyd T, et al. Robotic-assisted microvascular surgery: skill acquisition in a rat model. J Robot Surg. 2018;12(2):331–6.
8. Ghanem TA. Transoral robotic-assisted microvascular reconstruction of the oropharynx. Laryngoscope. 2011;121(3):580–2.
9. Gudeloglu A, Brahmbhatt JV, Parekattil SJ. Robotic-assisted microsurgery for an elective microsurgical practice. Semin Plast Surg. 2014;28(1):11–9.
10. Gundlapalli VS, Ogunleye AA, Scott K, et al. Robotic-assisted deep inferior epigastric artery perforator flap abdominal harvest for breast reconstruction: a case report. Microsurgery. 2018;38(6):702–5.
11. Hans S, Jouffroy T, Veivers D, et al. Transoral robotic-assisted free flap reconstruction after radiation therapy in hypopharyngeal carcinoma: report of two cases. Eur Arch Otorhinolaryngol. 2013;270(8):2359–64.
12. Katz RD, Rosson GD, Taylor JA, Singh NK. Robotics in microsurgery: use of a surgical robot to perform a free flap in a pig. Microsurgery. 2005;25(7):566–9.
13. Lai CS, Lu CT, Liu SA, Tsai YC, Chen YW, Chen IC. Robot-assisted microvascular anastomosis in head and neck free flap reconstruction: preliminary experiences and results. Microsurgery. 2019;39(8):715–20.
14. Maire N, Naito K, Lequint T, Facca S, Berner S, Liverneaux P. Robot-assisted free toe pulp transfer: feasibility study. J Reconstr Microsurg. 2012;28(7):481–4.
15. Manrique OJ, Bustos SS, Mohan AT, et al. Robotic-assisted DIEP flap harvest for autologous breast reconstruction: a comparative feasibility study on a cadaveric model. J Reconstr Microsurg. 2020;36(5):362–8.
16. Naito K, Imashimizu K, Nagura N, et al. Robot-assisted intercostal nerve harvesting: a technical note about the first case in Japan. Plast Reconstr Surg Glob Open. 2020;8(6):e2888.
17. Ozkan O, Ozkan O, Cinpolat A, Arici C, Bektas G, Can UM. Robotic harvesting of the omental flap: a case report and mini-review of the use of robots in reconstructive surgery. J Robot Surg. 2019;13(4):539–43.
18. Patel NV, Pedersen JC. Robotic harvest of the rectus abdominis muscle: a preclinical investigation and case report. J Reconstr Microsurg. 2012;28(7):477–80.
19. Selber JC. Transoral robotic reconstruction of oropharyngeal defects: a case series. Plast Reconstr Surg. 2010;126(6):1978–87.
20. Taleb C, Nectoux E, Liverneaux PA. Telemicrosurgery: a feasibility study in a rat model. Chir Main. 2008;27(2–3):104–8.
21. Stephenson ER Jr, Sankholkar S, Ducko CT, Damiano RJ Jr. Robotically assisted microsurgery for endoscopic coronary artery bypass grafting. Ann Thorac Surg. 1998;66(3):1064–7.
22. Yuh BE, Hussain A, Chandrasekhar R, et al. Comparative analysis of global practice patterns in urologic robot-assisted surgery. J Endourol. 2010;24(10):1637–44.
23. Zacharopoulou C, Sananes N, Baulon E, Garbin O, Wattiez A. [Robotic gynecologic surgery: state of the art. Review of the literature]. J Gynecol Obstet Biol Reprod 2010;39(6):444–52.
24. van der Hulst R, Sawor J, Bouvy N. Microvascular anastomosis: is there a role for robotic surgery? J Plast Reconstr Aesthet Surg. 2007;60(1):101–2.
25. Cau R. Design and realization of a master-slave system for reconstructive microsurgery Eindhoven: Technische Universiteit Eindhoven. 2014.
26. van Mulken TJM, Scharmga AMJ, Schols RM, et al. The journey of creating the first dedicated platform for robot-assisted (super)microsurgery in reconstructive surgery. Eur J Plast Surg. 2020;43(1):1–6.
27. Selber JC. The robotic DIEP flap. Plast Reconstr Surg. 2020;145(2):340–3.
28. Pedersen J, Song DH, Selber JC. Robotic, intraperitoneal harvest of the rectus abdominis muscle. Plast Reconstr Surg. 2014;134(5):1057–63.
29. Louis V, Chih-Sheng L, Chevallier D, Selber JC, Xavier F, Liverneaux PA. A porcine model for robotic training harvest of the rectus abdominis muscle. Ann Chir Plast Esthet. 2018;63(2):113–6.
30. Chung JH, You HJ, Kim HS, Lee BI, Park SH, Yoon ES. A novel technique for robot assisted latissimus dorsi flap harvest. J Plast Reconstr Aesthet Surg. 2015;68(7):966–72.
31. Garcia JC Jr, Torres MC, Fadel MS, Bader D, Lutfi H, Kozonara ME. Robotic transfer of the latissimus dorsi associated with levator scapulae and rhomboid minor mini-open transfers for trapezium palsy. Arthrosc Tech. 2020;9(11):e1721–6.
32. Lai HW, Chen ST, Lin SL, et al. Technique for single axillary incision robotic assisted quadrantectomy and immediate partial breast reconstruction with robotic latissimus dorsi flap harvest for breast cancer: a case report. Medicine. 2018;97(27):e11373.
33. Lai HW, Lin SL, Chen ST, et al. Robotic nipple sparing mastectomy and immediate breast reconstruction with robotic latissimus dorsi flap harvest - technique and preliminary results. J Plast Reconstr Aesthet Surg. 2018;71(10):e59–61.
34. Houvenaeghel G, El Hajj H, Schmitt A, et al. Robotic-assisted skin sparing mastectomy and immediate reconstruction using latissimus dorsi flap a new effective and safe technique: a comparative study. Surg Oncol. 2020;35:406–11.
35. Katz RD, Taylor JA, Rosson GD, Brown PR, Singh NK. Robotics in plastic and reconstructive surgery: use of a telemanipulator slave robot to perform microvascular anastomoses. J Reconstr Microsurg. 2006;22(1):53–7.

36. van Mulken TJM, Schols RM, Qiu SS, et al. Robotic (super) microsurgery: feasibility of a new master-slave platform in an in vivo animal model and future directions. J Surg Oncol. 2018;118(5):826–31.
37. van Mulken TJM, Boymans C, Schols RM, et al. Preclinical experience using a new robotic system created for microsurgery. Plast Reconstr Surg. 2018;142(5):1367–76.
38. Lai CS, Chen IC, Liu SA, Lu CT, Yen JH, Song DY. Robot-assisted free flap reconstruction of oropharyngeal cancer--a preliminary report. Ann Plast Surg. 2015;74(Suppl 2):S105–8.
39. Tsai YC, Liu SA, Lai CS, et al. Functional outcomes and complications of robot-assisted free flap oropharyngeal reconstruction. Ann Plast Surg. 2017;78(3 Suppl 2):S76–82.
40. Song HG, Yun IS, Lee WJ, Lew DH, Rah DK. Robot-assisted free flap in head and neck reconstruction. Arch Plast Surg. 2013;40(4):353–8.
41. van Mulken TJM, Schols RM, Scharmga AMJ, et al. First-in-human robotic supermicrosurgery using a dedicated microsurgical robot for treating breast cancer-related lymphedema: a randomized pilot trial. Nat Commun. 2020;11(1):757.
42. Alrasheed T, Liu J, Hanasono MM, Butler CE, Selber JC. Robotic microsurgery: validating an assessment tool and plotting the learning curve. Plast Reconstr Surg. 2014;134(4):794–803.
43. Selber JC, Alrasheed T. Robotic microsurgical training and evaluation. Semin Plast Surg. 2014;28(1):5–10.
44. Lee JY, Mattar T, Parisi TJ, Carlsen BT, Bishop AT, Shin AY. Learning curve of robotic-assisted microvascular anastomosis in the rat. J Reconstr Microsurg. 2012;28(7):451–6.
45. Piatkowski AA, Keuter XHA, Schols RM, van der Hulst R. Potential of performing a microvascular free flap reconstruction using solely a 3D exoscope instead of a conventional microscope. J Plast Reconstr Aesthet Surg. 2018;71(11):1664–78.
46. Schols RM, Connell NJ, Stassen LP. Near-infrared fluorescence imaging for real-time intraoperative anatomical guidance in minimally invasive surgery: a systematic review of the literature. World J Surg. 2015;39(5):1069–79.

Technical Tips in Microvascular Surgery

Marios Nicolaides and Georgios Pafitanis

9.1 Introduction

Over the past two decades, microvascular anastomosis has advanced remarkably, but there are still situations that challenge even the most experienced surgeons. Examples include extremely small or short vessels, large discrepancies in vessel diameter, and difficult anatomy that limits the operative field. In such situations, excessive manipulation of the vessel walls or substandard techniques can result in adverse effects. This chapter outlines several *tips* that can be used to overcome these challenges and lessen the frustration associated with the process. The suggested techniques have a steeper learning curve and necessitate proficiency in basic microsurgical skills, but once mastered they can lead to higher vessel patency, increased flap survival rate, and reduced operative time.

9.2 Modified Writing Position and Quadropod Grip

Correct handling of surgical instruments is fundamental in microsurgery to allow for minimal movements in the operative field. Maintaining manual dexterity while avoiding body fatigue is imperative given the long nature of most reconstructive operations. The microsurgeon should achieve a well-supported hand position to avoid hand tremor and allow for isolated finger movement. The hand is traditionally stabilized at the metacarpophalangeal joints by resting the lateral aspect of the hand on any flat surface in the operative field.

M. Nicolaides (✉)
Barts and The London School of Medicine and Dentistry, Queen Mary University of London, London, UK
e-mail: marios.nicolaides@nhs.net

G. Pafitanis
London Reconstructive Microsurgery Unit (LRMU), Department of Plastic Surgery, Emergency Care and Trauma Division, The Royal London Hospital, Barts Health NHS Trust, London, UK

There are two commonly used handling methods for microsurgical instruments: the "writing" position and the "quadrupod" grip.

The "writing" position, also known as the three-digit tripod grip, is achieved by using the index and middle fingers to manipulate the instrument against the thumb (Fig. 9.1a). Better stability and reduced resting tremor can be achieved by gently flexing the middle finger at the proximal and distal interphalangeal joints while resting the index finger and thumb on it (Fig. 9.1b). This position can be used in most cases of conventional microsurgery but is challenged in supermicrosurgery (vessels with diameter of <0.8 mm), where the resting motor tremor is exaggerated. The "quadrupod" grip can be used in such cases. This technique is achieved by using the index, middle, and ring fingers to manipulate the instrument against the thumb (Fig. 9.1c). The use of the ring finger decreases the distance from the tip of the instrument and, thus, allows for more delicate and balanced movements. In this four-finger technique, microsurgical suturing can be performed by just moving the ring finger and the other fingers follow.

9.3 Airborne Suture Tying

Suture tying in microvascular anastomoses is performed in a timely manner, but usually not rushed, as most flaps tolerate long ischemia periods without significant compromise to the flap—the first goal is an atraumatic anastomosis. However, in cases of intestinal flaps for pharyngoesophageal reconstruction, or compromised flaps of any type, time is of essence. The "airborne" suture tying technique aims to speed up the knot tying process by maintaining the free suture end always in the air.

- *Step 1:* First, the needle is passed through both vessels keeping the end on the right (free end) short. The short end is then grasped by the right forceps (two thirds of the

© Springer Nature Switzerland AG 2023
D. Nikkhah et al. (eds.), *Core Techniques in Flap Reconstructive Microsurgery*, https://doi.org/10.1007/978-3-031-07678-7_9

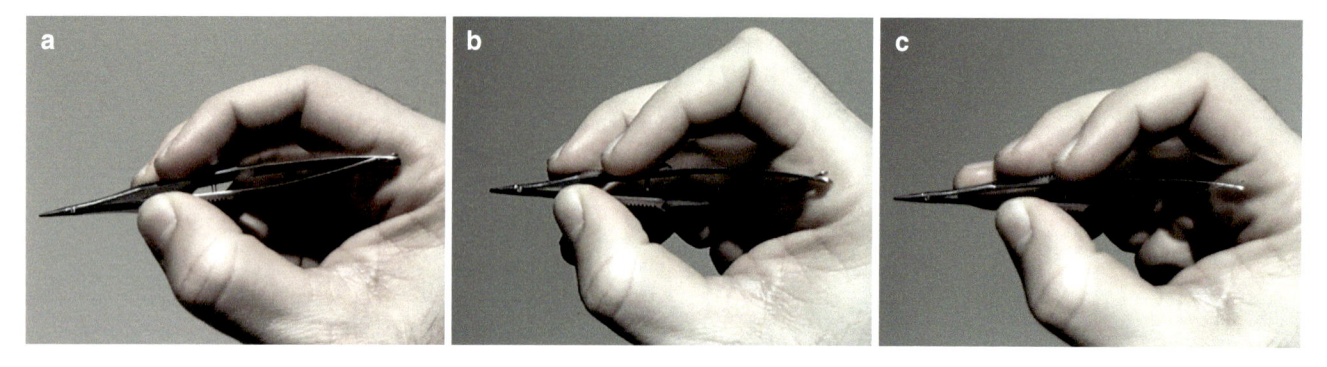

Fig. 9.1 (**a**) The "writing" position, also known as the three-digit tripod grip. (**b**) The "modified writing" position where the middle finger is flexed at the proximal and distal interphalangeal joints while the index finger and thumb rest on it. (**c**) The "quadrupod" grip is achieved by using the index, middle, and ring fingers to manipulate the instrument against the thumb

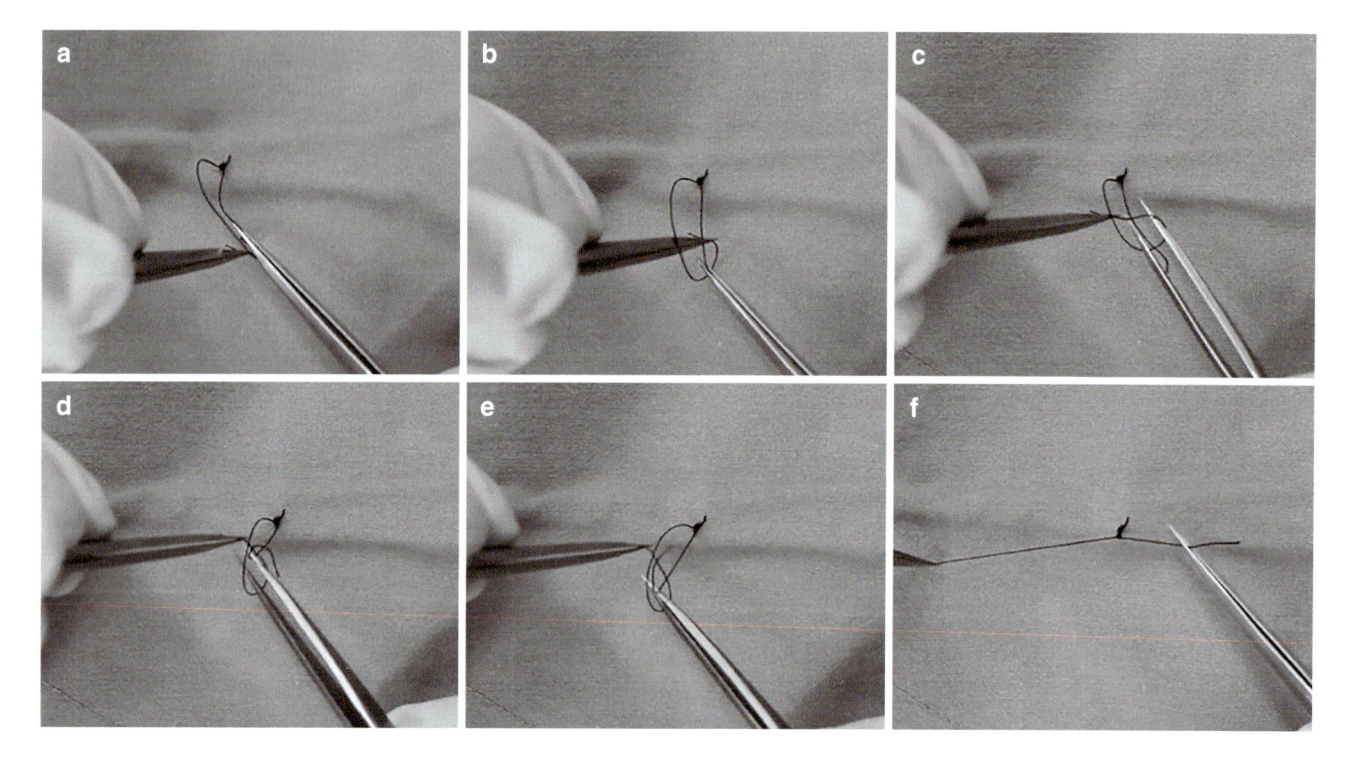

Fig. 9.2 (**a–f**) Airborne suture step-by-step microvascular tying

distance from vessel to tip) with the instrument tip pointing up (Fig. 9.2a).
- *Step 2:* The left end (suture end) is grasped by the left forceps (at a location so that it is double the size of the free end) with the instrument tip pointing down (Fig. 9.2b).
- *Step 3:* A C-loop (lasso loop) is created on the suture end and encircles the tip of the right instrument (Fig. 9.2c).
- *Step 4:* The right forceps releases the short end momentarily and moves down with the loop, allowing the short end to fall posterior to the C-loop, where it regrasps it (Fig. 9.2d). The first knot is then secured to complete the first throw. Both the long and short ends of the suture point at each other.
- *Step 5:* The left forceps holding the suture end (long) moves downward to form a vertical C-loop (concave side on top) which is wrapped under and around the tip of the right instrument (Fig. 9.2e).
- *Step 6:* The right instrument releases the short end momentarily and moves up to regrasp it and bring it back down through the loop to complete the second knot (Fig. 9.2f).

This technique, besides being quicker than conventional methods of knot tying, can also prevent damage caused to surrounding structures when trying to pick up the free end while also decrease the probability of lumen contamination when the free end collects debris. The airborne suture tying technique can be used in combination with the any suturing method.

9 Technical Tips in Microvascular Surgery

9.4 One-Way-Up Technique

In situations where the operative field is limited in space or the vessel is short, the "one-way-up" technique for microvascular end-to-end anastomoses becomes useful. In this technique, anastomosis can be achieved without lifting the clamp or maneuvering the vessel ends. The double clamp should be placed with the tips facing the surgeon to allow for better access and visualization.

- *Step 1:* The first and only stay suture is placed as further away from the surgeon as possible (at the back wall) outside in on the right side and inside out on the left side. The knot is tied, and the long end secured on the clamp, while the other end is cut short (Fig. 9.3a).
- *Step 2:* The one-way-up technique is then started at the most difficult point in the back wall by passing the needle outside in on the left wall and inside out on the right wall where the knot is tied (Fig. 9.3b).
- *Step 3:* The next sutures are placed proximally to the previous one in a similar fashion. Suturing is continued until the whole length of the inferior walls is sutured (Fig. 9.3c).
- *Step 4:* Then, the surgeon can change to their traditional method of suturing for the anterior wall or apply continuous-interrupted suturing (Fig. 9.3d, e).

One end should be kept always long to assist in securing the vessel ends while performing the one-way-up technique.

9.5 Continuous-Interrupted Suturing

Interrupted and continuous suturing are two widely accepted and traditional suturing techniques for microvascular end-to-end anastomoses. Interrupted suturing can be achieved by placing three sutures at equal distance and then placing interrupted sutures in between (triangulation method). Continuous suturing is faster but increases the risk of stricture. Continuous-interrupted suturing is a new technique that combines the advantages of both.

- *Step 1:* Two interrupted sutures are applied for the bi-angulation technique or the back wall of the vessel is already sutured as seen in Fig. 9.4a.
- *Step 2:* A loose running suture is then applied on the anterior wall next to the first suture and continuing until three or four consecutive loose loops are created—this step mimics continuous suturing, but the suture is left loose and untied instead (Fig. 9.4b).
- *Step 3:* Starting from the first, the loops are tied successively. The ends of each suture should be cut to avoid multiple long ends in the anastomotic field (Fig. 9.4c).

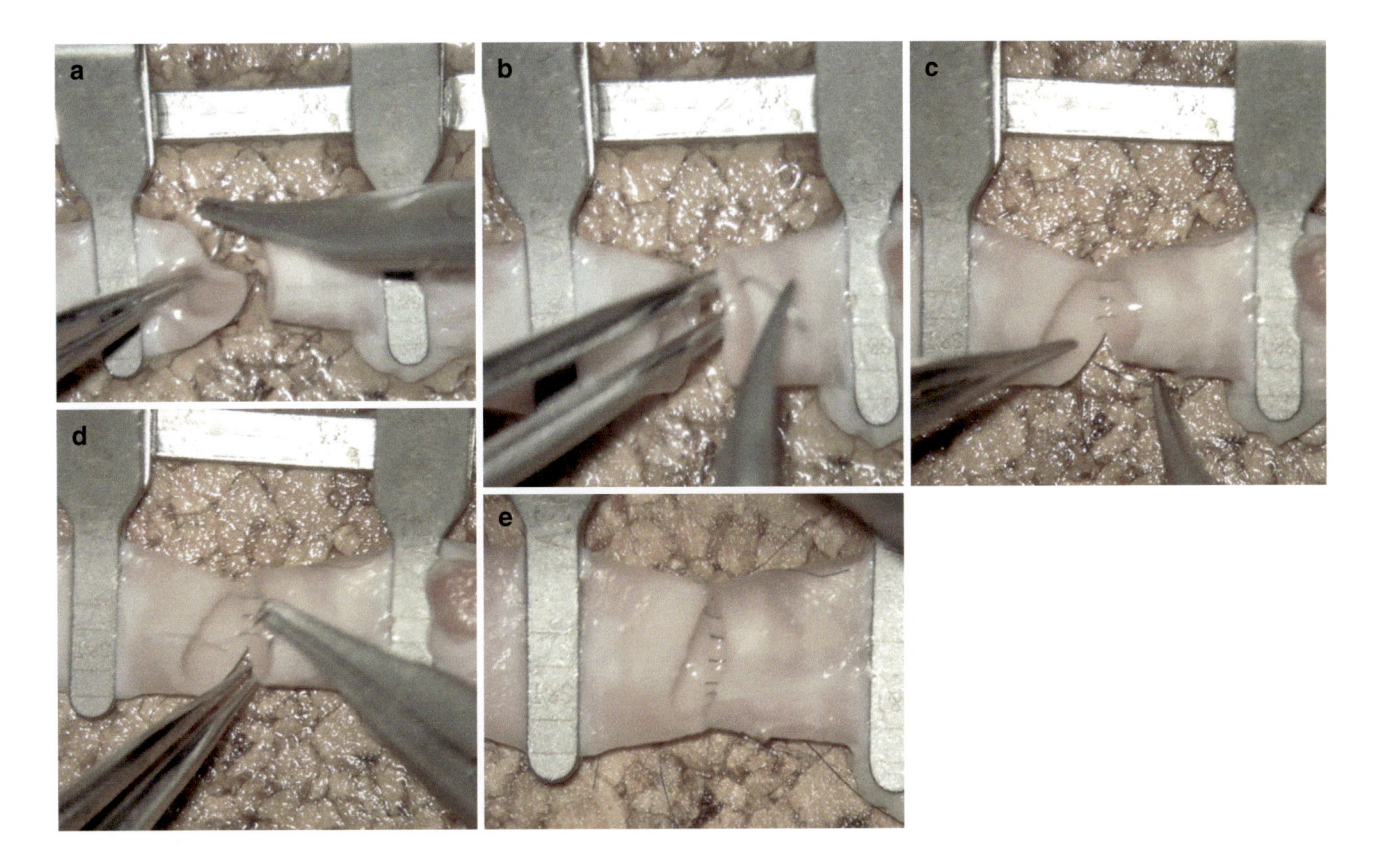

Fig. 9.3 (a–e) One-way-up microvascular anastomosis step-by-step technique

Fig. 9.4 (a–e) Continuous-interrupted suturing step-by-step technique

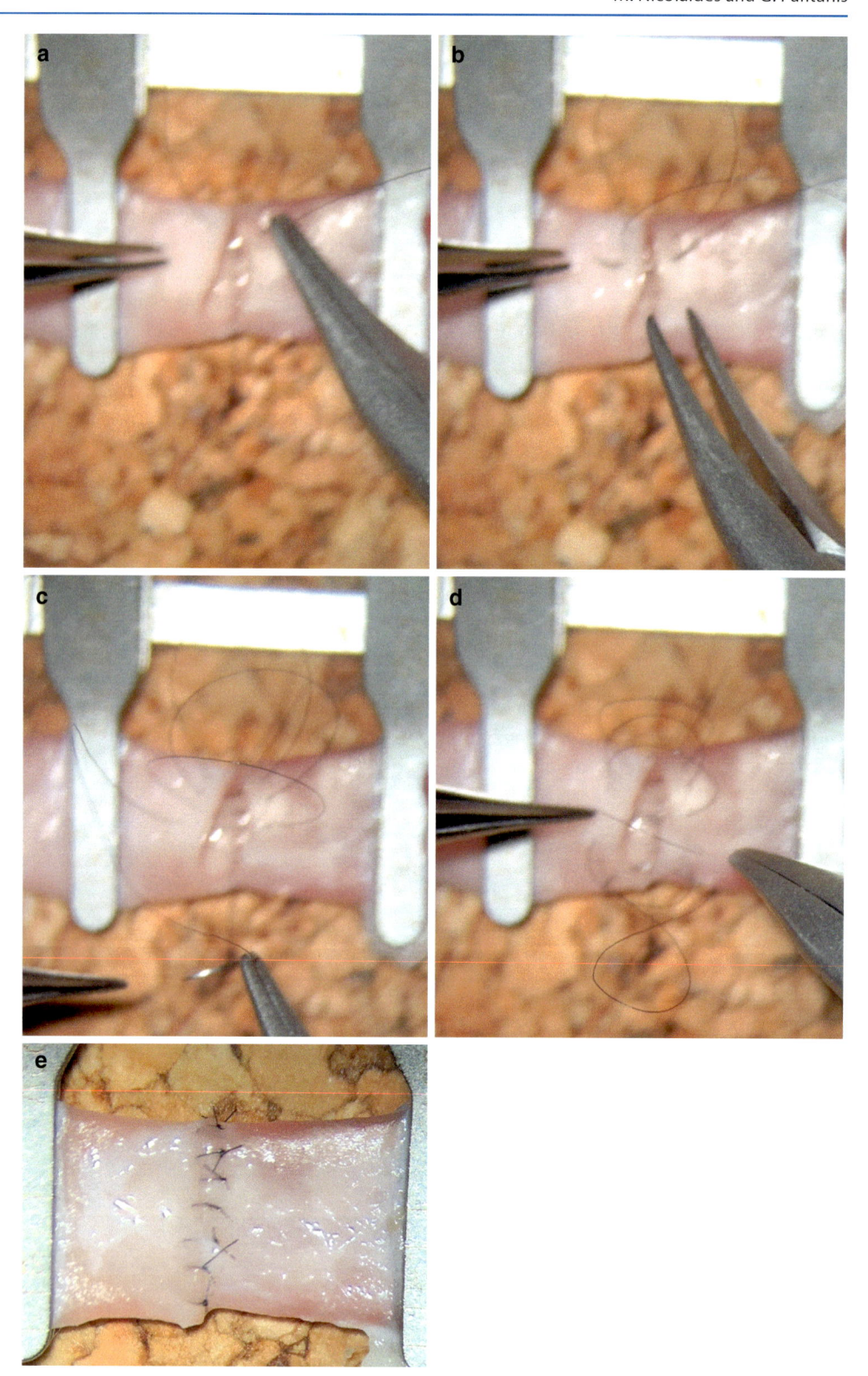

- *Step 4:* Finally, the previous two steps are repeated until all the anastomosis is completed (Fig. 9.4d, e).

The continuous-interrupted suturing method is quicker than the interrupted suturing method without risking stenosis of the anastomosis. Furthermore, the application of the sutures can be done in a very precise manner as the lumen and posterior wall of both vessels are visible throughout suturing without extensive manipulation of the vessel walls.

9.6 Needle-Splint Technique

The "needle-splint" technique is a modification of the continuous-interrupted suturing method described above (see Sect. 9.5). This technical refinement takes advantage of the suture needle to ensure optimal eversion and alignment of the vessel walls while maintaining visualization of the intima.

- *Step 1:* Two interrupted sutures are applied proximal (0°) and distal (180°) to the surgeon.
- *Step 2:* A loose running suture is then applied on the anterior wall next to the first suture and continuing until two or three consecutive loose loops are created—this step mimics continuous suturing, but the suture is left loose and untied instead (Fig. 9.5).
- *Step 3:* The needle is inserted both through vessel walls proximal to the created loose loops, but it is not passed completely through to create a "splint." The needle is then used to manipulate the vessel walls ensuring optimal positioning.
- *Step 4:* Starting from the first, the loops are tied successively. The ends of each suture should be cut to avoid multiple long ends in the anastomotic field (Fig. 9.5). The needle is pushed through completely and the final knot is tied.

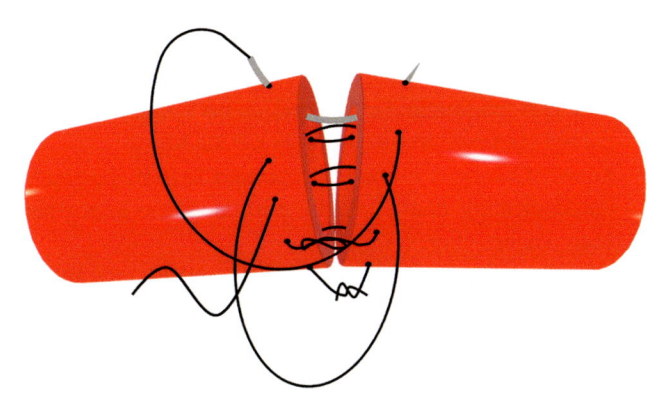

Fig. 9.5 The Needle-splint technique

9.7 Crater Arteriotomy Technique

In cases of vessel-size discrepancy, an end-to-side microvascular anastomosis is preferred over the conventional end-to-end method. The "crater" arteriotomy technique is a type of excision arteriotomy (from outside in) for the side vessel that allows direct visualization of the intimal surfaces during suturing. This technique can prevent complications resulting from intimal injury, such as thrombus formation and consequent flap failure.

- *Step 1:* The adventitia layer of the "side" vessel is dissected off using curved microsurgical scissors (Fig. 9.6a).
- *Step 2:* The vessel wall is gripped using the microsurgical forceps in left hand and tented upward. A V-shaped shallow cut is made at about a 30–45° angle using adventitia scissors in right hand. The cut is then deepened (30–50%

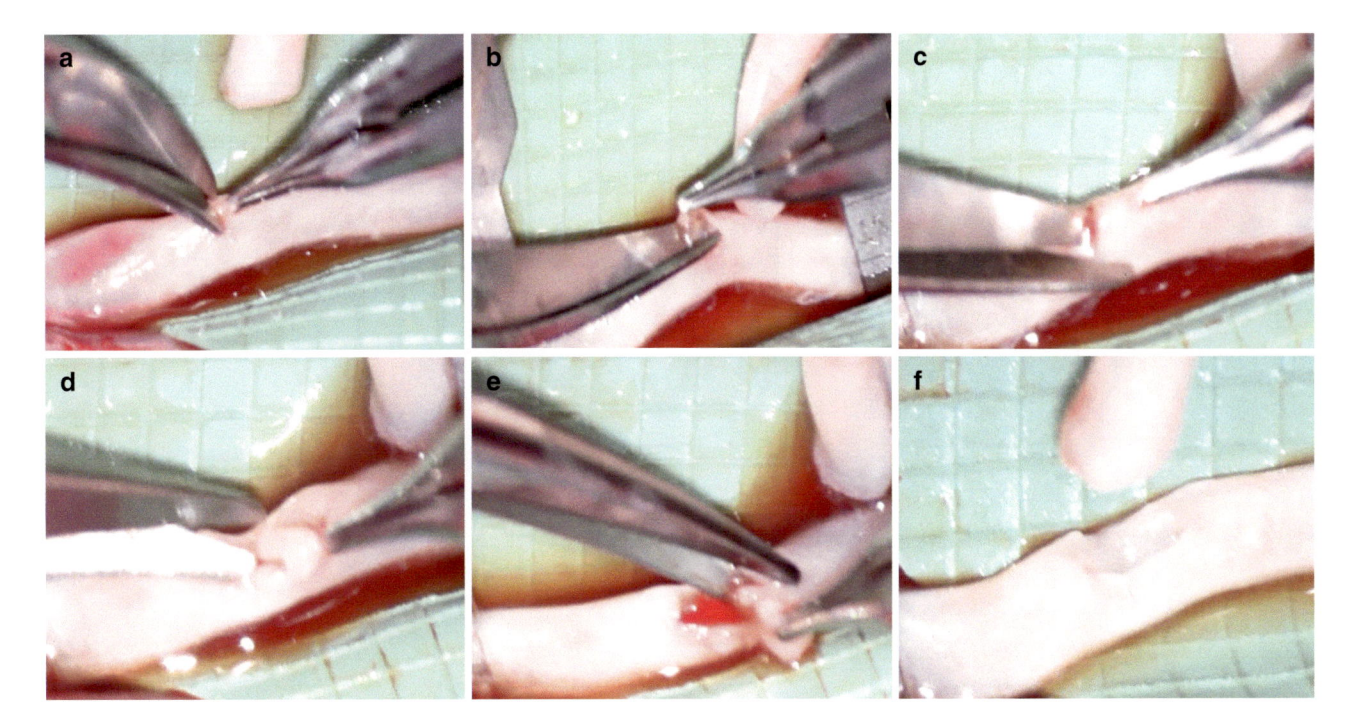

Fig. 9.6 (**a–f**) The crater arteriotomy step-by-step technique

of vessel thickness or until blood is seen to extravasate) (Fig. 9.6b, c).
- *Step 3:* The microsurgical forceps in left hand are used to gently lift the tip of the V-shaped cut and pull it to the left at a 45° angle. The scissors in right hand are used with the concave side down to extend the cut at each side of the "V" (Fig. 9.6d, e).
- *Step 4:* The two cuts should eventually meet, creating a biconvex/oval hole in the vessel wall (Fig. 9.6f).

9.8 End-to-Patch Technique

End-to-patch technique is a microvascular pedicle modification for free flap transfer that utilizes the "mother" vessel wall to enlarge and increase the caliber of the free flap pedicle. It can be used in either arterial or venous pedicles, and the technique can be used to upscale a pedicle caliber to any size vessel directed by the recipients provided they are smaller than the "mother" nominate vessel that gives off the flap pedicle.

- *Step 1:* The pedicle is marked along with an elliptical component of the "mother" vessels' wall.
- *Step 2:* A full thickness vessel wall is cut along with the pedicle to allow a perfect match to the recipient vessel.
- *Step 3:* The "mother" vessel is either sutured primarily—ideally with an 8/0 or 7/0 microvascular suture or patch grafted if this technique is applied to an arterial pedicle (Fig. 9.7).

9.9 Dealing with Non-spurting Recipient Arteries

Non-spurting recipient arteries are often encountered during free tissue transfer. These are conventionally shortened using straight scissors at an appropriate distance judged by the microsurgeon. This approach is usually successful but can result in excessive shortening as estimating an appropriate distance is challenging. Furthermore, it can cause intimal separation in atherosclerotic arterial stumps. An alternative technique has been described to minimize these limitations by using circumferential excision and stepwise shortening.

- *Step 1:* A longitudinal cut is made in the vessel wall using curved microsurgical scissors (Fig. 9.8a, b).
- *Step 2:* Cutting is *gradually* continued until blood spurts out, indicating that a healthy portion of the artery has been reached (Fig. 9.8c, d).
- *Step 3:* A microsurgical clamp is applied proximally (Fig. 9.8e).

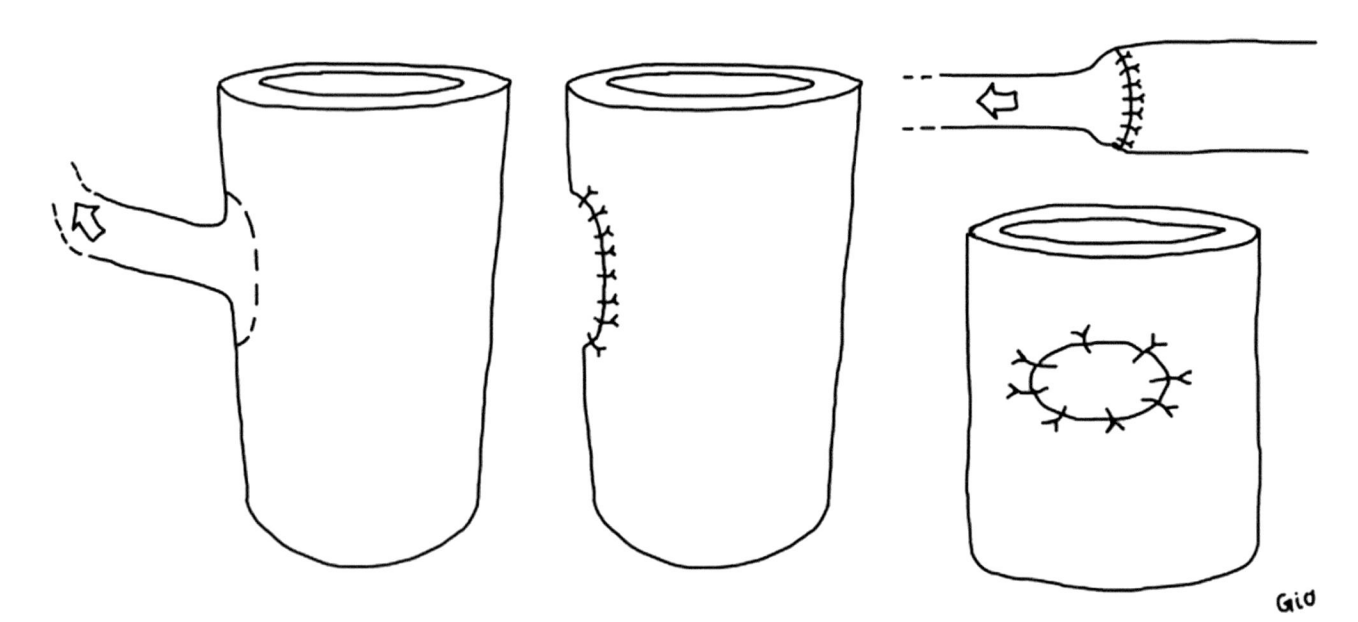

Fig. 9.7 The end-to-patch arteriotomy technique—a step-by-step guide

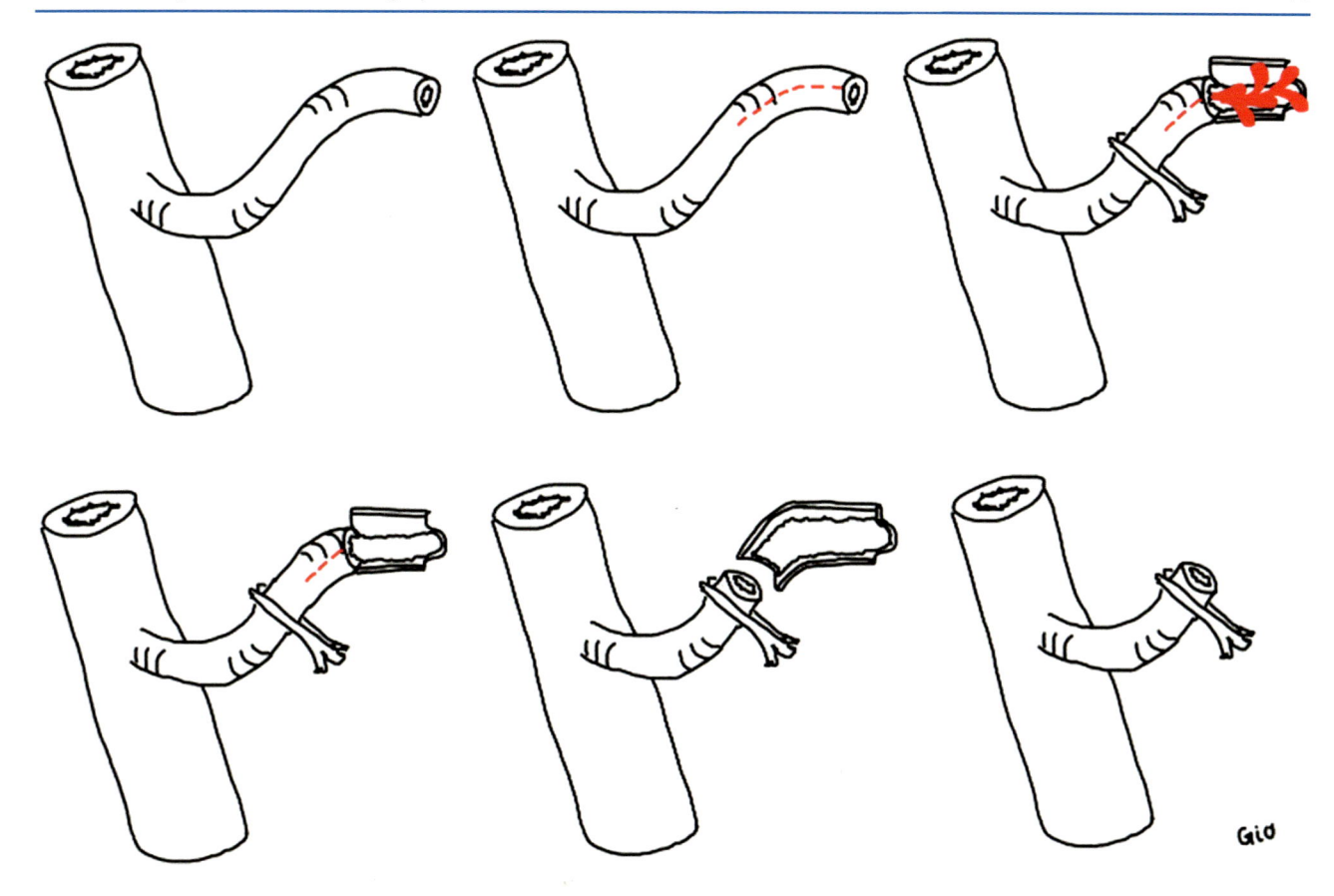

Fig. 9.8 (**a–f**) Step-by-step Miyamoto non-spurting test

- *Step 4:* The distal vessel wall is trimmed with circumferential excision (Fig. 9.8f).

9.10 Dealing with Large Vessel-Size Discrepancy

Vessel-size discrepancy is common in microvascular anastomosis. It interrupts laminal blood flow, predisposing the anastomotic site to thrombi formation. Several techniques have been described to address small- to medium-size discrepancy, including mechanical dilation, end-to-side anastomosis, sleeve anastomosis, and miscellaneous methods such as grafts, adhesives, and couplers. For large vessel-size discrepancies, geometrical techniques seem to be more promising. Below we describe the "fish-mouth" and "sliced-pants" geometrical techniques.

9.11 Fish-Mouth Microvascular Anastomosis Technique

- *Step 1:* Mark the 12 and 6 o'clock position on the vessel circumference in a similar manner as the bi-angulation technique (Fig. 9.9a).
- *Step 2:* With a sharp straight micro-scissors, cut full thickness to allow upscaling of the vessel caliber diameter (Fig. 9.9b).
- *Step 3:* The tiny sharp triangles are smoothened to allow a more linear vessel caliber diameter and unify the vessel circumference (Fig. 9.9c).
- *Step 4:* The vessel has been upscaled and allowed an increase in diameter (Fig. 9.9d).

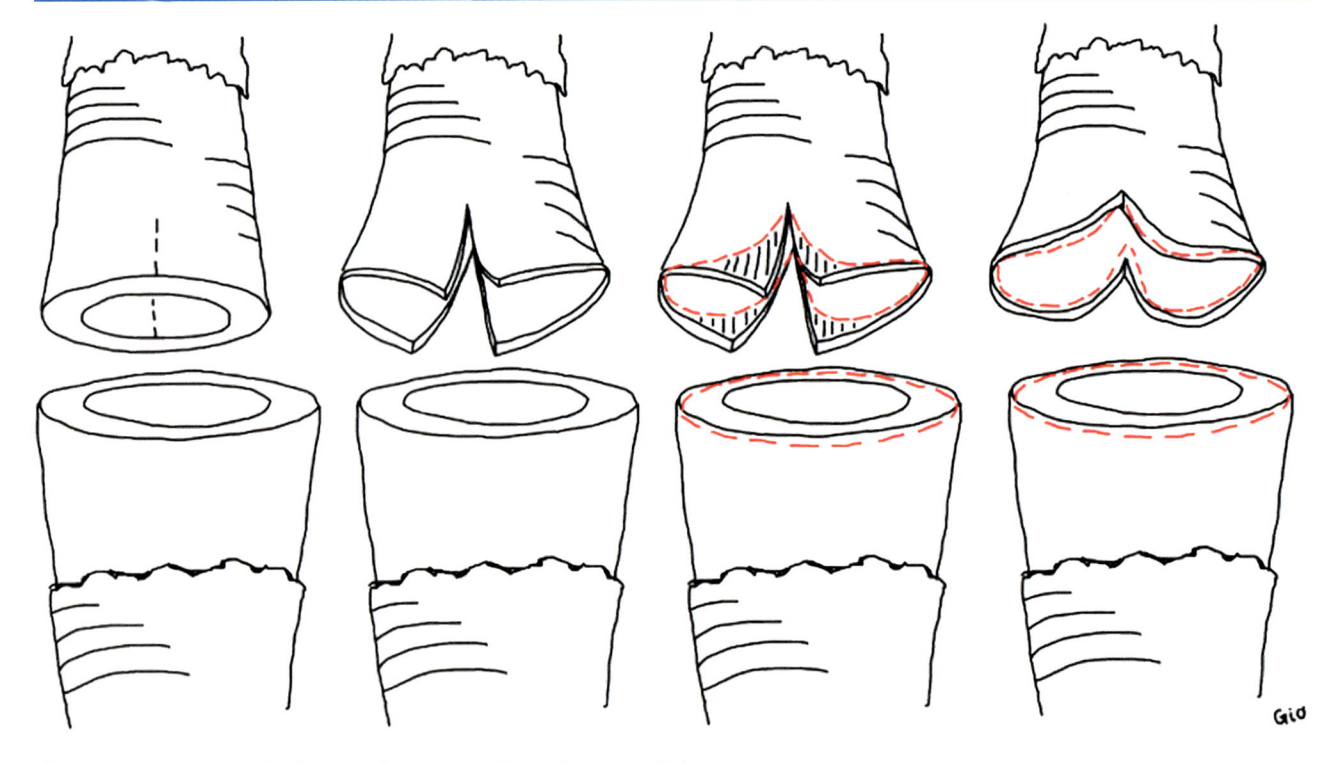

Fig. 9.9 (**a–d**) Fish-mouth microvascular anastomosis step-by-step technique

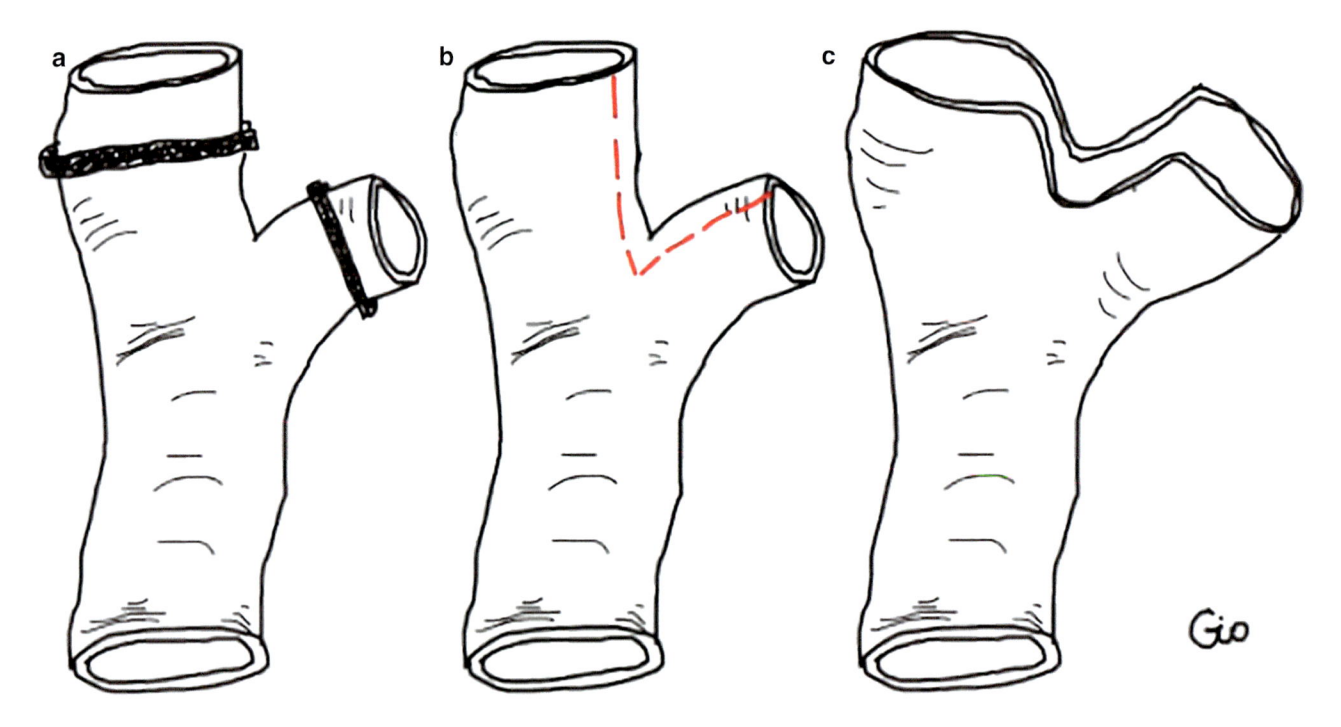

Fig. 9.10 (**a–c**) The sliced-pants technique

9.12 Sliced-Pants Technique

- *Step 1:* Identify a branched donor vessel. The total diameter of the two branches should be slightly larger than the diameter of the recipient vessel (Fig. 9.10a).

- *Step 2:* The adjacent vessel walls of the two branches are incised to remove about 15–20% of the diameter of each vessel (Fig. 9.10b).
- *Step 3:* The two open vessels are sutured together to produce a single vessel of larger caliber (Fig. 9.10c).

References

1. Lin SJ, Lee BT. The intrinsic tying platform in microsurgery. Plast Reconstr Surg. 2009;123(6):223e–4e.
2. Fuse Y, et al. "Quadrupod" Grip for Handling Supermicrosurgical Instruments. J Reconstr Microsurg. 2019;35(5):e1–2.
3. Chen H-C, et al. "Airborne" suture tying technique for the microvascular anastomosis. Plast Reconstr Surg. 2004;113(4):1225–8.
4. Agko M, et al. "Airborne" suture tying technique: simple steps to make it easy. Head Neck. 2017;39(12):2558–61.
5. Nikkhah D, Pafitanis G. Posterior wall first anastomosis for replantation. Plast Reconstr Surg. 2020;146(6):827e. https://journals.lww.com/plasreconsurg/Fulltext/2020/12000/Posterior_Wall_First_Anastomosis_for_Replantation.54.aspx.
6. Harris GD, et al. Posterior-wall-first microvascular anastomotic technique. Br J Plast Surg. 1981;34:47. https://www.jprasurg.com/article/0007-1226(81)90096-5/pdf.
7. Sapountzis S, et al. A novel "continuous-interrupted" method for microvascular anastomosis. Microsurgery. 2014;34(1):82–4.
8. Pafitanis G, et al. The "needle-splint" technique: a method of accurate apposition and eversion during microvascular anastomosis. Plast Reconstr Surg Glob Open. 2020;8(1):e2611.
9. Pafitanis G, et al. The "crater" arteriotomy: a technique aiding precise intimal apposition in end-to-side microvascular anastomosis. Plast Reconstr Surg Glob Open. 2020;8(10):e3014.
10. Lim SY, et al. End-to-patch anastomosis for microvascular transfer of free flaps with small pedicle. J Plast Reconstr Aesthet Surg. 2015;68(4):559–64.
11. Miyamoto S, Fukunaga Y, Sakuraba M. Technical tips to trim the stump of a nonspurting recipient artery. Plast Reconstr Surg Glob Open. 2014;2(11):e248.
12. Harashina T, Irigaray A. Expansion of smaller vessel diameter by fish-mouth incision in microvascular anastomosis with marked size discrepancy. Plast Reconstr Surg. 1980;65(4):502–3.
13. Nicolaides M, Pafitanis G. Overcoming size discrepancy in microvascular anastomosis: the 'sliced-pants' technique. Ann R Coll Surg Engl. 2022;104:234.

Part II
Core Flaps

Temporal Artery Flaps

Oliver J. Smith, Greg O'Toole, and Walid Sabbagh

10.1 Introduction

The superficial temporal artery (STA) is the terminal branch of the external carotid artery and it provides a rich arterial supply to the tissues of the temporal fossa, forehead, upper helix and scalp. The principal flap supplied by the STA is the temporoparietal fascia flap. The TP or TPF flap involves the tissue of the temporoparietal fascia (also known as the superficial temporal fascia). The use of fasciocutaneous tissue supplied by the STA for reconstruction was first described by Monks [1] in 1898 for reconstruction of the lower eyelid. However the TP flap was not popularised until the late twentieth century. It is a thin, pliable and richly vascular fascial flap with a broad arc of rotation making it a versatile flap for reconstruction of the scalp, face, mandible and oral cavity [2]. The TP flap is most commonly used in auricular reconstruction as soft tissue coverage for cartilage-based or synthetic frameworks. It can be raised as an ipsilateral turndown flap, or in rarer cases as a contralateral free tissue transfer. Its rich vascularity makes it an ideal flap to support cartilage and skin grafts and is therefore well suited to ear reconstruction. It can also be used as a pedicled fascial flap for intraoral defects [3] and has been described as a free flap in hand reconstruction to allow tendon glide in full-thickness defects [4]. The STA and accompanying vein can also be used as a vascular pedicle for fasciocutaneous island flaps of forehead and temporal skin to reconstruct a variety of facial [5] and scalp defects [6]. The flap can also be raised with calvarial bone in rare cases for midface reconstruction [7].

O. J. Smith (✉) · G. O'Toole · W. Sabbagh
Department of Plastic and Reconstructive Surgery, Royal Free Hospital, London, UK

10.2 Anatomy

The external carotid artery splits into the STA and the maxillary artery anterior to the ear and within the substance of the parotid gland. Before leaving the parotid gland, the STA gives off the transverse facial artery which runs inferior to the zygomatic arch to supply the masseter and lateral canthal skin. The STA then courses superiorly over the zygomatic arch within the substance of the temporoparietal (TP) fascia where it can be palpated anterior to the tragus, before giving off the middle temporal artery to the temporalis muscle. It then divides above the arch into anterior (frontal) and posterior (parietal) branches. The anterior branch runs forwards to supply the frontalis muscle and frontal scalp and is closely related to the temporal branch of the facial nerve. The posterior branch runs superiorly towards the scalp vertex to supply the parietal skin, periosteum and temporoparietal fascia. The level of bifurcation above the arch of the STA can vary considerably; however in 90% of cases, it is within 2 cm above the tragus [8]. Reconstructive surgeons of the ear should be aware that in the microtia ear, the STA has many anatomical variations and commonly passes more anteriorly over the zygoma than in the healthy ear [9]. The vessel in the microtia patient can be atrophic and therefore difficult to palpate making preoperative planning more challenging.

The course of the superficial temporal vein (STV) is less reliable and often runs apart from the artery. Bifurcation of the STV is also not reliable, and it may continue as a single branch, often running posterior to the artery after it has bifurcated [10]. Unreliability of the vein reduces the versatility of free tissue transfer based on the superficial temporal pedicle and is a consideration when planning to use the superficial temporal vessels as donors for microvascular reconstruction.

The temporoparietal fascia is a thin highly vascularised layer that lies deep to, and is firmly adhered to, the fibrofatty subdermal layer containing the hair follicles of the temporal region. The TP fascia is continuous with the superficial musculoaponeurotic system (SMAS) of the face, the galea superiorly and the frontalis and occipital muscle anteriorly and posteriorly. Deep to the TP fascia is a loose areolar layer within which runs the temporal branch of the facial nerve. This loose areolar layer separates the TP fascia from the deep temporal fascia which overlies the temporalis muscle and becomes continuous with the periosteum superiorly. At this point there is a rich network of anastomotic vessels between the superficial and deep temporal fascias, allowing incorporation of the deeper structures (muscle, periosteum, calvarium) into a flap based on the superficial temporal vessels [11].

Anatomical variation in the vascular supply of the TP fascia is common. An anatomical study by Park et al. found that the TP fascia was supplied by the STA as the dominant vessel in 88% of cases [12], with the remainder supplied by the posterior auricular artery and occipital artery as the dominant vessel. Venous drainage of the fascia is even more variable with only 67% drained by the STV as the dominant draining vessel. However, a TP flap is always raised on the STA as the vascular pedicle. In situations where the STA is not palpable, fascia could be raised on the other arteries, but these flaps would not be described as TP flaps.

10.3 Preoperative Investigation

It is important to take a comprehensive history prior to surgical planning to identify any contraindications to TP flap usage such as previous trauma, irradiation, surgery or carotid artery pathology. The superficial temporal artery can be identified preoperatively by digital palpation and the position confirmed with handheld Doppler. Care should be taken to identify the main pedicle and both the anterior and posterior branches. Preoperative imaging for the purposes of raising the flap is not necessary.

10.4 Flap Design and Markings

The positions of the main pedicle, anterior and posterior branches, and the hairline are marked. The hair is shaved along the course of the vessel and the planned incision sites, although it may be prudent to shave a larger area in ear reconstruction (Fig. 10.1). The fascial flap is most commonly raised via a 'Y'-shaped incision with a straight limb anterior to the ear extending into a 'Y' shape superiorly to allow good exposure of the fascia. However several other incisions are described including a zigzag incision favoured by one of our senior authors (Fig. 10.2) which has shown to improve postoperative scarring [13], a horizontal straight line (Fig. 10.3), two parallel lines, or an incision around the ear to lift the pocket. The size of

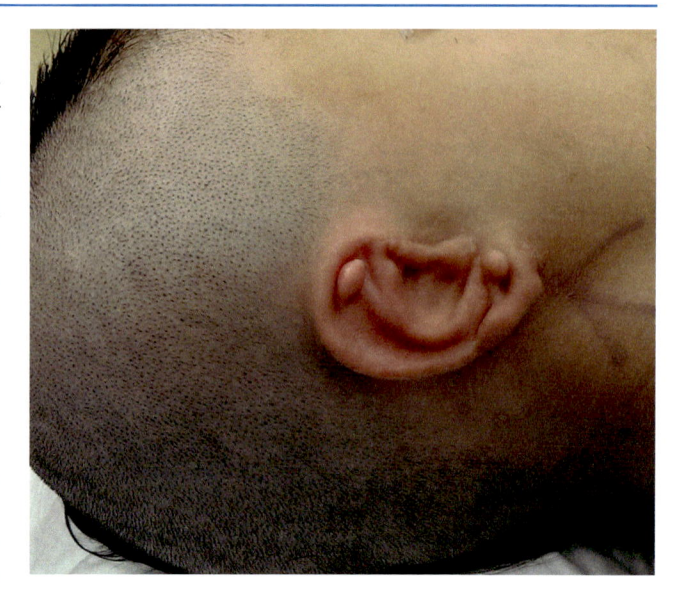

Fig. 10.1 Picture illustrating the degree of hair shaving required when using the TP flap for ear reconstruction

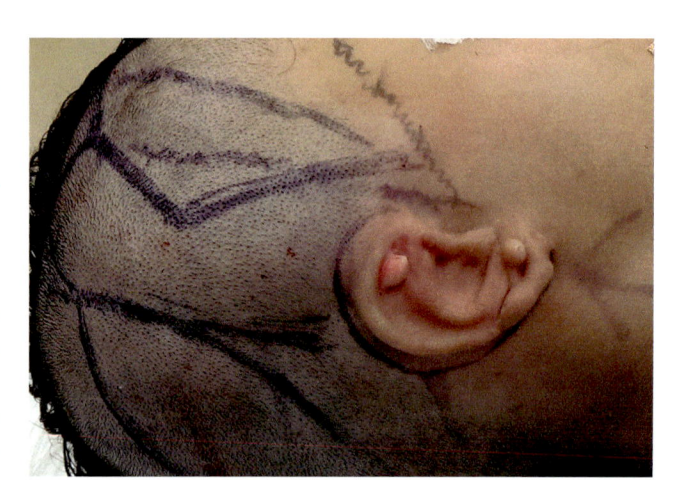

Fig. 10.2 Picture showing the preoperative markings for a zigzag incision. Also marked are the anterior and posterior temporal artery branches and the area of the TP fascia

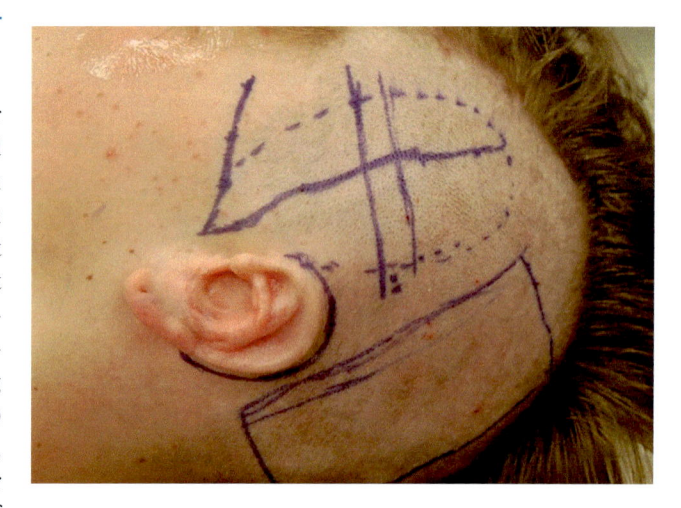

Fig. 10.3 Picture showing the preoperative markings for a transverse incision. Also marked are the anterior and posterior temporal artery branches and the area of the TP fascia

the flap required should be marked on the fascia after the initial skin raise and should be narrowed at the cephalic end to avoid damage to the temporal branch of the facial nerve. In rare instances where a fasciocutaneous flap is required for skin defects, this is designed and marked on the skin over the posterior branch. A TP flap based on the anterior branch is rare due to the risk of brow ptosis and unilateral forehead paralysis; however cutaneous island flaps can be raised on this vessel where non-hair bearing-skin is required. If reconstruction of hair-bearing skin is required, a 2–3-cm-wide pedicle can be easily closed, and defects of up to 4 × 5 cm have been described [14]; however skin defects larger than this may require preoperative expansion.

10.5 Flap Elevation

- Step 1: Local anaesthetic infiltration and hydro-dissection of the superficial plane

  Local anaesthetic is infiltrated along the marked incision lines and within the superficial plane. This is a difficult plane to inject due to the adherence of the subcutaneous fat to the fascia, but if the correct plane is found, this assists in the dissection of this plane at the next step. The key is to see subcutaneous spreading of the fluid under the skin. Hyalase can be added to the local anaesthetic mix to help in developing the plane.

- Step 2: Incision and skin elevation (Fig. 10.4)

  After the initial incisions are made sharp, dissection is commenced at the level just deep to the hair follicles. A plane can be found where the subcutaneous fat is adhered to the TP fascia, although identification of this plane can be difficult and care must be taken to avoid damaging the hair follicles which may lead to postoperative alopecia. The STA is located on the surface of the fascia, and great care should be taken in elevating the skin over the STA to ensure the vessel is not damaged and included in the flap. The veins (if present) are usually found within the subcutaneous fat.

- Step 3: Elevation of the posterior flap (Fig. 10.5)

  Once the TP fascia is exposed, the frontal branch of the artery and any veins not included in the flap are ligated or cauterised. Elevation of the posterior flap at the avascular deep plane is then straightforward. The posterior flap is raised superior to inferior, cauterising rare perforating vessels to the deeper tissues as the flap raise advances. The pedicle is then dissected caudally to the desired pivot point.

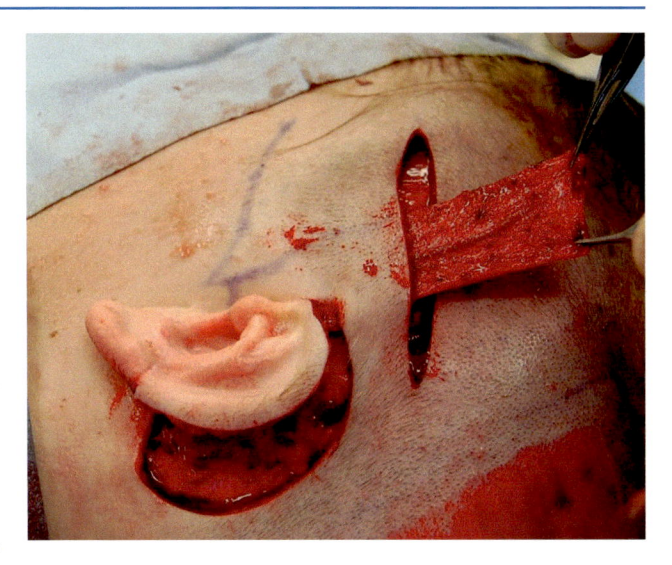

Fig. 10.4 Picture showing the flap dissected free from the overlying skin. Visible on the surface of the flap is the temporal artery

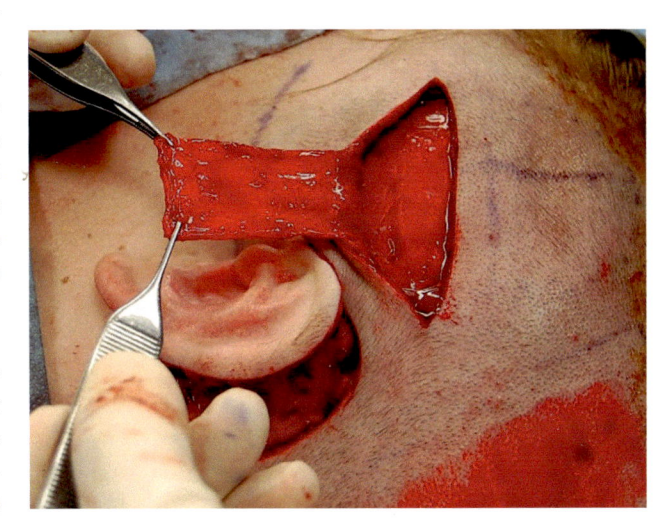

Fig. 10.5 Picture showing elevation of the posterior flap

10.6 Core Surgical Techniques in Flap Dissection

- Step 1: Hydro-dissection

  The authors' preference is to use a dental local anaesthetic such as Lignospan (lidocaine with adrenaline). A fine dental needle (30 G) should be used to avoid damage to vessels and the surgeon should not inject directly over the vessels. The adrenaline will help to reduce bleeding from the richly vascular subdermal scalp plexus during skin dissection and allow a better view of the operative field. Local anaesthetic should be infiltrated at least

30 min before surgery to give the adrenaline time to work. Hyalase may be added to assist in developing the superficial plane. Injection directly over the vessel should be avoided to prevent damage.
- Step 2. Skin elevation

    Identification and careful preservation of the superficial temporal vessels as they traverse the subcutaneous fat superficial to the fascia. The STV is especially vulnerable as these pass posterior to the artery and in a more superficial plane [5]. These vessels must be dissected and traced down to the pedicle anterior to the tragus. Therefore dissection under loupe magnification is recommended. The authors recommend skin elevation to be undertaken with a sharp scalpel or a Colorado needle on a low setting. Dissection should be at the level just deep to the hair follicles. The use of bipolar cautery should be minimised to avoid damaging hair follicles. If inclusion of an STV branch is not possible, then the fascial cuff enveloping the arterial pedicle should be kept a few centimetres wider to allow venous drainage via the fascial venous network.
- Step 3. Posterior flap raise

    The flap should be designed so that the caudal end is as narrow as possible but also ensuring incorporation of the pedicle and any veins. This allows the maximum arc of rotation whilst also ensuring adequate vascular supply. The pedicle should be dissected free of tethering tissue to ensure a tension-free transfer to the recipient site.

    If the surgeon requires bone, then this can be included in the flap by preserving the desired width of fascial connection to the periosteum and deep temporal fascia (which are continuous with each other) above the temporal line which can be palpated at the cephalic border of the temporalis muscle. The outer table is then harvested using a right-angled saw and curbed osteotome and the dissection is then continued below this as outlined in step 3.
- Step 4: Closure and postoperative care

    Direct, multilayered closure is achievable in most cases. The authors recommend a fine absorbable suture such as 5.0 monocryl to close the deep dermal tissue. Deep sutures should be kept to a minimum as these can damage hair follicles. An interrupted 5.0 nylon or prolene suture should be used for the skin and removed at 7 days. When direct closure would lead to undue tension on the skin, a V-Y skin flap advancement is used for closure. The authors recommend the use of a low suction drain to prevent haematoma which can be removed 24 h postoperatively.

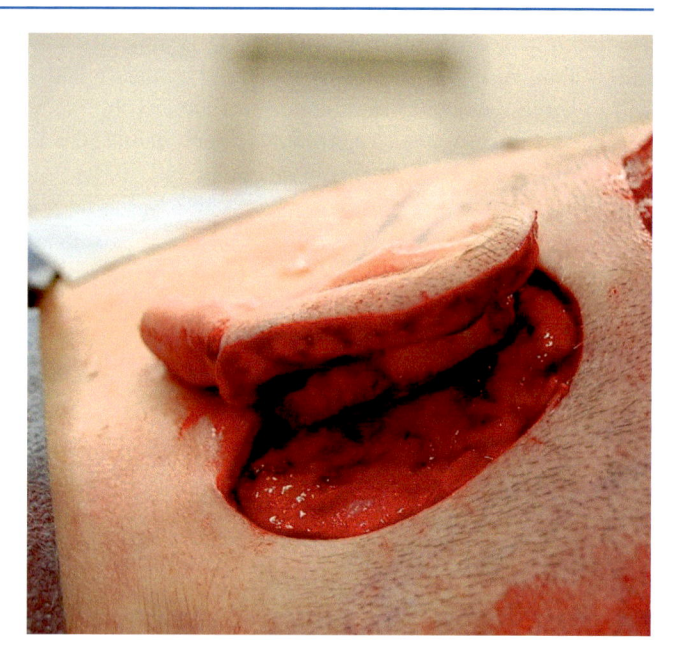

Fig. 10.6 Picture showing second stage ear reconstruction with cartilage framework release and skin insufficiency requiring TP flap coverage

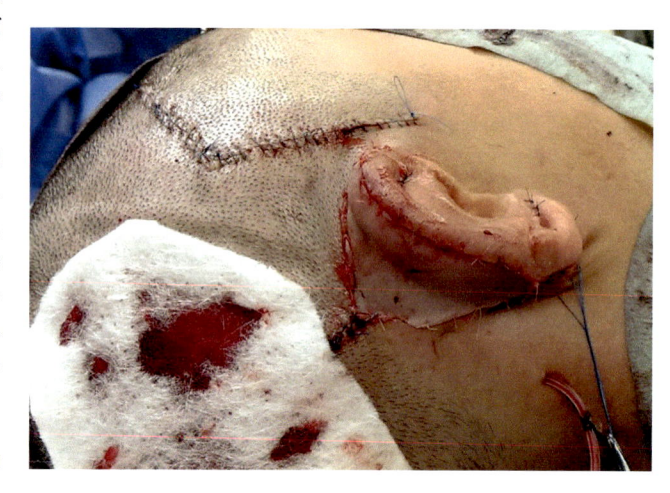

Fig. 10.7 Picture showing coverage of cartilage framework with TP flap and split skin graft

10.7 Clinical Scenario

A TP flap is most commonly used in the second stage of ear reconstruction where the auricular framework is elevated and the flap is used to provide additional soft tissue coverage, with a split thickness or full-thickness skin graft used to provide final skin coverage [15] (Figs. 10.6 and 10.7). This technique can also be used to cover a polyethylene implant [16] although it is the authors' preference to use an autologous technique. The flap may also be used in cases of ear reconstruction where there is inadequate local skin to cover the auricular framework. This may be the case in severe microtia where there is a deficiency of the skin, or in cases of low hairline, previous trauma, irradiation or secondary reconstruction where previous surgery has failed leaving heavily scarred tissue and a lack of skin.

10.8 Pearls and Pitfalls

Pearls

- Use Doppler to accurately mark the position of the vessels preoperatively due to the wide variation in vessel anatomy.
- Skin incision can be sloped in direction of hair follicles to minimise risk of alopecia.
- The undersurface of the flap is a safe zone and can be dissected very easily.
- Venous drainage often the problem therefore tries to include a posterior vein or keep the base of the flap as wide as possible.
- Take extra care during skin raise to avoid hair follicle damage. The use of hydro-dissection will assist this.

Pitfalls

- The flap may be more appropriate in girls with long hair as this helps to hide the scar and any alopecia. Boys with shorter hair are more likely to have more visible scarring.
- There is also a higher risk of unsatisfactory postoperative scarring in those with fairer hair compared to darker hair.
- Scars can stretch leaving an unsatisfactory cosmetic outcome.
- There is high risk of vessel damage during flap elevation.
- There is risk of temporal branch of facial nerve injury during elevation of the anterior flap.

10.9 Selected Readings

- Park C, Lew D-H, Yoo W-M. An analysis of 123 temporoparietal fascial flaps: anatomic and clinical considerations in total auricular reconstruction. Plast Reconstr Surg. 1999;104:1295–306.

  A comprehensive clinical and anatomical analysis of one units extensive experience in using TP flaps for auricular reconstruction.

- Nagata S. A new method of total reconstruction of the auricle for microtia. Plast Reconstr Surg. 1993;92(2):187–201.

  Seminal paper on microtia reconstruction.

- Nagata S. Secondary reconstruction for unfavorable microtia results utilizing temporoparietal and innominate fascia flaps. Plast Reconstr Surg. 1994;94:254–65.

  Pioneer of ear surgery discussing the use of TP flaps in complex and redo microtia surgery.

- Gillies HD. Plastic surgery of the face. New York, NY: Gower Medical Publishing Ltd; 1983.

  Classic text from the father of plastic surgery who outlines the use of pedicled island flaps based on the superficial temporal vessels for facial reconstruction.

References

1. Monks GH. The restoration of a lower lid by a new method. Bost Med Surg J. 1898;139:385–7.
2. Collar RM, Zopf D, Brown D, Fung K, Kim J. The versatility of the temporoparietal fascia flap in head and neck reconstruction. J Plast Reconstr Aesthet Surg. 2012;65:141–8.
3. Nayak VK, Deschler DG. Pedicled temporoparietal fascial flap reconstruction of select intraoral defects. Laryngoscope. 2004;114(9):1545–8.
4. Upton J, Rogers C, Durham-Smith G, Swartz WM. Clinical applications of free temporoparietal flaps in hand reconstruction. J Hand Surg. 1986;11(4):475–83.
5. Elbanoby TM, Zidan SM, Elbatawy AM, Aly GM, Sholkamy K. Superficial temporal artery flap for reconstruction of complex facial defects: a new algorithm. Arch Plast Surg. 2018;45:118–27.
6. Tenna S, Brunetti B, Aveta A, Poccia I, Perichetti P. Scalp reconstruction with superficial temporal artery island flap: clinical experience on 30 consecutive cases. J Plast Reconstr Aesthet Surg. 2013;66:660–6.
7. Davison SP, Mesbahi AN, Clemens MW, et al. Vascularized calvarial bone flaps and midface reconstruction. Plast Reconstr Surg. 2008;122:10e–8e.
8. Beheiry EE, Abdel-Hamid FA. An anatomical study of the temporal fascia and related temporal pads of fat. Plast Reconstr Surg. 2007;119(1):136–44.
9. Olcott CM, Simon PE, Romo T III, Louie W. Anatomy of the superficial temporal artery in patients with unilateral microtia. J Plast Reconstr Aesthet Surg. 2019;72:114–8.
10. Ausen K, Pavlovic I. Flaps pedicled on the superficial temporal artery and vein in facial reconstruction: a versatile option with a venous pitfall. J Plast Surg Hand Surg. 2011;45:178–87.
11. Nakajima H, Imanishi N, Minabe T. The arterial anatomy of the temporal region and the vascular basis of various temporal flaps. Br J Plast Surg. 1995;48:439–50.
12. Park C, Lew D-H, Yoo W-M. An analysis of 123 temporoparietal fascial flaps: anatomic and clinical considerations in total auricular reconstruction. Plast Reconstr Surg. 1999;104:1295–306.
13. Tanaka A, Hatoko M, Kuwahara M, Yurugi S, Lioka H, Niitsuma K. Evaluation of scars after harvest of the temporoparietal fascial flap depending on the design of the skin incision. Ann Plast Surg. 2002;48(4):376–80.
14. Algan S, Kara M, Cinal H, Barin EZ, Inaloz A, Tan O. The temporal artery island flap: a good reconstructive option for small to medium-sized facial defects. J Oral Maxillofac Surg. 2018;76:894–9.
15. Nagata S. A new method of total reconstruction of the auricle for microtia. Plast Reconstr Surg. 1993;92(2):187–201.
16. Tahir Y, Reinisch J. Porous polyethylene ear reconstruction. Clin Plast Surg. 2019;46(2):223–30.

Supraorbital and Supratrochlear Artery Flaps - Forehead Flap and Modifications

Daniel B. Saleh and Alex Dearden

11.1 Introduction

The first evidenced scripture of the forehead flap was believed to be around 600 BC, in India, in the ancient medical treatises the Sushruta Samhita [1]. Modern translation reveals the description of the total nasal reconstruction was derived from a cheek flap but nevertheless was the first description of a pedicled tissue transfer in contemporary reconstructive terms.

The Italian Antonio Branca brought the forehead flap to Europe in the fifteenth century [2], but it was not until 1794 when J. C. Carpue read an editorial in *The Gentleman's Magazine* where its journey to become the workhorse for nasal reconstruction began [3]. Following his intrigue in the novel technique, he practised on cadavers for over 20 years before utilising it on two soldiers in 1814 [4].

Further refinements were made, the most recent iterations of which have been popularised by Burget and Menick in the 1980s [5–7] by narrowing the base of the paramedian flap for greater arc of rotation and the safety of debulking the distal flap superficial to the frontalis muscle. These have largely been borne out of better anatomic understanding in conjunction with the reconstructive concepts of angiosomes, delay and dermal blood supply.

11.2 Anatomy

Typically, four paired arteries supply the forehead skin:

- Angular, branching into the dorsal nasal and central
- Supratrochlear
- Supraorbital
- Superficial temporal and its terminal branches

D. B. Saleh (✉)
Plastic and Reconstructive Surgery, Royal Victoria Infirmary, Newcastle Upon Tyne, UK

A. Dearden
Royal Victoria Infirmary, Newcastle Upon Tyne, UK

Although orientated in an axial direction, the arborising nature of these vessels makes a rich interconnecting network of vascularity orientated in the glabella and medial canthal region [8]. This has enabled the application of various flaps designs and their refinements over the past century to address a variety of reconstructive challenges in the facial, head and neck regions.

Mangold's injection study demonstrated that the median and paramedian flaps are positioned so that their main supply is from the supratrochlear artery with additional filling from the dorsal nasal and supraorbital arteries [9].

The supratrochlear artery is a terminal branch of the ophthalmic artery. It exits the superior medial orbit 1.7–2.2 cm lateral to the midline and continues a vertical course for approximately 3 cm at the medial position of the brow [8]. It initially lies superficial to the corrugator supercilii muscle but deep to the orbicularis and frontalis at the level of the brow then traversing the frontalis to lie in the subcutaneous tissues 1 cm above the brow where the option of flap debulking is possible.

The paired dorsal nasal arteries usually merge after 5 mm to form a single central artery supplying the glabella and inferior and middle transverse thirds of the central forehead [10]. A recent histological study [11] suggests it is the central artery to be the prominent blood supply of the medial forehead flap design challenging its nomenclature as a true axial flap of the supratrochlear artery. The central artery forehead flap is now well described in the contemporary literature [12].

The frontal (anterior) branch of the superficial temporal artery enters the forehead at different transverse levels at the lateral orbital rim. Once it crosses this line, it usually divides into an ascending branch and a transverse branch of smaller diameter at this level [10]. The anterior superficial temporal artery is superficial to the temporalis muscle, and as it medialises it gradually becomes more superficial to a subdermal level. The average diameter of the anterior superficial temporal artery is 2 mm at the level of the lateral orbital rim [10]. Care must be taken to preserve the temporal branch on the facial nerve which runs anteroinferiorly to the artery with

64% predictability; thus surgical precision is paramount in this region to avoid neural injury [13].

The venous system is formed from the parallel supratrochlear and central veins. They converge over the glabella to drain into the angular veins either side of the nose. The central vein is often larger on one side of the forehead and should also be incorporated into the flap design. Furthermore it can aid as a landmark to decide which side of the forehead to use to ensure optimal drainage.

11.3 Preoperative Investigation

Routine preoperative radiology is seldom required in planning these flaps unless there has been significant surgery in the region and axial vascular supply is in question. In such circumstances computed tomography with contrast can be useful for identification of enhancing vessels along their complete course and permits cross midline comparison to correlate with previous scars.

Handheld Doppler examination with intensity of at least 8 Hz in the clinic will determine the presence of suitable vessels that can be used for flap transfer. This can be augmented by use of infrared thermography (see stepwise flap raising).

We have successfully transferred forehead flaps in patients with superficial scars from cutaneous malignancy resection and even deep dermal/full-thickness burns. Specifically, if there is axial pulsation on Doppler examination, scars can be incorporated into flap design in absolutely necessary. However one must consider a delay procedure in the first incidence to maximise success in these rarer scenarios.

11.3.1 Flap Design and Markings: Multistage Forehead Flap

11.3.1.1 The Multistage Paramedian Forehead Flap

The relative focus of this description pertains to nasal reconstruction but can be translated to an array of periocular, cheek and upper labial defects. An ipsilateral flap is better suited to treating defects on the ipsilateral nose or face if available.

The exact defect dimensions should be templated, and if this is challenging due to major distortion and secondary cicatrix, if available, the contralateral normal side should be templated as a mirror image (Fig. 11.1).

The multistage forehead flap tends to offer better functional and cosmetic outcomes in nasal reconstruction and the opportunity to better control structural support introduced into the repair.

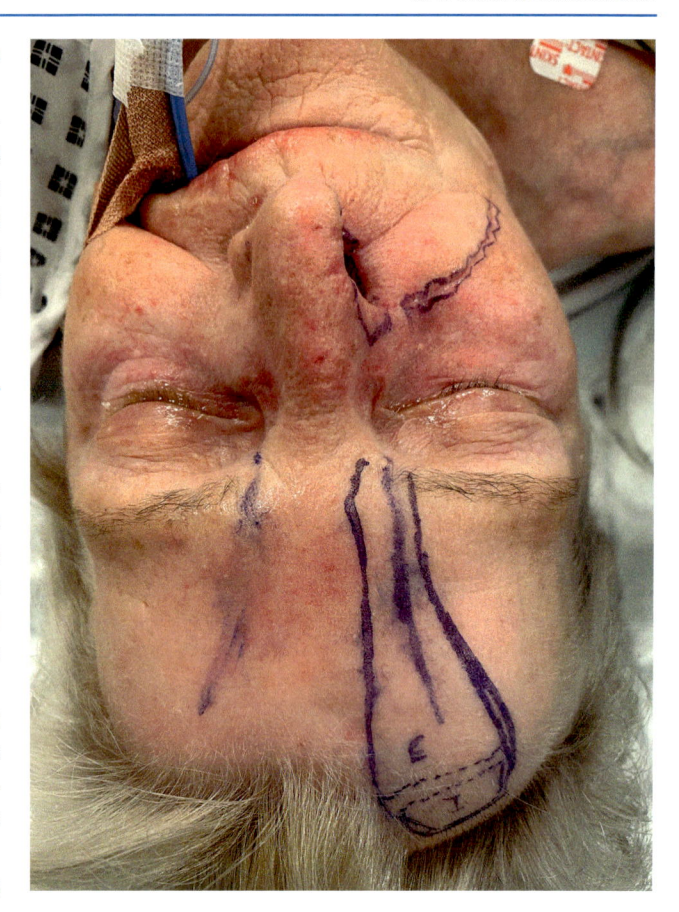

Fig. 11.1 A pre-templated and Dopplered paramedian forehead flap for a hemi-nasal reconstruction. Templates were taken from the normal contralateral side

11.3.2 The Anterior Superficial Temporal Artery Flap

This is a very useful forehead flap based on the anterior or frontal division of the superficial temporal artery (STA) flap. Lei and colleagues succinctly delineated the anatomy and that whilst the ASTA is essentially constant, it can vary in being a 'high' or 'low' type [13]. This flap incurs a scar in the suprabrow, or anterior temporal region, but has the versatility to reconstruct the periorbital and cheek region. This is a myocutaneous flap to ensure reliable vascularity as the vessels at its medial course can be intramuscular.

11.3.3 Flap Raise/Elevation: A Step-by-Step Guide

11.3.3.1 The Multistage Paramedian Forehead Flap

Where possible place the patient in marginal head down position supine to increase forehead blood flow and induce temporary venous filling.

1. Palpate the supratrochlear notch and place the handheld Doppler over this area in the medial brow region.
2. Follow the pulsation cranially to outline the exact pathway of the vessel (Fig. 11.1). In anaesthetised patients ensure they are normotensive. In the virgin forehead, it is not critical to do this, but it does allow much more accurate flap planning, reducing forehead wound morbidity and theoretically providing a more accurate wound repair.
3. Reverse plan using a gauze to ensure the correct length of flap is planned. Base your preformed template on the vessel axiality unless the hair pattern dictates a more lateral placement. This is less critical in cases whereby the distal flap is aimed at internal nasal lining, where hair growth is accepted (Fig. 11.1).
4. The proximal limits of the skin flap width need only to be approximately 1–2 cm centred over the Doppler signal; this also allows easier rotation of the flap to the defect (Fig. 11.1).
5. The flap is raised in a distal to proximal (cranial to caudal) fashion incising the skin, subcutaneous fat and frontalis muscle down to the periosteum. The upper two-thirds alone are incised initially. Blade dissection is preferable but monopolar cautery can also be used with low setting for the coagulation in order to protect the periosteum to permit maximal healing potential without desiccation.
6. Once this portion of the flap is raised, use the on-table Doppler to ensure the signal is present in the flap. Whilst this is not vital, with minimal fuss, it only takes 30–40 s to do and avoids the rare situation whereby anomalous anatomy is encountered.
7. Once the position of the vessel has been rechecked, the remaining skin incisions are made through the skin, and at the base of the wound, the periosteum is incised to continue in the sub-periosteal plane (Fig. 11.2). An Obwegeser elevator is gently used to lift the periosteum with the bevel facing the bone. Then blunt dissection with a Jameson or littler scissors will tease the fibres of the frontalis, procerus and corrugator supercilii to reveal the underlying periosteum at the medial and lateral extents of the flap edges. It is our preference to do this bluntly, because occasionally draining veins can be favourable placed in the arc of rotation for the flap; hence there is no need for ligation of these medial intramuscular veins unless they impede eventual flap transfer.
8. Once the skin and muscle dissection has reached the brow and the flap is liberated, the sub-periosteal dissection continues with care around the medial supraorbital bar where the vascular pedicle can be visualised in three typical configurations (Fig. 11.3):
   (a) Emerging from a supraorbital notch where the vessels are freely mobile with gentle caudal displacement

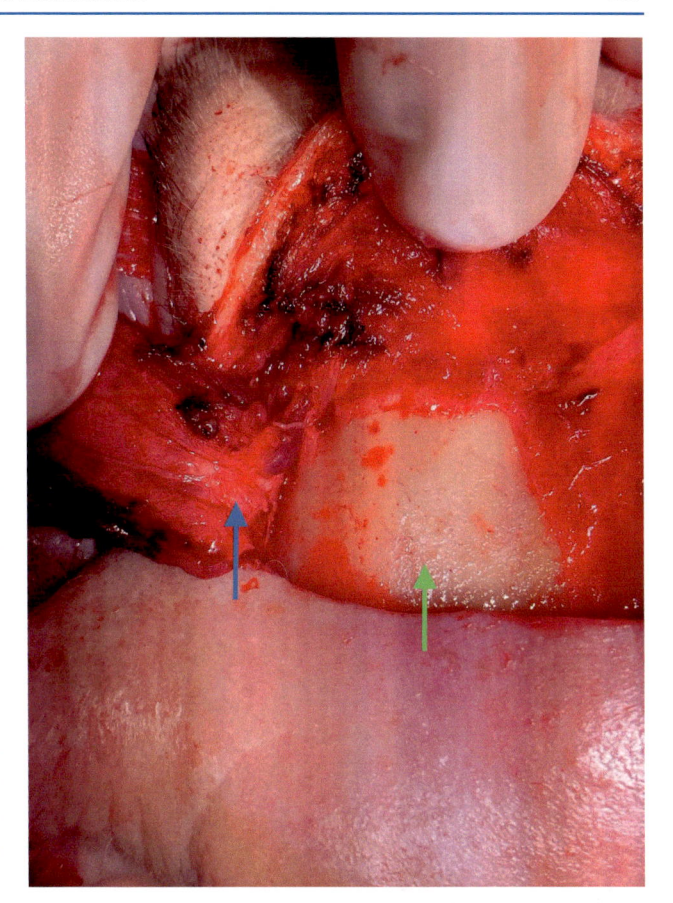

Fig. 11.2 The flap turned down caudally revealing the periosteum with denuded frontal bar and intact periosteum cranially

   (b) Emerging through a foramen, which may require a 2 mm osteotome to free the vessels (Figs. 11.4 and 11.5)
   (c) Emerging through a ligamentous foramen where the ligament can be divided with a Mitchell's trimmer

11.3.3.2 Point for Consideration

There is a variety of postulation, pontification and assertion regarding the need to see and mobilise the vessels in the above fashion. It is our preference to take the flap caudal to the brow to allow ease of rotation to the nasal defect. In the majority of cases, this requires one of the above manoeuvres to succeed. However, for cranial nasal defects, or eyelid/cheek resurfacing (for a contralateral forehead flap), a well-planned flap may avoid the need for dissection that involves seeing the pedicle, and thus, the flap could be regarded as agnostic with reference to the vascular pedicle. It is also reasonable to state avoiding dissection around (not of) the pedicle reduces the risk of inadvertent injury, compromising the reconstructive efforts. In general a cut as one goes principle for locoregional reconstruction is useful when one knows there is an axial supply within the flap.

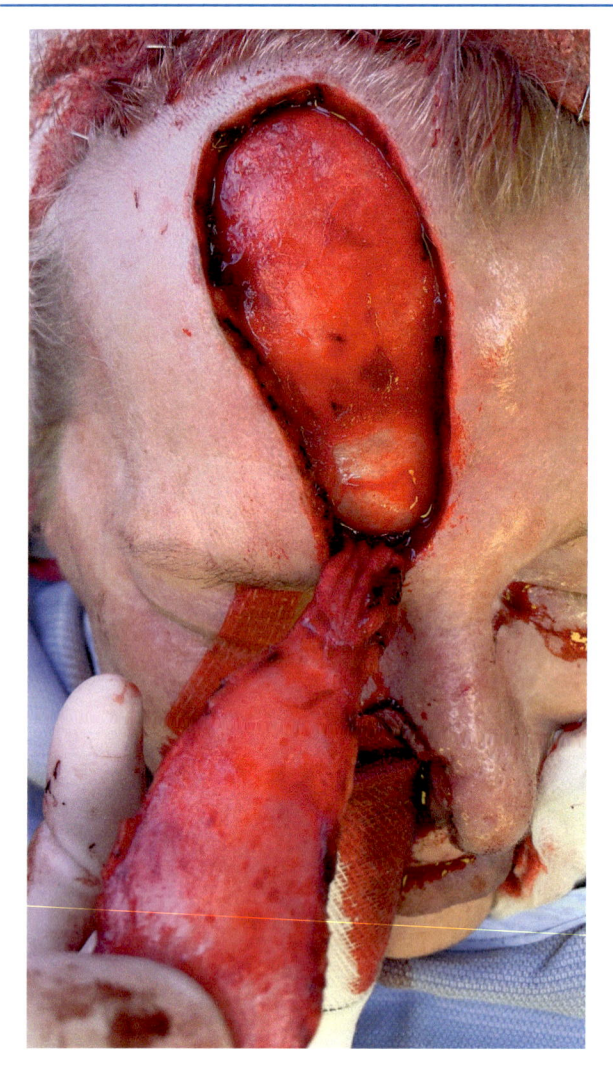

Fig. 11.3 Flap released from supraorbital bar over the medial brow

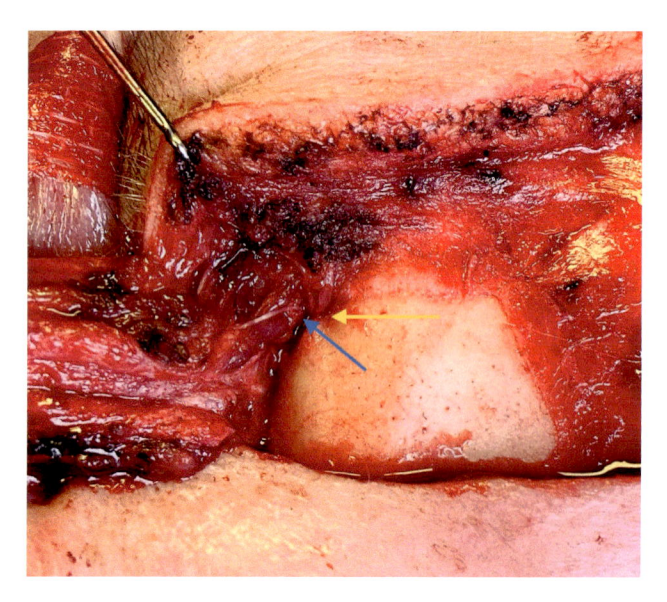

Fig. 11.4 Neurovascular structures emerging from a foramen; the yellow arrow depicts a retracted medial branch of the supratrochlear nerve, and the blue arrow shows the main vascular pedicle, with minor contributing venous branches laterally

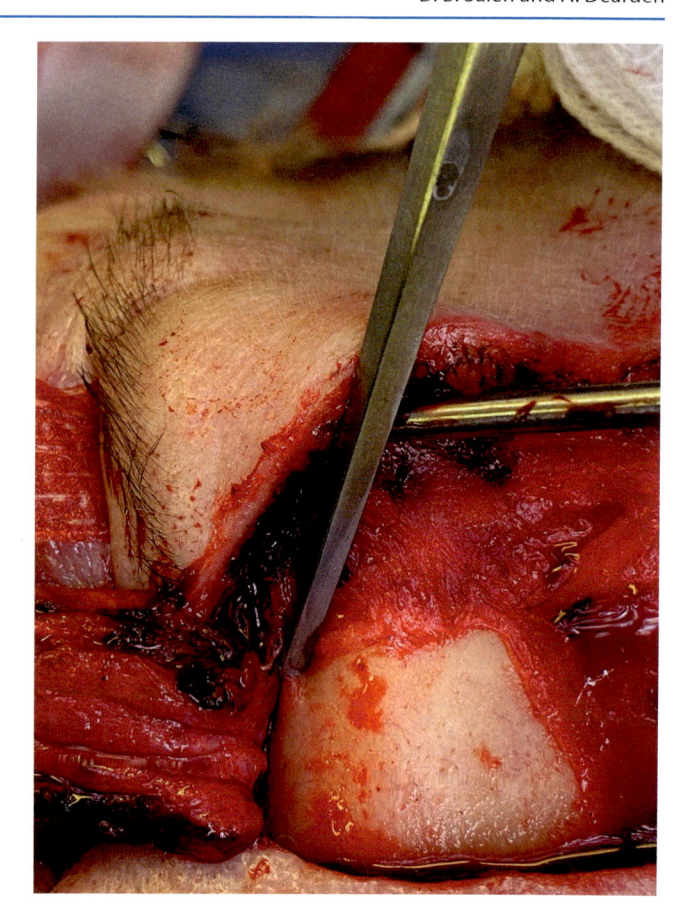

Fig. 11.5 2 mm osteotome to open the frontal foramen

A counterargument we, and others, would highlight is that in certain circumstances (e.g. a hemi-nasal reconstruction), inadequate caudal dissection and thus rotation of the flap may manifest itself as vascular (venous) kinking, also compromising the blood supply. So overall, with due care and attention, vascular visualisation, without overt pedicle dissection, is our preference.

9. The flap is now free to be transferred to the recipient site. We like to oppose the donor wound just above the brow first (Fig. 11.6), to align the brows correctly and ensure this does not cause any unusual flap compromise. It is frustrating to recognise the brows are mal-aligned following meticulous inset of the flap at the recipient site.

11.3.4 Anterior Superficial Temporal Forehead Flap

11.3.4.1 Patient Preparation, Marking and Surgery

1. Doppler examination starting pre-auricular and distal course is followed into the forehead/brow region depending on 'high/low' variant.

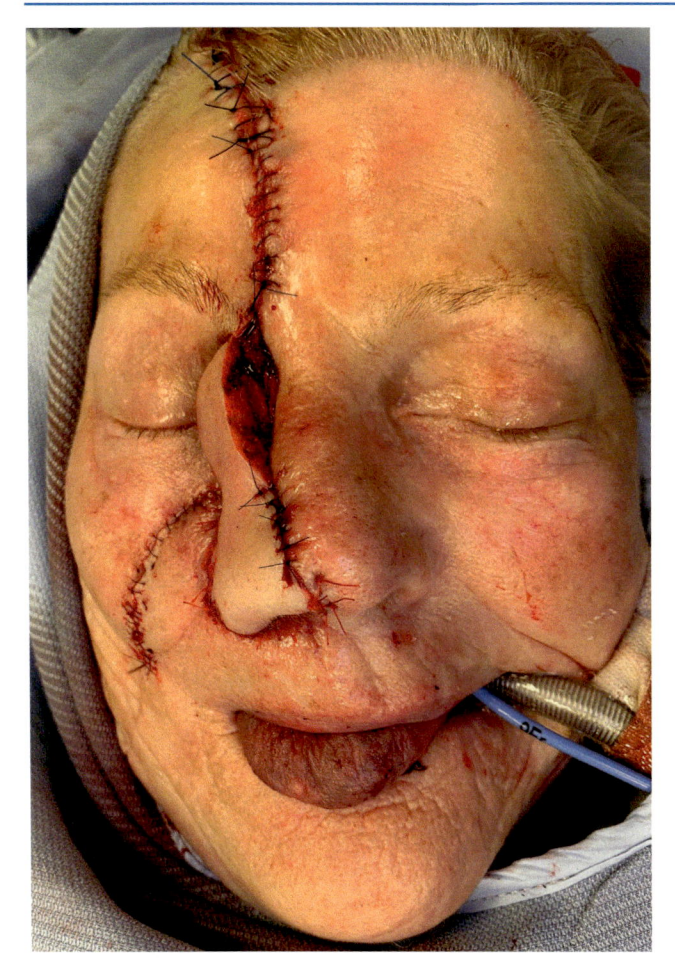

Fig. 11.6 Brow inset first (one or two sutures) followed by nasal inset

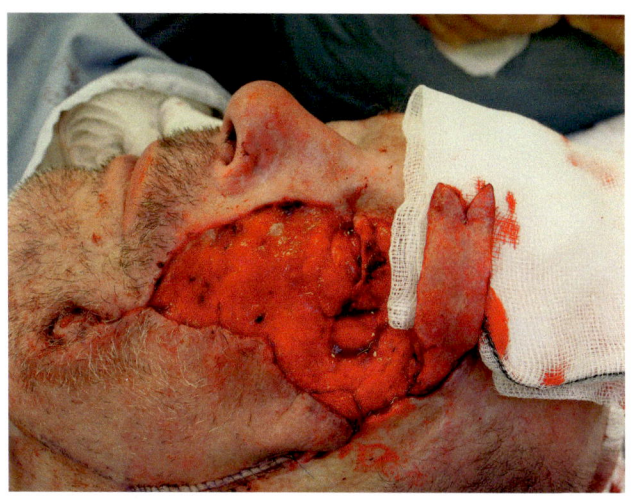

Fig. 11.7 Raised anterior superficial temporal artery flap in a facial reconstruction for a first-stage upper and lower eyelid reconstruction

11.3.5 Transverse Temporal Forehead Flaps

In keeping with the principles described above, the whole forehead (or parts of) unit can be raised in the submuscular plane for a variety of facial and intraoral defects, the latter typically being in a two-stage fashion requiring pedicle division after 3 weeks. This approach, whilst uncommon, has distinct advantages, in particular where facial salvage is paramount:

2. Ideally aim for direct closure—skin pinch to assess viability of direct closure and reverse plan the arc of the flap.
3. 'Zig-zag' or curvilinear incision over temporal course of the vessel, with skin flaps raised in subcutaneous plane until islanded incisions are made. Or in cases where lid reconstruction does not warrant significant pedicle mobilisation, we recommend a medial to lateral cut as you go approach to limit incisions made. This is preferred in case remedial facial procedures are required, or in patients in cutaneous malignancy where tissue preservation is more preferable (Fig. 11.7).
4. The islanded flap is then incised to include the caudal portion of the frontalis and bluntly dissect through the corrugator supercilii and orbital portions of the orbicularis oculi muscle to reach the areolar submuscle plane. Medially this plane is more adherent, and care must be taken to preserve the periosteum and supratrochlear/orbital neurovascular bundles.
5. The flap can then be raised in this plane from medial to lateral. At the lateral brow region, the dissection is blunt in the muscular plane to preserve terminating branches of the frontal nerve.

1. Midfacial and lower facial defects whereby the 'cranial' direction of scar and contracture of the flap is favourable to support the soft tissues and prevent unfavourable downward pull as seen in similar flaps from the upper chest to the lower face. Or from midfacial tissues to the lower eyelids.
2. In intraoral or facial tumour cases whereby a microsurgical solution is either not possible or has been used to maximal effect, for example, a patient who has had numerous oropharyngeal resections, free tissue transfers and radiation therapy (Figs. 11.8 and 11.9).

11.3.6 Core Surgical Techniques in Flap Dissection

11.3.6.1 Staged Considerations: Nasal Reconstruction

Prior to commencing nasal reconstruction, adjacent but contiguous defects in the eyelid(s), upper lip and cheek(s) must be repaired first to provide a stable surrounding framework for the nose. In certain cases, such as skin cancer cutaneopaths, in whom facial skin is in short supply, the forehead flap can be used for marginal medial cheek restoration at the

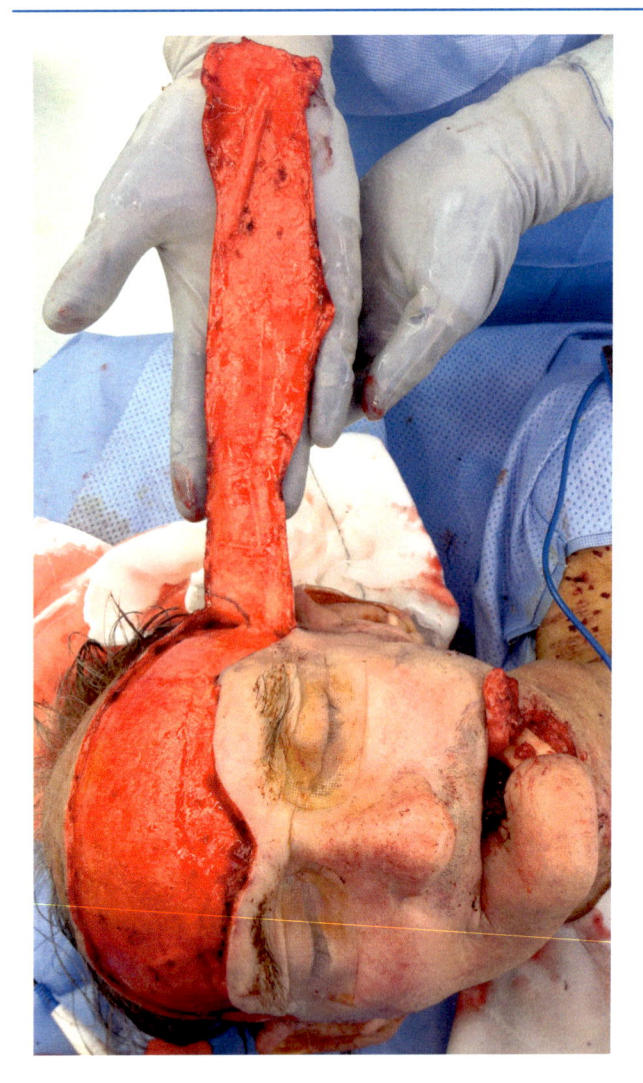

Fig. 11.8 A total forehead unit transverse flap raised on the left superficial temporal artery

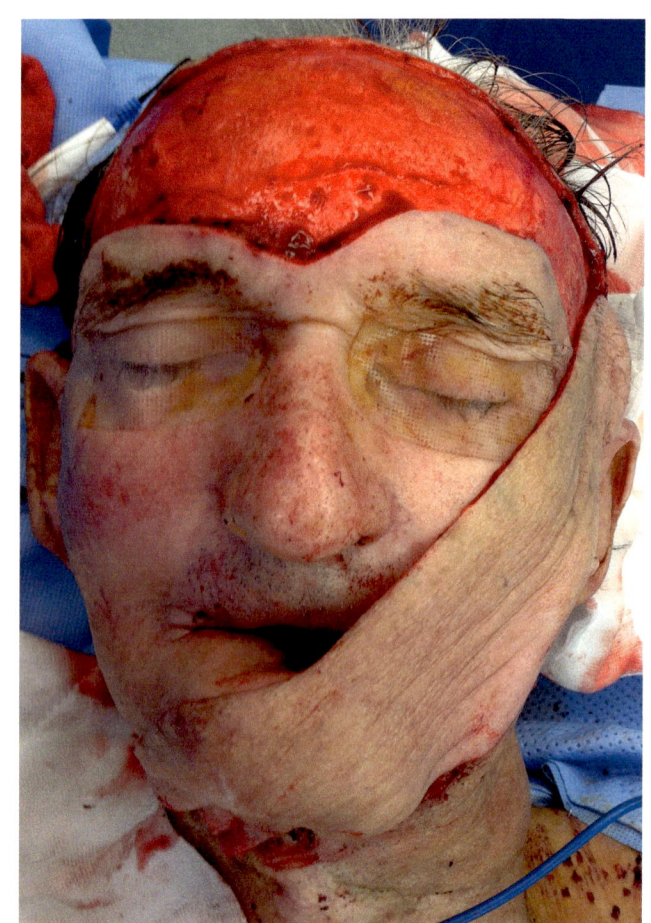

Fig. 11.9 Wide flap arc of rotation and can be tunnelled through the nasolabial region to close intraoral defects, such as the floor of the mouth in this case

same time as nasal reconstruction as a compromise (Figs. 11.10 and 11.11). However for the majority, it is better to restore surrounding anatomy in the first instance, or in the same procedure as the first nasal stage, but using alternate tissue sources (Fig. 11.12).

A particular consideration is the timing of cartilage grafting. In general it is our preference to:

1. Primarily place grafts where good lining already exists (Fig. 11.12)
2. Secondarily place grafts in intermediate stage(s) where the forehead flap or another form of tissue is deployed for lining in preliminary/first stages of reconstruction (Figs. 11.13, 11.14, and 11.15)

C

11.3.6.2 Intermediate Stages

After approximately 1 month, the flap at the recipient site can be safely elevated and thinned and allow the placement of cartilage grafts. Intermediate stages offer the excellent opportunity to sculpt soft tissue and accurately amend and augment structural support (Fig. 11.16).

11.3.6.3 Final Stage

Division of the pedicle often leaves a 'V'-shaped unit of tissue to interpose into the brow wound whilst making sure pre-marked brow height symmetry is retained.

11.3.6.4 Flap Delay

The rich blood supply in the forehead does permit transfer of a flap with surgical scars, particularly if the previous surgical intervention is known, for example, curettage, cryotherapy or a simple skin excision of a lesion. Deep scars to the periosteum or bone may have interrupted the axiality of the flap and design has to take this into account.

11 Supraorbital and Supratrochlear Artery Flaps - Forehead Flap and Modifications 111

Fig. 11.10 Large orbital exenteration, cheek resection and mid nasal resection for basal cell carcinoma. Planned reconstruction with cheek rotation flap and single-stage forehead with cheek extension

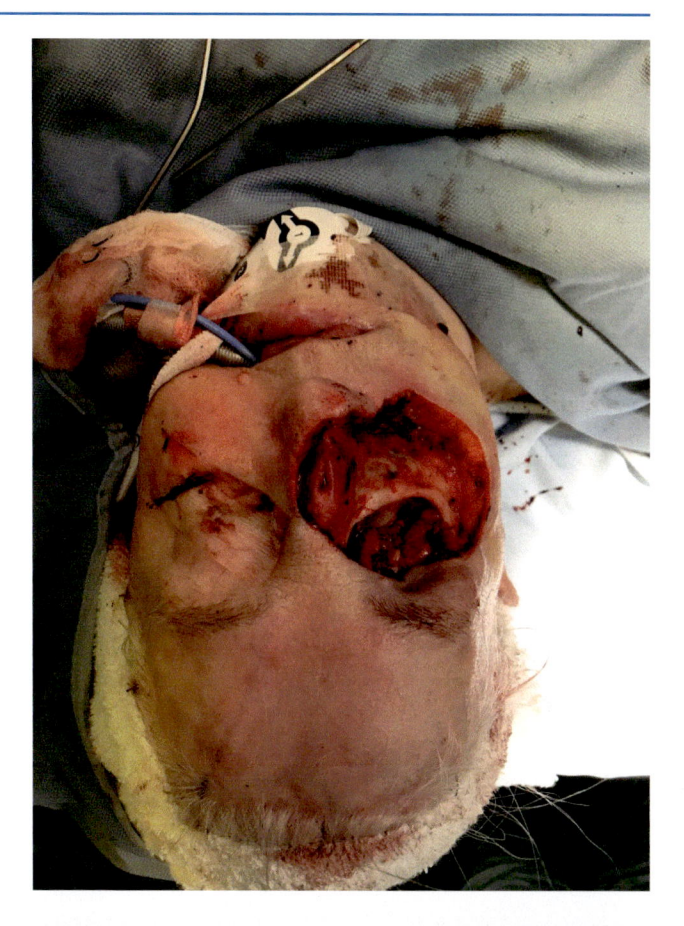

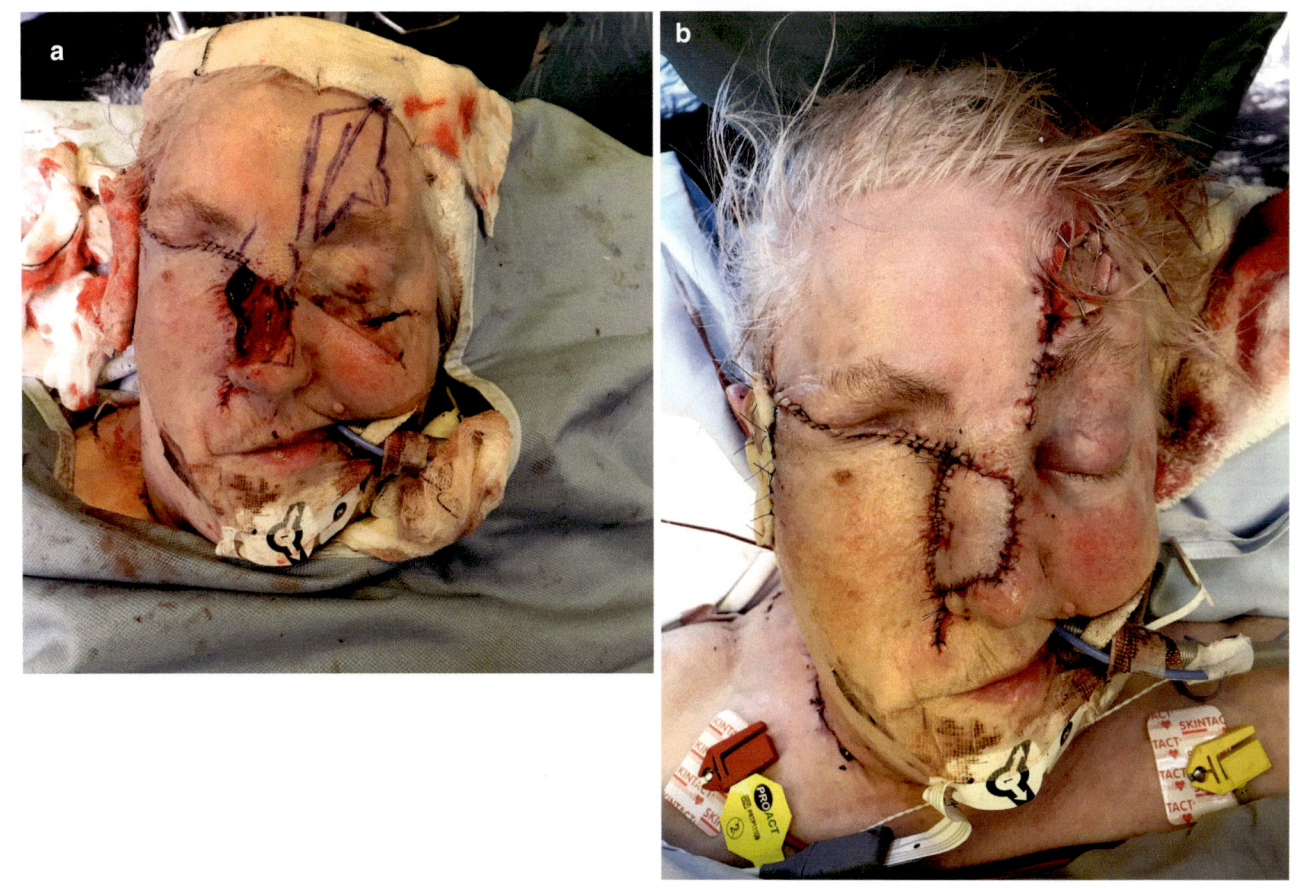

Fig. 11.11 Flap plan with cheek extension and final flap inset. (**a**) flap markings with cheek extension (**b**) final inset of single stage flap and cheek rotation

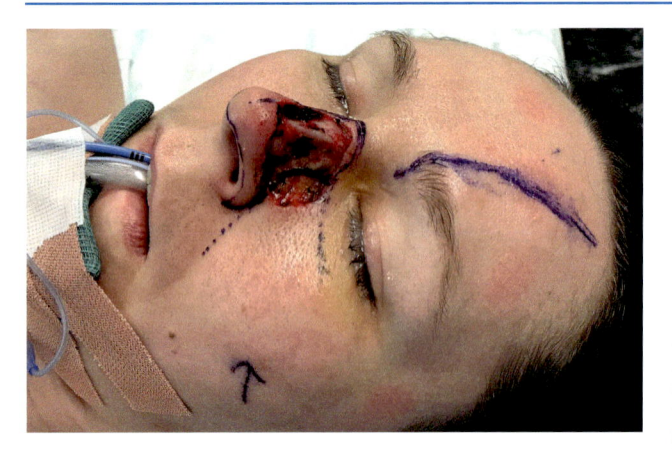

Fig. 11.12 Cheek and nasal floor reconstruction to restore a soft tissue platform for the nose in conjunction with first-stage nasal reconstruction. Cartilage grafts also placed for forehead flap transfer with modified subunit completion of the nasal defect

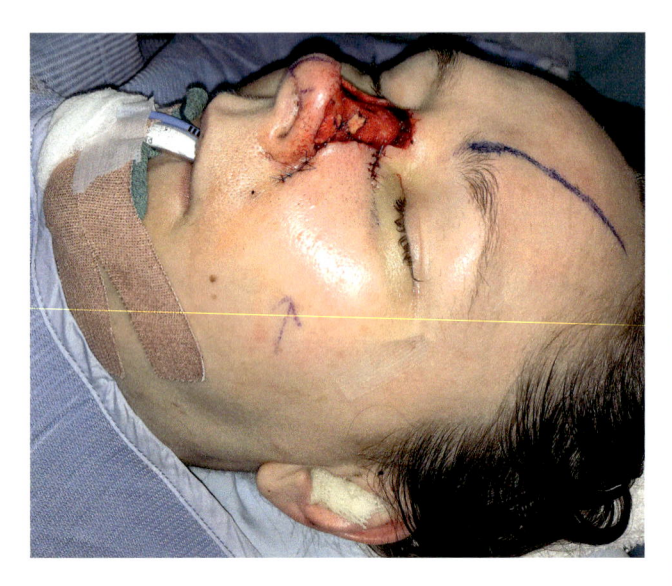

Fig. 11.13 Cheek and nasal floor reconstruction to restore a soft tissue platform for the nose in conjunction with first-stage nasal reconstruction. Cartilage grafts also placed for forehead flap transfer with modified subunit completion of the nasal defect

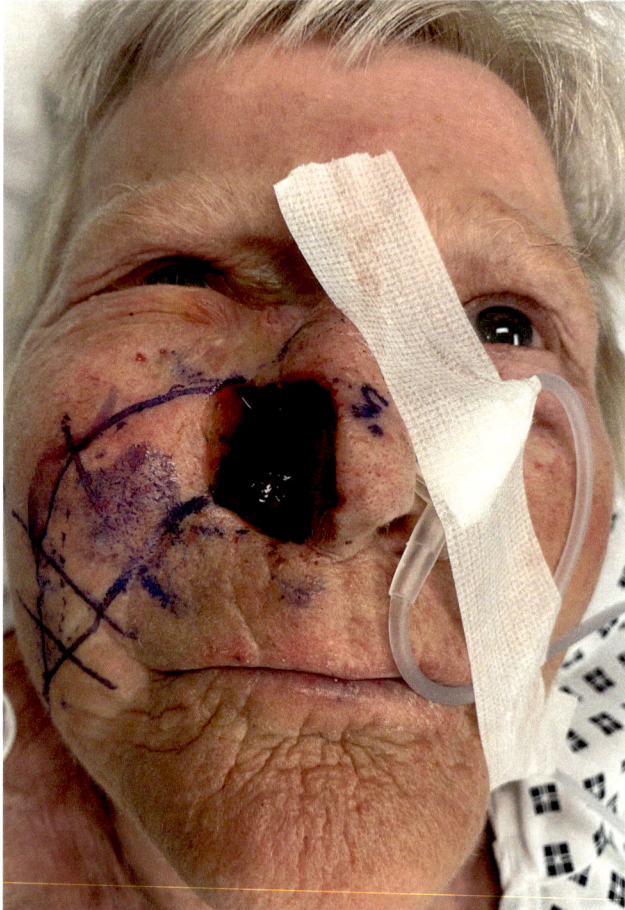

Fig. 11.14 Cheek and nasal floor reconstruction to restore a soft tissue platform prior to first-stage nasal reconstruction in a post-Moh's micrographic resection. V-Y advancement and full-thickness skin grafting to the right nasal defect rim

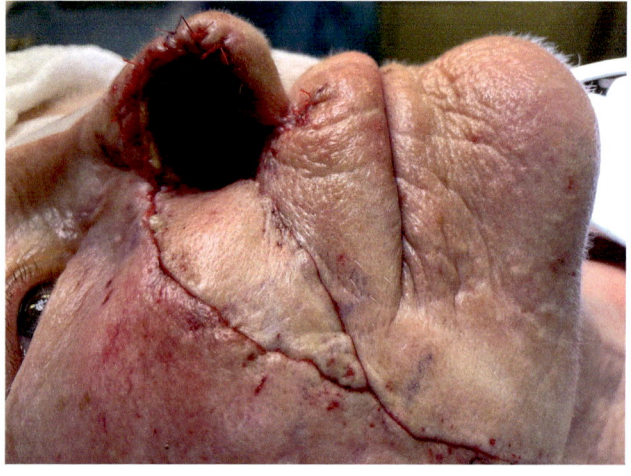

Fig. 11.15 Cheek and nasal floor reconstruction to restore a soft tissue platform prior to first-stage nasal reconstruction in a post-Moh's micrographic resection. V-Y advancement and full-thickness skin grafting to the right nasal defect rim

Where there is a good Doppler signal, but scarring (Fig. 11.17), we advocate delay manoeuvres to augment the flap prior to definitive elevation.

11.3.6.5 The Single-Stage Forehead Flap

Converse [2] popularised the islanded forehead flap for nasal reconstruction, and the broad principles of safe harvest are the same. We reserve this option in patients where:

1. Dual or multistage surgery is problematic.
   (a) Concurrent anticoagulant therapy where there is elevated risk associated with numerous episodes of stopping and starting between stages.

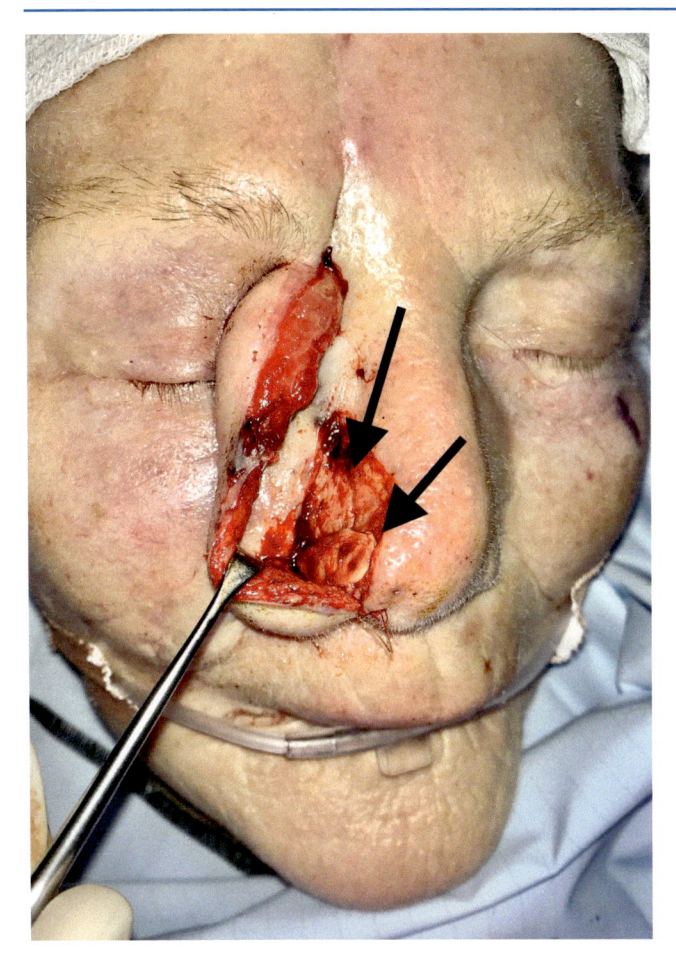

Fig. 11.16 Secondarily placed septal cartilage grafts with partial flap elevation and thinning

    (b) Concurrent oncological therapy.
    (c) Major anaesthetic risk/interventional risks with elevated frailty scores and advanced patient age.
    (d) Inability for regular visits to hospital for aftercare and repeated surgical episodes.
2. There is a mature defect where lining can be established with ease without the need for >1 cm folding of the flap—we find a larger requirement for lining and folding results in potential airway impedance.
3. The patient is unwilling to have pre-expansion of the forehead in previously scarred or very low hairline situations.

The key difference is the need to island the flap at the brow by only incising the skin and bluntly separating the skin and subcutaneous fat to allow rotation. Once the flap is mobilised enough, this dissection can stop. Then the next consideration is to split the glabellar skin or tunnel (Figs. 11.18 and 11.19). The latter is preferable and frequently possible. Both result in glabellar prominence which is less so in the elderly population where skin and muscle atrophy at the radix is more common. However this is disadvantage of this technique and patients must be counselled regarding this.

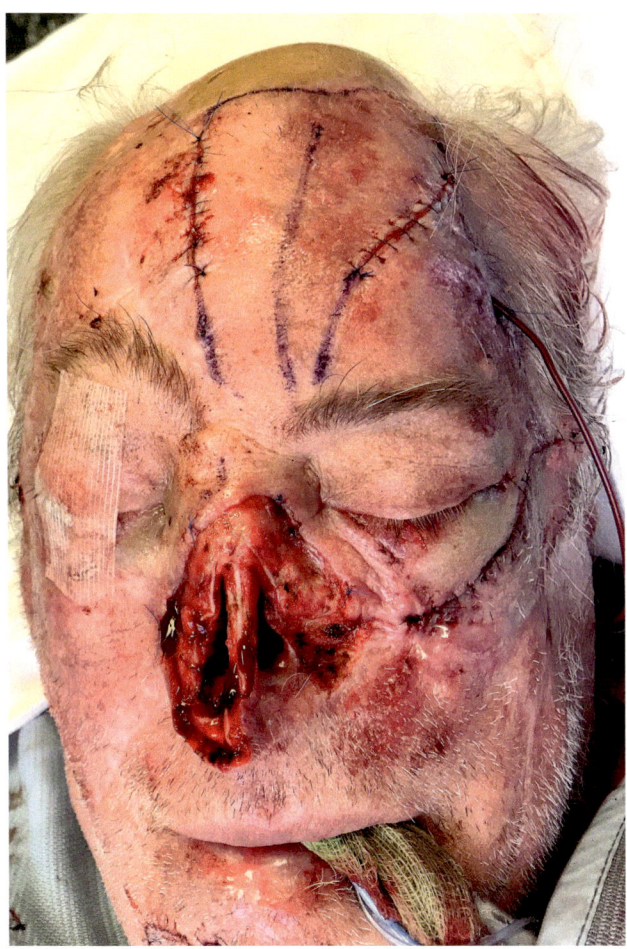

Fig. 11.17 A sub-total rhinectomy defect with a plan for delayed reconstruction post-radiotherapy. A scalp reconstruction with free anterolateral thigh flap limited the forehead donor flap. Previous BCCs resected from right forehead including deep excision of eyebrow region. Therefore delayed left paramedian forehead flap with division of superficial temporal vessels and vessels from the right forehead

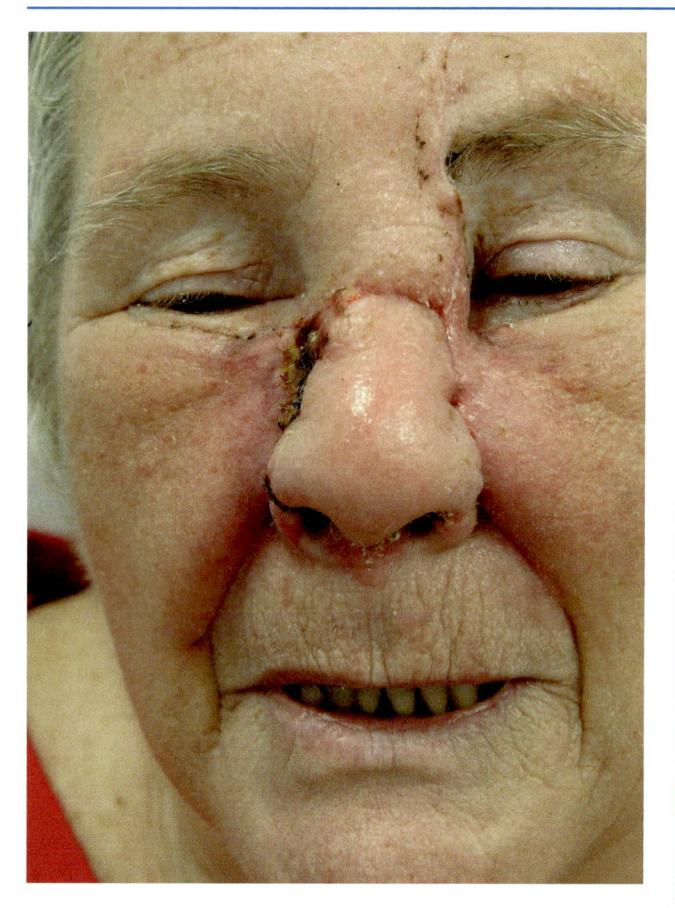

Fig. 11.18 A patient 2 weeks post-glabellar split to pass a bulky single-stage flap down to reconstruct a sub-total rhinectomy defect with costal cartilage construct

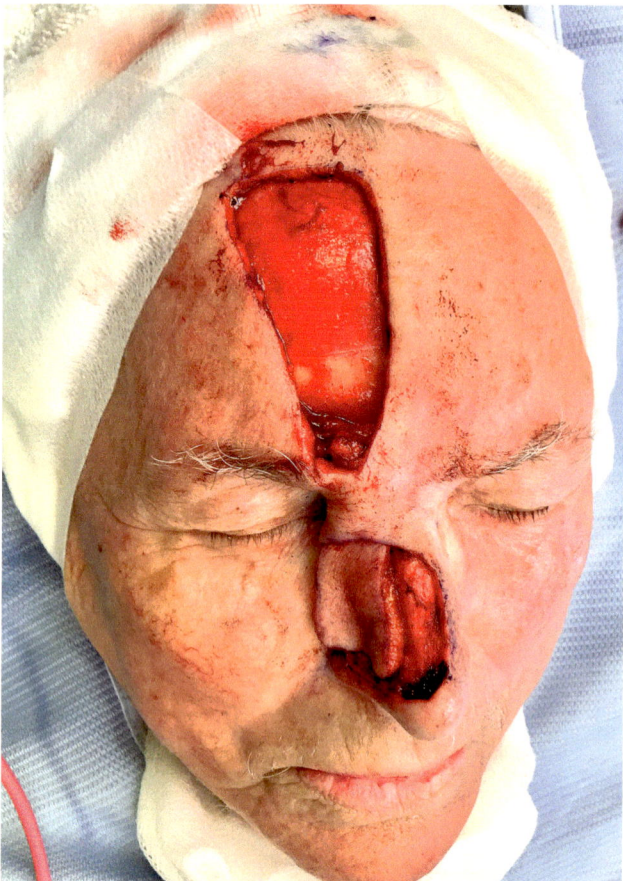

Fig. 11.19 A tunnelled flap where the glabellar bridge is soft and wide to prevent any pedicle compression

11.3.6.6 Donor Site Management

In general, a forehead unit donor site or hemi-forehead donor site is best replaced with a reconstruction such as a full- or split-thickness skin graft. In the majority of cases whereby the donor defect is secondary to paramedian harvest, the majority of most donor sites can be directly closed with careful attention to the brow height.

The most distal aspect of the donor site is often too wide to permit direct closure. There are three typical ways to close this part of the wound:

1. Leave to heal by secondary intent. We dress the wound with Jelonet gauze and foam tie-over and convert to antiseptic dressings after 1 week until the wound is less than approximately 4 cm^2, which can then be simply hydrated with petroleum jelly until completely healed. This method offers good aesthetics long term, and in many cases the patient's hair can conceal this area of the scar. If poor scar quality results, there is still the option of scar excision and reconstruction.
2. Skin graft reconstruction. This is offered to patients with photographic examples of secondary intent as a comparator. Some patients prefer a graft to achieve healing quicker and accept poorer aesthetics of the graft.
3. Pre-trichial forehead advancement flaps either side of the defect, or a similar form of scalp advancement anteriorly. These can work well, and give the best scar aesthetics, at the potential cost of 'burning' a salvage option of the contralateral forehead flap.

In cases where the periosteum desiccates (Fig. 11.20), there also remain a number of options to resurrect and close the wound, and we have deployed all of the following at some juncture:

1. Burring and direct or further partial closure if the cicatrix thus far allows; or advance the pre-trichial forehead skin in uni- or bilateral advancement flaps provided there is no need for further forehead flaps (i.e. the original reconstruction has been a success).
2. Our preferred method if the above is not possible is to perform a pericranial flap to provide a vascularised wound bed and apply a split skin graft, for later serial excision.

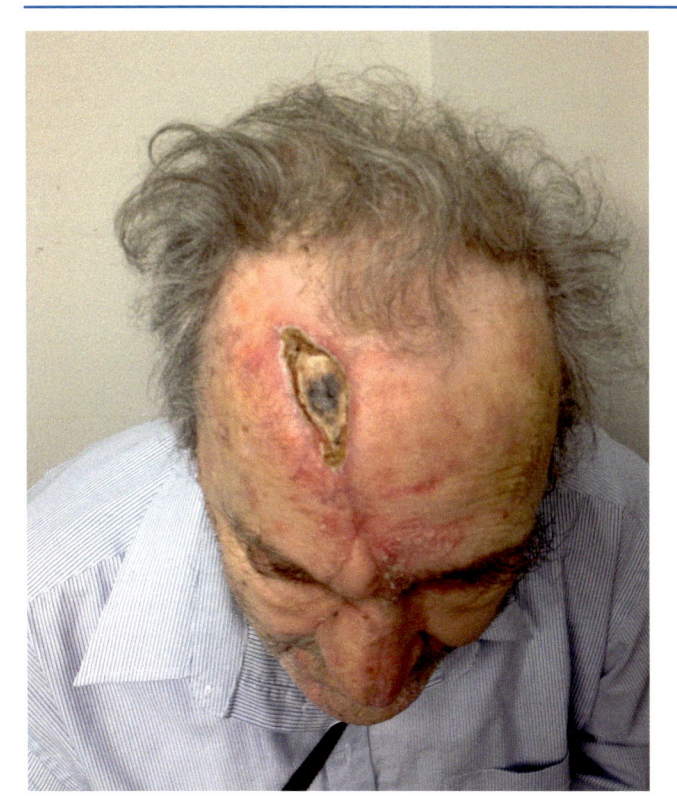

Fig. 11.20 Desiccated outer table of the calvarium

3. Burr the frontal bone to punctate bleeding and dress to heal with hydrocolloid dressings.
4. Burr as above and apply split skin graft, or regenerative templates and split skin graft (e.g. 1 mm Matriderm).

Burring and grafting is very useful if the pericranium is not available or not sensible for the particular patient one is faced with.

Expansion for the sake of donor closure is to be discouraged. The tissue quality is lacking, and rotation of the expanded forehead is challenging despite ample physical tissue. Expansion is only really merited when more forehead tissue is required for the reconstructive effort, or to augment a delay procedure to maximise blood supply.

11.3.6.7 Final Thoughts

In general, the forehead region has a rich, dependable, multi-faceted blood supply that is versatile and can be adapted to reconstruct large surface areas of all sections of the face. Whilst it is best known for nasal reconstruction, there are many other useful applications for this tissue, and it holds distinct advantages of reliable blood supply and good tissue match, with well-tolerated donor site morbidity in the vast majority of cases. Doppler examination and guidance in surgery is easy and cheap and ensures safe tissue units, for bespoke and controlled reconstructive efforts.

11.4 Pearls and Pitfalls

Pearls

- Plan properly and use adjuncts such as Doppler guidance to plan the flap.
- Use ipsilateral flaps where possible for easier arc of rotation and a shorter flap (helping avoid hairline).
- Template the defect exactly using the contralateral side—if a total rhinectomy is planned, get pre-ablative moulds of the nose where possible (or 3D prints).
- Ensure the patient understands what is required of them for multistage surgery and the journey concept of this surgery.
- In revision or complex anatomy, use delay principles safely to augment the remaining forehead tissue.

Pitfalls

- Try to avoid raising the flap in the subcutaneous plane.
- Inadequate release of the vessels at the supraorbital ridge can inhibit rotation of the flap and encourage venous kinking.
- Poor planning of the eyebrow incisions is key—offset eyebrows can detract from the reconstructive effort.
- Advancement flaps of the remaining forehead are tempting to avoid donor wounds, but this can burn salvage options in flap failure.

11.5 Selected Readings

- Menick FJ. Nasal Reconstruction. Plast Reconstr Surg. 2010;125:1–13.

  A comprehensive overview of the key tenets in nasal reconstructive surgery and planning.
- Lei T, Xu DC, Gao JH et al. Using the frontal branch of the superficial temporal artery as a landmark for locating the course of the temporal branch of the facial nerve during rhytidectomy: an anatomical study. Plast Reconstr Surg 2005;116:623–629.

  An excellent appraisal for the anatomy in relation to the superficial temporal artery and its terminal branches in the forehead.

- Kleintjes WG. Forehead anatomy: arterial variations and venous link of the midline forehead flap. J Plast Reconstr Aesthet Surg. 2007;60(6):593–606.

  An important discussion about anatomic variability and highlights the need for Doppler examination of the planned donor site to maximise results, avoid marginal necrosis and achieve reliable results.

- Saleh DB, Dearden AS, Smith J, Mizen KD, Reid J, Eriksen E, Fourie L. Single-stage nasal reconstruction with the islanded forehead flap.

  An overview and assessment of the suitability of single stage reconstructions and when best to consider deploying it as a reconstruction.

References

1. Yalamanchili H, Sclafani AP, Schaefer SD, Presti P. The path of nasal reconstruction: from ancient India to the present. Facial Plast Surg. 2008;24(1):3–10.
2. Baker SR. Interpolated paramedian forehead flaps. In: Principles of nasal reconstruction. New York, NY: Springer; 2011.
3. McDowell F. The 'B.L.' bomb-shell (B. Lucas). Plast Reconstr Surg. 1969;44:67–73.
4. Carpue JC. An account of two successful operations for restoring a lost nose from the integuments of the forehead. London: Longman, Hurst, Rees, Orme and Brown; 1816. p. 84.
5. Burget GC, Menick FJ. Nasal reconstruction: seeking a fourth dimension. Plast Reconstr Surg. 1986;78(2):145–57.
6. Burget GC, Menick FJ. Nasal support and lining: the marriage of beauty and blood supply. Plast Reconstr Surg. 1989;84(2):189–202.
7. Menick FJ. Aesthetic refinements in use of forehead for nasal reconstruction: the paramedian forehead flap. Clin Plast Surg. 1990;17(4):607–22.
8. Shumrick KA, Smith TL. The anatomic basis for the design of forehead flaps in nasal reconstruction. Arch Otolaryngol Head Neck Surg. 1992;118(4):373–9.
9. Mangold U, Lierse W, Pfeifer G. Die Arterien der Stirn als Grundlage des Nasenersatzes mit Stirnlappen [The arteries of the forehead as the basis of nasal reconstruction with forehead flaps]. Acta Anat (Basel). 1980;107(1):18–25.
10. Kleintjes WG. Forehead anatomy: arterial variations and venous link of the midline forehead flap. J Plast Reconstr Aesthet Surg. 2007;60(6):593–606.
11. Skaria AM. The median forehead flap reviewed: a histologic study on vascular anatomy. Eur Arch Otorhinolaryngol. 2015;272(5):1231–7.
12. Faris C, van der Eerden P, Vuyk H. The midline central artery forehead flap: a valid alternative to supratrochlear-based forehead flaps. JAMA Facial Plast Surg. 2015;17(1):16–22. https://doi.org/10.1001/jamafacial.2014.738. PMID: 25322444.
13. Lei T, Xu DC, Gao JH, et al. Using the frontal branch of the superficial temporal artery as a landmark for locating the course of the temporal branch of the facial nerve during rhytidectomy: an anatomical study. Plast Reconstr Surg. 2005;116:623–9.

Cervicofacial Flap 12

Luke Geoghegan, Dariush Nikkhah, and Tiew Chong Teo

12.1 Introduction

Esser first described a rotational cheek flap in 1918 [1], although Beare first described the cervicofacial flap in its modern form in 1969 [2]. Beare described the use of a laterally based advancement flap for reconstruction following exenteration of the orbit. Various modifications were described by Mustardé [3] and Converse [4] to overcome donor site issues, and a posteriorly based cervical advancement flap was first described in 1972 by Stark and Kaplan [5]. Juri and Juri refined the above techniques and described an anteriorly based flap that is both advanced and rotated forwards to cover cheek defects with primary closure of the donor site [6]. Anterior (or medially)-based flaps can be used to cover moderately sized defects of the anterior and *superior* cheek. Posterior (or laterally) based flaps can be used to cover moderate/large-sized defects of the anterior and *inferior* cheek.

12.2 Anatomy

The cheek is a laminated structure comprising, from superficial to deep, the epidermis, dermis, subcutaneous tissue and superficial muscular aponeurotic system (SMAS). The SMAS is an investing fibromuscular layer that encloses the platysma, risorius, triangularis, auricularis, occipitalis and frontalis. It connects the periosteum to the dermis and permits movement of the skin for facial expression. The SMAS serves as an important landmark, with the parotid gland and facial nerve lying deep to this tissue plane [7].

Roth described three anatomical subdivisions of the cheek [8]:

- Zone 1: Suborbital
- Zone 2: Pre-auricular
- Zone 3: Buccomandibular

Defects in each of the above zones are amenable to closure with the cervicofacial flap. Classically, the cervicofacial flap is raised in the subcutaneous plane superficial to the SMAS and is thus based on a random blood supply arising from the subdermal plexus. Arterial supply is dependent on whether the flap is anteriorly or posteriorly based. The anteriorly based flap is supplied by the perforating arteries from the facial and submental arteries; it facilitates closure of posterior or large anterior cheek defects through rotation and upward advancement of cervical tissue [9]. The posteriorly based flap is supplied by perforators from the superficial temporal artery; it facilitates closure of small- to moderately sized anterior cheek defects through rotation and advancement of the jowls and submental tissue [9].

The blood supply to the cervicofacial flap can be improved through dissection in a plane deep to the SMAS [10]. This flap is a myofascial cutaneous flap based on an axial blood supply via transverse facial artery perforators. During flap elevation of the cervical portion of the flap, perforators from the submental artery are preserved. An extension of the deep plane cervicofacial flap with an additional pectoral component has been described [11]. This cervicopectoral rotation flap is a fasciocutaneous flap supplied by the first four internal mammary perforators.

L. Geoghegan (✉)
Department of Plastic Surgery, John Radcliffe Hospital, Oxford University Hospitals NHS Trust, Oxford, UK
e-mail: luke.geoghegan13@imperial.ac.uk

D. Nikkhah
Royal Free Hospital, London, UK

T. C. Teo
Queen Victoria Hospital, East Grinstead, UK

12.3 Preoperative Investigation

Preoperative radiographic investigations are not routinely used in the planning of cervicofacial flaps. Consideration is instead given to patient-specific and injury-specific factors. The location and degree of local skin laxity should be assessed. Preoperative counselling should seek to identify patients who have risk factors for flap failure, including smoking, patients with a history of trauma or irradiation and those with pre-existing scars.

When examining the soft tissue defect, consideration should be given to the site, size, depth and underlying aetiology. The site of cheek defects will dictate the pedicle base location and required direction of skin flap motion. Generally, defects affecting more than 30% of the cheek will require coverage with rotation advancement flaps. Large defects of the anterior cheek and posterior defects can be covered with anterior-based rotation advancement flaps. Small-to-moderate defects affecting the anterior cheek are best covered with a posteriorly based rotation advancement flap. Vertical defects are amenable to closure via rotation advancement, whereas horizontal defects are best closed via superior advancement. Deeper defects have a higher risk of facial nerve injury and may require added soft tissue bulk to address contour defects. Extensive defects may necessitate reconstruction of the intraoral mucosal lining with either a free flap or a secondary local flap.

Clear margins should be ensured following oncologic resection. A history of burns or irradiation may necessitate creation of a larger defect due to poor laxity and vascularity of regional tissue. Infected or highly contaminated wounds may require delayed reconstruction following adequate debridement.

12.4 Flap Design and Markings

12.4.1 Anteriorly Based Flaps

Anteriorly based flaps are used to cover posterior and large anterior cheek defects through anterior advancement of soft tissue from the cheek, neck and anterior chest. The superior margin of the flap is marked in line with the defect to be covered, extending transversely towards the lateral canthus and inferiorly in the pre-auricular crease, around the earlobe buried in the occipital hairline. For large defects, markings can be extended along the anterior border of trapezius into the base of the neck. For considerably larger defects, a cervicopectoral flap can be implemented. Markings are extended inferiorly along the anterior border of the trapezius, along the deltopectoral groove before traversing medially across the chest wall in the third or fourth intercostal space.

12.4.2 Posteriorly Based Flaps

Posteriorly based flaps are used to cover small- to moderately sized anterior cheek defects through advancement of soft tissue from the jowl and neck. Markings are made from the defect inferolaterally either within or parallel to the nasolabial fold. For large defects, markings can be extended inferiorly into the neck, transversely and then postero-superiorly towards the mastoid, producing a curvilinear shape. Inclusion of the platysma increases the vascularity of the flap, with perfusion from the occipital artery, superficial cervical artery and transverse cervical artery. The modified skin-platysma rotation flap permits reconstruction following extensive ablative surgery of the head and neck [12]. For very large defects, the inferior vertical midline marking can be extended onto the sternum and then laterally across the anterior chest wall superior to the nipple areolar complex.

12.5 Flap Raise/Elevation: A Step-by-Step Guide

Outlined below are the steps for raising an anteriorly based cervicofacial flap:

1. Preparation
   (a) The patient should be positioned with the neck extended and head rotated towards the contralateral shoulder. The site should be marked (see Fig. 12.1), and the soft tissue defect size should be estimated. Betadine antiseptic is used to prepare the surgical field, extending onto the neck and chest for large soft tissue defects. The procedure can be performed under local or general anaesthesia; the use of lignocaine/adrenaline reduces bleeding in the operative field.

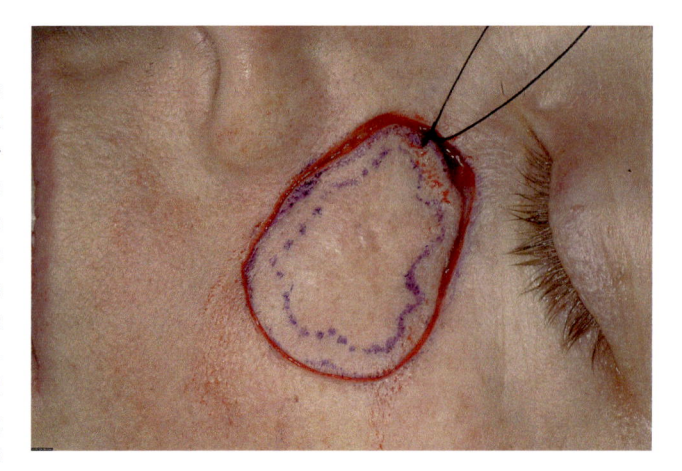

Fig. 12.1 Appearance of a left-sided morpheic basal cell carcinoma prior to resection

2. Incision Planning
   (a) The site of the defect should be used to guide whether an anteriorly or posteriorly based flap is used for soft tissue coverage. Anteriorly based flaps are used to cover posterior and large anterior cheek defects. Extension of the lateral flap border into the neck can be performed for large defects. Figure 12.2 illustrates markings for an anteriorly based flap. Care must be taken to ensure the base of the flap is appropriately broad as to not compromise vascular supply. If the defect is considerably large (between 6 and 10 cm), a clavipectoral flap should be marked via inferior extension along the deltopectoral groove and then transversely in the third or fourth intercostal space.
3. Incision
   (a) An incision is made along the superior aspect of the flap outline, extending transversely to the lateral canthus, inferior to the orbit in a sub-ciliary crease. The incision can then be extended slightly superior to the lateral canthus; see Fig. 12.3. This enables the flap to be fixed to underlying periosteum to minimise surface tension on the lower eyelid. The incision then extends inferiorly in the pre-auricular crease, around the earlobe to follow the occipital hairline. The incision can be extended inferiorly into the neck if the soft tissue defect is considerably large.
4. Elevation
   (a) The flap is raised in the subcutaneous plane, superficial to the SMAS. Dissection begins laterally and extends medially towards the defect; see Figs. 12.3, 12.4, 12.5, and 12.6. Care must be taken at the anterior border of the parotid gland due to the relatively superficial nature of the facial nerve at this point. Flap elevation continues medially until the defect is adequately covered by advancement and rotation with minimal tension; see Fig. 12.7. Once elevation is complete, adequate haemostasis is achieved using bipolar diathermy.

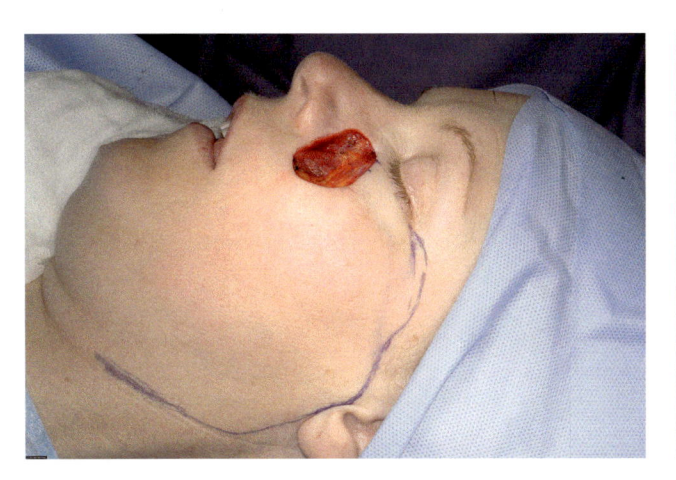

Fig. 12.2 Ovoid defect in the left infraorbital region following excision of the lesion. Markings for an anteriorly based cervicofacial flap are demonstrated

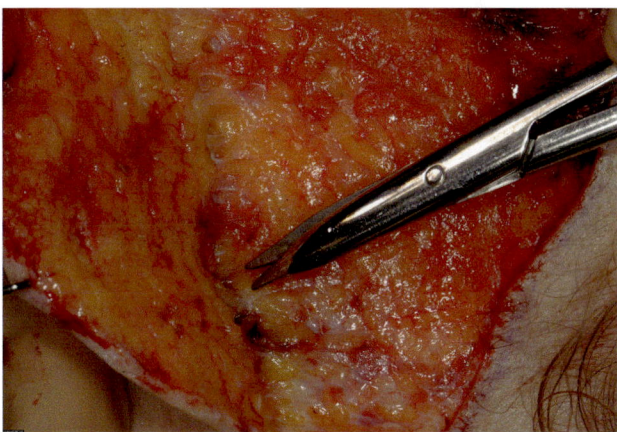

Fig. 12.4 Flap elevation at the anterior border of the parotid using blunt-tipped scissors

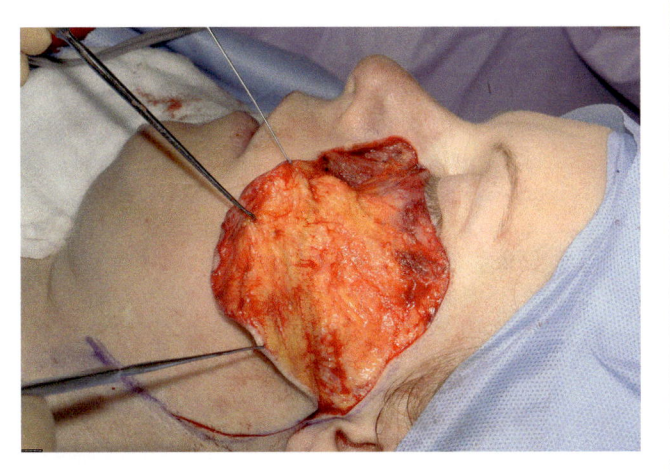

Fig. 12.3 Elevation of the cervicofacial flap in the subcutaneous plane superficial to the SMAS

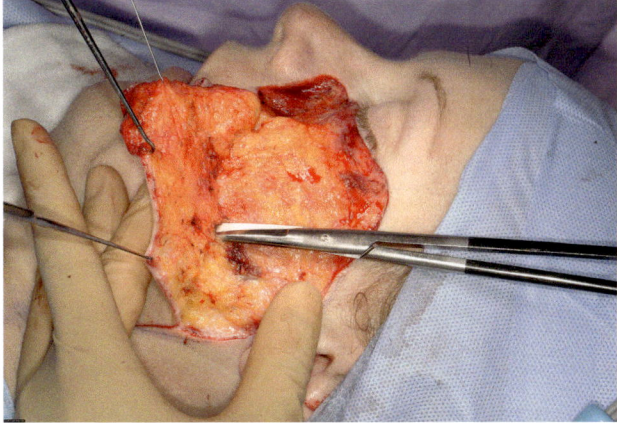

Fig. 12.5 Further dissection of the flap in the subcutaneous plane using blunt-tipped Gorney scissors over the anterior margin of the parotid gland

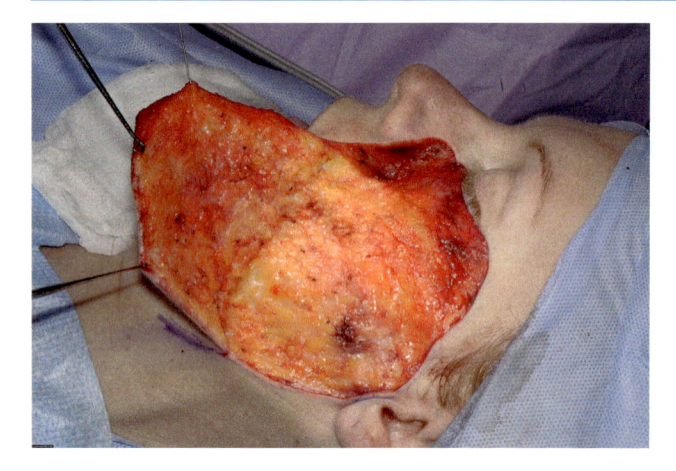

Fig. 12.6 Full elevation of the flap prior to advancement and forward rotation

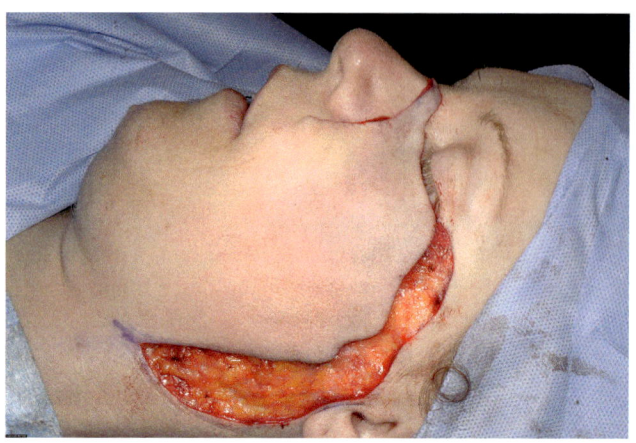

Fig. 12.7 Rotation and forward advancement of the flap to cover the infraorbital defect

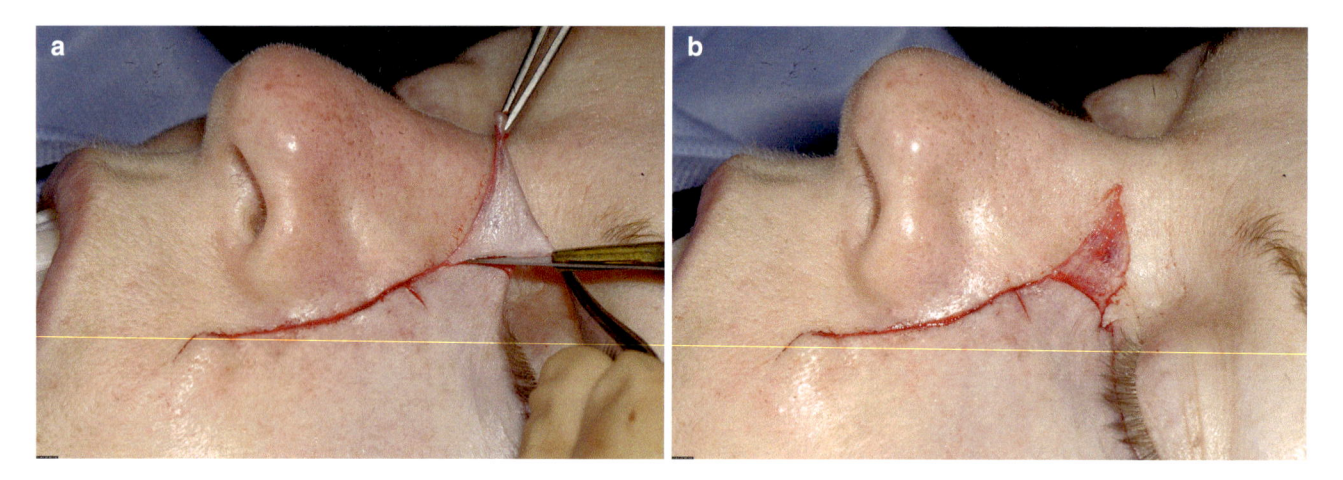

Fig. 12.8 (**a**) Excess soft tissue noted at the superomedial aspect of the flap. (**b**) This excess tissue can be de-epithelised and used as an autologous space filler

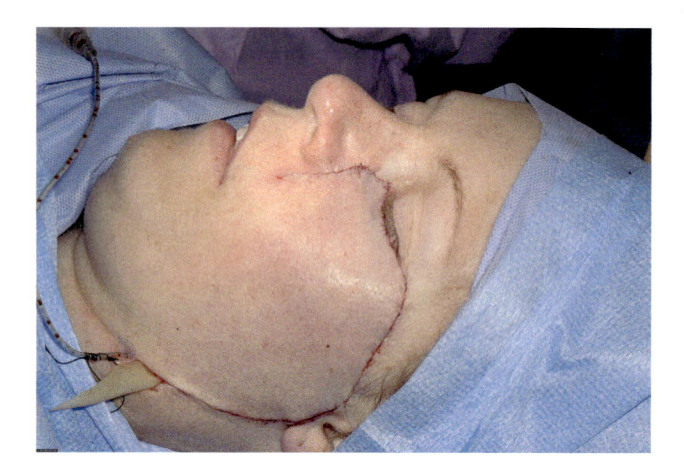

Fig. 12.9 Inset of the flap to cover the infraorbital defect. A Penrose and Jackson-Pratt drain are left in situ with no tension placed on the lower eyelid

5. Closure
    (a) Once the flap is rotated to fill the defect, excess tissue can be utilised as an autologous space filler following de-epithelisation; see Figs. 12.7 and 12.8. The flap is anchored superiorly to the periosteum of the zygoma using 4-0 polydioxanone to reduce tension and the incidence of both ectropion and scleral show. Soft tissue closure is achieved using interrupted 4-0 monocryl deep dermal sutures and a running 6-0 monocryl suture for epidermal closure. The lower eyelid is closed last to ensure tension-free closure. Any resultant dog ears are primarily excised, and closure around the eye is achieved using 6-0 nylon in a simple interrupted fashion. Both suction and passive drains can be sited at the inferior edge of the flap to minimize haematoma and seroma formation; see Fig. 12.9. The authors advocate drain removal 48 h post-operatively regardless of volume.

12.6 Core Surgical Techniques in Flap Dissection

The cervicofacial flap is raised in the subcutaneous plane, superficial to the SMAS. During flap elevation, care should be taken to ensure atraumatic tissue handling which improves flap survival and cosmesis. Sharp skin hooks should be used to provide vertical countertraction and permit sharp dissection using a ten-blade scalpel initially; see Fig. 12.3.

Dissection and elevation in the subcutaneous plane proceeds superior to the parotidomasseteric fascia; here the facial nerve is well-protected. Once dissection proceeds anteriorly to reach the anterior border of the parotid gland, approximately 2 cm anterior to the tragus, care must be taken as the facial nerve and its branches emerge from the parotid gland. Careful dissection using blunt-tipped Gorney scissors should be used in a plane perpendicular to the skin to ensure safe anterior dissection; see Figs. 12.4 and 12.5.

The risk of distal flap necrosis is minimised by avoiding closure under tension. Closure of the incision should be performed in layers, the authors' preference being interrupted 4-0 monocryl deep dermal sutures followed by a running subcuticular closure using 6-0 monocryl. Once again, atraumatic tissue handling techniques should be implemented using toothed forceps. Tension placed on the distal tip of the flap can be reduced by anchoring the superior margin of the flap to the periosteum of the zygoma using a 4-0 polydioxanone suture. Areas around the lower eyelid are closed last to ensure minimal tension is placed on the flap tip using simple interrupted 6-0 nylon sutures. Any resultant dog ears should be primarily excised. Excess tissue can be de-epithelialised and used to fill volumetric defects; see Fig. 12.8.

12.7 Clinical Scenario

A 42-year-old Caucasian female with Fitzpatrick skin type I was referred for the management of morpheic basal cell carcinoma affecting the left infraorbital region of the medial cheek (Roth zone 1); see Fig. 12.1. Following complete excision, the patient was left with a 2 × 1.5 cm ovoid soft tissue defect; see Fig. 12.2. An anteriorly based cervicofacial rotation advancement flap was planned (see Fig. 12.2), extending down to the angle of the mandible. The flap was raised in the subcutaneous plane superficial to the SMAS, advanced and rotated to fill the medial defect with minimal tension placed on the flap tip; see Fig. 12.7. Both a Penrose and Jackson-Pratt drain were left in situ post-operatively for 48 hours; see Fig. 12.9.

12.8 Pearls and Pitfalls

Pearls

- Failing to plan is planning to fail. Consider patient- and injury-specific factors when deciding whether to pursue anterior- or posterior-based flaps as well as the plane of flap elevation prior to surgery.
- Adequate vertical countertraction with skin hooks during flap elevation permits sharp dissection in the appropriate plane. Adequate illumination of the field using a headlight aids identification of the correct plane.
- Avoid injury to the facial nerve at the anterior border of the parotid through careful dissection using blunt-tipped scissors in a plane perpendicular to overlying skin.
- Superior anchoring of the flap to the periosteum of the zygoma prevents excessive tension and minimises risk of post-operative ectropion and scleral show.
- Begin epidermal closure along the postero-inferior edges of the flap to minimise tension placed upon the flap tip.

Pitfalls

- Facial nerve injury: Sound knowledge of regional anatomy and careful dissection using blunt-tipped scissors are the mainstay of prevention.
- Post-operative ectropion: Extending the flap superiorly at the lateral canthus and anchoring of the superior edge of the flap to the periosteum of the zygoma minimises tension placed on the lower eyelid. A frost suture can be placed for 24 h post-operatively; this reduces chemosis and provides upward tension on the lower eyelid where post-operative oedema may result in downward pull.
- Distal tip necrosis: Ensure minimal tension is placed on the flap; for patients at high risk of flap necrosis, consider raising in a plane deep to the SMAS. Additional skin grafts may be required to cover bare areas in particularly large defects.

- Haematoma: Haematoma formation may compromise cutaneous flow due to increased surface tension placed on the flap. Adequate haemostasis should be ensured intraoperatively with the use of bipolar diathermy and adequate post-operative drainage should be ensured. A single dose of intravenous tranexamic acid may also be given as an adjunct to minimise risk of haematoma formation.
- Infection: Ensure appropriate intravenous antibiotics effective against skin flora are given at induction.

12.9 Selected Readings

- Beare R. Flap repair following exenteration of the orbit. Proc R Soc Med. 1969;62(11):1087–90.

  The first modern technical description of the cervicofacial flap. Beare described the use of a posteriorly based cervicofacial advancement flap used to cover soft tissue defects secondary to exenteration of the orbit. Beare advocated cervical extension of the flap to provide adequate soft tissue for definitive coverage.

- Juri J, Juri C. Advancement and rotation of a large cervicofacial flap for cheek repairs. Plast Reconstr Surg. 1979;64(5):692–6.

  The first technical description of combined upward advancement and forward rotation to cover cheek defects using a cervicofacial flap. Juri and Juri advocated use of a flap which extends inferiorly in the pre-auricular crease around into the retroauricular hairline with elevation in the subcutaneous plane down to the clavicle for large flaps. They described advancement of the cervical portion of the flap with rotation of the superomedial edge to cover the anterior cheek defect.

- Quimby A, Fernandes R. The cervicofacial flap in cheek reconstruction: a guide for flap design. J Oral Maxillofac Surg. 2017;75(12):2708e1–6.

  Retrospective cohort study of 28 patients who underwent cervicofacial flap reconstruction for cheek defects. The mean soft tissue defect size was 44.5 cm²; all flaps were elevated in the subcutaneous plane superficial to the SMAS. Cervicofacial flap reconstruction was indicated following oncologic resection in 68% of patients; 39% were smokers and 11% underwent previous radiotherapy. Collectively, two patients developed wound complications (partial necrosis and dehiscence) at a mean of 4.6 months post-operatively.

- Tan ST, MacKinnon CA. Deep plane cervicofacial flap: a useful and versatile technique in head and neck surgery. Head Neck. 2006;28(1):46–55.

  Case series of 18 patients who underwent reconstruction of cheek defects using cervicofacial flaps raised in a plane deep to the SMAS. The mean soft tissue defect size was 29.7 cm². All defects were secondary to oncologic resection; 11 patients underwent simultaneous parotidectomy. Complications were reported in four patients at a mean of 21 months and included marginal flap necrosis, haematoma, ectropion and lower eyelid retraction.

- Liu FY, Xu ZF, Li P, et al. The versatile application of cervicofacial and cervicothoracic rotation flaps in head and neck surgery. World J Surg Oncol. 2011;9:135.

  Case series of 21 patients who underwent cervicofacial and cervicothoracic flaps for the reconstruction of cheek defects. Cervicothoracic flaps were defined as those whose base extended beyond the clavicle; all flaps were raised superficial to the SMAS and deep to platysma. Post-operative function was graded using a subjective rating scale which assessed speech and swallowing, and patient satisfaction scores were recorded. One patient had a poor subjective functional outcome and 95% of patients were satisfied. Three patients suffered distal flap epidermolysis and two developed full-thickness necrosis of the distal flap. No patients experienced total flap loss.

References

1. Esser J. Die Rotation der Wange. Leipzig: FVC Vogel Verlag; 1918.
2. Beare R. Flap repair following exenteration of the orbit. Proc R Soc Med. 1969;62(11 Pt 1):1087–90.
3. Mustardé JC. The use of flaps in the orbital region. Plast Reconstr Surg. 1970;45(2):146–50.
4. Converse J. Reconstructive plastic surgery. Philadelphia: WB Saunders; 1977.
5. Stark RB, Kaplan JM. Rotation flaps, neck to cheek. Plast Reconstr Surg. 1972;50(3):230–3.
6. Juri J, Juri C. Advancement and rotation of a large cervicofacial flap for cheek repairs. Plast Reconstr Surg. 1979;64(5):692–6.
7. Broughton M, Fyfe GM. The superficial musculoaponeurotic system of the face: a model explored. Anat Res Int. 2013;2013:794682.
8. Roth DA, Longaker MT, Zide BM. Cheek surface reconstruction: best choices according to zones. Oper Tech Plast Reconstr Surg. 1998;5(1):26–36.
9. Mureau MA, Hofer SO. Maximizing results in reconstruction of cheek defects. Clin Plast Surg. 2009;36(3):461–76.
10. Becker FF, Langford FP. Deep-plane cervicofacial flap for reconstruction of large cheek defects. 1996(0886-4470 (Print)).
11. Garrett WS Jr, Giblin TR, Hoffman GW. Closure of skin defects of the face and neck by rotation and advancement of cervicopectoral flaps. Plast Reconstr Surg. 1966;38(4):342–6.
12. Hakim SG, Jacobsen HC, Aschoff HH, Sieg P. Including the platysma muscle in a cervicofacial skin rotation flap to enhance blood supply for reconstruction of vast orbital and cheek defects: anatomical considerations and surgical technique. Int J Oral Maxillofac Surg. 2009;38(12):1316–9.

Bowel Flaps - Jejunum Flap

Georgios Pafitanis, Shin-Heng Chen, and Hung-Chi Chen

13.1 Introduction

Bowel flap harvesting requires general surgery principles to allow the harvesting of intra-abdominal-based structures that enable complex defect reconstructions, for example, a head and neck circumferential hypopharyngeal defect reconstructed with a free small bowel flap. The commonest intra-abdominal bowel flap used is the jejunum flap. The free jejunum flap is unique because it was the first free flap performed (1957) and it was the first intestinal free flap described in literature by Seidenberg in 1959 [1]. The jejunum free flap is normally harvested from the small bowel, starting from 30 cm distally from the ligament of Treitz. It provides a small bowel of diameter between 3 and 4 centimeters and could vary in the segment length between 7 and 25 cm. Harvesting of a small segment of the small bowel does not affect intestinal absorption function; however, intra-abdominal anastomotic complications may affect the patient systemically; therefore, a general/gastrointestinal surgery skill set is required to provide a swift end-to-end small bowel anastomosis [2].

13.2 Anatomy

The jejunum flap is supplied via segmental branches arising from the superior mesenteric artery. Its dominant pedicle starts from the origin of the selected segmental branch in the retroperitoneum and, when followed distally toward the arterial arcades, runs within the double layer of the mesentery. In the visceral nomenclature, each artery is accompanied by a single vein. The patients' body mass index and body habitus change the amount of fat tissue surrounding the flap pedicle, and the length of that pedicle becomes shorter as the mesentery approaches the ligament of Treitz. All segmental arteries are branching with one arch from where the vasa recta radiate toward the mesenteric border of the jejunum. At the distal part of the mesentery, the major arcade arteries supply directly the jejunum. The dominant segmental arterial diameter at the level of its origin varies between 2 and 3 mm, and the accompanying vein varies between 2 and 2.5 mm.

13.3 Preoperative Investigation

A preoperative computerized tomographic angiogram (CTA) is indicated in cases where there is a history of previous abdominal surgeries. The vascular anatomy of the free jejunum flap is constant and has some minor anatomical variations that do not alter the surgical technique. Radiological investigations do not provide clarity in the pedicle selection or the segmental artery if selected. Instead, this is only decided intraoperatively during the extracorporeal examination of the mesentery and the bowel segment of choice.

13.4 Flap Design and Markings

The flap harvesting and flap transfer occurs while the patient is in supine position with the arms in 90 degrees abduction or tucked on the side of the patient's body. A vertical midline laparotomy or a superior mini-laparotomy allows access to the abdominal cavity. Hand-assisted laparoscopic harvesting is also possible but not recommended by the authors as it holds hidden challenges in the pedicle choice, length, and critical decision-making during the jejunum extracorporeal examination.

G. Pafitanis (✉)
London Reconstructive Microsurgery Unit (LRMU), Department of Plastic Surgery, Emergency Care and Trauma Division (ECAT), The Royal London Hospital, Barts Health NHS Trust and University College Hospital London (UCLH), London, UK

S.-H. Chen · H.-C. Chen
Department of Plastic Surgery, China Medical University Hospital, Taichung, Taiwan

13.5 Flap Raise/Elevation: A Step-by-Step Guide

- For open approach, the vertical laparotomy incision allows access to the abdominal cavity through the linea alba (Fig. 13.1a, blue marking; Fig. 13.1b, black vertical laparotomy marking). The laparotomy incision requires to be slightly longer in obese patients to allow ease to access the bowel, and most times it requires infraumbilical extension.
- Exploration of the small bowel and identification of the proximal origin at the mesentery where the ligament of Treitz is located. The origin of the segmental pedicles and their orientation at a distance greater than 30 cm from the ligament of Treitz is located and carefully examined extracorporeally (Fig. 13.2). The maximum segment of the jejunum could be up to 25–30 cm depending on the pedicle blood supply and the reconstructive defect.
- The segmental pedicle of choice along with the arcades branching toward the vasa recti is carefully chosen to match the defect length. The mesentery circular sector is marked along with the jejunum transection margins.
- The pedicle of interest from the segmental origin toward the arcades that supply the jejunum segment is separated from the remaining vascular branches via the loop-ligation hand tie technique. The authors prefer not to use any modern energy-based tools (i.e., harmonic scalpel) for these ligations to minimize collateral heat damage (Figs. 13.3 and 13.4).
- When the jejunum sector wedge's blood supply is islanded on the chosen segmental artery pedicle, the bowel has to be prepared for resection. Two bowel clamps are used to isolate the jejunum segment after gentle push over of any bowel content proximal and distal to the chosen jejunum flap. Anastomotic linear stapling devices can be used; however, care should be invested in identifying a small gap between two consecutive vasa recti, to allow best possible jejunum flap edge perfusion. The authors prefer sharp bowel transection with blade which would be followed by a manual double layer Vicryl suture bowel anastomosis to reconstruct small bowel continuity (Fig. 13.5).
- The jejunum flap is only transected when the recipient vessels are fully prepared and ready for microvascular anastomoses to minimize ischemic time. Careful and ideal transfixion suture ligation of the segmental artery on the donor site is performed to avoid catastrophic hemorrhage. The free jejunum flap is then washed carefully and transferred to the defect site (Figs. 13.6 and 13.7).

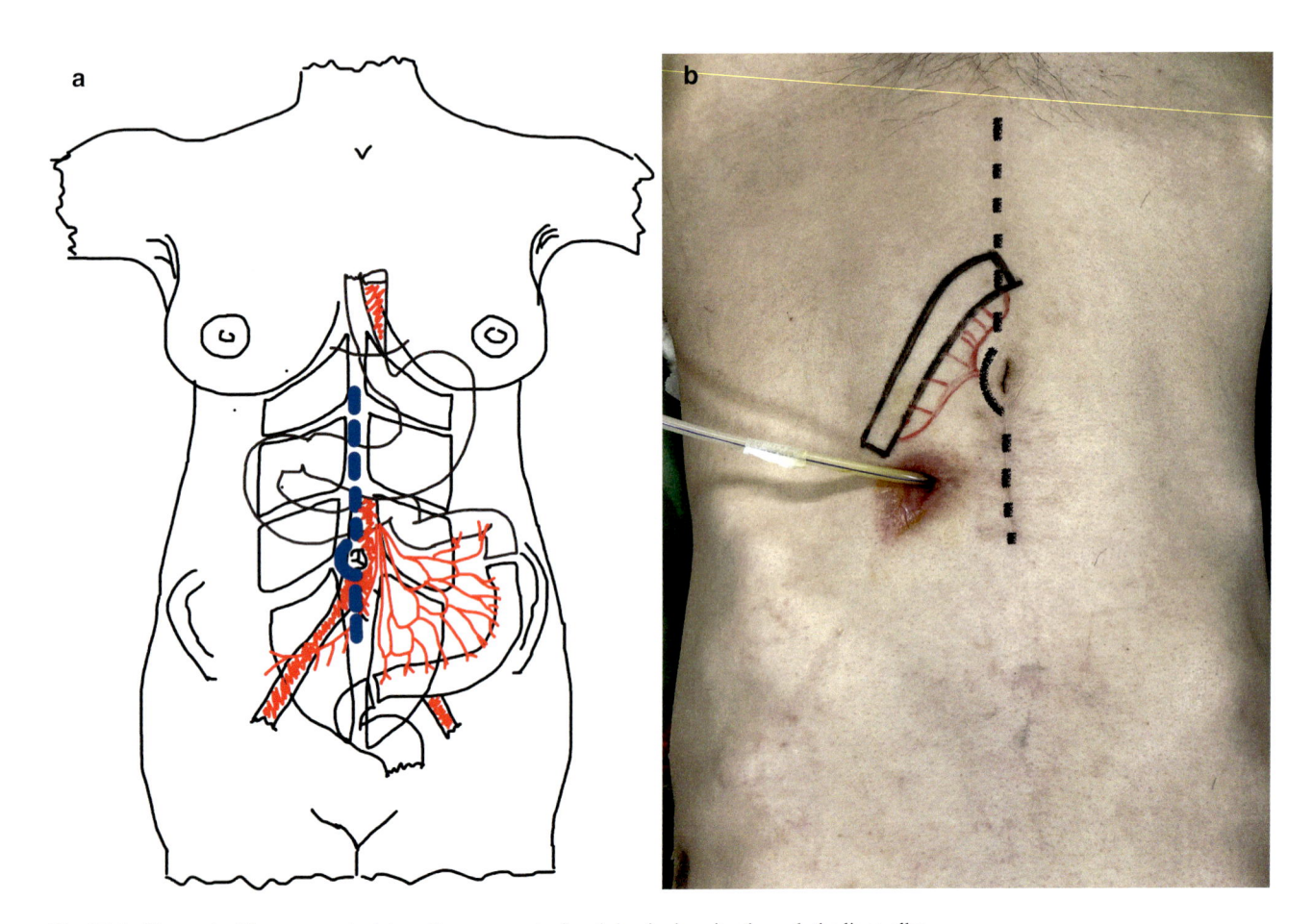

Fig. 13.1 The vertical laparotomy incision allows access to the abdominal cavity through the linea alba

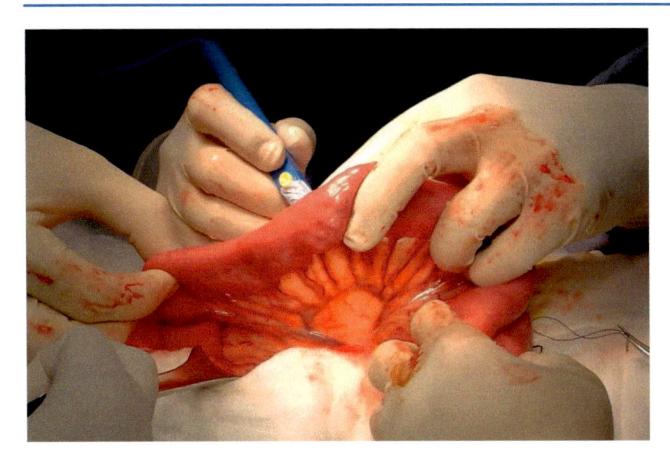

Fig. 13.2 The maximum segment of the jejunum flap could be up to 25–30 cm depending on the pedicle blood supply and the reconstructive defect

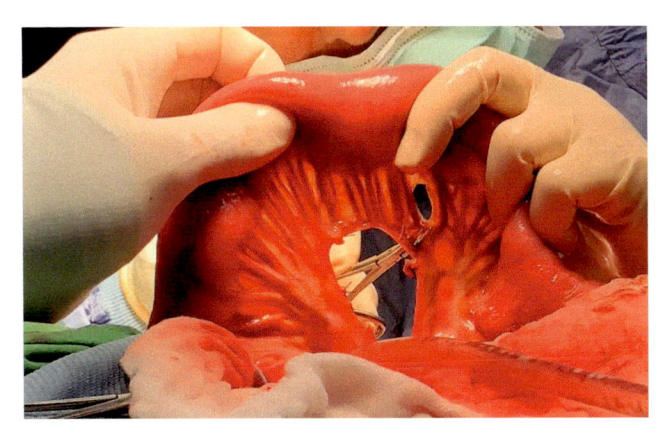

Fig. 13.3 The pedicle of interest from the segmental origin toward the arcades that supply the jejunum segment is separated from the remaining vascular branches via the loop-ligation hand tie technique

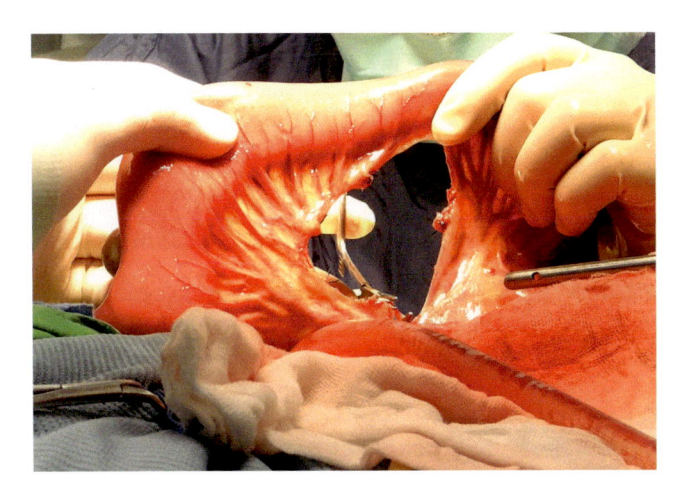

Fig. 13.4 The jejunum flap pedicle is dissected to its origin

- For hypopharyngeal and esophageal defects, a nasogastric feeding tube is inserted to allow easy identification of the neo-pharyngeal lumen and enable easier jejunum bowel anastomosis (Fig. 13.8).

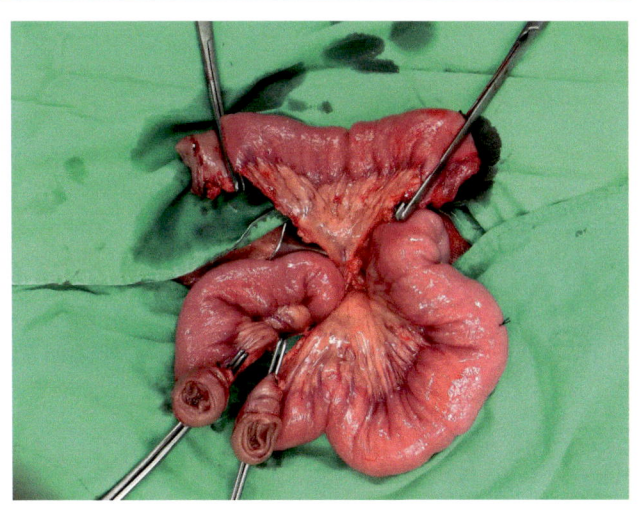

Fig. 13.5 When the jejunum sector wedge's blood supply is islanded on the chosen segmental artery pedicle, the bowel has to be prepared for resection

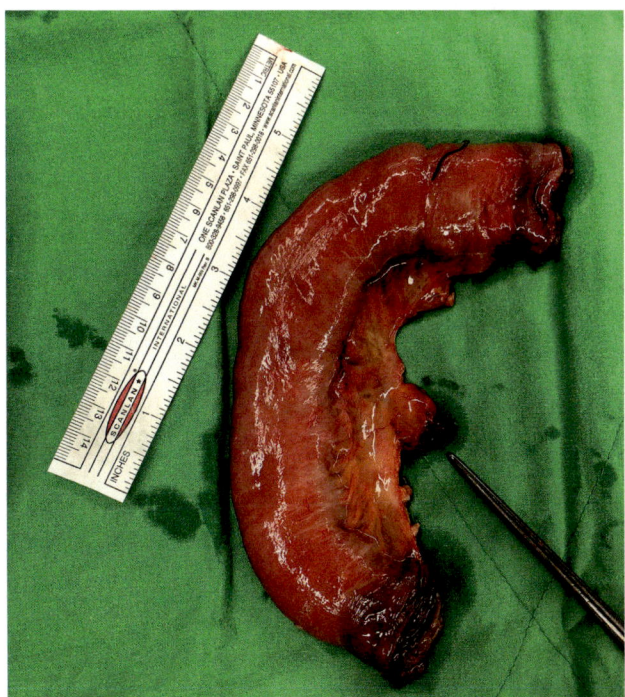

Fig. 13.6 The free jejunum flap is then washed carefully

- The microvascular anastomoses are performed under the microscope (i.e., superior thyroid, internal mammary or transverse cervical arteries). The jejunum inset and position should not cause any tension to the microvascular pedicle, and ideally a full-thickness fasciocutaneous skin flap deep to deep subcutaneous fascia should be able to cover the microvascular anastomosis for protection (Fig. 13.9a, b). Jejunum flap requires primary skin closure to allow wound healing; however, the authors have previously used split thickness skin grafting on the anti-mesenteric border of the bowel in extremely complex cases.

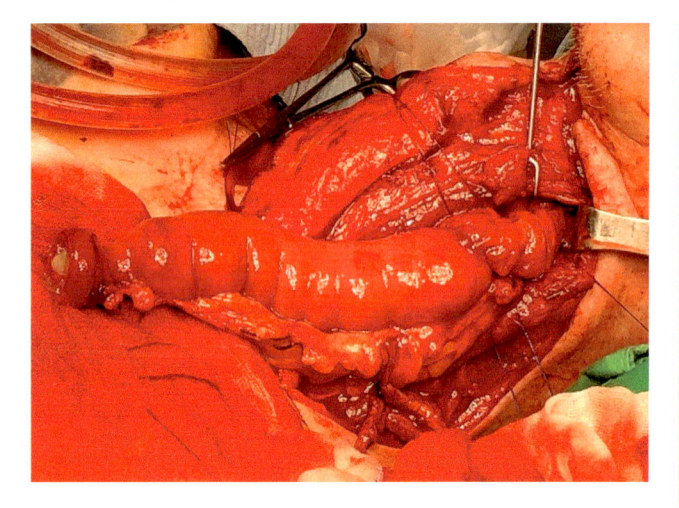

Fig. 13.7 The free jejunum flap is then transferred to the defect site and secured proximally

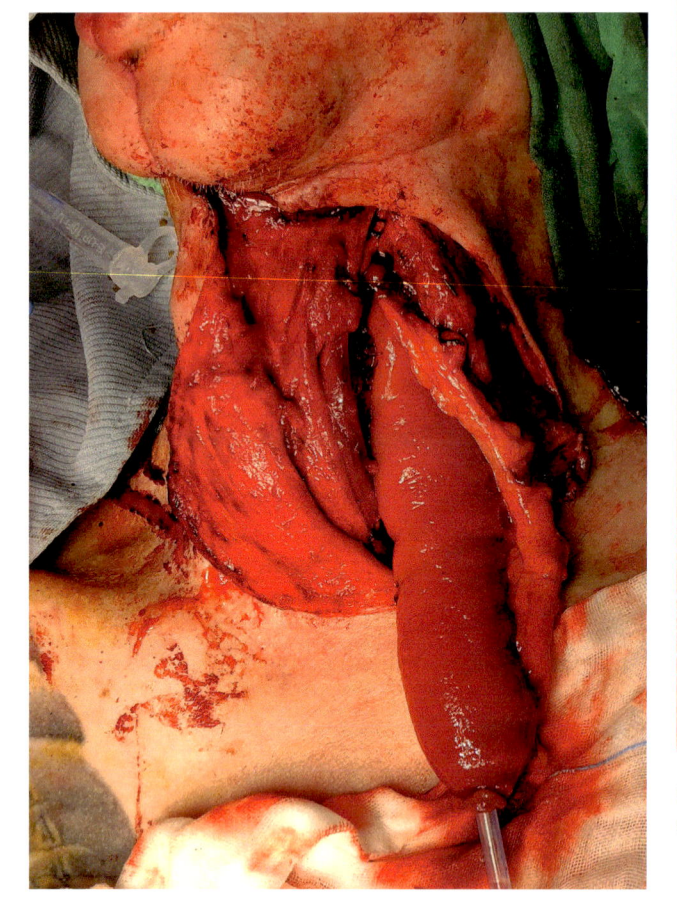

Fig. 13.8 A nasogastric feeding tube is inserted to allow easy identification of the neo-pharyngeal lumen and enable easier jejunum bowel anastomosis

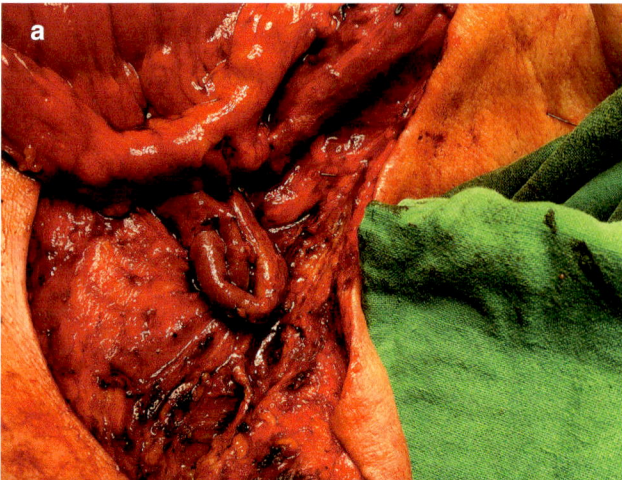

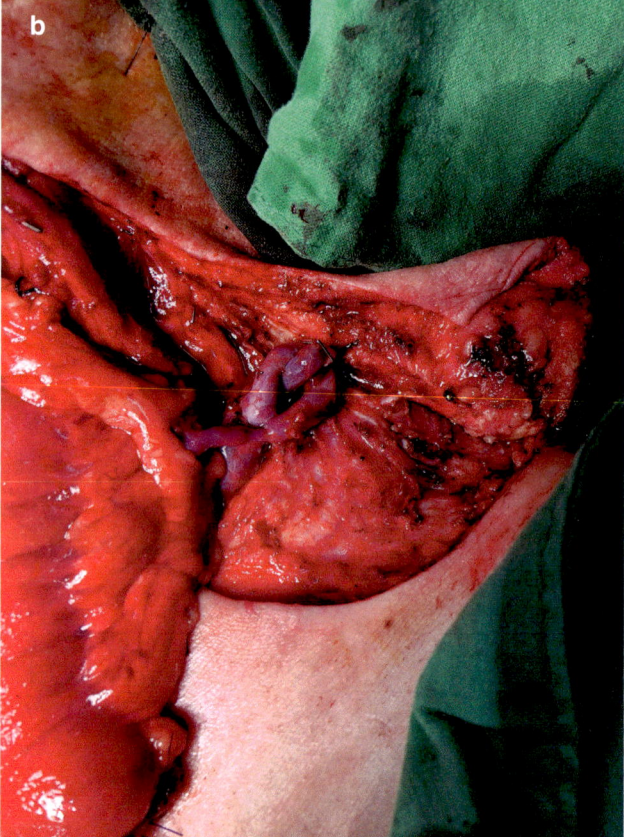

Fig. 13.9 The microvascular anastomoses are performed under the microscopic magnification without tension during jejunum flap inset

- The mesentery is sutured and examined to avoid internal herniation or other bowel-related complications. Abdominal wall mass closure is performed with a loop permanent 1–0 monofilament suture.

13.6 Core Surgical Techniques in Flap Dissection

- During careful examination of the mesentery; the transillumination is a very helpful way to allow clear visualization of vascular pedicles especially when there is a larger amount of fat between the double layers of the mesentery.

- It is very useful for hypopharyngeal and esophageal reconstruction while marking the length of the jejunum to add few centimeters of excess length to allow trimming and provide healthy viable edges prior to neo-pharyngeal anastomosis.
- A satellite segmental pedicle branch could be separated from the jejunum flap to supply a small segment of jejunum <5 cm in length to enable externalization during skin inset for flap monitoring.
- During arcades and mesenteric branching, ligation – extra care and meticulous hemostasis – can prevent postoperative intra-abdominal bleeds. The author-preferred ligation technique is via Vicryl 2/0 or 3/0 double loop ligations and for larger branches Vicryl transfixion sutures. Energy-based vessel ligation is recommended to be avoided.
- When the amount of mesentery fat is profuse, bi-digital gentle pressure of the double layer of mesentery peritoneum allows thinning of the fat tissue at the mesenteric transection wedge lines and also enables easier ligation of the arcade branches.
- Split jejunum flap modification: The jejunum tube is sharply divided to allow a split sero-mucosa flat design. This could be performed during inset while evaluating the exact patch pharyngoesophageal defect measurements; however, careful calculations are required to allow enough jejunum length.
- The jejunum segmental vessel pedicle is short. There is a limited arc of rotation or transposition of the jejunum during inset, and therefore this should be taken into consideration during flap length markings. The authors suggest that the recipient vessels are in the very immediate area of the esophageal defect and ideally in the middle of its length for tension-free flap inset.
- The authors choose to perform the proximal bowel anastomosis first before the microvascular anastomoses; however, this should not compromise the survival of flap due to extended ischemia time. Immediate after the microvascular anastomosis, the jejunum flap should be allowed to be perfused for few minutes, which would demonstrate an elongating effect. Only then the distal bowel anastomosis can be performed.

13.7 Clinical Scenarios

Case 1: Free Jejunum Flap for Hypopharyngeal Reconstruction

A 54-year-old male patient had hypopharyngeal carcinoma for which he underwent total laryngo-pharyngectomy and bilateral lymph node dissections. He had a family history of colorectal cancer, and therefore, not a candidate for ileocolon free flap reconstruction, due to the risk for future development of colon cancer in the reconstructed neck. The defect of the pharynx, cervical esophagus, and upper part of the trachea with loss of the larynx is demonstrated in Fig. 13.10. The segment of the free jejunum flap is demonstrated during flap dissection, and the chosen pedicle is confirmed with transillumination (Fig. 13.11). The jejunum free flap of equivalent length was transferred to reconstruct the esophageal defect (15 cm) (Fig. 13.12). Figure 13.13 demonstrates the postoperative esophagogram with smooth passage of the contrast medium from the mouth through the jejunum flap toward thoracic esophagus.

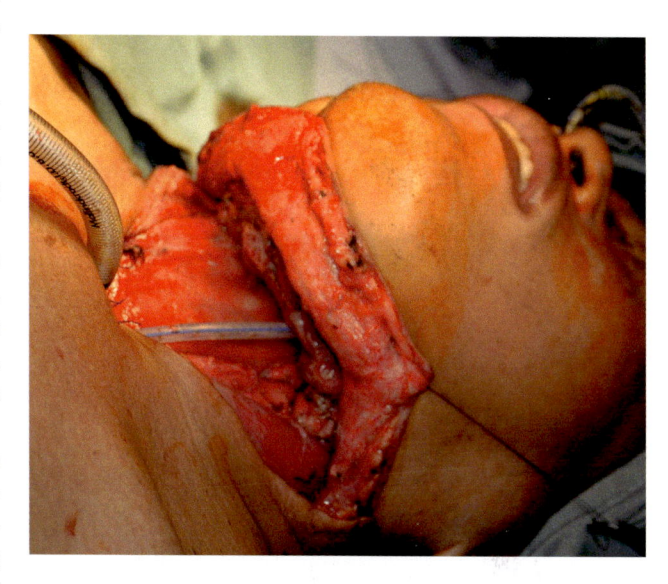

Fig. 13.10 The defect of the pharynx, cervical esophagus, and upper part of the trachea with loss of the larynx

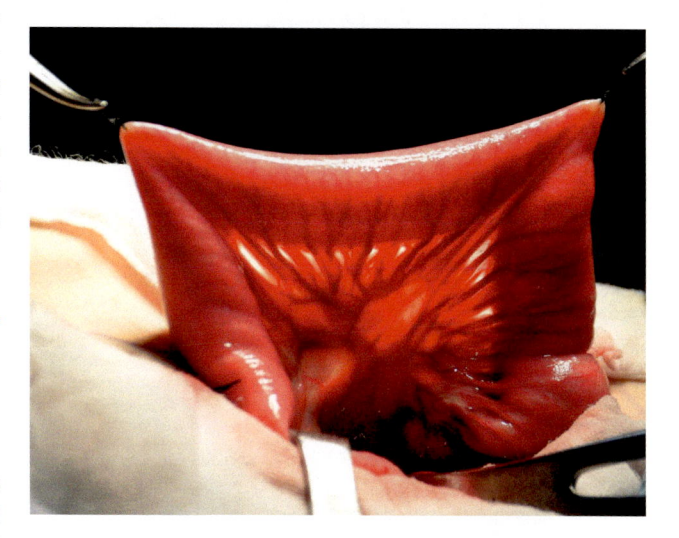

Fig. 13.11 The segment of the jejunum flap is identified and the chosen pedicle is confirmed with transillumination

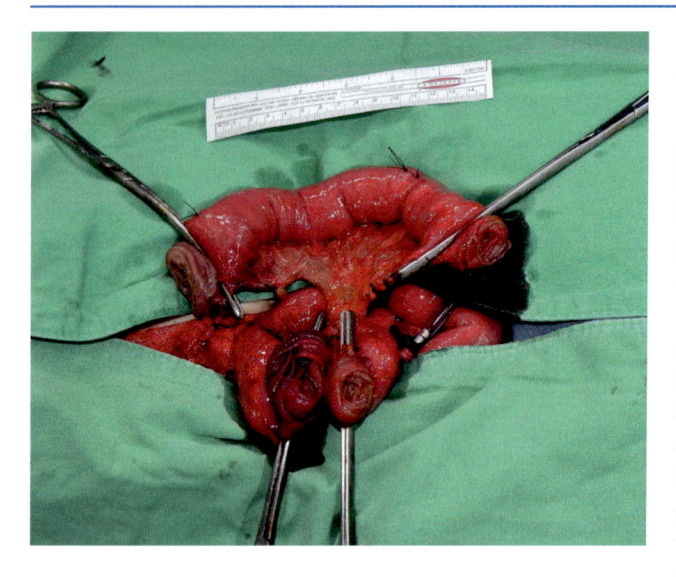

Fig. 13.12 The jejunum free flap of equivalent length following bowel transection and the microvascular pedicle fully dissected to its origin

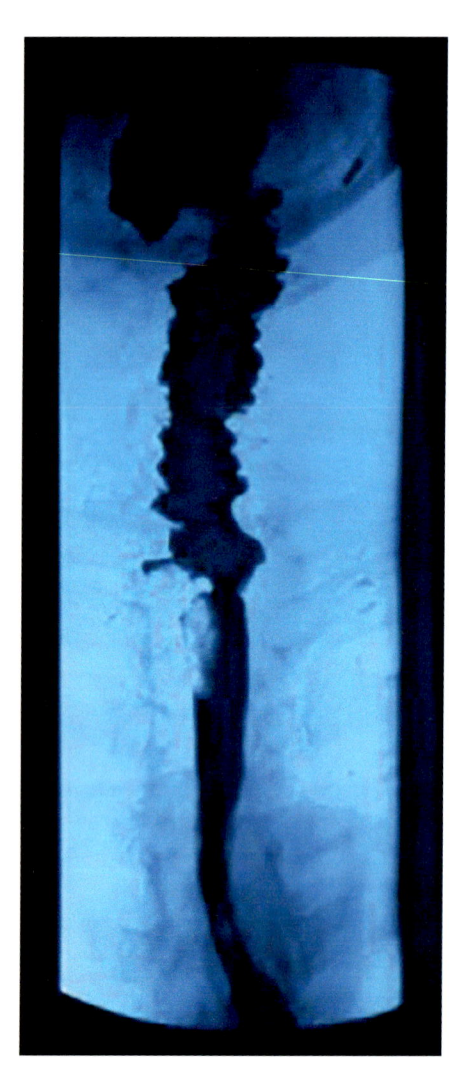

Fig. 13.13 Postoperative esophagogram (swallow test) of the contrast medium from the mouth through the jejunum flap toward thoracic esophagus

Case 2: Free Ileocolon Flap for Total Laryngopharyngeal Reconstruction

A 55-year-old male patient with hypopharyngeal cancer had a previous tracheostomy due to difficulty in breathing due to progressive airway obstruction. Total laryngopharyngectomy, bilateral lymph node dissection with postoperative radiotherapy, and chemotherapy were the management of choice (Fig. 13.14). Figure 13.15 demonstrated the expected pharyngeal defect, cervical esophagus, as well as laryngeal defect. An ileocolon free flap reconstruction was designed for total larynx and pharynx reconstruction (Fig. 13.16). The ileocolon free flap was after dissection, demonstrating a segment of ascending colon, along with the cecum and the ileocolic valve, that would allow simultaneous reconstruction of the pharynx and cervical esophagus. The segment of the ileum with ileocecal valve can be optimized to provide functional reconstruction of voice (Fig. 13.17). At immediate postoperative period, a swallowing function test showed continence of the swallowing tube, in the shape of the terminal ileum and colon flap (Fig. 13.18).

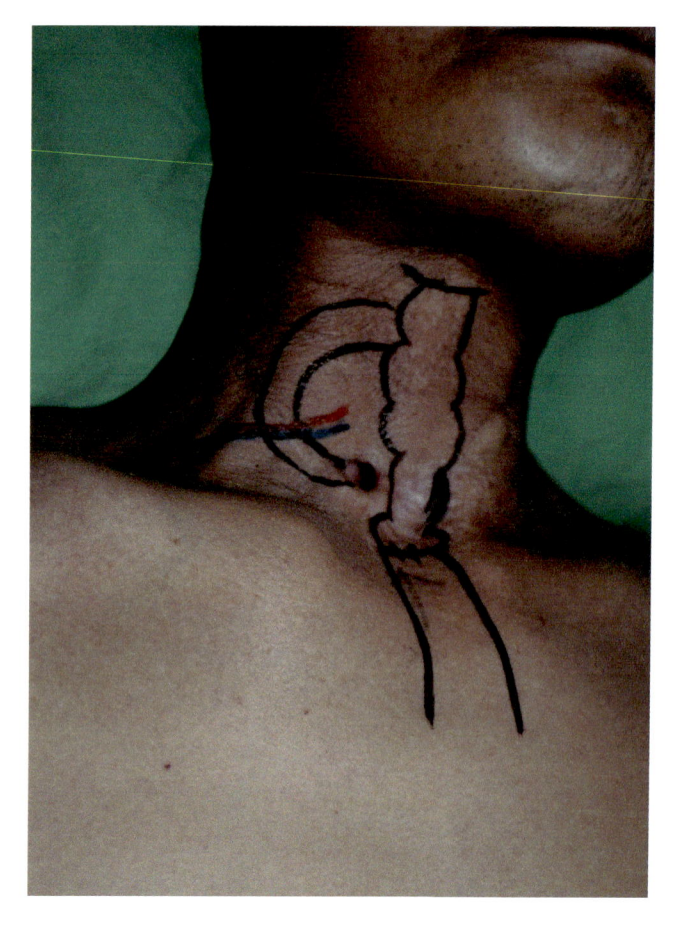

Fig. 13.14 Ileocolon flap design and markings

13 Bowel Flaps - Jejunum Flap

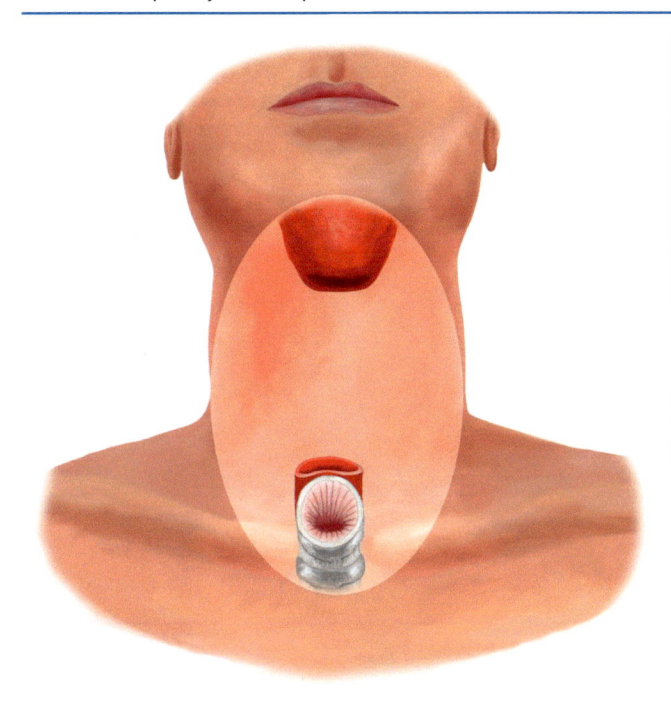

Fig. 13.15 Total layngopharyngectomy defect

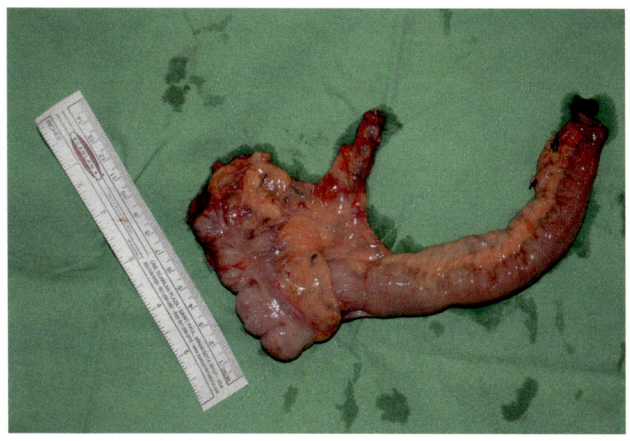

Fig. 13.17 The Ileocolon free flap following dissection

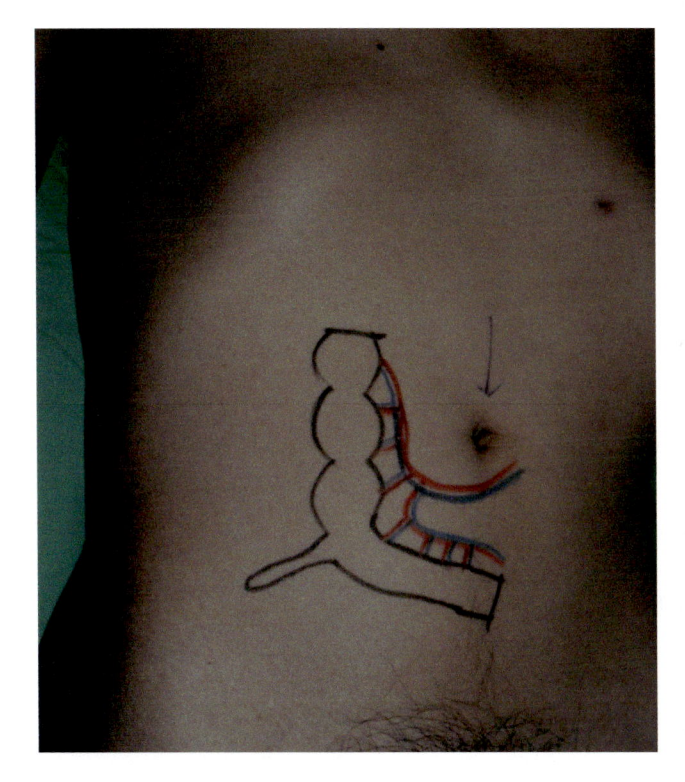

Fig. 13.16 The ileocolon flap design with the pedicle markings

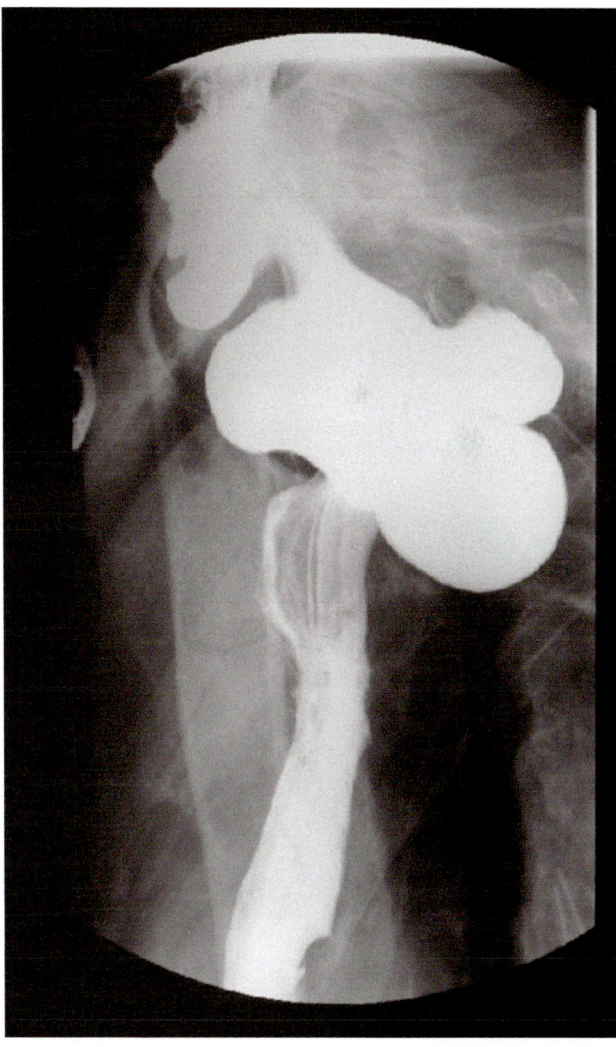

Fig. 13.18 Postoperative swallow test demonstrating the smooth passage of the dye through the ileocolon flap

Case 3: Free Ileum Flap for Urethral Reconstruction

A 34-year-old male patient had severe hypospadias. He underwent several previous operations utilizing local scrotal skin; however, he still had urethral stricture and was suffering several episodes of urinary infections and difficulty in voiding. Figure 13.19 shows a lateral view with a contracture of ventral side skin of the penis. Figure 13.20 demonstrates intraoperative dissection and resection of the contracture which was removed leaving a 7 cm urethral defect. A segment of free ileum flap was transferred for reconstruction of the urethra. A smooth passage of urine after surgery is demonstrated with the patient in standing position (Fig. 13.21).

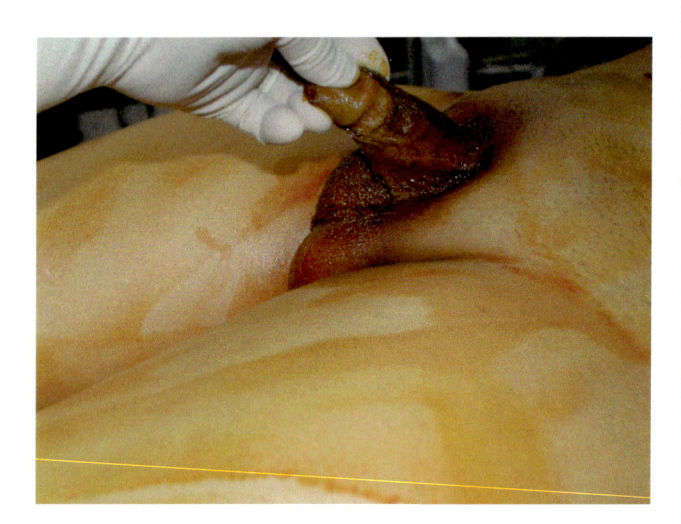

Fig. 13.19 Contracted penis and urethra from multiple revision hypospadias reconstructive procedures

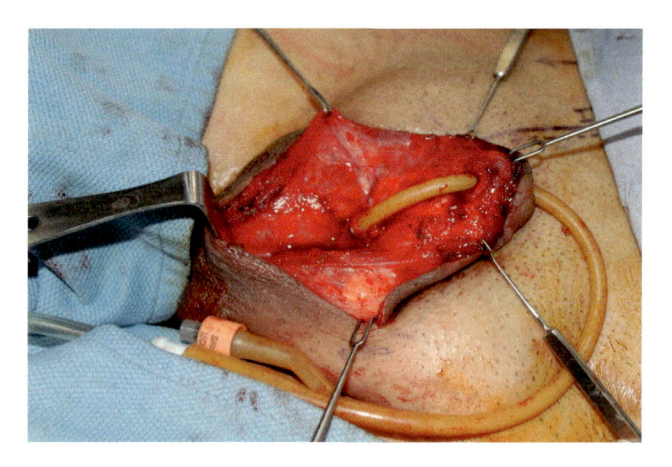

Fig. 13.20 Intraoperative dissection and resection of the contracture which left a 7 cm urethral defect

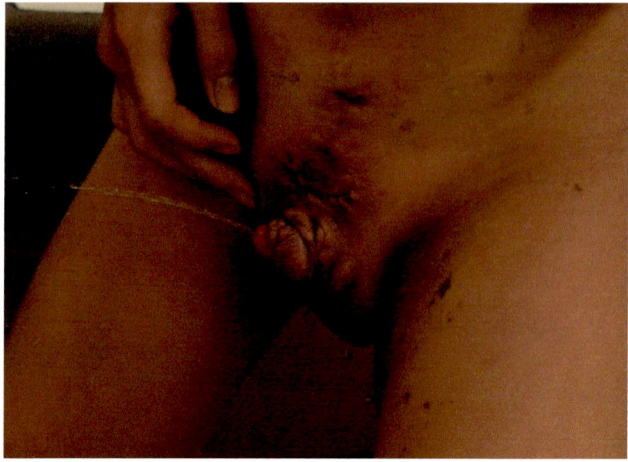

Fig. 13.21 A smooth passage of urine through the ileum flap in standing position

13.8 Pearls and Pitfalls

Pearls
- The jejunum segment should be made ideally at a distance 30 cm distal from the ligament of Treitz but should also be distal enough to allow accessible pedicle length and mesentery along with the adequate length of the jejunum flap to cover the defect.
- The choice of the segmental artery should be placed after careful examination of the anastomotic arcades. This would dictate the exact jejunum segment with the most robust mesenteric vascular supply, especially at its edges where healing of the bowel anastomosis will take place.
- A marking suture should be placed at the peristaltic direction of motion during harvesting to ensure appropriate inset for the neo-esophagus.
- The jejunum anastomosis is preferred to be performed with a two-layer suture closure, and if an anastomotic staple is used, an extra overlay seromuscular Vicryl mattress suture layer should be performed to reduce leaks.
- The jejunum serves as an excellent tubular structure option for reconstruction of vaginal defects; it offers a self-lubricated tube with peristalsis and has benefits over fasciocutaneous flaps for vaginal reconstructions.

Pitfalls

- The vasa recta, the distal branches of the arcade pedicles of the jejunum flap, are approximately 5 cm in length and enter the mesenteric border of the jejunum to supply a zone of approximately 1 cm of bowel – forming the vasa recti unit. This is paramount in flap manipulation as these vessels are very delicate, especially the veins. Care should be considered during harvesting and while deciding the level of jejunum transection to allow optimal edge perfusion.
- Surgical flow and flap harvest are simple and quick but should be performed with extra care in every step. All recipient vessels must be prepared before the flap is disconnected to avoid troublesome delay in microvascular anastomosis.
- The most difficult bowel anastomosis in the defect should be performed first, prior to microvascular anastomosis, and this should be quick to reduce ischemia time.
- The jejunum does not tolerate venous congestion as other fasciocutaneous flaps do; therefore, extra care should be put into optima microvascular suture line for the venous anastomosis. The authors prefer to complete the venous anastomosis first. If the arterial anastomosis has been performed first, the clamp should not be removed while performing the venous anastomosis as this will cause intra-flap congestion.
- Strictures and stenosis are recognized complications of neo-pharyngeal reconstruction with jejunum flap, especially in the inferior anastomotic line. Spatulating the jejunum lower edge allows larger circumference and lowers the risk for constriction during healing. Similarly, a double-barrel jejunum superior configuration may allow larger opening in the oropharyngeal anastomosis. Always aim for watertight closure.

13.9 Selected Readings

- Kim EKF, Mardini S, Salgado CJ, Chen H-C. Esophagus and hypopharyngeal reconstruction. Sem Plast Surg. 2010.

  The authors reviewed the literature on esophageal reconstruction. The most common methods used are gastric pull-up, pectoralis major flap, colon interposition, fasciocutaneous flaps (radial forearm free flap or anterolateral thigh flap), and free jejunum and colon flaps. The stricture rates, fistula rates, morbidity, and mortality of each flap were also reviewed.

- Razdan SN, Albornoz CR, Matros E, Paty PB, Cordeiro PG. Free jejunal flap for pharyngoesophageal reconstruction in head and neck cancer patients: an evaluation of donor-site complications. J Reconstr Microsurg. 2015.

  This article portrays the authors' critical appraisal on free jejunal transfer for pharyngoesophageal reconstruction and the associated donor site morbidity. Conversely, they discuss on the argument that support the use of fasciocutaneous flaps, given their low incidence of donor site complications. This study documented donor site complication rate with free jejunal flaps for pharyngoesophageal reconstruction, in the hands of an experienced surgeon. They concluded that free jejunal transfer is associated with minimal and acceptable donor site complication rates. The choice of flap for pharyngoesophageal reconstruction should be determined by the type of defect, potential recipient site complications, and the surgeon's familiarity with the flap. Potential donor site complications should not be a deterrent for free jejunal flaps given the low rate described in this study.

- Chen H-C, Rampazzo A, Gharb BB, Wong MTC, Mardini S, Chen H-Y, Salgado CJ. Motility differences in free colon and free jejunum flaps for reconstruction of the cervical esophagus. Plast Reconstruct Surg, 2008;122(5):1410–6.

  In this study the free colon and jejunal flaps are described as reliable and safe conduits for pharyngoesophageal reconstruction. According to the authors, compared with free colon flaps, free jejunum flaps have a smaller diameter and intrinsic peristaltic movement, both of which are considered possible causes of dysphagia. The authors evaluated the motility differences in free jejunum and colon flaps using radionuclide esophageal scintigraphy. Although neither flap showed normal swallowing characteristics, free jejunum flaps displayed greater esophageal clearance and should represent the first choice in hypopharyngeal reconstruction. Free colon and ileocolon flaps should be reserved for very proximal oropharyngeal defects and when simultaneous voice reconstruction is desired.

- Disa JJ, Pusic AL, Hidalgo DA, Cordeiro PG. Microvascular reconstruction of the hypopharynx: defect classification, treatment algorithm, and functional outcome based on 165 consecutive cases. Plast Reconstr Surg. 2003;111(2):652–60.

  The aims of this study were threefold: to develop a scheme for classification of hypopharyngeal defects, to establish a reconstructive algorithm based on this system, and to assess the functional outcome of such reconstruction. The authors report a retrospective review of a 14-year experience with 165 consecutive microvascular reconstructions of the hypopharynx in 160 patients. Their overall free flap success rate was 98%. They also report a treatment algorithm for microvascular hypopharyngeal reconstruction based on the type of defect with partial defects with radial forearm flaps, circumferential defects reconstructed with free jejunal flaps, and extensive, multilevel defects reconstructed with rectus abdominis myocutaneous flaps. This article concludes that microvascular reconstruction of pharyngeal defects is highly successful with few postoperative complications.

- Chen H-C, Kim EKF, Salgado CJ, Mardini S. Methods of voice reconstruction. Semin Plast Surg. 2010.

  The authors reviewed methods of voice reconstruction. Nonsurgical methods of voice reconstruction include electrolarynx, pneumatic artificial larynx, and esophageal speech. Surgical methods of voice reconstruction include neoglottis, tracheoesophageal puncture, and prosthesis. Tracheoesophageal puncture can be performed in patients with pedicled flaps such as colon interposition, jejunum, or gastric pull-up or in free flaps such as the perforator flaps, jejunum, and colon flaps. Other flaps for voice reconstruction include the ileocolon flap and jejunum. Laryngeal transplantation was also reviewed and discussed.

References

1. Seidenberg B, Rosenak SS, Hurwitt ES, Som ML. Immediate reconstruction of the cervical esophagus by a revascularized isolated jejunal segment. Ann Surg. 1959;149(2):162–71.
2. Razdan SN, Albornoz CR, Matros E, Paty PB, Cordeiro PG. Free jejunal flap for pharyngoesophageal reconstruction in head and neck cancer patients: an evaluation of donor-site complications. J Reconstr Microsurg. 2015;31(9):643–6.

Thoracodorsal Artery Flap: Latissimus Dorsi Flap

14

Mohammed Farid, Dariush Nikkhah, and Jeremy Rawlins

14.1 Introduction

The latissimus dorsi (LD) is a muscle name originated from Latin (latus = broad, dorsum = back) which means the "broadest muscle of the back" [1]. One of the first descriptions for LD use as a flap was apparent from drawings by anatomist and physician Vesalius (sixteenth century) who demonstrated the muscle division from origin and lateral rotation [2]. The LD flap was first reported as a pedicled flap (axial pattern) for a mastectomy defect by Tansini in 1906 [3]. Then, the clinical application was sporadic until Olivari in 1976 used LD for chest wall defects post-radiation exposure [4]. A year later in 1977, Schneider elaborated the concept to use LD flap with an implant-based breast reconstruction following radical mastectomy, which helped replace breast tissue and restore shape [5]. The year 1978 witnessed a number of advancements in LD flap reconstruction. Bostwick developed the principle for an island-based LD flap in breast reconstruction [6]. The versatile nature of the LD flap marked its use as a pedicled flap in head and neck reconstruction by Quillen. This was a rotational island flap tunnelled above pectoralis major muscle to reconstruct the lateral neck and cheek defects from resection of a mandibular defect [7]. Maxwell was the first who used the LD muscle as a free flap for scalp reconstruction [8]. A year later in 1979, May reported the use of free LD flaps in lower limb reconstruction [9]. In 1982, one of the first free LD reported cases in upper limb for hand reconstruction was performed by Bailey [10]. The further refinement of microsurgical concepts led to the expansion and diverse use of LD flaps over the past 40 years.

14.2 Anatomy

The latissimus dorsi is the most superficial and largest muscle of the posterior trunk [1]. The superomedial part is covered by trapezius muscle, and LD muscle covers part of the paraspinal and majority of serratus anterior muscle [11]. The origin is from the lower six thoracic vertebrae, tenth to 12th posterior ribs, superior angle of scapula, lower sacral vertebrae, thoracolumbar fascia and posterior iliac crest forming the roof of the superior lumbar triangle [12, 13]. The fibres span as a triangular and flat muscle to become a broad tendon [11]. The muscle has an aponeurotic attachment to the lower border of the serratus anterior and meets the teres major superiorly forming the posterior axillary fold before inserting into the lesser tubercle and the intertubercular groove of the humerus [13].

According to the Mathes and Nahai classification, the LD is a type V muscle with a dominant artery (thoracodorsal (TD)) and secondary segmental vessels from lumbar (medial paraspinal) and posterior intercostal (lateral) perforators [14]. The thoracodorsal artery is a branch of the subscapular artery forming a pedicle to enter the LD muscle 8–12 cm proximal to the humeral insertion. The neurovascular bundle is on the deep surface of LD muscle found 4 cm distal to inferior border of the scapula and 2.5 cm lateral to medial border of LD muscle [15]. At this point, the pedicle then divides into two branches (medial and lateral) parallel to the superior and anterior edge of the LD muscle. This concept forms the basis of splitting the LD muscle. Within the muscle, these branches divide into smaller ones which anastomose with lumbar and intercostal perforators [12, 14, 16]. The pedicle length is 8 cm on average (range 6–12 cm) and has a mean diameter of 3 mm (range 2–4 mm). The venous drainage

---

Supplementary Information The online version contains supplementary material available at https://doi.org/10.1007/978-3-031-07678-7_14.

M. Farid (✉)
Department of Plastic Surgery, Royal Stoke University Hospital, Stoke-on-Trent, UK

D. Nikkhah
Department of Plastic, Reconstructive and Aesthetic Surgery, Royal Free Hospital, London, UK

J. Rawlins
Department of Plastic Surgery, Royal Perth Hospital, Perth, WA, Australia

accompanies arteries, namely, the thoracodorsal vein with a similar average length and diameter to the thoracodorsal artery. Secondary venous drainage with concomitant veins follows perforating secondary arteries [11]. The motor supply is from the thoracodorsal nerve (posterior cord brachial plexus) which runs parallel to the vascular pedicle and innervates the LD muscle [16]. The sensory supply to the muscle is from the posterior branches of the lateral cutaneous branches of intercostal nerves laterally, and lateral branches of posterior rami (VI-XII) posteriorly. These branches are valuable to preserve sensation when raising a reverse LD flap based on intercostal perforators [11].

14.3 Preoperative Investigation

The free or pedicled LD flap is not associated with particular preoperative investigations or imaging modalities [11]. This is predominantly related to the consistent anatomy of the pedicle. The underlying factor to determine the feasibility of raising LD flap is a thorough examination to rule out any potential contraindications. Palpation of the muscle bulk with shoulder extension, medial rotation and adduction against examiner's hand is indicated [1]. A pinch test for skin paddle orientation is crucial for the myocutaneous LD flap to determine if primary closure is feasible. If the muscle function is thought to be compromised due to previous injury (damage to the thoracodorsal pedicle), pathology or surgery (posterolateral thoracotomy), then preoperative imaging (Doppler ultrasound) would be essential to determine adequate LD perfusion. Nonetheless, a recent study indicated the benefit of reduction in surgical time and identifying thoracodorsal pedicle with a preoperative CT-A in those with previous axillary surgery or irradiation. Other relative contraindications to perform LD flap is insufficient donor LD bulk, hobbies like climbing causing shoulder weakness and inability to achieve lateral decubitus position to harvest the flap [16, 17, 18, 19, 20].

14.4 Flap Design and Markings

Flap design is based on LD landmarks, muscle harvest, skin paddle and indication for reconstruction. Preoperatively, the LD muscle is palpated along its anterior border with a pinch test for skin paddle and forceful contraction to visualise it.

All markings in standing position preoperatively are checked intraoperatively. Anteriorly, a vertical line is drawn from mid-axillary point to mid-point between ASIS and PSIS to mark the most anterior border of the LD muscle. Another line is oblique above the inferior border of the scapula from the posterior axillary fold and along tip of the scapula to meet vertebral column, where a vertical line is drawn marking the most posterior border of thoracolumbar fascia. A horizontal line marking the iliac crest identifies the most inferior part of the LD flap. The variability in marking is based on whether a skin paddle is raised or a muscle-only flap. Intraoperatively, the patient is in the lateral decubitus position with arm rested on a board at 90 degrees shoulder and elbow flexion [21]. The skin paddle is safely marked within the borders of the LD muscle (tip of the scapula superiorly, iliac crest inferiorly, vertebral column posteriorly). Design of the paddle is either transverse (horizontal), oblique or vertical (Figs. 14.1, 14.2 and 14.3) [1]. Thoracodorsal perforators can be mapped with handheld Doppler to be incorporated within the skin paddle [14].

Fig. 14.1 Marking of the inferior border (iliac crest), posterior border (vertebral column) of LD flap and an oblique skin paddle

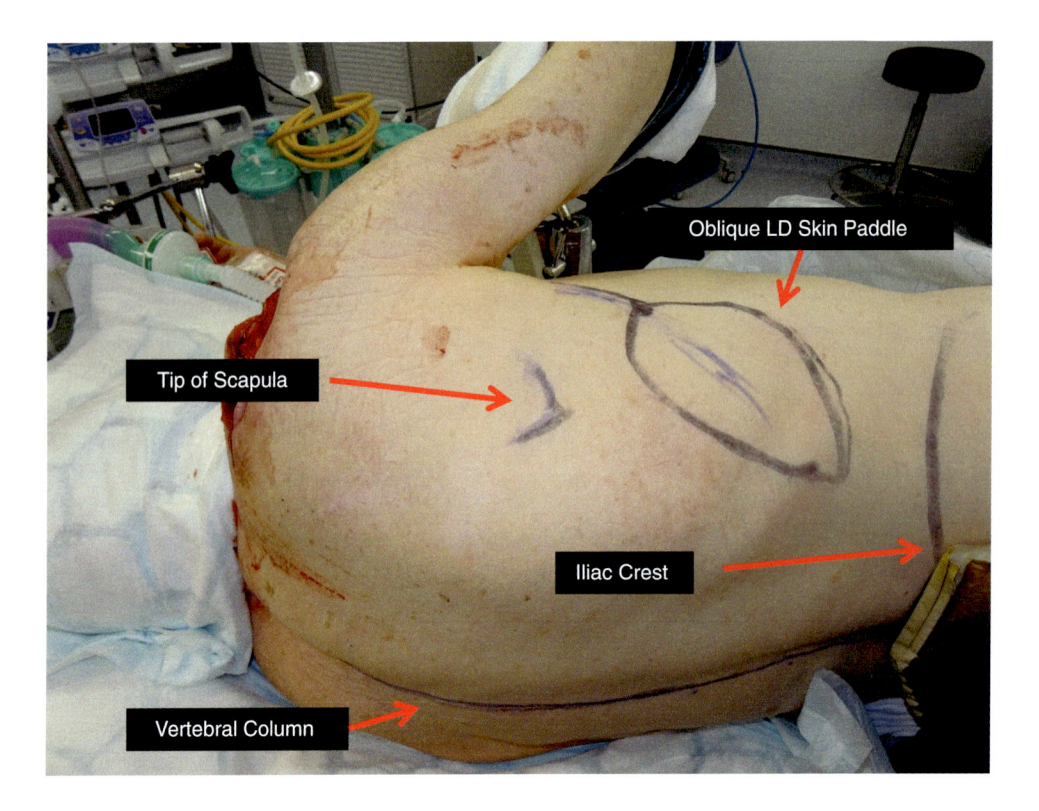

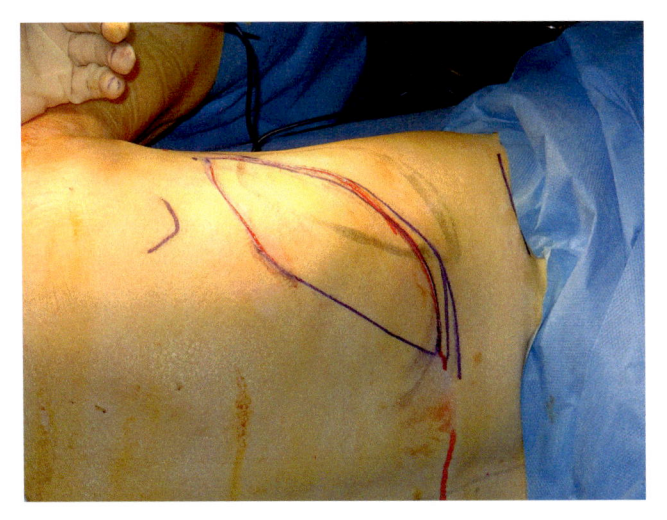

14 Thoracodorsal Artery Flap: Latissimus Dorsi Flap

Fig. 14.2 Large skin paddle over LD muscle design to correspond to defect size

14.5 Flap Raise/Elevation: A Step-by-Step Guide

Step 1. Incision and Anterior Flap Dissection The exact incision is based on either a muscle-only flap or a myocutaneous flap. The first incision is along the posterior axillary fold and corresponding to the anterior border of the skin paddle (Fig. 14.4) reaching above the iliac crest margin. Dissection to the fascial plane (Fig. 14.5) is continued and a subcutaneous flap is raised anterior to the skin paddle to identify the anterior border of the LD muscle (Fig. 14.6).

Step 2. Posterior Flap Dissection A subcutaneous flap is raised posterior to the skin paddle edge to further define the posterior border of LD muscle (Fig. 14.7). The muscle edges are identified below the flaps and the skin paddle is located

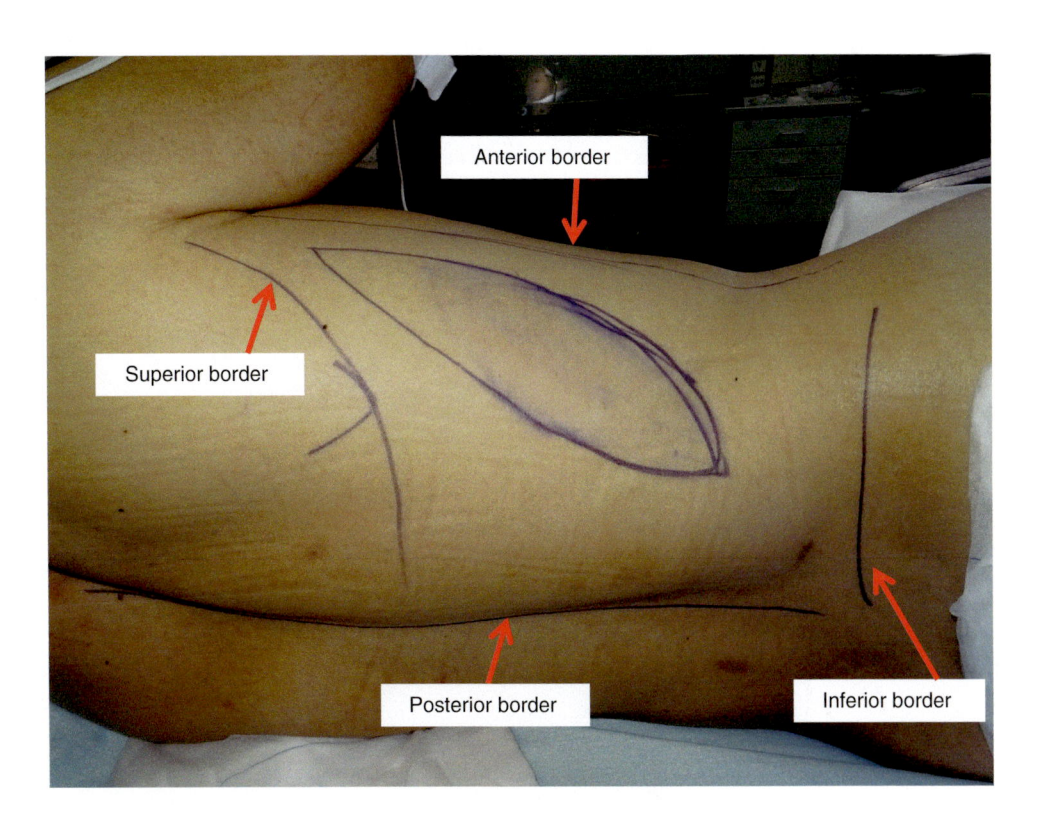

Fig. 14.3 Borders of LD muscle flap

Fig. 14.4 LD skin paddle anterior incision along posterior axillary fold

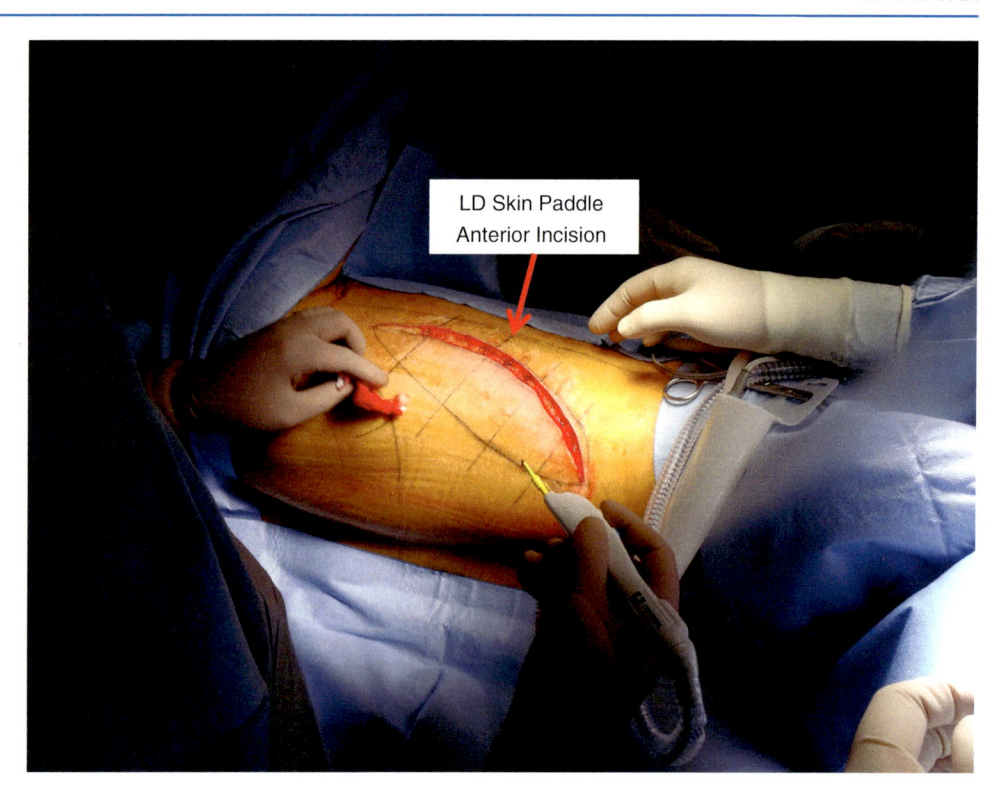

Fig. 14.5 LD skin paddle anterior incision down to fascial plane

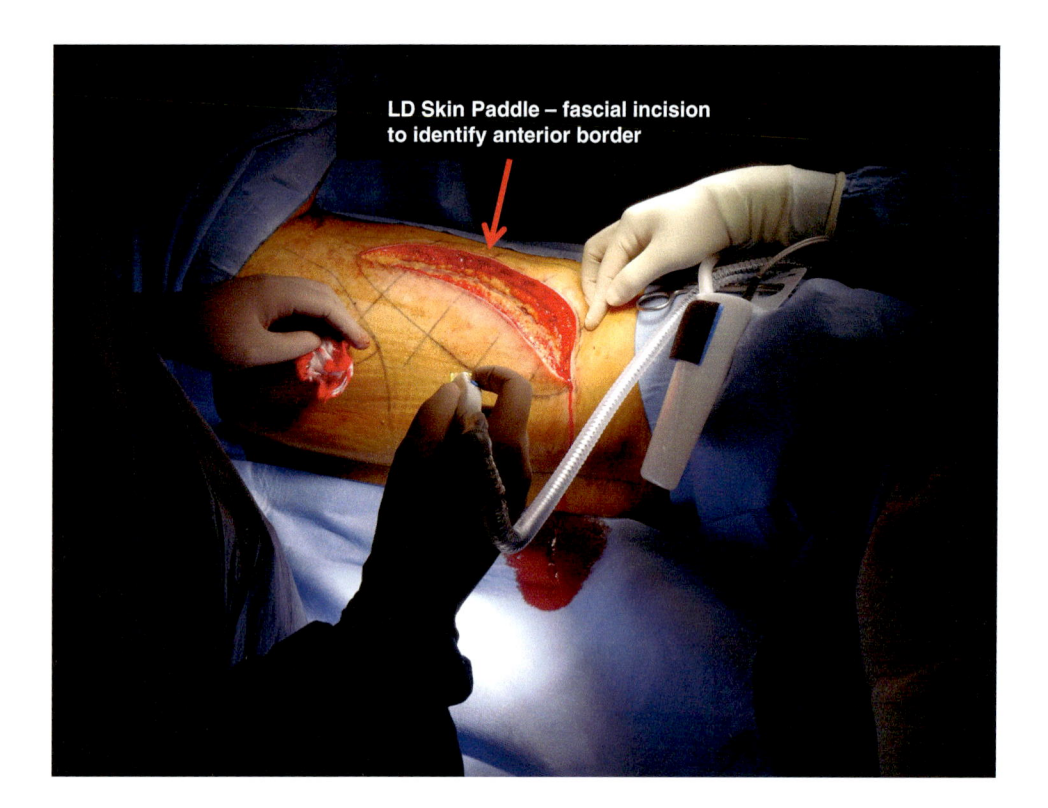

Fig. 14.6 LD skin paddle anterior subcutaneous border raised to reveal LD anterior border

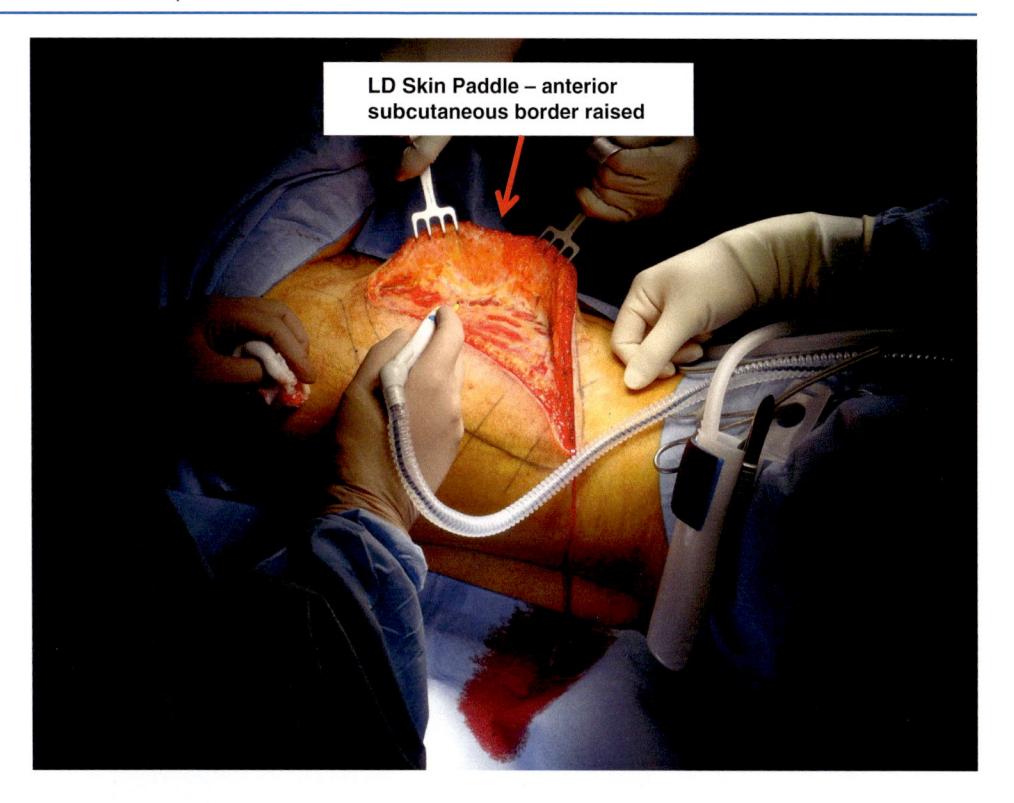

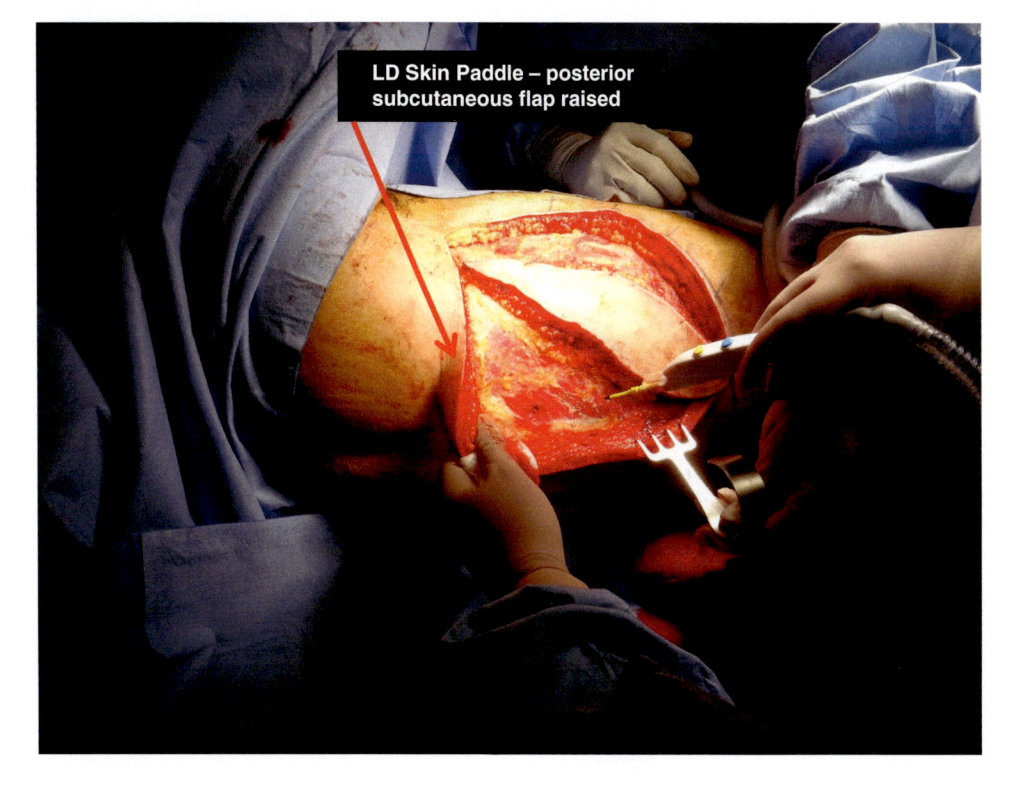

Fig. 14.7 LD skin paddle posterior subcutaneous border raised to reveal LD posterior border

on the LD muscle. Multiple perforators from the posterior intercostal arteries are encountered and isolated with ligaclips throughout LD dissection posteriorly (Fig. 14.8).

Step 3. LD Muscle Raising The LD muscle is detached anteriorly along the posterior axillary line. Teres major and serratus anterior muscles are identified by observing the muscle contraction and the orientation of the fibres. The teres major is noted above the tip of the scapula while the serratus anterior is between the latissimus dorsi and pectoralis major muscle. Then, the lower edge is separated from the iliac crest and thoracolumbar insertion. The posterior border along midline is divided (Fig. 14.9), so the skin paddle with the LD muscle is free along the anterior, inferior and posterior borders (Fig. 14.10).

Fig. 14.8 LD posterior border and undersurface demonstrating intercostal perforators

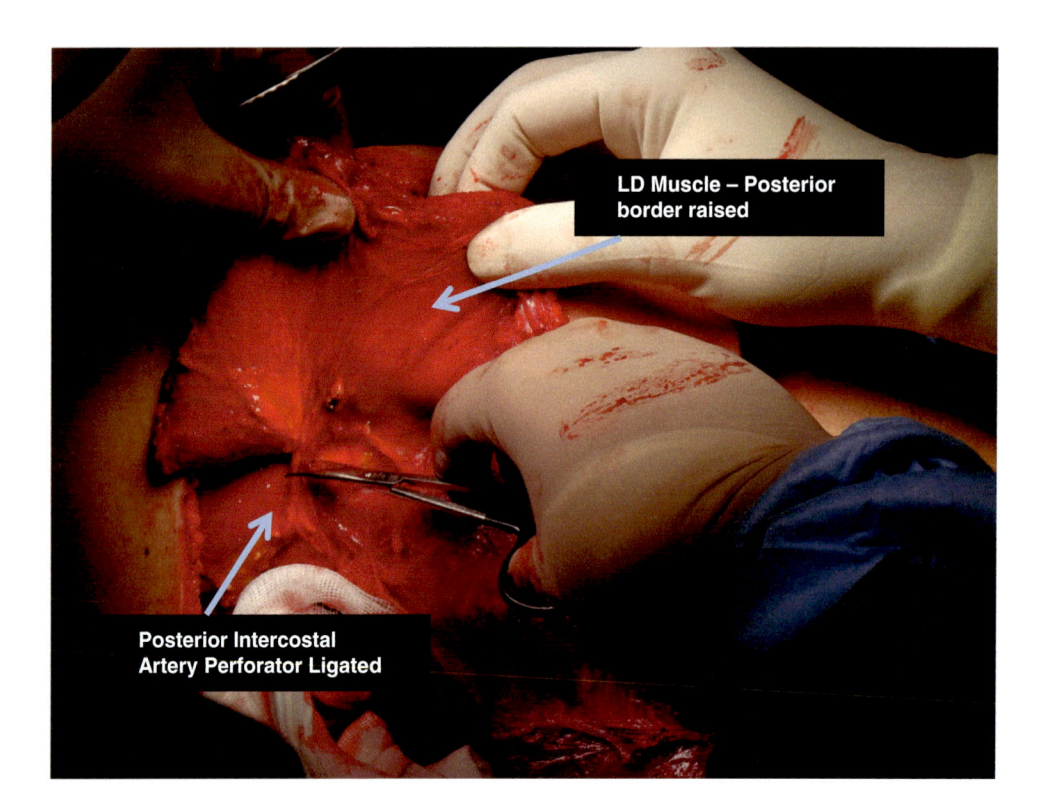

Fig. 14.9 LD posterior and inferior borders raised with skin paddle

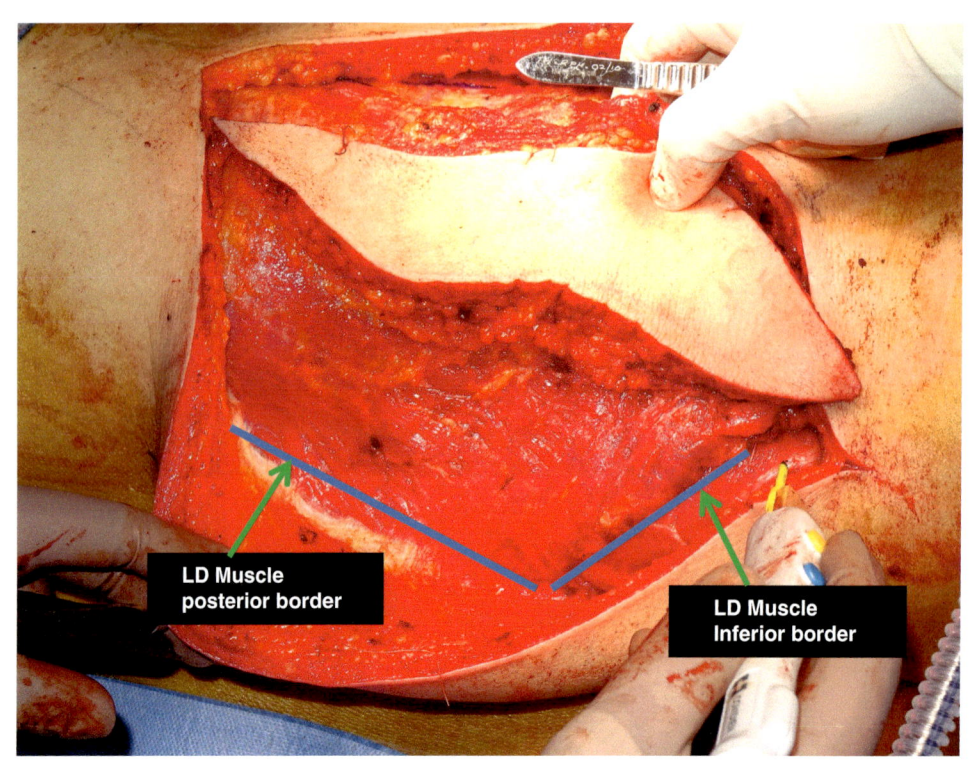

14 Thoracodorsal Artery Flap: Latissimus Dorsi Flap

Step 4. Identification of Thoracodorsal Pedicle Continue to raise the LD myocutaneous flap from caudal to cranial. The plane is identified along a layer of loose areolar tissue. Dissection is away from the LD muscle, ensuring the vascular pedicle is preserved (Fig. 14.11). The pedicle location is consistent being few centimetres from the anterior edge of LD muscle cranially. Retraction of the pedicle allows visualisation of the remaining LD muscle and its attachment.

Step 5. Muscle Separation As dissection progresses caudally, identify the tip of the scapula which marks the superior border of LD flap. Continue dissection of the LD from the inferior border of the trapezius muscle. Anteriorly, ensure that the serratus anterior is separated from LD muscle on the inferior-posterior margin (Fig. 14.12). Careful attention is needed when reaching this point to separate muscles rather than en bloc dissection of both muscles which is a common pitfall.

Step 6. Flap Division/Isolation The proximal humeral insertion is identified through careful dissection along a tunnelled plane. The vascular pedicle underneath the LD tendon is protected with operating surgeon's fingers while carefully dividing the tendon at insertion. The flap is raised with its vascular supply at this level as free flap or kept attached as a pedicled flap (Fig. 14.13). A headlight or lighted retractor is useful in this phase of the operation to clearly identify the tendon insertion and the pedicle.

Step 7. Closure The donor site is closed in a tensionless fashion; multilayered (2/0 PDS and 3/0 Monocryl) and two drains are left in situ (Fig. 14.14). Towel clips are used to help facilitate closure sequentially (Figs. 14.15 and 14.16).

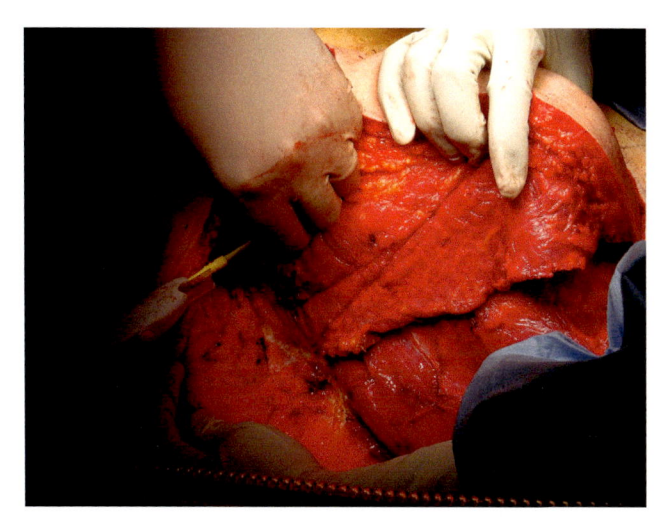

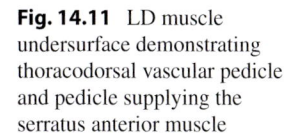

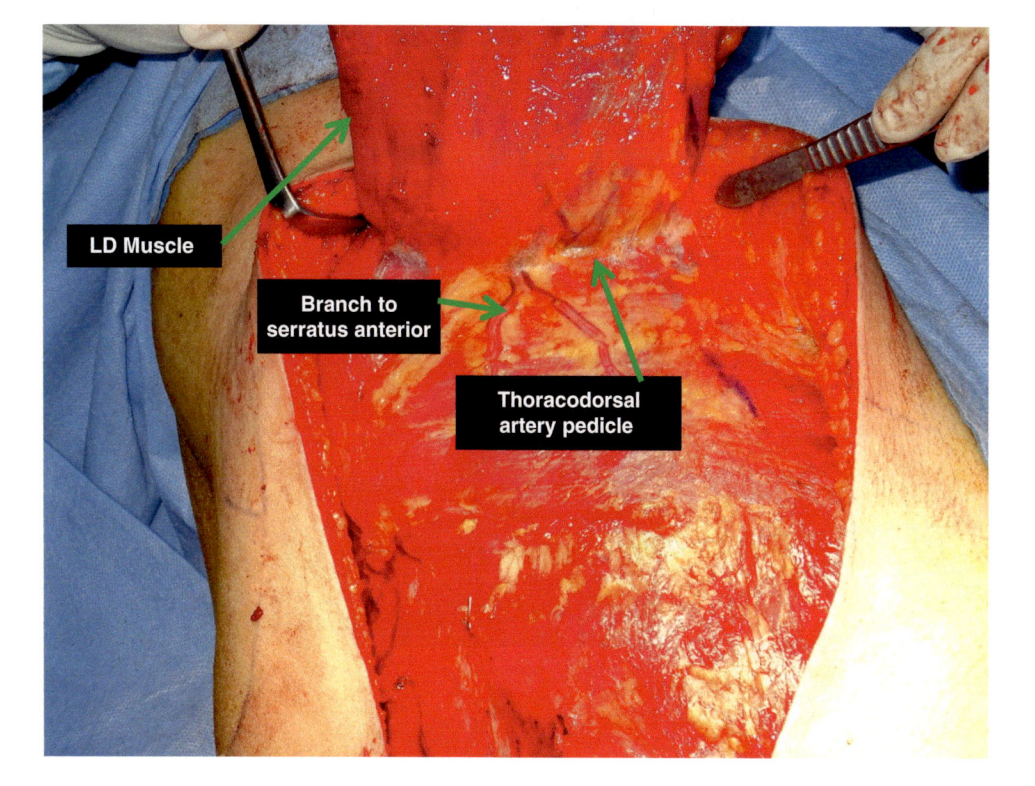

Fig. 14.10 LD posterior, inferior, anterior border elevation

Fig. 14.11 LD muscle undersurface demonstrating thoracodorsal vascular pedicle and pedicle supplying the serratus anterior muscle

Fig. 14.12 Continuation of anterior-superior LD muscle and separation from the serratus anterior

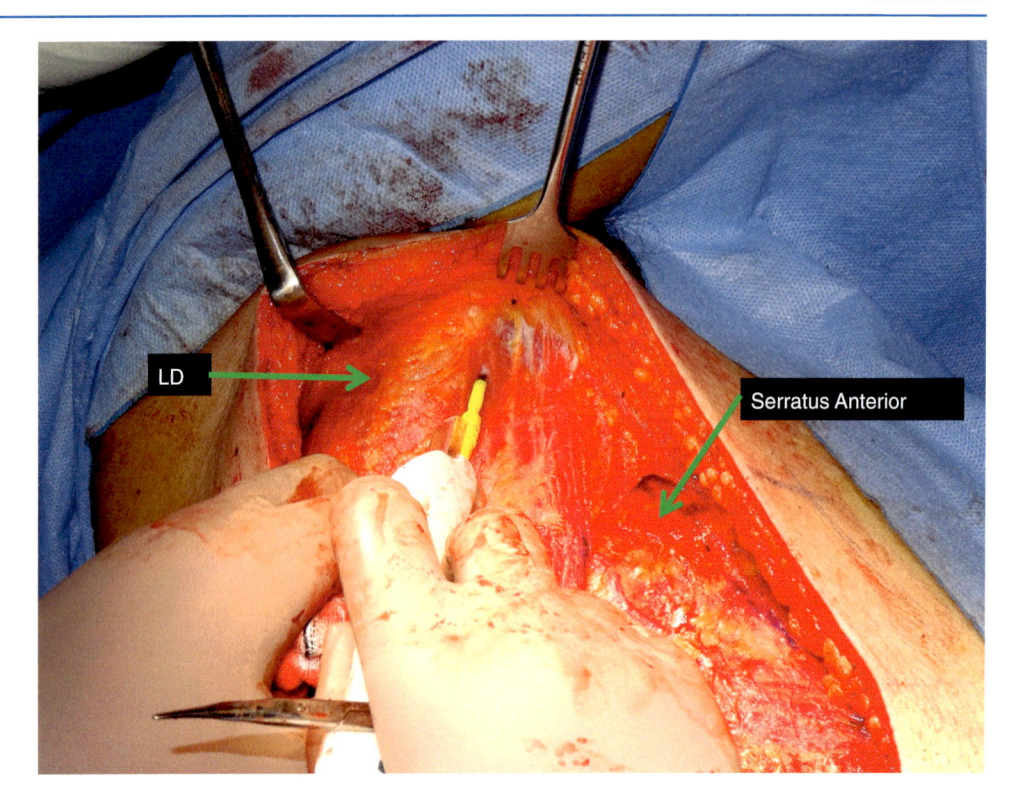

Fig. 14.13 LD flap raised reaching superior border of tendinous insertion

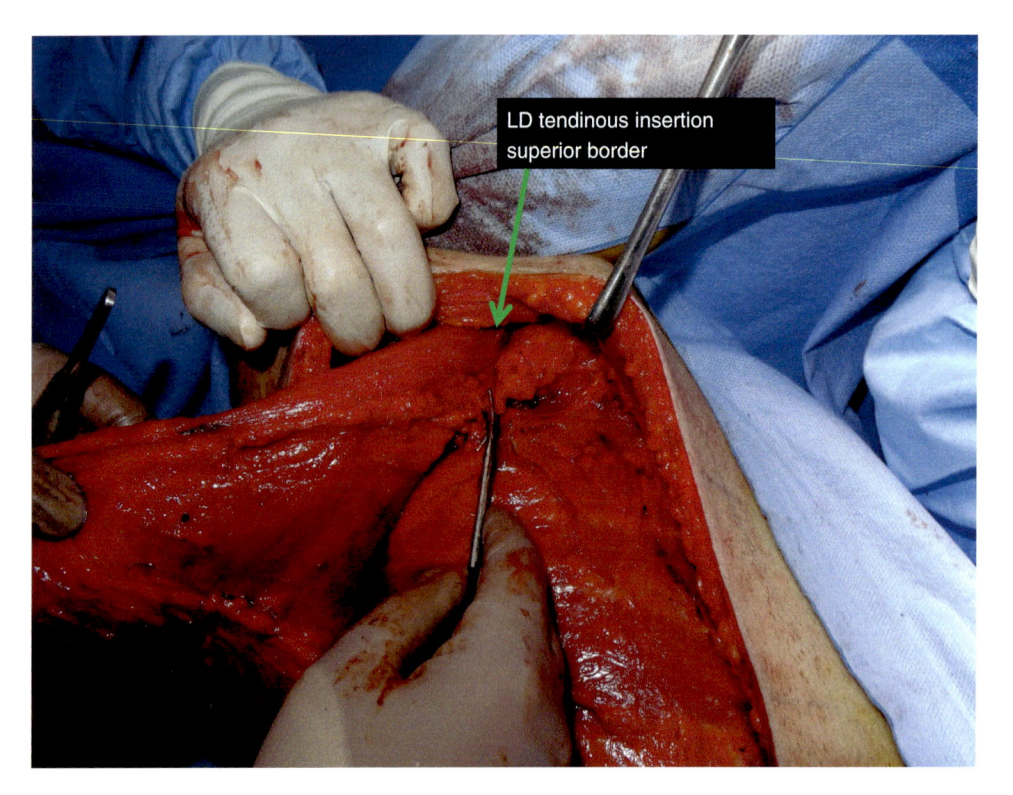

Fig. 14.14 Insertion of two drains and sequential closure of donor site

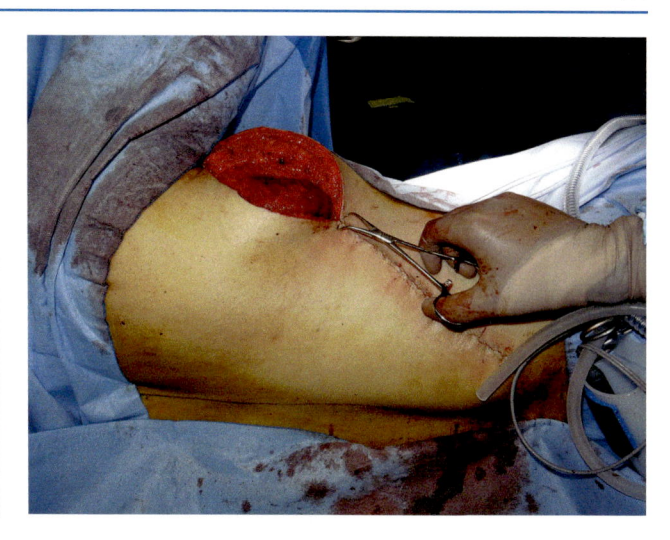

Fig. 14.15 Use of towel clip to facilitate tensionless closure of donor site

Fig. 14.16 LD donor site closure, dressing applied and drains secured

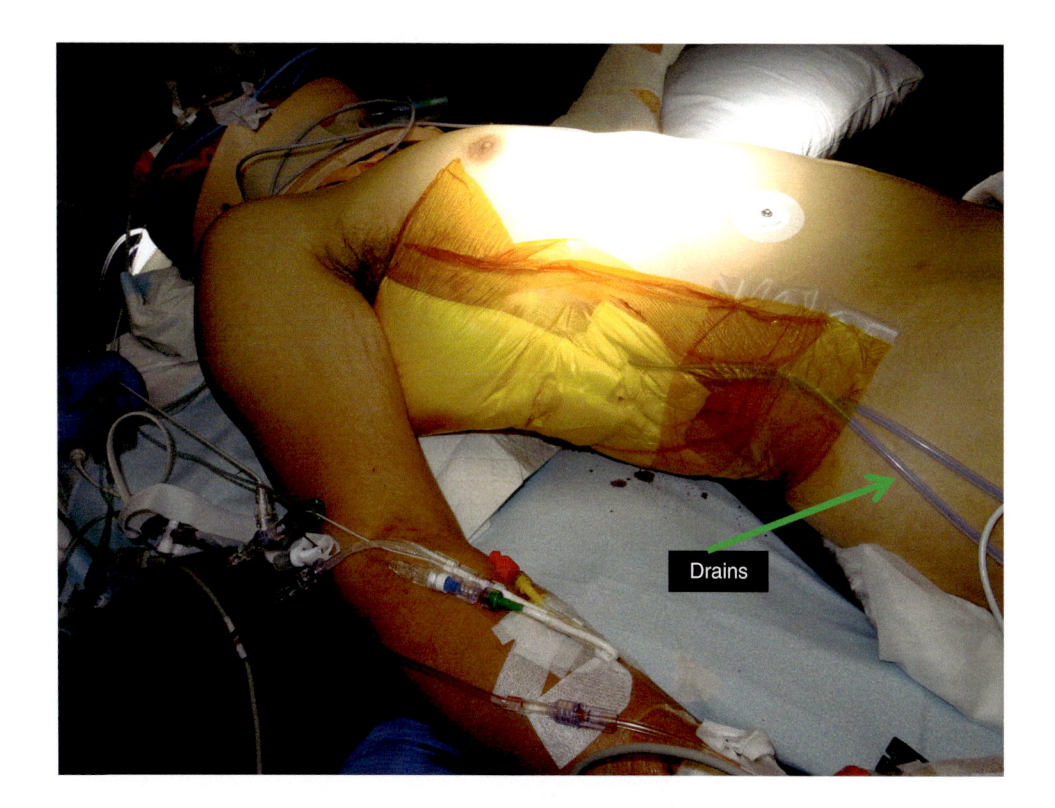

14.6 Core Surgical Techniques in Flap Dissection

Skin Paddle Temporary interrupted sutures are placed between the skin paddle and LD muscle to prevent shear that may injure perforators (Fig. 14.17). The orientation of the skin paddle is ideally based on perforators along the perforators of the thoracodorsal artery.

Thoracodorsal Pedicle Protection A cuff of the fascia and fat is to be kept around the pedicle to prevent kinking or compression in the axillary tunnel. The thoracodorsal nerve may be divided to avoid muscle contraction at recipient site and animation from shoulder movement.

Venous Congestion The creation of the tunnel should allow for the surgeon's hand to fit at least prior to detachment of humeral insertion of the LD. The main issue with a narrowed tunnel is risk of venous congestion secondary to vascular compression of a pedicled flap.

Arc of Rotation The anterior arc allows the flap to reach the trunk and neck while posterior arc for vertebral defects

Fig. 14.17 Interrupted temporary sutures to stabilise skin paddle to LD muscle

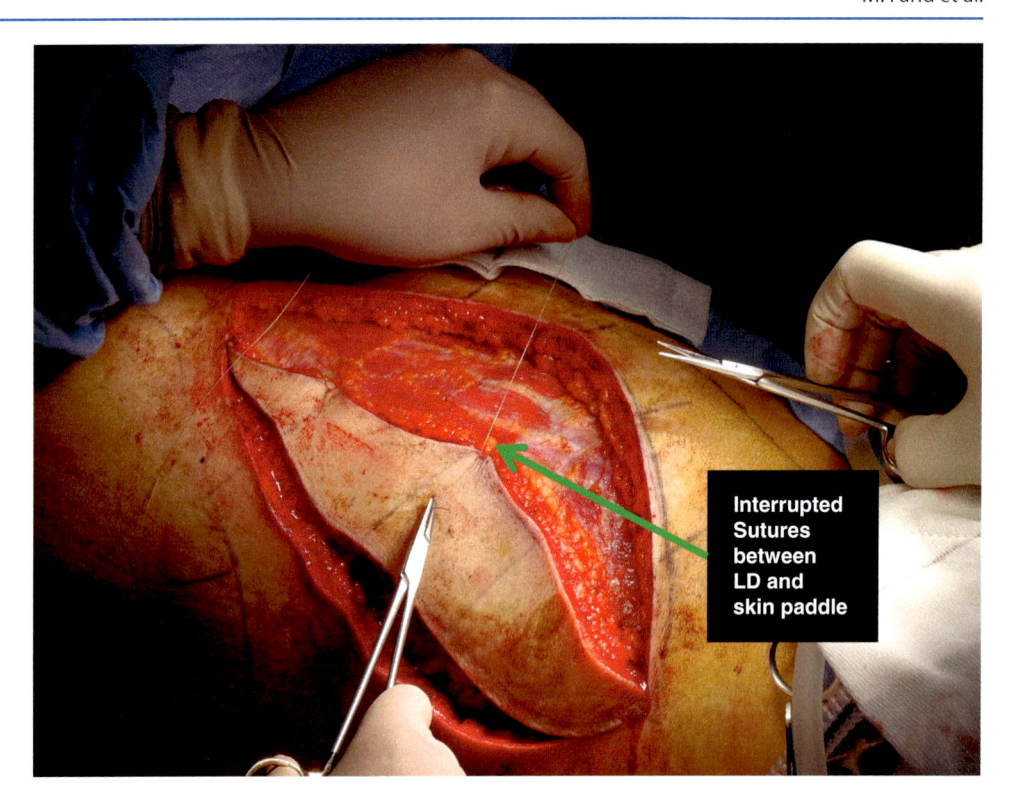

Fig. 14.18 Division of LD muscle tendinous humeral insertion

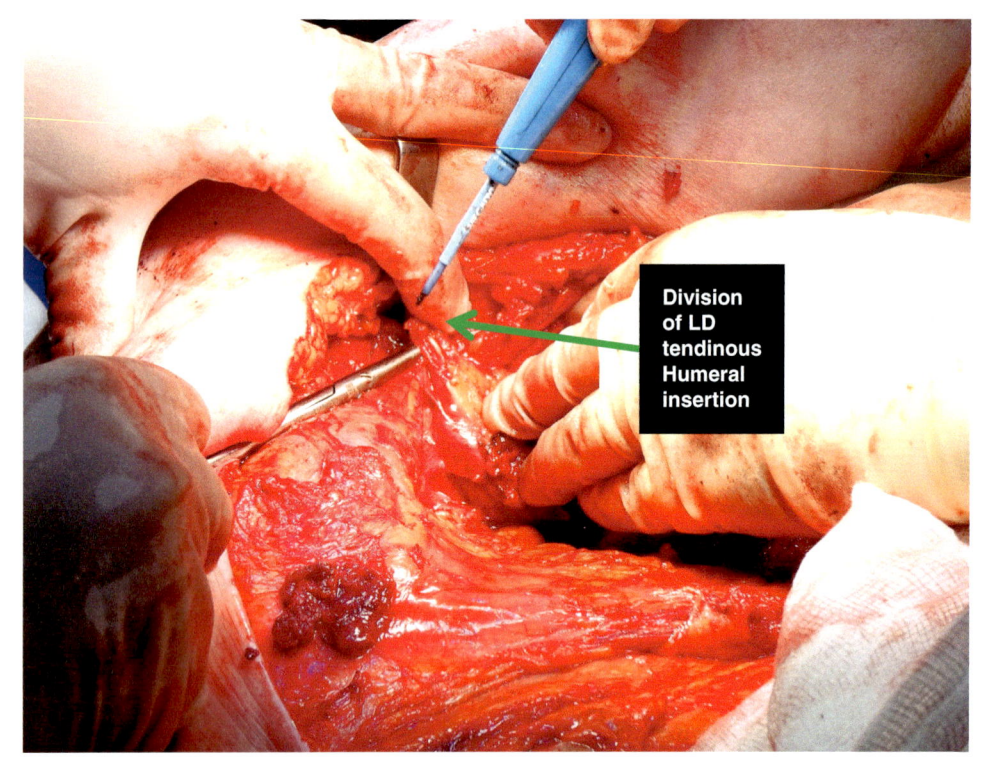

(cervical to lumbar). This is determined by humeral attachment, other muscle insertion (pectoralis minor) and vascular perforators of lumbar, intercostal or serratus anterior muscles. The subscapular artery recruitment would increase the length and diameter of the pedicle. The length and size of the flap also determine arc of rotation in reaching defect.

Humeral Insertion Division This constitutes one of the final steps allowing the flap to mobilise further or detach as a free flap. This is particularly crucial for ipsilateral shoulder defect reconstruction or breast reconstruction as a pedicled flap (Fig. 14.18).

14.7 Clinical Scenario

Case 1 Right shoulder reconstruction with pedicled LD flap. This 67-year-old gentleman had a total shoulder arthroplasty. The prosthesis became infected and was subsequently removed by the orthopaedic team. After debridement a pedicled myocutaneous LD flap was performed to cover exposed shoulder joint. The patient had an uneventful recovery (Figs. 14.19, 14.20, 14.21, and 14.22).

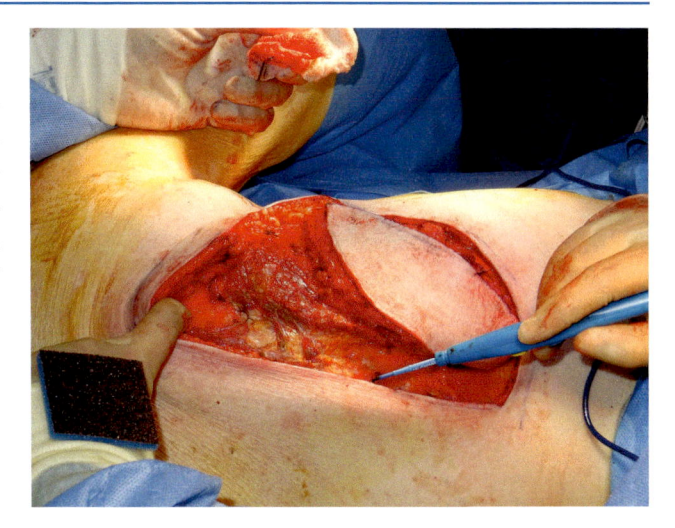

Fig. 14.20 LD myocutaneous flap islanded

Fig. 14.19 Right shoulder defect post-debridement and removal of prosthesis

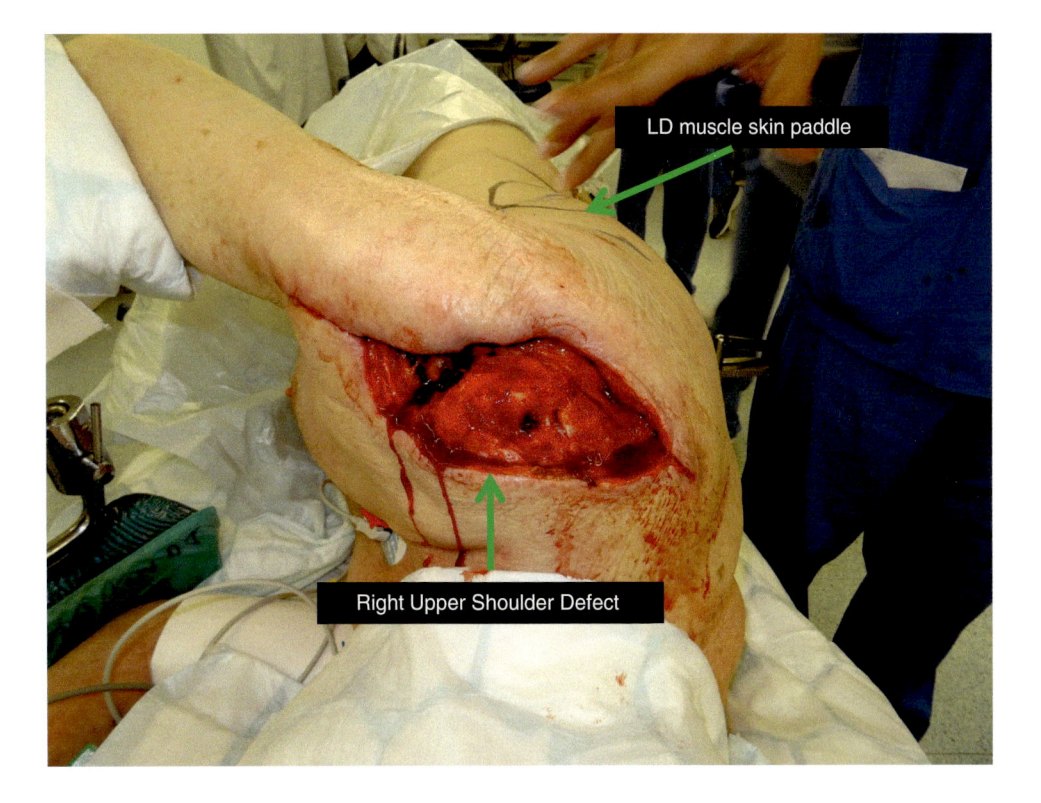

Fig. 14.21 Pedicled LD myocutaneous flap tunnelled through the axilla to reach shoulder defect

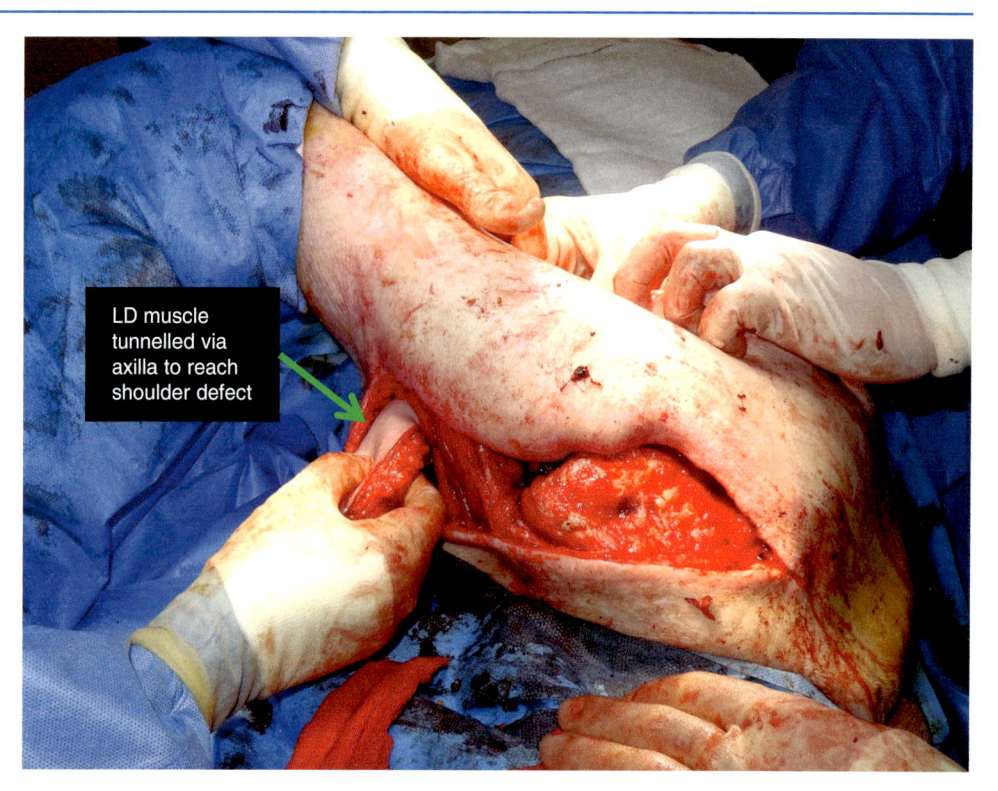

Fig. 14.22 LD myocutaneous flap inset and closure to cover shoulder defect

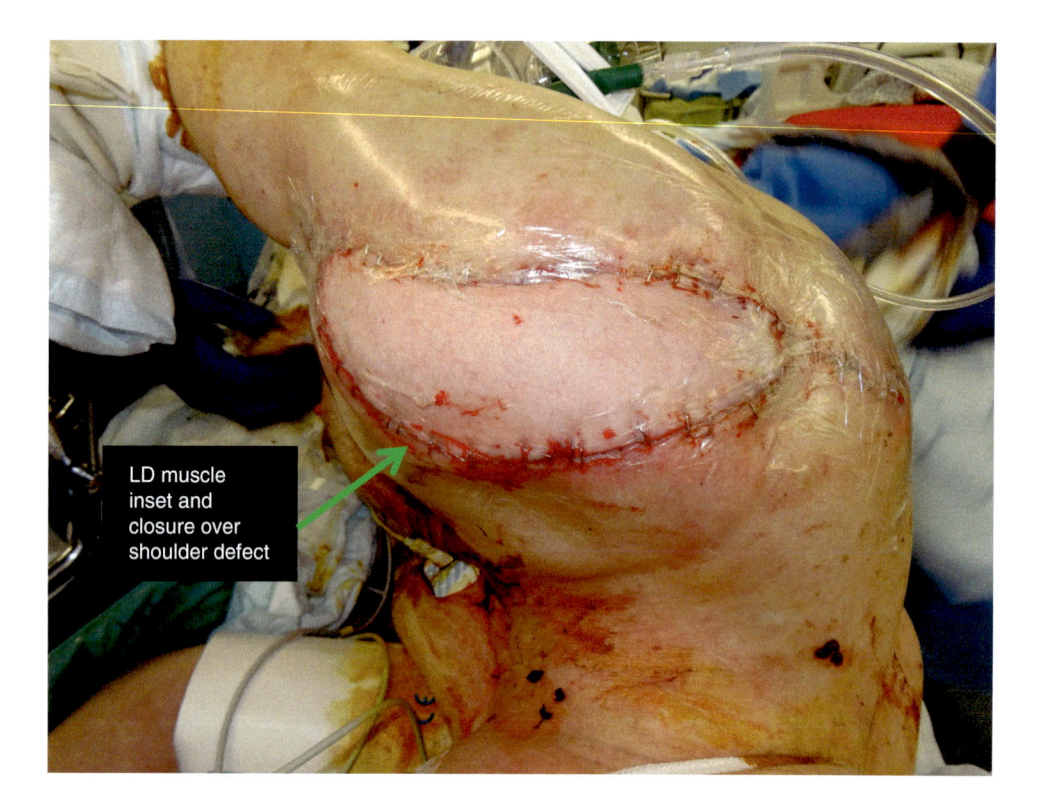

Case 2 Amputated contralateral left forearm stump resurfaced with Free myocutaneous LD flap. This 37-year-old man had a crush avulsion injury to the arm during an industrial accident. His forearm was avulsed and he sustained segmental fractures of the radius, ulna and humerus. Replantation was not feasible due to the poor condition of the amputated part and the significant crush avulsion mechanism. To salvage his exposed radius and ulna and to preserve function of his elbow joint, a contralateral free myocutaneous LD flap was performed. This was anastomosed to the brachial artery and associated venae comitantes. He made an excellent recovery and was fitted with an upper limb prosthesis (Figs. 14.23, 14.24, 14.25, 14.26, 14.27, 14.28, 14.29, and 14.30).

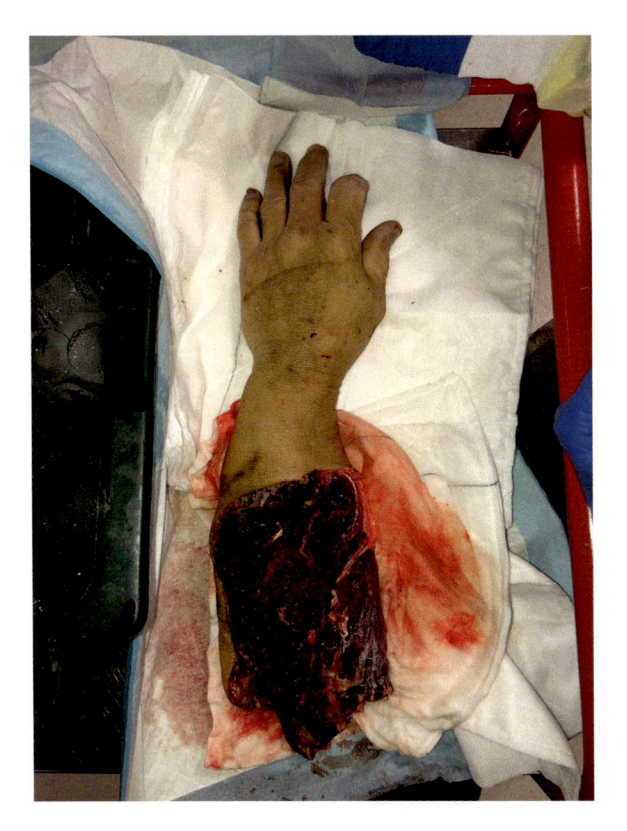

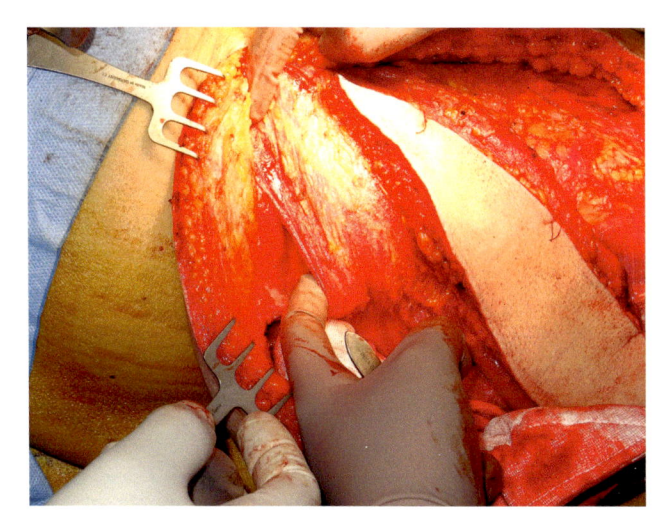

Fig. 14.25 LD myocutaneous flap raised demonstrating superior insertion

Fig. 14.23 Left forearm avulsion/amputation injury

Fig. 14.24 Left forearm post-debridement with exposed radius

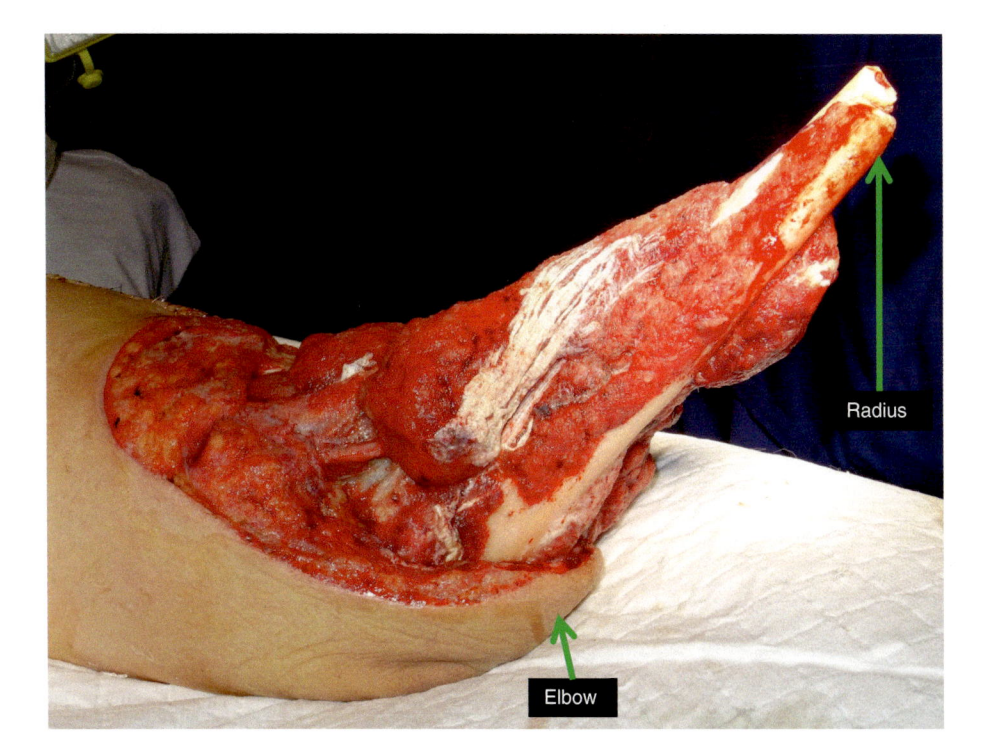

Fig. 14.26 Preparation of recipient vessels in right forearm showing brachial artery

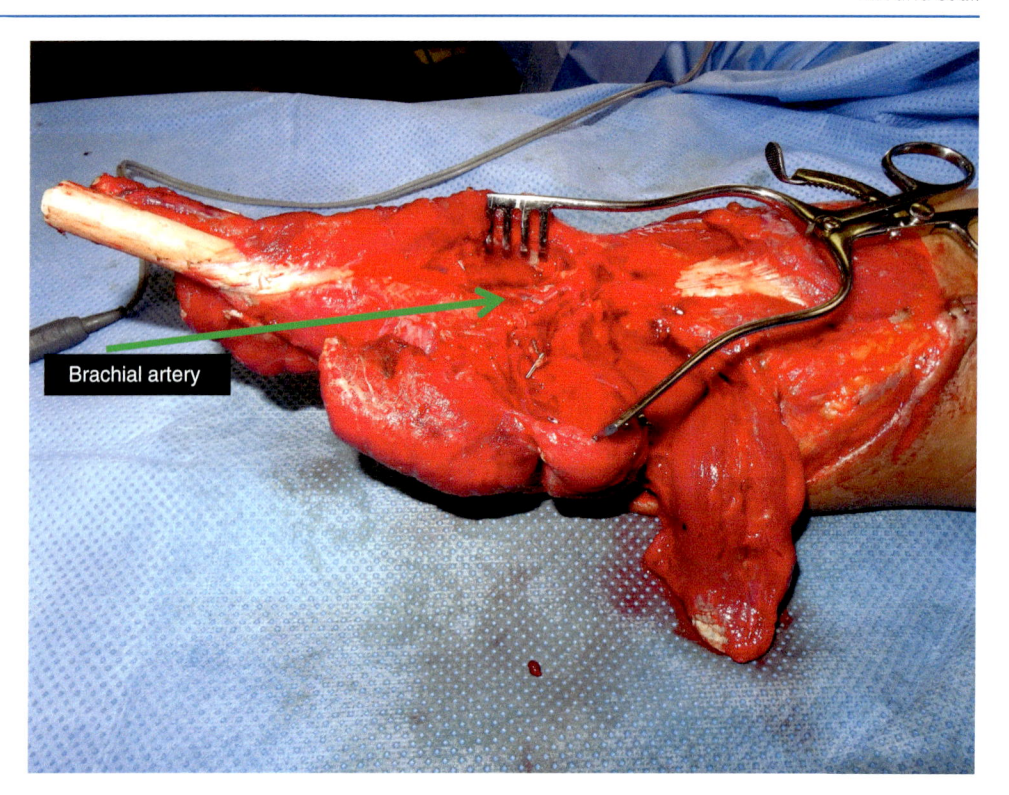

Fig. 14.27 Intraoperative LD flap inset and covered with SSG and skin paddle to cover radius

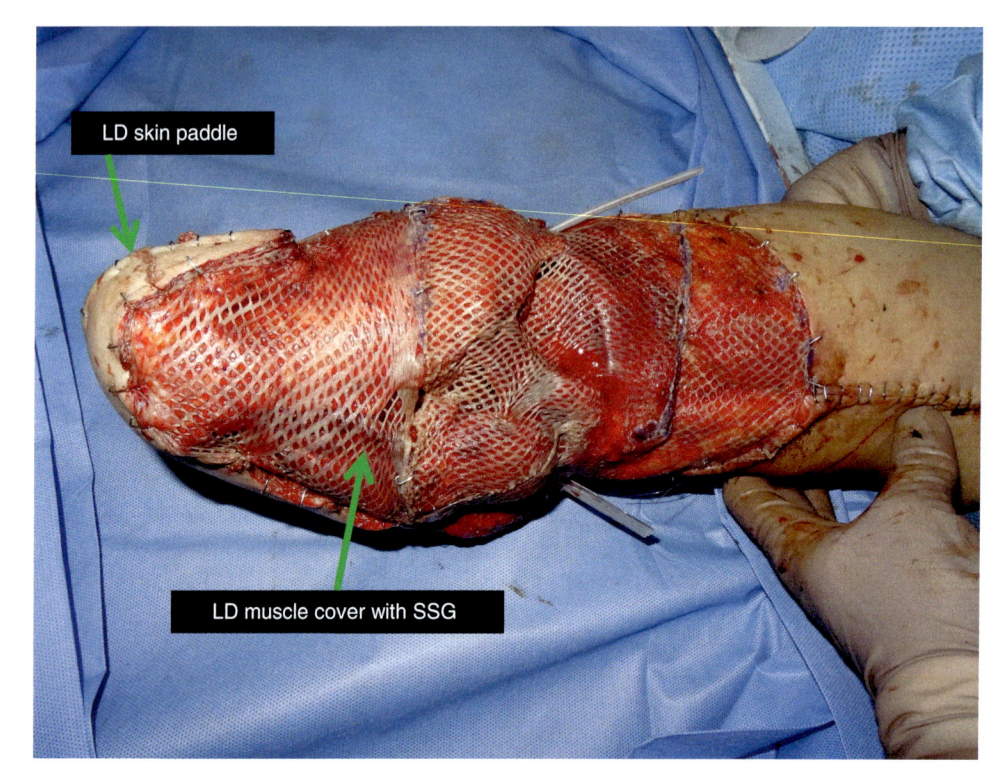

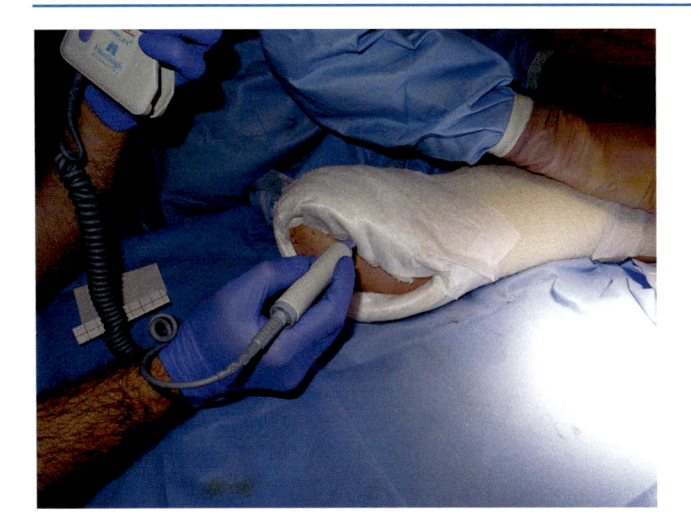

Fig. 14.28 Intraoperative check for US Doppler signal on skin paddle for LD flap

Fig. 14.29 Post-operative SSG take and early results for LD myocutaneous flap

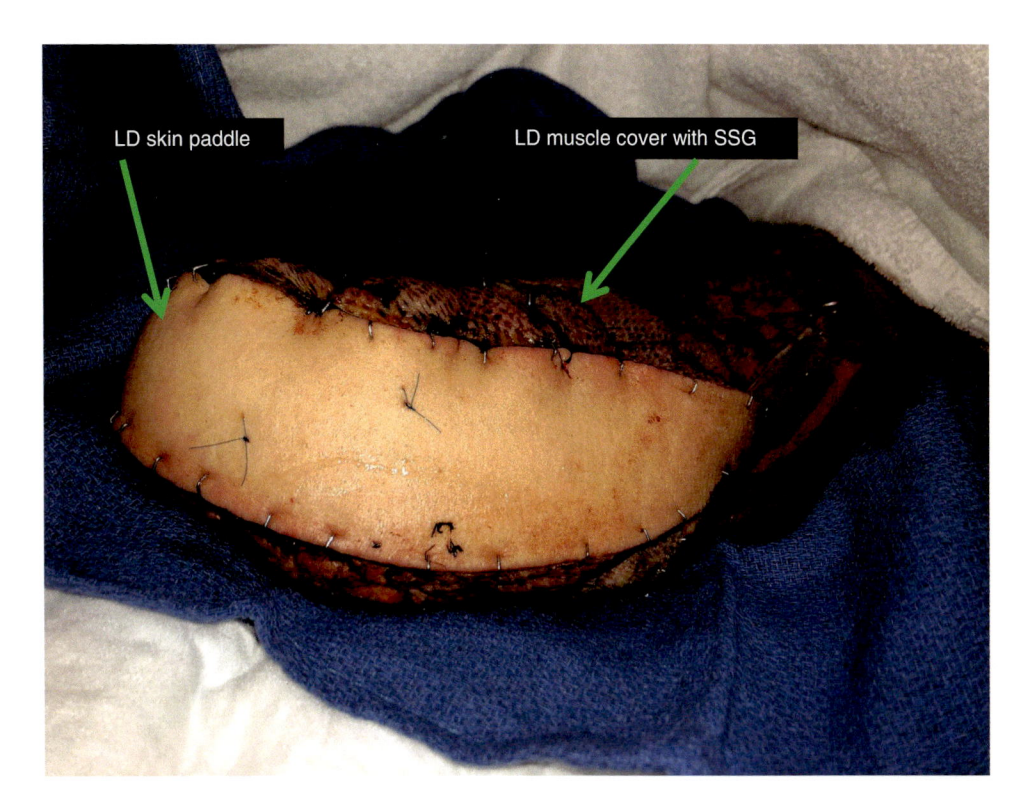

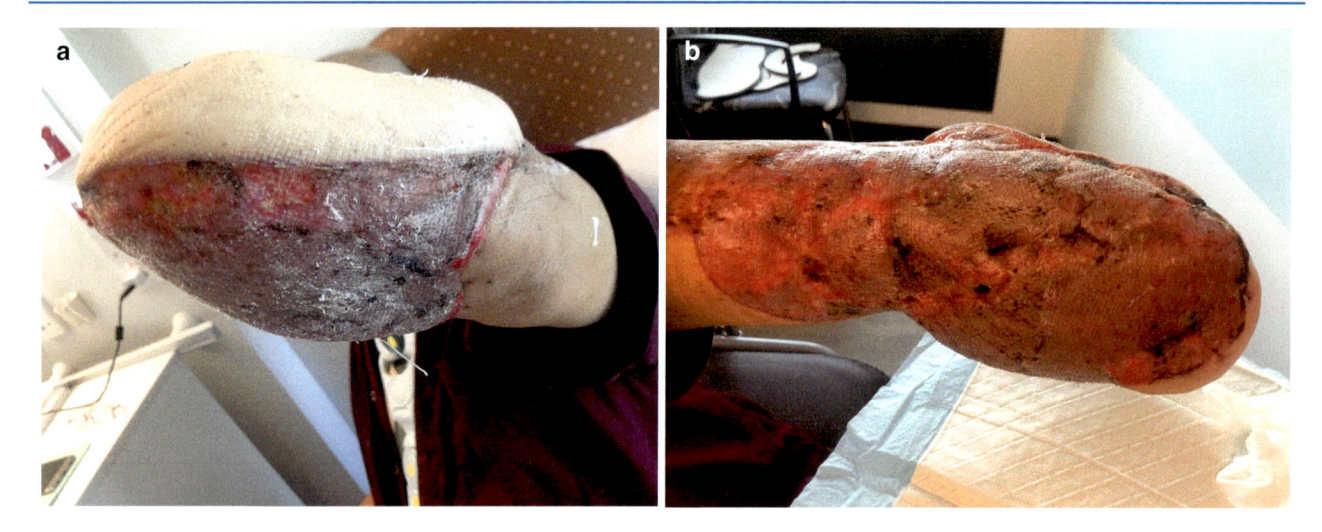

Fig. 14.30 (**a**) Post-operative follow-up showing SSG take and LD skin paddle (**b**) Post operative appearance if LD over arm

Fig. 14.31 Right lower limb open tibial fracture, soft tissue debridement and ex-fix stabilisation

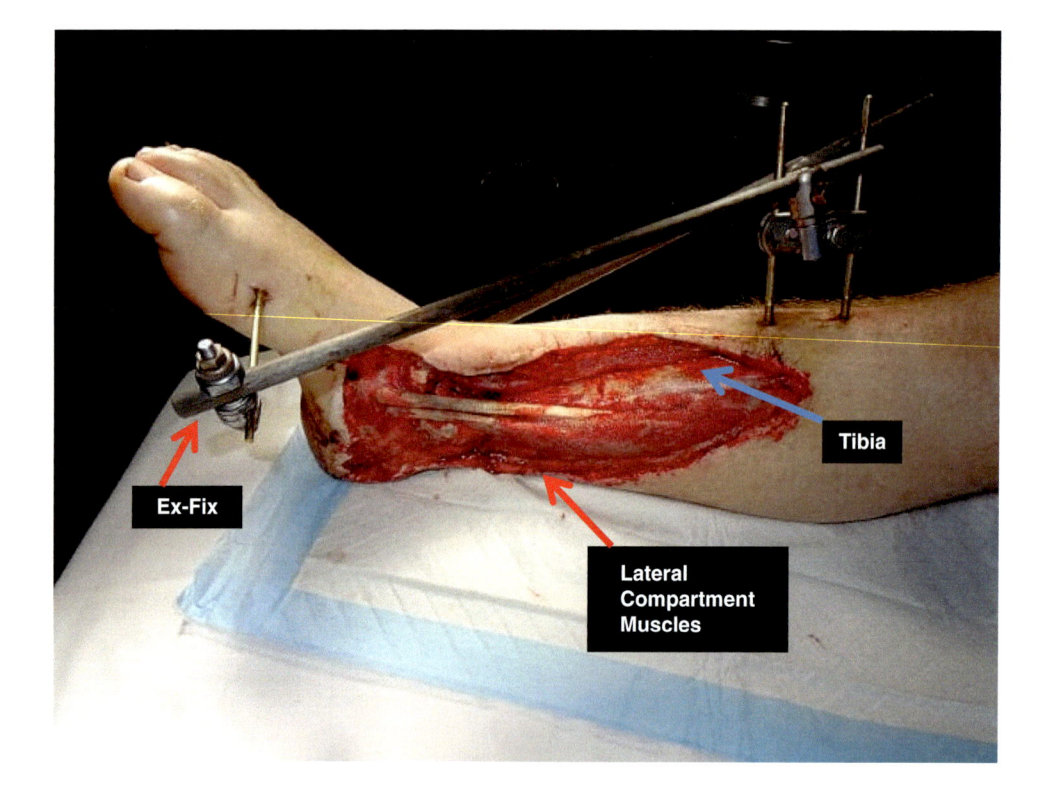

Case 3 Right lower limb open fracture resurfaced with a free LD flap. This 57-year-old man had a right lower limb injury from a road traffic accident. The right leg had open tibia fracture (Gustilo-Anderson IIIB) with compromised posterior compartment muscles. The initial operation involved debridement of devitalised muscles and bony stabilisation with an external fixator. This was followed by definitive fracture fixation, soft tissue coverage with LD muscle flap and split thickness skin graft. The extensive nature of the wound with bony exposure and large soft tissue defect necessitated the need for LD muscle flap. A three-vessel run-off confirmed on CT-A and anastomosis was performed end to end (thoracodorsal to posterior tibial artery) (Figs. 14.31, 14.32, and 14.33).

Fig. 14.32 LD muscle free flap inset into right lower limb defect

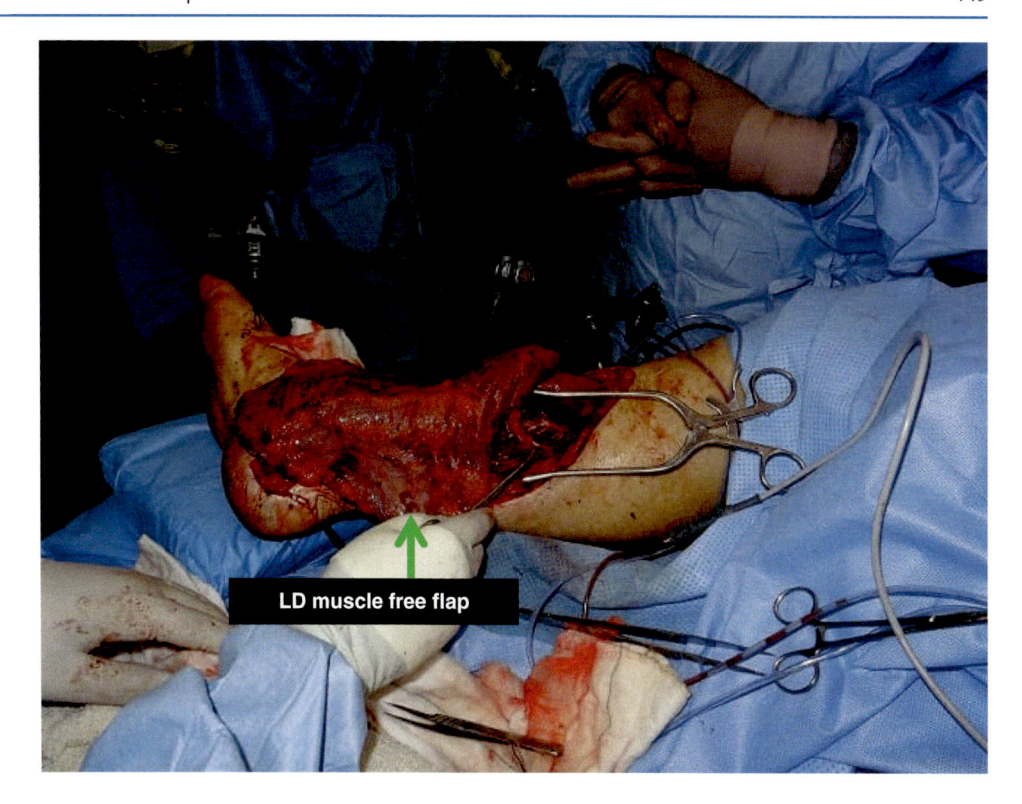

Fig. 14.33 LD muscle covered with SSG post-operatively

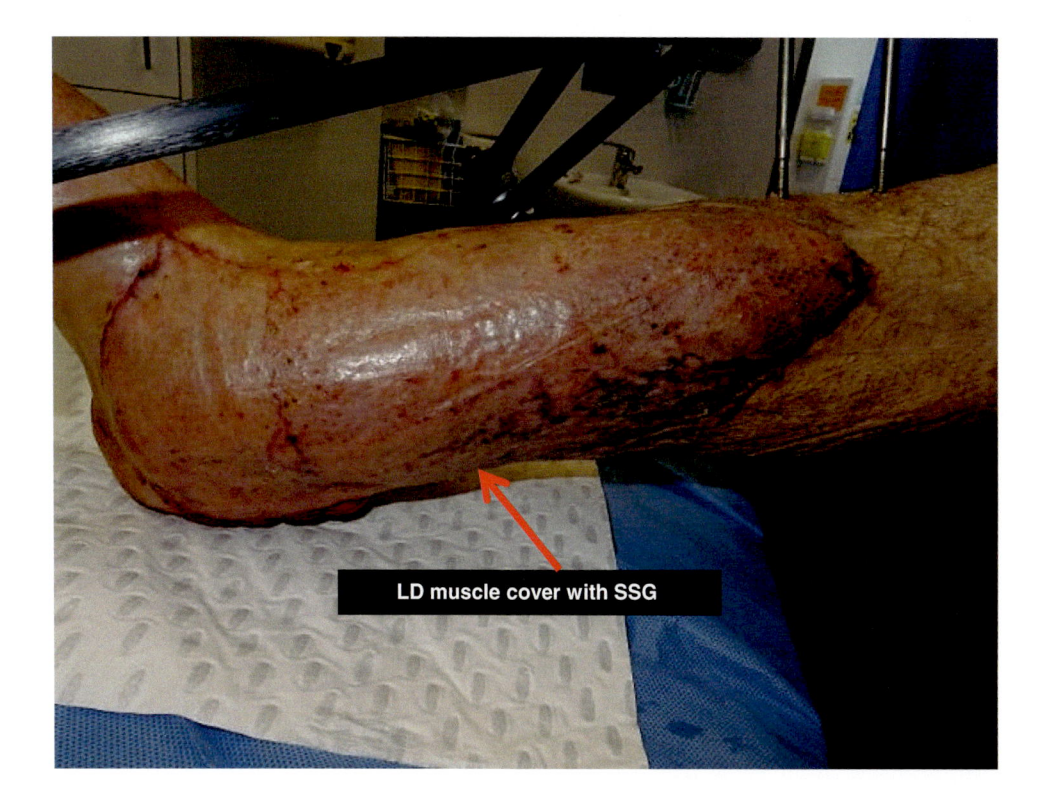

14.8 Pearls and Pitfalls

Incision The orientation of the scar should be attempted to be covered by clothes. A horizontal scar can be hidden along bra straps for women allowing a better cosmetic result of donor site.

Vascular Pedicle Dissection The pedicle is identified and protected when progressing into caudal LD insertion. Identify the branch to the serratus anterior to prevent injury to the vascular pedicle to the LD flap. The vascular pedicle can expand to include branch to the serratus anterior or tip of the scapula when raised as a chimeric flap.

Anatomy Preservation The surgeon should ensure there is clear identification of the surrounding muscles and vasculature throughout dissection. Allow orientation of fibres to orientate LD from other muscles.

Donor Site Towel clips are used to help facilitate closure sequentially (Fig. 14.18). Drains are to be kept until output volume <30 mls in each. Quilting is recommended to reduce the risk of seroma formation on donor site [22].

Flap Harvest The LD flap can be raised in an extended fashion recruiting subcutaneous tissue to increase volume. Subcutaneous tissue fat pads are distributed in the posterolateral thoracic region in five zones. This corresponds to area under cutaneous crescent of LD skin paddle (Zone 1), the entire flap between the muscle and fascia (Zone 2), scapular hinge flap above superomedial of LD muscle (Zone 3), anterior hinge flap on the external forward part of LD (Zone 4) and suprailiac fat zone above iliac crest on lower aspect of LD flap (Zone 5) [23]. This is particularly useful in breast reconstruction for a satisfactory volume replacement, avoidance of implant and better cosmetic appearance.

Flap Inset Aim for tensionless inset of pedicled flap by releasing any fascial attachment that prevents advancement of the flap. Observe the flap for any evidence of venous congestion once inset into defect.

Patient Positioning The lateral position with arm up on the LD side harvest allows good planning. Patients may need to be repositioned to allow flap inset into defect. Nonetheless, a trans-axillary approach is feasible with the patient in a supine position also described to harvest a portion of LD muscle flap in facial reanimation [24]. The option for prone positioning is noted for bilateral breast reconstruction or even unilateral [25].

Flap Size The broad size of LD muscle and its thickness allow coverage for large defects in the lower or upper limb, head and neck or trunk defects. The LD muscle can provide a better option than fasciocutaneous flaps particularly in overweight patients where fasciocutaneous flaps would be bulky in comparison to the more slender LD muscle.

14.9 Selected Readings

- Watanabe K, Kiyokawa K, Rikimaru H, Koga N, Yamaki K, Saga T. Anatomical study of latissimus dorsi musculocutaneous flap vascular distribution. J Plast Reconstr Aesthetic Surg. 2010; 63:1091–1098.

  This cadaveric study provides the basis for safe myocutaneous LD flap harvest based on vascular angiosomes to prevent skin necrosis in peripheral areas. First vascular territory is by direct anastomosis of perforating branches of the thoracodorsal artery and branches of the ninth, tenth and eleventh intercostal and scapular circumflex arteries. A second vascular territory is based on perforating branches of the subcostal artery and perforating branches of the first and second lumbar arteries. If the skin above LD muscle is recruited, this would extend into a third vascular territory caudally from the inferior border of the twelfth rib. These vascular territories are connected with choke vessels for overlapping angiosomes. We advocate the use of intraoperative adjuncts to further illustrate the vascular territories intraoperatively.

- Winter R, Steinböck M, Leinich W, Reischies FMJ, Feigl G, Sljivich M, et al. The reverse latissimus dorsi flap: An anatomical study and retrospective analysis of its clinical application. J Plast Reconstr Aesthetic Surg. 2019;72:1084–90.

  This is an interesting anatomical and clinical study demonstrating a new concept based on reverse LD flap harvest. Blood supply is based on perforators from sixth intercostal to subcostal area, defined as a "hotspot" as 7 cm broad area over eighth to eleventh intercostal vessels. Reconstruction of the lateral thoracic chest wall and sacral area is deemed feasible based on this concept.

- Clemens MW, Kronowitz S, Selber JC. Robotic-assisted latissimus dorsi harvest in delayed-immediate breast reconstruction. Semin Plast Surg. 2014;28:20–5.

  The innovative concept of robotic microsurgery is demonstrated in LD flap harvest for delayed and immediate breast reconstruction following radiotherapy. Minimal donor site morbidity with three port sites access required for instruments without an incisional site. Long-term outcome (>1 year) is part of future research for robotic LD flap in breast reconstruction. The senior author first described the technique in 2012 and advocates the need to be selective in choosing suitable patients for this technique.

- Lu J, Chavanon V, Margulies I, Yao AS. Cross-leg latissimus dorsi free flap with chimeric serratus anterior bridge for lower extremity trauma: Case report and reconstructive algorithm. J Clin Orthop Trauma. 2019;10(5):867–72.

  Lower limb defects for Gustilo-Anderson IIIB and IIIC open fractures require complex reconstruction. Due to vascular injury, limited reconstructive options were available from the ipsilateral leg. Limb salvage was subsequently achieved with a chimeric cross-leg latissimus dorsi-serratus anterior (LD-SA) free flap based off the contralateral healthy leg.

- Sarifakioglu N, Bingül F, TerzioǦlu A, Ates L, Aslan G. Bilateral split latissimus dorsi V-Y flaps for closure of large thoracolumbar meningomyelocele defects. Br J Plast Surg. 2003;56::303–6.

  Neural tube defects including meningomyelocele require careful choice of flaps for adequate coverage. This case illustrates the use of bilateral split LD muscle to cover a lumbar defect in a 2-month-old baby. The flaps are based on the thoracic and lumbar perforators advanced towards midline without tension. Bilateral LD flaps were advanced along the orientation of muscle fibres with primary closure of donor site as V-Y advancement flap.

References

1. Neligan P. Chapter 19: Latissimus dorsi flap breast reconstruction. In: Gart M, Kim J, Fine N, editors. Plastic surgery (aesthetic), vol. II, 4th ed, Section II: (reconstructive breast surgery). 2018. p. 300–20.
2. Bostwick J III. Latissimus dorsi flap: current applications. Ann Plast Surg. 1982;9(5):377–80.
3. Tansini I. Sopra il mio nuevo processo di amputazione della mammella. Gazz Med Ital; 1906.
4. Olivari N. The latissimus flap. Br J Plast Surg. 1976;29(2):126–8.
5. Schneider WJ, Hill HL Jr, Brown RG. Latissimus dorsi myocutaneous flap for breast reconstruction. Br J Plast Surg. 1977;30(4):277–81.
6. Bostwick J 3rd, Vasconez LO, Jurkiewicz MJ. Breast reconstruction after a radical mastectomy. Plast Reconstr Surg. 1978;61(5):682–93.
7. Quillen CG, Shearin JC, Geogiade NG. Use of the latissimus dorsi myocutaneous island flap for reconstruction in the head and neck area. Plast Reconstr Surg. 1978;62:113–7.
8. Maxwell GP, Sueber K, Hoopes JE. A free latissimus dorsi myocutaneous flap. Plast Reconstr Surg. 1978;62:462–6.
9. May J, Lukash F, Gallico G. Latissimus dorsi free muscle flap in lower-extremity reconstruction. Plast Reconstr Surg. 1981;68(4):603–7.
10. Bailey B, Godfrey A. Latissimus dorsi muscle free flaps. Br J Plast Surg. 1982;35(1):47–52.
11. Samir M, Fu-Chen W. Chapter:41: Latissimus dorsi flap. In: German G, Reichenberger M, editors. Flaps and reconstructive surgery, 2nd ed. 2016. p. 446–63.
12. Wolfe S, Hotchkiss R, Pederson W, Kozin S, Cohen M. Chapter 45: Free flaps to the hand and upper extremity. In: Jones N, Lister G, editors. Green's operative hand surgery, 7th ed. 2016. p. 1575–610.
13. Sood R, Easow J, Konopka G, Panthaki Z. Latissimus dorsi flap in breast reconstruction: recent innovations in the workhorse flap. Cancer Control. 2018;25(1):1–7.
14. Pu L, Karp N. Chapter 8: Latissimus dorsi flap breast reconstruction. In: Abraham J, Saint-Cyr M, editors. Atlas of reconstructive breast surgery, 1st ed. 2019. p. 94–104.
15. Heitmann C, Pelzer M, Kuentscher M, et al. The extended latissimus dorsi flap – revisited. Plast Reconstr Surg. 2003;111:1697–701.
16. Myers E, Snyderman C. Chapter 172: Trapezius and latissimus dorsi regional flaps. In: Howard B, Hackman T, editors. Operative otolaryngology: head and neck surgery, 3rd ed. 2017. p 1199–207.
17. Kademani D, Tiwana P. Chapter 113: The latissimus dorsi free flap. In: Bonin G, Makhoul NM, editors. Atlas of oral and maxillofacial surgery, 1st ed. 2015. p. 1174–82.
18. Mayer H, Buena P, Petersen M. The value of preoperative computed tomography angiography (CT-A) in patients undergoing delayed latissimus dorsi flap breast reconstruction after axillary lymph node dissection or irradiation and suspicion of pedicle injury. J Plast Reconst Aesth Surg. 2020;73(11):2086–102.
19. Bonomi S, Settembrini F, Salval A, Gregorelli C, Musumarra G, Rapisarda V. Current indications for and comparative analysis of three different types of latissimus dorsi flaps. Aesthetic Surg J. 2012;32(3):294–302.
20. Laitung JKG, Peck F. Shoulder function following the loss of the latissimus dorsi muscle. Br J Plast Surg. 1985;38:375–9.
21. Engdahl R, Disa J, Athanasian EA, Healey JH, Cordeiro PG, Fabbri N. Pedicled latissimus dorsi flap for shoulder soft-tissue reconstruction after excision of a musculoskeletal neoplasm. JBJS Essent Surg Tech. 2016;6(2):e16.
22. Daltrey I, Thomson H, Hussien M, Krishna K, Rayter Z, Winters Z. Randomized clinical trial of the effect of quilting latissimus dorsi flap donor site on seroma formation. Br J Surg. 2006;93(7):825–30.
23. Delay E, Gounot N, Bouillot A, Zlatoff P, Rivoire M. Autologous latissimus breast reconstruction: a 3-year clinical experience with 100 patients. Plast Reconstr Surg. 1998;102:1461–78.
24. Leckenby J, Butler D, Grobbelaar A. The axillary approach to raising the latissimus dorsi free flap for facial re-animation: a descriptive surgical technique. Arch Plast Surg. 2015;42(1):73–7.
25. Hammond D. Latissimus dorsi flap breast reconstruction. Plast Reconstr Surg. 2009;124(4):1055–63.

Thoracodorsal Artery Perforator Flap

15

Youn Hwan Kim and Lan Sook Chang

15.1 Introduction

The conventional latissimus dorsi muscle or myocutaneous flap is considered the workhorse flap for large defect coverage in the fields of reconstruction, and it has been well-described in numerous reports. However, sacrifice of the latissimus dorsi muscle can cause donor damage affecting shoulder function. Recently, donor function effects and morbidities have been increasing where substantial amounts of muscle are sacrificed. Koshima and Soeda introduced the "perforator flap" concept when using deep inferior epigastric flaps in 1989. The perforator concept reduces donor morbidities and creates thin flaps without the need for any debulking procedures. Angrigiani later described the thoracodorsal artery perforator flap in the lateral thoracic region, and the use of this flap was developed and expanded by the authors Y.H. Kim and J.T. Kim.

Unfortunately, the thoracodorsal artery perforator flap has not achieved the popularity of the anterolateral thigh flap due to a lack of exact surface landmarks for perforator mapping and the lateral position needed for flap harvesting. However, accumulated knowledge of regional anatomy and clinical experience has facilitated perforator mapping and provided an easy route for obtaining thoracodorsal artery perforator flaps in a supine position. As a result, the thoracodorsal artery perforator flap now provides as good an option for soft tissue resurfacing as the anterolateral thigh flap.

15.2 Anatomy

15.2.1 Arterial Supply

Previously, two types of perforator, septocutaneous and musculocutaneous, were recognized at the same donor site of the flank area, and two perforator flaps based on these two perforators were clinically available. With more experience and the accumulation of anatomical knowledge, it is clear that more rows of perforators originate from the lateral thoracic artery as direct cutaneous perforators in the lateral thoracic region. Thus, three longitudinal rows of perforator groups in the lateral thoracic region, the anterior, middle, and posterior rows, run at intervals and parallel to the anterior border of the latissimus dorsi muscle and lateral border of the pectoralis major muscle, and these provide surface landmarks for flap design (Fig. 15.1).

The anterior row of perforators is located along the lateral border of the pectoralis major and on the surface of the serratus anterior muscle. Most of these are derived from the lateral thoracic artery and are direct cutaneous perforators from the axillary artery. In some cases the lateral thoracic artery originates from the subscapular arterial system, but regardless of its origin, this artery is relatively small compared to the other rows of perforators. Also the venous drainage is not the same as the arterial drainage, and the unique lateral thoracic vein should be included once the lateral thoracic artery perforator has been chosen. In addition, the pedicle is relatively short because of the absence of an intramuscular course. Several reports highlight the usefulness of lateral thoracic artery perforator flaps. The ease of finding and dissecting these perforators is a great merit, but nevertheless they are not necessarily the first option since other reliable musculocutaneous or septocutaneous perforators are known to exist.

The middle row of perforators lies anterior to the latissimus dorsi muscle border and arises from branches of the thoracodorsal system. The thoracodorsal artery penetrates the latissimus dorsi muscle about 8–14 cm from the bifurcation of the subscapular artery. Shortly before it enters the muscle, a branch is given off to the serratus anterior muscle. The latissimus dorsi muscle is supplied by two main muscular branches from the thoracodorsal artery, horizontal or transverse branches of the thoracodorsal artery and descending

Y. H. Kim (✉) · L. S. Chang
Department of Plastic and Reconstructive Surgery, School of Medicine, Hanyang University, Seoul, South Korea

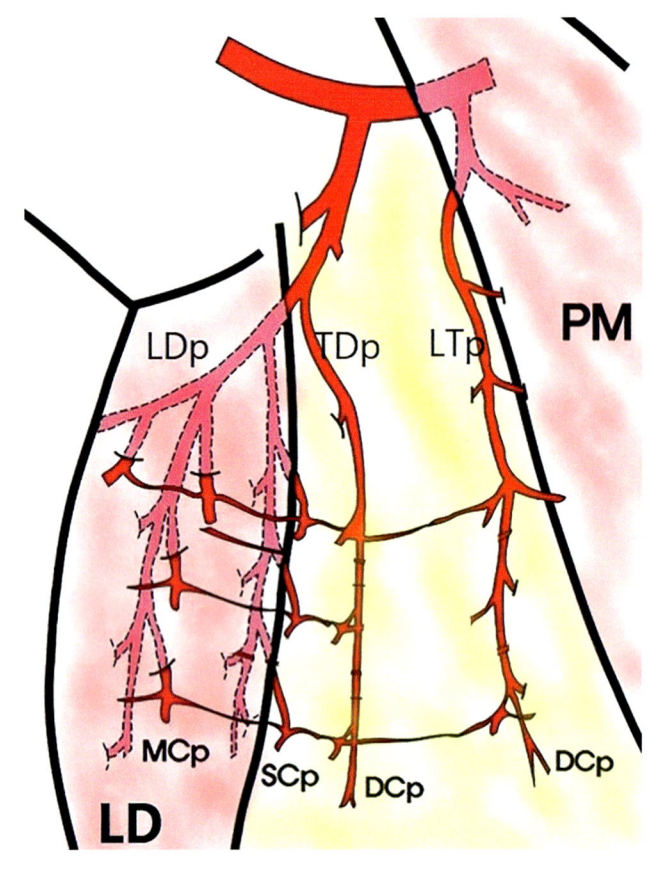

Fig. 15.1 Schematic drawing of the right lateral thoracic area. The anterior row of direct cutaneous perforators (DCp) is from the lateral thoracic artery, while the middle rows of the septocutaneous perforators (SCp) and direct cutaneous perforators originate from the cutaneous branch, which are from the thoracodorsal artery or serratus anterior branch. The posterior row of musculocutaneous perforators (MCp) sprout from the latissimus dorsi muscle, and those three perforator rows are horizontally connected with three perforator rows. Flaps based on the three types of perforator are named lateral thoracic perforator flaps (LTp), thoracodorsal perforator flaps (TDp) and latissimus dorsi perforator flaps (LDp), respectively

branches of the thoracodorsal artery, and numerous musculocutaneous or septocutaneous perforators arise from each branch. The descending branches run parallel to the anterior border, and the horizontal branches run obliquely to the dorsal and medial part of the muscle.

The most posterior row is made up of musculocutaneous perforators passing through the latissimus dorsi muscle. These perforators often originate from posterior horizontal branches of the thoracodorsal artery and are widely distributed over the large area of latissimus dorsi muscle. They are quite difficult to dissect intramuscularly so it is better to choose a perforator near the muscle border or in a thin area of muscle. Not all perforators can be dominant, and dominance is variable, but if a reliable perforator can be selected, it can provide nourishment to a 25 cm length of flap.

15.2.2 Venous Drainage

All venous branches drain into the axillary vein, except for occasional branches draining into the subclavian or brachial vein. The important thing about the venous anatomy is the course of the lateral thoracic vein. All the perforators in the lateral thoracic region except the lateral thoracic artery have the same course as the arterial and venous branches. But the lateral thoracic artery and vein often drain in a different way. So venous dissection should be performed with care when the lateral thoracic artery is selected as the dominant perforator.

15.2.3 Nerves

The thoracodorsal motor nerve accompanies the pedicles, and it is easy to preserve this nerve during dissection of a pedicle. The intercostal nerves are the dominant sensory nerves in this region and are useful for harvesting sensate flaps. The other sensory nerves of the proximal region of the armpit, including the costo-brachial and lateral thoracic nerves, should be saved.

15.3 Preoperative Investigation

The handheld Doppler provides a simple and easy way to detect reliable perforators. However, it can get confused by the source vessels and serratus anterior branches or lateral intercostal perforators. Therefore the use of preoperative mapping using a handheld Doppler is now decreasing.

High-resolution ultrasonograms have recently been used to detect perforators. They provide the locations and sizes of vessels and blood flow information. A skillful radiologist is required to detect reliable perforators and a lot of time is needed for preoperative mapping.

CT angiography requires less labor and time than sonograms, but radiation exposure and cost problems remain. Preoperative CT angiography is mandatory for preparation of recipient vessels in lower extremity reconstruction, while it is not suitable for perforator mapping in the lateral thoracic region. Mun et al. introduced multidetector-row computed tomographic angiography for thoracodorsal artery perforator mapping. Although a very small number of perforators were missed on the computed tomography images, the ones missed were always smaller than the ones identified and did not affect the validity of their study. However, the difficulty in interpreting the computed tomography images was greater than with abdominal donors because the perforators were smaller and the back occasionally has little subcutaneous tissue.

15.4 Flap Design and Markings

To harvest a thoracodorsal artery perforator flap, the patient is placed in a supine position with the arm abducted and elevated. Redundant flank tissue is pinched to estimate the point of primary closure of the donor site, and the anterior border of the muscle is identified. The surface landmarks used are the border of the pectoralis major muscle and the anterior border of the latissimus dorsi muscle, along which the midportion is outlined. A parallel incision is made along the midportion between the anterior border of the latissimus dorsi and pectoralis major muscles (Fig. 15.2).

15.5 Flap Raise/Elevation: A Step-by-Step Guide

1. Skin Traction
   After skin incision, traction toward the surgeon is applied to the skin flap, along with countertraction to the muscle toward the chest, to avoid missing very small latissimus dorsi perforators (Fig. 15.3).
2. Finding the Latissimus Dorsi Muscle
   Finding the anterior border of the latissimus dorsi muscle is the quintessential step in successful flap harvest. Since the anterior border of the latissimus dorsi muscle is easier to find on the distal part, it is better to elevate the flap from the distal part. After finding the anterior border, flap is raised while maintaining the suprafascial layer.
3. Finding Reliable Perforators.
   There are numerous perforators along the anterior border of the latissimus dorsi muscle, and we try to include reliable "pulsatile" perforators that enter to the skin paddles. If there are no visible perforators piercing the latissimus dorsi, reliable septocutaneous or direct cutaneous perforators are often used instead.

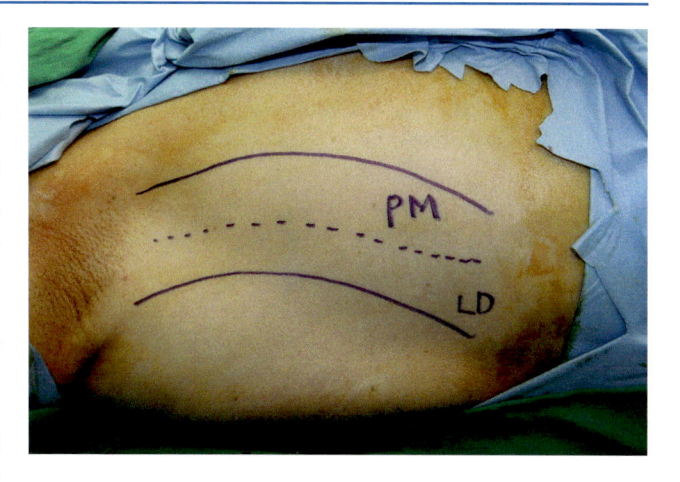

Fig. 15.2 Surface marking and flap design. The surface landmarks used are the border of the pectoralis major muscle and the anterior border of the latissimus dorsi muscle, along which the midportion is outlined. A parallel incision is made along the midportion between the anterior border of the latissimus dorsi and pectoralis major muscles (*PM* pectoralis major, *LD* latissimus dorsi)

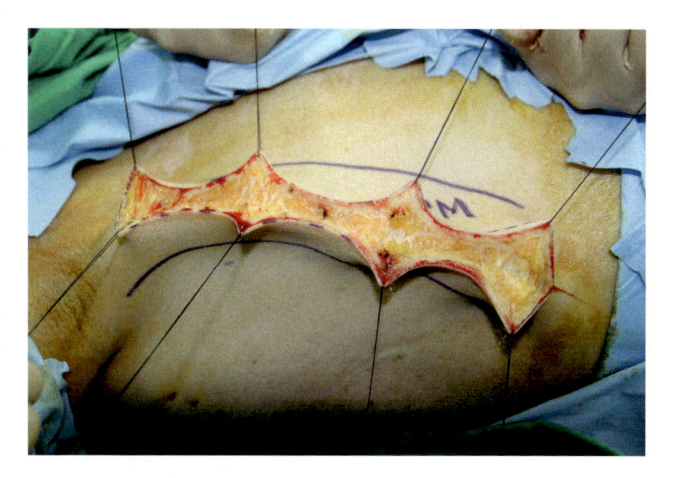

Fig. 15.3 Skin traction. After skin incision, traction towards the surgeon is applied to the skin flap, along with counter-traction to the muscle towards the chest, to avoid missing very small latissimus dorsi perforators

15.6 Core Surgical Techniques in Flap Dissection

Once a suitable perforator is identified, we continue the dissection of the thoracodorsal artery branches using bipolar electrocauterization while preserving the thoracodorsal nerve. In the case of thoracodorsal perforator flaps, branches of the thoracodorsal vessel, the serratus anterior vessels, and the circumflex scapular vessels are often ligated to achieve a longer vascular pedicle. Once the pedicle dissection is complete, an outline that matches the defect is made, and the flap is harvested from caudal to cephalad. Since the intramuscular dissection is important, the detailed technique is described below:

1. Conventional Intramuscular Pedicle Dissection

    Using the conventional method, further intramuscular dissection is made following the perforator from the muscle entry point to the thoracodorsal vessels. The avascular plane between the latissimus dorsi muscle and the fascia of the serratus anterior muscle is dissected, and the subscapular arterial system including the serratus anterior branch, the circumflex scapular branches, and several muscular branches from the thoracodorsal vessels is located. Apart from the vessels that are harvested, other vascular branches are ligated during proximal dissection of the main pedicle. This dissection is performed immediately below the axillary vessels.

2. Modified Intramuscular Pedicle Dissection

    The quality of the intramuscular dissection of the perforator is the key to success or failure. Intramuscular dissection requires great care until the diameter of the perforator increases where it enters the descending or transverse branch of a thoracodorsal vessel. We have introduced a modified technique for intramuscular dissection that makes it easier and safer than the classical method and decreases operative time.

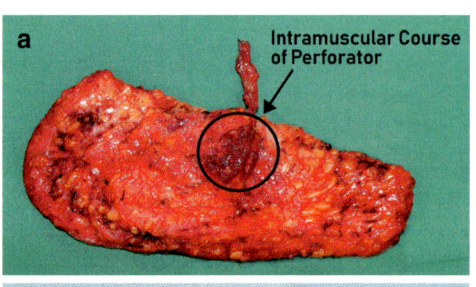

In the modified method, after a reliable perforator that pierces the latissimus dorsi muscle is found, the perforator is marked using a vessel loop. The anterior border of the latissimus dorsi muscle is detached from the serratus anterior muscle and chest wall. The thoracodorsal vessels are then dissected to the bifurcation point of the transverse and descending branches and followed proximally to the axillary vessels. After that, the thoracodorsal vessel branches are traced distally to their points of entry into the muscle before intramuscular dissection.

With the latissimus dorsi muscle stretched in the anterior direction, transillumination makes it easy to trace a perforator from its point of entry, past the muscle to the branch of the thoracodorsal vessels. The point where the perforator is illuminated at the inner portion of the latissimus dorsi is marked, and a cuff of muscle about 2 cm width is harvested intact by bipolar electrocautery (Fig. 15.4).

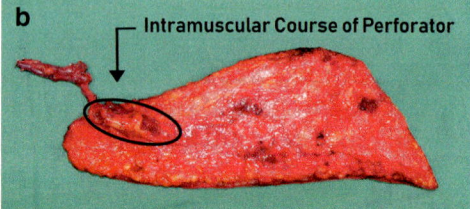

15.7 Clinical Scenario

A 73-year-old man with a history of diabetes presented with necrosis of the right fifth toe and a 5×6 cm^2 sized ulcer over the dorsum of the right foot, with exposure of the tendon (Fig. 15.5a). Preoperative CT angiography showed segmental occlusion of the anterior tibial artery, posterior tibial artery, and peroneal arteries of the right lower limb (Fig. 15.5b). Percutaneous angioplasty was performed.

Fig. 15.4 Various showcases of modified method of intramuscular dissection. (**a–c**) Modified method of intramuscular dissection of a thoracodorsal artery perforator flap. The pedicle incorporated a small muscle cuff during intramuscular dissection using bipolar cauterization

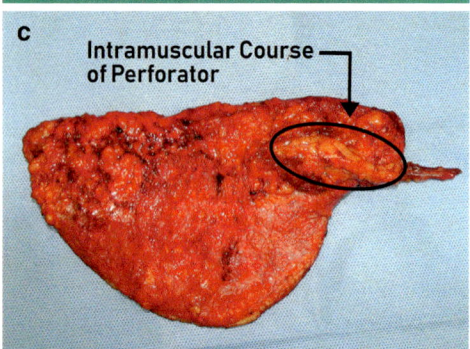

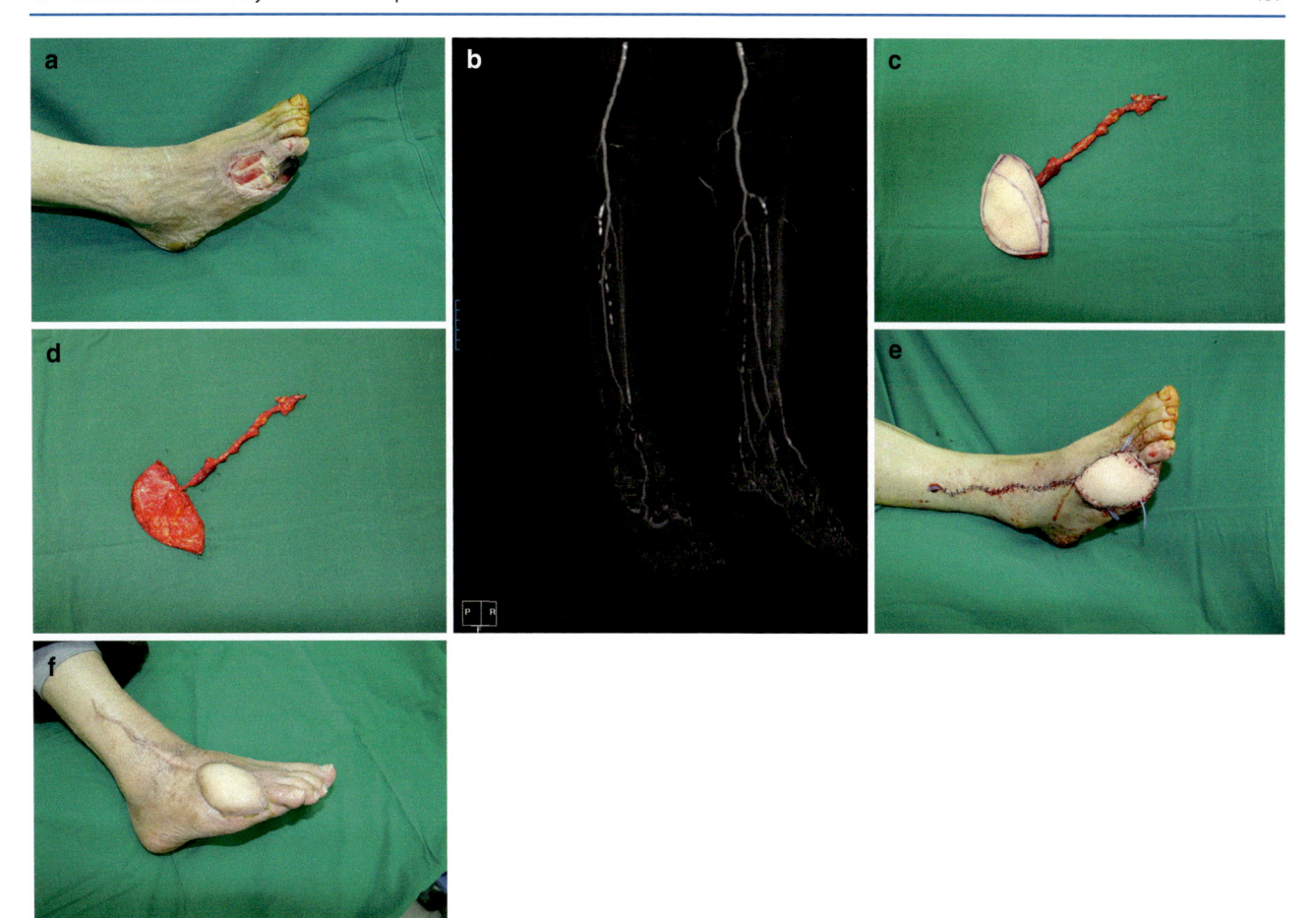

Fig. 15.5 Case. (**a**) A 73-year-old male with diabetes presented with necrosis of the right fifth toe and a 5 × 6 cm² sized deep ulcer exposing extensor tendon. (**b**) Preoperative CT angiography showed segmental occlusion of the anterior tibial artery, posterior tibial artery, and peroneal arteries of the right lower limb. (**c, d**) 8 × 5 cm² sized thoracodorsal artery perforator had an 18 cm pedicle with an eccentrically located perforator. (**e**) The thoracodorsal vessels were anastomosed to the anterior tibial vessels above the ankle in an end-to-side manner. (**f**) The flap survived completely and there was no recurrence of ulcer during 2 years of follow up. Without additional debulking surgery, the patient has no difficulty putting on shoes

However, only the anterior tibial artery was successfully cleared above the ankle. One week after revascularization, debridement of the dorsal foot was performed with ray amputation of the fifth toe. The defect was reconstructed using an 8 × 5 cm² sized thoracodorsal artery perforator free flap. The length of the pedicle reached 18 cm to reach above the ankle, and the perforator was positioned eccentrically to the flap to secure the long pedicle (Fig. 15.5c, d). The thoracodorsal vessels were anastomosed to the anterior tibial vessels above the ankle in an end-to-side manner (Fig. 15.5e). The flap survived completely and there was no recurrence of ulcer during 2 years of follow-up. Without additional debulking surgery, the patient has no difficulty putting on shoes (Fig. 15.5f).

15.8 Pearls and Pitfalls

Pearls

- How to Product a Long Vascular Pedicle
  When CT angiography reveals no suitable recipient vessels near a defect, the long vascular pedicle technique is used in order to approach above the ankle level to seek reliable recipient vessels.
  - Choose a Distally Located Perforator
    To obtain a long vascular pedicle, a distally located perforator from the descending branches of the thoracodorsal vessels should be selected. Proximal perforators from descending branches or perforators from transverse branches are not good candidates.
  - Make the Perforator in the Eccentric Position of the Flap
    If a much longer vascular pedicle is required, we position the perforator close to the margin of the flap and design the flap eccentrically. The actual pedicle length can be affected by the flap size and the entry point of the perforator to the skin flap. Assuming that the pedicle is harvested with the same length, the flap where the perforator is located in the center has a shorter length of the actual pedicle than located in the edge by the size of the skin flap. Perforators can be located eccentrically using the free-style flap harvesting technique as described by Wei FC. A reliable perforator is first located, and the flap is designed around it such that it can be elevated safely and the location of the perforator can be controlled. A maximum actual pedicle length was achieved with this technique in our hands. Pedicle length can often be extended from 15 cm to 20 cm by this modification (Fig. 15.6). Concerns about perfusion in flaps where the perforator is eccentric have been demonstrated in our previous study that if the perforator is reliable, sufficient perfusion is provided. However, the flap should be harvested parallel to the anterior border of the latissimus dorsi muscle because vascular networks and the subdermal plexus are connected parallel to the latissimus dorsi muscle according to the perforasome theory.
- How to Manage Multiple Defect?
  When multiple or distant defects require reconstruction simultaneously, a chimeric pattern flap is harvested (Fig. 15.7). After finding reliable perforator, the subscapular arterial system including the serratus anterior branch, the circumflex scapular vessel branches, and several muscular branches from the thoracodorsal vessels can be located in the avascular plane under the latissimus dorsi muscle. The other branches of the thoracodorsal vessels such as the transverse branch can be harvested together with the latissimus dorsi muscle, and the serratus anterior branch and muscle can also be harvested, if required. The skin paddle is first inset into the defect and fixed in position, and then the latissimus dorsi or serratus anterior muscle components are carefully positioned over the remaining defect avoiding twisting or kinking the pedicle.
- How to Harvest a Thin Flap?
  Suprafascial dissection is the norm for raising perforator flaps. However, elevation along the superficial fascial layer between the superficial and deep adipose tissue can provide a thin flap (Fig. 15.8). Preserving the linking vessels and orienting the flap in the direction of linking vessels make it possible to harvest long and thin flaps. In addition, the flap can be thinned further by defatting procedure with sharp Metzenbaum scissors until the superficial fat tissue is all removed except around the perforator. Great care should be taken to avoid injury to perforators and subdermal plexus. These superthin flaps can be used for head and neck resurfacing and are often used for finger and toe resurfacing.

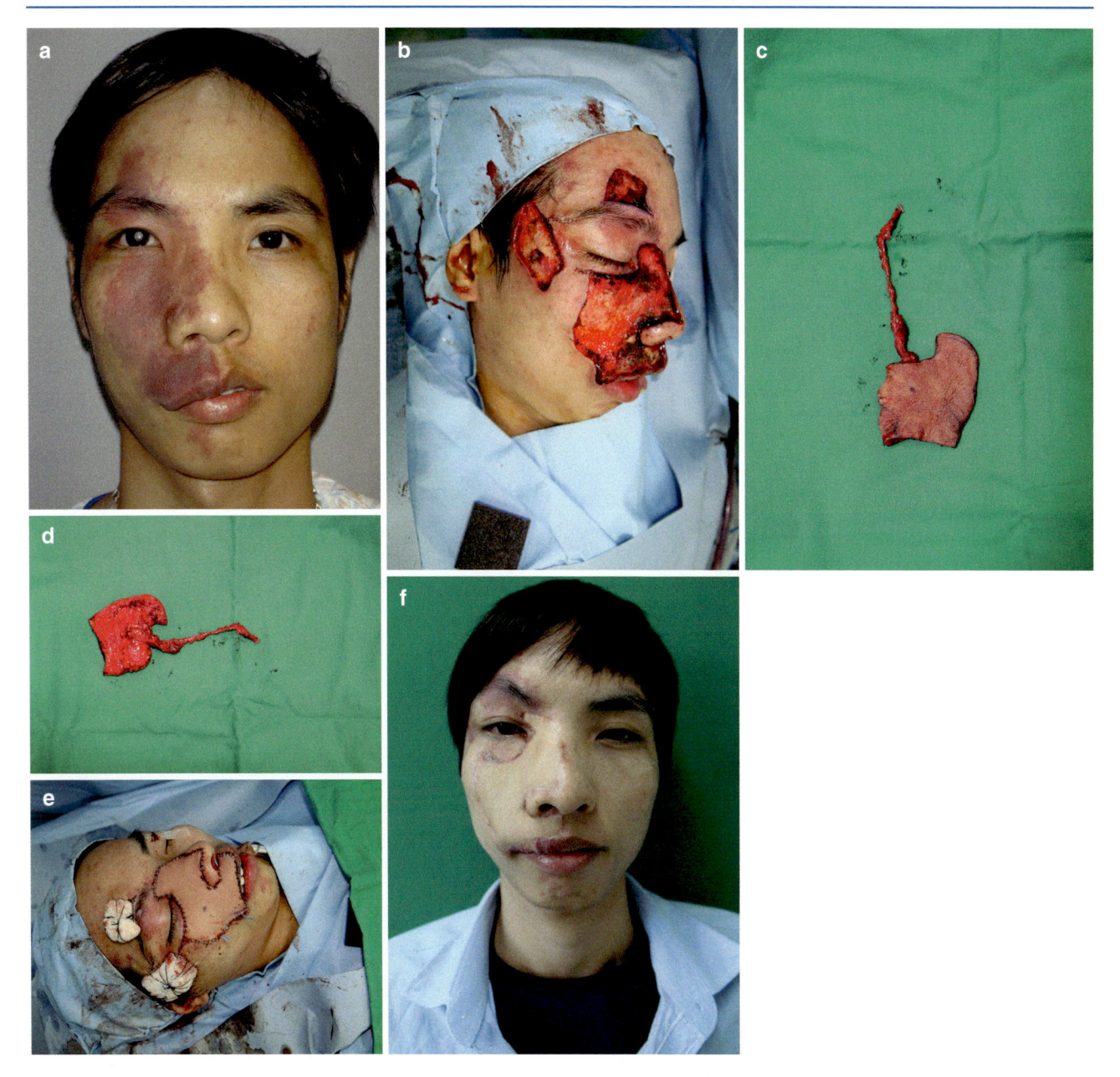

Fig. 15.6 TDAP free flap with long pedicle. (**a**) A 20-year-old male suffered capillary malformation on his right hemiface. (**b**) A severe pigmented lesion was removed and superficial temporal vessels were selected as recipient site. Required pedicle length was more than 18 cm. (**c, d**) A distal perforator from the lateral thoracic region was selected and the perforator was eccentrically located. So we harvested a TDAp flap with a pedicle of more than 18 cm in length. (**e**) Immediate postoperative view showing good color match with contours. (**f**) Long-term follow-up view

Fig. 15.7 TDAP free flap with chimeric pattern. (**a**) Post cranioplasty infection with skin loss. (**b**) Radical debridement and dead tissues were removed. (**c**) TDAp chimeric flap including a skin paddle and latissimus dorsi muscle flap. (**d**) The skin paddle was resurfaced to the scalp defects, and the latissimus dorsi muscle was used for dead space obliteration of temple region. (**e**) Long-term follow-up view shows no recurrence of infection

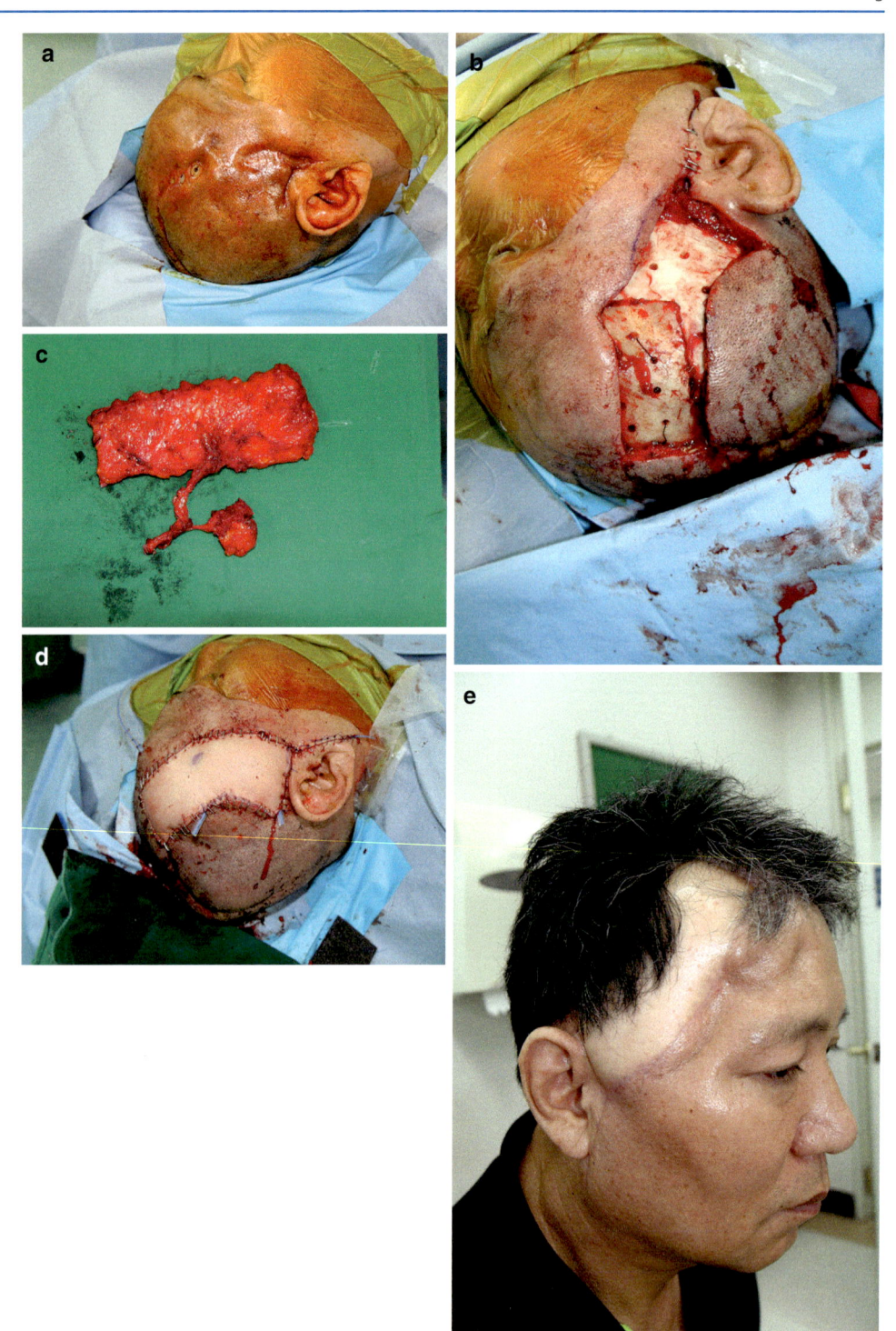

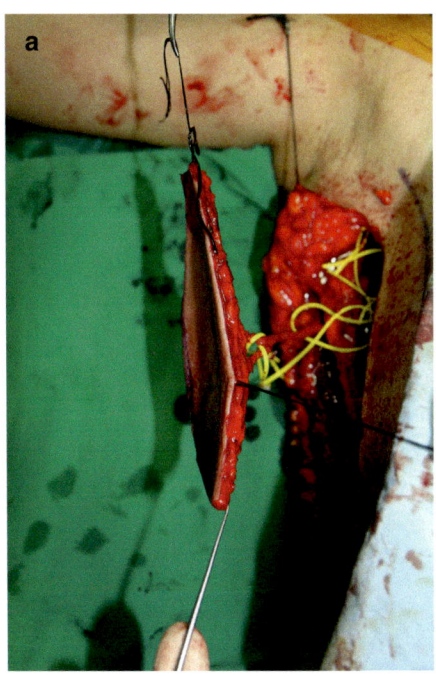

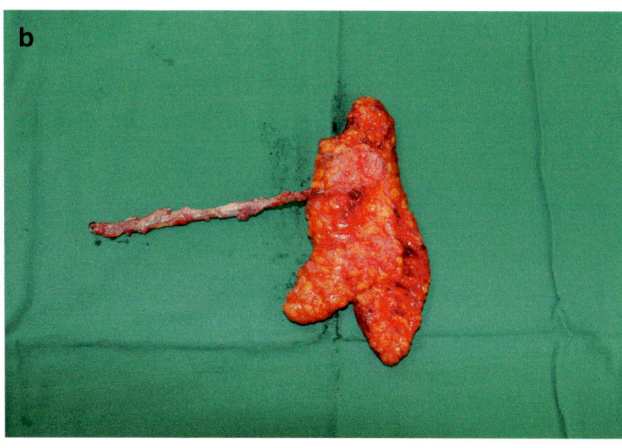

Fig. 15.8 Thin TDAP flap. (**a**) Suprafascial dissection is the norm for raising perforator flaps. Dissection in the plane between the superficial and deep adipose layers provides a very thin flap. (**b**) The flap is thinned further by monopolar electrocautery, with the flap held under tension with skin hooks, and with special care at the entrance of the perforator into the skin envelope

Pitfalls

- To Avoid Missing Perforator
  - Traction
    Traction of both sides of the skin of the incisional margin helps perforators to stand out. Perforators naturally run vertically toward the skin, but following a surgical access incision, they "lie down," so traction perpendicular to the skin plane makes them easier to find.
  - Dissection Plane
    If the dissection is started in the superficial fat layer, perforators are likely missed. Initial dissection for finding perforators should start in the suprafascial layer of the latissimus dorsi muscle. A sharp vertical dissection is performed down to the plane of the deep fascia until a pulsating perforator is detected. This dissection should run from distal to proximal.
  - Distinguish the Thoracodorsal Perforators from the Intercostal Perforators
    Once a reliable musculocutaneous perforator is identified, it is first traced distally to establish its point of entry to the fat and skin. Some perforators follow a horizontal course above the fascia for a few centimeters before piercing the overlying fat. Intercostal perforators in the distal area are often regarded as thoracodorsal musculocutaneous perforators. If we follow and dissect an intercostal perforator, we waste a lot of time as its short length and small diameter make it unsuitable as a flap perforator. Intercostal perforators run distally unlike thoracodorsal perforators, which run proximally. So you can distinguish a few dissection of intramuscular dissection of the latissimus dorsi.
- Exceptional Situation Without Reliable Perforator
  If the thoracodorsal artery perforator is small or not reliable, there are several reliable alternatives. In one approach, a small portion of muscle around bifurcation point of the transverse and descending branch can be harvested with the skin paddle in what we call the muscle-sparing technique. Another option is to combine latissimus dorsi muscle flaps with skin grafts because thinner flaps can be achieved with this approach. However, if we need skin flap, this method is not suitable. Finally, most surgeons look for other perforators. Fortunately, another dominant nourishing artery, such as the intercostal artery, is often available. In such situations we tend to find reliable perforators in the intercostal area (ninth to eleventh intercostal grooves), which enables us to harvest lateral intercostal artery perforator (LICAP) flaps. Deep dissection is performed to obtain suitable vessels for anastomosis. In our experience the maximal pedicle length is approximately 5 cm (Fig. 15.9).

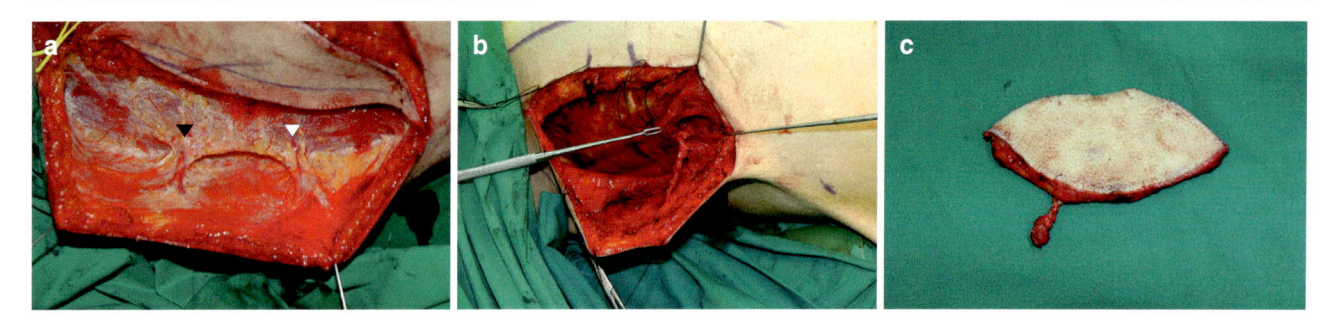

Fig. 15.9 Lateral intercostal artery perforator (LICAP) flap. (**a**) Black triangular arrow shows the thoracodorsal artery perforator and the white triangular arrow shows the lateral intercostal artery perforator (LICA p). (**b, c**) The initial plan was TDAP flap resurfacing; unfortunately there were no suitable reliable thoracodorsal perforators in the lateral thoracic region, but there was a reliable perforator in the distal region. We dissected into the rib cage and harvested a LICAP flap with a pedicle of 5 cm length instead of a TDAP flap

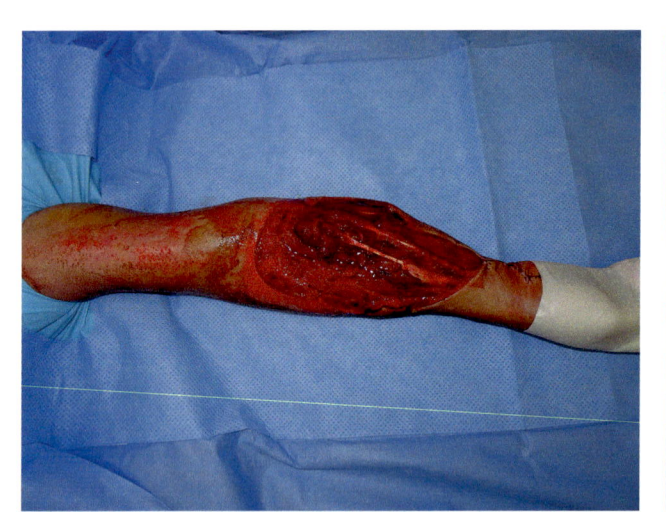

Fig. 15.10 Degloving injury to the forearm, radius, and ulna fixed with plate

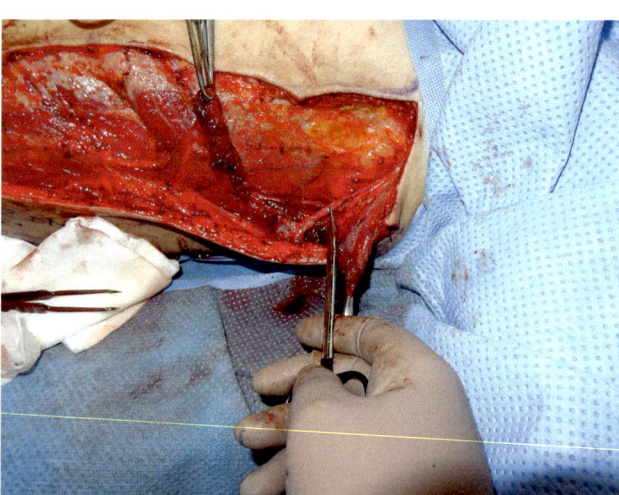

Fig. 15.11 Perforator dissection through the latissimus dorsi muscle

Case Scenario B: TDAP Flap for Extremity Reconstruction

Dariush Nikkhah Consultant Plastic Surgeon Royal Free Hospital

Jeremy Rawlins Consultant Plastic Surgeon Royal Perth Hospital

A 27-year-old man was struck by a lorry while on his motorbike. He sustained open fractures of his radius and ulna and soft tissue loss of his right forearm. After surgical debridement and fixation, an immediate free flap was planned for coverage (Fig. 15.10). The patient was placed supine and the most dominant perforator was marked with handheld Doppler. A 9 by 25 cm thoracodorsal artery perforator flap was raised, and the main perforator was dissected through the anterior border of the latissimus dorsi muscle (Fig. 15.11). The flap was anastomosed end to side to the brachial artery and two veins were repaired end to end with venous couplers. The donor site was closed primarily, and the patient made a full recovery and had an excellent outcome at 3 months with full function of his right extremity (Figs. 15.12 and 15.13).

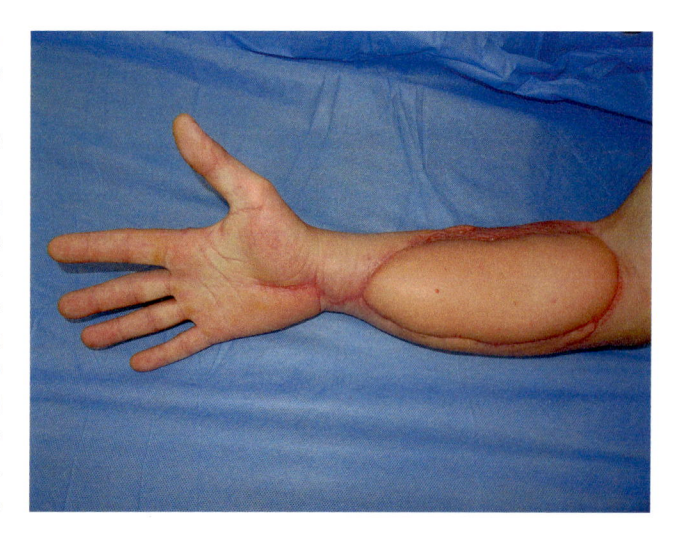

Fig. 15.12 Extremity outcome at 3 months

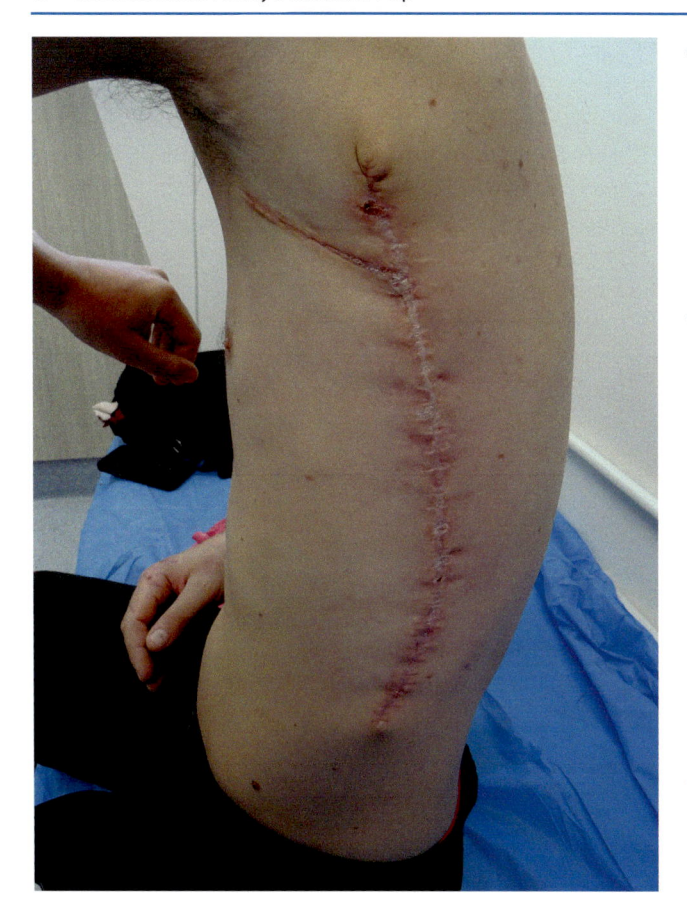

Fig. 15.13 Donor site outcome at 3 months

15.9 Selected Readings

- Koshima I, Soeda S. Inferior epigastric artery skin flaps without rectus abdominis muscle. Br J Plast Surg. 1989;42:645–8.

  The author harvested inferior epigastric artery skin flap without the rectus abdominis muscle, pedicled on the muscle perforators and the proximal inferior deep epigastric artery. They suggested the possibility of a perforator flap by showing that a large flap without muscle could survive on only a single muscle perforator.

- Abgrigiani C, Grilli D, Siebert J. Latissimus dorsi musculocutaneous flap without muscle. Plast Reconstr Surg. 1995;96:1608–14.

  The possibility of raising the cutaneous island of the latissimus dorsi musculocutaneous flap without muscle based on only one cutaneous perforator is presented in this paper. An anatomic study performed in 40 fresh cadaver specimens demonstrated that the vertical intramuscular branch of the thoracodorsal artery gives off two to three cutaneous branches (perforators) that are consistently present.

- Kim JT. Two options for perforator flaps in the flank donor site: Latissimus dorsi and thoracodorsal perforator flaps. Plast Reconstr Surg. 2005;115:755–63.

  The author summarized the confused nomenclature of the perforator flap in the lateral flank area. The difference between latissimus dorsi perforator flap and thoracodorsal perforator flap was explained, and its clinical application was reported.

- Mun GH, Kim HJ, Cha MK, Kim WY. Impact of perforator mapping using multidetector row computed tomographic angiography on free thoracodorsal artery perforator flap transfer. Plast Reconstr Surg. 2008;122:1079–88.

  Preoperative perforator mapping of thoracodorsal artery perforator flap was performed using multidetector-row computed tomographic angiography. The computed tomographic findings were compared with the acoustic Doppler flowmetric and intraoperative findings. Perforator mapping with preoperative multidetector-row computed tomographic angiography is valuable for both planning and executing thoracodorsal artery perforator flap transfer.

- Colohan S, Wong C, Lakhiani C, Cheng A, Maia M, Arbique G, Saint-Cyr M. The free descending branch muscle sparing latissimus dorsi flap: vascular anatomy and clinical applications. Plast Reconstr Surg. 2012;130:776e–87e.

  The authors investigate the vascular anatomy of the muscle-sparing variant and describe its application as a free flap based on the descending branch of the thoracodorsal artery. Computed tomography angiography demonstrated perfusion of the latissimus dorsi muscle by the transverse and descending branches, with overlap of vascular territories via cross-linking vessels. In the clinical study, the free muscle-sparing latissimus dorsi flap provided excellent coverage with no flap complications or seroma.

- Kim SW, Youn S, Kim JT, Kim YH. A modified method for harvesting thoracodorsal artery perforator flaps in a simple and time-saving approach. Microsurgery. 2016;36:642–6.

  The authors propose a modified method for harvesting the thoracodorsal perforator flap during lower extremity reconstruction and compare it with the conventional method. Using the modified method for flap harvest, a reliable perforator was found, and a cuff of muscle was left around the perforator without intramuscular dissection. When the modified method was used, total operating time was reduced from 311 to 272 min.

- Kim YH, Lee HE, Lee JH, Kim JT, Kim S. Reliability of eccentric position of the pedicle instead of central position in a thoracodorsal artery perforator flap. Microsurgery. 2017;37:44–8.

The aim of this study was to compare the safety and reliability of thoracodorsal artery perforator flaps harvested with centrally or eccentrically located perforators. There have been concerns regarding flap perfusion and distal vascularity in eccentrically located perforators. However, authors suggest that both eccentric and central perforators are safe options in thoracodorsal artery perforator flap.

- Saint-Cyr M, Wong C, Schaverien M, Mojallal A, Rohrich RJ. The perforasome theory: vascular anatomy and clinical implications. Plast Reconstr Surg. 2009;124:1529–44.

The authors investigated the three-dimensional and four-dimensional arterial vascular territory of a single perforator, termed a "perforasome," in major clinically relevant areas of the body. A vascular anatomy study was performed using 40 fresh cadavers. Each perforasome is linked with adjacent perforasomes by means of two main mechanisms that include both direct and indirect linking vessels. Every clinically significant perforator has the potential to become either a pedicle or free perforator flap.

The Scapular Axis Flaps: An Expendable Direct Cutaneous Perforator with Many Options

16

Daniel Saleh and John Henton

16.1 Introduction

The scapular axis provides an abundance of tissue options in reconstruction. Both the scapular and parascapular flaps were described in 1982 by Dosantos and Nassif, respectively.

These cutaneous flaps are less favored than the nearby latissimus dorsi, but they do offer versatility without sacrificing a muscle unit.

Scapular axis flaps can provide large skin/fasciocutaneous flap options and an osseous flap. The osseous component which largely is the lateral border of the scapula receives a nonpenetrating periosteal vascular (NPPV) supply [1]. Thus for cortical reconstructions with little reliance on endosteal blood supply, these units of bone can be very useful for an array of applications.

Pedicled scapular and parascapular cutaneous flaps are commonly used for defects in the axilla or posterior trunk. As free flaps they are widely used in extremity reconstruction alongside the head and neck. These skin flaps offer excellent versatility for reconstructive needs, for large surface areas with acceptable donor morbidity, largely confined to stretched scars. Moreover no motor units to regional musculature are affected by flap dissection, and parascapular flap harvest can be performed in the supine position.

16.2 Anatomy

The scapular axis flaps all derive from the subscapular artery, which arises from the third part of the axillary artery. The subscapular artery gives rise to the thoracodorsal artery and the circumflex scapular artery. The circumflex scapular passes through the triangular space where it becomes the superficial circumflex scapular artery (SCSA). The SCSA gives off several cutaneous branches including the transverse branch (scapular flap) and the descending (parascapular flap).

The scapula bone is enveloped by a plexus of communicating vessels. Several of these on the lateral edge of the scapula are given off by the subscapular artery before it becomes the SCSA. Scapula bone can therefore be taken as a flap in isolation or combined with other flaps in the scapular axis. Furthermore, if the subscapular artery is included, flaps based on the thoracodorsal artery may be taken on the same pedicle (latissimus dorsi, scapular tip bone flap, and the serratus).

Any of these can be taken in isolation or in combination as chimeric flaps. To include the thoracodorsal-based flaps, the teres minor needs disinsertion or sectioning; Fig. 16.5 depicts a raised latissimus dorsi and parascapular flap with the intervening teres muscle still intact between the pedicles.

Both the scapular and parascapular flaps must incorporate the skin overlying the triangular space to capture the SCSA and its key branches.

If dissected back to the subscapular artery, a pedicle up to 7 cm long with an arterial diameter of up to 4 mm may be obtained. There are usually two venae comitantes.

The scapular flap can be taken horizontally up to the midline of the back, although flaps crossing the midline are possible especially if a delay procedure is used. Around 10 cm flap width in the vertical plane may be closed directly.

The parascapular flap can be up to 30 cm long, and flap width can vary between 15 and 25 cm for direct closure, depending on the patient's habitus. Larger flaps can be harvested but require secondary closure. The osseous component of the lateral scapular border can be 2–3 cm wide and approximately 12 cm long.

Anatomical variants: sometimes the circumflex scapular artery can arise directly from the axillary artery, and it is important to recognize the midline is not a "boundary" for these flaps.

D. Saleh (✉) · J. Henton
Newcastle University Hospitals NHS foundation Trust, Newcastle upon Tyne, UK

© Springer Nature Switzerland AG 2023
D. Nikkhah et al. (eds.), *Core Techniques in Flap Reconstructive Microsurgery*, https://doi.org/10.1007/978-3-031-07678-7_16

16.3 Preoperative Investigation

Outpatient vascular assessment can be performed with handheld Doppler examination to confirm the presence and location of the SCSA cutaneous perforator in the skin over the triangular space. It is also possible to trace the courses of the transverse branch and the descending branches with the Doppler to plan flap dimensions.

To locate the perforator, with the patient's arm abducted, feel for the point where there is an indentation between the bulk of the superior border of the teres major and the inferior border of the teres minor on the lateral edge of the scapular.

Cross-sectional computed tomography (CT) with contrast will delineate the vascular anatomy, and while we routinely do this, the recognized anatomical variations described above may mean some would take benefit from radiographic anatomy.

CT is helpful in patients where a virtually planned osseous flap is desired. This allows clear three-dimensional (3D) reconstruction of the scapula and the desired osseous component for the purpose of intraoperative jigs to perform accurate osteotomies. In such cases we do add the contrast component to the CT examination to assess the vascular pedicles.

16.4 Flap Design, Markings, and Positioning

Flaps can be individual, conjoined, or chimerized. We describe below raising of individual parascapular and scapular flaps. The obliquely oriented parascapular flap is sometimes referred to as the "inframammary extended circumflex scapular flap" or IMECC. For the purpose of this description, we describe a conventional parascapular flap, but the skin markings can be obliquely oriented from the posterior axillary fold toward the pectoral crease and chest if needed/desired.

These flaps are generally hairless in females and many males, but lack good cutaneous nerves to allow for coaptation to restore sensibility. The osseous component is confined to the lateral border of the scapula and is best incorporated into a parascapular skin flap.

Depending on the complexity of the reconstructive effort, variable components of the thoracodorsal axis can also be incorporated into these flaps.

16.5 Positioning

The best positioning in our experience is lateral or "lazy" supine with a soft bolster across the posterior-inferior costal margin on the ipsilateral side (Fig. 16.1).

The key to positioning is allowing movement of the shoulder girdle. Irrespective of whether the patient is lateral or lazy supine, we prep the skin down to the elbow and sterile wrap the hand and forearm to lie in a sterile trough assembled at 90 degrees to the operating table (Fig. 16.2). This allows easy movement of the arm and shoulder to open up the triangular space and ease pedicle visualization and dissection depending on the components of the flap.

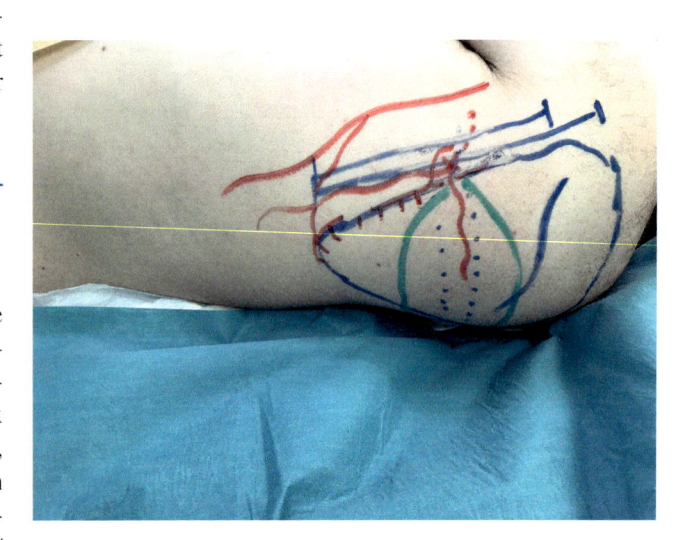

Fig. 16.1 An example of supine positioning with a small bolster under the ipsilateral hemitrunk lying approximately parallel with the posterior costal margin. The green markings show a small scapular flap can easily be raised in this position across the midline. The red cross hatches showing the lateral border portion of an osseus flap. All red markings depict Dopplered vessels in the operative position

Fig. 16.2 The positioning of the forearm and arm allows shoulder girdle movements to allow fluid raising and exposure of the triangular space. A dual team limb reconstruction and osseo-cutaneous parascapular flap being harvested in the supine position. The forearm is sterile wrapped and placed in a sterile trough when needed

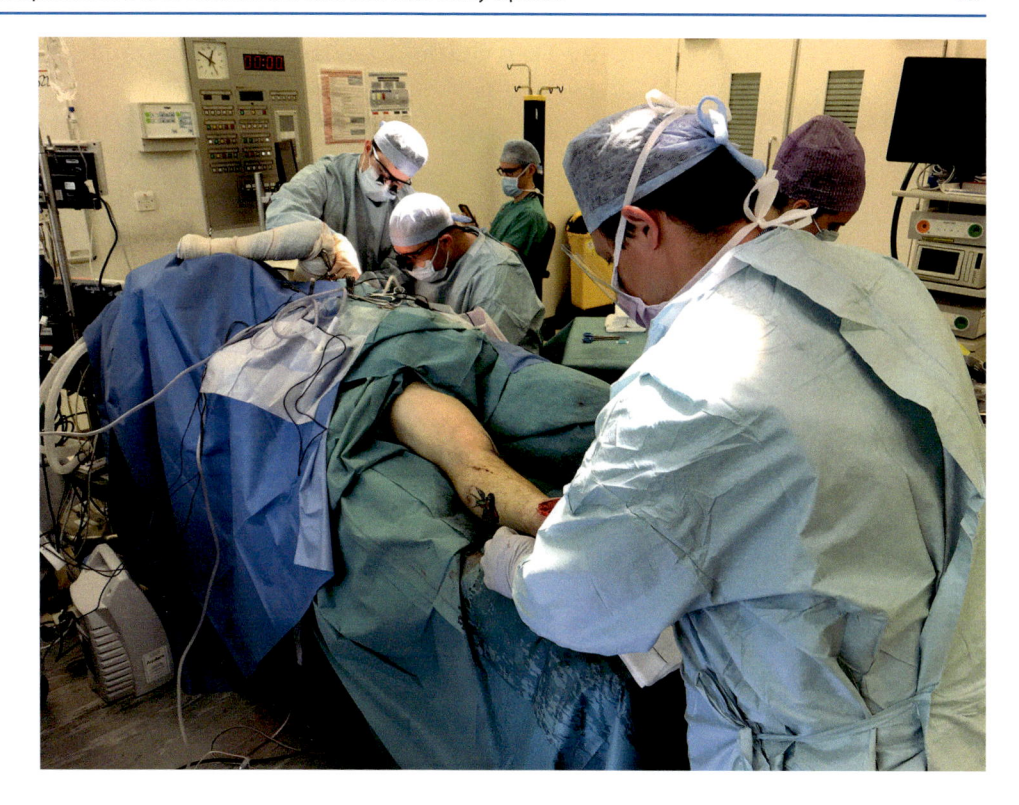

16.6 Flap Markings

It is our experience that marking the patient in the planned operative position is preferred. We advise positioning as above, so, for example, placing the patient in the lateral decubitus position with the ipsilateral arm abducted to 90° and supported by a colleague by the bedside will allow accurate marking presurgery. The scapula is very mobile and given the mobility of the truncal skin on the flank and back – vascular anatomy and Doppler signal can vary.

Mark the scapular outline and the scapular spine. The main pedicle emerges from the triangular space **above** the teres major. It is difficult to clinically isolate and clearly identify the teres major in many patients. Thus, we draw a line parallel to the lateral scapular border limited to its cranio-caudal axis (Fig. 16.3) and also a similar line running from the scapular spine to the inferior tip of the scapula. At approximately the midpoint of these lines at the lateral scapular border—the Doppler signal of the main pedicle can be found as it emerges above the teres major. Here the vascular signal can be followed for either branch. In general the parascapular flap branch runs roughly parallel to the lateral scapular border with the arm **abducted to 90°; similarly** the scapular branch runs parallel to the scapular spine. Given the variability in patient positioning and mobility of the truncal skin, we prefer to follow the vascular signal with a Doppler in the **primary operative position.**

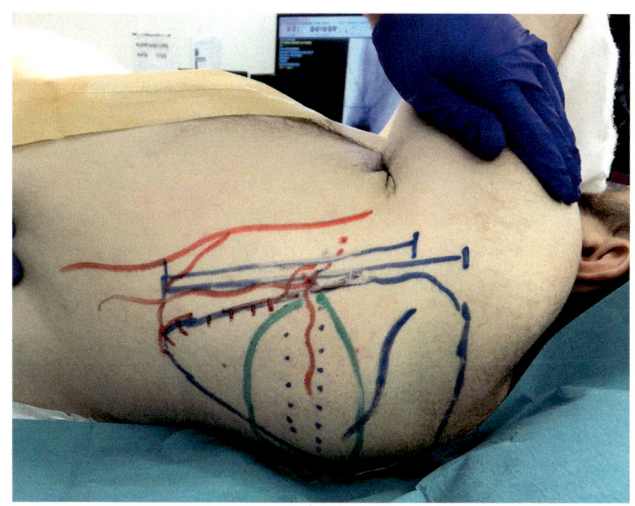

Fig. 16.3 Two parallel lines on the lateral border, from the spine to tip, and upper border to tip of the scapular and their respective midpoints. Around this midpoint the exit of the main pedicle from the triangular space can be Dopplered

Figure 16.1 highlights the markings with a green scapular flap outlined, the red cross hatch delineating the lateral border osseous component and the parascapular branch running immediately lateral to the lateral scapular border. These vessels were all Dopplered.

16.7 Flap Elevation: A Step-by-Step Guide

16.7.1 Scapular Flap

Our preference is to medially expose the vessels and therefore raise the flap from medial to lateral.

Mark the ellipse desired and to directly close by pinch. A relatively avascular plane exists in the suprafascial plane. Incise all the markings except the lateral quarter until the vascular pedicle is visualized. This avoids being compromised by variable anatomy whereby the medial aspect of the ellipse does not include the vessel.

The sharp dissection with monopolar cautery proceeds over the trapezius, infraspinatus (and possibly rhomboid major), and teres minor.

Once over the surface of the teres minor, it is common to see the pedicle in the subcutaneous tissue. The dissection can now proceed subfascially using a blade or Jameson scissor dissection, as this makes it easier to include the fibrofatty tissue around the pedicle as the triangular space is approached. The remainder of the flap can now be incised knowing the vasculature is within the flap tissue.

Once the vessel and surrounding fat is released from the most lateral surface of the teres minor, move the arm into the trough (or across the anterior trunk), and retract the teres minor with a Czerny retractor medially. This opens the triangular space and will allow accurate ligation of the many small venous branches draining the surrounding musculature. As more tissue is released, a Norfolk-Norwich self-retainer can be placed between the teres minor and the long head of triceps to allow dissection of the pedicle with the surrounding anatomy relatively **static**.

Larger-caliber arterial vessels an also be ligated and the pedicle dissected to the desired point.

16.7.2 Parascapular Flap

This flap is similar to the scapular flap and is preferred often because it provides a larger skin paddle, with ease of patient positioning.

Once the flap markings are complete, incise the distal three quarters of the flap to preserve the proximal part, which can be incised once the vessels are visualized at the entry point to the flap.

The flap is lifted in the suprafascial plane, using monopolar cautery, over the latissimus dorsi until the teres major muscle comes into view. The dissection then proceeds in the subfascial plane which will also bring the teres minor into view medially. At this juncture it is common to see the vessels across the free upper edge of the teres major as the fibrofatty tissue comes into the surgical field. A Travers self-retainer can be placed between the teres minor and major to better identify side branches going to the lateral scapula and muscles.

The dissection follows the free edge of the teres major gradually advancing the dissection well into the triangular space. Figure 16.4 demonstrates a retracted teres major exposing the length of the pedicle in the triangular space.

16.7.3 Osseus Flaps

Either skin flap can be incorporated into taking the lateral border of the scapular for an osteocutaneous reconstruction.

The major difference in technique arises once entering the triangular space. The medial vessels, which are numerous, running from the main pedicle to the lateral border of the scapula must be preserved. Thus, the main release of the pedicle occurs primarily on its lateral aspect. Once the lateral

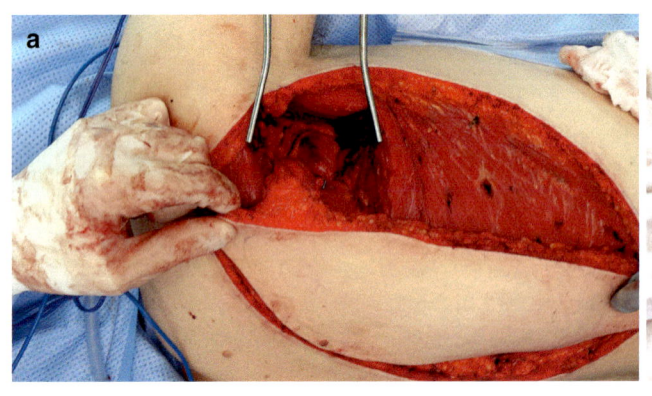

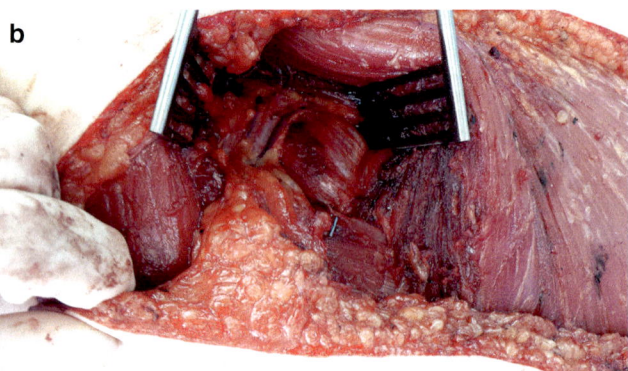

Fig. 16.4 (**a**, **b**) Teres major retracted and the pedicle dissection complete in a parascapular flap

pedicle dissection is complete, all that should be tethering the skin flap to the triangular space is the soft tissue (small vessel) attachments to the scapula.

Reflect the skin flap laterally, and incise the musculature (infraspinatus), along the desired length of the scapula border – this does not typically include the bone cranial (superior) to the scapular spine. Similarly it is advisable to avoid taking the tip of the scapula with this pedicle as it has separate axial blood supply from the thoracodorsal axis; therefore if desired additional pedicle dissection would be required.

Once the muscle is incised, lift the periosteum from medial to lateral but not to denude the bone flap portion.

Our preference is to use a sagittal saw for a uniform step-wise bone cut which allows control once through the deep cortical aspect of the bone. Once the cuts are complete, an Obwegeser elevator can be passed on the deep surface of bone to "lever" it free from the subscapularis fibers which are now the only soft tissue attachments remaining.

16.8 Pearls and Pitfalls

Be wary of the venous branches that require ligation once in the triangular space. Typically these flaps have two venae draining the tissue, and so one must be cautious as to not ligate a main vein of the flap. There can be variability in our experience in the venous anatomy.
Once the axial vessels come into view in the "fast" phase of raising the flap, switch to more delicate dissection with scissors.
When ligating the venous branches in the triangular space, attempt to preserve the length of one additional branch in case of flap drainage problems (Fig. 16.5 ligated side branch of good caliber).
When using the osseus flap, re-tensioning the subscapularis and infraspinatus muscles is important. We prefer to place 2 mm drill holes in the neo-lateral border of the scapula and use a 2.0 Ethibond suture passed through the now free edge of the infraspinatus, through the hole, and through the deeper free edge of subscapularis to then be tied.
When combining thoracodorsal flaps and scapular flaps, release the teres muscle to allow conjoined pedicle dissection (Fig. 16.5).

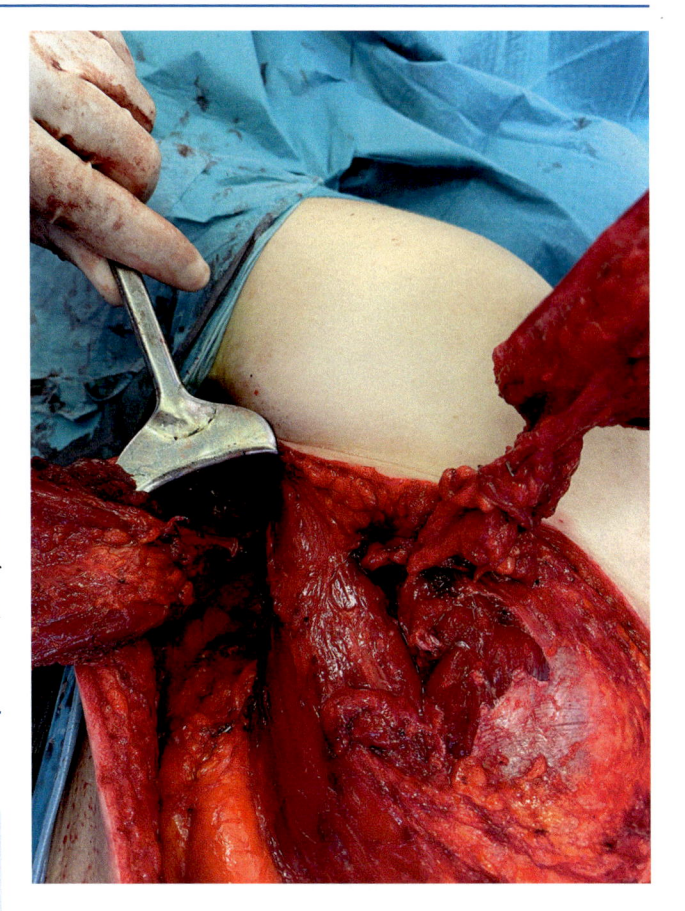

Fig. 16.5 A latissimus dorsi and parascapular flap raised with the intervening teres minor still intact which requires sectioning or disinsertion to chimerize

16.9 Clinical Example

A 47-year-old woman was involved in a cycling accident and denuded the soft tissues of the dorsomedial foot and sustained a midfoot fracture dislocation (Fig. 16.6). Following osteosynthesis soft reconstruction was performed. The patient desired a discrete donor site, and given the dimensions were felt to exceed those appropriate for a groin flap, a scapular flap was advocated to allow the scar to be concealed by underwear and clothing.

The flap was raised in the lateral position allowing access to the foot for osteosynthesis and reconstruction. A skin flap was preferred in this patient because it was felt by the orthopedic team skeletal revision was a risk given the severity of the midfoot injury, and so having a skin flap would more easily permit reaccessing the midfoot if ever needed (Fig. 16.7).

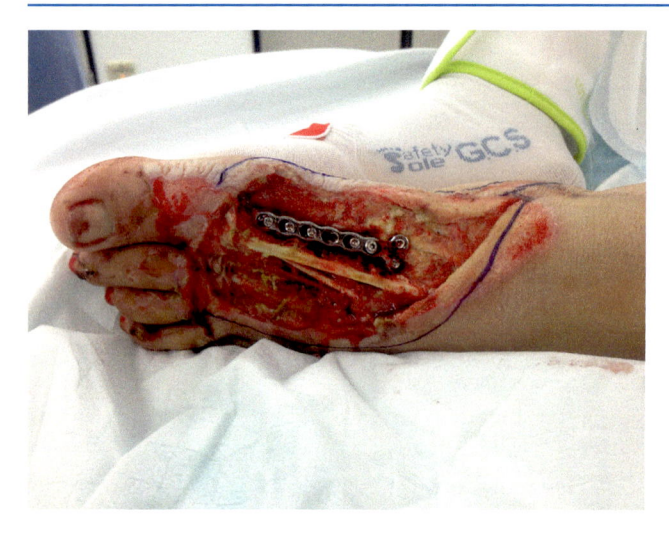

Fig. 16.6 A left foot injury in a 47-year-old woman

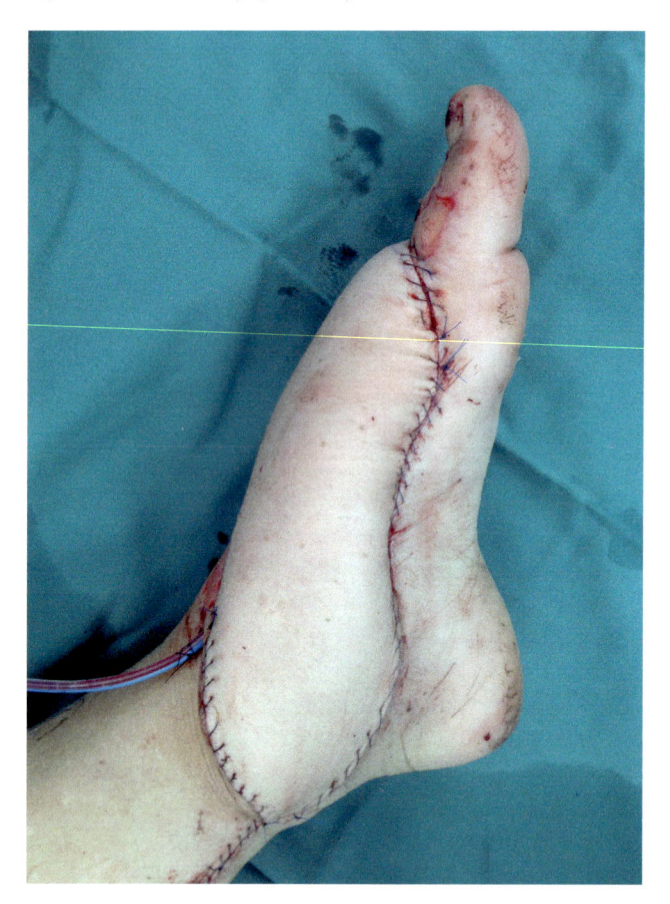

Fig. 16.7 Parascapular flap reconstruction of a dorsal and medial foot defect following trauma

16.10 Selected Readings

- Tang AL, Bearelly S, Mannion K. The expanding role of scapular free-flaps. Curr Opin Otolaryngol Head Neck Surg. 2017;25:411–5.
- Mayou BJ, Whitby D, Jones BM. The scapular flap – an anatomical and clinical study. Br J Plast Surg. 1982;35:8–13.
- Klinkenberg M, Fischer S, Kremer T, Hernekamp F, Lehnhardt M, Daigeler A. Comparison of anterolateral thigh, lateral arm, and parascapular free flaps with regard to donor-site morbidity and aesthetic and functional outcomes. Plast Reconstr Surg. 2013;131:293–302.
- Izadi D, Paget JTEH, Haj-Basheer M, Khan UM. Fasciocutaneous flaps of the subscapular artery axis to reconstruct large extremity defects. J Plast Reconstr Aesthet Surg. 2012;65:1357–62.

Reference

1. Sparks DS, Saleh DB, Rozen WM, Hutmacher DW, Schuetz MA, Wagels M. Vascularised bone transfer: history, blood supply and contemporary problems. JPRAS. 2017;70:1–11.

Thoracoacromial Artery Flap: Pectoralis Major Muscle Flap

Jonathan A. Dunne, Ian C. C. King, Dariush Nikkhah, and Jeremy Rawlins

17.1 Introduction

The pectoralis major flap was first described by Hueston and McConchte [1] in 1968 as a means of ensuring adequate blood supply for a skin flap to reconstruct the chest wall; Brown et al. further modified the use of the flap for sternal defects to make the repair more robust [2]. Maruyama first reported its use in head and neck surgery in 1977 to reconstruct an oral cavity defect [3], and it was subsequently popularised by Ariyan [4]. The flap comprises the pectoralis major muscle, with or without overlying skin, and can include the rib to reconstruct mandibular defects. It is most frequently used as a pedicled flap but can also be utilised as a free flap and remains a workhorse flap in head and neck reconstruction and is frequently used for sternal defects secondary to infection, tumours or trauma.

17.2 Anatomy

The pectoralis major is an anterior muscle of the pectoral girdle with two origins. The clavicular head originates from the antero-medial portion of the clavicle and sternal head from the anterior manubrium, sternum, costal cartilages 1–6 and external oblique aponeurosis. The two heads converge as one muscle, occasionally with a small gap, to form a tendon inserting into the inter-tubercular groove. The medial and lateral pectoral nerves innervate the muscle and are commonly divided during elevation of the flap.

The pectoralis major muscle flap is a Mathes and Nahai type V flap, with a dominant vascular pedicle and multiple minor pedicles. The major vascular supply is from the pectoral branch of the thoracoacromial artery. The pectoral branch emerges from the main trunk lateral to the pectoralis minor, lying deep to the pectoralis major, and traverses deep to it before emerging medial to its tendon and piercing the clavipectoral fascia. It runs on the muscle's deep surface in a distinct fascial plane, before dividing into muscular and cutaneous perforators.

The clavicular branch of the thoracoacromial artery almost exclusively supplies the clavicular head of the pectoralis major. Minor segmental supply is from the internal mammary artery perforators through intercostal spaces 1–3 medially and the long thoracic artery laterally. A cadaveric study by Freemean demonstrated a rich anastomosis between major and minor pedicles, with significant vascular contributions by all pedicles to the muscle, which in turn supplies the skin paddle via perforators [5]. The rich vasculature allows flap elevation on a major or minor pedicle. Accompanying venae comitantes provide venous drainage from the muscle, and an overlying skin paddle has drainage into the cephalic vein. A skin paddle extending inferior to the muscle has a random blood supply, as opposed to axial vasculature.

17.3 Preoperative Investigation

Clinical assessment is the mainstay of preoperative work-up for the pectoralis major flap, and determining the requirements of the defect is imperative in flap planning. For head and neck reconstruction, the necessity of a skin paddle must be considered with the knowledge it will create a bulkier flap. In addition, in female patients in particular, a skin paddle may carry increased donor site morbidity with breast distortion. Chest wall defects may be reconstructed with an

J. A. Dunne (✉)
Imperial College Healthcare NHS Trust, London, UK

I. C. C. King
Queen Victoria Hospital NHS Foundation Trust, East Grinstead, UK

D. Nikkhah
Department of Plastic, Reconstructive and Aesthetic Surgery, Royal Free Hospital, London, UK

J. Rawlins
Department of Plastic Surgery, Royal Perth Hospital, Perth, WA, Australia

advancement-rotation flap based on the pectoral branch, or a turnover flap vascularised by the internal mammary artery perforators. Consideration of previous cardiac surgery, which may have utilised the ipsilateral internal mammary vessels, should be considered and will preclude use of a turnover flap.

17.4 Flap Design and Markings

The surface marking of the pectoral branch of the thoracoacromial artery is from the midpoint of the clavicle descending inferiorly and continued as a line bisecting it from the acromioclavicular joint to the xiphoid process. The internal mammary artery perforators emerge from intercostal spaces one to three, 1 to 2 cm lateral to the sternum with the second perforator usually the largest.

The boundaries of the muscle are the clavicle superiorly, sternum medially and anterior axillary fold laterally. Mediastinal defects are commonly reconstructed without a skin paddle, with overlying skin closed directly or with a split-thickness skin graft. A unilateral pectoralis major muscle flap will cover most sternal defects, although may struggle to cover the xiphoid process. Options include a contralateral turnover flap or a different flap such as omentum or rectus abdominis flaps.

A number of skin paddle designs have been reported, and a paramedian skin paddle is frequently used in head and neck reconstruction, beginning inferior to the second intercostal space to permit use of a deltopectoral flap as a backup, acknowledging the defensive approach proposed by MacGregor [6].

17.5 Flap Raise/Elevation: A Step-by-Step Guide

17.5.1 Head and Neck Reconstruction

Step 1 Flap Design
Mark the surface anatomy of the vascular pedicle and the skin incision.

A paramedian skin flap overlying muscle is frequently used. The arc of rotation from the inferior border of the clavicle to the distal edge of the skin paddle should be measured and be equal to or greater than the distance from the inferior clavicle and the distal edge of the defect (Figs. 17.1 and 17.2).

Step 2
The skin paddle should be incised down to the muscle fascia and undermining avoided, as it may damage musculocutaneous perforators. The pedicle lies deep to the muscle, and therefore the superficial surface of the pectoralis major

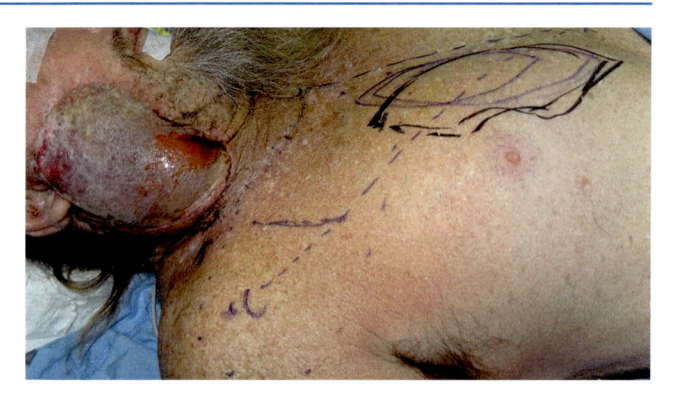

Fig. 17.1 Markings: note the necrotic free flap on the right neck. Markings for the pectoralis major myocutaneous flap don't cross the midline

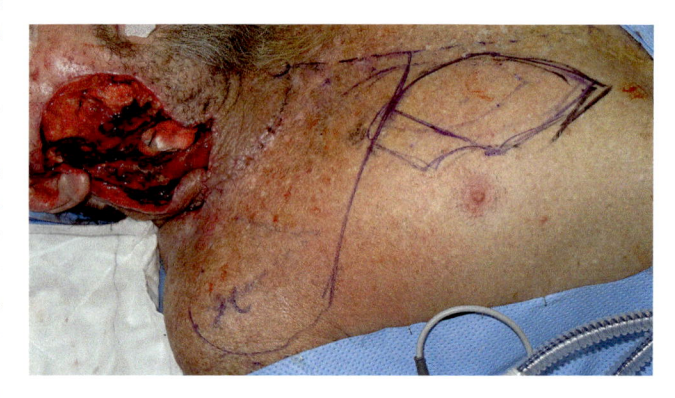

Fig. 17.2 Defensive markings: preserving the upper intercostal perforators enables the deltopectoral flap to be protected in case of further difficulties with the reconstruction (a final lifeboat). Note the design of this flap goes just lateral to the deltopectoral groove where the blood supply becomes random pattern rather than axial

should be dissected and exposed without concern. The skin paddle may be tacked to the muscle to avoid damage due to shear (Fig. 17.3).

Step 3
The lateral border of the muscle is identified and the deep surface of the muscle elevated from minimal attachments in this region. The muscle is incised with cautery from its medial and inferior origin, leaving the superior muscle intact. Internal mammary artery perforators are cauterised when dividing the muscle from its medial origin except when performing a turnover flap (Figs. 17.3, 17.4, and 17.5).

Step 4
Continued flap elevation should leave the fascia on the deep surface intact. With ongoing dissection of the flap away from the pectoralis minor, the pedicle will be seen on the deep surface of the muscle within the fascia. Branches of the medial pectoral nerve and lateral thoracic artery traverse the pectoralis minor and will be divided as they enter the deep surface of the flap (Fig. 17.6).

17 Thoracoacromial Artery Flap: Pectoralis Major Muscle Flap

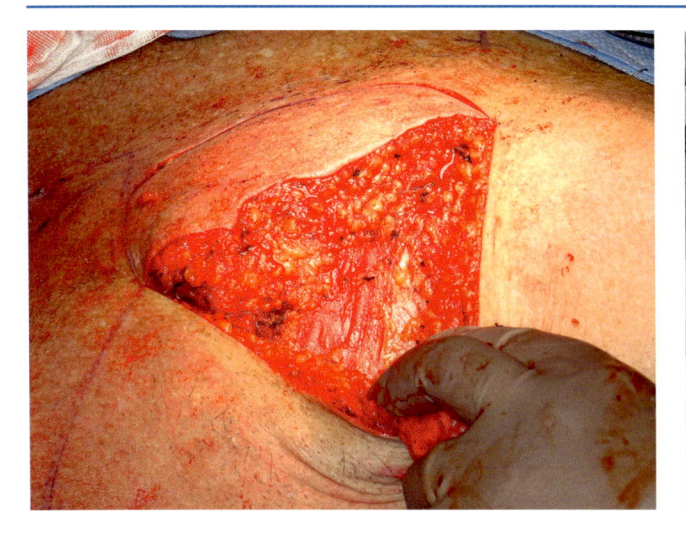

Fig. 17.3 Identify inferior border of the pectoralis major muscle: this allows the surgeon to adjust markings of the flap if required prior to complete elevation. Defining boundaries is key

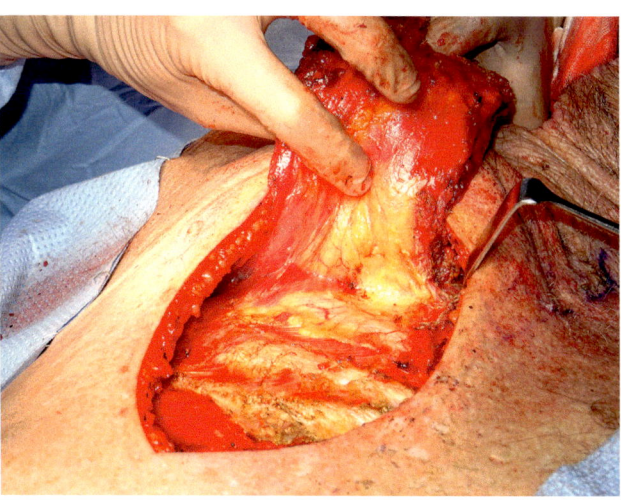

Fig. 17.6 Medial release: carefully dissect the muscle from the chest wall, taking care to look out for the pedicle which will appear on the deep side of the pectoralis major muscle

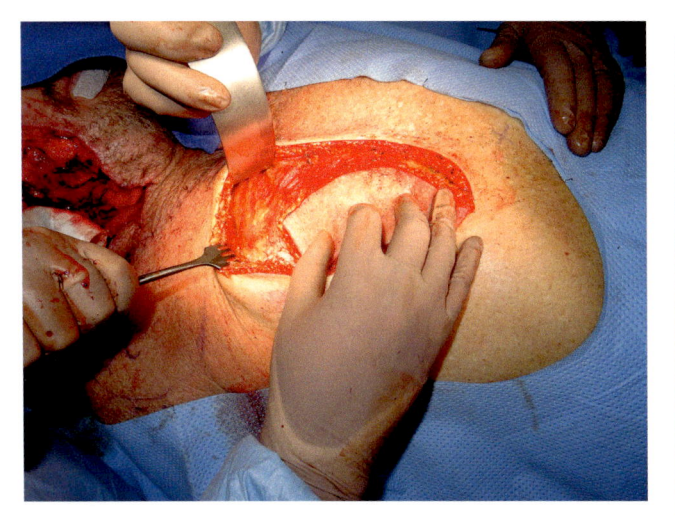

Fig. 17.4 Medial dissection: release from sternal attachments is key: take care to carefully control the medial intercostal perforators if present; these can be large

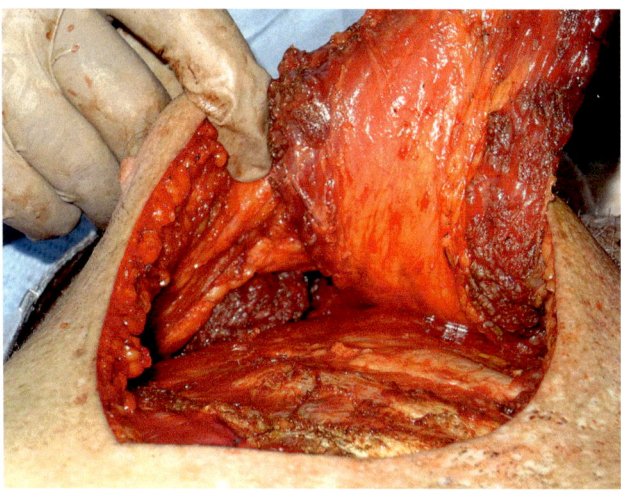

Fig. 17.7 Lateral release: dividing the tendinous insertion is essential to being able to mobilise this flap

Step 5

Lateral to the pedicle, the insertion of the flap into the intertubercular groove is divided (Fig. 17.7).

Step 6

Further muscular fibres at the origin are released until adequate movement is achieved, which can necessitate islanding the flap on the vascular pedicle (Fig. 17.8).

The flap is passed superiorly via a wide subcutaneous tunnel into the neck, usually superficial to the clavicle, ensuring there is no twisting of the pedicle (Figs. 17.9 and 17.10).

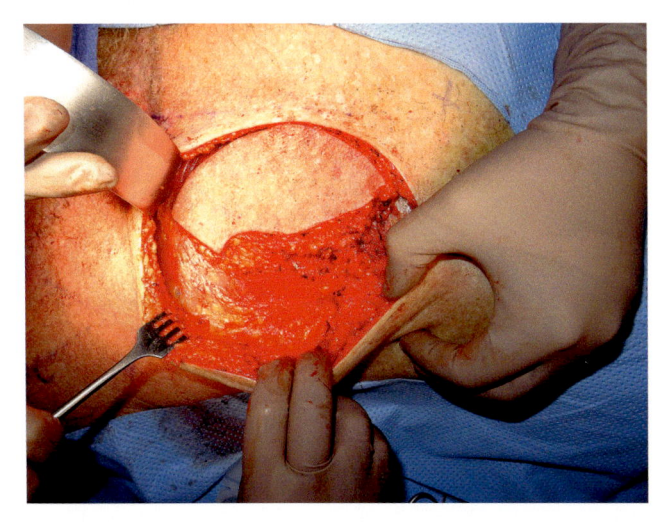

Fig. 17.5 Lateral dissection: further defining the boundaries and insertion of the muscle, allowing visualisation of the released tissue and donor sites

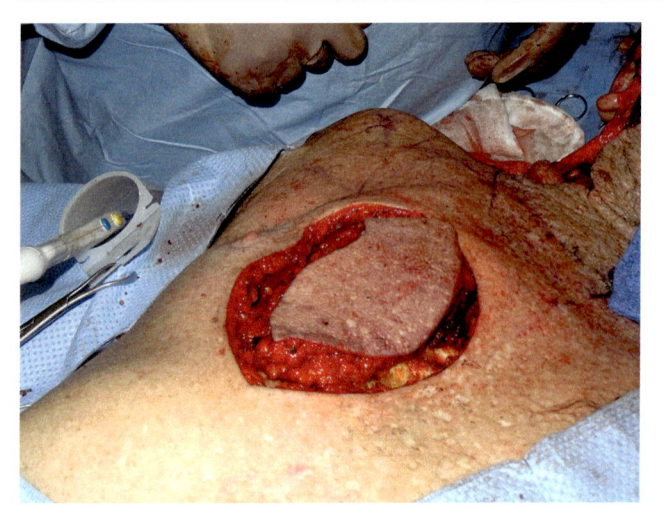

Fig. 17.8 Wide subcutaneous undermining: closure of the donor site is dependent on wide undermining of the surrounding soft tissue

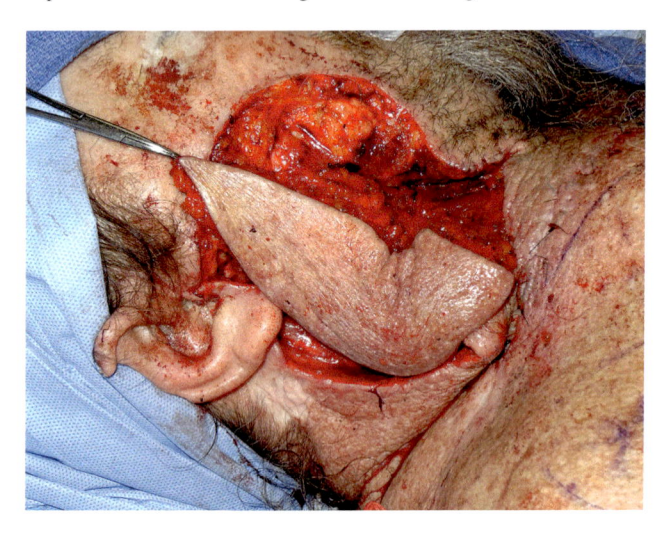

Fig. 17.9 Flap turn-up: the flap can be tunnelled and turned through a subcutaneous tunnel, positioning the flap in the position which puts least tension on the pedicle and enables optimal skin flap placement

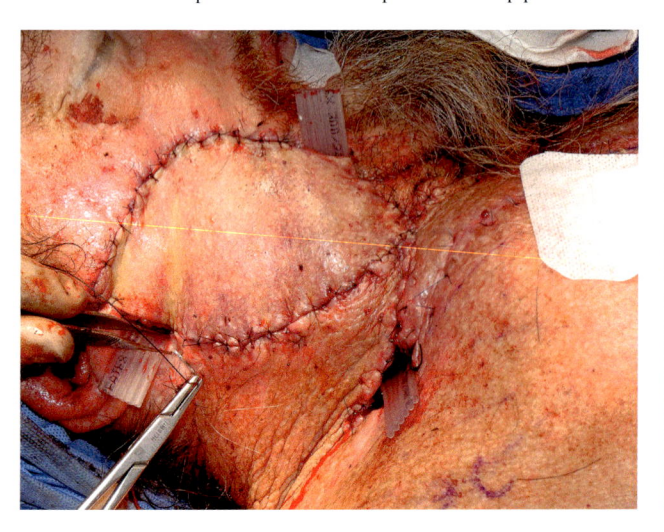

Fig. 17.10 Flap inset: the pectoralis major flap is sutured in place in layers with care to ensure a drain is placed at the inferior aspect to allow for swelling and any blood to escape as required

17.5.2 Sternal Reconstruction

The approach for the coverage of midline defects such as those involving the sternum is slightly different from the above. The movement required is less significant and the vector differs. The technique below is for an advancement-rotation flap, not a turnover flap.

Step 1
Comprehensive debridement of the wound is vital, including removal of metalwork and devitalised bone. Infected sternal bone is soft, whereas bone which is viable is firm and makes a characteristic clicking sound on debridement (Fig. 17.11).

Step 2
The pectoralis major muscle can be accessed from the wound edges and is dissected free from the subcutaneous tissue plane. A lighted retractor is helpful for dissection in the subcutaneous plane (Fig. 17.12).

Step 3
The muscle is then undermined and dissected from the chest wall, taking care to control intercostal perforators with Ligaclips. The muscle is elevated off the pectoralis minor:

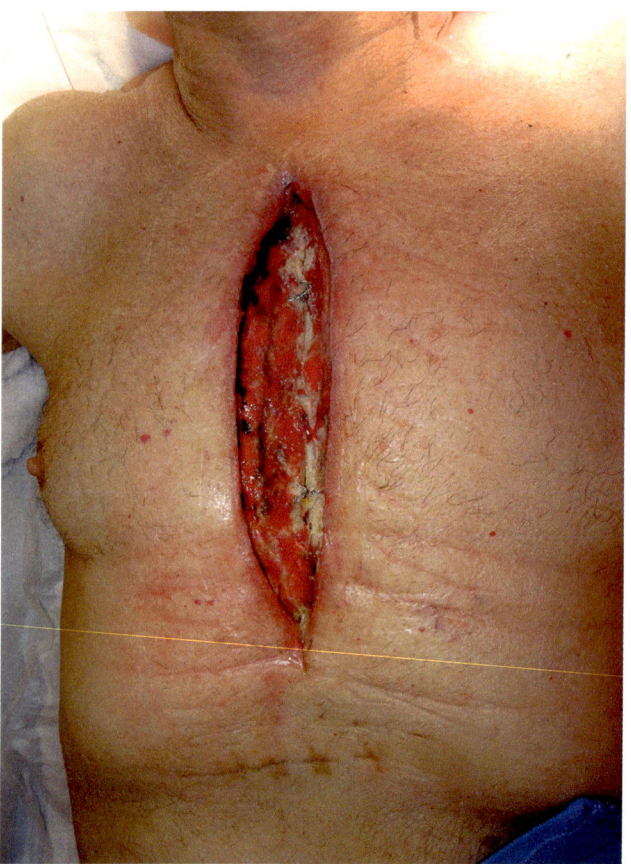

Fig. 17.11 Sternal dehiscence: note exposed wires, devitalised sternum and undebrided soft tissue along dehisced median sternotomy incision

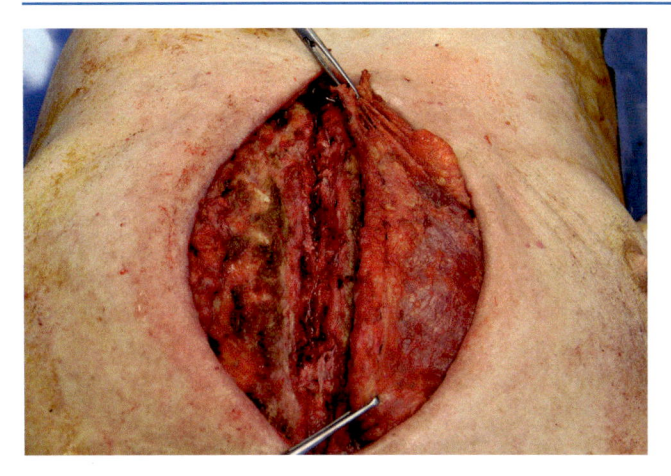

Fig. 17.12 Defining the border of the pectoralis major. Allis forceps hold the muscle up to free it from the underlying chest wall once it is free from the cutaneous plane

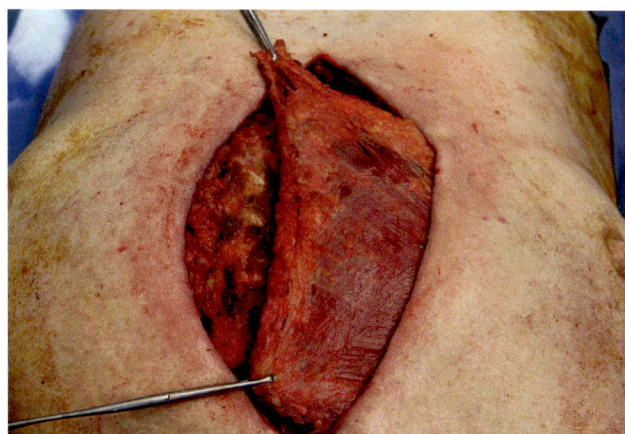

Fig. 17.13 Mobilisation of the pectoralis major: demonstrating the advancement of the completely released muscle

retraction with a Deaver is essential here. Care is taken to preserve the feeding vessels to the muscle.

Step 4
Two Allis forceps are attached to the leading edge of the muscle adjacent to the wound, and traction is placed on the freed up muscle by an assistant. Movement and flap reach can be increased by releasing the tendinous insertion of the muscle. Access to this is most safely achieved through a separate incision in the anterior axillary line; however some surgeons prefer to approach this through the sternal wound (Fig. 17.13).

Step 5
The process is repeated as necessary on the contralateral pectoralis major muscle (if available).

Step 6
Both pectoralis muscles are advanced. The leading edge of the muscle to be used to fill the dead space is sutured in place with parachuted 2/0 PDS mattress sutures. The second muscle flap is then double-breasted over the buried flap for security with 2/0 PDS. Mediastinal and subcutaneous 16Ch drains are placed bilaterally. This double breasting of

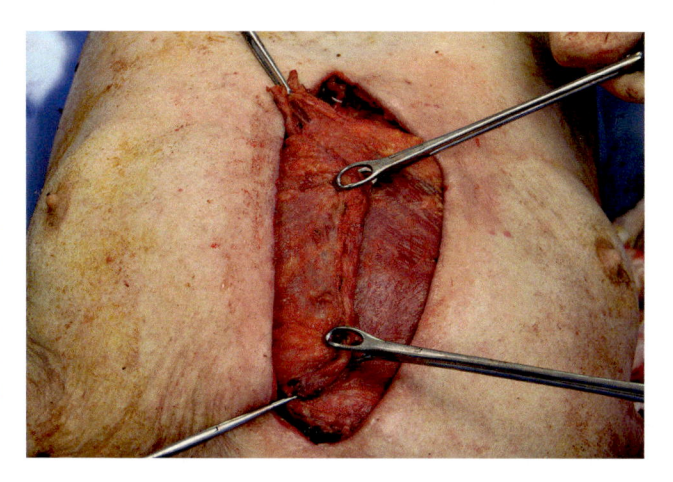

Fig. 17.14 Double-breasting of the pectoralis major muscles: this serves to reinforce the stability of the sternum and eliminate residual dead space

the pectoralis flaps provides some sternal stability (Fig. 17.14).

Step 7
The skin wound is finally closed in layers to achieve a sound and watertight closure. Topical negative pressure dressing application can help splint these wounds (Fig. 17.15).

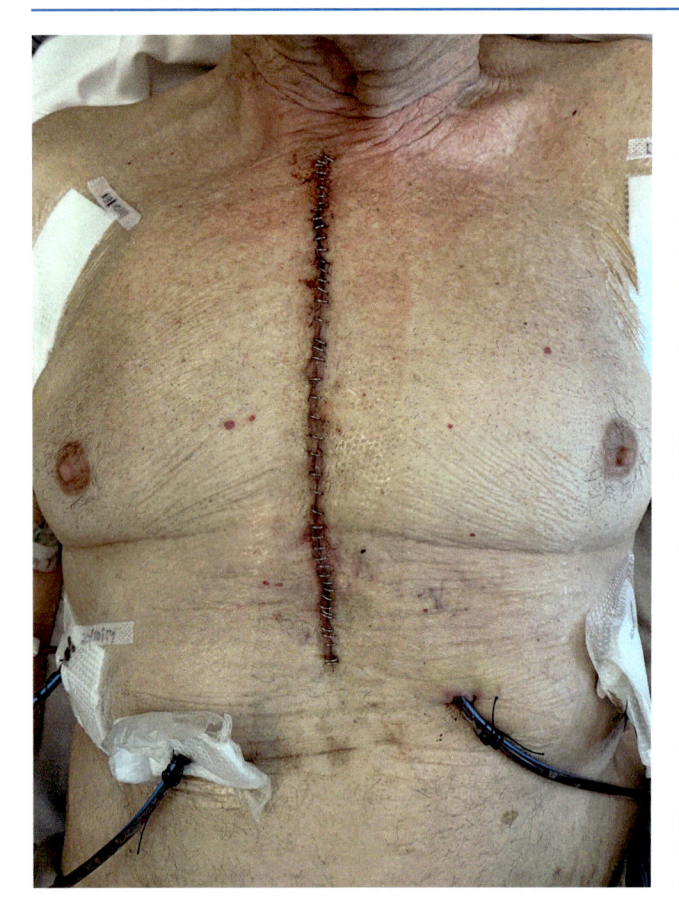

Fig. 17.15 Closure of median sternotomy: the skin incision close well and judicious use of drains is recommended

17.6 Core Surgical Techniques in Flap Dissection

Step 1 Flap Design
Preserve the first two intercostal vessels when designing the skin paddle in case a deltopectoral flap is required in the event of flap failure—the 'defensive approach' described by MacGregor.

Many cutaneous paddles have been described, and they have the most reliable vasculature when located over muscle.

In female patients, the skin paddle can be located at the infra-mammary crease—this may be inferior to the pectoralis major, and the blood supply is no longer axial and should be considered as random pattern with a 1:1 length-to-width ratio.

Step 2 Superficial Muscle Flap Dissection
Monopolar diathermy and a lighted retractor permit swift dissection of the superficial muscle surface.

Steps 3, 4, 5 Flap Elevation
The distal extent of the flap can be elevated with monopolar diathermy. Dissecting scissors or bipolar provide more cautious dissection near the pedicle.

Rotation-advancement muscle flaps for sternal defects may be challenging to visualise and dissect at the lateral edge. A separate skin incision over the tendon may facilitate its division at the inter-tubercular groove.

Step 6
Additional length for transfer to the neck may be gained by dividing the muscle origin at the clavicle and isolating the flap on the pedicle alone. In addition, excising a cuff of muscle so the upturned flap is applied directly to the clavicle without an intervening muscular bridge can increase length.

Passing the flap deep to the clavicle can increase length by up to 4 cm, allowing caution for adjacent vascular structures.

17.7 Clinical Scenario

Clinical Scenario A **Head and neck salvage**
    Surgeon: Jeremy Rawlins Dariush Nikkhah
A 54-year-old man with failed free anterolateral thigh flap to right mandibular SCC secondary to thrombus. Following flap debridement, vessels, bone and nerves lie exposed. The pectoralis major flap is ideal for this salvage operation where microsurgical options have failed and a robust myocutaneous flap with a reliable blood supply is required.
    Clinical Scenario B **Sternal mediastinitis**
    Surgeon: Dariush Nikkhah
A 74-year-old diabetic male with sternal wound breakdown 10 days following coronary artery bypass grafting where both internal mammary arteries had been harvested. Following preoperative optimisation and debridement by the cardiothoracic team, sternal wires had been removed, and there is a soft tissue defect comprising the skin, fat, and mediastinum, and the pericardium is exposed beneath. Advancement of bilateral pectoralis major flaps is appropriate in such a scenario.

17.8 Pearls and Pitfalls

Pearls

- The larger the skin paddle harvested, the higher the likelihood of skin survival.
- Additional length of skin paddle can be obtained beyond the edge of the paddle as a random-pattern flap, but this has higher risk of skin necrosis.
- The defensive approach for head and neck reconstruction defines a paddle of skin marked from the second and third intercostal spaces bounded cranially along the clavicle, laterally by the deltopectoral groove. This permits a deltopectoral flap to be

raised if required as a lifeboat flap. Preservation of this tissue necessitates subcutaneous tunnelling of the myocutaneous flap to reach the clavicle.
- If access is particularly challenging or the skin defect is significant, the deltopectoral flap can be raised concurrently for access and to allow soft tissue advancement for closure. This serves to delay the deltopectoral flap for future use if required.
- Division of the clavicular pectoralis muscle fibres above the pedicle, division of the lateral thoracic artery and/or splitting and removing the middle one-third of the clavicle can increase flap reach.

Pitfalls

- Judicious use of Ligaclips to control chest wall muscle perforators is important to control bleeding.
- Adequate retraction using a Deaver is key to identifying and protecting the vessel on the underside of the muscle.
- Division of the clavicle or passing the flap below the clavicle increases operative time, morbidity and complications.
- When insetting the flap into the neck, avoid overly rotating, compressing or kinking the proximal flap, taking particular care where the flap crosses the clavicle.

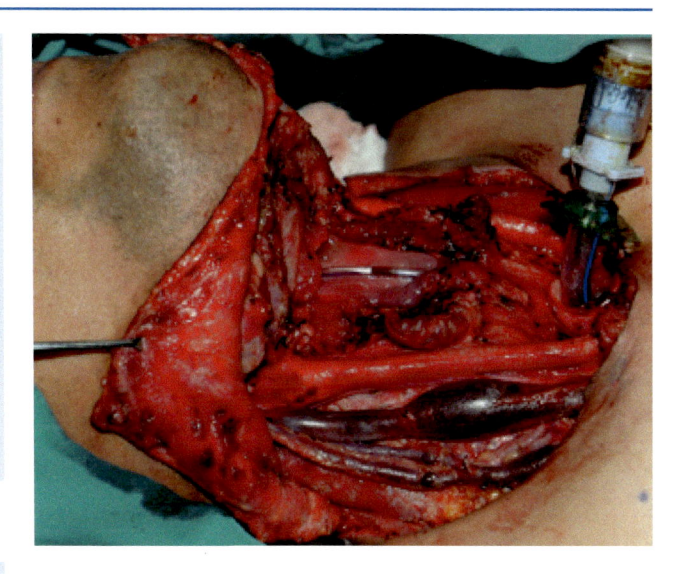

Fig. 17.16 Circumferential hypopharyngeal and oesophageal defect following total laryngopharyngectomy requiring tubular flap reconstruction

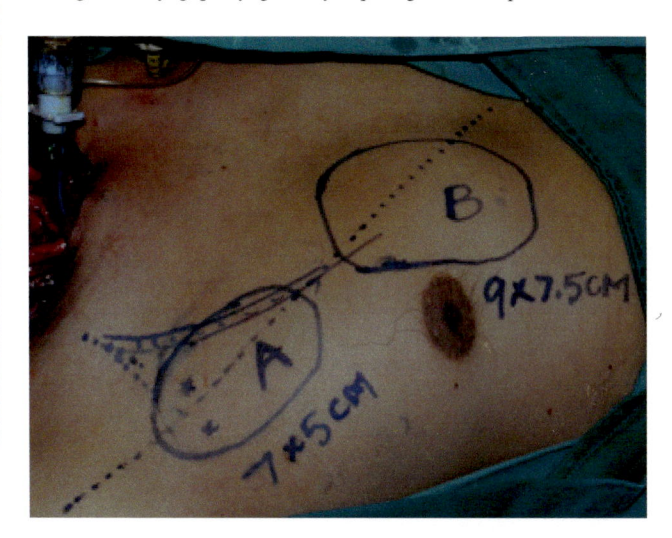

Fig. 17.17 Surgical markings for the chimeric myocutaneous pectoralis major flap (**B**) and the perforator-based thoracoacromial flap (**A**)

17.9 Chimeric Thoracoacromial Pectoralis Major Flap

The chimeric pectoralis major flap allows simultaneous raise of a myocutaneous component and fasciocutaneous flap [7] to allow versatility in the flap inset, especially in pharyngeal circumferential defects (Fig. 17.16). It is based both on the clavicular branch of the thoracoacromial artery and occasionally the fasciocutaneous perforators arising from the long thoracic artery laterally [8]. Freemean et al. demonstrated a rich anastomosis link between thoracoacromial, internal mammary and when present the lateral thoracic artery [5]. The rich muscle vasculature allows myocutaneous flap elevation at any axis longitudinal to the thoracoacromial artery branches and a separate perforator-based fasciocutaneous skin flap based on a cutaneous perforator.

The accompanying venae comitantes provide enough venous drainage for the myocutaneous component; however, the fasciocutaneous flap raising requires extra care to preserve venous drainage to the overlying skin paddle through venous networks of the cephalic vein [5]. The thoracoacromial artery may require to be dissected allowing ease during inset and the two skin components.

Design, Flap Dissection and Inset

- The surface markings according to the cutaneous perforators from the pectoral branch of TAA, using a handheld Doppler. A 4-cm^2 area around the located perforator was drawn along the line joining the acromion to the xiphoid process intersection with the perpendicular line drawn from the midclavicular line (Fig. 17.17).

- The chimeric TAAP flap raised from medial to lateral. The fasciocutaneous perforator constantly arises from the septum between the clavicular and the sternocostal heads of PM muscle. The fasciocutaneous component dissection proceeds along the subfascial plane. The thoracoacromial pedicle with the two chimeric components could be lengthened by superior retraction under the clavicle.
- During the dissection, the pectoral branch of the thoracoacromial pedicle is preserved to harvest the myocutaneous flap component (Fig. 17.18). The two flaps can then pass under the clavicular head of the pectoralis major muscle and through either a subcutaneous tunnel or even under the clavicle bone, to allow inset in a pharyngoesophageal defect (Fig. 17.19).
- A spiral inset configuration of the two skin paddles allows slightly lengthening and less tension neo-pharyngeal suturing.
- Both transverse (fasciocutaneous component) and the vertical (myocutaneous component) could be primarily closed.

Chimeric Pectoralis Major Flap (Figs. 17.16, 17.17, 17.18, and 17.19).

A total laryngopharyngectomy defect with a 10-cm pharyngeal circumferential defect in a 58-year-old male was reconstructed with the chimeric pectoralis major regional flap. The bilobe flap was raised using the thoracoacromial fasciocutaneous (transverse) component and the myocutaneous (vertical) component.

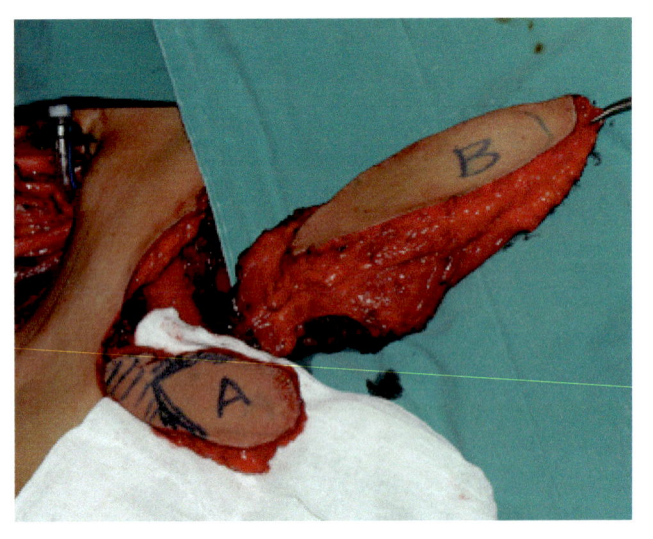

Fig. 17.18 Both the myocutaneous pectoralis major flap and the TAAP flap dissected and islanded on the thoracoacromial pedicle

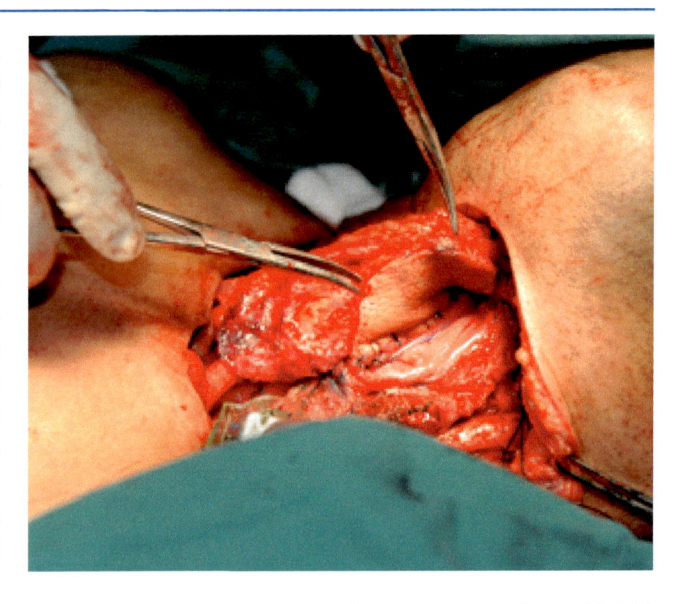

Fig. 17.19 Chimeric pectoralis major myocutaneous flap and TAAP flap inset to form the neo-oesophageal tube

17.10 Selected Readings

- Hueston JT, McConchie IH. A compound pectoral flap. Aust N Z J Surg. 1968;38(1):61–3.

  Description of including the pectoralis major in chest flap for repair of large chest wall defects, including medial ends of clavicles and sternum.

- Brown RG, Fleming WH, Jurkiewicz MJ. An island flap of the pectoralis major muscle. Br J Plast Surg. 1977;30:161–5.

  Case report describing the use of bilateral pectoralis major muscles for sternal reconstruction. Both flaps were advanced with division of the tendinous insertion and lateral thoracic arteries and were double-breasted for reinforced closure. The skin was tacked to the muscle and the remaining defect grafted.

- Maruyama Y, Fujino T, Aoyagi F, et al. One stage reconstruction of oral cavity by use of pectoralis major myocutaneous island flap. Keio J Med. 1978;27:47–52.

  Describes the transfer of the flap through a midline section of the clavicle for oral cavity reconstruction using the pedicled pectoralis major flap for a one-stage reconstruction of the oral defect.

- Ariyan S. The pectoralis major myocutaneous flap. A versatile flap for reconstruction in the head and neck. Plast Reconstr Surg. 1979;63:73–81.

  Seminal paper widely credited (incorrectly) as describing the pectoralis major myocutaneous flap first. Ariyan

describes the anatomical landmarks based on cadaveric dissection. He further describes the pectoralis major myocutaneous flap as having a combined skin-muscle pedicle and discusses modifications such as islanding the flap by dividing the clavicular muscular attachments.

- McGregor IA. 1980 Fundamental techniques of plastic surgery, 7th ed. Edinburgh: Churchill Livingstone.

  Describes the use of a combined pectoralis major myocutaneous flap and deltopectoral flap in intra-oral reconstruction.

- McGregor IA. A "defensive" approach to the island pectoralis major myocutaneous flap. Br J Plast Surg. 1981;34:435–7.

  Proposes the preservation of the deltopectoral flap during the elevation of the pectoralis major flap, advocating the raising of this flap as an islanded flap and utilising a subcutaneous tunnel for flap dissection and delivery.

- Palmer JH, Batchelor AG. The functional pectoralis major musculocutaneous island flap in head and neck reconstruction. Plast Reconstr Surg. 1990; 85(3):363–7. https://doi.org/10.1097/00006534-199003000-00004.

  Describes a modification of islanding the pectoralis major myocutaneous flap to maintain maximal donor-site function, facilitate closure of the donor site defect, increase pedicle length and the arc of rotation, reduce pedicle bulk and improve cosmesis.

Acknowledgements We thank Georgios Pafitanis, Dajiang Song and Zan Li for writing this case scenario section.

References

1. Hueston JT, McConchie IH. A compound pectoral flap. Aust N Z J Surg. 1968;38(1):61–3.
2. Brown RG, Fleming WH, Jurkiewicz MJ. An island flap of the pectoralis major muscle. Br J Plast Surg. 1977;30:161–5.
3. Maruyama Y, Fujino T, Aoyagi F, et al. One stage reconstruction of oral cavity by use of pectoralis major myocutaneous island flap. Keio J Med. 1978;27:47–52.
4. Ariyan S. The pectoralis major myocutaneous flap. A versatile flap for reconstruction in the head and neck. Plast Reconstr Surg. 1979;63:73–81.
5. Freeman JL, Walker EP, Wilson JS, Shaw HJ. The vascular anatomy of the pectoralis major myocutaneous flap. Br J Plast Surg. 1981;34:3–10.
6. McGregor IA. A "defensive" approach to the island pectoralis major myocutaneous flap. Br J Plast Surg. 1981;34:435–7.
7. Zhang YX, Li Z, Grassetti L, et al. A new option with the pedicle thoracoacromial artery perforator flap for hypopharyngeal reconstructions. Laryngoscope. 2015;126:1315.
8. Zhang YX, Yongjie H, Messmer C, et al. Thoracoacromial artery perforator flap: anatomical basis and clinical applications. Plast Reconstr Surg. 2013;131:759e–70e.

Transverse Cervical Artery Flap - Supraclavicular Flap

Pedro Ciudad, Juste Kaciulyte, Georgios Pafitanis, and Hung-Chi Chen

18.1 Introduction

The supraclavicular region represents a fetching donor site for several flaps for its cutaneous features and easy-to-hide location. In 1842, Mutter [1] was the first to introduce a random shoulder-based flap for a neck burn contracture. A century later, in 1958, Kirschbaum [2] described the acromial or "in charretera" flap, as the ornamental military patch placed on shoulders. The "in charretera" fasciocutaneous flap was renamed as cervicohumeral flap by Mathes and Vasconez [3], who were the first to study the supraclavicular region's vascular anatomy in 1970.

Lamberty et al. [4] followed this lead and in 1979 reported the supraclavicular artery being a branch of the transverse cervical artery in most cases, and they described the supraclavicular artery flap as an axial flap. Nevertheless, the flap's popularity witnessed a quick fall as the use of excessively long tissues' portions led to frequent distal necrosis.

Almost 20 years had to pass until Pallua et al. [5] gave new revival to the flap, by reporting its successful use in cervicomental scar contractures treatment in 1997. Since then, it has been used as a pedicled fasciocutaneous flap mostly, in various cervicofacial district reconstructions.

The first to introduce the idea of free muscle perforator flaps' harvest from the supraclavicular region were Mizerney et al. [6] and Cordova et al. [7] in 1995 and 2008, respectively. Finally, in 2012 Becker described supraclavicular lymph node transfer technique for limb lymphedema management [8].

18.2 Anatomy

The transverse cervical artery (TCA) and the supraclavicular artery are the main vessels of the supraclavicular region. They are both found in the lateral triangle of the neck which is delimitated by the anterior clavicular part inferiorly, the sternocleidomastoid muscle anteriorly, and the trapezius muscle posteriorly.

After its origin from the subclavian artery, the TCA runs posteriorly and laterally passing under the omohyoid muscle, toward the trapezius muscle. In this path, TCA passes superficially to the scalene muscles and the brachial plexus and traverses the fibro-adipose tissue of the supraclavicular fossa. Close to the trapezius muscle, the TCA splits into its two final branches, superficial and deep. One or two committing veins travel alongside the TCA.

The supraclavicular artery emerges from the TCA after its passage under the omohyoid muscle, at the middle third of the clavicle in 90% of cases and at the lateral third in the other 10% [9]. This origin from the TCA has been observed from 62.9% to 100% of cases, according to various anatomical studies [10]. In the remaining cases, it arises from the suprascapular artery. During its course, the supraclavicular artery presents a diameter of 1–1.5 mm and it divides into two branches [11]. The main lateral deltoid branch passes through the deep fascia while running laterally over the cap of the shoulder, toward the acromioclavicular joint and the deltoid muscle. It supplies the overlying skin from the neck to upper chest, including the shoulder and the deltoid region. One or two committing veins travel alongside toward the external jugular vein (EJV). The anterior thoracic branch directs to the anterior thoracic region.

P. Ciudad (✉)
Department of Plastic, Reconstructive and Burn Surgery, Arzobispo Loayza National Hospital, Lima, Peru

Academic Department of Surgery, Federico Villarreal National University, Lima, Peru

J. Kaciulyte
Department of Surgery "P. Valdoni", Unit of Plastic and Reconstructive Surgery, Sapienza University of Rome, Policlinico Umberto I, Rome, Italy

G. Pafitanis
Department of Plastic Surgery, Emergency Care and Trauma Division (ECAT), The Royal London Hospital, Barts Health NHS Trust, London, UK

H.-C. Chen
Division of Plastic Surgery, China Medical University Hospital, Taichung, Taiwan

Finally, the venous drainage of the supraclavicular area is provided by the superficial cervical vein (SCV) too. The SCV emerges anteriorly from the trapezius muscle and stays under the superficial cervical fascia while coursing parallel to the clavicle. After receiving perforators from the overlying skin, the SCV reaches the EJV.

18.3 Preoperative Investigation

Doppler exam represents the most frequent preoperative investigation in supraclavicular flap planning [12]. The exam can easily locate the emergence of supraclavicular artery in the lateral neck triangle. Moreover, it may be useful intraoperatively, to follow the flap's pedicle during its harvest.

Computed tomography angiography (CTA) is considered a valid preoperative exam to study the vascular regional system, for cases of free flap planning in particular [13].

These two most used techniques have been compared to triplex ultrasound, magnetic resonance angiography, digital subtraction angiography, and indocyanine green (ICG) angiography in a study on preoperative supraclavicular mapping capacity by Sheriff et al. [14] Despite that handheld Doppler showed perforators in 80% of cases, CTA results were considered the best of the series, as it identified 60% of perforators and it traced the supraclavicular artery's course in 45% of cases. For the ICG showed similar mapping efficacy, it was named as a feasible alternative to CTA, with the advantage of no radiation-related risks. ICG exam has proven its validity intraoperatively, even in confirming flap's blood perfusion and being predictive for flap's survival [15].

Before supraclavicular lymph node harvest, ICG is used to reverse mapping upper limb's lymph flow and to identify the sentinel lymph nodes to be spared [16].

18.4 Flap Design and Markings

The best exposure is obtained with the patient in supine position with a shoulder roll placed to create neck hyperextension. The left side should be avoided in order to prevent risk of iatrogenic injury to the thoracic duct. The anatomical landmarks of the pedicle's origin correspond to the lateral triangle of the neck: the clavicle inferiorly, the sternocleidomastoid (SCM) muscle anteriorly, and the medial border of the trapezius muscle posteriorly (Fig. 18.1). Lymph node harvest is performed within these triangle borders. In fasciocutaneous flaps, skin paddle is drawn along an axis traced from the center of the triangle toward the acromioclavicular joint and the deltoid muscle. With no pre-expansion, maximum flap's measures are about 30 × 10 cm, with possible primary closure [17].

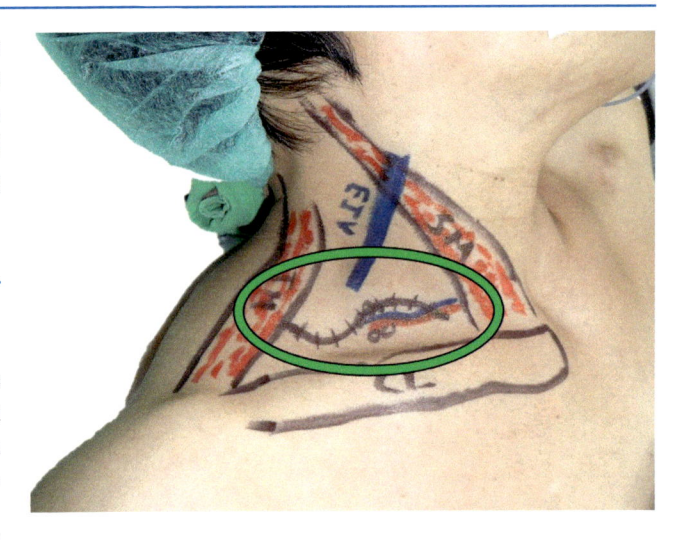

Fig. 18.1 Anatomical landmarks of the transverse cervical artery-based flap correspond to the lateral triangle of the neck with the clavicle (CL) inferiorly, the sternocleidomastoid muscle (SM) anteriorly, and the medial border of the trapezius muscle (TM) posteriorly

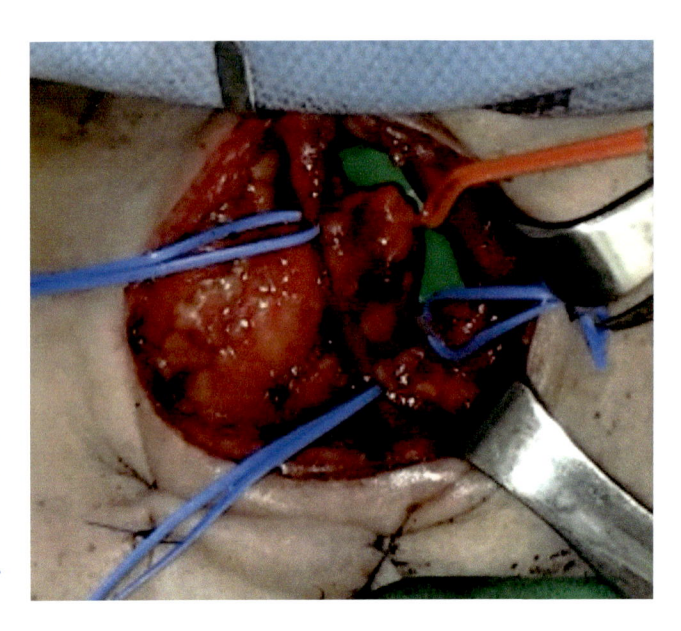

Fig. 18.2 After skin incision and dissection up to the platysma muscle, the EJV is identified (proximal and distal blue laces) and ligated proximally and distally

18.5 Flap Raise/Elevation: A Step-by-Step Guide

In right neck's lateral triangle, skin incision deepens up to the platysma muscle close to the lateral border of the SCM. The EJV is identified and ligated proximally and distally (Fig. 18.2).

After EJV ligation, dissection continues medially until the TCA with its committing veins are visualized (Fig. 18.3).

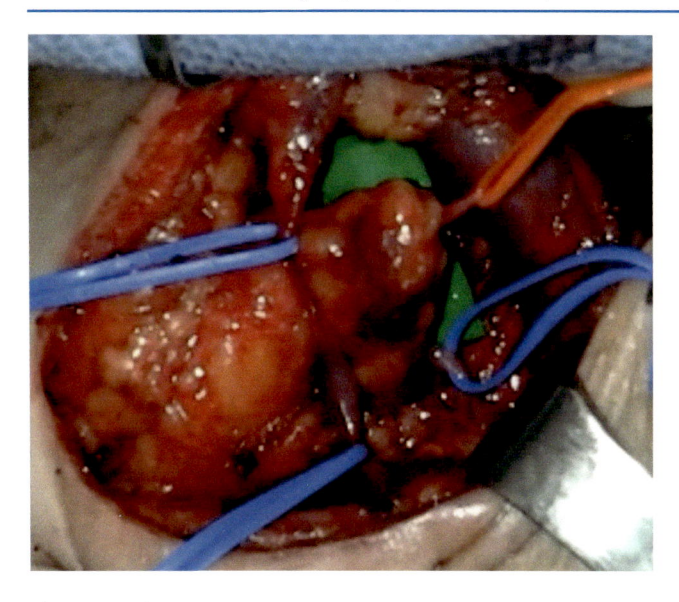

Fig. 18.3 After EJV ligation (double blue laces), dissection is carried out deeper and medially until the TCA (red lace) with its committing veins (single blue lace) are visualized

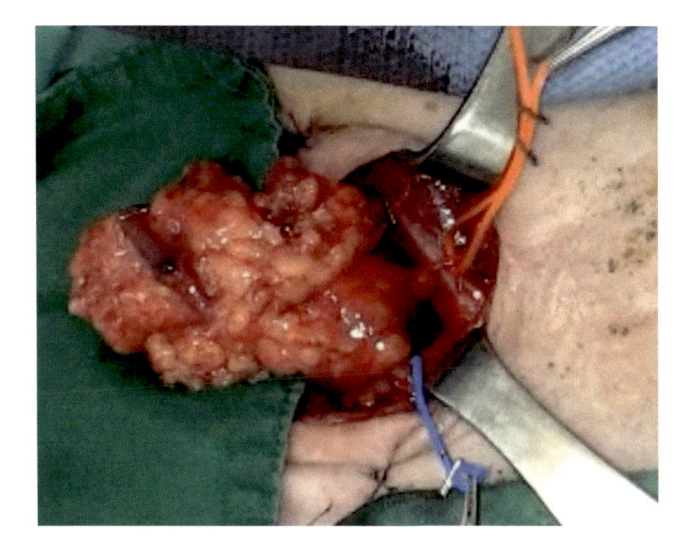

Fig. 18.4 The supraclavicular lymph node flap appears ready for harvest, together with its pedicle that consists in TCA (red lace) and one committing vein (blue lace)

TCA and its veins form the flap's pedicle that is followed toward the trapezius muscle direction. Care is taken to preserve lymph nodes that surround the TCA in a fibro-adipose tissue envelope (Fig. 18.4).

18.6 Core Surgical Techniques in Flap Dissection

1. Surgery is performed under general anesthesia, with the patient in supine position and neck hyperextension, thanks to a shoulder roll to favor right side exposure. The anatomical landmarks to identify are those of the lateral triangle of the neck: the clavicle inferiorly, the SCM anteriorly, and the medial border of the trapezius muscle posteriorly. Handheld preoperative Doppler exam may show the exact location of the anterior perforating branch of the supraclavicular artery.

2. Fasciocutaneous paddle dissection is started from the lateral-distal edge. The vessels run within the subcutaneous plane, so rising can be carried out above the muscle fascia to the clavicle, with no risk to harm the pedicle. When required, the clavicle's periosteum may be included to perform a chimeric osteocutaneous flap.

3. At the clavicle level, intraoperative handheld Doppler or direct visual exam may show the pedicle within the subcutaneous tissues of the flap. The supraclavicular artery and its committing veins are followed including a soft tissue cuff, to their origin from the transverse cervical vessels. After omohyoid muscle visualization, it has to be preserved with its cephalic reflection. In this way, between the reflected omohyoid muscle and the scalenus muscles, TCA can be identified within the adipose tissue of the supraclavicular fossa. The TCA is transected posteriorly and followed anteriorly to obtain a vessel diameter of almost 1.5 mm.

4. When feasible, the SCV should be included in the flap in order to supercharge its venous drainage and prevent congestion. The SCV runs superficially from the trapezius muscle in the deltopectoral fossa toward the EJV. The dissection is performed in retrograde direction, after the main pedicle identification.

5. The dissection is slightly different when supraclavicular lymph nodes are harvested. A 4-cm S-shaped incision is performed 1.5 cm above the clavicle, within the lateral neck triangle.

6. Sub-platysmal flaps are raised to the triangle anatomical landmarks and the dissection deepens at the lateral border of the SCM. Particular care is taken to identify and preserve the EJV.

7. The dissection continues until the omohyoid muscle is identified and reflected cephalad and the TCA with its committing veins are visualized and followed in a plane above the scalene muscles, toward the trapezius muscle direction. Care is taken to preserve a consistent fibro-adipose tissue surrounding the TCA, thus including the lymph nodes.

8. The SCV is constantly superficial and posterolateral to the TCA. It should be preserved and included in the flap, together with the EJV that is ligated proximally and distally.

9. The fibro-adipose tissue harvested can be crossed by a prominent cutaneous sensory nerve. As the majority of

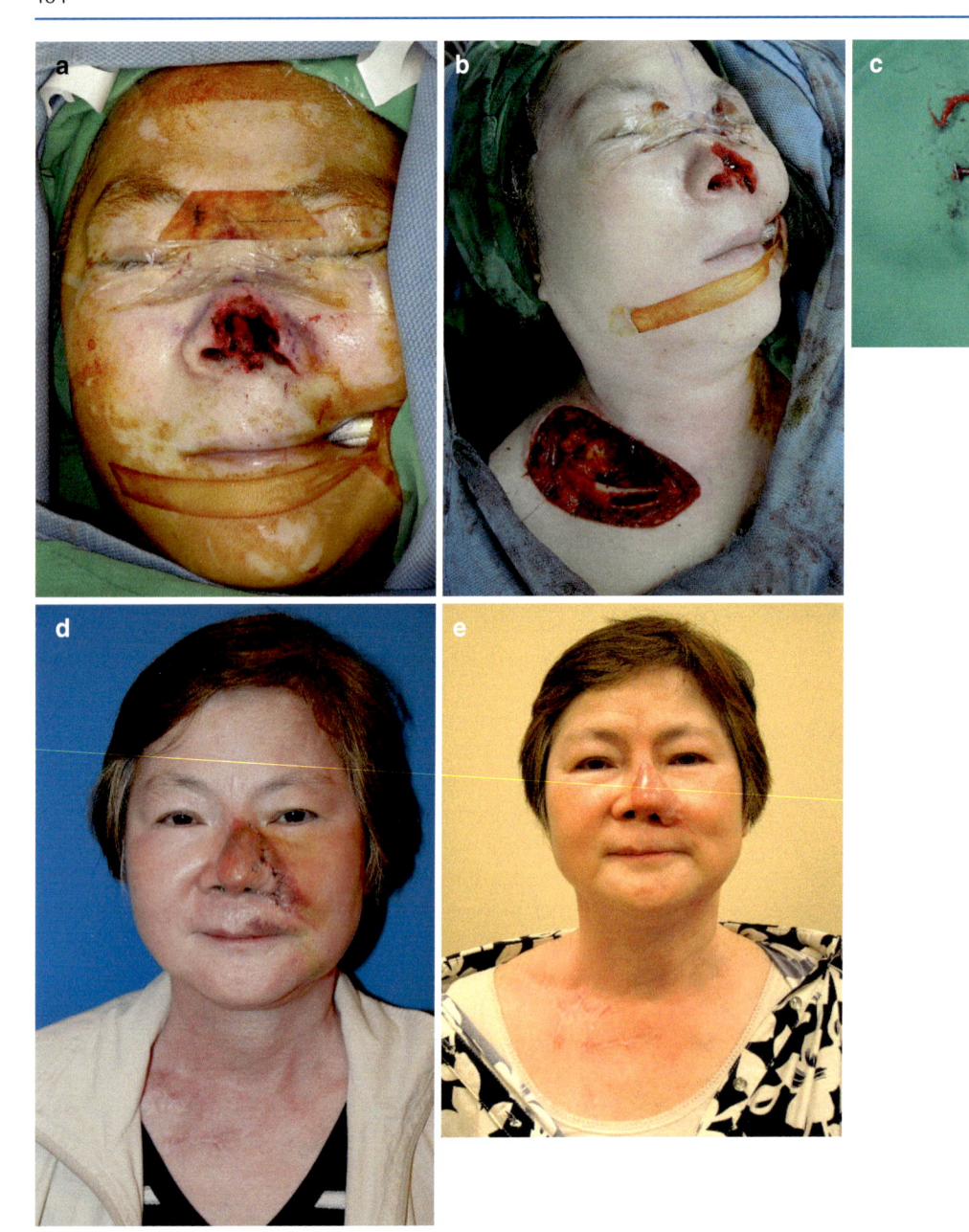

Fig. 18.5 (**a**) Nasal bone and tip, part of the lateral walls and septum, and both soft triangles loss consequent to squamous cell carcinoma resection. (**b**) Intraoperative picture that shows the donor site from which the SOC free flap with a skin paddle of 6 x 4 cm has been harvested. (**c**) SOC free flap with a skin paddle of 6 × 4 cm and a clavicle's corticoperiosteal segment of 3 × 0.4 cm, ready for the inset. (**d**) Postoperative picture taken 6 days after surgery. (**e**) Postoperative picture taken 5 months after reconstructive and revision surgeries

   the lymph nodes are deeper, the nerve can be spared usually. Nevertheless, there can be cases in which a lymph node may be present superficially to the nerve. If the superficial lymph node has to be included in the flap, the nerve can be accurately divided and re-anastomosed immediately after.
10. The donor site is closed primarily, with multilayer stitches and performing z-plasty technique. A suction drain is placed to avoid hematoma and seroma.

18.7 Clinical Scenario

18.7.1 Supraclavicular Osteocutaneous (SOC) Free Flap

A 62-year-old female presented with ulcerated 1.5 × 1 cm squamous cell carcinoma of the nasal dorsum.

Wide local excision was performed and resulted in nasal bone and tip, part of the lateral walls and septum, and both soft triangles resection (Fig. 18.5a). Immediate reconstruction was achieved with SOC free flap with a skin paddle of 6 × 4 cm and a clavicle's corticoperiosteal segment of 3 × 0.4 cm (Fig. 18.5b, c).

TCA and its committing vein were anastomosed to the left facial vessels with vein graft interposition (Fig. 18.5d).

No postoperative complications occurred, and flap debulking procedures were carried out at 10 weeks and 4 months postoperatively (Fig. 18.5e).

18.7.2 Supraclavicular Vascularized Lymph Node Transfer (VLNT)

Here we present a case of right lower limb I stage lymphedema according to the International Society of Lymphology (ISL) (Fig. 18.6a). A 48-year-old female presented it after ablative surgery for cervical cancer and groin lymph node dissection, performed 1.5 years before.

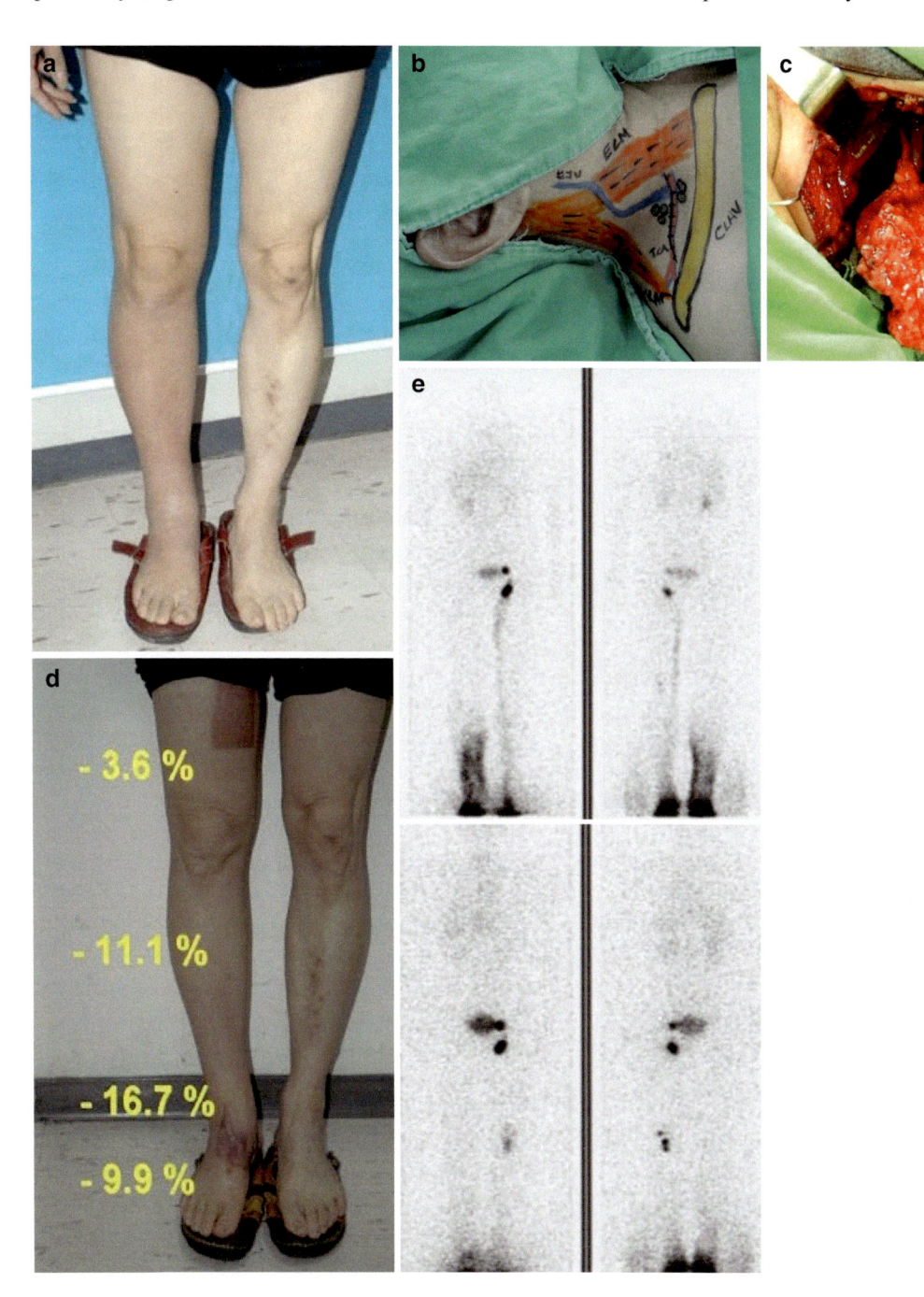

Fig. 18.6 (a) Right lower limb lymphedema assessed as stage I according to ISL, subsequent to groin lymph node dissection surgery. Intraoperative pictures of VLN flap harvest from the right supraclavicular region (b): the lymph nodes were harvested together with the TCA, one committing vein, and the EJV (c). Postoperative pictures at 6 months after surgery that show circumference reduction rates achieved with the VLNT (d) and the lymph flow improvement at lymphoscintigraphy exam (e)

After right supraclavicular VLN flap harvest together with the TCA, one committing vein, and the EJV, anastomoses were performed to the dorsum of the foot.

The anastomoses were performed to the dorsalis pedis artery, its committing vein, and a superficial vein of the foot dorsum. Coverage was achieved with a local flap and split-thickness skin graft. Follow-up lasted 7 months, and limb circumference reduction was registered together with lymph flow improvement at postoperative lymphoscintigraphy (Fig. 18.6d, e).

18.8 Pearls and Pitfalls

Pearls
- The supraclavicular flap demands for inevitable learning curve. Anatomical variations of the TCA have to be kept in mind: most often it origins from the thyrocervical trunk (80%) or directly from the subclavian artery (20%), but cases of its rise from the internal mammary artery have been reported [18, 19].
- According to the authors' experience, when the TCA arises directly from the subclavian artery, the pedicle's dissection is more tedious as it must be performed deeper and adjacent to the clavicle.
- The inclusion of SCV and EJV in the flap is important in order to avoid venous congestion.
- Primary repair of the cutaneous sensory nerve results in faster recovery of sensation.
- The supraclavicular lymph node flap is a buried flap with no skin island included. Its postoperative monitoring can be easily done through the skin graft.

Pitfalls
- Harvest must be done from the right side of the neck in order to avoid potential traumatic injury to the main lymphatic duct.
- Ipsilateral neck scars and upper extremity lymphedema are considered contraindications.
- Reverse ICG mapping, meticulous ligation of lymphatic vessels, and close suction drainage will reduce donor site lymphedema or lymphorrhea.
- Obese patients will present an increase amount of fat tissue in the neck, so a deeper dissection is required.
- Thoughtful recipient site selection is fundamental in VLNT.

18.9 Selected Readings

- Lamberty BG. The supra-clavicular axial patterned flap. Br J Plast Surg. 1979;32:207–12.
- *Important from a historical point of view: the first description of the axial supraclavicular flap based on vascular studies of the supraclavicular artery as a branch of the TCA.*
- Cordova A, Pirrello R, D'Arpa S, Jeschke J, Brenner E, Moschella F. Vascular anatomy of the supraclavicular area revisited: feasibility of the free supraclavicular perforator flap. Plast Reconstr Surg. 2008;122:1399–409.
- *It was one of the first studies to introduce the idea of the possibility to harvest a free flap based on supraclavicular artery.*
- Pallua N, Wolter TP. Moving forwards: the anterior supraclavicular artery perforator (a-SAP) flap: a new pedicled or free perforator flap based on the anterior supraclavicular vessels. J Plast Reconstr Aesthet Surg. 2013;66:489–96.
- *The paper presents an overview of the current indications and outcomes of the flap. Moreover, the authors describe the innovative use of anterior supraclavicular pedicle.*
- Kokot N, Kim JH, West JD, Zhang P. Supraclavicular artery island flap: critical appraisal and comparison to alternate reconstruction. Laryngoscope. 2020.
- *A thorough literature review shows flap's complications rates in head and neck oncologic reconstruction, with examination of risk factors and comparisons to alternative flaps often considered the gold standard: the pectoralis myocutaneous flap, radial forearm free flap, and anterolateral thigh flaps.*
- Ciudad P, Manrique OJ, Date S, Sacak B, Chang WL, Kiranantawat K, Lim SY, Chen HC. A head-to-head comparison among donor site morbidity after vascularized lymph node transfer: Pearls and pitfalls of a 6-year single center experience. J Surg Oncol. 2017;115:37–42.
- *The authors discuss general pearls and pitfalls for VLN harvest from supraclavicular site and compare it to the other donor sites in terms of morbidity and complications.*
- Ciudad P, Agko M, Perez Coca JJ, Manrique O, Chang WL, Nicoli F, Chen SH, Chen HC. Comparison of long-term clinical outcomes among different vascularized lymph node transfers: 6-year experience of a single center's approach to the treatment of lymphedema. J Surg Oncol. 2017;116:671–682.
- *This study evaluates the long-term clinical outcomes among different VLNT, showing their individual pearls and pitfalls.*

- Nicoli F, Orfaniotis G, Gesakis K, Lazzeri D, Ciudad P, Chilgar RM, Sapountzis S, Sönmez TT, Maruccia M, Constantinides J, Sacak B, Chen HC. Supraclavicular osteocutaneous free flap: clinical application and surgical details for the reconstruction of composite defects of the nose. Microsurgery. 2015;35:328–32.
- *This is the first description of a chimeric osteocutaneous supraclavicular free flap, used to reconstruct a composite nasal defect.*
- Sapountzis S, Singhal D, Rashid A, Ciudad P, Meo D, Chen HC. Lymph node flap based on the right transverse cervical artery as a donor site for lymph node transfer. Ann Plast Surg. 2014;73:398–401.
- *The authors present their experience in VLN harvest together with the right TCA. A thorough surgical technique description is offered.*

References

1. Mütter TD. Case of deformity from burns relieved by operation. Am J Med Sci. 1842;4:66–80.
2. Kirschbaum S. Mentosternal contracture: preferred treatment by acromial (in charretera) flap. Plast Reconstr Surg Transplant Bull. 1958;21:131–8.
3. Mathes SJ, Vasconez LO. The cervicohumeral flap. Plast Reconstr Surg. 1978;61:7–12.
4. Lamberty BG. The supra-clavicular axial patterned flap. Br J Plast Surg. 1979;32:207–12.
5. Pallua N, Machens HG, Rennekampff O, Becker M, Berger A. The fasciocutaneous supraclavicular artery island flap for releasing postburn mentosternal contractures. Plast Reconstr Surg. 1997;99:1878–84, discussion 1885–6.
6. Mizerny BR, Lessard ML, Black MJ. Transverse cervical artery fasciocutaneous free flap for head and neck reconstruction: initial anatomic and dye studies. Otolaryngol Head Neck Surg. 1995;113:564–8.
7. Cordova A, Pirrello R, D'Arpa S, et al. Vascular anatomy of the supraclavicular area revisited: feasibility of the free supraclavicular perforator flap. Plast Reconstr Surg. 2008;122:1399–409.
8. Becker C, Vasile JV, Levine JL, et al. Microlymphatic surgery for the treatment of iatrogenic lymphedema. Clin Plast Surg. 2012;39:385–98.
9. de Carvalho FM, Correia B, Silva Á, Costa J. Versatility of the supraclavicular flap in head and neck reconstruction. Eplasty. 2020;5(20):e7.
10. Kokot N, Kim JH, West JD, Zhang P. Supraclavicular artery island flap: critical appraisal and comparison to alternate reconstruction. Laryngoscope. 2020;132(Suppl 3):1–14.
11. Ma X, Zheng Y, Xia W, et al. An anatomical study with clinical application of one branch of the supraclavicular artery. Clin Anat. 2009;22:215–20.
12. Gao Y, Yuan Y, Li H, Gu B, Xie F, Herrier T, Li G, et al. Preoperative imaging for thoracic branch of supraclavicular artery flap: a comparative study of contrast-enhanced ultrasound with three-dimensional reconstruction and color duplex ultrasound. Ann Plast Surg. 2016;77:201–5.
13. Adams AS, Wright MJ, Johnston S, et al. The use of multislice CT angiography preoperative study for supraclavicular artery island flap harvesting. Ann Plast Surg. 2012;69(3):312–5.
14. Sheriff HO, Mahmood KA, Hamawandi N, et al. The supraclavicular artery perforator flap: a comparative study of imaging techniques used in preoperative mapping. J Reconstr Microsurg. 2018;34:499–508.
15. Suzuki Y, Shimizu Y, Kasai S, Yamazaki S, Takemaru M, Kitamura T, Kawakami S, Tamura T. Indocyanine green fluorescence video-angiography for reliable variations of supraclavicular artery flaps. Arch Plast Surg. 2019;46(4):318–23.
16. Dayan JH, Dayan E, Smith ML. Reverse lymphatic mapping: a new technique for maximizing safety in vascularized lymph node transfer. Plast Reconstr Surg. 2015;135:277–85.
17. Pallua N, Wolter TP. Moving forwards: the anterior supraclavicular artery perforator (a-SAP) flap: a new pedicled or free perforator flap based on the anterior supraclavicular vessels. J Plast Reconstr Aesthet Surg. 2013;66(4):489–96.
18. Read WT, Trotter M. The origins of transverse cervical and of transverse scapular arteries in American Whites and Negroes. Am J Phys Anthropol. 1941;28:239–47.
19. Huelke DF. A study of the transverse cervical and dorsal scapular arteries. Anat Rec. 1958;132:233–45.

Inferior Epigastric Artery Flap: Deep Inferior Epigastric Artery Perforator Flap

Alexandra O'Neill, Dariush Nikkhah, Ahmed M. Yassin, and Bernard Luczak

19.1 Introduction

The deep inferior epigastric artery perforator (DIEP) flap nicely demonstrates the evolution of free flap reconstruction from myocutaneous flaps to the perforator-based fasciocutaneous flaps that are the preferred technique today. This refinement in flap technique was driven by the desire to achieve gold standard reconstruction, based on reliable vasculature with reproducible results all while reducing donor site morbidity.

The rectus abdominis myocutaneous flap was first described by Drever in 1977. Two years later, Hartrampf demonstrated that the skin island could be designed transversely across the lower abdomen for a more aesthetically pleasing donor site. The transverse rectus abdominis myocutaneous (TRAM) flap became the standard in autologous breast reconstruction and remained so until Koshima, Allen and Blondeel popularised the DIEP flap.

In an attempt to overcome the donor site morbidity associated with muscle sacrifice, Koshima and Soeda expanded on the earlier work of Taylor exploring the skin territory of the rectus abdominis muscle and described the "inferior epigastric artery skin flap without rectus abdominis muscle" which they initially described for floor of mouth reconstruction [1]. Allen and Treece demonstrated comparable results in breast reconstruction to the traditionally used TRAM flap without the muscle sacrifice and the DIEP flap for autologous breast reconstruction quickly gained traction as the new gold standard [2].

While the DIEP is a versatile flap, it is most commonly used in autologous reconstruction of the breast, both immediate and delayed. It can additionally be used in any large defect requiring fasciocutaneous resurfacing.

19.2 Anatomy

The deep inferior epigastric artery originates from the external iliac artery (EIA) just superior to the inguinal ligament directly opposite the origin of the deep circumflex iliac artery. The artery courses superomedially towards the linea semilunaris with paired venae comitantes piercing the transversalis fascia and coursing between the posterior rectus sheath and the undersurface of the rectus abdominis muscle. The main trunk of the DIEA commonly branches at the arcuate line into one of three distinct branching patterns: single intramuscular artery (no branching), double intramuscular artery and triple intramuscular arteries occurring 29%, 57% and 14%, respectively [3]. This branching pattern corresponds with the number of branches of the deep superior epigastric artery and the number of anastomoses between the deep superior and deep inferior epigastric arteries (Fig. 19.1).

On average four to five large (>0.5 mm) perforators are present each side of the midline with the highest concentration within a paramedial rectangular area 2 cm cranial and 6 cm caudal to the umbilicus and 1–7 cm lateral to the umbilicus [4] (Fig. 19.2).

In type II branching patterns, medial row perforators are seen coursing towards and crossing the midline connecting to the contralateral medial row perforators via a subdermal plexus [5]. The lateral row perforator branches however are directed predominately laterally, and while studies demonstrate they will reliably perfuse the ipsilateral medial row perforators and less reliably contralateral medial row perforators, they will not perfuse contralateral lateral row perforators [6].

Supplementary Information The online version contains supplementary material available at [https://doi.org/10.1007/978-3-031-07678-7_19].

A. O'Neill (✉) · B. Luczak
Department Plastic and Reconstructive Surgery, Royal Perth Hospital, Perth, WA, Australia
e-mail: Alexandra.O'Neill@health.wa.gov.au

D. Nikkhah
Division of Surgery and Interventional Science, University College London UCL, London, UK
e-mail: d.nikkhah@nhs.net

A. M. Yassin
Plastic Surgery Department, Royal Free Hospital, London, UK

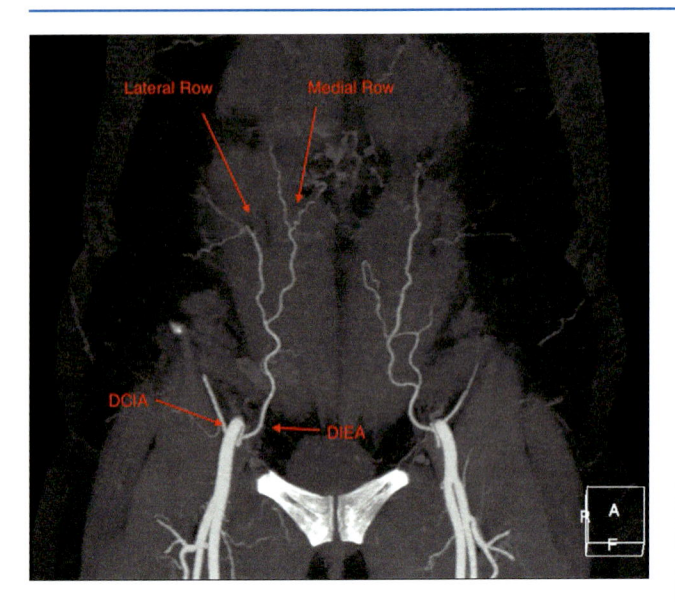

Fig. 19.1 Moon and Taylor type II branching pattern of the deep inferior epigastric artery (DIEA). The origin of the DIEA and deep circumflex iliac artery (DCIA) from the external iliac artery (EIA) is nicely demonstrated in this image

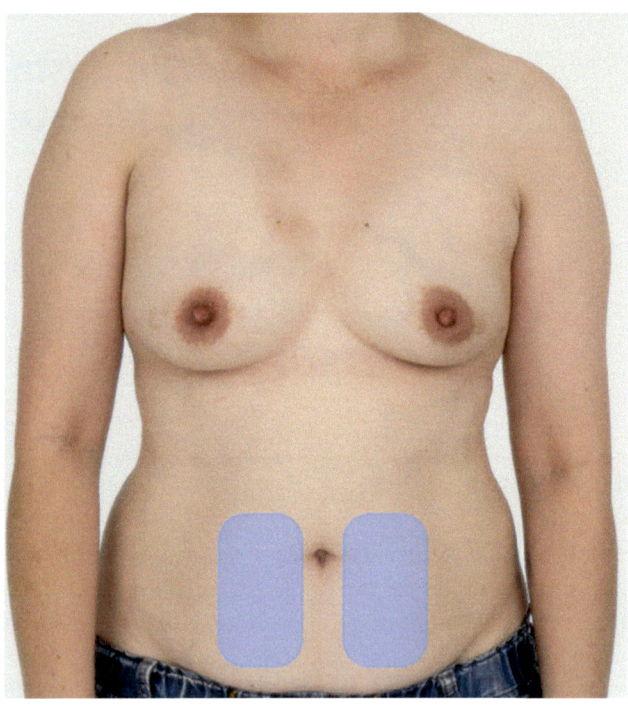

Fig. 19.2 Zone of the highest concentration of perforators, 2 cm cranial/6 cm caudal, 1 cm lateral, 7 cm lateral

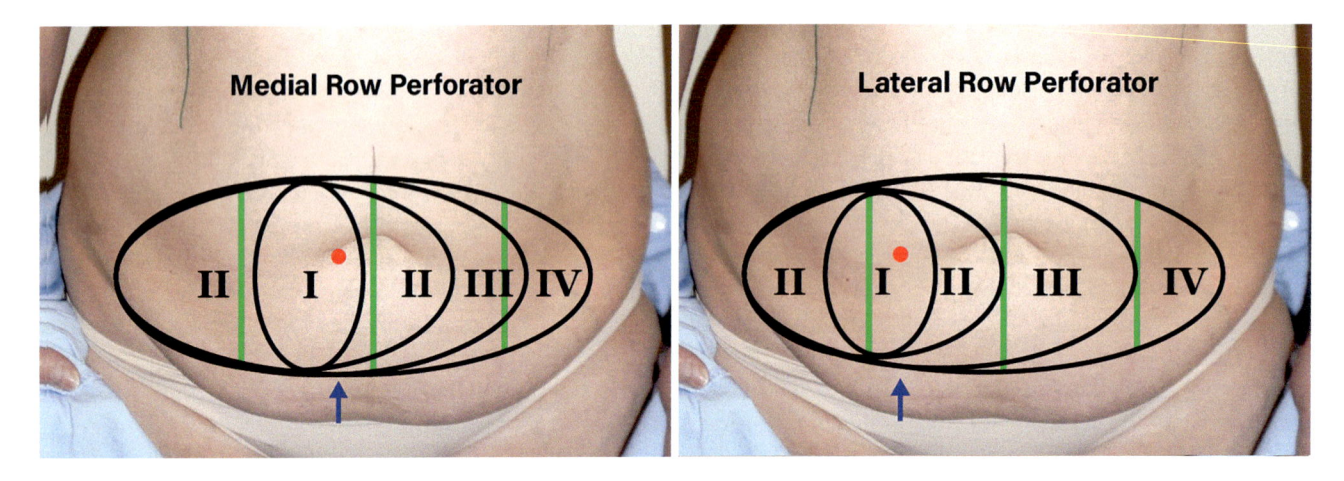

Fig. 19.3 Perfusion zones of the DIEP flap based on a medial row perforator (left) and lateral row perforator (right)

Classically described perfusion zones of the abdominal wall were based on filling of the entire DIEA system as occurs in the TRAM flap; however with the transition to perforator-based surgery as in the DIEA perforator flap, a revision was necessary. Rozen et al. proposed a new model based on the perforator angiosome concepts which better illustrates the least poorly perfused zones based on medial versus lateral row perforator flaps [7] (Fig. 19.3).

Mixed segmental intercostal nerves pass from lateral to medial below rectus abdominis, penetrating the mid-portion of the muscle where it courses over the lateral row perforators of the DIEA at which point it divides into two motor branches, one medial and one lateral, and a sensory branch. The majority of nerves are small and supply a narrow strip of muscle; however there are larger, type II nerves, commonly at the level of the arcuate line that innervate the entire width of the muscle [8].

19.3 Preoperative Investigation

Multidetector-row computed tomography (MDCT) is the gold standard preoperative assessment of choice, providing accurate evaluation of the vascular anatomy of the abdomi-

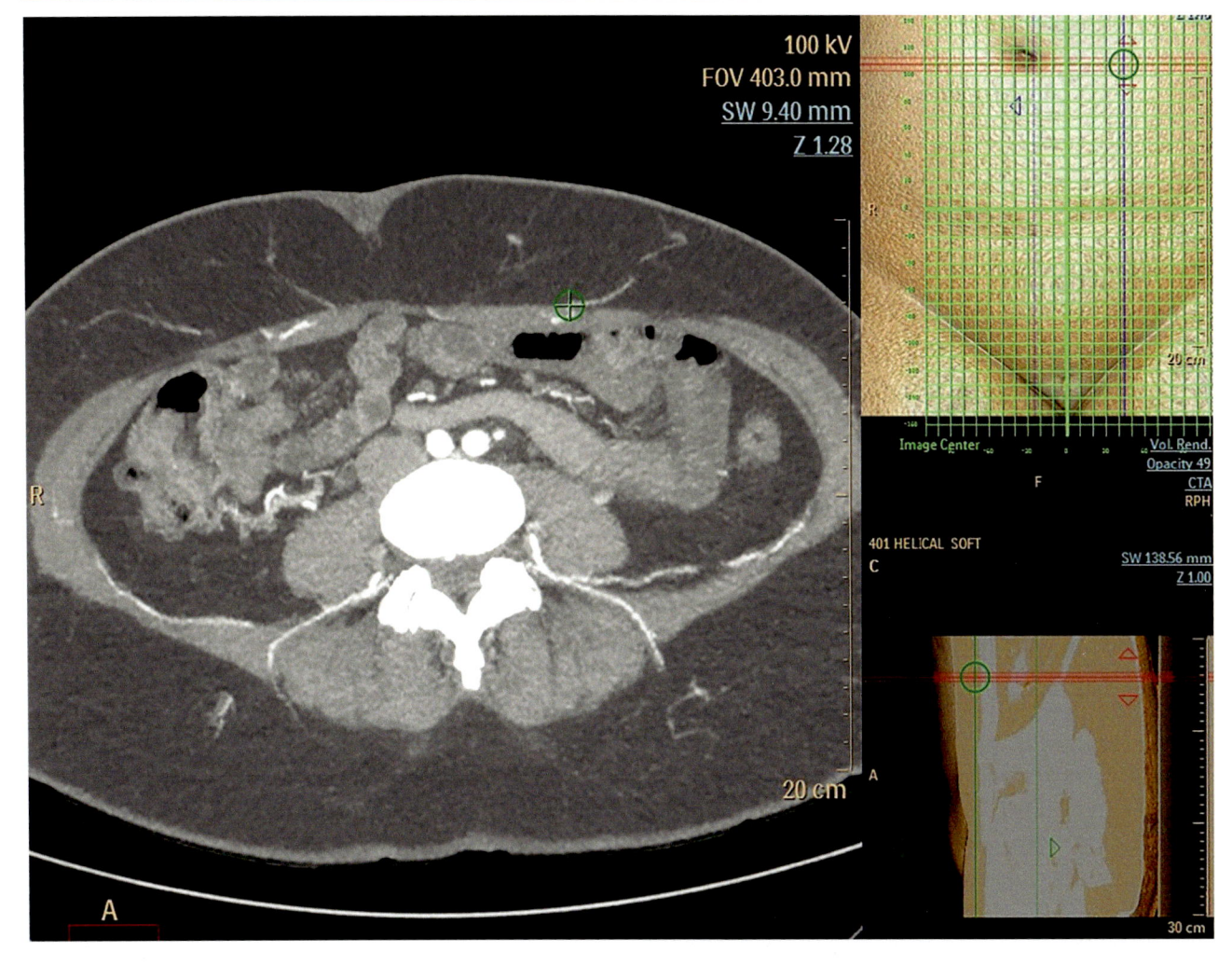

Fig. 19.4 CT preoperative planning

nal wall, thereby reducing operating time by allowing expedient dissection of the dominant perforator [9]. MDCT identifies three-dimensional positioning of perforators, perforator number, calibre and course, facilitating surgical planning and a hierarchy for perforator selection. Additional information about the relative dominance of the deep and superficial systems is demonstrated, allowing surgical consideration of the superficial inferior epigastric artery (SIEA) flap as an alternative (Fig. 19.4).

Conventional handheld Doppler ultrasound with 8 MHz probe is used immediately preoperatively for surface localisation and marking of perforators with correlation to the MDCT-identified perforator. Additionally, thermal imaging is emerging as a useful adjunct to handheld Doppler for surgical planning. Indocyanine green laser angiography has shown promise when used intraoperatively at aiding analysis of flap perfusion and reduction in fat necrosis [10, 11].

19.4 Flap Design and Markings

Initial simple markings are done with the patient standing, typically in concert with breast markings (Fig. 19.5). The midline is marked from the sternal notch, through the xiphisternum to the labial cleft. The suprapubic fold is marked plus any additional scars on the lower abdomen. Attempts should be made to utilise Pfannenstiel scars if present; however this is not always possible without compromising flap volume or abdominal closure in which case the incision should be made a safe distance above the existing scar.

With the patient supine, markings proceed symmetrically laterally from the marked midline. The inferior incision extends 7 cm laterally if placed in an ideal low position, followed by a variable distance 3–5 cm superior and parallel to the inguinal crease. The transverse 7 cm component is lengthened into the oblique line as the inferior incision is

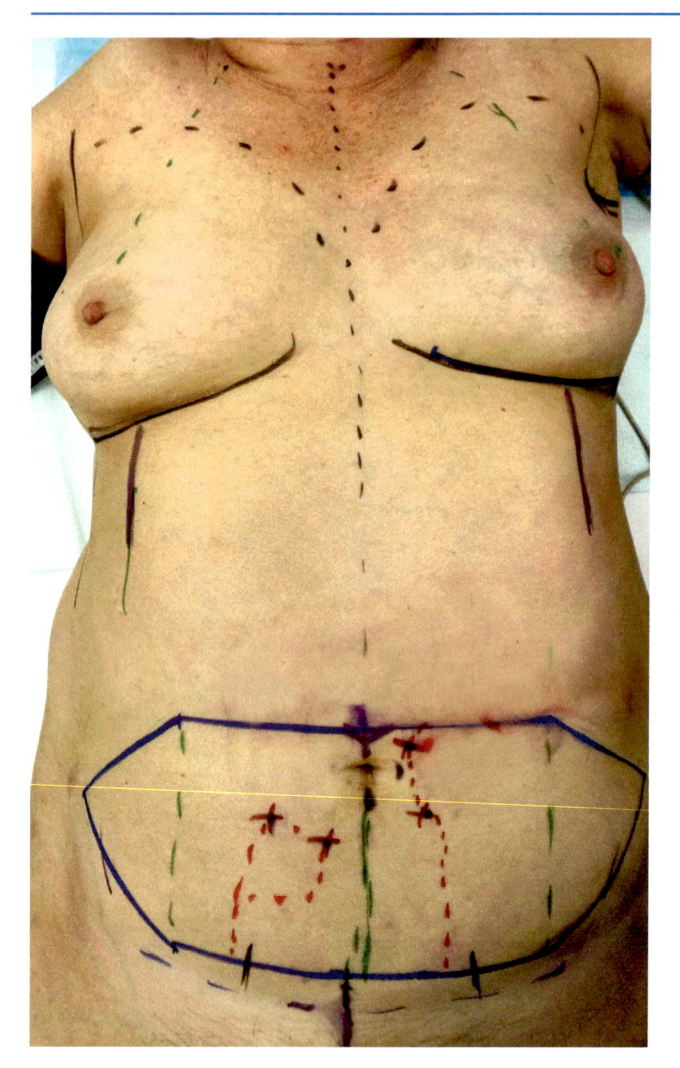

Fig. 19.5 Preoperative markings of the flap and breast footprint. Red crosses indicate Doppler-identified perforators with a medial and lateral row marked on the left abdomen and two medial row perforators on the right. The red dotted line marks the vessel course as seen on bedside thermal imaging. Flap incision (unbroken blue line) is marked above the suprapubic crease (blue dashes) to increase flap volume and facilitate abdominal closure

elevated. The lateral extent is dependent on the extent of abdominal excess fat, with a typical total inferior incision length of 22–28 cm.

Doppler identification of the perforators is performed which allows appropriate positioning of the superior incision, commencing with a 10 cm transverse component. The oblique incision is angled to meet the most lateral extent of the inferior incision.

We suggest including a soft cupid's bow curve in the central aspect of both the upper and lower markings to reduce tension on the central abdominal wound. The volume of subcutaneous tissue in the flanks is assessed and can be included with the flap if required within the constraints of the zonal perfusion.

Symmetry is confirmed with height at the midline, 10 cm lateral points and incision lengths.

19.5 Flap Raise/Elevation: A Step-by-Step Guide

1. *Incision*
   (a) Incise the superior margin of the flap, chamfering as required by volume, and raise the superior abdominal flap all the way to the xiphisternum. This will enable concurrent abdominal closure during flap inset. Once raised the superior abdominal flap is retracted and secured to the upper abdominal wall with staples to aid exposure during the flap raise (Fig. 19.6).
   (b) Inferior incision is then completed, and time is taken to dissect a length (approximately 3–5 cm) of superficial inferior epigastric vein (SIEV) which can be used as a lifeboat if the situation of venous congestion arises (Fig. 19.7).
2. *Perforator Identification*
   (a) Monopolar diathermy on a coagulation setting is utilised to raise the flap from lateral to medial above the external oblique fascia up to and slightly beyond the linea semilunaris (Fig. 19.8).
   (b) Monopolar diathermy on a lower cut setting is utilised to the proximity of the perforator and then changed to bipolar forceps in a dissecting fashion in the perforator's immediate proximity. Be guided by the pre-op perforator markings during this stage of the flap raise. Gentle traction on the flap while dissecting will also help in the identification of perforators (Fig. 19.9). If a single perforator is possible, our preference is to utilise the medial row in a unilateral DIEP or the lateral row in a bilateral reconstruction; however if the perforator is small, it may be necessary to include a second perforator from the same row (Fig. 19.10).
3. *Perforator Dissection*
   (a) Incise the fascia immediately adjacent to the perforator, commencing cranially, and encircle the perforator (Fig. 19.11). Identify the point of origin in the muscle and follow through its intramuscular course to the DIE vessels with tenotomy scissors or heat sink bipolar. The superior continuation needs to be ligated early to allow perforator mobilisation. The pedicle is then followed to its origin being cautious to ligate any muscular side branches (Fig. 19.12). A narrow cuff of fascia may be left around the perforator in the case of small perforators. It is useful to have the abdominal wall muscles relaxed during dissection and until abdominal wall closure is complete. Fish hooks can be used to retract the fascia during perforator dissection.
   (b) If the perforator is felt to be too small, an additional perforator from the same row can be dissected, and

Fig. 19.6 Clinical illustration demonstrating initial incisions and superior abdominal flap raise which is subsequently secured to the upper abdominal wall

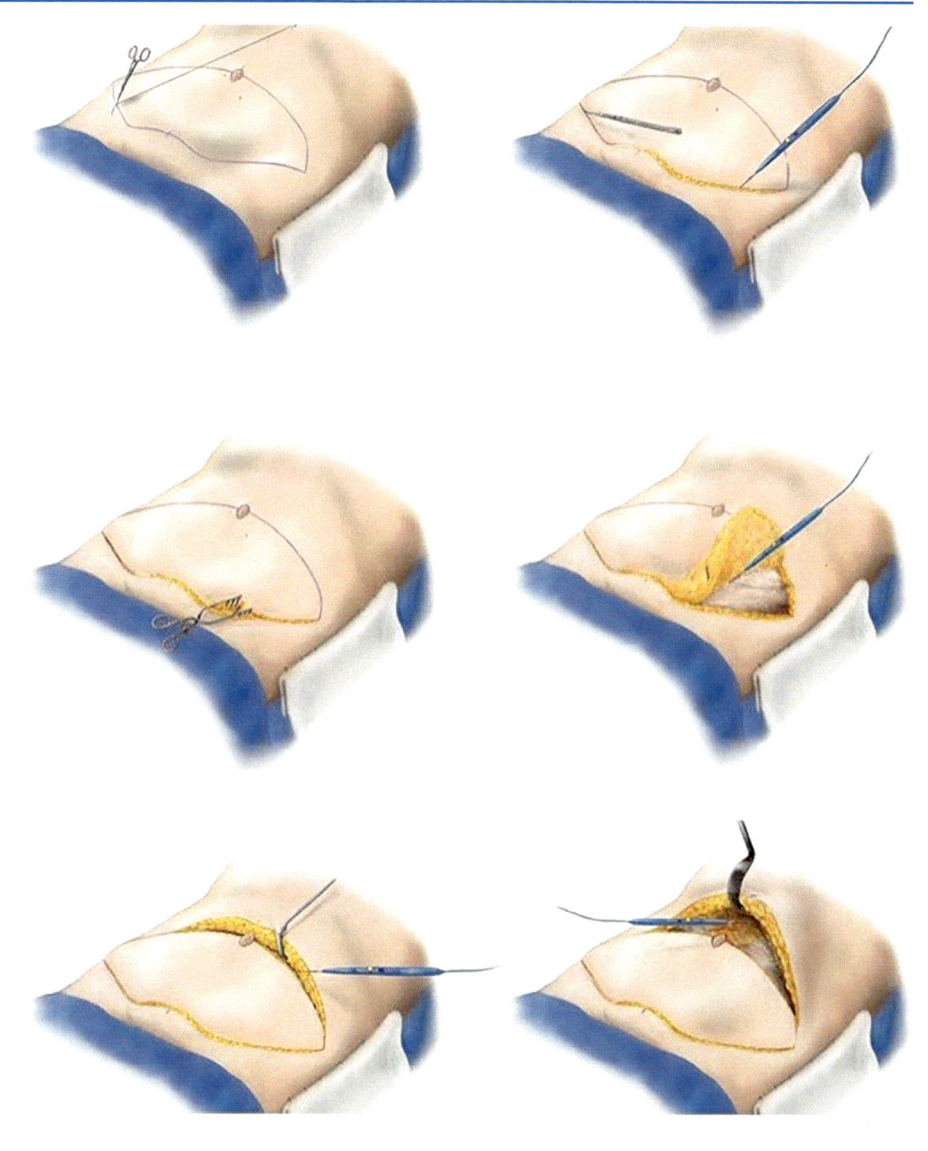

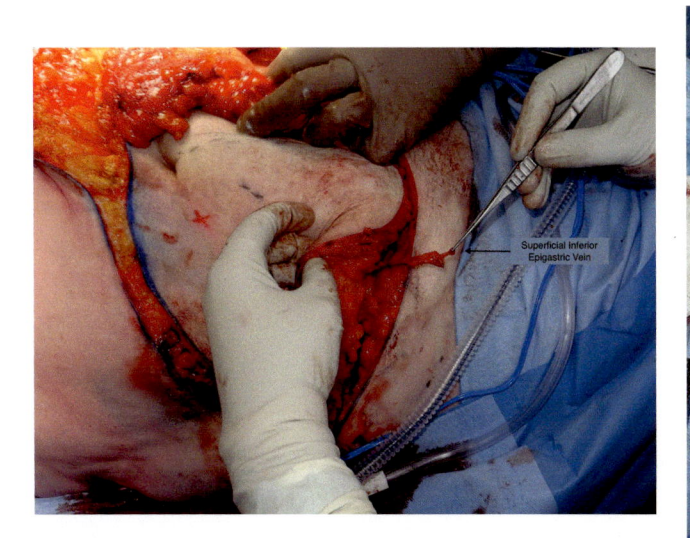

Fig. 19.7 Superficial inferior epigastric vein, located approximately one-third from the pubic symphysis to the anterior superior iliac spine (ASIS), is dissected for use as a lifeboat

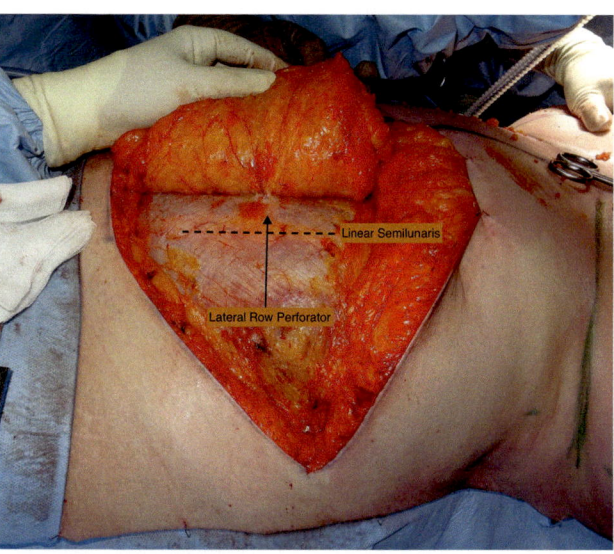

Fig. 19.8 Suprafascial flap raise until the lateral row perforators are reached just beyond the linea semilunaris

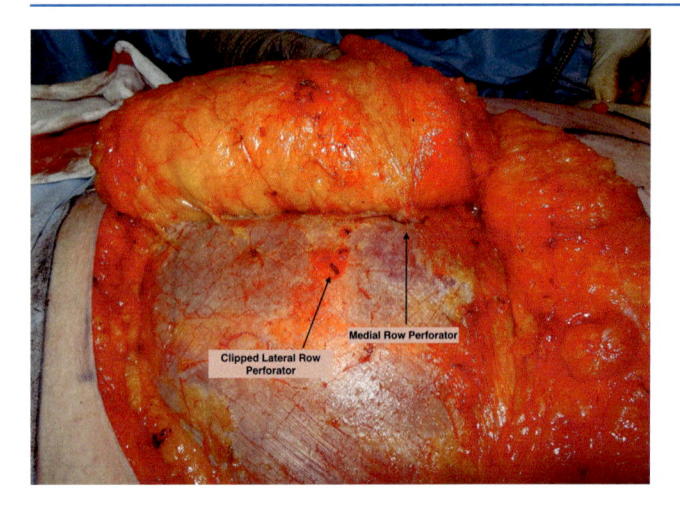

Fig. 19.9 Medial row perforator is seen tethering the fascia to the undersurface of the flap. Gentle traction on the flap aids in demonstrating this tethering

Fig. 19.10 Clinical illustration demonstrating lateral to medial suprafascial flap raise (top left), perforator identification (top right), fascia incision with small cuff around perforator (middle left) and perforator dissection through its intramuscular course (middle right and bottom left) to the DIEA origin at the EIA

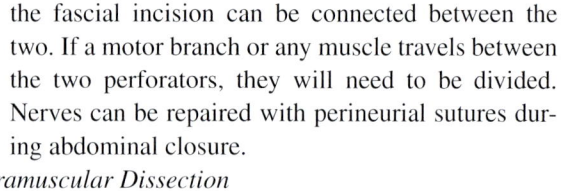

the fascial incision can be connected between the two. If a motor branch or any muscle travels between the two perforators, they will need to be divided. Nerves can be repaired with perineurial sutures during abdominal closure.

4. *Intramuscular Dissection*
   (a) The rectus abdominis muscle is split longitudinally and held open with self-retainers to facilitate perforator dissection to the main branch of the DIEA at the posterior surface of the rectus.
   (b) The lateral edge of the rectus muscle is elevated exposing the DIEA, if adequate access through the longitudinal split does not expose the origin.

5. *Pedicle Dissection*
   (a) Dissect the pedicle inferiorly to its origin, applying ligature clips to side branches so as to isolate the main DIEA. Ensure adequate control of large

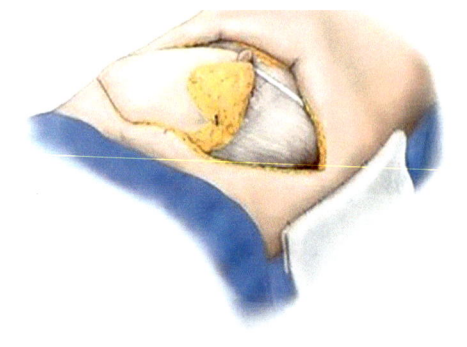

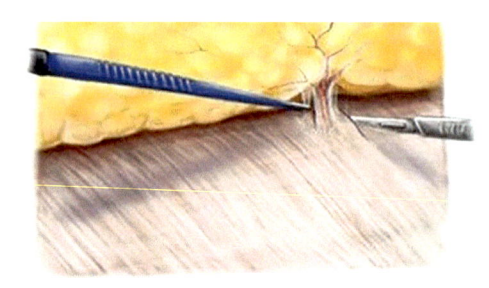

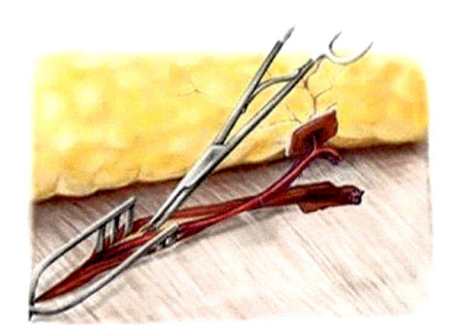

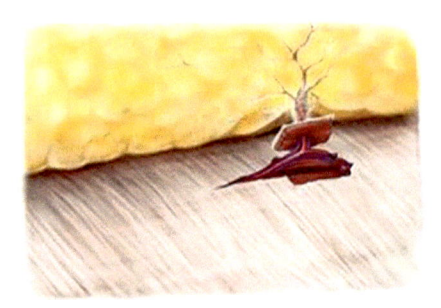

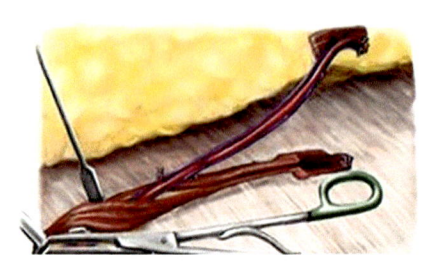

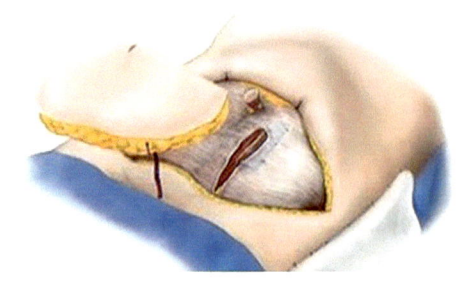

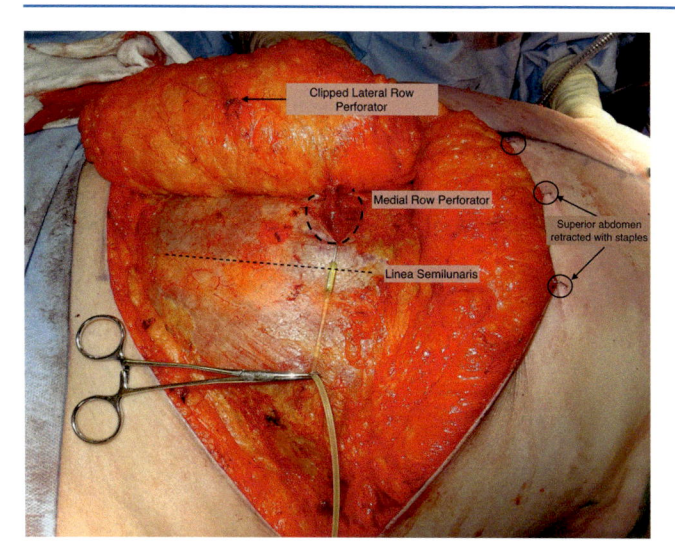

Fig. 19.11 Fascial incision circumferentially around the dominant perforator allows visualisation of the perforator exiting the rectus abdominis muscle. The previously identified lateral row perforator is seen with a ligature clip in the lateral aspect of the flap

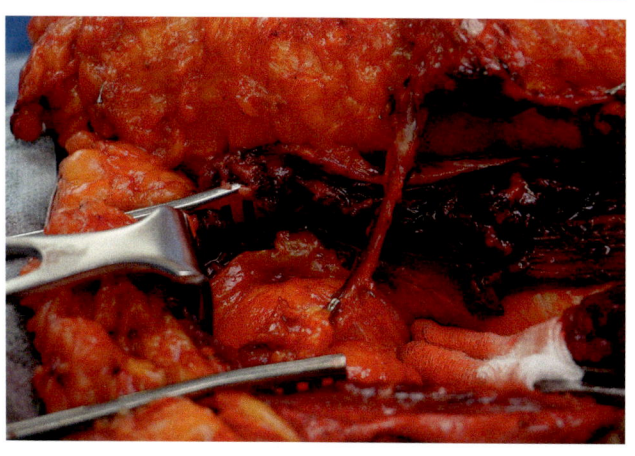

Fig. 19.13 The flap perforator is dissected through its intramuscular course to the deep inferior epigastric artery origin from the external iliac artery with its adjacent venae comitantes. A Czerny retractor is used to expose the vessel origin and a swab on a stick is used to displace the bulging peritoneal fat

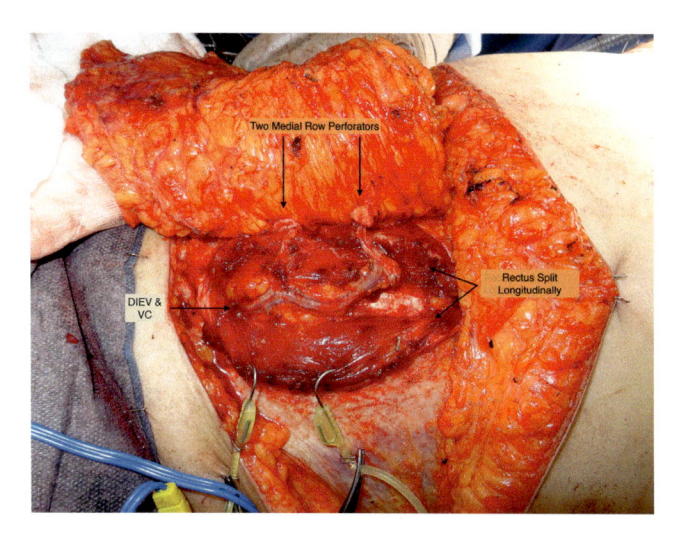

Fig. 19.12 Two medial row perforators have been dissected through the longitudinally split rectus abdominis which is retracted using fish hooks

branches to other rows of perforators. A Czerny is often needed for exposure of the DIEA origin, and a peanut or similar is useful to compress bulging peritoneum if the full length of the DIEA is required (Fig. 19.13). Both the pedicle length and size can be tailored to the given case.

6. *Umbilicus Preparation*
   (a) Incise the umbilicus circumferentially to subcutaneous tissue; then with the aid of skin hooks elevating the umbilicus from the abdominal pannus, dissect the umbilical stalk down to the anterior rectus sheath (Fig. 19.14). Mark the superior aspect of the umbilicus with a suture left long; this will aid umbilicus retrieval during closure. (Some units like to perform this step at the very beginning; however we opt to isolate the umbilicus only once the perforators are dissected as the periumbilical perforators can cause staining of the surrounding tissue making dissection more difficult.)

7. *Preparation for Transfer*
   (a) Once the flap is islanded on its pedicle, it should be secured to the abdominal wall until the recipient site is ready for inset to prevent any unintended avulsion.
   (b) Preparation of the flap is easier and more efficient on the abdomen. The skin requirement is overestimated and partial de-epithelialisation is performed. Doppler marking sutures are inserted. Excess and non-perfused zones are discarded (Fig. 19.15).

8. *Flap Transfer and Inset*
   (a) The flap is divided and weighed, prior to transfer with attempts to correlate this to the mastectomy specimen (Fig. 19.16).

9. *Donor Site Closure*
   (a) The fascia is repaired with care taken to include both internal and external oblique aponeuroses. We advocate a two-layer fascial closure with a betadine-dipped non-absorbable suture with or without an underlay mesh, which can be used if nerve division was required but is otherwise rarely required. An umbilicoplasty is performed with the surgeon's preferred technique, and if there is any uncertainty about the umbilical location, the ASIS can be used to guide placement (Fig. 19.17).

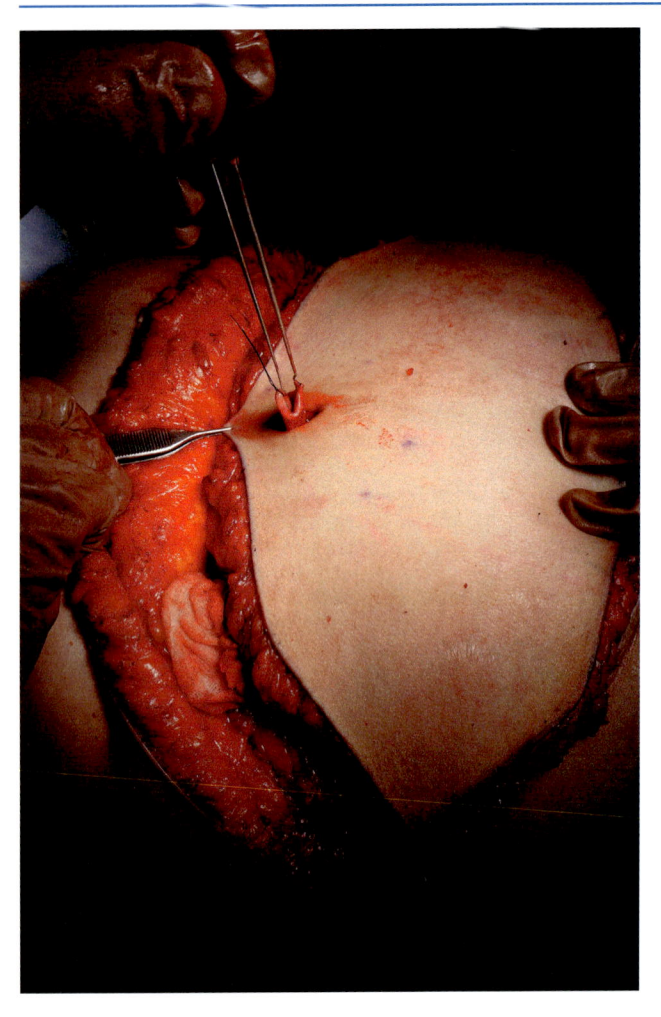

Fig. 19.14 The umbilicus is incised circumferentially and the stalk is dissected with the aid of two skin hooks

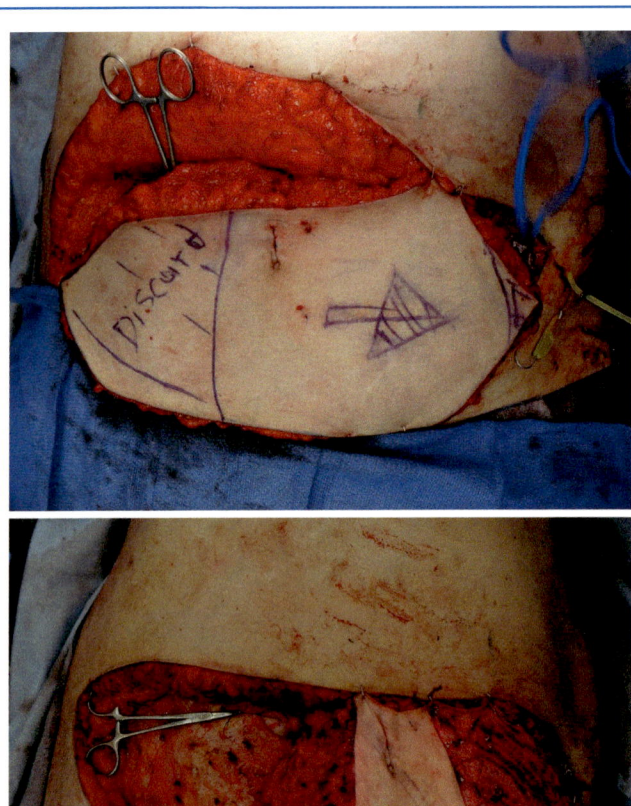

Fig. 19.15 The flap is prepared while still perfused on the abdominal wall with excision of zone IV plus any excess flap volume and preliminary de-epithelialisation of the flap

Fig. 19.16 Flap shape and volume is guided by the patient's pre-marked breast footprint and mastectomy weight

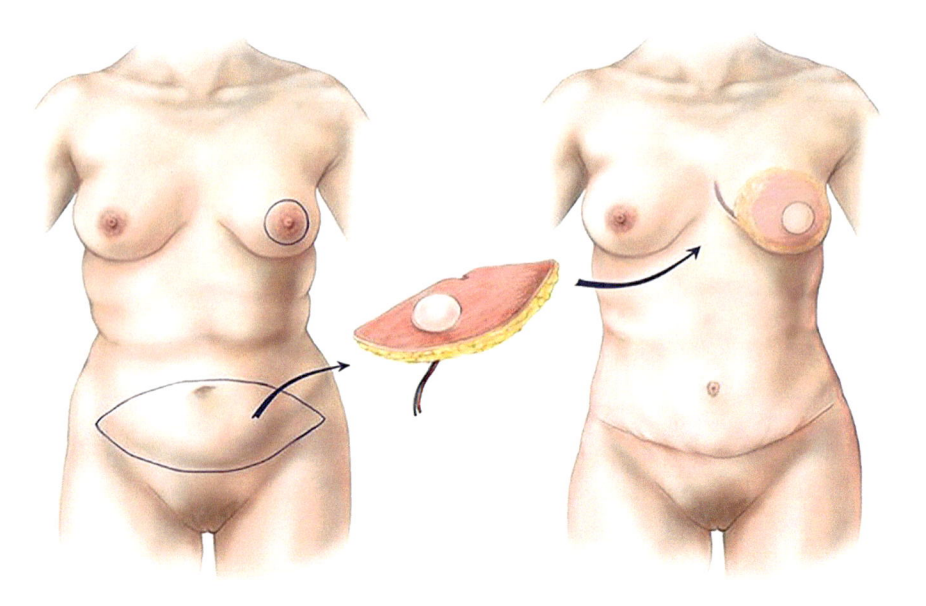

Fig. 19.17 Clinical illustration demonstrating drain placement, fascial closure, umbilicus retrieval and abdominal wall closure

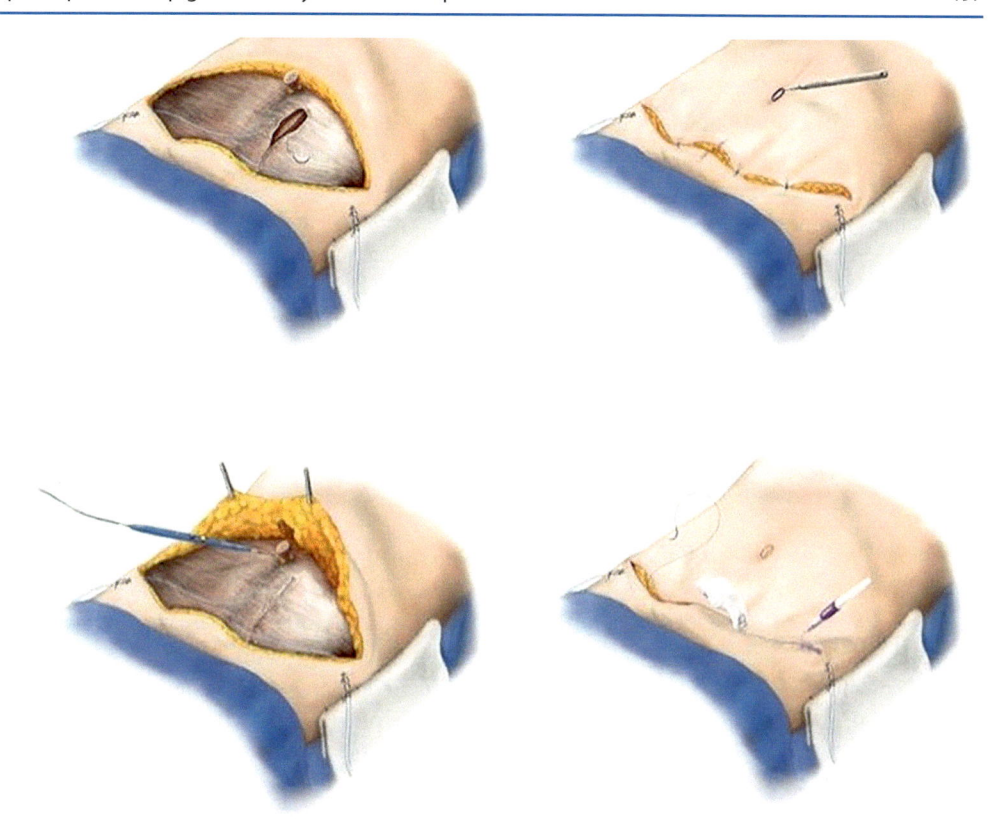

(b) Rectus sheath catheters or TAP blocks can be used to reduce systemic postoperative analgesic requirements [12].

19.6 Core Surgical Techniques in Flap Dissection

19.6.1 Perforator Dissection

When in close proximity to the anticipated perforators, transition to bipolar cautery. Meticulous dissection and haemostasis are essential at this stage as even a small amount of bleeding can cause tissue staining which renders the dissection much more difficult. With guidance from preoperative imaging, the dominant perforator is approached; however care should be taken to identify and preserve adjacent perforators which may be required in the event of smaller than anticipated dominant perforators. A suprafascial dissection is performed circumferentially around the dominant perforator and adjacent perforators in the event of a small dominant perforator, before the fascia is incised. This creates a zone of safety around the perforator and prevents future injury during the final stages of flap raise. A small vascular clamp can be applied to the back-up perforator(s) to assess adequate perfusion and aid decision-making regarding the required number of perforators.

Bipolar cautery at low current of the planned fascial incision can reduce the risk of blood staining. Care must be taken when incising the fascia as the perforator can travel obliquely under the fascia before commencing its intramuscular course. When the fascia is firmly adherent to the perforator, it is safest to leave a small cuff of fascia around the vessel. The perforator must be circumferentially dissected in the subfascial plane as was performed suprafascially, and then intramuscular dissection can begin. The fascia is now incised parallel to the rectus abdominis fibres. The muscle fibres overlying the pedicle are gradually divided allowing adequate exposure of the entire pedicle length. Care is taken to identify and ligate or coagulate all side branches throughout the intramuscular course, a distance of 1–2 mm from the main pedicle to prevent unintended vessel injury, thereby isolating the pedicle from the surrounding rectus muscle. The vessel runs in a loose areolar plane allowing blunt dissection and resistance is indicative of a side branch requiring ligation. The pedicle dissection proceeds until adequate length or ideal calibre vessel for anastomosis has been reached. Typically one artery and two venae comitantes are included in the pedicle. Ligation of the smaller vein at the end of the dissected pedicle diverts flow through the large vein prior to transfer and avoids confusion once the veins have collapsed post transfer.

19.6.2 Nerve Preservation

Nerves enter the rectus with the lateral row perforators of the DIEA placing them at risk particularly when multiple lateral row perforators are harvested. When perforator dissection necessitates motor nerve division, we advocate a perineurial repair under loupe magnification with 9/0 nylon sutures once the flap has been harvested. Division of type II nerves results in larger segments of muscle denervation and potential for abdominal wall complications. Underlay mesh should be considered in this situation.

19.6.3 Bipedicled and Stacked DIEP

Bipedicled and stacked DIEP flaps are useful in women with a paucity of abdominal tissue, those requiring large volume reconstructions and those with midline abdominal scars. Bipedicled/stacked flaps involve raising the entire abdominal pannus on two pedicles for a unilateral reconstruction. Murray et al. described a classification system for the use of the bipedicled flap, the pedicle options and the four types of intraflap anastomotic configurations [13]. The internal mammary artery/vein (IMA/V) antegrade or large intercostal perforator remains the primary recipient; however in type 4 anastomosis, where pedicles are independently anastomosed, the IMA/V retrograde is also used. Shaping the entire abdominal flap has been described in four different configurations involving folding, dividing and coning the tissue to achieve best aesthetic outcomes [14].

19.7 Breast Neurotisation

Post-mastectomy breast numbness has a significant impact on postoperative quality of life with patients now seeking not only reconstruction of the breast mound but also restoration of cutaneous sensation. The value of nerve coaptation has been debated in the literature with some arguing collateral ingrowth from surrounding nerve fibres is sufficient for protective sensation; however a recent study of bilateral autologous breast reconstruction with unilateral sensory nerve coaptation demonstrates improved sensory recovery in the neurotised breast compared to the contralateral non-neurotised breast [15, 16].

19.8 Clinical Scenario

Case 1: Immediate Unilateral Breast Reconstruction

A 56-year-old female underwent unilateral skin sparring, nipple sacrificing mastectomy and sentinel lymph node biopsy for a grade 2 invasive ductal carcinoma of the left breast. Mastectomy weight was 914 g. She underwent immediate reconstruction with stacked DIEP flaps with a total flap weight of 1029g (Fig. 19.18a, b).

Case 2: Bilateral Delayed Reconstruction

A 58-year-old lady underwent bilateral breast reconstruction with DIEP free flaps 4 years post bilateral mastectomy and left sentinel lymph node biopsy (SLNB) for left breast grade III IDC and high-grade DCIS; concurrent SLNB was negative for malignancy. Mastectomy weights were right 700 g and left 990 g and DIEP reconstructions weighed 676 g and 862 g. Post-op day 1 the flap was noted to be venously congested, and she underwent return to theatre for a cephalic turn-up and anastomosis to the SIEV with a successful outcome (Fig. 19.19). (See Video 19.1—demonstrating another case of a delayed DIEP with cephalic turndown.)

Case 3: Bilateral Immediate Reconstruction with Mastectomy Skin Reduction for Ptosis Correction

A 44-year-old lady underwent a bilateral nipple-sacrificing mastectomy for strong family history and BRCA1 genetic mutation with immediate breast reconstruction with DIEP free flap. Mastectomy weights were right 531 g and left 676 g, and her respective flap reconstructions weighed 484 g and 525 g. She was noted to have grade III ptosis and was subsequently planned for bilateral skin reduction with an inverted T technique to be performed simultaneously (Fig. 19.20a, b).

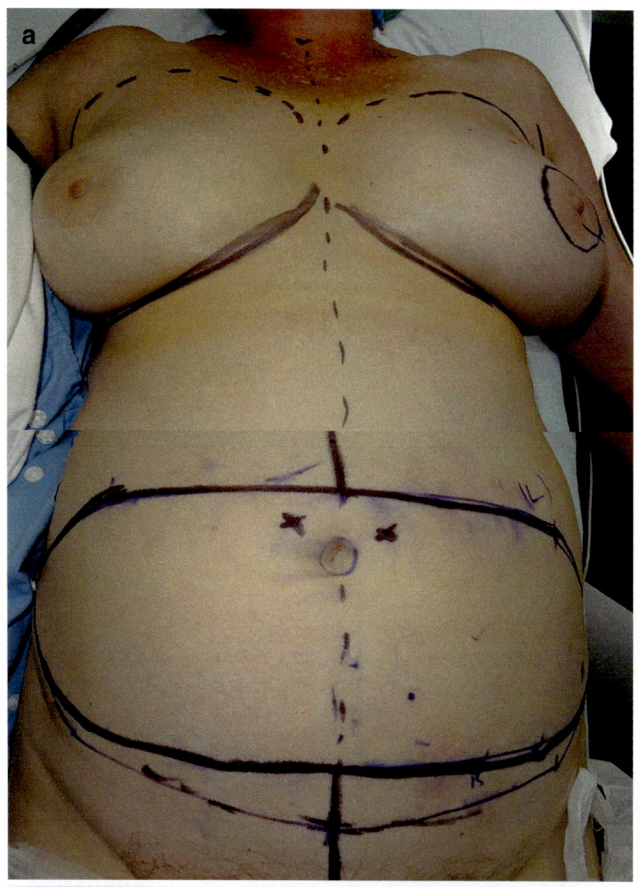

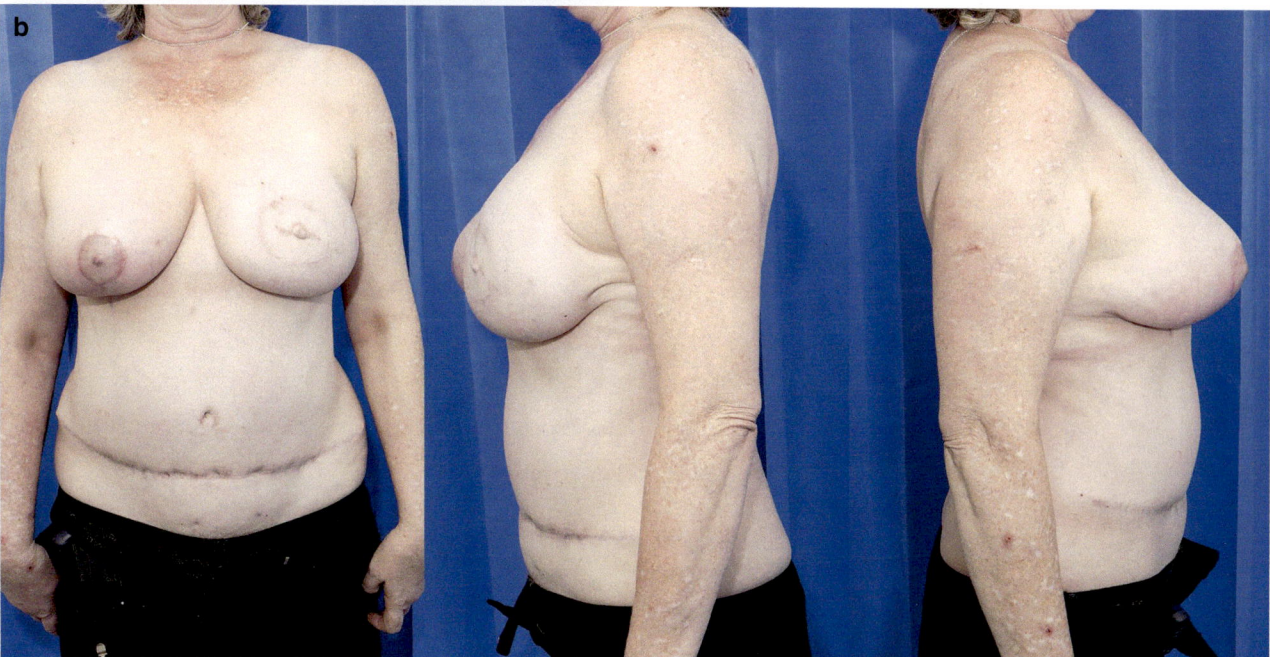

Fig. 19.18 (**a**) A 56-year-old lady underwent a unilateral immediate breast reconstruction with stacked DIEP flap. Preoperative photographs. (**b**) Post reconstruction

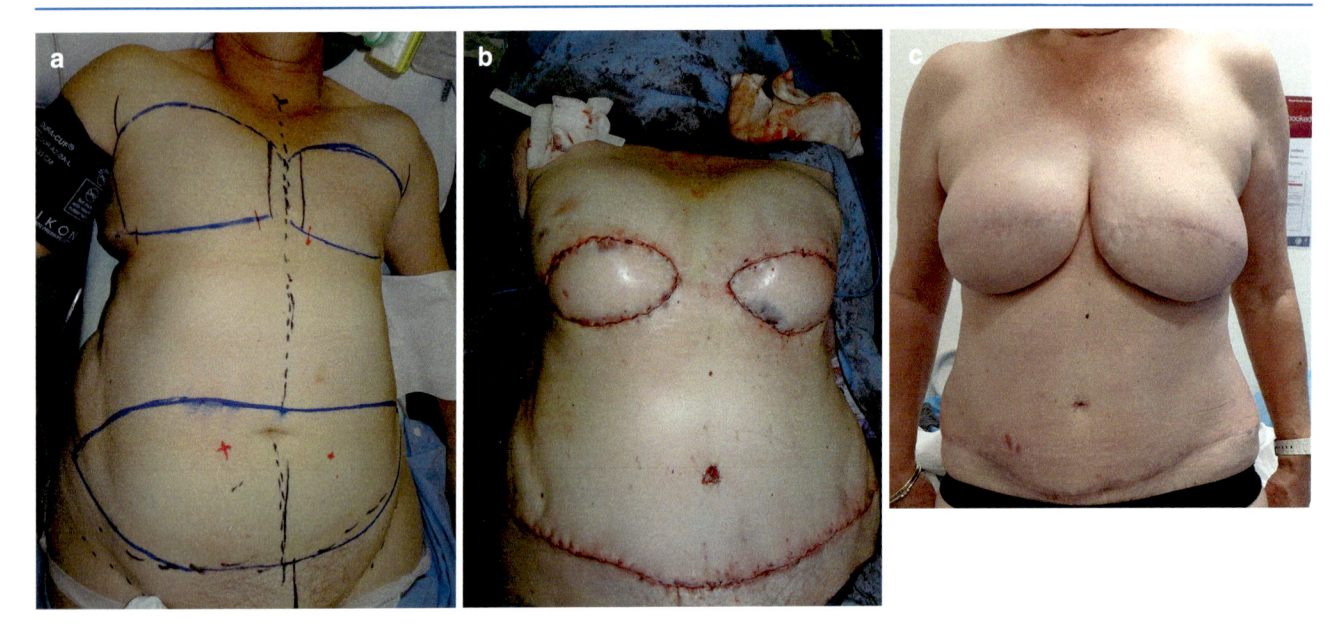

Fig. 19.19 (**a**) Case 2: Preoperative markings of a 58-year-old lady undergoing delayed breast reconstruction 4 years following bilateral mastectomy. Note the template of the new breast footprint, with care taken to prevent symmastia of the reconstructed breasts. (**b**) On table appearances immediately following bilateral delayed breast reconstruction with DIEP free flaps. (**c**) 12 months following bilateral delayed breast reconstruction with DIEP flaps, very faint scars from the cephalic turn-up procedure can be seen

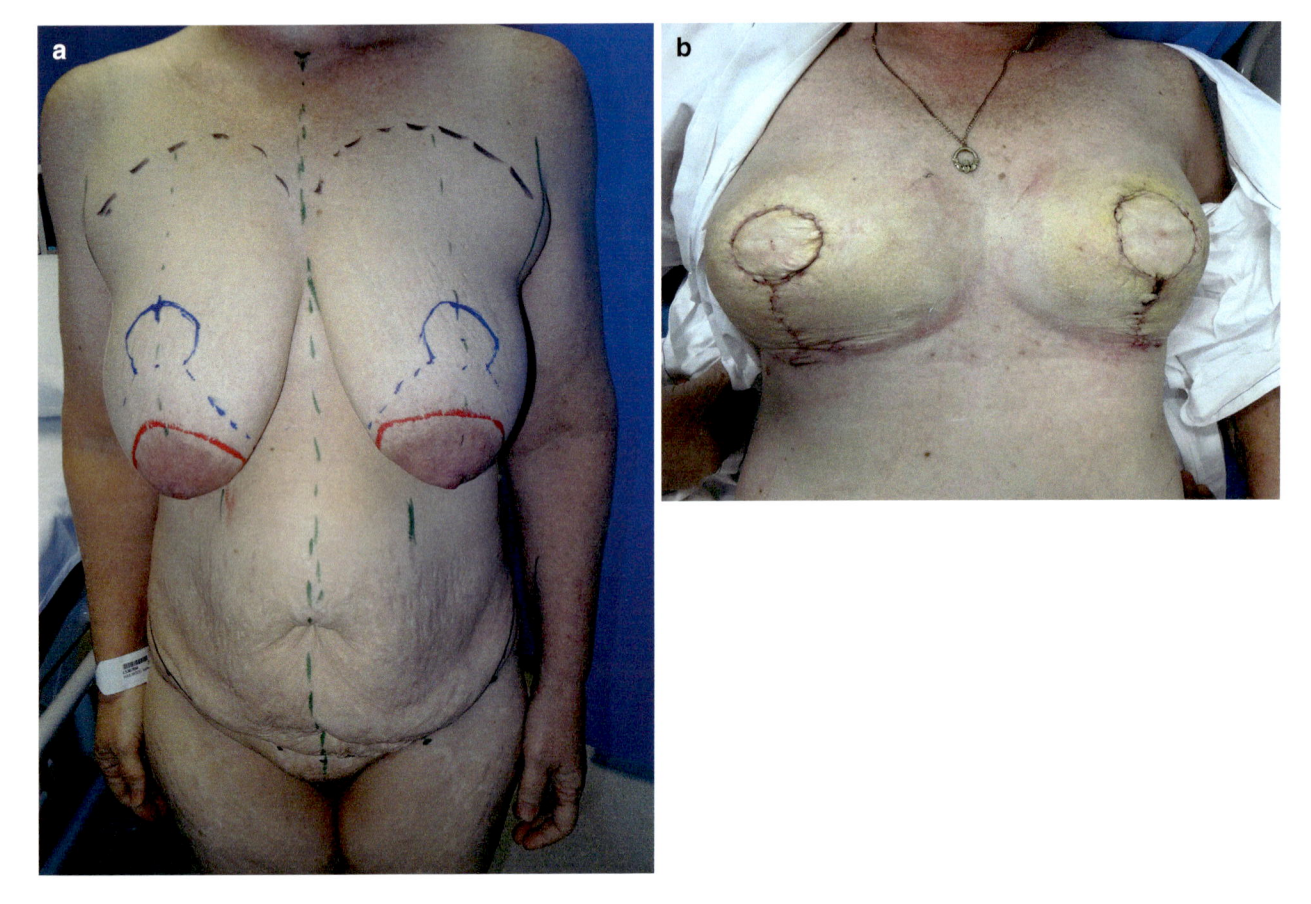

Fig. 19.20 (**a**) Case 3: Preoperative markings for a 44-year-old woman undergoing bilateral breast reconstruction, requiring simultaneous reduction of the skin envelope. (**b**) Day 2 post-bilateral breast reconstruction with wise pattern skin reduction

19.9 Pearls and Pitfalls

Patient selection is key to success.
Patient understanding of expected volume, abdominal scarring that is typically higher than a cosmetic abdominoplasty and the transfer of abdominal wall features such as striae, moles, etc. is key to patient satisfaction. Numerous studies demonstrate increased complications in both active and ex-smokers, and patients should be counselled to cease smoking 6 weeks either side of surgery [17]. Although significant interunit variability exists, extrapolated evidence suggests a BMI over 30 is associated with increased morbidity, predominantly donor site morbidity. Reconstruction is generally afforded to women with a BMI up to 32; however, immediate cases can be considered judiciously up to a BMI of 35 [18].

Dual consultant team has been shown to reduce surgical time and also provides an ideal opportunity for training and mentorship of junior surgeons [19, 20]. In delayed breast reconstruction, one team can prepare the breast pocket and recipient vessels, while the second team raises the DIEP flap from the contralateral abdominal wall. In bilateral breast reconstruction, while one team is performing the microvascular anastomoses, the second team can proceed with the second DIEP flap raise.

Adjustment of flap markings
The inferior and superior flap incisions can be moved superiorly to increase tissue capture and ensure tension-free closure of the abdominal wound.

Perforator selection
Preoperative CT angiogram provides an excellent guide to perforator selection. If the perforator is small, then a second perforator should be included in the flap. If there is uncertainty about the perfused skin territory, adjacent perforators can be preserved and vascular clamps applied to assess the flap perfusion. If deemed adequate, then the perforators can be ligated with haemoclips. Similarly, in unilateral DIEPs the contralateral DIEA perforators can be dissected suprafascially and microvascular clamps applied on the dominant perforators as a contingency plan.

Venous lifeboat
Time should be taken to preserve a 3–5 cm length of the superficial epigastric vein which can provide a secondary venous outflow in the event of venous congestion. The SIEV can be dissected into the flap in the event it is required.

Nerve preservation
Motor nerve preservation is essential for preserving function of the rectus abdominis muscle but should not compromise flap perfusion. If a second perforator is required at the cost of a nerve, then the perforator takes precedence, and mesh should be considered to augment the rectus abdominis.

Flap preparation on the abdomen
Mark and excise zone IV plus any obvious flap excess so that the flap is marginally bigger than anticipated. Judicious de-epithelialisation can occur prior to transfer. Delayed reconstructions can be more difficult in predicting the extent of de-epithelialisation and are often easiest if done during flap inset.

Abdominal closure
Elevation of the superior abdominal skin early in the operation facilitates abdominal wall closure during the flap inset.

Identify abdominal scars
Pfannenstiel incisions don't preclude the use of the DIEP flap, consideration should be made regarding incorporating the scar in the inferior incision versus placing the flap incision a safe distance from the scar, and the surgeon should be aware of the increased scarring in this region.

Flap inset—immediate versus delayed breast reconstruction—flap orientations (Fig. 19.21).

Delayed breast reconstruction requires recreation of the breast footprint and reestablishment of the inframammary fold (IMF). In cases of unilateral delayed reconstruction, the contralateral breast can be used to guide IMF placement, typically 2 to 3 cm higher than the contralateral side unless there is significant skin fibrosis and contraction at the mastectomy site, in which case the IMF should be positioned higher. The scar is excised, and the skin between the scar and IMF is de-epithelialised which aids creation of lower pole projection. The breast pocket above the scar is raised according to the preoperative footprint markings superiorly, medially and laterally. The flap then needs to be fashioned into a three-dimensional asymmetric conus to replicate the native breast. Although not essential, we routinely utilise the contralateral abdomen which is rotated 180 degrees as originally recommended by Blondeel which places the bulk of the flap in the inferior pole of the breast. Once the anastomoses are performed, shaping of the breast begins. Techniques such as removing a wedge of tissue from the periumbilical region to create greater inferior fullness and suture techniques are described for creating the breast conus.

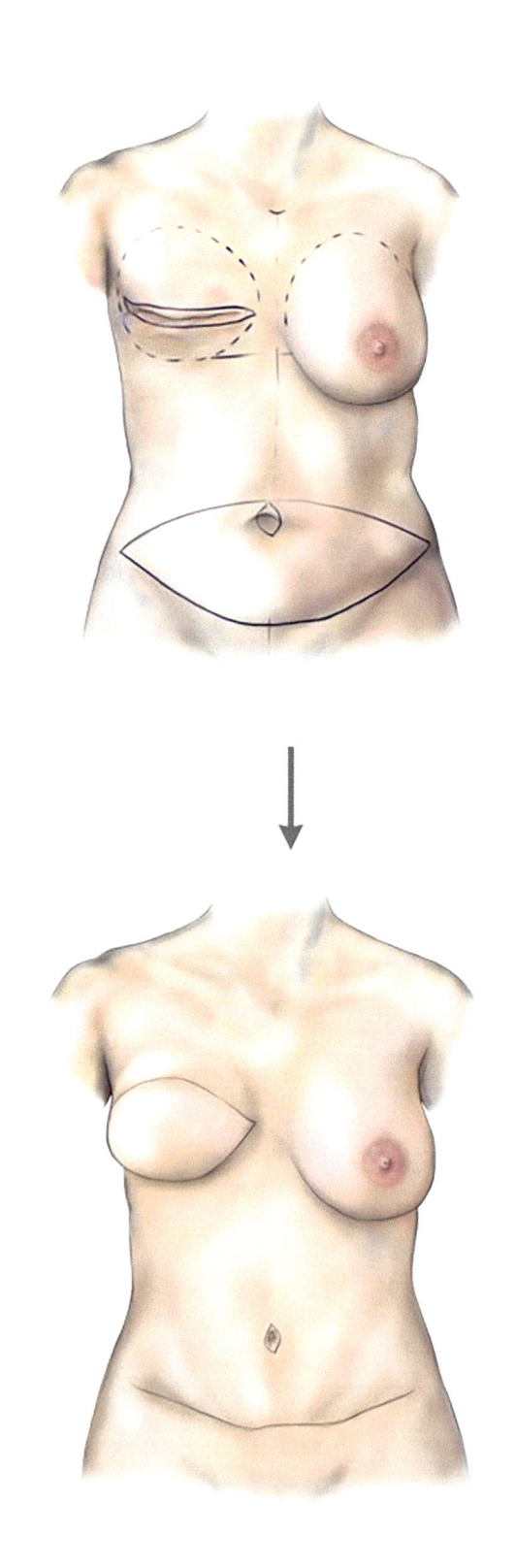

Fig. 19.21 Preoperative marking and postoperative skin paddle differences between immediate and delayed unilateral breast reconstructions

We recommend making the reconstructed breast 10% larger than the native breast to account for resolution of swelling postoperatively and to create an appropriate scaffold that can be liposculpted during a future procedure.

In immediate reconstructions, the flap weight is guided by the mastectomy weight. In particularly ptotic breasts or where the patient requests a breast reduction at the time of reconstruction, the excess skin envelope can be addressed with a keyhole or wise pattern skin reduction. It is essential to mark the breast footprint preoperatively and reconstruct any borders that are violated during the mastectomy, the most common being the IMF and the lateral border. Sutures are again used to fashion the breast conus, with the skin gently draped over the flap and the final result assessed.

19.10 Selected Readings

- Koshima I, Soeda S. Inferior epigastric artery skin flaps without rectus abdominis muscle. Br J Plast Surg. 1989;42(6):645–8.
- *The original paper demonstrating a large fasciocutaneous flap based on a single rectus abdominis muscle perforator was possible, thereby addressing the donor site morbidity associated with rectus abdominis sacrifice and the bulk issues that were sometimes undesired with the TRAM flap.*
- Dancey A, Blondeel PN. Technical tips for safe perforator vessel dissection applicable to all perforator flaps. Clin Plast Surg. 2010;37(4):593–606, xi–vi [21].
- *A comprehensive stepwise approach to DIEA perforator dissection accompanied by detailed intraoperative photography and numerous technical tips learned throughout the senior authors' extensive career.*
- Rozen WM, et al. The perforator angiosome: a new concept in the design of deep inferior epigastric artery perforator flaps for breast reconstruction. Microsurgery. 2010;30(1):1–7.
- *This paper identifies fundamental differences in the medial and lateral row perforators of the DIEA and proposes a new model of abdominal wall perfusion based on a single perforator.*
- Blondeel PN, et al. Shaping the breast in aesthetic and reconstructive breast surgery: an easy three-step principle. Plast Reconstr Surg. 2009;123(2):455–62 [22].
- *The first of a four-part series addressing the aesthetics of breast reconstruction. While not directly related to microvascular breast reconstruction, this paper is essential reading for all surgeons reconstructing the breast as it simplifies a complex reconstructive problem into three key anatomic features, thereby providing an algorithm of sorts to produce consistent and aesthetically pleasing reconstructive results.*
- Blondeel PN, et al. Shaping the breast in aesthetic and reconstructive breast surgery: an easy three-step principle. Part II--Breast reconstruction after total mastectomy. Plast Reconstr Surg. 2009;123(3):794–805 [23].
- *Part two of the four-part series builds on the anatomic features discussed in part one and provides an approach to analysing the post-mastectomy breast. It explores differences in unilateral and bilateral breast reconstruction as well as primary* versus *delayed reconstruction providing key steps to addressing the breast footprint, conus and skin envelope. This is a must-read paper for any surgeon embarking on a career in breast reconstruction.*
- Hembd AS, et al. Intraoperative assessment of DIEP flap breast reconstruction using indocyanine green angiography: reduction of fat necrosis, resection volumes, and postoperative surveillance. Plast Reconstr Surg. 2020;146(1):1e–10e.

Acknowledgements We thank Julia Ruston for her illustrations in this chapter for the text and also the video.

References

1. Koshima I, Soeda S. Inferior epigastric artery skin flaps without rectus abdominis muscle. Br J Plast Surg. 1989;42(6):645–8.
2. Allen RJ, Treece P. Deep inferior epigastric perforator flap for breast reconstruction. Ann Plast Surg. 1994;32(1):32–8.
3. Moon HK, Taylor GI. The vascular anatomy of rectus abdominis musculocutaneous flaps based on the deep superior epigastric system. Plast Reconstr Surg. 1988;82(5):815–32.
4. Blondeel PN, et al. Doppler flowmetry in the planning of perforator flaps. Br J Plast Surg. 1998;51(3):202–9.
5. Bailey SH, et al. The single dominant medial row perforator DIEP flap in breast reconstruction: three-dimensional perforasome and clinical results. Plast Reconstr Surg. 2010;126(3):739–51.
6. Schaverien M, et al. Arterial and venous anatomies of the deep inferior epigastric perforator and superficial inferior epigastric artery flaps. Plast Reconstr Surg. 2008;121(6):1909–19.
7. Rozen WM, et al. The perforator angiosome: a new concept in the design of deep inferior epigastric artery perforator flaps for breast reconstruction. Microsurgery. 2010;30(1):1–7.
8. Rozen WM, et al. Avoiding denervation of rectus abdominis in DIEP flap harvest: the importance of medial row perforators. Plast Reconstr Surg. 2008;122(3):710–6.
9. Masia J, et al. Multidetector-row computed tomography in the planning of abdominal perforator flaps. J Plast Reconstr Aesthet Surg. 2006;59(6):594–9.
10. Hembd AS, et al. Intraoperative assessment of DIEP flap breast reconstruction using indocyanine green angiography: reduction of fat necrosis, resection volumes, and postoperative surveillance. Plast Reconstr Surg. 2020;146(1):1e–10e.

11. Momeni A, Sheckter C. Intraoperative laser-assisted indocyanine green imaging can reduce the rate of fat necrosis in microsurgical breast reconstruction. Plast Reconstr Surg. 2020;145(3):507e–13e.
12. Zhong T, et al. Transversus abdominis plane (TAP) catheters inserted under direct vision in the donor site following free DIEP and MS-TRAM breast reconstruction: a prospective cohort study of 45 patients. J Plast Reconstr Aesthet Surg. 2013;66(3):329–36.
13. Murray A, et al. Stacked abdominal flap for unilateral breast reconstruction. J Reconstr Microsurg. 2015;31(3):179–86.
14. Patel NG, et al. Stacked and bipedicled abdominal free flaps for breast reconstruction: considerations for shaping. Gland Surg. 2016;5(2):115–21.
15. Slezak S, McGibbon B, Dellon AL. The sensational transverse rectus abdominis musculocutaneous (TRAM) flap: return of sensibility after TRAM breast reconstruction. Ann Plast Surg. 1992;28(3):210–7.
16. Bijkerk E, et al. Breast sensibility in bilateral autologous breast reconstruction with unilateral sensory nerve coaptation. Breast Cancer Res Treat. 2020;181(3):599–610.
17. Klasson S, et al. Smoking increases donor site complications in breast reconstruction with DIEP flap. J Plast Surg Hand Surg. 2016;50(6):331–5.
18. Lee KT, Mun GH. Effects of obesity on postoperative complications after breast reconstruction using free muscle-sparing transverse rectus abdominis myocutaneous, deep inferior epigastric perforator, and superficial inferior epigastric artery flap: a systematic review and meta-analysis. Ann Plast Surg. 2016;76(5):576–84.
19. Butler DP, Woollard A, Grobbelaar AO. Dual-consultant led elective microsurgery: the implications on service provision and training. J Plast Reconstr Aesthet Surg. 2013;66(10):1435–6.
20. Canizares O, et al. Optimizing efficiency in deep inferior epigastric perforator flap breast reconstruction. Ann Plast Surg. 2015;75(2):186–92.
21. Dancey A, Blondeel PN. Technical tips for safe perforator vessel dissection applicable to all perforator flaps. Clin Plast Surg. 2010;37(4):593–606, xi–vi.
22. Blondeel PN, et al. Shaping the breast in aesthetic and reconstructive breast surgery: an easy three-step principle. Plast Reconstr Surg. 2009;123(2):455–62.
23. Blondeel PN, et al. Shaping the breast in aesthetic and reconstructive breast surgery: an easy three-step principle. Part II--Breast reconstruction after total mastectomy. Plast Reconstr Surg. 2009;123(3):794–805.

20. Inferior and Superior Epigastric Artery Flaps: The Rectus Abdominis Muscle Flap

Matthew Wordsworth, Dariush Nikkhah, Alex Woollard, and Norbert Kang

20.1 Introduction

The deep inferior epigastric artery is a workhorse of reconstructive plastic surgery. It can be raised as a muscle flap or as a myofasciocutaneous flap with a wide range of skin paddles; the inferior epigastric artery supplies the largest skin area on the body. It is most commonly used as a fasciocutaneous flap in breast reconstruction (the DIEP flap) or as a transverse rectus abdominis myofasciocutaneous flap (the TRAM flap). As an inferiorly based pedicled flap, the tissue pivots at the level of the pubis, and the flap is used for perineal, groin and lower trunk reconstruction, usually with a vertically orientated skin paddle (the VRAM flap). The rectus abdominis muscle can also be raised on the superior epigastric artery, as a pedicled flap to reconstruct chest wall and midline sternal defects.

In the 1970s a number of surgeons had published on using a superiorly based pedicled rectus muscle flap for breast and chest wall reconstruction, but the first use of the inferior epigastric artery free rectus muscle flap was by published by Pennington et al. [1]. The work of Taylor et al. [2] demonstrated the dense anastomotic network between the superficial and deep inferior epigastric vessels and reliability of the skin perforators. The rectus abdominis flap has been described in both limb and head and neck reconstruction, but it is most commonly used when the abdomen has been opened as part of the resection surgery. Pedicled VRAMs in perineal reconstruction have been shown to reduce wound healing complications in irradiated abdominoperineal resection defects [3].

20.2 Anatomy

The rectus abdominis muscle can be easily palpated and visualised in slim patients. The medial border is the midline, the linea alba, and the lateral border is the linea semilunaris. The rectus abdominis muscle is 7–10 cm wide and is a long muscle stretching from its origin at the cartilaginous union of the lower ribs and xiphisternum to the insertion at the symphysis and crest of the pubis bone. The muscle is segmented by three (rarely four) tendinous insertions running horizontally creating the colloquially named 'six-pack' appearance. Anterior to the rectus muscle throughout its length is the anterior rectus sheath consisting of the aponeurosis of the external oblique muscle and the anterior aponeurosis of the internal oblique muscle. The posterior rectus sheath consists of the posterior aponeurosis of the internal oblique and the aponeurosis of the transversus abdominis muscle until that sheath ends at the horizontal level of the anterior superior iliac spine: the arcuate line. Caudal to the arcuate line, the rectus muscle therefore only lies on the transversalis fascia and parietal peritoneum (Fig. 20.1). The rectus abdominis muscle is innervated segmentally by terminal branches of the intercostal nerves from the sixth to twelfth ribs; these nerves enter the muscle posteriorly on the lateral third of the muscle.

The rectus abdominis flap has a Mathes and Nahai type III arterial supply with two dominant and minor pedicles. The dominant pedicles are the superior and inferior epigastric arteries. The internal mammary artery and vein become the superior epigastric vessels and insert into the superior third of the rectus muscle posteriorly and medially. The superior epigastric vessels anastomose in the middle third of the muscle with the inferior epigastric artery and vein, a branch of

---

M. Wordsworth (✉)
Royal Centre for Defence Medicine, Birmingham, UK
e-mail: matt.wordsworth1@nhs.net

D. Nikkhah · A. Woollard · N. Kang
Royal Free Hospital, London, UK
e-mail: d.nikkhah@nhs.net

© Springer Nature Switzerland AG 2023
D. Nikkhah et al. (eds.), *Core Techniques in Flap Reconstructive Microsurgery*, https://doi.org/10.1007/978-3-031-07678-7_20

Fig. 20.1 Rectus sheath anatomy

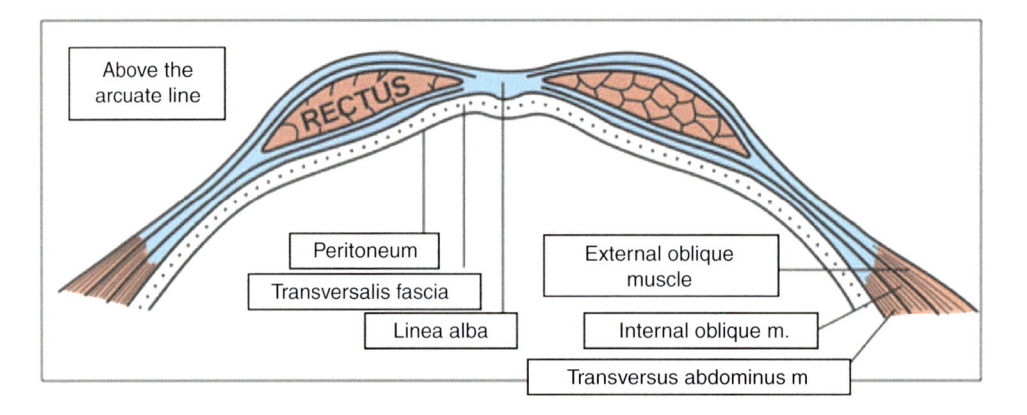

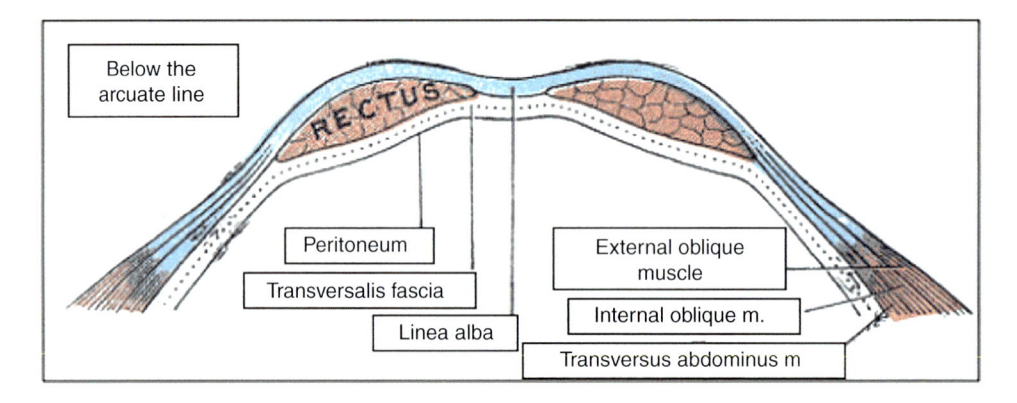

the external iliac artery and vein. The inferior epigastric artery pierces the transversalis fascia and enters the muscle at the inferior aspect of the middle third, posteriorly and in the lateral aspect of the muscle. The minor pedicles are six small intercostal arteries and one subcostal artery that enter the deep aspect of the muscle and anastomose with the epigastric arteries. Anatomical variability exists with the number of anastomoses between the superior and inferior epigastrics and where the deep inferior epigastric vessels enter the muscle (usually 3 cm caudally to the arcuate line)—see Moon and Taylor [4] for more detail. The inferior epigastric artery is typically 2–4 mm diameter and 5–10 cm pedicle length can be harvested. Venous drainage is from two venae comitantes with one vein usually similar in size to the artery.

20.3 Preoperative Investigation

Skin perforators in the rectus abdominis flap can be simply identified using handheld Doppler. CT angiography is not mandated but is recommended in instances where previous surgery may have affected the normal vascular anatomy of the inferior and superior epigastric arteries. Preoperative CT angiography reduces the duration of surgery in DIEP breast reconstruction, and this may be applicable when mobilising the inferior epigastric artery in the setting of a rectus abdominis flap.

20.4 Flap Design and Markings

The design of the rectus abdominis flap depends on which components are required. The flap can be raised as a muscle-only flap but it is more commonly used with a skin paddle. The skin paddle can be orientated vertically, horizontally or obliquely. The para-umbilical perforators are the most crucial for skin perfusion, and therefore the fasciocutaneous portion of the flap should not be dissected from the central portion of the rectus muscle belly. An extended VRAM that incorporates a vertical skin paddle with an oblique extension to the costal margin has been described by Villa et al. [5]. The size of the skin paddle is determined by the requirements of the defect and what can be closed directly in the donor site.

20.5 Flap Raise/Elevation

In this description a pedicled myocutaneous flap is used with a vertical skin paddle over the middle and upper portion of the rectus for a perineal reconstruction after an open abdominoperineal resection, for example, for the excision of a low rectal carcinoma.

Step 1: Skin Marking Choose the side, contralateral to any planned or current stoma or significant scars. Mark the midline, and curve around the umbilicus so that it is not incorpo-

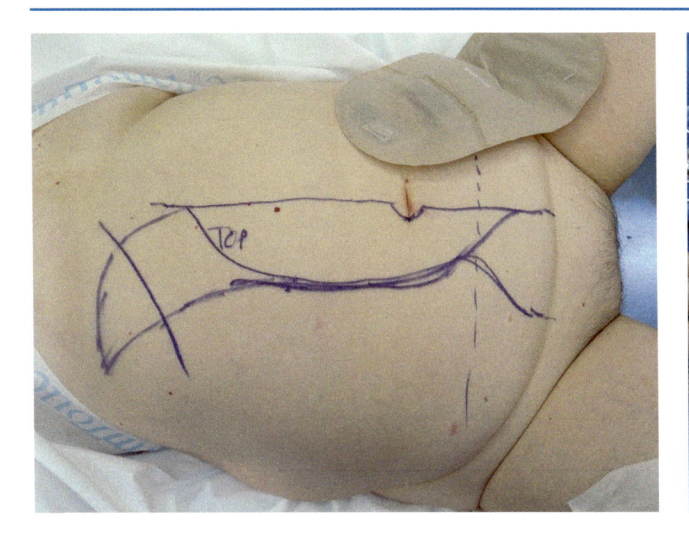

Fig. 20.2 Skin marking for a vertical rectus abdominis myocutaneous flap

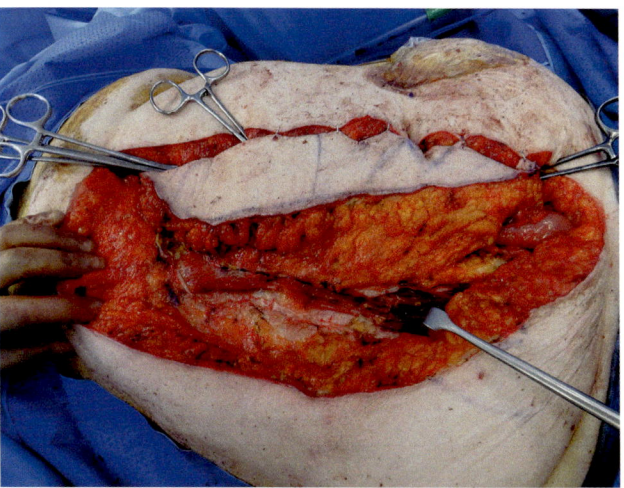

Fig. 20.3 Incision to the anterior rectus sheath

rated in the flap. Palpate and mark 7–10 cm laterally to mark the linea semilunaris which is the lateral border of the rectus muscle. Draw the costal margin to mark the superior limit of the muscle, and draw a horizontal line across from ASIS to ASIS to mark the arcuate line. Check the degree of skin laxity in the abdomen for direct closure and draw the skin paddle over the rectus muscle. The size of the skin paddle can be templated on the defect. Ensure the base of the skin paddle is located over the periumbilical perforators (Fig. 20.2).

Step 2: Identifying the Perforators Incise the midline skin and subcutaneous fat down to the anterior rectus sheath fascial layer. Blunt dissect at the periumbilical region to carefully visualise perforators coming through the rectus fascia into the skin and fat of the flap.

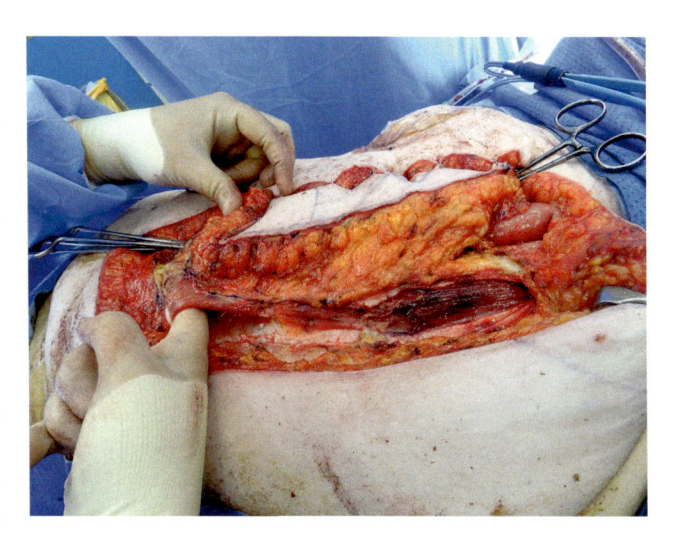

Fig. 20.4 Raising the cranial end of the rectus abdominis muscle prior to dividing it

Step 3: Raising the Anterior Sheath Incise the lateral skin and subcutaneous edge of the flap down to the semilunaris (Fig. 20.3). The portion of rectus sheath containing the perforators is islanded from the rest of the rectus sheath by extending the sheath incision vertically on the medial and lateral edge of the sheath. A fascial incision inferior and superior to the perforators to join the lateral and medial incisions completes the island of the rectus fascia. The rectus sheath should ideally not be cut below the arcuate line as this risks a hernia due to a lack of posterior rectus sheath below this point. Vertically incise the rectus sheath in the middle of the muscle superior to the perforators, and divide the muscle horizontally (Fig. 20.4). Identify and clip the superior epigastric vessels within the rectus muscle.

Step 4: Mobilising the Rectus Muscle The flap is freed from the remaining rectus sheath. There are adhesions at the tendinous intersections of the rectus muscle, but the muscle belly is otherwise easily mobilised off the sheath. Start by completing the dissection of the muscle off of the sheath anteriorly, then around the medial edge and onto the posterior sheath towards the lateral edge. The pedicle will be visible on the posterior surface of the muscle. Medially is an avascular plane, laterally there are anastomoses between the pedicle and the lower intercostal vessels and the segmental nerve innervation will also need dividing.

Step 5: Mobilising the Pedicle Once the rectus muscle is free from the sheath, the deep interior epigastric artery pedicle and venae comitantes should be mobilised into the pelvis (Fig. 20.5). The pivot point for the pedicled flap is the origin at deep inferior epigastric artery from the external iliac artery at the inguinal ligament. For pedicled perineal reconstruction, the flap is to be rotated medially and passed down

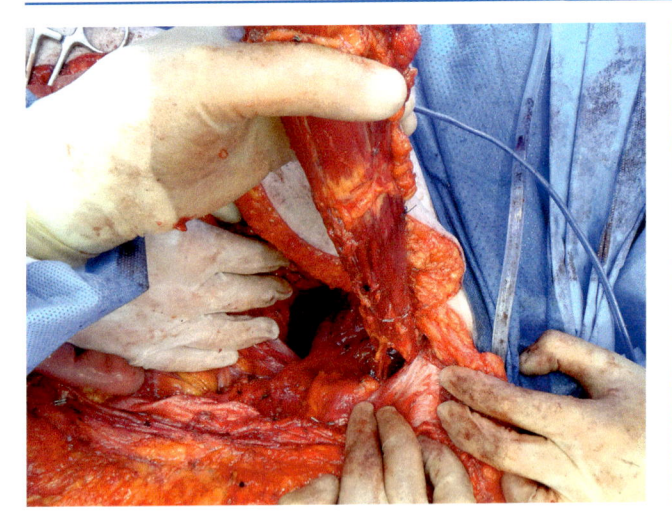

Fig. 20.5 Mobilising the pedicle into the pelvis

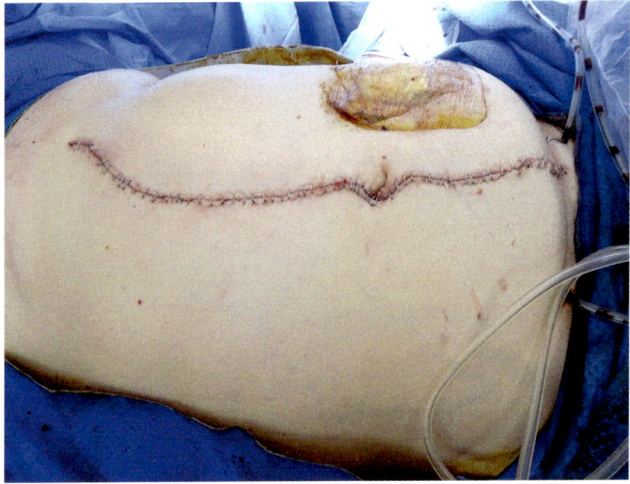

Fig. 20.7 Donor site closed

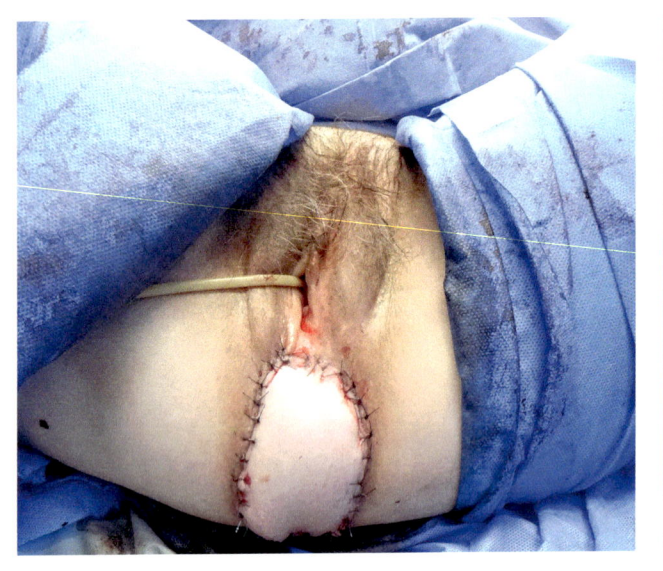

Fig. 20.6 An inset flap

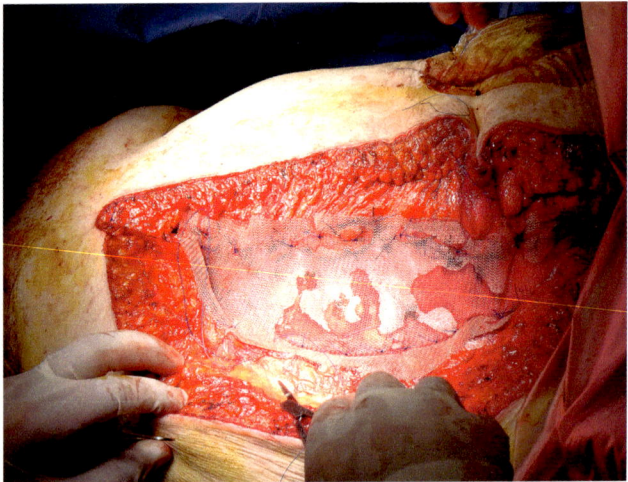

Fig. 20.8 Onlay mesh closure of the anterior sheath

through the pelvis to fill the defect. The transversalis defect needs to be sufficient to prevent constriction of the pedicle. If the flap is being used as a free flap, then the pedicle is divided close to the origin which provides 5–10 cm of pedicle length and usually a 2–3 mm diameter artery.

Step 6: **Insetting the Flap and Closing the Donor Site** For the pedicled reconstruction, the flap is passed down into the pelvis under direct vision and brought through the perineal defect. The inferior insertion of the rectus muscle can be partially or completely divided if it is limiting the pedicle's reach. The skin island can be temporarily stapled in position to adjust the size of the skin island if required and to check that there is no tension on the pedicle. The flap can then be inset in layers (Fig. 20.6). Where possible the anterior rectus sheath should be closed directly. An onlay mesh may be indicated to strengthen the anterior rectus sheath repair (Fig. 20.7). The donor site skin can be closed directly (Fig. 20.8).

20.6 Core Surgical Techniques in Flap Dissection

Step 1 When marking the midline, check the rectus abdominis has not been lateralised by a diastasis; the degree of diastasis can be assessed preoperatively on CT.

Step 2 Incise the skin with a blade and the subcutaneous tissue with a monopolar diathermy.

Step 3 Dividing the superior rectus muscle can be done quickly and cleanly with a linear stapler. When mobilising the rectus muscle off the sheath, keep gentle traction on the

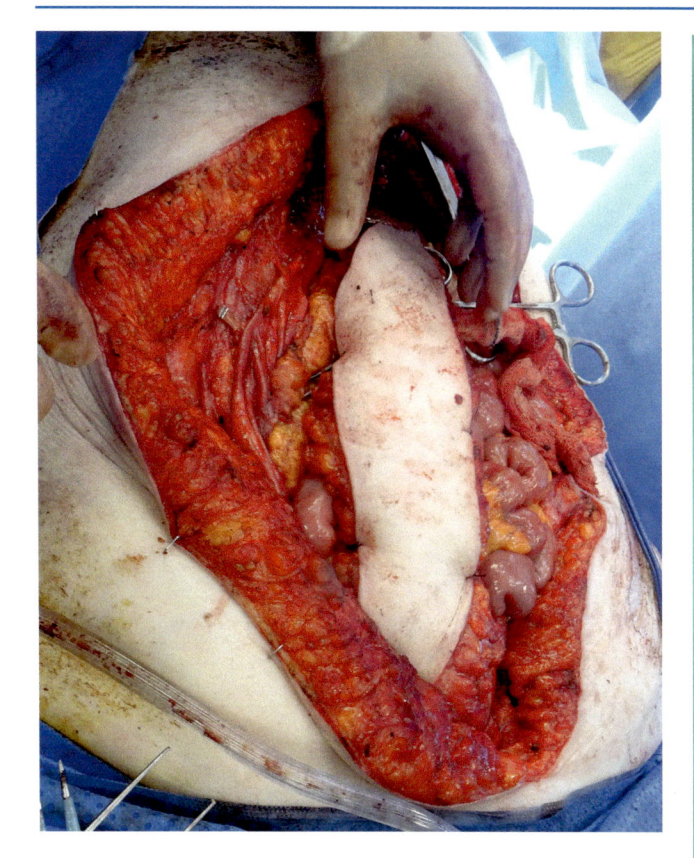

Fig. 20.9 Suturing the skin island to the muscle to prevent shearing

edge of the sheath with Allis clamps. When incising the sheath, leave a cuff of rectus sheath adjacent to the linea alba and linea semilunaris to facilitate direct closure (or mesh attachment if needed).

When mobilising the muscle to prevent shear forces on the perforators, a tacking suture can be placed from skin island edge through the muscle edge to the cut fascial edge (Fig. 20.9).

Step 4 The lateral edge of the rectus abdominis muscle is best delineated from a posterior approach. Branches can be clipped, and smaller branches can be cauterised with bipolar.

Step 5 The pedicle can kink on the transversalis fascia when rotated down into the pelvis so it should be fully mobilised. Partial division of the medial attachments of the rectus abdominis pelvic insertion allows for increased reach, whilst leaving the lateral musculotendinous fibres intact protects the pedicle from excessive traction.

Step 6 A layered and meticulous closure is critical to a good outcome. The rectus abdominis muscle can be inset as a sling to obliterate the dead space; the Scarpa's fascia can be

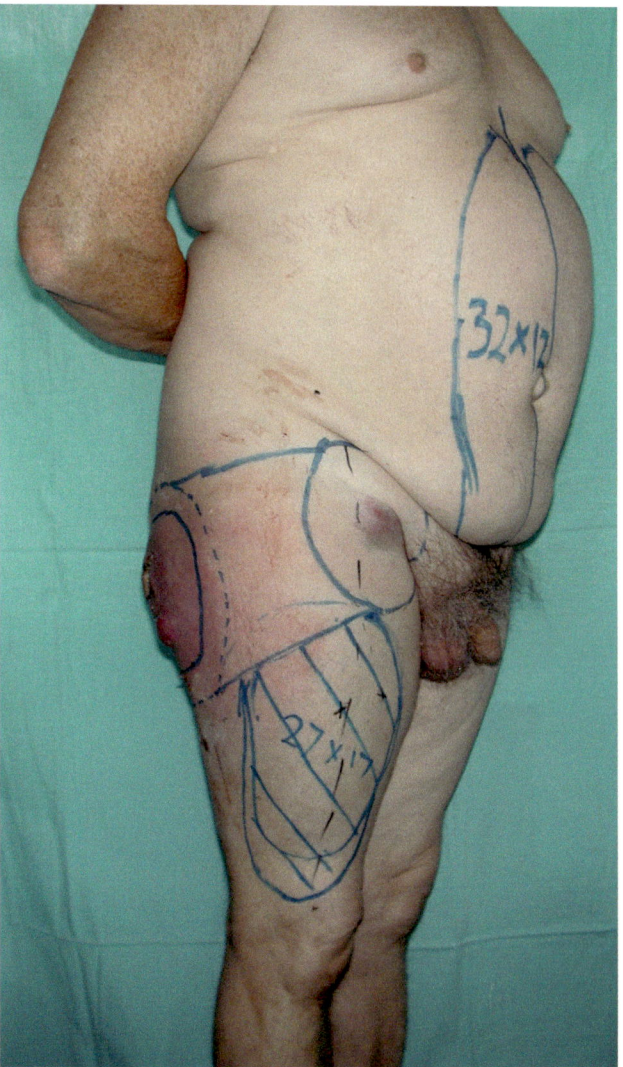

Fig. 20.10 An example of flap planning for a combined pedicled VRAM and ALT flaps to reconstruct the planned excision of a Merkel cell carcinoma and lymph node

sutured to the levator ani muscle layer. It is easier to de-epithelialise any areas of the skin if required prior to delivering the flap into the perineum.

20.7 Clinical Scenario

The patient pictured has a Merkel cell carcinoma of the right gluteal skin region with a metastatic lymph node in the right groin. The lesion and node are excised en bloc with appropriate margins leaving a large soft tissue defect (Fig. 20.10).

A pedicled anterolateral thigh flap was used to reconstruct the lower half (Fig. 20.11). The rectus abdominis flap donor site was closed directly, and the anterolateral thigh flap donor site was grafted with a split thickness skin graft (Fig. 20.12).

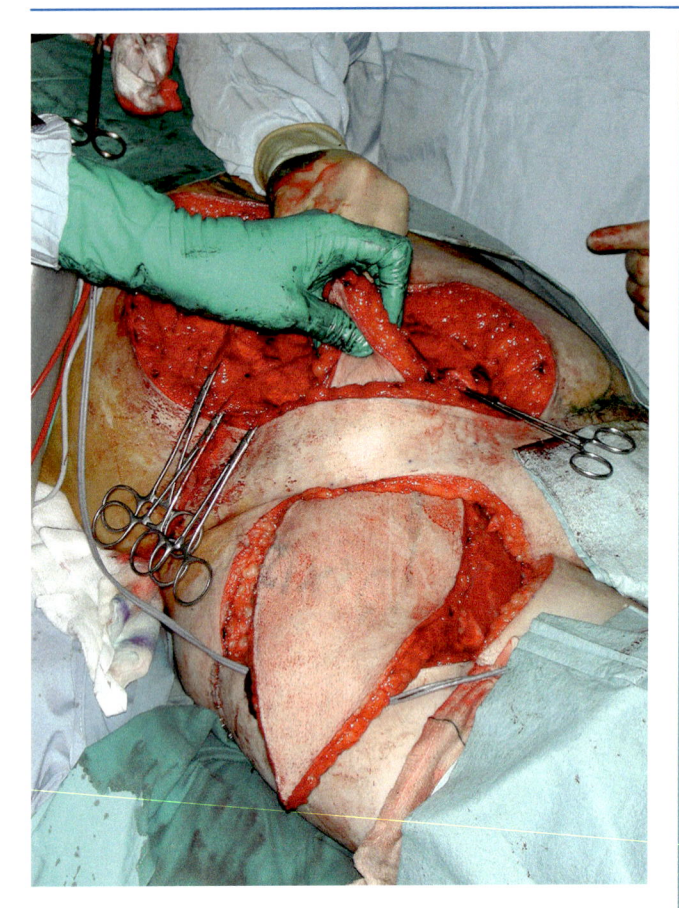

Fig. 20.11 Intraoperative reconstruction using a pedicled rectus abdominis flap passing under a tunnel of lower abdominal skin to reconstruct the superior half of the defect

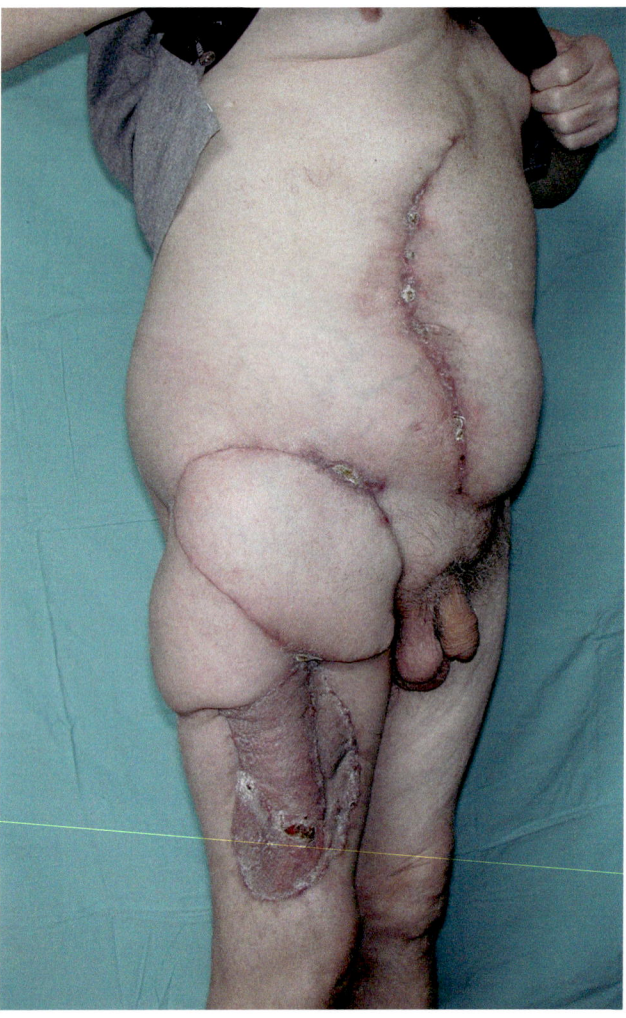

Fig. 20.12 Postoperative appearance of the inset flaps

20.8 Pearls and Pitfalls

Pearls
- The male pelvis is longer than the female and will therefore require a longer length of the VRAM flap to reconstruct a perineal defect.
- The arcuate line is not visible directly so mark the skin and respect the boundary to reduce the risk of postoperative hernia.
- The easiest way to find the pedicle is approaching the vessels from medial to lateral on the posterior surface of the rectus muscle and following it caudally.
- A strip of muscle lateral to the pedicle can be left as it will remain innervated and vascularised by the lateral supply of the intercostal neuromuscular bundle. The dissection is more challenging and time-consuming.
- If there is difficulty closing the donor site, consider a component separation to achieve tension-free closure.

Pitfalls
- If the superior epigastric artery is not identified and clipped during the division of the superior portion of the rectus muscle, it may retract into the proximal muscle and bleed.
- If the skin paddle is not carefully handled, it can shear on the anterior rectus sheath damaging the perforators.
- The inferior insertion of the rectus prevents traction injury to the pedicle as the flap is moved into the pelvis. If the muscle is released inferiorly, take care not to stretch the pedicle.
- If the anterior rectus sheath is incised below the arcuate line, a postoperative hernia is more likely so a mesh reinforcement is necessary.
- If the pedicle is not fully mobilised, it can be compressed by the transversalis fascia when the flap is pedicled into the perineum.

20.9 Selected Readings

- McMenamin DM, et al. Rectus abdominis myocutaneous flaps for perineal reconstruction: Modifications to the technique based on a large single-centre experience. Ann R Coll Surg Engl. 2011;93(5):375–81.
- *A British case series with useful pearls and technical discussion.*
- Rai R, et al. Tendinous inscriptions of the rectus abdominis: a comprehensive review. Cureus. 2018;10(8)e3100.
- *Detail on tendinous inscription and discusses the muscular anatomy and segmental innervation of the rectus abdominis.*
- Lejour M, Dome M. Abdominal wall function after rectus abdominis transfer. Plast Reconstr Surg. 1991;87(6):1054–68.
- *Discussion and data on donor site morbidity.*
- Campbell CA, Butler CE. Use of adjuvant techniques improves surgical outcomes of complex vertical rectus abdominis myocutaneous flap reconstructions of pelvic cancer defects. Plast Reconstr Surg. 2011;128(2):447–58.
- *Six technical modification to reduce wound healing complications.*
- Cordeiro PG, Santamaria E. A classification system and algorithm for reconstruction of maxillectomy and midfacial defects. Plast Reconstr Surg. 2000;105(70):2331–46.
- *An algorithm for mid facial reconstruction using the rectus muscle free flap.*

References

1. Pennington DG, Lai MF, Pelly AD. The rectus abdominis myocutaneous free flap. Br J Plast Surg. 1980;33(2):277–82.
2. Taylor GI, et al. The extended deep inferior epigastric flap. Plast Reconstr Surg. 1983;72(6):751–65.
3. Butler CE, Gündeslioglu AÖ, Rodriguez-Bigas MA. Outcomes of immediate vertical rectus abdominis myocutaneous flap reconstruction for irradiated abdominoperineal resection defects. J Am Coll Surg. 2008;206(4):694–703.
4. Moon HK, Taylor GI. The vascular anatomy of rectus abdominis musculocutaneous flaps based on the deep superior epigastric system. Plast Reconstr Surg. 1988;82(5):815–32.
5. Villa M, et al. Extended vertical rectus abdominis myocutaneous flap for pelvic reconstruction: three-dimensional and four-dimensional computed tomography angiographic perfusion study and clinical outcome analysis. Plast Reconstr Surg. 2011;127(1):200–9.

21

Superficial Inferior Epigastric Artery and Superficial Circumflex Iliac Artery Perforator Combined Flaps

Hidehiko Yoshimatsu, Yuma Fuse, Ryo Karakawa, and Akitatsu Hayashi

21.1 Introduction

The superficial inferior epigastric artery (SIEA) flap has been widely used in autologous breast reconstruction for small to medium breasts. Dissection of the pedicle does not entail intramuscular dissection, thus resulting in low donor site morbidity. The SIEA flap is also indicated for coverage of a small- to medium-sized defect, especially when the superficial circumflex iliac artery (SCIA) perforator (SCIP) flap cannot be used due to scars from previous surgeries.

A unique application of the SIEA flap is combining the flap with the SCIP flap to cover a large defect. For coverage of large defects, using multi-lobed flaps, KISS flap, and multi-lobed latissimus dorsi musculocutaneous flap have been reported by Zhang et al. A combined bilobed flap consisting of the SCIP flap and the SIEA flap allowed a flap coverage strategy that can be applied in a prone position with minimal donor site morbidity (with no muscular sacrifice and little or no muscular dissection). Using this strategy of combined flaps, a large flap up to 20 x 20 cm can be obtained with primary closure of the donor site. The bilobed design allows coverage of three-dimensional convex defects, especially useful for coverage of the knee, the elbow, and the scalp, while maintaining minimal donor site morbidity.

21.2 Anatomy (Fig. 21.1)

The SIEA takes off from the femoral artery 1–3 cm below the inguinal ligament, sharing a common branch with the SCIA in 33–48% of cases (Fig. 21.2). After penetrating the Scarpa's fascia just superior to the inguinal ligament, the SIEA ascend lateral to the linea semilunaris. The branches from the SIEA do not cross the midline in most cases, thus limiting its angiosome. Unlike the deep inferior epigastric artery (DIEA), which runs beneath the rectus abdominis muscle giving off perforators to the adipose layer and the skin paddle, the SIEA runs toward the superficial layer of the adipose tissue as it travels in the superior direction. This peculiar characteristic allows a fairly thin axial-pattern flap. Although a high absence rate (35%) of the SIEA was reported in historical works, a recent study using modern imaging

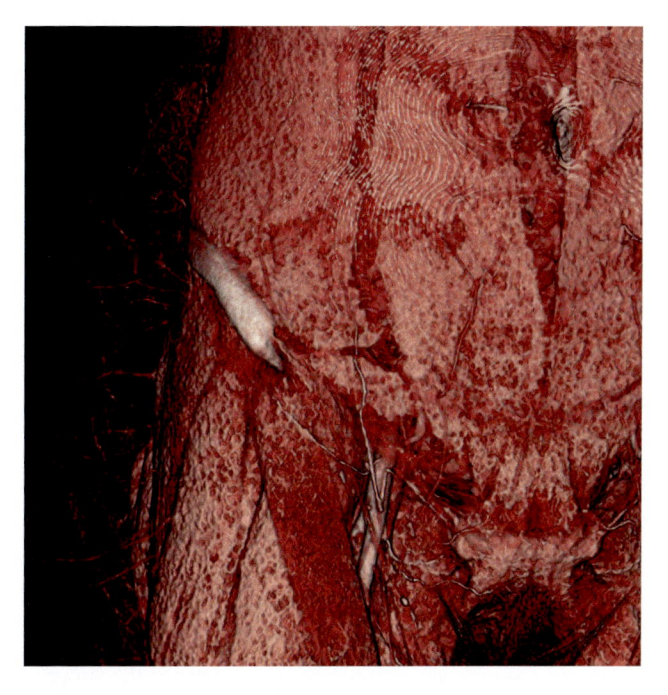

Fig. 21.1 Reconctructed image of CT anigography of the groin arteries

H. Yoshimatsu (✉) · Y. Fuse · R. Karakawa
Department of Plastic and Reconstructive Surgery, Cancer Institute Hospital of the Japanese Foundation for Cancer Research, Tokyo, Japan

A. Hayashi
Lymphedema Center, Kameda General Hospital, Chiba, Japan

© Springer Nature Switzerland AG 2023
D. Nikkhah et al. (eds.), *Core Techniques in Flap Reconstructive Microsurgery*, https://doi.org/10.1007/978-3-031-07678-7_21

Fig. 21.2 Anatomical variations of the SIEA and the SCIA

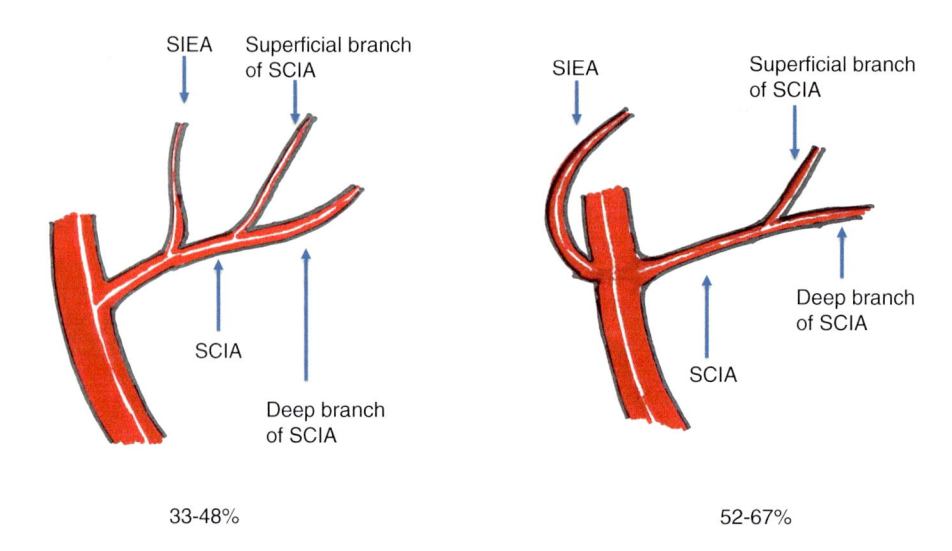

33–48%   52–67%

techniques identified the SIEA in 94% of cases. The average diameter of the SIEA is 1.4 mm (0.6–2.0 mm). The superficial inferior epigastric vein (SIEV) and the superficial circumflex iliac vein (SCIV) consist of the main venous drainage system in the lower abdomen and the groin area. The venae comitantes of the SIEA and the SCIA work as additional drainage. The SIEV runs with the SIEA in some cases, but in many cases, the SIEV runs parallel to and 4 cm medial to the SIEA at the inguinal ligament level.

After branching off from the femoral artery, the superficial circumflex iliac artery (SCIA) bifurcates into the superficial branch and the deep branch. While the superficial branch gives off perforators to the skin, the deep branch runs beneath the deep fascia, giving off branches to the sartorius muscle and the iliac bone. The transverse branch of the deep branch, which runs in the lateral direction, is given off from the deep branch of the SCIA approximately 2.5 cm caudal to the ASIS. The transverse branch can be used as a guideline to identify the deep branch.

21.3 Preoperative Investigation

Preoperative CT angiography is highly recommended to identify the SIEA and the SIEV. If CT angiography cannot be used, Doppler ultrasonography or handheld Doppler should be used to mark the course of the SIEA and the SIEV. When planning a SCIP-SIEA combined flap, the use of CT angiography or Doppler ultrasonography is highly recommended to evaluate whether the SCIA and the SIEA share a common trunk. For elevation of the SCIP flap, handheld Doppler should suffice. The course of the superficial branch of the SCIA can be detected with handheld Doppler.

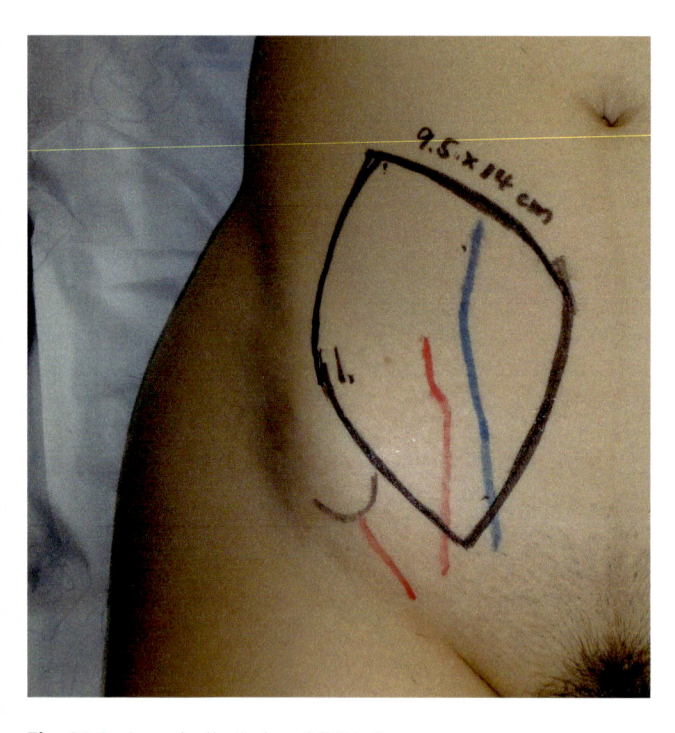

Fig. 21.3 A vertically designed SIEA flap

21.4 Flap Design and Markings

For use in autologous breast reconstruction, the SIEA flap is designed similar to the DIEP flap, in an abdominoplasty-like fashion. The perfusion of the flap should be evaluated with intraoperative indocyanine (ICG) angiography after the elevation, and malperfused regions should be discarded.

For use in other purposes, a vertically designed SIEA flap, which allows direct closure of the donor site, should be designed with the SIEA and the SIEV situated in the middle of the skin

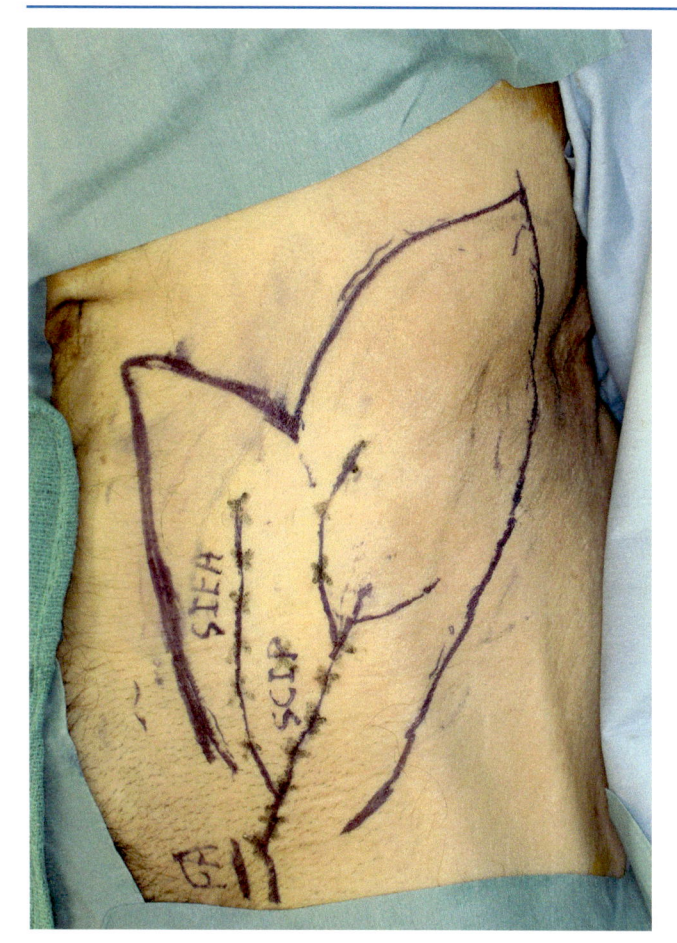

Fig. 21.4 A SIEA-SCIP combined bilobed flap for coverage of larger defects

paddle (Fig. 21.3). The width of the flap is determined by the laxity of the abdominal tissue, usually between 9 and 12 cm. The length of the flap can exceed the umbilicus, reaching 20 cm, but the perfusion should be confirmed intraoperatively using the ICG angiography. When a certain pedicle length is required, the skin paddle should be designed superiorly. The pedicle length should be expected to be around 5 cm in these cases.

To cover a large defect with minimal donor site morbidity, the SIEA flap can be combined with the SCIP flap (Fig. 21.4). For this bilobed flap, the preoperative examination should be performed with CT angiography or color Doppler ultrasonography to evaluate whether the SIEA and the SCIA share a common trunk. The width of each flap is determined by the laxity of the tissue, but in many cases, a 10 cm width can be achieved in both flaps, resulting in a combined width of 20 cm.

21.5 Flap Raise/Elevation: A Step-by-Step Guide

21.5.1 Vertical SIEA Flap (Figs. 21.5, 21.6, 21.7, and 21.8)

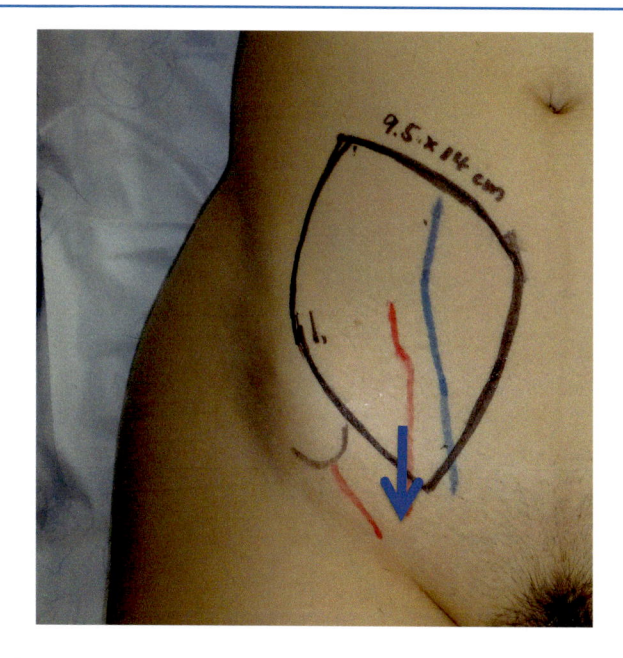

Fig. 21.5 An incision (blue arrow) is placed over the inferior markings of the SIEA and the SIEV

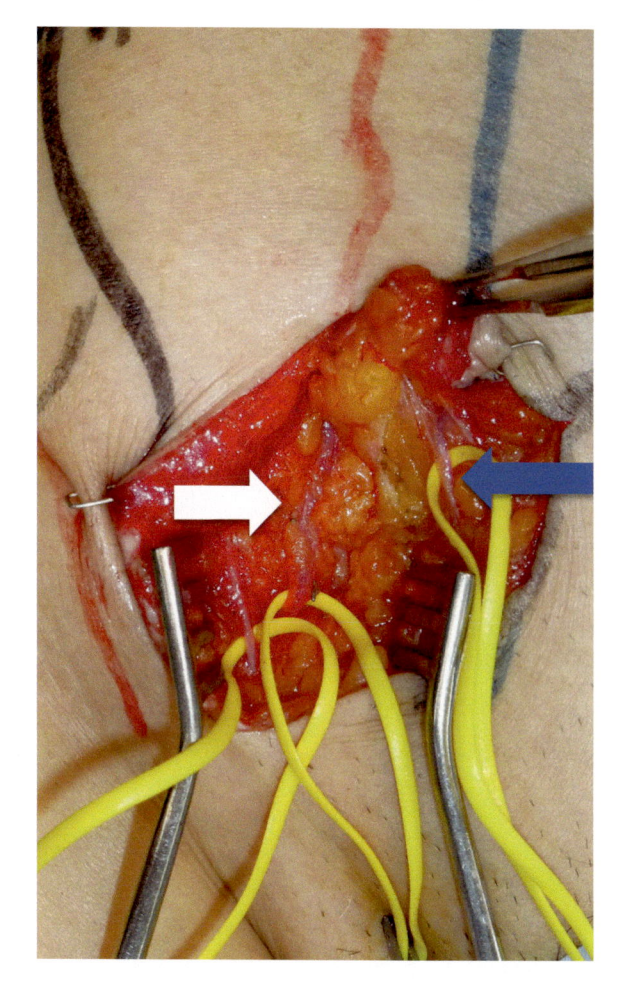

Fig. 21.6 The SIEA and the SIEV are looked for in the adipose tissue. The SIEA (white arrow) and the SIEV (blue arrow) are found and dissected

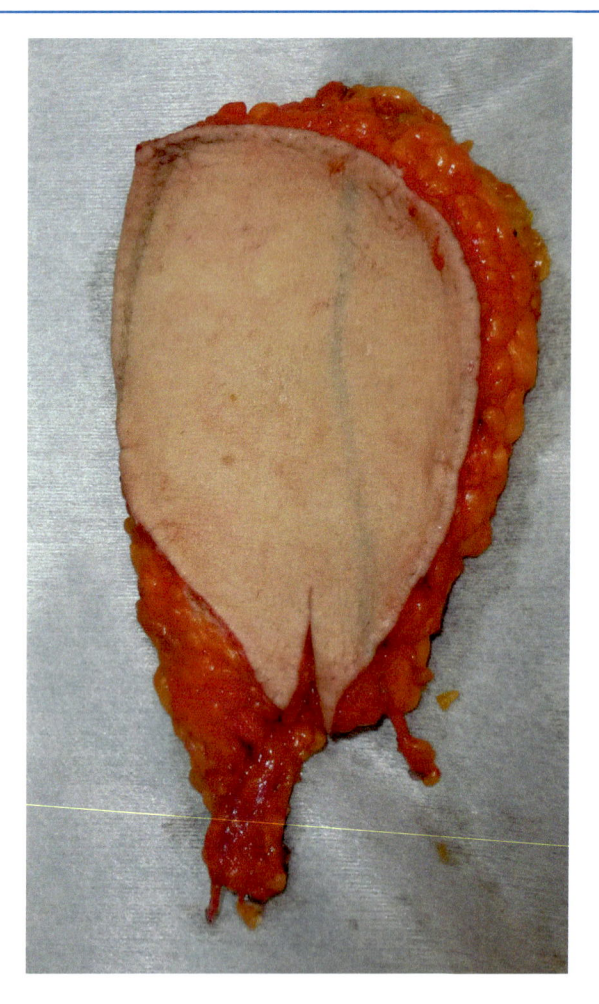

Fig. 21.7 An incision is made around the flap design. The flap can be elevated from the cephalad to the caudal at a dissection plane immediately above the deep fascia

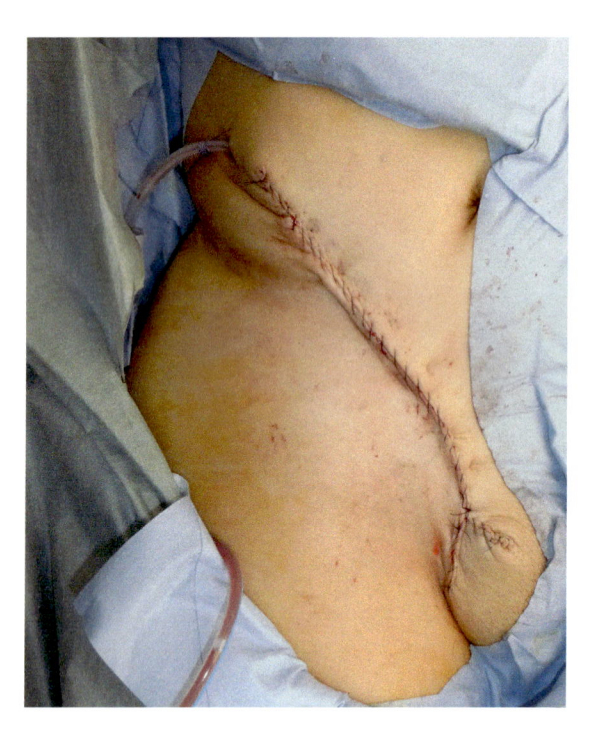

Fig. 21.8 The donor site is closed primarily in a multilayer fashion over a drain

21.5.2 SCIP-SIEA Combined Flap (Figs. 21.9, 21.10, 21.11, and 21.12)

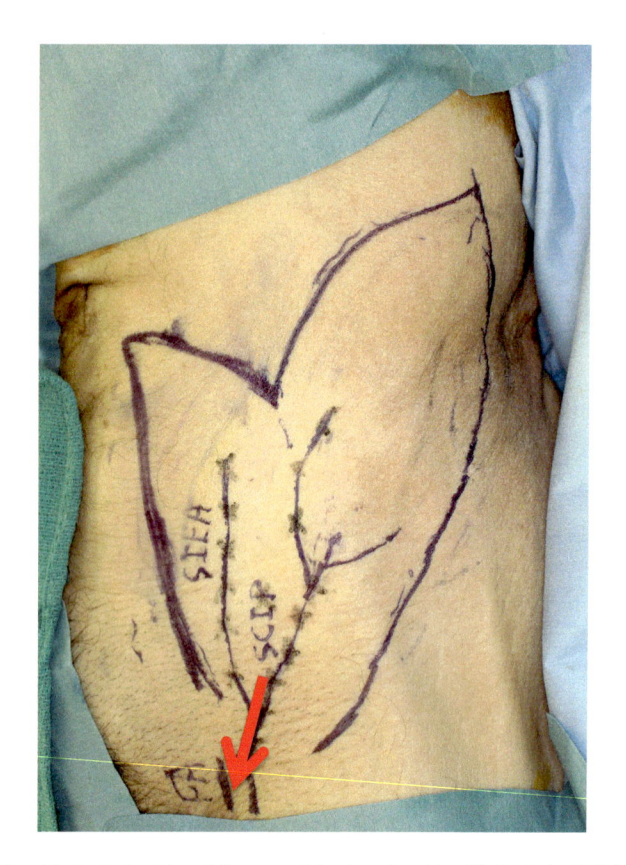

Fig. 21.9 An incision (blue arrow) is placed to identify both the SIEA and the SCIA

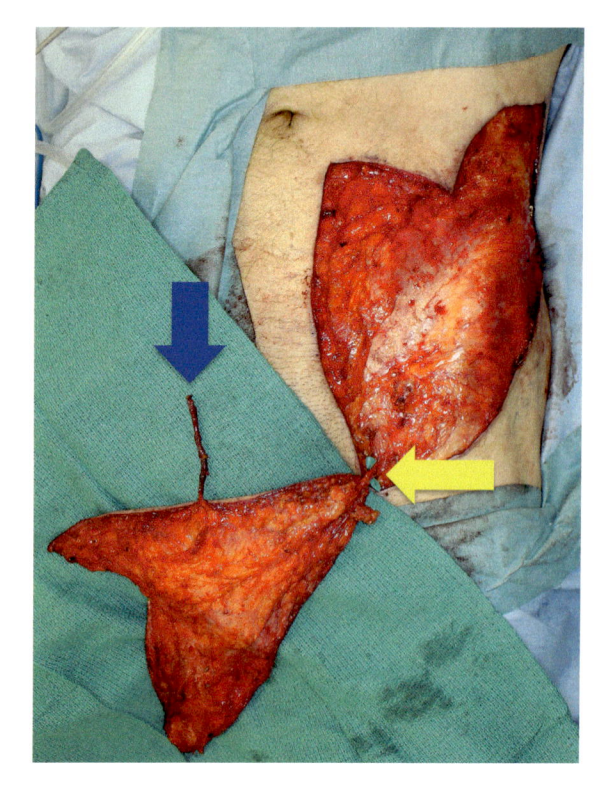

Fig. 21.10 After identification of the SIEA, the SCIA (yellow arrow), the SIEV (blue arrow), and the SCIV (yellow arrow), the flap is elevated above the deep fascia

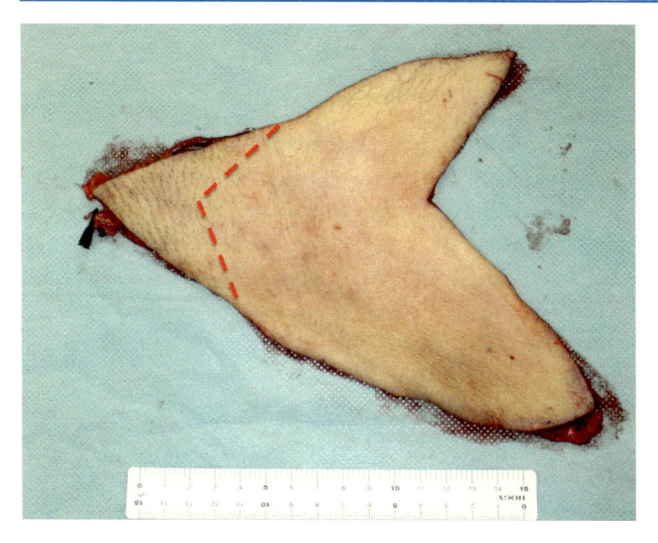

Fig. 21.11 A longer pedicle can be obtained by placing the caudal edge of the skin paddle superiorly (red dotted line)

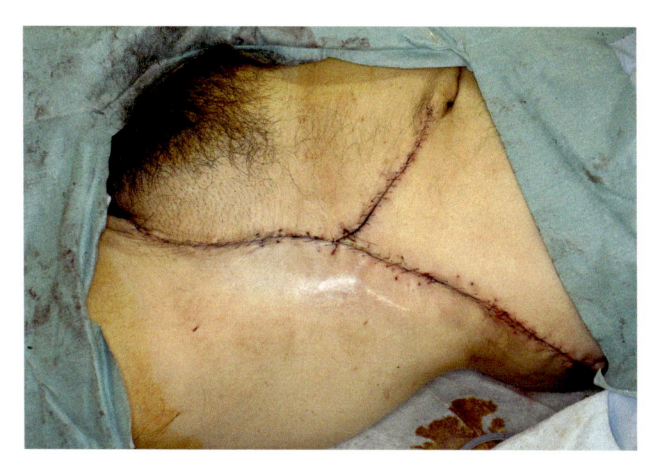

Fig. 21.12 The donor site is directly closed in a multilayer fashion over a drain

21.6 Core Surgical Techniques in Flap Dissection

21.6.1 Vertical SIEA Flap

1. Preoperative identification of the SIEA is critical for success. Precise markings of the pedicle are possible when Doppler ultrasonography is used.
2. Identification and dissection of the SIEA is the crux of the elevation. Meticulous care should be taken at this step since the SIEA can be located at a superficial layer, usually just beneath the Camper's fascia. The authors prefer using a monopolar cautery device set at 15/15 for this purpose. Meticulous hemostasis maintains a clear surgical field and thus is the key to the successful identification of the vessels. The depth of the SIEA should be confirmed with preoperative CT angiography or Doppler ultrasonography. If the identified SIEA is not pulsating or its diameter is smaller than 1.0 mm at its takeoff from the femoral artery, conversion to other flaps (e.g., DIEP flap or SCIP flap) should be considered.
3. The SIEA runs superficially as it takes its cephalad course; the flap can be elevated safely including the SIEA and the SIEV if the dissection plane is set at the layer where the SIEA and the SIEV were found. The authors use a monopolar cautery device set at 30/30 for this procedure.
4. The patient should be informed of the displacement of the umbilicus.

21.6.2 SCIP-SIEA Combined Flap

1. The side where the SIEA and the SCIA share a common trunk should be selected as the donor site when possible. If they do not share a common trunk, two arterial anastomoses will be necessary. As for the SCIA, either the superficial branch or the deep branch of the SCIA can be used as the pedicle.
2. If the diameter of the SIEA is smaller than 0.5 mm, a deep inferior epigastric artery perforator (DIEP) found within the flap design can be used. For minimal donor site morbidity, the DIEP dissection can be limited to its takeoff point from the DIEA. If the SCIA and the SIEA share origins, a single arterial anastomosis is made. If they do not, both arteries are anastomosed. The anastomosis of both the SIEV and SCIV is recommended, which will sometimes require intra-flap anastomosis.
3. The same pedicle elongation method can be applied in vertically designed SIEA flaps.
4. The patient should be informed of the displacement of the umbilicus.

21.7 Clinical Scenario

The SIEA flap is indicated for coverage of small- to medium-sized defect, when the SCIP flap cannot be used due to previous surgical history, etc. The flap can be converted from the SCIP flap to the SIEA flap if the SIEA is larger than the SCIA.

The SCIP-SIEA combined flap is indicated for coverage of large defects (up to 20 × 20 cm). The bilobed design allows coverage of three-dimensional convex defects, especially useful for coverage of the knee, the elbow, and the scalp.

21.8 Pearls and Pitfalls

Pearls
- When an adequate pedicle is found, the elevation of the SIEA is rather simple since it does not involve intramuscular dissection of the pedicle.
- A relatively thin skin paddle can be expected even in obese patients because the SIEA runs in a superficial layer.
- When the SIEA and the SCIA do not share a common trunk, either the superficial or the deep branch of the SCIA can be used for the recipient artery for the SIEA.
- The DIEP can serve as the backup flap for the SIEA in the SIEA-SCIP combined flap.
- Because the anatomy can be complicated at times, the dissection of the proximal portion of the SIEA and the SCIA should be done under a surgical microscope.

Pitfalls
- Conversion to other flaps (e.g., DIEP flap or SCIP flap) should be considered when the exposed SIEA is not pulsating or its diameter is smaller than 1.0 mm at its takeoff from the femoral artery.
- The SIEA runs in a superficial layer as it goes superficially. When performing a vertical SIEA flap, the initial incision for the pedicle dissection should not be placed too high.
- The superior region of the SIEA flap can go higher than the umbilicus, but its perfusion should always be confirmed with ICG angiography when available.
- Damage to the lymph nodes and the lymphatic vessels can result in postoperative lymphorrhea or seroma. Meticulous coagulation of the lymphatic vessels, along with hemostasis, should be performed before donor site closure.
- Non-pulsating SIEA should not be used as the pedicle of the flap. Conversion to the SCIP flap or the DIEP flap should be considered.

21.9 Selected Readings

- Hester TR Jr., Nahai F, Beegle PE, Bostwick J 3rd. Blood supply of the abdomen revisited, with emphasis on the superficial inferior epigastric artery. Plast Reconstr Surg. 1984;74(5):657–70.
- Rozen WM, Chubb D, Grinsell D, Ashton MW. The variability of the Superficial Inferior Epigastric Artery (SIEA) and its angiosome: a clinical anatomical study. Microsurgery. 2010;30(5):386–91.
- Kita Y, Fukunaga Y, Arikawa M, Kagaya Y, Miyamoto S. Anatomy of the arterial and venous systems of the superficial inferior epigastric artery flap: a retrospective study based on computed tomographic angiography. J Plast Reconstr Aesthet Surg. 2020;73(5):870–5.
- Yoshimatsu H, Hayashi A, Karakawa R, Yano T. Combining the superficial circumflex iliac artery perforator flap with the superficial inferior epigastric artery flap or the deep inferior epigastric artery perforator flap for coverage of large soft tissue defects in the extremities and the trunk. Microsurgery. 2020.
- Coroneos CJ, Heller AM, Voineskos SH, Avram R. SIEA versus DIEP arterial complications: a cohort study. Plast Reconstr Surg. 2015;135(5):802e–7e.
- Zhang YX, Hayakawa TJ, Levin LS, Hallock GG, Lazzeri D. The economy in autologous tissue transfer: part 1. The kiss flap technique. Plast Reconstr Surg. 2016;137(3):1018–30.
- Zhang YX, Messmer C, Pang FK, Ong YS, Feng SQ, Qian Y, Spinelli G, Agostini T, Levin LS, Lazzeri D. A novel design of the multilobed latissimus dorsi myocutaneous flap to achieve primary donor-site closure in the reconstruction of large defects. Plast Reconstr Surg. 2013;132(5):886e–7e.

Superior Gluteal Artery Perforator Flap

22

Mohammed Farid and Mohamed Shibu

22.1 Introduction

The superior gluteal artery perforator (SGAP) flap evolved in its composition and application over the past four decades. A myocutaneous SGAP free flap was first used in breast reconstruction by Fujino in 1975 [1]. In 1984, Remirez then described the use of sliding myocutaneous gluteal flaps for sacral defect reconstruction [2]. The evolution of perforator flaps happened with the introduction of fasciocutaneous flap concept in reconstructive microsurgery. This led to reduced morbidity associated with SGAP muscle flaps. The turning point was when Koshima in 1993 described up to 25 perforators in the gluteal region and the first to use gluteal fasciocutaneous pedicled flaps in sacral reconstruction [3]. Verpaele and Blondeel et al. modification led to the selection of a single-perforator superior gluteal artery to be the choice for sacral reconstruction in 1999 [4]. Within the same period in 1995, Allen et al. utilised SGAP fasciocutaneous flap in breast reconstruction [5]. The current state is the use of predominately SGAP as a fasciocutaneous pedicled flap for sacral reconstruction and a free flap in breast reconstruction. The use of gluteal muscle should be reserved to patients with extensive sacral defects for dead space obliteration.

22.2 Anatomy

The superior gluteal artery (SGA) is one of the terminal branches of the internal iliac artery [6, 7]. A continuation of the posterior trunk of this vessel appears complete in the majority of cases, but can arise from a common stem (truncus glutealis) with the inferior gluteal artery [8]. The SGA courses posteriorly between the lumbosacral trunk and the first sacral ventral ramus and then exits through the greater sciatic foramen [9]. It leaves the pelvis above the upper border of the piriformis muscle, to divide into superficial and deep branches [6]. The superficial branch of SGA passes between gluteus maximus and medius in a septal plane. It gives off three branches either muscular (supplies gluteus maximus), septocutaneous (skin and subcutis) and musculocutaneous (run through the gluteus muscle to reach skin) [9]. Cormack and Lamberty described a posterior, intermediate and anterior branch (synonymous to septocutaneous) for the superficial part of SGA [8]. The deep branch gives off superior (supplies gluteus medius) and inferior (supplies gluteus medius and minimus). Musculocutaneous perforators for the deep branch are difficult to dissect and should not be used as a pedicle for SGA. A large venous network (caput medusa) is found where superficial and deep branches of SGA branch superior to the piriformis [9].

Particular anatomical landmarks are described to locate the SGAP topographically. With the hip flexed and internally rotated, the SGAP exit from the pelvis corresponds to the junction of the upper and middle third between the posterior superior iliac spine (PSIS) and greater trochanter [6]. The exit point corresponds anatomically to 6 cm below the posterior superior iliac spine and 4.5 cm lateral to the midline of the sacrum [10]. The piriformis is located half-way between the greater trochanter and the sacrum. Perforators are located lateral to SGA and above the piriformis. An average of three perforators are found to supply the skin (Fig. 22.1) [6, 7, 11]. A more detailed anatomical study by Ahmadzadeh et al. [12] described a mean of 5 ± 2 myocutaneous perforators from SGA in the gluteal region. He described that the average cutaneous SGA vascular area was 69 ± 56 cm^2 which corresponds to the angiosome territory. The diameter of the SGA ranges from 0.6 to 3.5 mm [11, 13, 14]. The pedicle length is short with an average of 3 to 7 cm (range 2–10 cm) [6, 13]. Venous drainage is through the

---

Supplementary Information The online version contains supplementary material available at https://doi.org/10.1007/978-3-031-07678-7_22.

M. Farid (✉)
Department of Plastic Surgery, Royal Stoke University Hospital, Stoke-on-Trent, UK

M. Shibu
Department of Plastic Surgery, The Royal London Hospital, London, UK

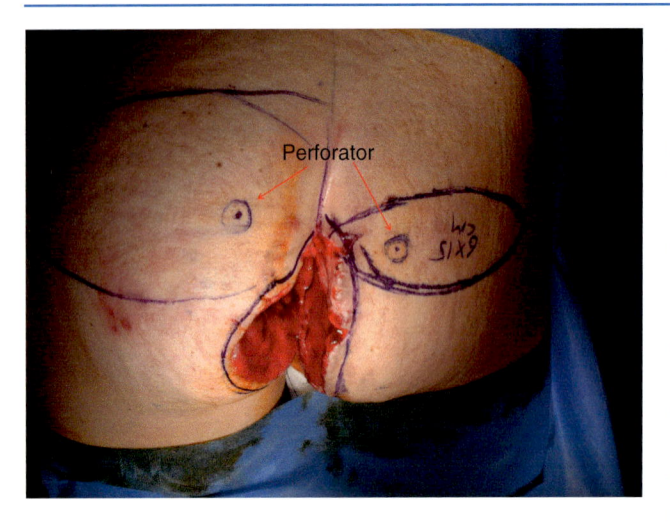

Fig. 22.1 Bilateral SGAP flaps to reconstruct a perineal defect from pelvic exenteration (anal SCC)

superior gluteal vein (SGV) (venae comitantes) with many tributaries from pelvic veins. The average length of SGV is 2.5 cm and diameter of 3 mm [13].

22.3   Preoperative Investigation

Preoperative imaging is one of the crucial steps to allow safe surgical planning prior to raising the SGAP flap. The perforators for SGA can be localised using either a handheld Doppler ultrasound (US), duplex US, computed tomography angiography (CTA) or magnetic resonance angiography (MRA) imaging. All imaging should be performed while the patient is in the prone position.

Handheld Doppler US is routinely used in the immediate preoperative period and determines location and number of SGA perforators. Angiography combined with CT or MR identifies the perforator pathway (musculocutaneous or septocutaneous), location and calibre of vessels [6, 10, 15]. MRA imaging identifies perforator branches, has no ionising radiation compared to CT and offers excellent soft tissue detail. CTA also allows 3-D reconstruction of the images to add more detail into the course of perforator [9].

The investigation of choice is based on the resources available, surgeon's preference and intended operation whether pedicle or free SGA flap. The choice we propose is the use of handheld Doppler for pedicled SGAP flaps to be combined with MRA or CTA if a free SGAP flap is planned. The ultimate goal is to safely identify and isolate the perforator without flap compromise at any point during the operation.

22.4   Flap Design and Markings

The SGA perforator is identified at the junction between the proximal and middle third of a line drawn from PSIS and greater trochanter of the femur. Flap design is in a fusiform shape, oriented from 0° to 90°, on the area surrounding the perforator (Fig. 22.2). Flap dimension is based on the defect size and location in the gluteal region or the desired size for free flap breast reconstruction. The maximum flap size by one SGAP perforator can be 14 cm wide and up to 30 cm long [11, 16]. The length of the flap is based on reverse planning for defect size. The skin paddle length should be made a few centimetres longer than the defect size to reach the distal end of defect once rotated. Bilateral SGAP flaps can be planned based on the clinical indication in terms of defect dimensions (Fig. 22.3).

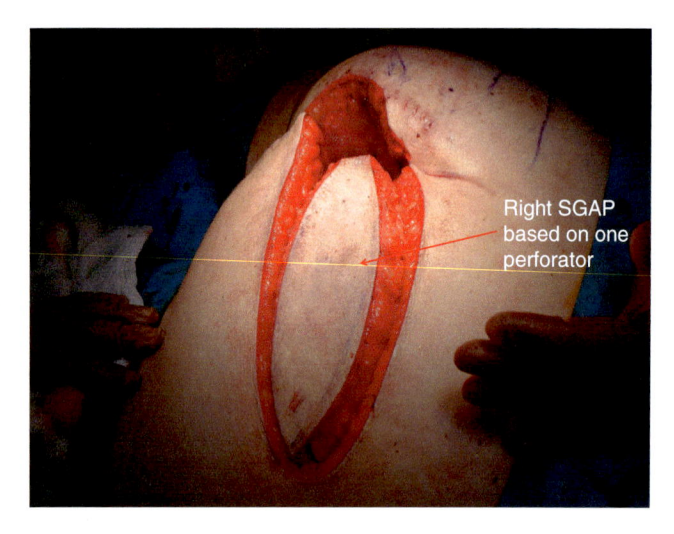

Fig. 22.2 Right SGAP flap islanded based on a single perforator

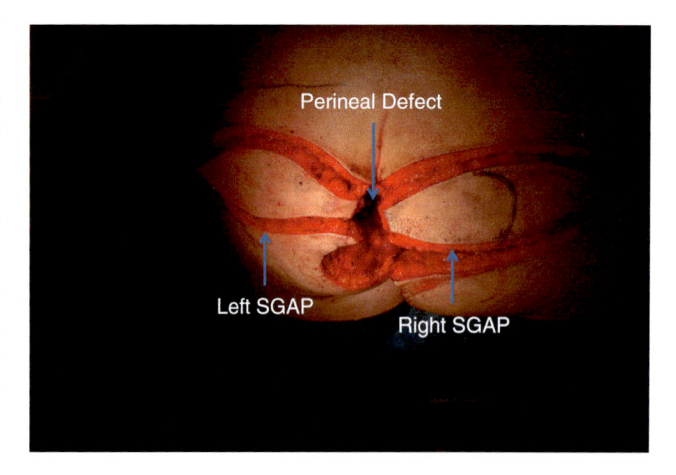

Fig. 22.3 Bilateral SGAP islanded and perineal defect post debridement

22.5 Flap Raise/Elevation: A Step-by-Step Guide

Step 1: Incision. An incision is made through the marked area for flap skin paddle. The depth of the incision is down to gluteal subfascial plane. Dissection can be beveled at an angle to recruit more subcutaneous tissue and volume.

Step 2: Raising Flap. The flap is raised supero-laterally and then inferiorly in the gluteal subfascial plane. Once the correct plane is identified, the flap is raised lateral to medial towards the SGA perforator (Fig. 22.4). When the perforator is visualised, the dissection is moved superomedially towards the perforator towards the perforator. Intraoperative Doppler is used to confirm the flow of the perforator and can be palpated for pulsatile flow.

Step 3: Islanding the Flap (propeller). Once the perforator is identified from all angles, the pedicle is traced by gluteal muscle dissection. The flap is mobilised and would rotate on a perforator axis as a propeller flap (Fig. 22.5).

The following steps would depend on the size and the depth of the defect. Two SGAP flaps are raised in large perineal defects as in the case demonstrated.

Step 4: Flap De-epithelialised. The contralateral SGAP flap to the defect side is de-epithelialised and inset deep into the defect (Figs. 22.6 and 22.7).

Step 5: Second SGAP Flap Raised. The ipsilateral SGAP flap to defect is raised similar to Steps 1–3. This flap is inset on top of de-epithelialised SGAP flap (Figs. 22.8, 22.9, 22.10, and 22.11). This is followed by insertion of two suction drains prior to closure.

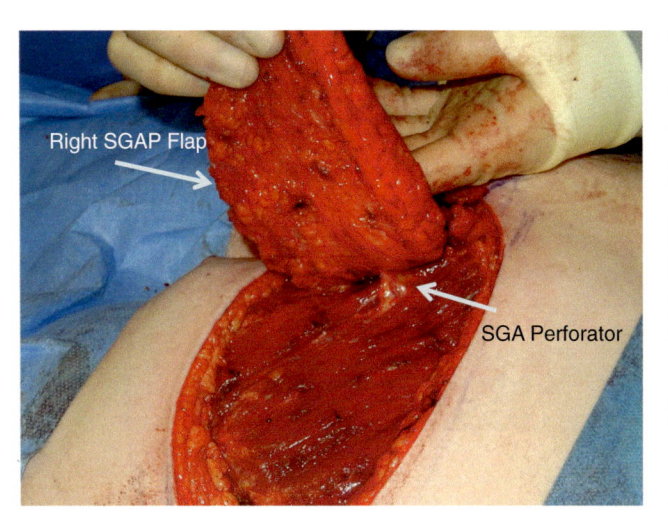

Fig. 22.4 Right SGAP flap demonstrating the perforator once flap islanded

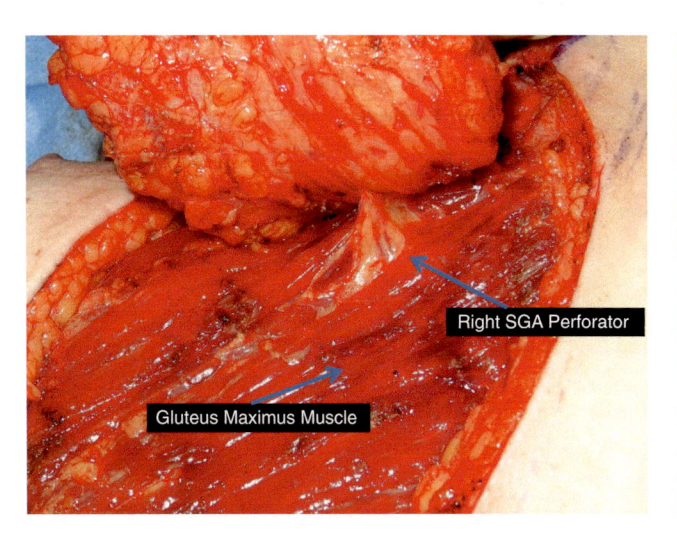

Fig. 22.5 Right SGA perforator close-up and underlying gluteus maximus muscle

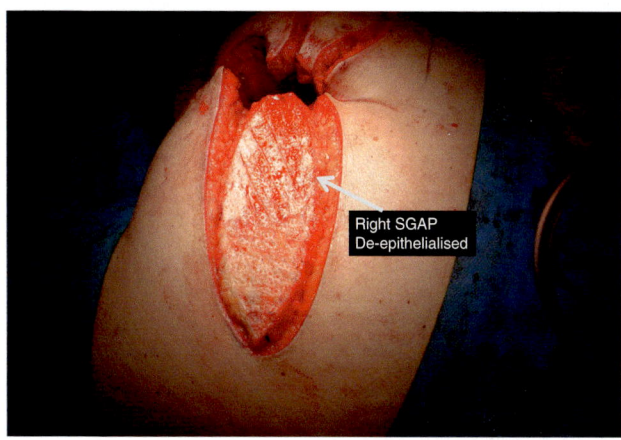

Fig. 22.6 Right SGAP flap de-epithelialised to fill in deep into the defect

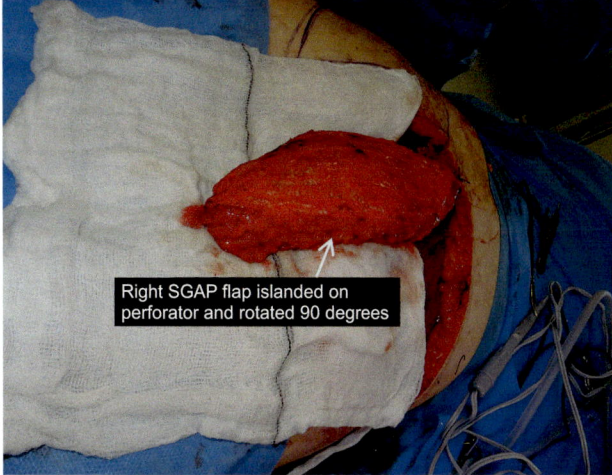

Fig. 22.7 Right SGAP flap islanded on a single perforator, de-epithelialised and rotated 90 degrees

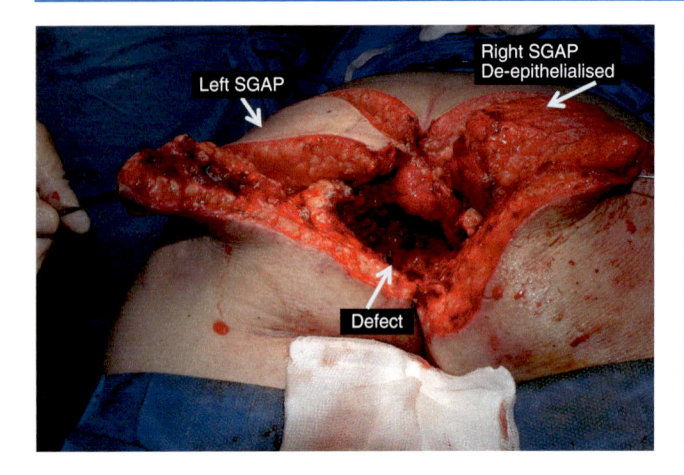

Fig. 22.8 Bilateral SGAP flap to reconstruct perineal defect

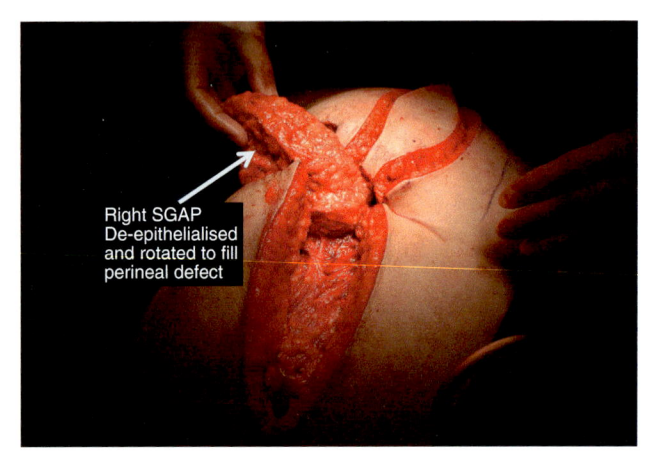

Fig. 22.9 Right SGAP flap rotated to fill perineal defect

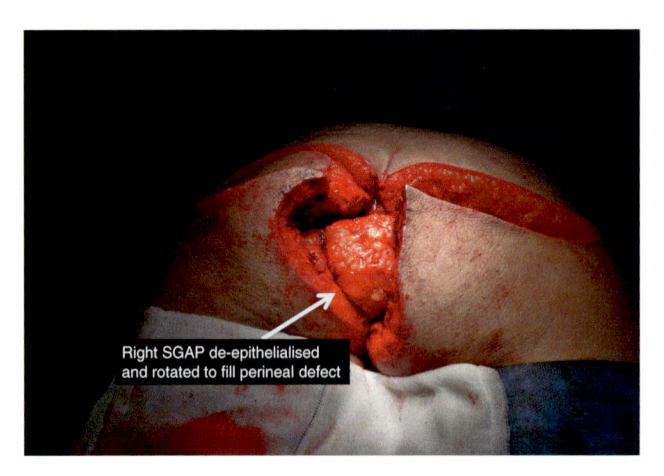

Fig. 22.10 Right SGAP flap rotated and mobilised to fill perineal defect

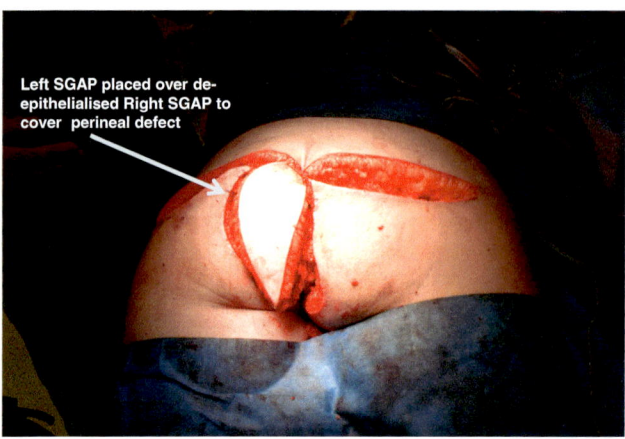

Fig. 22.11 Left SGAP flap over de-epithelialised right SGAP to cover perineal defect

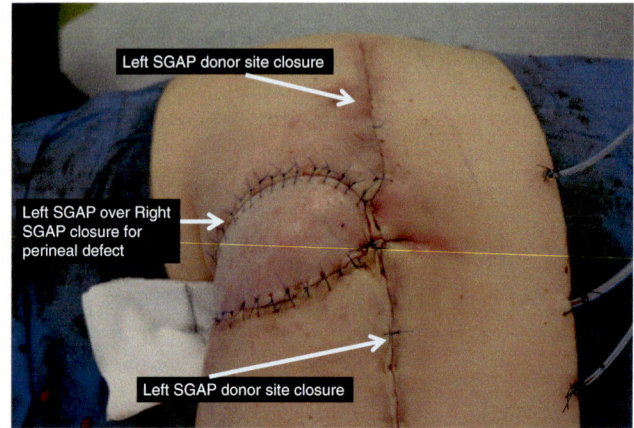

Fig. 22.12 Bilateral SGAP closure of donor and recipient site

Step 6: Closure Post Inset. Three-layer closure from deep to superficial. The deepest layer would be above the gluteal fascial planes (3/0 PDS suture), deep dermal layer (3/0 Monocryl) and skin (3/0 Nylon Interrupted) (Fig. 22.12).

22.6 Core Surgical Techniques in Flap Dissection

Step 1: Perforator Checkpoint: The flap relies on one main SGAP perforator. Adequate attention and step-by-step approach when raising flap. Regular checkpoint throughout dissection using handheld Doppler to ensure pedicle is not compromised at any point.

Step 2: Perforator Dissection: Careful gluteal muscle dissection to obtain longer SGAP pedicle which can reach up to 10–12 cm [14]. This is important for free flap cases to reduce the tension on the pedicle and ensure adequate length to reach the recipient site. The SGAP pedicle length can be further extended with the use of a vein graft [16]. The length of the pedicle would increase the arc of rotation to reach the defect.

Step 3: Perforator Torsion: Perforator to be isolated from surrounding tissue to allow flap rotation. Perforator torsion or kinking would cause flap venous congestion. This is commonly seen in SGAP flaps with poor planning related to perforator dissection. The pedicle is dissected down without any kink on rotation to adhere to the principles of the propeller flap concept [17].

Step 4: Flap Inset: Pedicled SGAP flap, inset should be tensionless without any pull or traction on the pedicle. This may lead to vessel spasm and flap compromise.

Step 5: Closure: The aim is to close the donor site primarily. This is dependent on the laxity of surrounding soft tissue and the width of the flap harvest (less than 10 cm).

Instrumentation: A number of smaller vessel branches along the SGAP pedicle should be Ligaclipped safely. Lone stars can be used to retract the tissue margins either side of the flap which facilitate dissection. Safe use of bipolar diathermy when dissecting the pedicle is advised. The setting we recommend is 6–8 watts. DeBakey forceps are placed 2 mm from the pedicle when cauterising small vessel branches off the pedicle (heat-sink principle) [18].

22.7 Clinical Scenario

Scenario A: M Shibu and D Nikkhah A 53-year-old man with Crohn's disease underwent a pelvic exenteration for anal SCC (Fig. 22.13). He had had multiple previous abdominal operations and was not a suitable candidate for an abdominal-based flap. Decision was made to perform an SGAP flap to obliterate the dead space (Figs. 22.1, 22.2, 22.3, 22.4, 22.5, 22.6, 22.7, 22.8, 22.9, 22.10, 22.11, 22.12, and 22.13). This flap was raised in the standard fashion and the perforator isolated and the skin de-epithelialised and placed into the perineal defect. A second flap was designed on the contralateral side. An IGAP flap with its leading edge de-epithelialised was advanced to cover the first flap. The patient had an uneventful recovery and was discharged at 1 week.

Scenario B: M Shibu and D Nikkhah A 26-year-old woman underwent a pelvic exenteration for rectal cancer. Decision was made to perform bilateral SGAP flaps, one to obliterate the dead space and the second to cover the soft tissue defect (Figs. 22.14, 22.15, 22.16, 22.17, and 22.18 and Video 22.1).

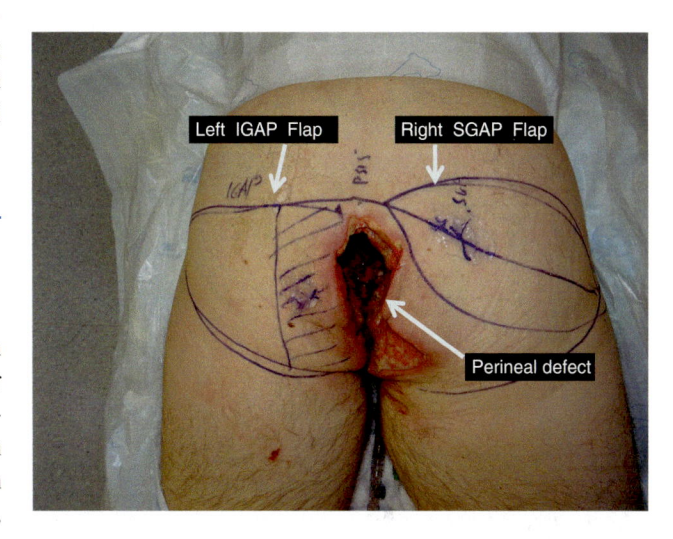

Fig. 22.14 A 26-year-old woman underwent a pelvic exenteration for rectal cancer

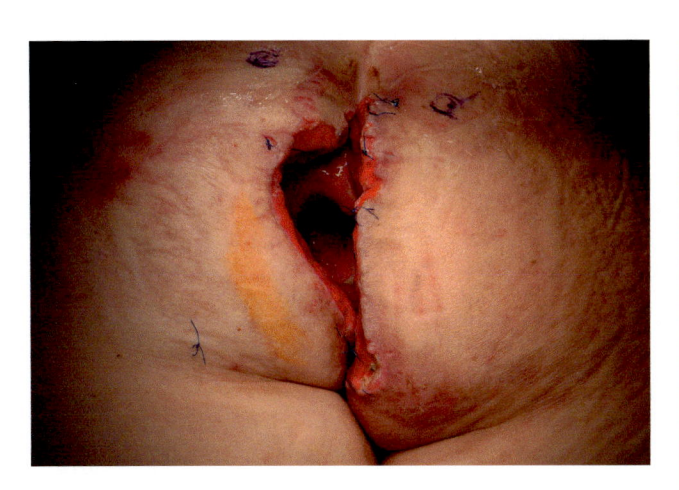

Fig. 22.13 A 53-year-old man with Crohn's disease underwent a pelvic exenteration for anal SCC

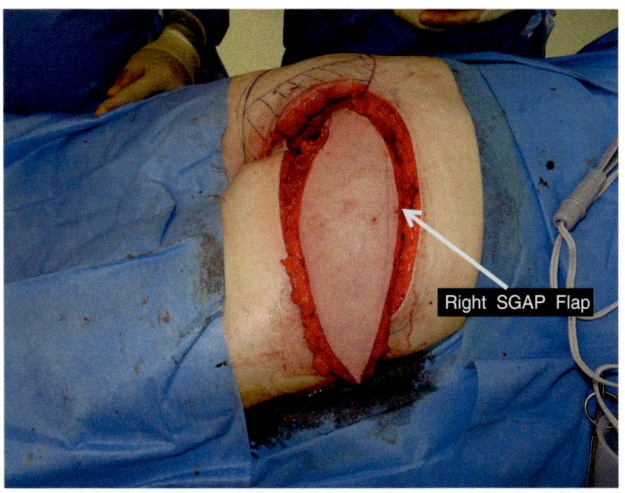

Fig. 22.15 Right SGAP flap islanded

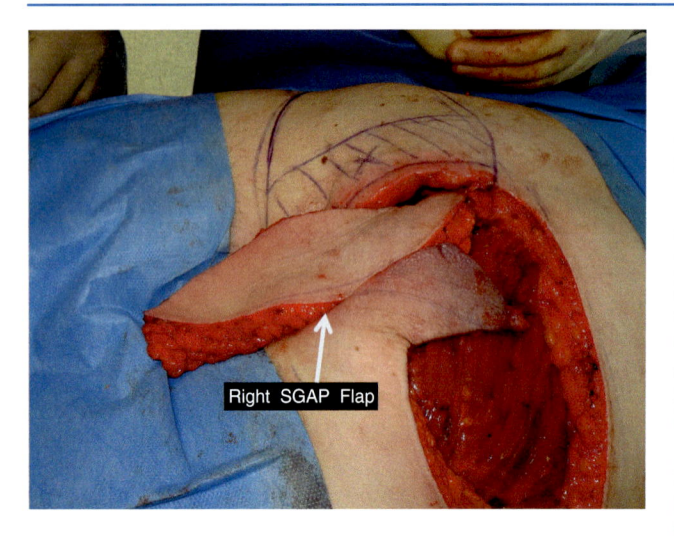

Fig. 22.16 Right SGAP flap rotated into perineal defect

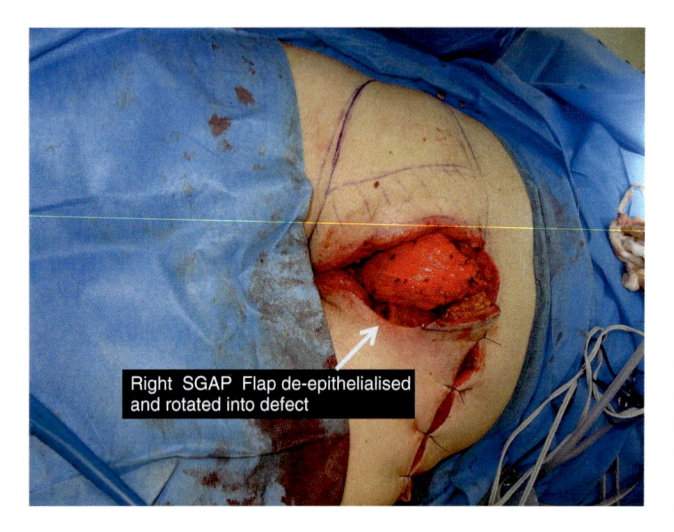

Fig. 22.17 Right SGAP flap de-epithelialised, rotated and placed in perineal defect

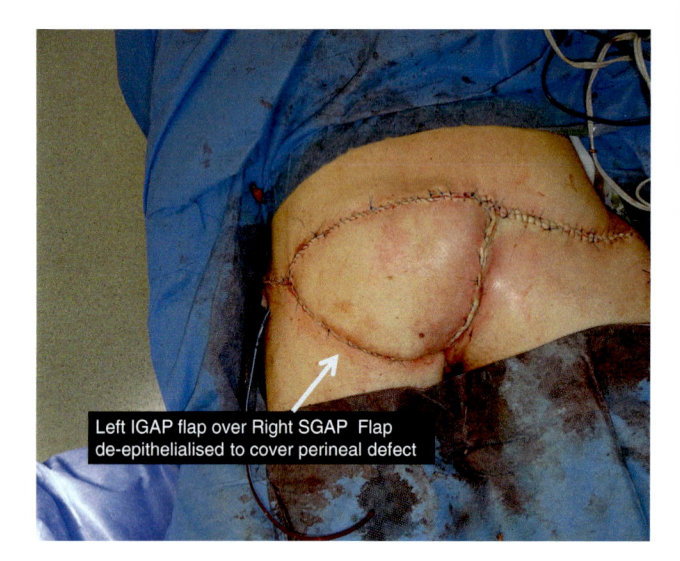

Fig. 22.18 Left IGAP flap over de-epithelialised right SGAP flap and closure of donor sites

22.8 Pearls and Pitfalls

- **Venous congestion:** Linked mainly to perforator kinking or twisting. This risk is reduced with raising the flap as a propeller, hence freeing the pedicle. The other technical tip is to rotate the flap on pedicle in a clockwise/anticlockwise based on visualising the pedicle to rule out kinking (Video 22.2).
- **Flap tip necrosis:** Based on the angiosome concept, the distal end of the flap may suffer necrosis. The perforator branches may not reach the distal end of the flap. Intraoperative mapping with indocyanine green fluorescence (ICG) angiography may help in viewing under-perfused flap areas which can then be excised.
- **Flap wound dehiscence:** Wound edges of the SGAP flap may break down with pressure or swelling postoperatively. Removal of continuous undissolved sutures for 2–3 weeks, nurse laterally or prone, wound care and regular reviews all reduce this risk.
- **Intraoperative pedicle/flap compromise:** Meticulous attention to flap dissection and perforator identification is crucial to prevent immediate complications. Using intraoperative handheld Doppler, careful muscle dissection and appropriate inset all help in minimising complications.
- **Breast reconstruction:** The SGAP is used as a free flap in breast reconstruction. Preoperatively, patients ideally are made aware that gluteal fat is thicker and less malleable than normal breast tissue. Intraoperatively, patient positioning is variable either lateral decubitus or then changed to supine depending whether unilateral or bilateral breast reconstruction. The short pedicle length can be a limiting factor to being first choice in breast reconstruction. Shaping of SGAP to breast form is challenging due to the nature of the tissue. Postoperatively, secondary surgery to re-contour gluteal regions may be indicated as patients report unaesthetic look of their buttocks.

22.9 Selected Readings

- Ahmadzadeh R, Bergeron L, Tang M, Morris SF. The superior and inferior gluteal artery perforator flaps. Plast Reconstr Surg. 2007.

    This paper is a cadaveric anatomical study specific to SGAP and IGAP perforators. It gives an accurate description of the perforator landmarks and maps their territory based on the angiosome principle. This information provides the basis for safe surgical dissection and planning to minimise flap compromise.

- Blondeel PN, Beyens G, Verhaeghe R, Van Landuyt K, Tonnard P, Monstrey SJ, et al. Doppler flowmetry in the planning of perforator flaps. Br J Plast Surg. 1998.

The authors support this paper to describe the use of handheld Doppler and duplex US in perforator planning. Preoperative and intraoperative US help reduce operating time and decision-making for suitable perforators. SGAP perforator anatomy is consistent, and identification using handheld Doppler US has a high positive predictive value (91.9%) which confirms its reliability in perforator planning.

- Gagnon A, Blondeel P. Superior gluteal artery perforator flap. Semin Plast Surg. 2006.

   This paper offered a comprehensive and specific encounter for SGAP flaps. It highlighted the anatomical landmarks, marking, perforator dissections and indications. There was a clear distinction for the use as pedicled flap for loco-regional defects or free flap in breast reconstruction.

- Verpaele AM, Blondeel PN, Van Landuyt K, Tonnard PL, Decordier B, Monstrey SJ, et al. The superior gluteal artery perforator flap: An additional tool in the treatment of sacral pressure sores. Br J Plast Surg. 1999.

   The paper highlighted the known concepts introduced previously by Koshima (first SGAP) and Ramirez (sliding SGAP flap). The main recommendation is the dissection of the pedicle from the muscle to allow longer pedicle length and flap translation without perforator torsion. Another technical tip was the avoidance of tunnelling SGAP flap and utilising of ipsilateral SGAP for sacral defects.

- Acartürk TO, Parsak CK, Sakman G, Demircan O. Superior gluteal artery perforator flap in the reconstruction of pilonidal sinus. J Plast Reconstr Aesthetic Surg. 2010.

   The paper showed the detailed planning for SGAP flap in pilonidal sinus surgery. This was based on transposing the flap without perforator dissection, visualisation or skeletonisation from the gluteal muscle. No complications reported by the author based on their technique.

- Zeng A, Jia Y, Wang X, Liu Z. The superior gluteal artery perforator flap for lumbosacral defect repair: A unified approach. J Plast Reconstr Aesthetic Surg. 2013.

   This is interesting short correspondence describing a new technique in raising pedicled SGAP flap. The perforator was not identified with handheld Doppler but based on an exploratory incision. This incision was 2 cm below and parallel to middle of a line between the PSIS and greater trochanter. The technique applied flap tunnelling to reach lumbosacral defect without any suggested complications. A long pedicled SGAP advancement flap would help reach a distant defect site.

- Zoccali G, Mughal M, Giwa L, Roblin P, Farhadi J. Breast reconstruction with Superior Gluteal Artery Perforator free flap: 8 years of experience J Plast Reconstr Aesthetic Surg. 2019.

   This is one of the largest studies in the literature for the use of free SGAP flaps in breast reconstruction. It addresses the indications, complications and outcomes for SGAP breast reconstruction. The paper also looked at re-operation rates and reasons behind it. It describes flap inset prior to anastomosis to prevent vessel avulsion considering the short pedicle length. For immediate breast reconstruction, flap was harvested on lateral position at the same time as mastectomy. One of the main recommendations is appropriate patients' selection and takes into account cultural belief about aesthetics.

References

1. Fujino T, Harashina T, Aoyagi F. Reconstruction for aplasia of the breast and pectoral region by microvascular transfer of a free flap from the buttock. Plast Reconstr Surg. 1975;56:178–81.
2. Ramirez OM, Swartz WM, Futrell JW. The gluteus maximus muscle: experimental and clinical considerations relevant to reconstruction in ambulatory patients. Br J Plast Surg. 1987;40(1):1–10.
3. Koshima I, Moriguchi T, Soeda S, et al. The gluteal perforator-based flap for repair of sacral pressure sores. Plast Reconstr Surg. 1993;91(4):678–83.
4. Verpaele AM, Blondeel PN, Van Landuyt K, Tonnard PL, Decordier B, Monstrey SJ, et al. The superior gluteal artery perforator flap: an additional tool in the treatment of sacral pressure sores. Br J Plast Surg. 1999;52:385–91.
5. Allen RJ, Tucker C. Superior gluteal artery perforator free flap for breast reconstruction. Plast Reconstr Surg. 1995;95:1207–12.
6. Samir M, Fu-Chen W. Chapter:58: Superior and inferior gluteal artery perforator flaps. In: Levine J, Allen R, editors. Flaps and reconstructive surgery. 2nd ed; 2016. p. 687–99.
7. Lin C-T, Dai N-T, Chang S-C, Chen S-G, Chen T-M, Wang H-J, Tzeng Y-S. Ten-year experience of superior gluteal artery perforator flap for reconstruction of sacral defects in tri-service general hospital. J Med Sci (Taiwan). 2014;34(2):66–71.
8. Cormack G, Lamberty B. Chapter 6: Buttock. In: The arterial anatomy of skin flaps. 2nd ed; 1996. p. 220–6.
9. Spiegel A. Chapter 9: Septocutaneous gluteal artery perforator (Sc-GAP) flap for breast reconstruction: how we do it. In: Tuinder S, Van Der Hulst R, Lobbes M, Versluis B, Lataster A, editors. Breast reconstruction - current perspectives and state of the art techniques. 1st ed; 2013. p. 135–50.
10. Pu L, Karp N. Chapter 5: free gluteal perforator flap breast reconstruction. In: Levine J, Conde-Green A, Andrade P, editors. Atlas of reconstructive breast surgery. 1st ed; 2019. p. 61–72.
11. Lin CT, et al. Modification of the superior gluteal artery perforator flap for reconstruction of sacral sores. J Plast Reconstr Aesthet Surg. 2014;67(4):526–32. https://doi.org/10.1016/j.bjps.2013.12.031.
12. Ahmadzadeh R, et al. The superior and inferior gluteal artery perforator flaps. Plast Reconstr Surg. 2007;120(6):1551–6. https://doi.org/10.1097/01.prs.0000282098.61498.ee.
13. Samir M, Fu-Chen W. Chapter: 28: Gluteus flap. In: Hamdi M, Gagnon A, editors. Flaps and reconstructive surgery. 2nd ed; 2016. p. 377–95.
14. Elizabeth Hall-Findlay E, Evans G. Chapter 11: Gluteal flap breast reconstruction. In: Cheng M-H, Huang J-J, editors. Aesthetic and reconstructive surgery of the breast. 1st ed; 2010. p. 161–70.
15. Sakuraba M, Asano T, Yano T, Yamamoto S, Moriya Y. Reconstruction of an enterocutaneous fistula using a superior gluteal artery perforator flap. J Plast Reconstr Aesthet Surg. 2009;62(1):108–11. https://doi.org/10.1016/j.bjps.2007.09.009.
16. Gagnon A, Blondeel P. Superior gluteal artery perforator flap. Semin Plast Surg. 2006;20(2):79–88.
17. Teo TC. The propeller flap concept. Clin Plast Surg. 2010;37(4):615–26, vi.
18. Allan J, Dusseldorp J, Rabey NG, Malata CM, Goltsman D, Phoon AF. Infrared evaluation of the heat-sink bipolar diathermy dissection technique. J Plast Reconstr Aesthet Surg. 2015;68(8):1145–51.

Inferior Gluteal Artery Perforator Flap

Maleeha Mughal and Paul Roblin

23.1 Introduction

The inferior gluteal artery perforator (IGAP) flap was first described for use in ischial pressure sores by Higgins et al. in 2002 [1]. It has since gained in popularity for perineal reconstructions due to its technical simplicity and reliability.

In clinical practice the IGAP flap is a workhorse flap for sacral and pelvic defects following pelvic oncological resections, pressure sores, and traumatic injuries [2].

The perforators in the lower gluteal region are relatively constant; therefore, preoperative and even intraoperative identification (for a number of cases) of perforators is unnecessary. If extensive mobility is required (more than can be achieved with the myocutaneous flap), this flap can be completely isolated on a single or two perforators only. In a majority of cases, sufficient mobility can be achieved with the retention of multiple perforators. This robust vascular supply allows larger flaps to be harvested reliably, and it can also be elevated with sensory innervation from the posterior cutaneous nerve of the thigh.

It is also important to note that in suitable patients, for disease involving the vaginal vault, the IGAP flap (uni- or bilateral) can reliably be used for simultaneous closure of the perineal defect and vaginal reconstruction, thus permitting earlier discharge, return to daily living, and sexual activity in a single-stage operation.

23.2 Anatomy

Both the inferior gluteal artery and superior gluteal artery are terminal branches of the internal iliac artery. They exit the pelvis through the greater sciatic foramen. The inferior gluteal artery travels inferior to the piriformis muscle and is accompanied by the internal pudendal vessels, the pudendal nerve, the greater sciatic nerve, and the posterior cutaneous nerve of the thigh. The perforators from the inferior gluteal artery traverse the caudal half of the gluteus maximus muscle, in a more oblique fashion than the course of the superior gluteal vessels. Cutaneous perforators ultimately reach the external border of the gluteal musculature. Therefore, the length of the IGAP pedicle is typically longer than that of the SGAP. Between two and four perforating vessels from the inferior gluteal artery will be located in the lower half of each gluteal muscle.

23.3 Preoperative Investigation

Due to constant anatomy of the perforators in the region, preoperative imaging is not essential when using the IGAP for perineal reconstruction. However magnetic resonance imaging (MRI) of the gluteal perforators is preferred by the authors when utilizing the flap for breast reconstruction. In that instance our flap of choice is the superior gluteal artery perforator (SGAP) flap which has been discussed further in the remit of this book.

23.4 Flap Design and Markings

23.4.1 Markings

The patient is positioned prone as the specimen is delivered through the wound. The IGAP flap is designed in a V-Y fashion, with the lower border placed in the buttock crease and the lateral extension medial to the greater trochanter. A line is drawn from the greater trochanter to the posterior superior iliac spine; the inferior gluteal artery perforators are inferior to this line; these can be mapped with a Doppler probe if required, but with more experience this step is not necessary (Fig. 23.1). Bilateral IGAPs mirror each other.

M. Mughal (✉) · P. Roblin
Guy's and St. Thomas Hospital, London, UK

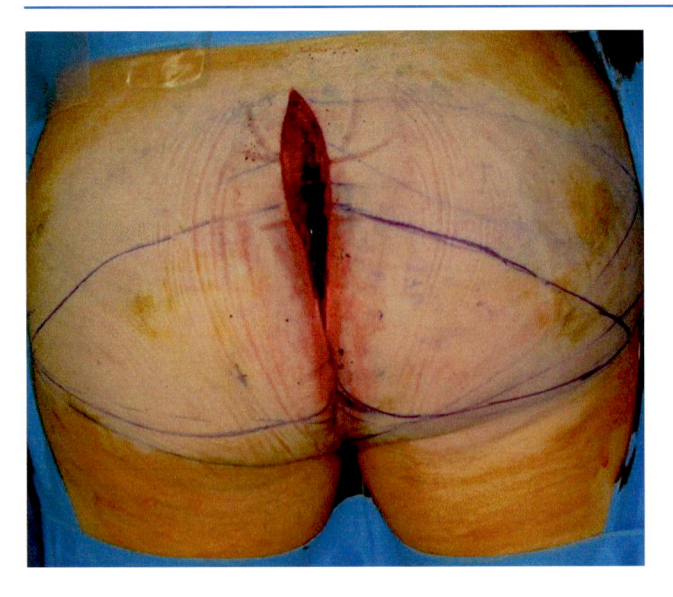

Fig. 23.1 Bilateral IGAP flap markings. The inferior edge is kept above the gluteal crease

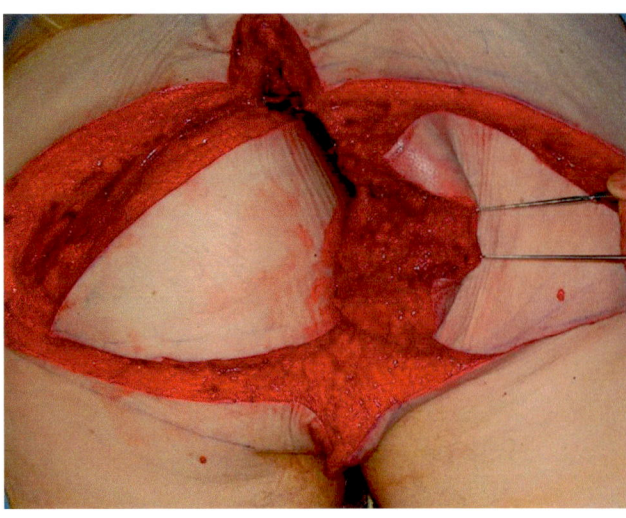

Fig. 23.2 Subfascial raise of both IGAP flaps, medial edge of the right IGAP elevated to show medial dissection

23.5 Flap Raise/Elevation: A Step-by-Step Guide

1. The flap is raised from lateral to medial in a subfascial plane using a monopolar diathermy. This approach allows identification of the perforating vessels passing through the gluteal muscle into the flap (Fig. 23.2). A consistent perforating vessel is usually identified at the junction between the lateral and middle third of the flap. This perforator is isolated and can be traced down through the muscle to allow adequate mobilization.
2. Once the perforator has been isolated and dissected, the medial border of the flap is raised in a subfascial plane. Perforators from the medial and central areas can then be isolated and dissected dependent on the degree of medial transposition required.
3. The flap is advanced medially; the medial edge is de-epithelialized and buried to fill the dead space in the pelvis (Fig. 23.3).
4. In cases where bilateral flaps are required, the first flap is inset as mentioned above, the second flap is advanced medially and de-epithelialized, and this is then closed in a double-breasted fashion (Fig. 23.4).
5. Two lateral suction drains are placed under the upper and lower borders of the flap. The wound is closed in layers with absorbable sutures.

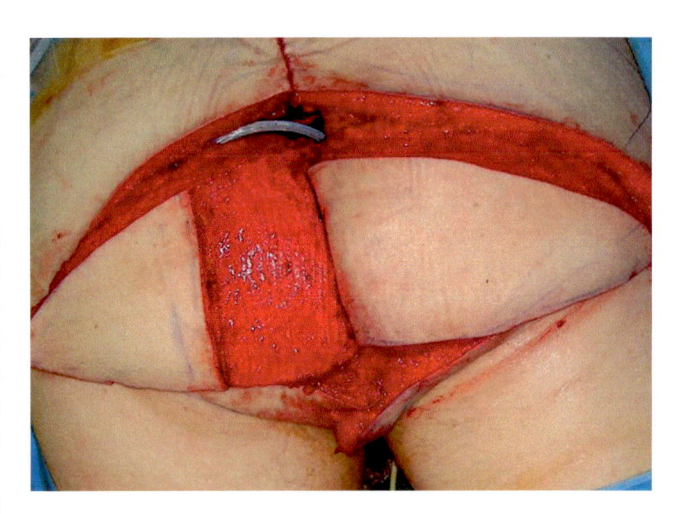

Fig. 23.3 Medial edge of flap de-epithelialized to allow inset into pelvic cavity

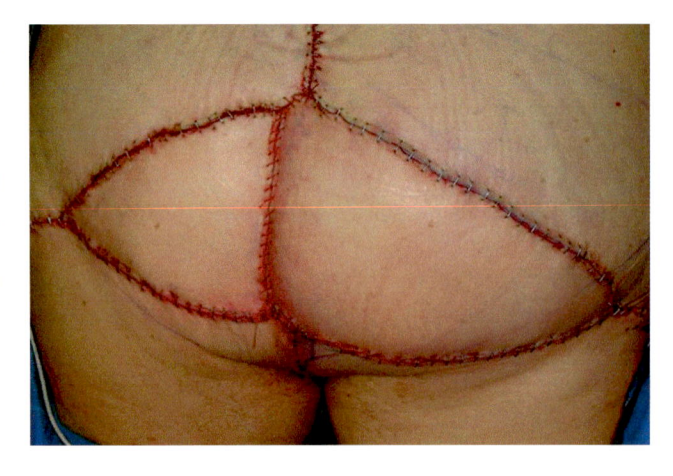

Fig. 23.4 Closure of bilateral IGAPs

23.6 Core Surgical Techniques in Flap Dissection

The flap design should allow adequate closure of the resulting donor site; in some cases undermining of the superior and inferior borders will be required to ensure a tension-free closure.

Once the flap is raised and medially mobilized, it is crucial to secure the de-epithelialized superior edge of the flap to the anterior surface of the sacrum. The surgeon should be vigilant in ensuring that the sacral venous plexus is not damaged at this stage; this can lead to hemorrhage which is difficult to control.

The de-epithelialized medial edge then should be secured to the lateral pelvic outlet to ensure a complete seal of the pelvic cavity to avoid herniation of pelvic contents. This is done with 0'Vicryl suture.

In addition to the aforementioned flap drains, a non-suction pelvic drain is used. This is placed through the opposite buttock in case of unilateral IGAPs and through the inferior border of a flap if bilateral IGAPs have been used.

The authors also utilize this flap for reconstruction of vaginal defects in addition to closing the perineal wound. When a posterior vaginal reconstruction only is required, the defect is measured, and a template created. The template is transferred to the medial edge of the IGAP, and that portion of skin is preserved when de-epithelializing the flap. This area is then inset using parachute suture technique to close the vaginal defect. Care must be taken in deciding where the de-epithelialization commences on the flap as well as its width as this will dictate the vaginal diameter, thereby reducing the risk of subsequent stenosis but must still allow a tension-free midline closure of the perineal defect.

23.7 Clinical Scenario

Unilateral IGAP flap marked for closure of perineal defect following abdominoperineal excision (APE) for rectal cancer (Fig. 23.5). The perforators are marked with a handheld Doppler. The flap is elevated and two perforators dissected along their course to achieve adequate medial advancement (Fig. 23.6). The flap is inset by using 0'Vicryl for anchoring sutures to the sacrum and the pelvic walls. Dermal and skin closure is carried out with dissolvable sutures (Fig. 23.7).

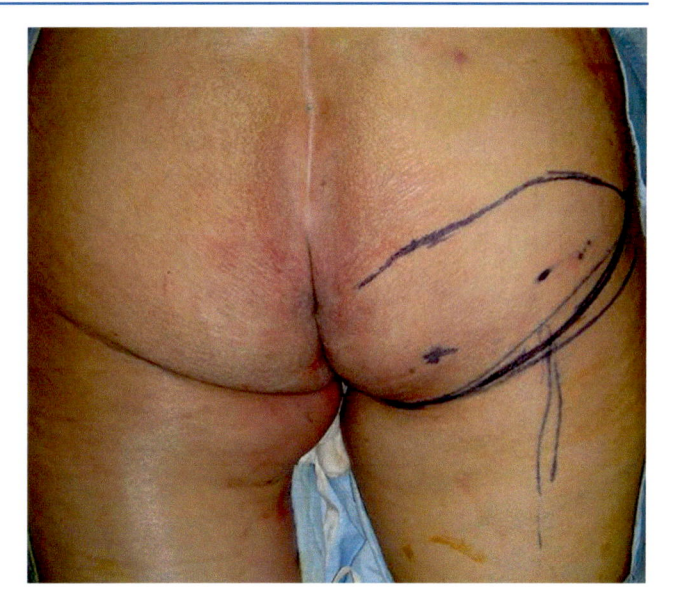

Fig. 23.5 Unilateral IGAP flap perforators, marked with handheld Doppler

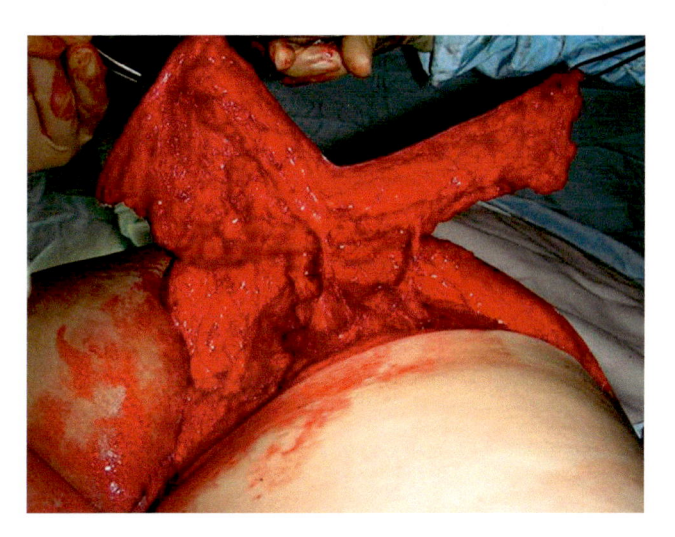

Fig. 23.6 Perforator dissection complete and flap elevated, this flap can be rotated at 90 degrees to allow closure of the defect if required

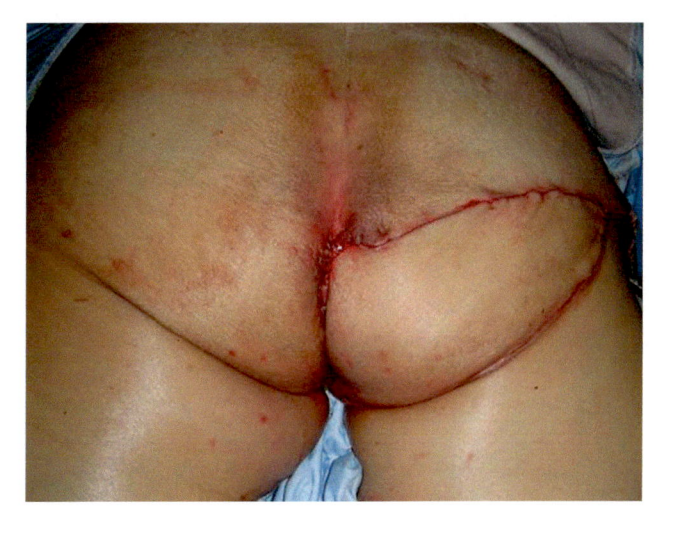

Fig. 23.7 Unilateral IGAP flap inset into perineal defect

23.8 Summary

Bilateral IGAPs provide enough bulk in our experience, in dealing with extensive defects resulting from total pelvic exenteration (TPE) with high sacrectomies. It is documented that gluteal fasciocutaneous flaps provide sufficient tissue for even significant sacrectomy defects over 2000 cm^3 in volume [3].

The IGAP is a robust flap, which is technically simple and reproducible. It has minimal donor site complications and postoperative pain. The constant anatomy allows ease in planning and design, and in the modern era of minimally invasive surgery, i.e., robotic and laparoscopic resections, it remains a compatible local option for perineal reconstruction.

23.9 Pearls and Pitfalls

Pearls
- The surgeon needs to ensure that the flap raise is in the subfascial plane, dividing the fascia completely facilitates medial mobilization and in patients with laxity of tissue planes, the medial mobilization of the flap can be achieved without dissecting the pedicle.
- Medial edge should also be raised in the subfascial plane to aid advancement.
- The middle one third of the flap will contain the maximum number of perforators. Care must be taken not to elevate this area unless perforator dissection is planned.
- In patients with less buttock laxity, undermining of the superior and inferior aspect will be required to aid closure of the donor site.
- One advantage of the V-Y pattern is that in the event of wound dehiscence, the flap can be readvanced to close the defect.

Pitfalls
- Delayed wound healing is a common complication especially in the midline due to pelvic collections. In our experience the pelvic drain is kept in for at least 2 weeks postoperatively to aid drainage.
- Postoperative compliance for nursing side to side for 48 hours is important; in our experience patients requiring prolonged intensive care admission after surgery are at higher risk of wound healing complications.

23.10 Selected Readings

- Mughal M, et al. Reconstruction of perineal defects. Ann R Coll Surg Engl. 2013;95(8):539–44.
- *Overview of principles of perineal reconstruction with management options.*
- Niranjan NS, et al. Perforator flaps for perineal reconstructions. Semin Plast Surg. 2006;20:133–44.
- *Key paper describing the anatomy and technical aspects of local flap reconstruction options in the perineum.*
- Higgins JP, et al. Ischial pressure sore reconstruction using an inferior gluteal artery perforator (IGAP) flap. Brit Journ Plast Surg. 2002;55(1):83–5.
- *Description of the inferior gluteal artery perforator flap and its use in perineal reconstruction.*
- Hainsworth A, et al. Perineal reconstruction after abdominoperineal excision using inferior gluteal artery perforator flaps. BJS. 2012;99:584–8. https://doi.org/10.1002/bjs.7822.
- *Clinical outcomes of Abdominoperineum excision reconstruction with IGAP flaps.*
- Garvey PB, Rhines LD, Feng L, Gu X, Butler CE. Reconstructive strategies for partial sacrectomy defects based on surgical outcomes. *Plastic and reconstructive surgery.* [Online] United States; 2011;127(1):190–199. Available from: https://doi.org/10.1097/PRS.0b013e3181f95a19.
- *Surgical outcomes of large pelvic exenterations and reconstruction with IGAP flaps.*

References

1. Higgins JP, et al. Ischial pressure sore reconstruction using an inferior gluteal artery perforator (IGAP) flap. Br J Plast Surg. 2002;55(1):83–5.
2. Mughal M, et al. Reconstruction of perineal defects. Ann R Coll Surg Engl. 2013;95(8):539–44.
3. Garvey PB, Rhines LD, Feng L, Gu X, Butler CE. Reconstructive strategies for partial sacrectomy defects based on surgical outcomes. Plast Reconstr Surg. 2011;127(1):190–9. https://doi.org/10.1097/PRS.0b013e3181f95a19.

The Lumbar Artery Perforator Flap: A True Alternative in Autologous Breast Reconstruction

Filip B. J. L. Stillaert, Phillip Blondeel, and Koenraad Van Landuyt

24.1 Introduction

The lumbar artery perforator (LAP) flap is designed around the love-handle region and incorporates skin and an ample amount of subcutaneous fat tissue. Its use in autologous breast reconstruction was initially described in 2003 [1].

Obviously, autologous breast reconstructions are superior to implant-based reconstructions as they yield long-term, natural results and avoid complications related to implant-based surgery.

The reference in autologous breast reconstruction is the deep inferior epigastric artery perforator flap (DIEP flap), and alternatives such as the SGAP flap (superior gluteal artery perforator), TMG flap (transverse myocutaneous gracilis), or PAP flap (profunda artery perforator) have been reported. These substitutes are selected when the DIEP flap is not suitable due to inadequate volume or compromised tissue after previous surgery.

Yet, none of these flaps offer the convenience of the DIEP flap. The SGAP flap was our second choice, but the firmness of the gluteal fat can be an annoying hitch to shape an aesthetically pleasing breast. Differently, a great benefit of the LAP flap is the pliable and moldable fat tissue overlying the gluteus medius muscle.

The LAP flap is an excellent choice in slender, "pear-shaped" patients, as an alternative or surrogate for the DIEP flap or in patients that prefer not to have an abdominal scar.

Filip B. J. L. Stillaert (✉) · P. Blondeel · K. Van Landuyt
Department of Plastic and Reconstructive Surgery, University Hospital Gent, Ghent, East Flanders, Belgium
e-mail: Filip.stillaert@ugent.be; Phillip.blondeel@ugent.be; Koenraad.vanlanduyt@ugent.be

24.2 Anatomy

The four-paired lumbar arteries arise from the aorta and the majority pass posterior to psoas major muscle. The upper three lumbar arteries course between the quadratus lumborum muscle and the erector spinae muscle. The lumbar arteries arising from L4 run directly anterior to the quadratus lumborum muscle. The arteries pierce the aponeurosis of the transversus abdominis lateral to the erector spinae muscle or have an intramuscular course through the erector spinae. Once the vessels perforate the thoracolumbar fascia, they immediately branch into smaller vessels to supply the subcutaneous fat. Perforators arising from the fourth lumbar artery follow a more septocutaneous course and emerge between the erector spinae muscles and the quadratus lumborum (Fig. 24.1).

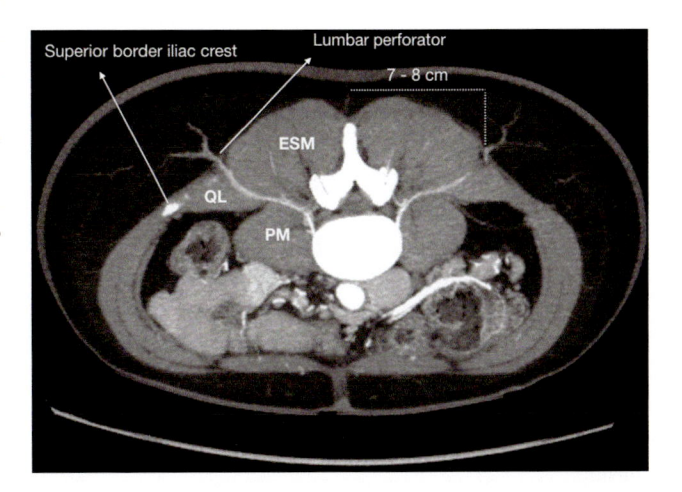

Fig. 24.1 CT scan showing the anatomy of the lower back region. The lumbar artery perforator L4 has a septocutaneous course and runs posteriorly to the psoas major muscle (PM). It then travels in between the quadratus lumborum muscle (QL) and the erector spinae muscle (ESM) and pierces the thoracolumbar fascia

© Springer Nature Switzerland AG 2023
D. Nikkhah et al. (eds.), *Core Techniques in Flap Reconstructive Microsurgery*, https://doi.org/10.1007/978-3-031-07678-7_24

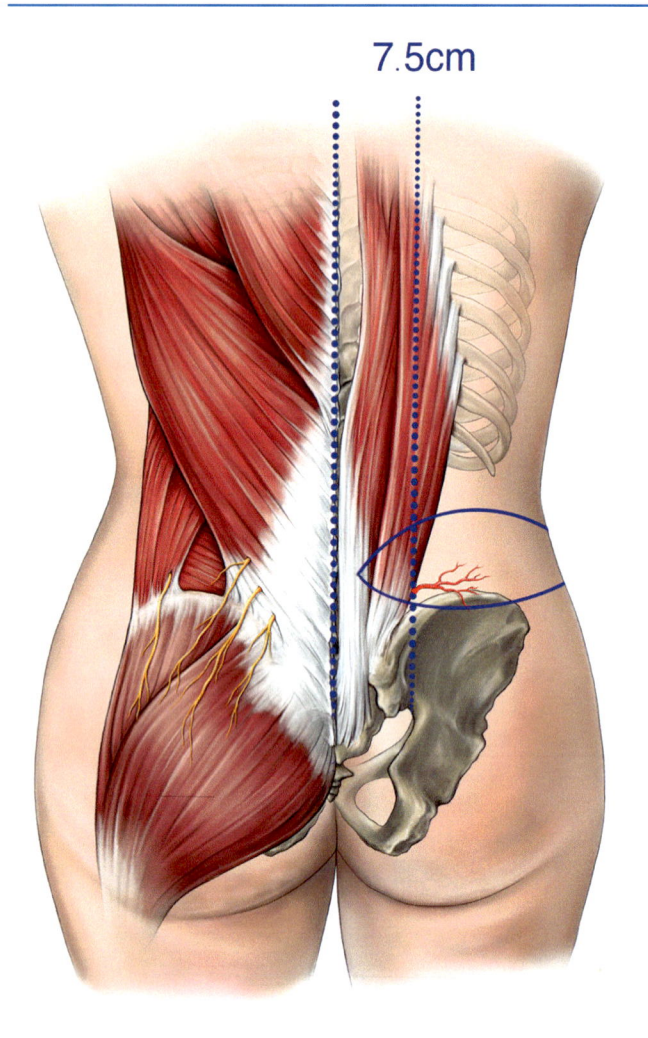

Fig. 24.2 The cluneal nerves innervate the upper part of the buttock region. These nerves are included in the LAP flap dissection and can be used to restore the sensibility of the newly reconstructed breast

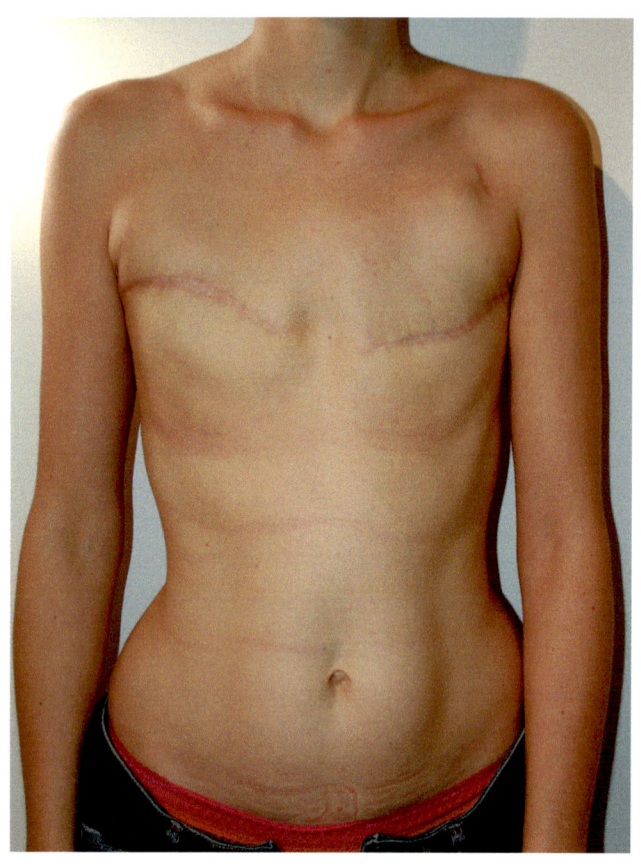

Fig. 24.3 A 33-year-old, slender patient with a medical history of bilateral mastectomy. Insufficient abdominal tissue excludes the use of a DIEP flap to perform an autologous breast reconstruction

Anatomical studies revealed an average of 5 ± 2 lumbar artery perforators [2–5]. The mean diameter of the lumbar artery and vein perforator ranges between 2.1 and 2.8 ± 0.3 mm [2, 4]. It is generally accepted that the lower lumbar vessels give off more and larger perforators with a dominancy of L3 and L4 perforators in more than 90 percent of the patients [2]. The mean point of perforation of the lumbar fascia is at an average distance of 7.5 cm from the midline [2, 5] (Fig. 24.2). This length is measured from a bird's eye view (CT scan findings). The real anatomical distance will be at 8–9 cm seen the convex shape of the erector spinae muscle.

The superior cluneal nerves innervate the skin of the upper part of the buttock region (Fig. 24.2). They are the first structures that are encountered intraoperatively and pierce the thoracolumbar fascia. The nerves can be incorporated in the LAP flap to restore breast sensation.

24.3 Preoperative Investigation

The ideal case for a breast reconstruction with a LAP flap is a slender patient with a pear-shaped body morphology that presents with surplus tissue in the love-handle region (Figs. 24.3 and 24.4). Medical history should exclude clotting diseases, smoking habits, allergy, lower spine surgery, or lower spine conditions.

A preoperative computed tomography (CT) angiography is performed of the lumbar and thoracic region (Fig. 24.5). This examination is performed in prone position and visualizes the size, branching pattern, pedicle length, patency, exact anatomical course, and position of the lumbar perforators.

It also displays the available donor tissue in the love-handle region. Permeability of the deep inferior epigastric vascular pedicle should be investigated whenever a previous breast reconstruction with a DIEP flap has been performed. Perforators are marked by the radiologist using a grid system with the midline being the Y-axis and the iliac crest being the X-axis.

24.4 Flap Design and Markings

The LAP flap is designed around the excess tissue in the love-handle region (Fig. 24.2). The initial markings are made in a standing position. Markings include the midline, the superior border of the iliac crest, and a vertical line drawn at 7.5 cm from the midline (Fig. 24.6). The skin island is designed around the perforator and the flap design starts medially at approximately 2 cm from the midline. A pinch test is performed to evaluate for a tension-free closure of the donor site. It is obvious that a primary reconstruction requires a smaller skin paddle compared to secondary reconstructions.

The flap is redesigned with the patient in prone position and marked more inferiorly due to the change in position (Fig. 24.7). The location of the perforator is confirmed by Doppler examination, and usually the L4 perforator is

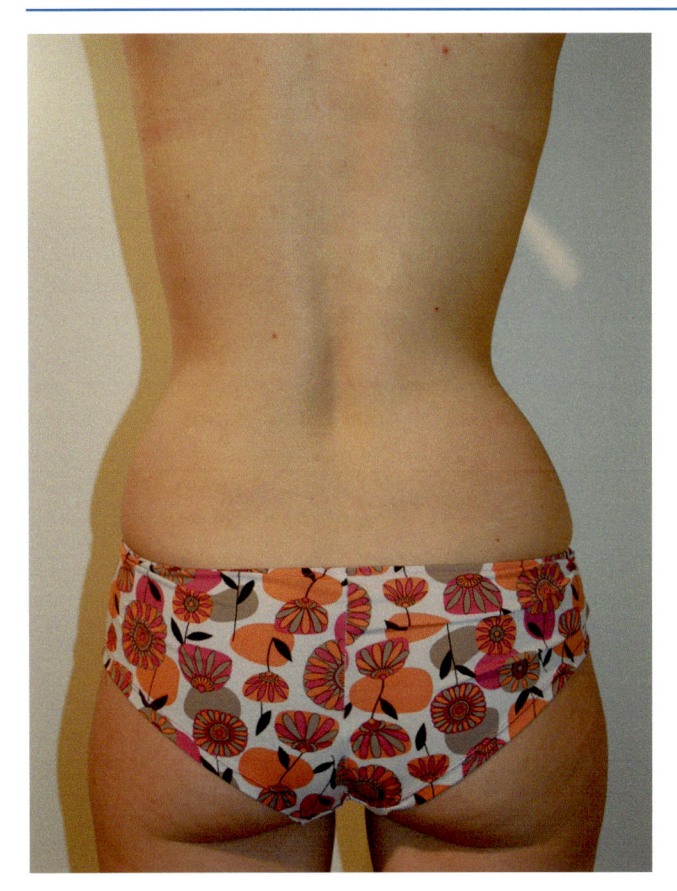

Fig. 24.4 The patient has a typical pear-shaped body morphology with excess tissue in the love-handle region. She is a good candidate for a bilateral, autologous breast reconstruction with a LAP flap. A bilateral LAP procedure is performed in a two-staged approach with an interval of 6 weeks

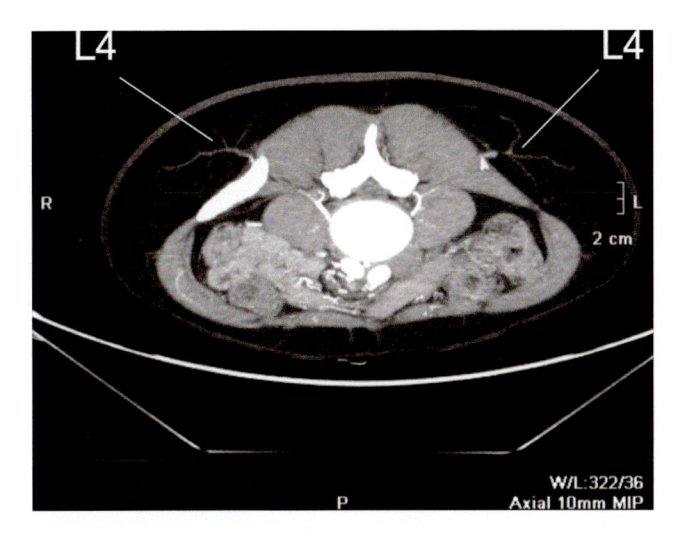

Fig. 24.5 The CT scan of the patient mentioned in Figs. 24.2 and 24.3 shows acceptable lumbar artery perforators to perform a LAP flap breast reconstruction. Notice the ample amount of subcutaneous tissue in the love-handle region compared to the subcutaneous abdominal tissue

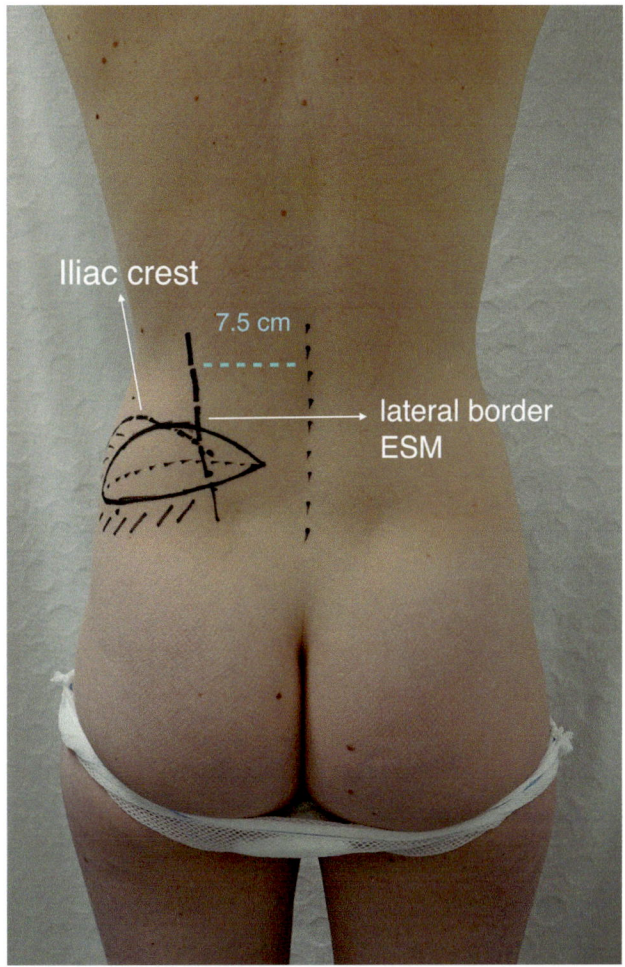

Fig. 24.6 The flap is designed in the lower back region and includes skin and subcutaneous fat tissue of the love-handle region. The midline is marked and a vertical line at 7.5 cm from the midline is drawn. Additional markings include the superior border of the posterior iliac crest and the presumed position of the final scar. The lateral border of the erector spinae muscle is marked (ESM)

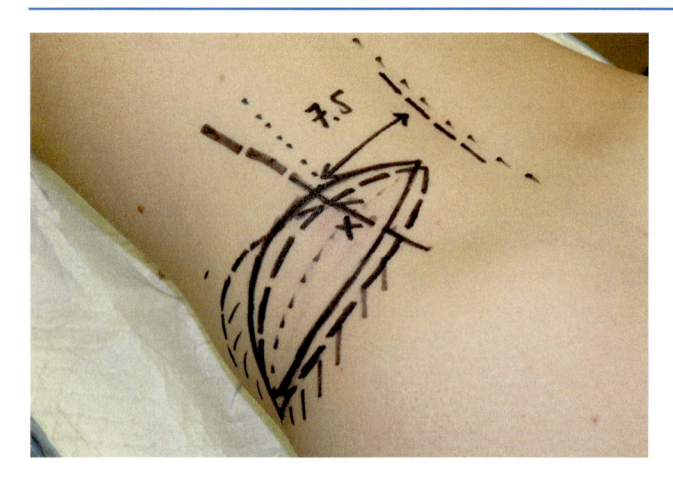

Fig. 24.7 The flap is redesigned more inferiorly with the patient in prone position (interrupted line)

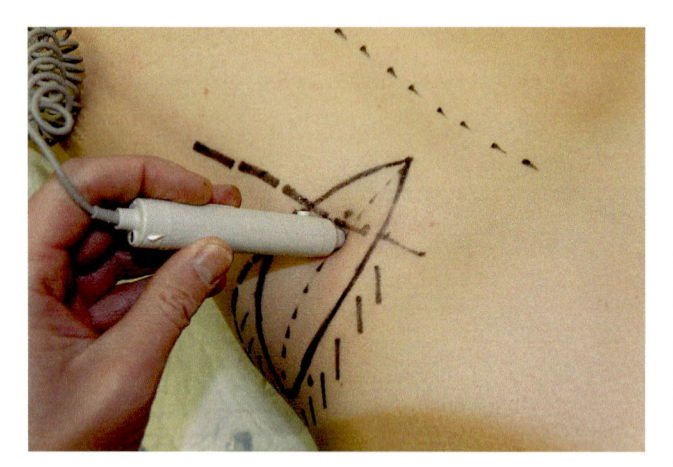

Fig. 24.8 The location of the perforator is confirmed with Doppler examination and marked

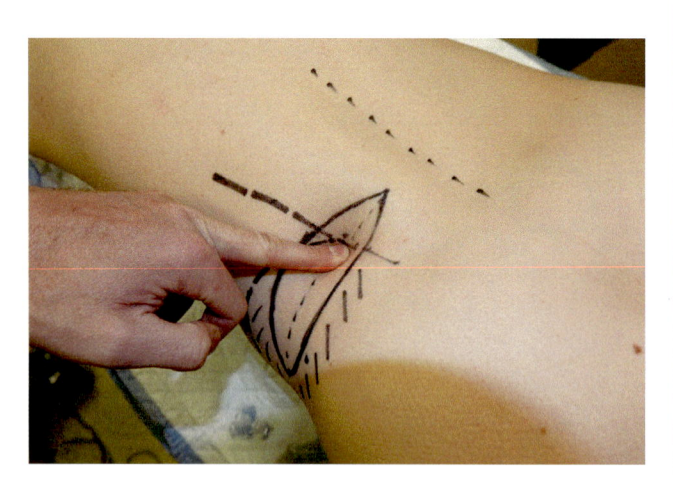

Fig. 24.9 Usually the L4 perforator is located where the lateral border of the erector spinae muscle meets the superior border of the iliac crest

located at the point where the vertical line meets the superior iliac crest (lateral border of the erector spinae muscle) (Figs. 24.8 and 24.9).

24.5 Flap Raise/Elevation: A Step-by-Step Guide

24.5.1 Supine Position

24.5.1.1 Mastectomy and Recipient Vessels
(Fig. 24.10)

The mastectomy is performed in primary cases with dissection of the recipient, parasternal mammary vessels. In secondary cases the skin inferiorly to the mastectomy scar is undermined and not desepidermised. This will recover part of the original skin envelope and minimizes the surface of the skin island of the LAP flap. Whenever feasible the mammary vessels are isolated through an intercostal approach without resection of the costochondral cartilage.

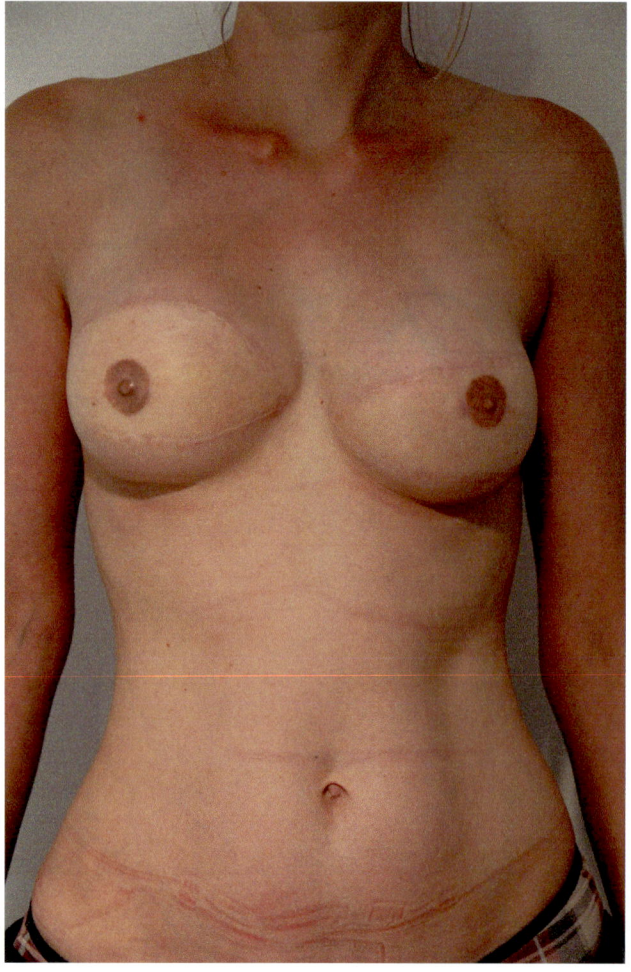

Fig. 24.10 Postoperative result of a bilateral breast reconstruction with the LAP flap (patient presented in Fig. 24.3). The skin inferiorly to the mastectomy scar has been recovered in order to minimize the surface of the skin island of the LAP flap

24 The Lumbar Artery Perforator Flap: A True Alternative in Autologous Breast Reconstruction

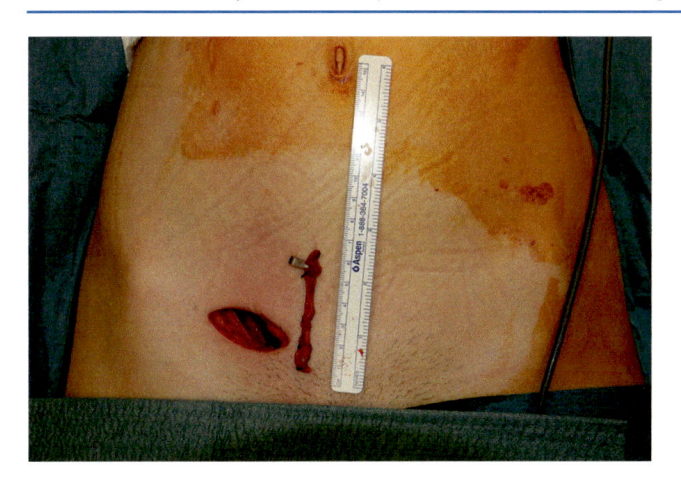

Fig. 24.11 A vascular interposition graft is harvested through a small incision in the groin region. The deep epigastric artery and vein are suitable vessels to lengthen the perforator. This facilitates flap inset, avoids traction on the anastomosis with the recipient vessels, and overcomes the size discrepancy between the perforator and the recipient (mammary vessels). Usually, the vascular interposition graft has a length of approximately 7 cm

24.5.1.2 Vascular Interposition Graft
(Fig. 24.11)

Meanwhile, the deep inferior epigastric artery and vein are harvested through a small incision in the inguinal region. The pedicle is divided as distal as possible in order to deal with the vessel discrepancy between the perforator and vascular graft. The graft is kept aside in a sterile heparin gauze. The convenience of harvesting the interposition graft at this stage is that the anastomosis with the perforator can be completed during the time when the patient is repositioned in supine position after flap harvest.

24.5.2 Prone Position

24.5.2.1 Flap Harvest from Medial to Lateral
(Figs. 24.12, 24.13, 24.14, 24.15, 24.16, 24.17, and 24.18)

The patient is installed in prone position for flap harvest. Flap margins are infiltrated with a xylocaine 1%-adrenaline solution to minimize intraoperative bleeding.

The flap is incised completely, and beveling is performed superiorly and more extensively in the inferior part of the flap to include the fat overlying the gluteus medius muscle.

Dissection starts from **medial to lateral** on top of the thoracolumbar fascia and continues over the concave contour of the erector spinae muscle. The superior border of the iliac crest is palpated and acts a reference point during the dissection.

The **superior cluneal nerves** are visualized and perforate the thoracolumbar fascia medially to the perforators. They can be used to restore breast sensation.

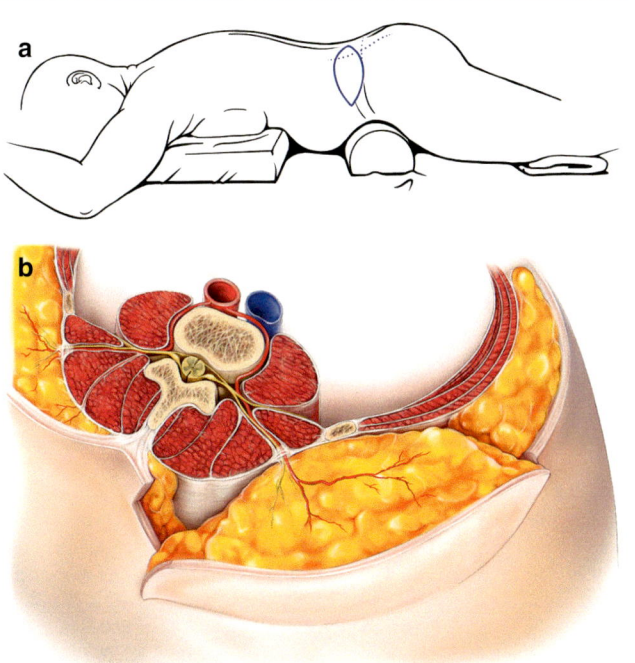

Fig. 24.12 (a–b) Dissection is performed in prone position and runs from medial to lateral on top of the thoracolumbar fascia. The subcutaneous tissue layer in the medial part of the flap is less voluminous compared to the lateral part. This facilitates dissection and exposure. The thoracolumbar fascia runs over the erector spinae muscle and the quadratus lumborum muscle. In between those two muscles, the fascia consists of two layers which could be confusing during dissection

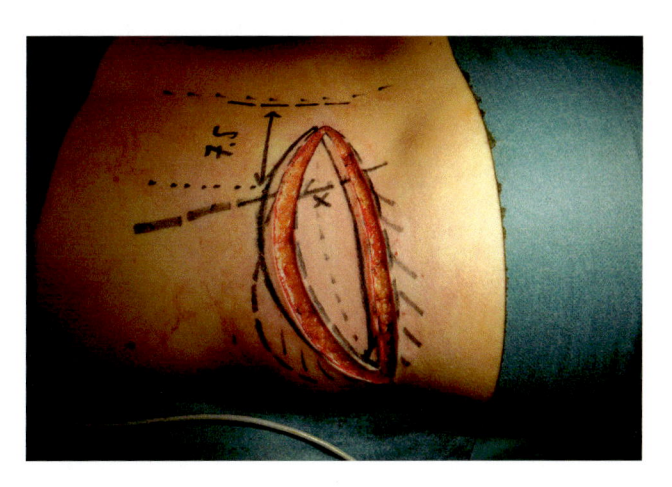

Fig. 24.13 The flap is completely incised circumferentially to allow for maximal exposure during dissection

The thoracolumbar fascia is incised and the cluneal nerve is isolated. Lateral to the cluneal nerve, the perforator is visualized: L4 runs adjacent to the upper margin of the iliac crest, and often L3 can be incorporated as well (can be used as a backup in case of damage to L4).

The perforator is progressively dissected out, and all side branches are carefully clipped to obtain maximal hemostasis. The dissection proceeds until a length of approximately 4–5 cm is obtained with an **artery that has a suitable diam-**

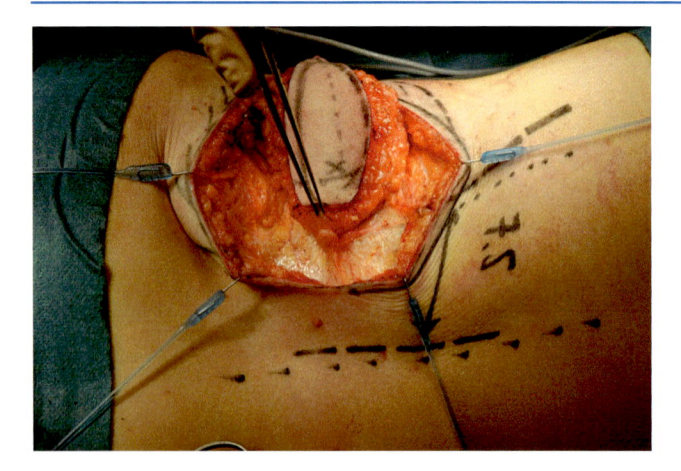

Fig. 24.14 Flap harvest starts at the medial side with the patient in prone position. The medial part has a thin subcutaneous layer and provides better exposure compared to a lateral approach. Dissection continues over the thoracolumbar fascia, and the superior border of the iliac crest is palpated (blue interrupted line). The iliac crest margin is a guidance as the L4 perforator will pierce the thoracolumbar fascia near this border at the lateral border of the erector spinae muscle. The first anatomical structures that are encountered are the superior cluneal nerves (*) that pierce the thoracolumbar fascia. These nerves are included in the flap and used for later anastomosis to the intercostal nerve

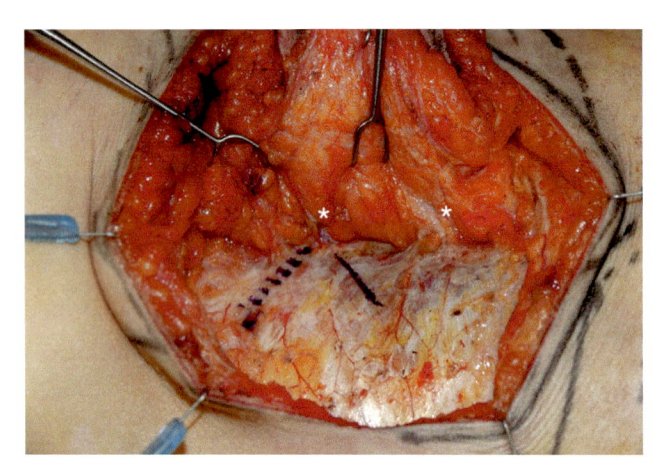

Fig. 24.15 Flap harvest starts at the medial side with the patient in prone position. A medial to lateral dissection provides better surgical exposure. Dissection is continued over the thoracolumbar fascia and continued to the lateral border of the erector spinae muscle

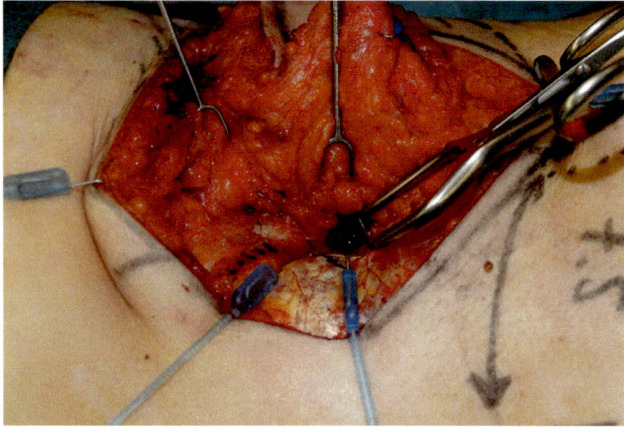

Fig. 24.16 The thoracolumbar fascia is incised, and the perforator is isolated. One can observe the L4 perforator that runs against the superior border of the iliac crest

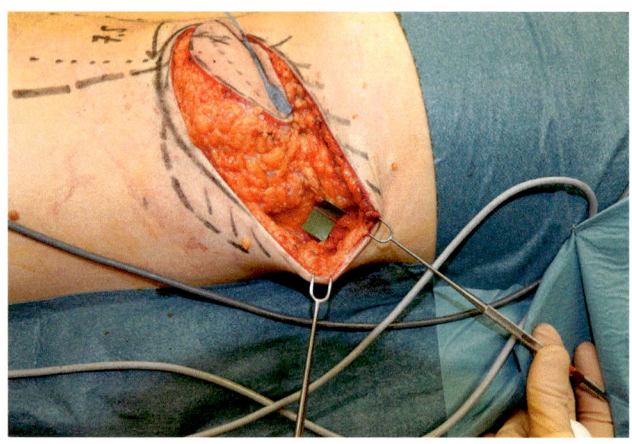

Fig. 24.17 Lateral dissection often reveals the descending branch of the iliohypogastric nerve

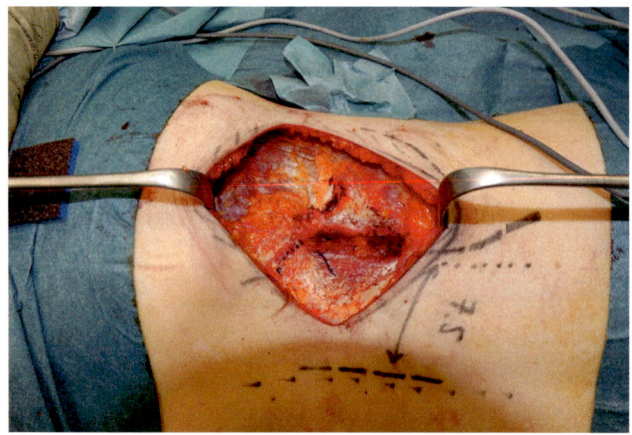

Fig. 24.18 Intraoperative view on the donor site and incision in the thoracolumbar fascia

eter to perform the anastomosis with the interposition graft. One should avoid a dissection toward the processus spinosus in order to avoid nerve damage.

Finally, the LAP flap is fully freed and includes the fat tissue overlying the gluteus medius muscle which has a unique, soft, and moldable consistency. In the lateral region of the flap, one should try to avoid damage to the iliohypogastric nerve (lateral cutaneous branch).

The incision in the thoracolumbar fascia is closed with a running Prolene 2/0 suture. Drains are inserted and the donor site is closed with Vicryl 2/0 tacking sutures. Subcutaneous sutures with Vicryl 3/0 close the donor site and the skin is closed with a running Monocryl 4/0 suture.

24.5.3 Supine Position

The patient is repositioned in supine position to perform the actual breast reconstruction. Meanwhile, the anastomosis between the vascular interposition graft and the perforator is carried out on a side table.

24.5.3.1 Anastomosis Between the Perforator of the LAP Flap and the Vascular Interposition Graft (Fig. 24.19)

The flap is transferred to a side table, and an end-to-end anastomosis is performed with an Ethilon 10/0 suture between the perforator and the vascular interposition graft. This is an important step in the procedure and requires specific attention: the anastomosis should be perfect as it will be difficult to place additional sutures once the flap has been anastomosed to the recipient vessels.

24.5.3.2 Flap Transfer to the Chest and Flap Insertion (Figs. 24.20 and 24.21)

The LAP flap is transferred to the mastectomy site. An end-to-end anastomosis is performed with an Ethilon 9/0 suture in between the vascular interposition graft and the recipient vessels (in most cases the parasternal mammary vessels in the intercostal space III). An additional nerve anastomosis is performed between the cluneal nerve and the intercostal nerve with an Ethilon 9/0 suture. The flap is positioned to shape the breast: the gluteal part with the moldable fat can be positioned superiorly to achieve upper-pole fullness and cleavage definition or can be positioned inferiorly to achieve lower-pole fullness.

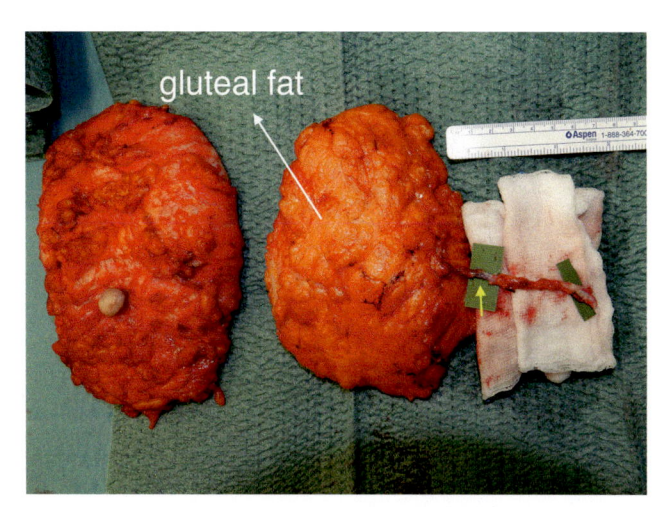

Fig. 24.19 The mastectomy specimen is seen on the left side. The LAP flap has the same shape and volume of the breast. A vascular interposition graft is anastomosed to the perforator to lengthen the pedicle, avoid traction, and facilitate flap inset (arrow). Most of the volume of LAP flap consists of gluteal fat overlying the gluteus medius muscle

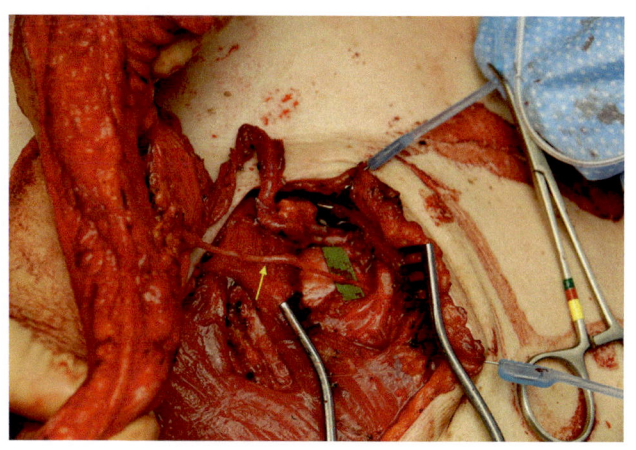

Fig. 24.20 An intraoperative view on the anastomosis between the vascular interposition graft and the mammary vessels. Notice the tension-free appearance of the pedicle of the LAP flap. An additional anastomosis is seen between the cluneal nerve and the intercostal nerve (arrow)

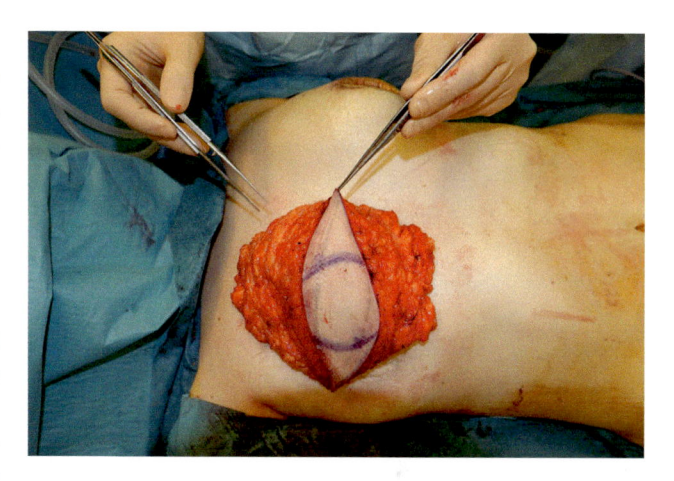

Fig. 24.21 The LAP flap is seen on the chest wall and has ideal volume and contours to reconstruct a breast. It has a conic shape. The gluteal fat can be positioned inferiorly to have lower-pole fullness or can be positioned superiorly to have a well-defined cleavage. In this case the gluteal fat is seen superiorly

24.6 Core Surgical Techniques in Flap Dissection

1. Harvest of the deep inferior epigastric pedicle as an interposition graft (Fig. 24.22).

   The vascular interposition graft plays a crucial role in a breast reconstruction using the LAP flap. It lengthens the vascular pedicle of the LAP flap, avoids tension on the anastomosis with the recipient vessels, and overcomes the discrepancy between the perforator and the recipient vessels. It is important to harvest this interposition graft as distal as possible to match vessel diameter between perforator and graft.

2. Dissection proceeds from medial to lateral in prone position (Fig. 24.23).

   Instead of a lateral decubitus approach, we prefer to perform flap harvest in prone position from medial to lateral. The advantage is a less voluminous tissue bulk on the medial part of the LAP flap. A dissection from lateral to medial in lateral decubitus position will result in a more difficult approach and intraoperative view due to the tissue in the lateral part of the LAP flap.

3. The perforator is located at the lateral border of the erector spinae muscle (Fig. 24.12).

   The CT scan measures the position of the perforator in a bird eye's view (normally 7.5–8 cm) from the midline. Remember that the contour of the erector spinae muscle is a concave contour and the real location of the perforator will be at approximately 9 cm. The border of the iliac crest is also a good reference point to guide your dissection.

4. The cluneal nerve.

   The cluneal nerves are the first identifiable anatomical structures to be encountered. They are located medially to the perforator and should be included in the LAP flap. They are anastomosed to the intercostal nerve to restore sensation in the breast.

5. Do not proceed your dissection too deep until the processus spinosus.

   The moment the artery of the perforator has an acceptable diameter (2 mm), the perforator can be clipped. A

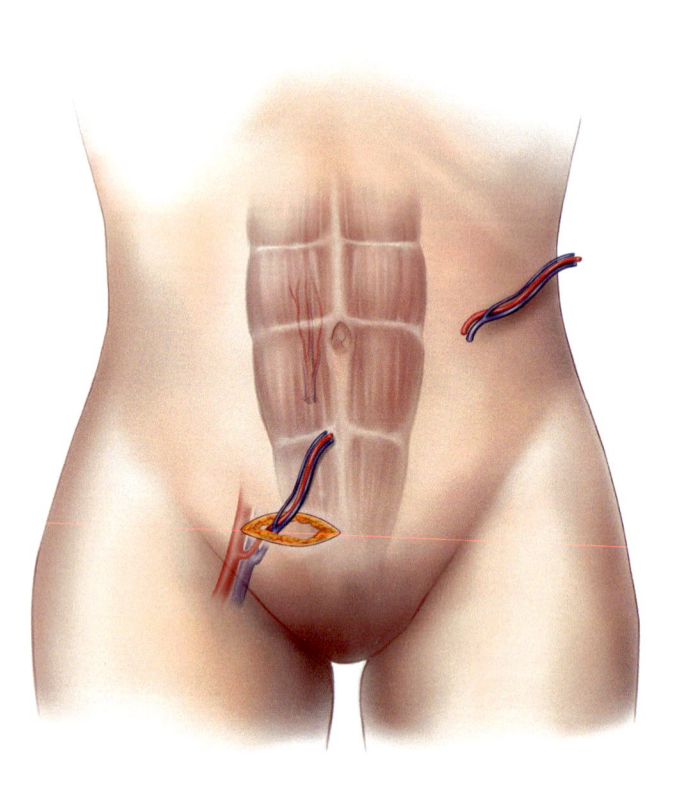

Fig. 24.22 Our first choice for an interposition graft is the deep inferior epigastric vessels. They are harvested through a small incision in the inguinal region. Dissection should proceed as distal as possible to overcome the vessel diameter discrepancy. Alternatives whenever they are not available are the thoracodorsal vessels or the descending branch of the lateral circumflex femoral vessels

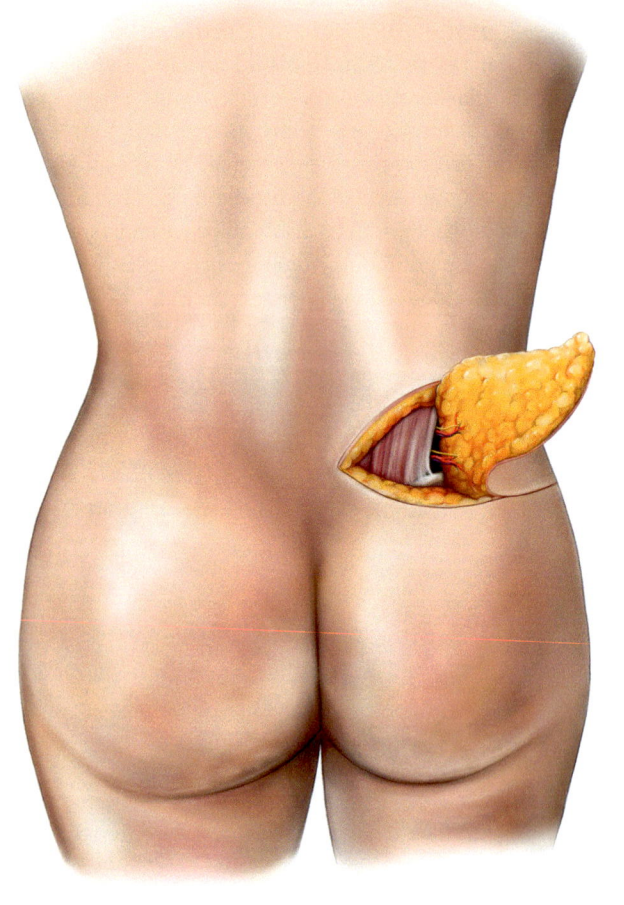

Fig. 24.23 The LAP flap is harvested in prone position and dissection starts medial. The subcutaneous tissue bulk in this region is less voluminous compared to the lateral part and facilitates dissection and surgical exposure

dissection that goes too deep will increase the risk of nerve root damage, and an intraoperative bleeding will be too difficult to handle.
6. Try to avoid a dissection too laterally to avoid damage to the iliohypogastric nerve.

   Whenever feasible, especially in slender patients, one should identify the descending branch of the iliohypogastric nerve to avoid postoperative discomfort in the lateral part of the buttock region or upper thigh region.
7. Include the fat overlying the gluteus medius muscle.

   The fat overlying the gluteus medius has an ideal consistency to shape the breast. It is moldable and has a softer consistency compared to subcutaneous fat.
8. The vascular interposition graft is anastomosed to the perforator on a side table (Fig. 24.24).

A crucial step that requires attention is the anastomosis between the perforator and the interposition graft. An Ethilon 10/0 suture is used to anastomose the artery and vein. Often a second vein can be anastomosed. This anastomosis should be perfect as it will be challenging to add additional sutures once the vascular clamps are released on the recipient vessels.

24.7 Clinical Scenario

Case 1

Post-bariatric 48-year-old patient with a history of gastric bypass surgery and a circumferential abdominoplasty procedure. One year later she had a prophylactic bilateral mastectomy with immediate implant-based reconstruction. She developed an infection of the right implant and both implants were removed with the insertion of new implants. She had a recurrence of the infection on the right side with wound dehiscence and was referred to our department for a second opinion (Fig. 24.25).

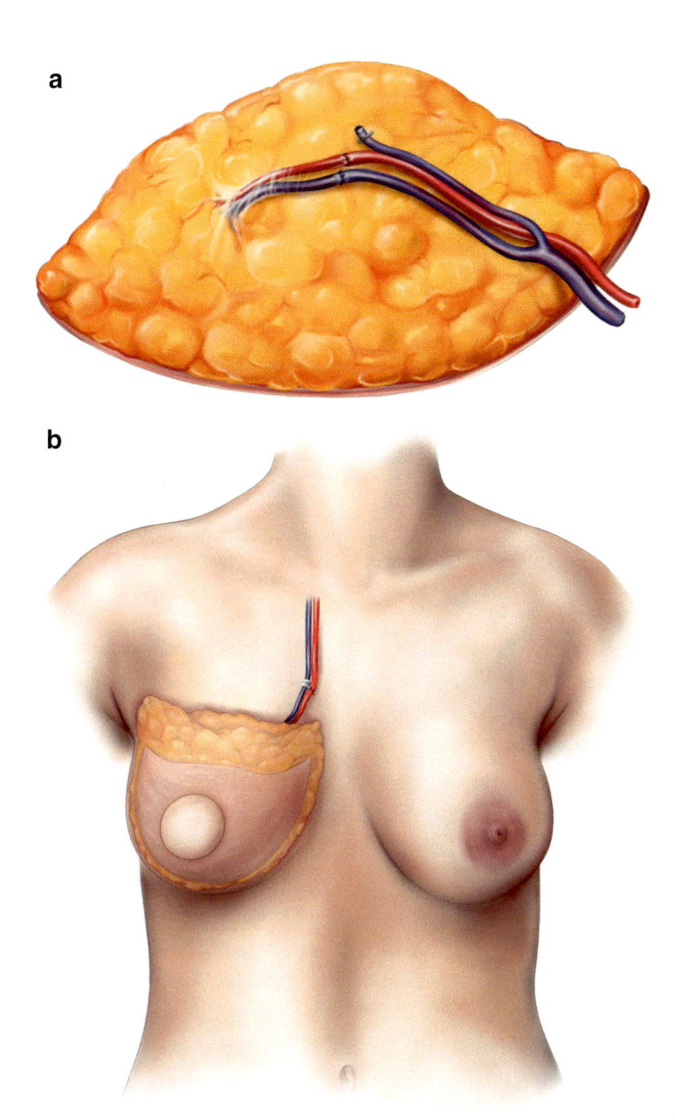

Fig. 24.24 (**a**, **b**) It is mandatory to lengthen the perforator with an interposition graft. The anastomoses are done on a side table with a 10/0 Ethilon suture. Lengthening the perforator avoids traction on the anastomosis with the recipient vessels and facilitates flap inset

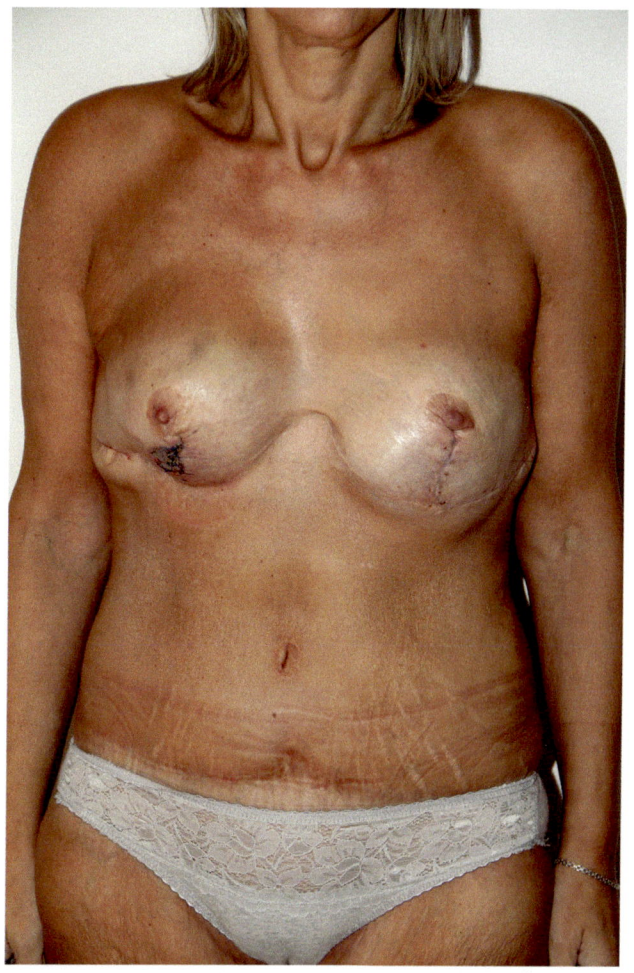

Fig. 24.25 History of bilateral mastectomy with complicated implant-based reconstruction. She presented at our outpatient with implant exposure, footprint deformity, and excessive scarring. She had a history of gastric bypass surgery and circumferential abdominoplasty

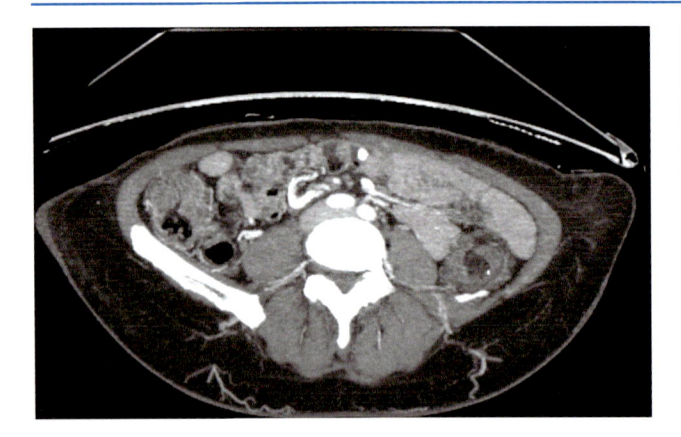

Fig. 24.26 Angio-CT scan examination revealed acceptable and non-scarred lumbar artery perforators to perform a LAP flap breast reconstruction procedure

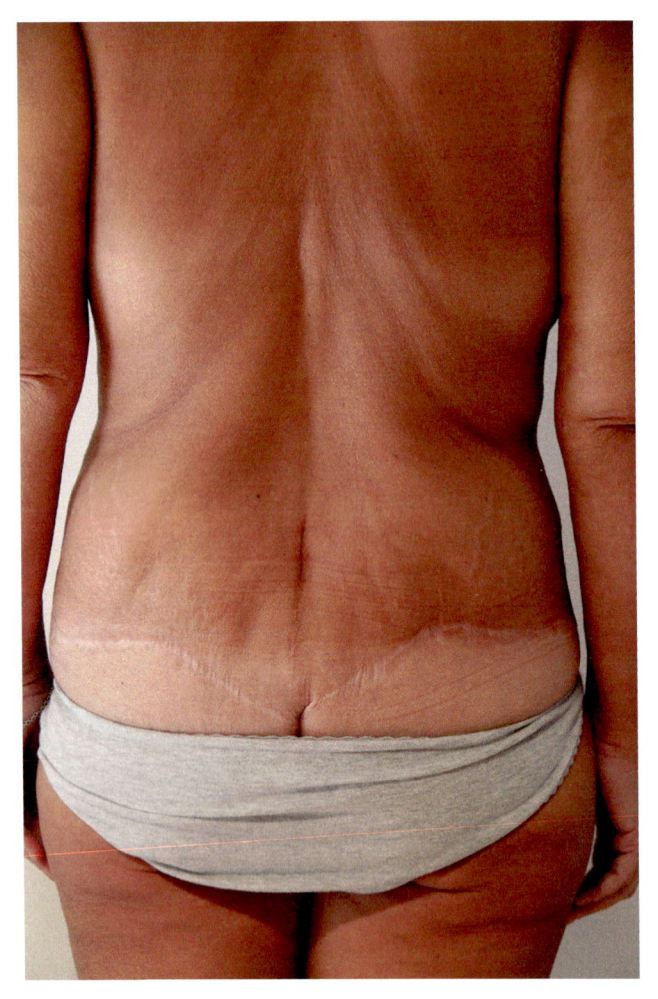

Fig. 24.27 The LAP flap was chosen to avoid additional scarring, and we used the existing scars of the circumferential abdominoplasty procedure

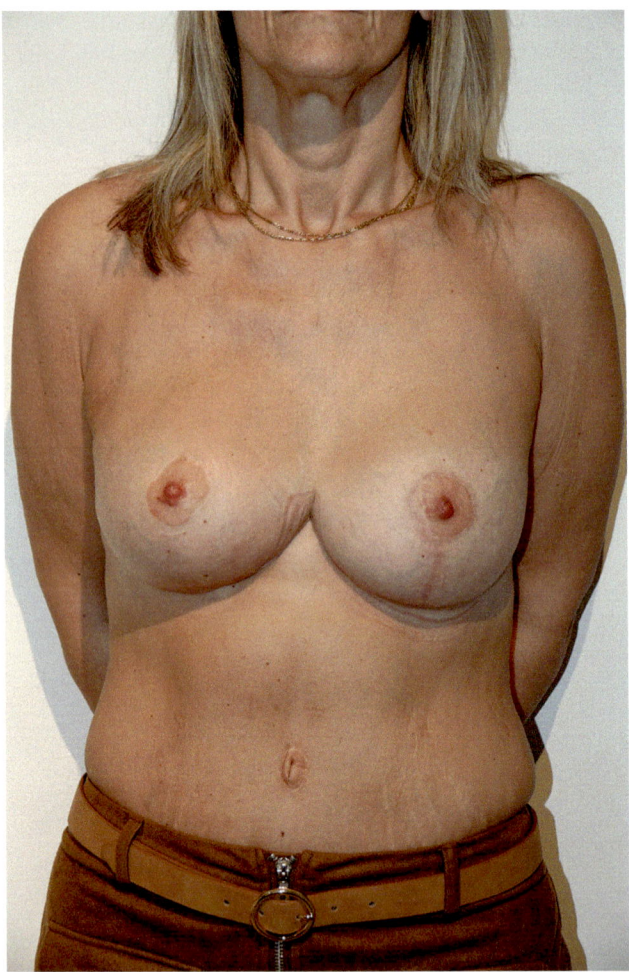

Fig. 24.28 Postoperative view at 2 years with bilateral LAP flap reconstruction and an additional implant of 185 mL. Restoration of breast projection, breast volume, footprint, and symmetry

Her angio-CT scan showed well-developed lumbar artery perforators (Fig. 24.26). To avoid additional scarring, we opted to use the existing scars in the lower back region and choose a LAP flap to reconstruct both breasts (Fig. 24.27). The weight of the right and left LAP flap was 395 gr and 365 gr, respectively.

Postoperatively the patient requested for additional volume, and an additional silicon ergonomic implant was inserted of 185 mL (Fig. 24.28).

Case 2

A 34-year-old patient diagnosed with BRCA1 mutation. History of right breast cancer with mastectomy and prophylactic left mastectomy (Fig. 24.3). She refused a reconstruction with implants and came to our department for a second opinion. She is an ideal candidate for a breast reconstruction with a bilateral LAP procedure (Fig. 24.4). The angio-CT scan examination revealed acceptable lumbar artery perforators to perform the breast reconstruction (Fig. 24.5). She is seen 2 years postoperatively (Fig. 24.29).

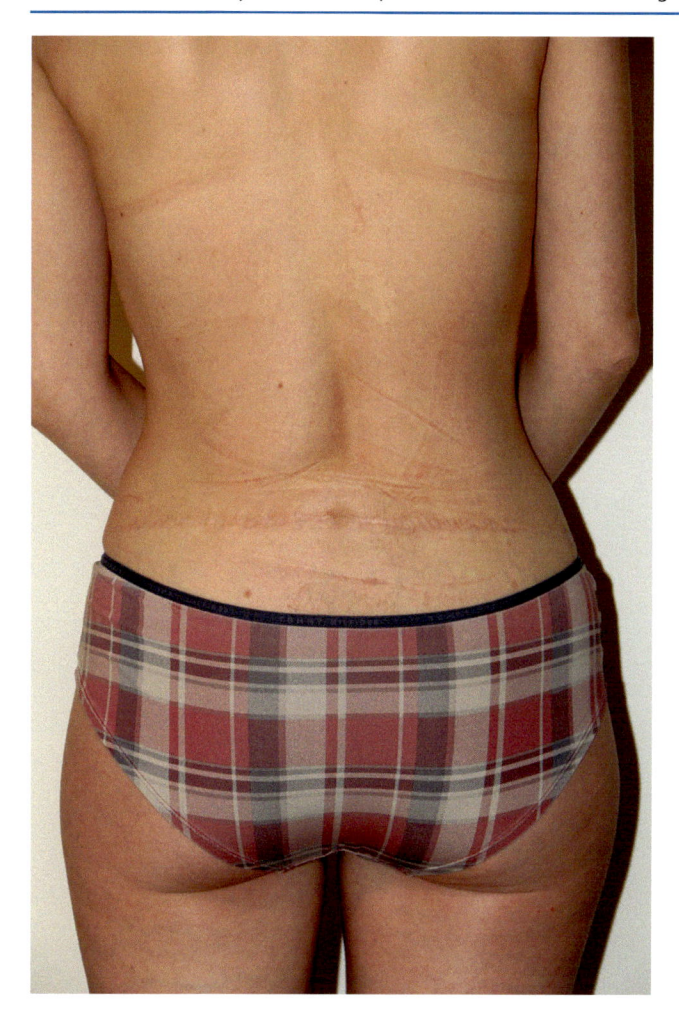

Fig. 24.29 View on the donor site of a bilateral LAP breast reconstruction (patient presented in Fig. 24.3)

24.8 Pearls and Pitfalls

Pearls
- Dissection in prone position not lateral decubitus position.
- Dissection from medial to lateral.
- Harvest the deep epigastric inferior vessels as an interposition graft (alternatives are thoracodorsal vessels or descending branch of the lateral circumflex femoral artery/vein).
- Include the cluneal nerve to restore sensation.
- Use the operating microscope to dissect the perforators.

Pitfalls
- Harvest the interposition graft as distal as possible to match vessel diameter.
- Include the fat overlying the gluteus medius muscle.
- Avoid damage to the iliohypogastric nerve that crosses the lateral border of the iliac crest.
- Do not proceed the perforator dissection too deep to avoid nerve damage or uncontrolled bleeding; as long as the artery diameter is sufficient you should stop the dissection.
- Try to limit the size of the skin island in order to perform a tension-free closure of the donor site.

24.9 Selected Readings

- de Weerd L, Elvenes OP, Strandenes E, Weum S. Autologous breast reconstruction with a free lumbar artery perforator flap. Br J Plast Surg. 2003;56(2): 180–3.
- Opsomer D, Stillaert F, Blondeel P, Van Landuyt K. The Lumbar artery perforator flap in autologous breast reconstruction: initial experience with 100 cases. Plast Reconstr Surg. 2018;142(1):1e–8e.
- Sommeling CE, Colebunders B, Pardon HE, Stillaert FB, Blondeel PN, van Landuyt K. Lumbar artery perforators: an anatomical study based on computed tomographic angiography imaging. Acta Chir Belg. 2017;117(4): 223–6.
- Peters KT, Blondeel PN, Lobo F, van Landuyt K. Early experience with the free lumbar artery perforator flap for breast reconstruction. J Plast Reconstr Aesthet Surg. 2015;68(8):1112–9.
- Offman SL, Geddes CR, Tang M, Morris SF. The vascular basis of perforator flaps based on the source arteries of the lateral lumbar region. Plast Reconstr Surg. 2005;115: 1651–9.

References

1. de Weerd L, Elvenes OP, Strandenes E, Weum S. Autologous breast reconstruction with a free lumbar artery perforator flap. Br J Plast Surg. 2003 Mar;56(2):180–3.
2. Hamdi M, Craggs B, Brussaard C, Seidenstueker K, Hendrickx B, Zeltzer A. Lumbar artery perforator flap: an anatomical

study using multidetector computed tomographic scan and surgical pearls for breast reconstruction. Plast Reconstr Surg. 2016;138(2):343–52.
3. Lui KW, Hu S, Ahmad N, Tang M. Three-dimensional angiography of the superior gluteal artery and lumbar artery perforator flap. Plast Reconstr Surg. 2009;123:79–86.
4. Offman SL, Geddes CR, Tang M, Morris SF. The vascular basis of perforator flaps based on the source arteries of the lateral lumbar region. Plast Reconstr Surg. 2005;115:1651–9.
5. Kato H, Hasegawa M, Takada T, Torii S. The lumbar artery perforator based island flap: anatomical study and case reports. Br J Plast Surg. 1999;52:541–6.

Right Gastroepiploic Artery: Omental Flap

25

Vladimir Anikin and Katherine de Rome

25.1 Introduction

The greater omentum is a well-vascularized fatty apron, coined the "abdominal policeman" in 1906 by the surgeon Rutherford Morrison (1). Its use as a flap has evolved with time, ever since its first described use in the protection of intestinal anastomosis in 1888. The first free omental flap was performed by McLean and Buncke in 1972 where a large scalp defect was reconstructed with omentum and covering skin graft (2). This greatly expanded its potential indications for recipient sites which were previously limited by pedicle length.

The omentum has unique properties which convey specific advantages to its use as a flap. It has the ability to promote neo-angiogenesis and tissue healing in regions to which it is applied, a critical benefit to ischemic and inflamed tissues. Studies have demonstrated the omentum to be a rich source of growth factors, inflammatory mediators, and pluripotent stem cells (3). Another favorable characteristic is its high lymphoedema absorptive capacity and amorphous structure, easily able to fill cavity defects.

The indications for free or pedicled omental flaps are vast. Common recipient sites include head and neck defects, locally advanced breast cancer, prevention of lymphoedema in radical lymph node dissections, and treatment of deep sternal wound infections. It is also important to note a number of important relative contraindications for the use of the omentum, for instance, previous major abdominal operations, portal hypertension, and a history of gastric outlet obstruction.

25.2 Anatomy

The omentum is a double layer of the peritoneum, attached to the greater curvature of the stomach and transverse colon, hanging to cover the contents of the abdominal cavity. Its blood supply is derived from the branches of celiac trunk, namely, the right and left gastroepiploic arteries (Fig. 25.1). The right gastroepiploic artery is typically dominant compared to the left and is the largest terminal branch of the gastroduodenal artery (GDA). The gastroepiploic veins accompany the gastroepiploic arteries and drain into the portal system.

The GDA arises from the common hepatic artery in 75% of cases; it may also branch from the right or left hepatic artery and can rarely arise from the superior mesenteric artery. It runs posterior to the proximal duodenum, along the lower margin of the pylorus, and then along the greater curvature of the stomach between the layers of the omentum as the right gastroepiploic artery (RGEA). Its termination is variable; most commonly it terminates at the middle of the gastric curvature; however, in 30% of patients, there is a well-developed continuous arcade with the left artery. There are several gastric and omental branches arising from the gastroepiploic arcade. The omental branches course inferiorly providing the omentum with its arterial supply and forming secondary anterior and posterior arcades. The right gastroepiploic vein (RGEV) runs parallel to the RGEA along the greater curvature of the stomach joining the superior mesenteric vein near its junction with the splenic vein.

Anatomical studies have demonstrated a variation in size of the RGEA along its course. The diameter varies from 3.0 mm at origin to 1.5 mm at middle of the greater curvature. Its flow rate also varies considerably between patients, with an average of 55.78 ml/min (4). This corresponds to a

V. Anikin (✉)
Department of Thoracic Surgery, Harefield Hospital, Royal Brompton and Harefield Hospital NHS Foundation Trust, London, UK

Department of Oncology and Reconstructive Surgery, Sechenov First Moscow State Medical University, Moscow, Russia
e-mail: v.anikin@rbht.nhs.uk

K. de Rome
Department of Thoracic Surgery, Harefield Hospital, Royal Brompton and Harefield Hospital NHS Foundation Trust, London, UK

© Springer Nature Switzerland AG 2023
D. Nikkhah et al. (eds.), *Core Techniques in Flap Reconstructive Microsurgery*, https://doi.org/10.1007/978-3-031-07678-7_25

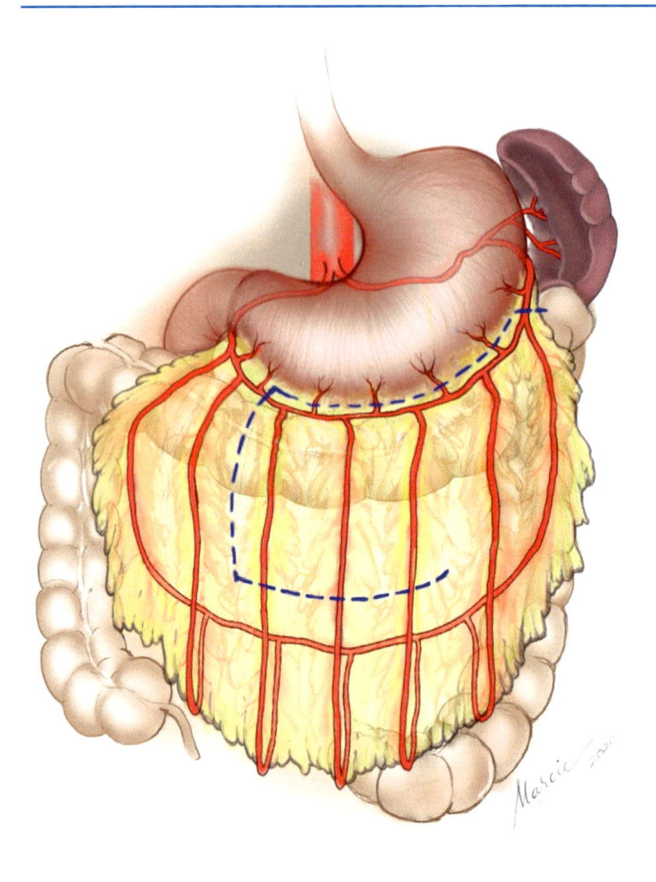

Fig. 25.1 Anatomical overview of anatomy of the greater omentum (Courtesy of Marcie Bunalade, 2020, All rights retained)

greater flow rate than other commonly used flaps, for example, the latissimus dorsi flap based on the thoracodorsal artery with an estimated in situ flow rate of 16.6 ml/min (5).

25.3 Preoperative Investigation

To date it has not been possible to calculate omental volume from preoperative investigations. Anatomical studies in cadavers have demonstrated considerable variation in its size with average dimensions of 34 cm wide by 24 cm in length (6). The omental flap size, however, correlates roughly with patient's height and weight but not significantly enough to accurately predict flap volume. The best predictor of omental volume is total body fat content, and obese individuals will have excessive volumes when compared to a malnourished cachectic patient. Some groups have suggested the use of a diagnostic laparoscopy prior to reconstruction in order to gauge omental volume and any conflicting abdominal pathology such as significant adhesions from prior surgery or trauma.

Preoperative evaluation of the omental blood supply is recommended if easily accessible. CT angiography has been shown to be an effective tool in the assessment of the anatomical properties of the RGEA (7). It can ensure suitability for its use as a flap prior to mini laparotomy is performed. Alternative ultrasonographic evaluation of the GEA is also feasible (8). Pulsatile flow and diameter can be recorded from upper median views of the abdomen, negating the need for IV contrast when contraindicated.

25.4 Flap Design and Markings

Flap design and arterial supply are determined by distance to the recipient site. If the pedicled flap does not have sufficient length to reach the site via the right gastroepiploic artery and primary arcade, the flap can be lengthened further. This is done through division of the primary arcade and use of the secondary arcade. The feeding arcade can be further skeletonized to aid delivery of the flap. Delivery route must also be taken into consideration preoperatively; a window may be made in the diaphragm for this purpose but must be of sufficient size to prevent torsion or compression of the pedicle.

25.5 Core Surgical Techniques in Flap Dissection

An upper midline laparotomy is a standard access for the greater omentum. Previous abdominal surgeries or disease may have resulted in adhesions which need to be divided and taken down before the omentum can be fully assessed. Integrity and blood flow through the omentum can be assessed through manual pulse check or with a handheld Doppler probe.

Mobilization of the omentum from the transverse colon is first achieved through dissection along the avascular embryonic fusion plane; care is taken to avoid damage to middle colic arterial branches. This dissection is aided by cephalad retraction of the omentum with countertraction on the transverse colon (Fig. 25.2). The omentum can then be delivered through the midline incision to aid planning of the size of the graft.

The left gastroepiploic artery and vein are commonly ligated near the spleen, if basing the flap blood supply on the dominant right gastroepiploic artery. However, in some situations, e.g., left-sided chest wall defects, excessive stretch on the right-sided pedicle may dictate the use of the left gastroepiploic artery instead. The omentum is carefully dissected from the stomach along the greater curvature in a left to right direction, dividing tributaries between the arcade and gastric wall (Fig. 25.3). We prefer to divide these vessels with ligation rather than use powered instruments to avoid thermal injury to the arcade. The arcade is mobilized to the level of the pylorus. An optional running stitch along the greater cur-

Fig. 25.2 Separation of the greater omentum from the transverse colon (Courtesy of Marcie Bunalade, 2020, All rights retained)

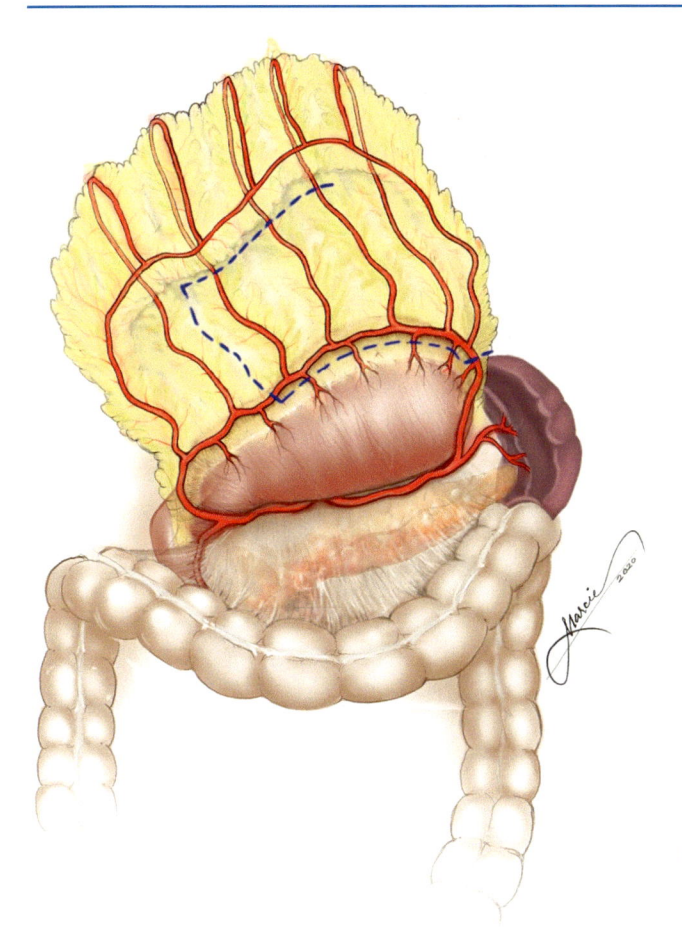

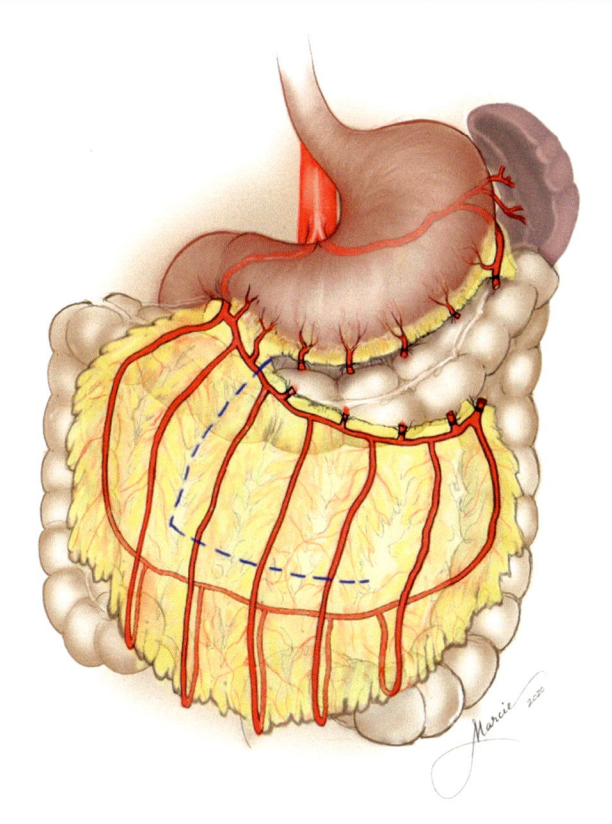

Fig. 25.3 Mobilization of the greater omentum from the stomach (Courtesy of Marcie Bunalade, 2020, All rights retained)

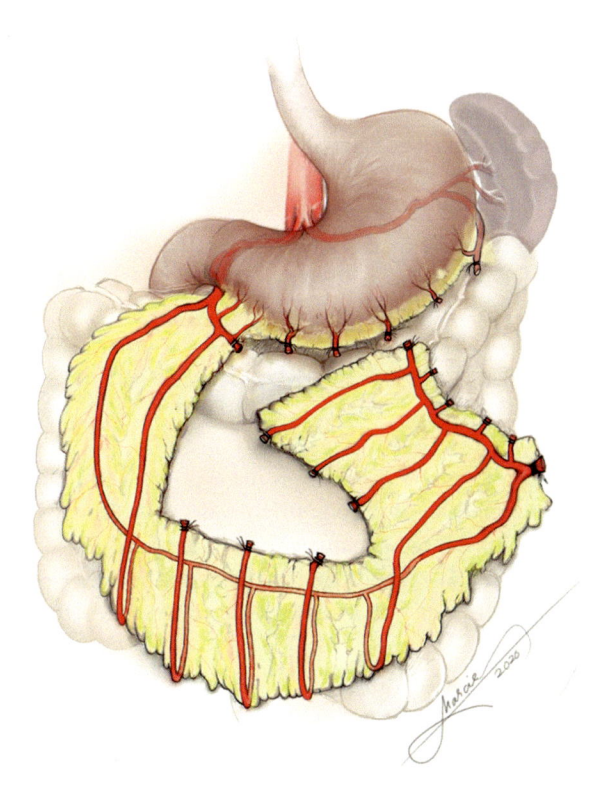

Fig. 25.4 Elongation of the pedicled greater omentum flap (Courtesy of Marcie Bunalade, 2020, All rights retained)

vature is recommended to peritonize the denuded area and provide additional security to ligated stumps.

The omentum can now be assessed as to whether it will reach the desired recipient site. If this is not possible, the pedicled omental flap can be lengthened through the division of the anterior epiploic arteries basing the blood supply on the secondary anterior and posterior omental arcades (Fig. 25.4). Passing the omentum through the laparotomy wound should be avoided, for target sites within the thorax creation of a window in the anterior diaphragm can be created to allow passage of the flap (Fig. 25.5). A free omental flap is possible for remote coverage. In these instances, the right gastroepiploic artery and vein are carefully denuded under magnification. Once the recipient site is ready, the vascular pedicle can be divided between ligatures and re-anastomosed at the distant site. Following transposition, the flap can be secured along its perimeter with absorbable interrupted or a running stitch.

Although open harvesting of the omental flap is described above, it is important to mention laparoscopic harvesting of the omental flap (LHOF) which was first described by Costa

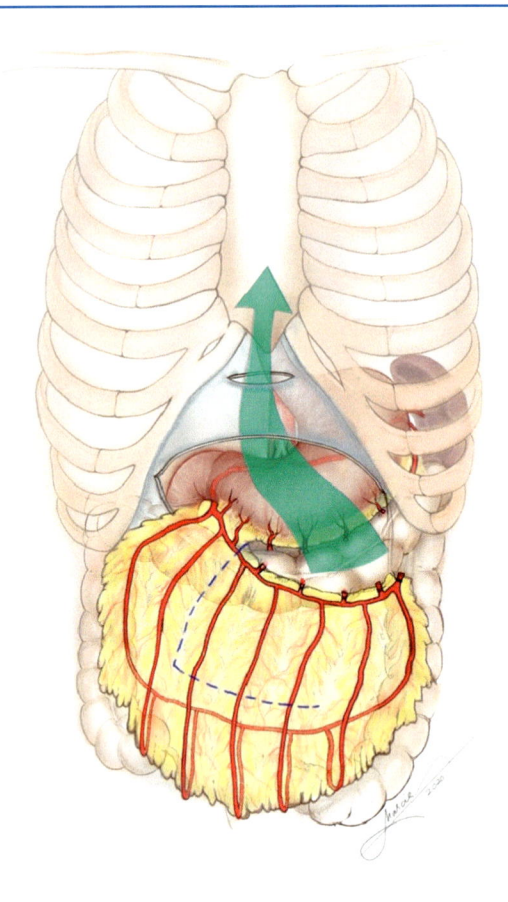

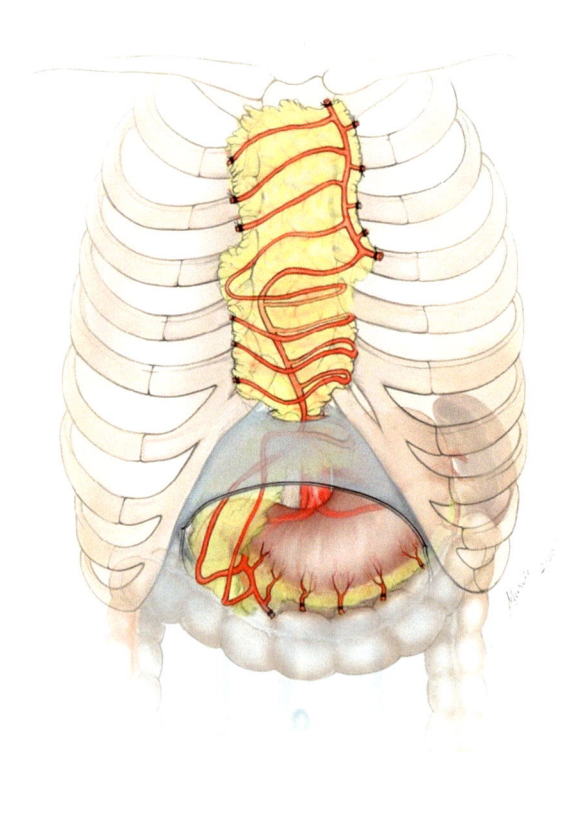

Fig. 25.5 (**a**, **b**) Delivery of pedicled omental flap to recipient site (Courtesy of Marcie Bunalade, 2020, All rights retained)

in 1998. It has since become a popular technique in breast reconstructive surgery with evidence supporting its safety and success rates (9). Laparoscopic harvesting significantly reduces donor site morbidity, with no midline scar and reduction in adhesions and incisional hernias rates, and therefore may be preferable if the requisite laparoscopic skills are available to the harvesting team.

25.6 Flap Raise: A Step-by-Step Guide

Step 1 Upper midline incision is made or less commonly a transverse incision over epigastric quadrant. Adhesions are taken down and omentum carefully separated from the abdominal wall. Its blood supply via the right and left gastroepiploic arteries can be assessed with a handheld Doppler probe.

Step 2 The greater omentum is then separated from the transverse colon along embryologic fusion plane. In this way the omentum is fully mobilized and graft size can be planned.

Step 3 If basing the flap off of the dominant right gastroepiploic artery, the left can be ligated near the spleen. The greater omentum is then dissected from the stomach along the greater curvature preserving gastroepiploic arcade.

Step 4 The pedicled flap can be lengthened by dividing anterior epiploic arteries and maintaining its blood supply through secondary anterior and posterior omental arcades. Blood supply maintained through first two omental branches from the primary arcade.

Step 5 Greater omentum flap can be delivered through a window in the anterior portion of the diaphragm into thoracic cavity to avoid risk of hernias. The omental flap is secured with an absorbable interrupted or running stitch around its perimeter, with additional stitches to secure the pedicle taking care not to damage the feeding vessels.

25.7 Clinical Scenario: The Use of the Greater Omentum in Deep Sternal Wound Infections (DSWI) and Nonunion of the Sternum

Deep sternal wound infections (DSWI) are a rare (1%) but devastating complication of cardiac surgery. The use of the greater omentum as a salvage flap in DSWI is well described in the literature. We include here the case of a 64-year-old patient with chronic sternal nonunion and infection following coronary artery bypass surgery. The patient required bilateral internal mammary arteries for grafting which limited the options for sternal reconstruction with a pectoralis or rectus flap. He underwent sternal fixation with insertion of titanium StraTos bars (MedXpert, Germany) and an overlying pedicled omental flap (in Fig. 25.6) to promote healing. He made a complete and uneventful recovery, with no evidence of further infection of instability.

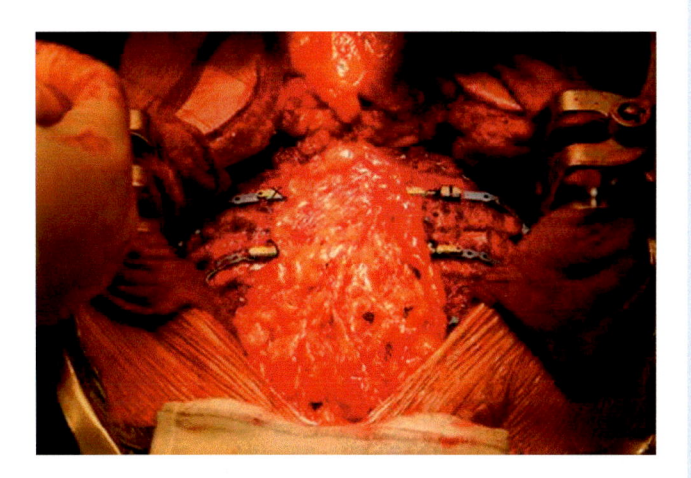

Fig. 25.6 An omental flap placed over titanium StraTos bars for chronic sternal nonunion

25.8 Pearls and Pitfalls

Pearls
- The omentum's unique angiogenic and immunological properties can promote wound healing even in hostile recipient sites with prior radiation exposure and infection.
- Perioperative antibiotics are deemed necessary in omental flaps due to transfer of fat tissue which increases risk of infection.
- Heparinization of patients for 5 days to preserve flap microcirculation in free flaps is recommended.
- When dividing small gastric branches, it may be advisable to use traditional ties and ligation over electrocautery to prevent inadvertent damage to the primary arcade.
- Postoperative use of portable Doppler sonography is particularly useful as a flap monitoring tool.

Pitfalls
- It is advisable to avoid use of the omentum in previous abdominal surgery or disease.
- Be mindful of omental atrophy (can be up to 50% in 3 months) when considering the size of flap required for the defect.
- The omentum is considered a "salvage flap" by many given the perceived donor site morbidity associated with harvesting.
- Common intra-abdominal complications following omental harvesting include ventral incisional hernias, gastric outlet obstruction, and intra-abdominal abscess formation; these may be reduced with laparoscopic harvesting technique.
- Free transfer of the omentum enables definitive closure of the peritoneal cavity, which can reduce abdominal complications.

25.9 Selected Reading

- Rutherford Morrison in 1906. British Journal of Surgery Br Med J. 1906;1:76.
- *Term "abdominal policeman" when referring to the omentum first used in 1906. He likened the structure to a jellyfish taking care of "whatever mischief is brewing."*
- McLean DH, Buncke HJJ. Autotransplant of omentum to a large scalp defect, with microsurgical revascularization. Plastic Reconstruct Surg. 1972;49(3):268–74.
- *First successful free transfer of greater omentum flap to a distant site.*
- Vernik J, Singh AK. Omentum: power to heal and regenerate. Int J Artif Organs. 2007;30(2):95–9.
- *Review article on the unique properties of the omentum and its application to surgical practice.*
- Tavilla G, Jackimovicz J, Berreklouw E. Intraoperative blood flow measurement of the right gastroepiploic artery using pulsed Doppler echocardiography. Ann Thorac Surg. 1997;64(2):426–31.
- *The average flow rate through RGEA calculated in bypass grafting as 55 ml/min (where no postoperative ischemic events occurred).*
- Lorenzetti F, Giordano S, Tukiainen E. Intraoperative hemodynamic evaluation of the latissimus dorsi muscle flap: a prospective study. J Reconstr Microsurg. 2012;28(4):273–8.
- *Study investigating the hemodynamic changes in the donor vessel of the free latissimus dorsi flap before and after denervation in free flap transfer.*
- Das SK. Assessment of the size of the human omentum. Acta Anatomica. 1981;110(2):108–12.
- *Extensive study on human omentum size in 200 cadavers and 100 laparotomies – highlighting rough correlation with height and weight of patient, but not significant enough to enable predication of omental volume.*
- Settembre N, Bouziane Z, Mandry D, Braun M, Malikov S. The omental free flap and flow-through flap: preoperative evaluation of right gastro-omental artery on multidetector computed tomography. Abdomin Radiol. 2020.
- *This recent study has provided evidence for the preoperative use of CT angiography in the assessment of RGEA blood flow.*
- Minakawa M, Fukuda I, Wada M. Preoperative Evaluation of the Right Gastroepiploic Artery Using Abdominal Ultrasonography. 1131–3.
- *This study demonstrated significant positive correlation between abdominal ultrasonographical evaluation of the RGEA diameter and postoperative angiography following use of the RGEA in bypass grafting.*
- Zaha H, Abe N, Sagawa N, Unesoko M. Oncoplastic surgery with omental flap reconstruction: a study of 200 cases. Breast Cancer Res Treat. 2017;162(2):267–74.
- *Assessment of safety and long-term complication rate in 200 patients with laparoscopic harvesting of the omental flap (LHOF) – 99% were successful, however 12% insufficient flap volume.*

Acknowledgments We thank Marciano Bunalade (Harefield Hospital) for providing the illustrations for this chapter.

Dorsal Metacarpal Artery Flaps

Prateush Singh, Andreas Georgiou, Julia Ruston, and Dariush Nikkhah

26.1 Introduction

Dorsal metacarpal artery flaps are vascularized skin flaps from the dorsum of the hand, based on either the first to the fourth dorsal metacarpal arteries or their perforators. Multiple variations have been described, differing based on their location, pedicle, and anterograde or reverse flow. In general, they provide a thin, pliable flap suitable for reconstruction of dorsal defects of the hand and digits (up to and even beyond the PIPJ), as well as the webspace and the thumb. Although the flaps can reach volar defects of proximal digits, they are not ideal, being non-glabrous and less of a color match than volar skin.

The first dorsal metacarpal artery (FDMA) flap is an anterograde neurovascular island flap, where robust skin from the dorsum of the proximal index finger is transferred to the thumb. It was initially described by Foucher and Braun in 1979 [1], with terminal branches of the radial nerve to provide sensation to the flap. Various techniques of elevation of the FDMA flap have been described, the Holevich technique gives the flap a tennis racquet form, and the skin island over the pedicle is smaller [2]. The FDMA flap is indicated in volar or dorsal thumb defects. It should be used with caution when resurfacing thumb pulp defects, as it may not reach the most distal thumb tip without resultant IPJ flexion and it does not provide glabrous tissue.

Quaba and Maruyama both described the reverse dorsal metacarpal artery (DMCA) flaps utilizing skin overlying the intermetacarpal space to reconstruct the webspace or the dorsum of digits, up to the proximal interphalangeal joint (PIPJ) [3, 4]. The Maruyama flap incorporates the main DMCA, while the Quaba flap is based on a DMCA perforator, which occurs just distal to the juncturae tendinae, and facilitates a slightly longer arc of rotation. Modifications based on the more dorsal communicating perforators of the common digital artery allow a more distally based pivot point and thus reconstruction of dorsal digital defects beyond the PIPJ. The primary indications described for the Quaba flap include reconstruction of webspace, dorsal metacarpal, dorsal phalangeal skin, and distal palmar defects [4]. Maruyama describes similar uses to reconstruct small soft tissue defects in the hand; however as the main DMCA is incorporated, the reach of this flap can extend beyond the PIPJ [3].

26.2 Anatomy

The dorsal metacarpal arteries run over the dorsal interosseous muscles to supply the skin and soft tissue over the dorsum of the hand and digits. Dorsal branches of the radial and ulnar arteries form the dorsal carpal arch, and from this the dorsal metacarpal arteries arise. The FDMA arises usually from the dorsal radial artery itself, and the second to fourth DMCA may also exhibit variations, such as arising direct from the radial artery or from adjacent metacarpal arteries. The fifth DMCA often arises direct from the ulnar artery. The anatomy can become less predictable toward the ulnar side (fourth and fifth metacarpal arteries may be completely absent). Each DMCA communicates with the deep palmar arch through intermetacarpal connections. Cutaneous perforators arise along the length of the DMCA. The perforator upon which the Quaba flap is based is around 1 cm proximal to the corresponding metacarpophalangeal joint (MCPJ) or 1.5 cm proximal to the leading edge of the interdigital web. With each DMCA there are two venae comitantes (0.2–0.3 mm diameter) which provide venous drainage for the flaps. Quaba et al. found on dissections of 18 cadaveric specimens that in the distal third, there was a consistent leash of blood vessels, however a paucity of vascular connections in

P. Singh · A. Georgiou · J. Ruston · D. Nikkhah (✉)
Royal Free Hospital, London, UK

the proximal two-thirds. The perforating vessels were seen entering the skin 0.5–1 cm proximal to the MCPJ. This pattern was found to be less consistent on the radial and ulnar border of the hand, but reliable between the second and fourth metacarpals [4].

The FDMA gives branches to the thumb and first webspace and terminates as the external dorsal artery of the index finger, supplying the skin over the dorsum of the index finger's proximal phalanx. The FDMA anatomy is relatively constant, with a diameter up to 1 mm and few collateral branches. Two dorsal veins run superficially to the artery alongside radial nerve branches [1]. In a study by Magdi Sherif in 21 cadaveric hands, they found 3 patterns of division of the FDMA [5]. It constantly gave three fascial branches: a radial branch, an ulnar branch, and an intermediate branch. A cutaneous branch was also observed, which may arise either from the radial artery or from the FDMA. It runs with the radial nerve supplying dorsal hand skin. This branch may supplement the vascularization of FDMA flap. Due to variation in the division pattern of the FDMA, it is safer to raise the whole first DIO fascia in the pedicle of the flap. This preserves the three branches of the artery without the dissection of FDMA or exposure of the artery of its origin.

The fourth DMCA does not reliably give off cutaneous perforators; however it consistently has a distal recurrent branch running superficial to the extensor digitorum communis tendon to the little finger, upon which flaps can be based [4].

Composite flaps for functional reconstruction include the incorporation of extensor tendon for tendon defects, which are not uncommon in cases of dorsal digital skin loss. Neurotized DMCA flaps can incorporate the dorsal cutaneous branches of the radial and ulnar nerves which run across the dorsum of the hand.

The arrangement of the DMCA and its cutaneous perforators are demonstrated in Fig. 26.1. The first diagram demonstrates the normal anatomy. The second diagram is a flap raised on the distal most cutaneous perforator of the DMCA. In the last diagram, the flap is raised on the main DMCA and its perforators (Fig. 26.1).

26.3 Preoperative Investigation

A preoperative handheld Doppler ultrasound can be used to identify the position of the perforators and to delineate the FDMA pedicle. This is especially useful where the anatomy is less consistent, toward the ulnar digits. Further imaging is not required.

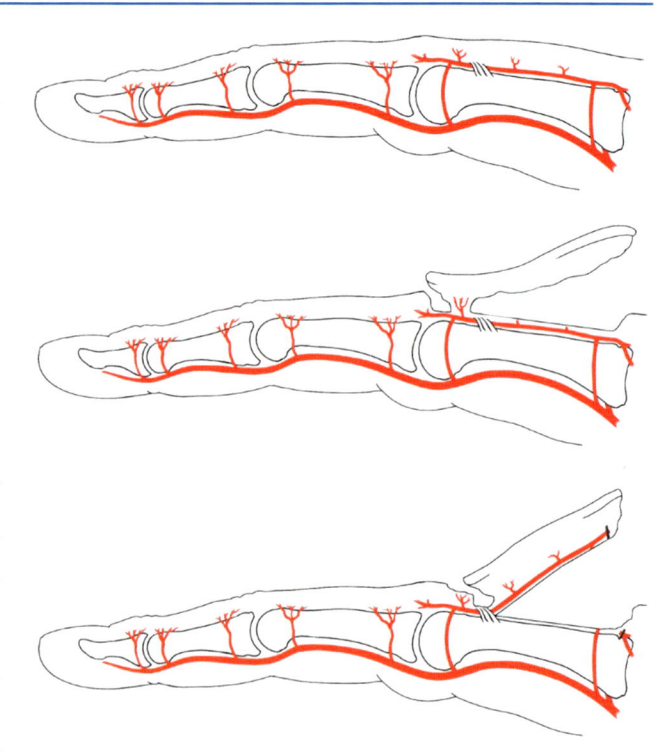

Fig. 26.1 Reverse Island DMCA flap based on single perforator (Quaba) or encorporating entire DMCA (Maruyama)

26.4 Flap Design and Markings

FDMA markings for thumb tip defect after Squamous Cell Carcinoma excision (Fig. 26.2).

The excision margins of the neoplasm on the thumb are marked, and this intended defect is used to template the required flap size over the proximal phalanx of the index finger (from MCPJ proximally to PIPJ distally and as wide as the mid-lateral lines if necessary). The FDMA is identified with handheld Doppler and marked. A curvilinear skin incision is marked over the pedicle.

Quaba flap markings for a defect on the dorsum of the left ring finger (Fig. 26.3).

The third webspace perforator is identified with Doppler and marked with a dot. This is the pivot point around which the flap will be rotated. The proximal tip of the marked flap should be the same distance from the perforator, as the distance to the distal defect edge. The maximum flap width is determined by the pinch test, to assess laxity for primary closure. The shaded area on the flap in this example illustrates where the skin will be de-epithelialized to go under the skin bridge at the recipient site (this is not usually required).

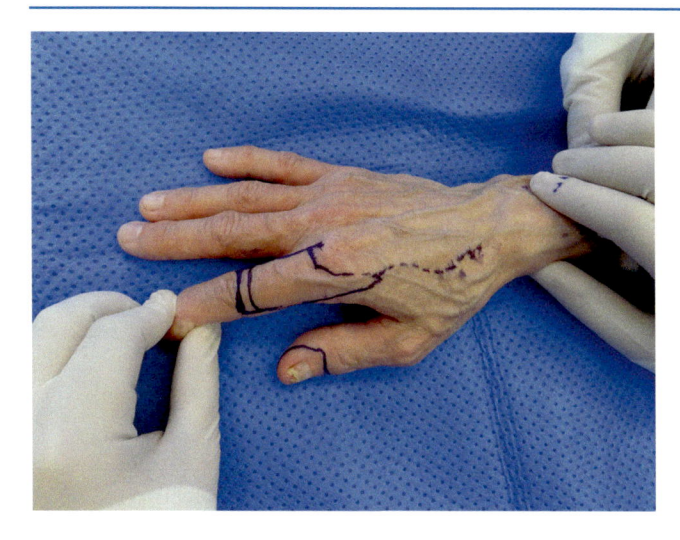

Fig. 26.2 The FDMA flap marked on the index

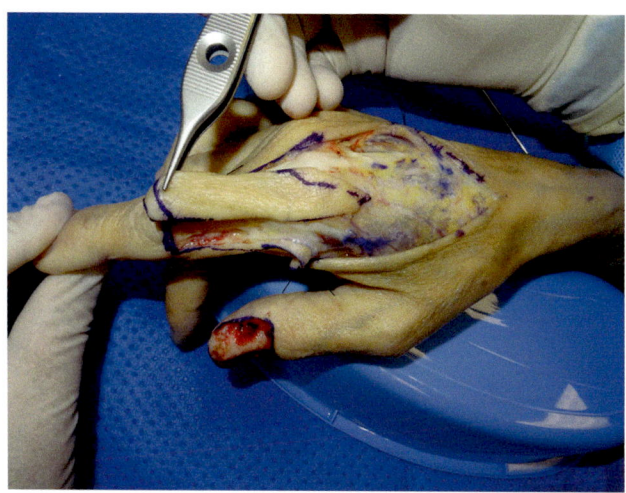

Fig. 26.4 Skin flaps are raised in a the subdermal plane

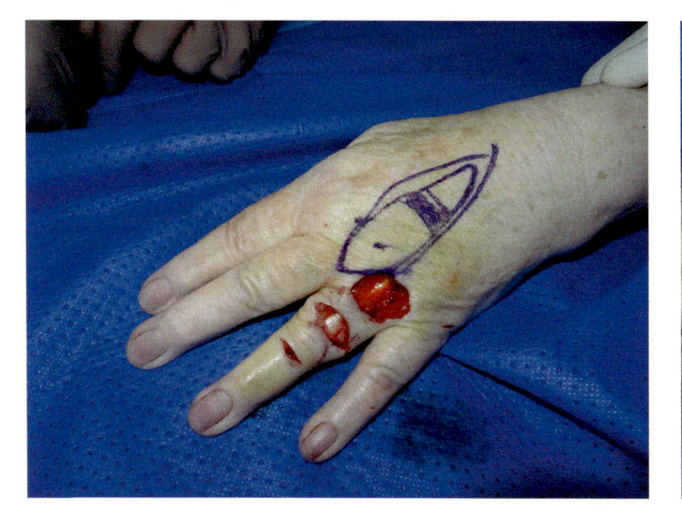

Fig. 26.3 Reverse DMCA Flap markings on the dorsum of the Left Ring Finger

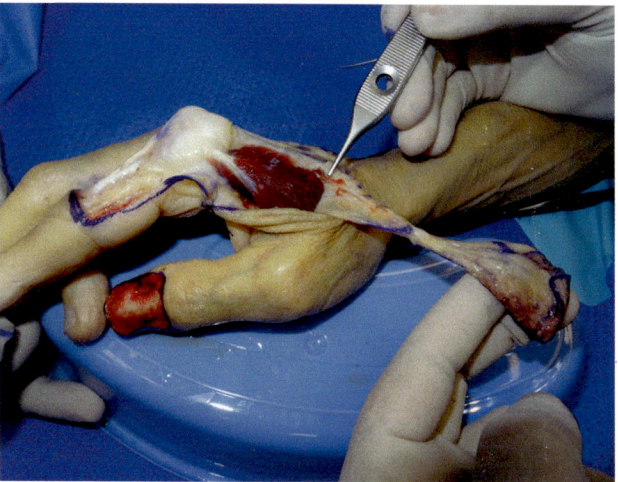

Fig. 26.5 Flap raised from distal to proximal under tourniquet control without exsanguination. Adson forceps demonstrating FDMA pedicle at the base of the flap

26.5 Flap Raise/Elevation: A Step-by-Step

DMCA flaps are raised using a size 15 blade under loupe magnification (2.5x), under tourniquet control without exsanguination (so the vessels are still visible).

26.5.1 FDMA Flap (Foucher Flap)

- Flap Raising.
  (a) Skin is incised over the pedicle (curvilinear) and skin flaps raised in the subdermal plane (to preserve underlying veins) and reflected (Fig. 26.4).
  (b) The flap itself is then raised from distal to proximal (Fig. 26.5). The skin paddle is raised in a plane superficial to the paratenon. Care must be taken at the MCPJ not to injure the FDMA or cutaneous branches that supply the skin island. We incorporate a small cutaneous tail to the skin island to avoid injury to the pedicle at the MCPJ (Fig. 26.6). Then upon reaching the insertion of the first dorsal interosseous muscle, the plane of dissection deepens to incorporating the entire epimysium and fascia of the first dorsal interosseous muscle with the FDMA pedicle. A wide cuff of adipofascial tissues over the first dorsal interosseous with additional veins are taken.
  (c) No attempt is made to skeletonize or visualize the main FDMA pedicle until the end of flap elevation (Fig. 26.5).
  (d) The proximal extent of pedicle dissection depends on required flap reach. The muscle branches will bleed and can be coagulated with bipolar diathermy.
- Flap Inset (Fig. 26.7).

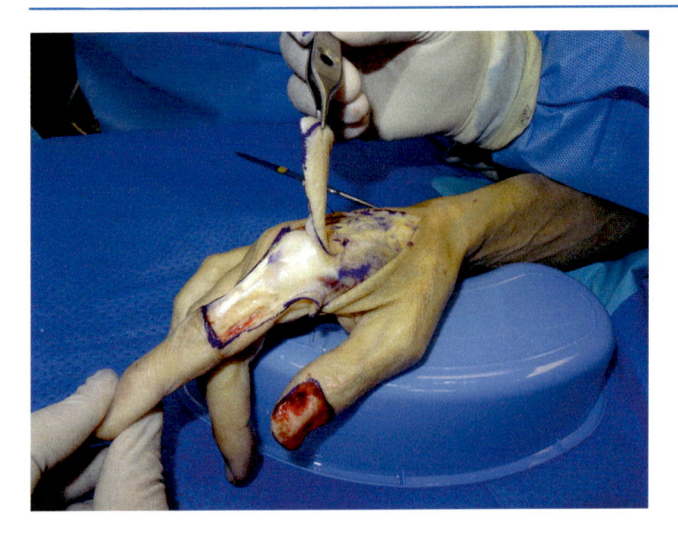

Fig. 26.6 Care must be taken at the MCPJ not to injure the FDMA or cutaneous branches that supply the skin island

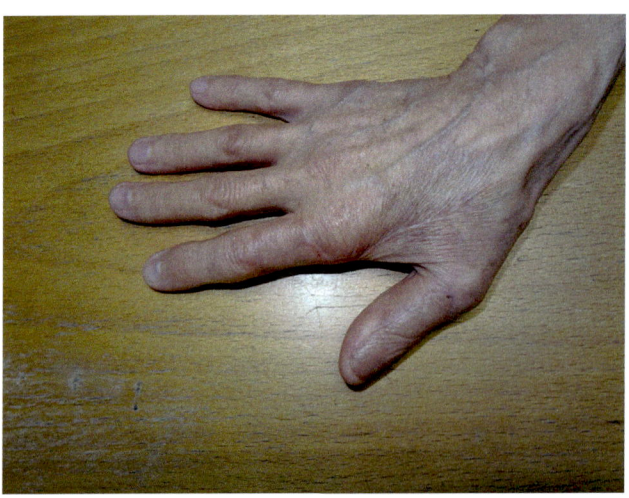

Fig. 26.8 Long term follow up of patient with FDMA flap to reconstruct dorsal thumb defect post SCC excision

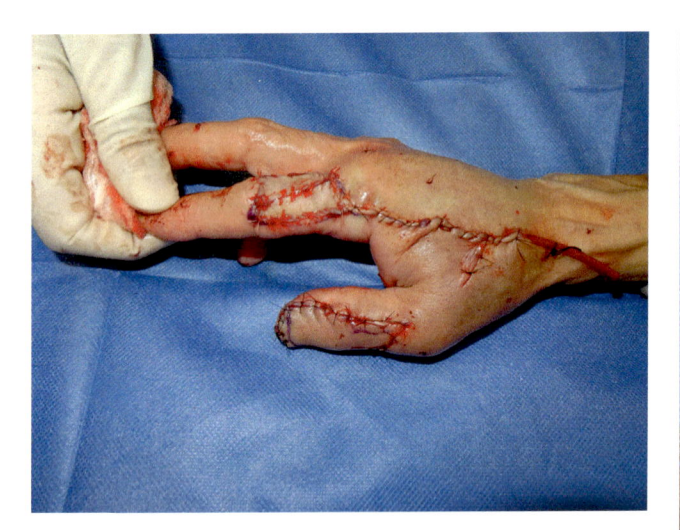

Fig. 26.7 Flap tunnelled and inset to cover dorsal thumb defect. Full thickness skin graft used to cover the donor site

(a) The flap is tunneled under the skin and inset to cover the recipient site. Vascular congestion can be minimized in flap inset in volar defects by dividing the skin and avoiding tunneling.
(b) A full- thickness skin graft is used to resurface the donor site.
- Outcome (Fig. 26.8).

(a) The patient had an excellent outcome with full function of the hand; the result is shown at 12 months.

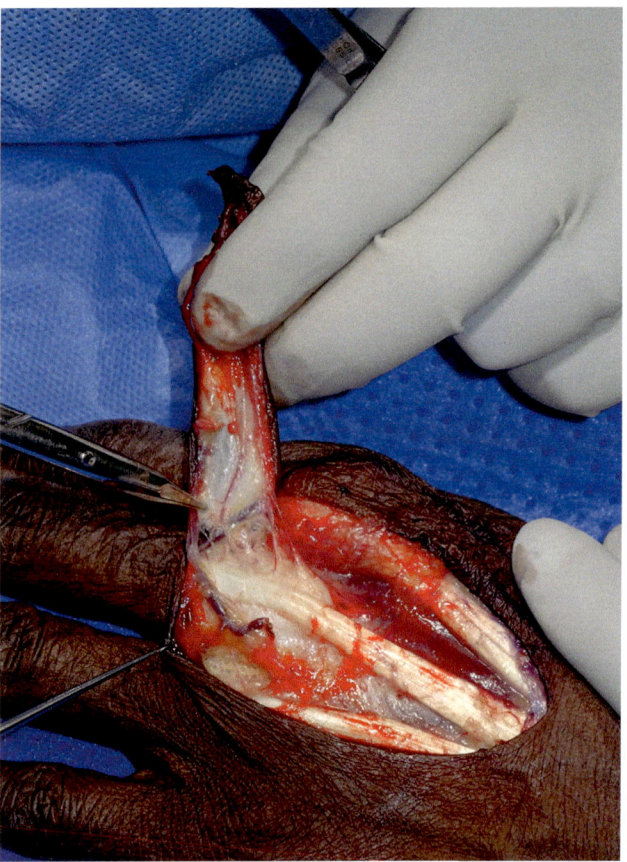

Fig. 26.9 Reverse dorsal metacarpal artery flap raised from proximal to distal. The tenotomies demonstrate the encorporation of an extra dorsal vein to reduce congestion

26.5.2 Reverse Dorsal Metacarpal Flap.

1. Flap Raising (Fig. 26.9)
   (a) The reverse dorsal metacarpal artery flap is raised here on the third DMCA. Raising starts proximally in a plane superficial to the paratenon. The dissection continues until the junctura is reached, as the perforator is just distal to this and should not be skeletonized.

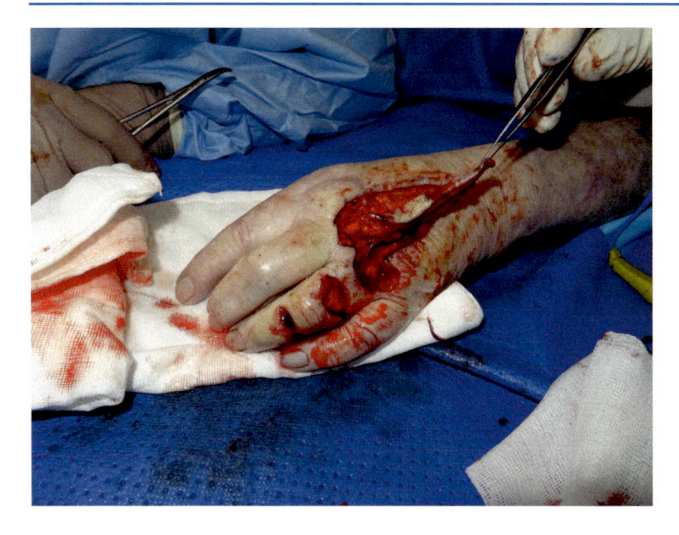

Fig. 26.10 Reverse DMCA flap raised on the 3rd DMCA perforator

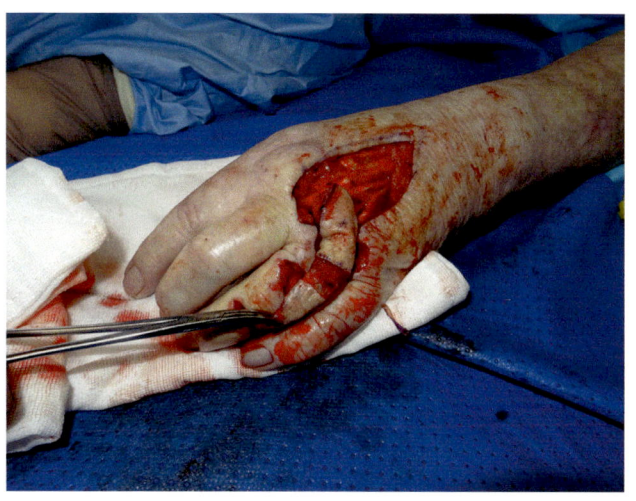

Fig. 26.12 Flap propelled through 180 degrees

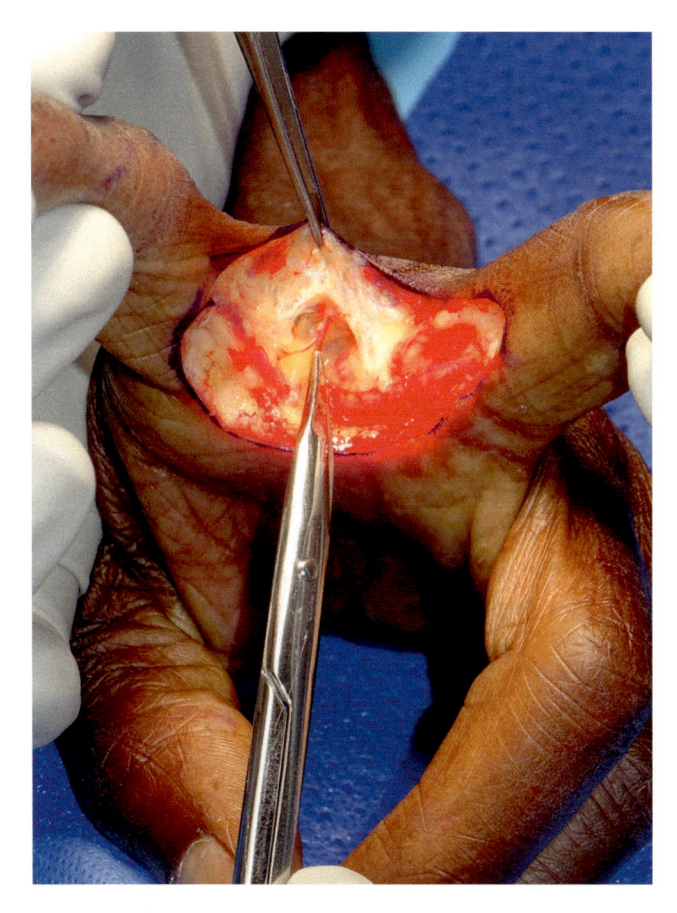

Fig. 26.11 DMCA perforator approached through a retrograde dissection after resection of a squamous cell carcinoma (SCC) in the webspace

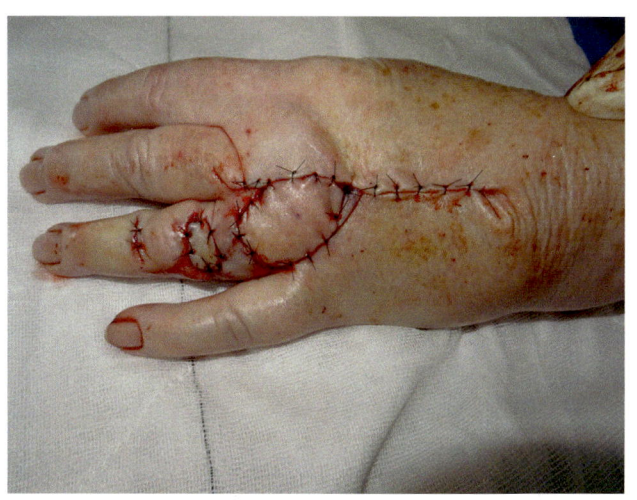

Fig. 26.13 3rd reverse DMCA flap inset to dorsal phalangeal skin defect

(b) The distal tip of the flap is raised, with careful dissection around the perforator (Figs. 26.10 and 26.11). An adipofascial cuff around the perforator is preserved, to maintain venous drainage. Dorsal veins are also included in the flap to reduce venous congestion (Fig. 26.9). Quaba also described a modification of this flap being raised with a "vascularized" tendon graft, which can be used to bridge an extensor gap.

(c) The flap is propelled through 180 degrees and the areas corresponding to the skin bridge de-epithelialized (Fig. 26.12).

1. Flap Inset (Fig. 26.13).
   (a) Here the tip of the flap has been tunneled to the distal defect (Fig. 26.8). In the majority of cases, the flap is simply rotated into the defect and inset, with primary closure of the donor site.
2. Outcome (Fig. 26.14).
   (a) The patient is shown here at 3-month follow-up with full range of motion (Fig. 26.15).

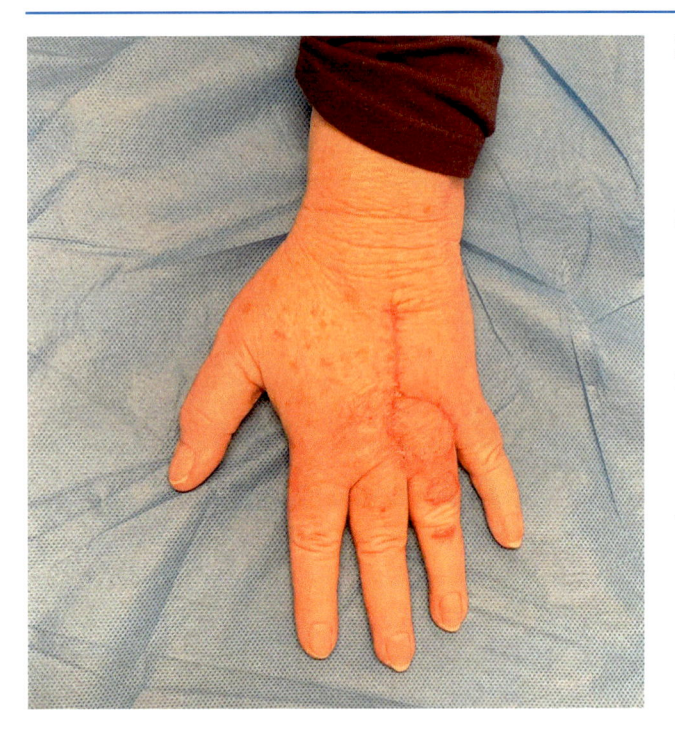

Fig. 26.14 3-month Follow-up

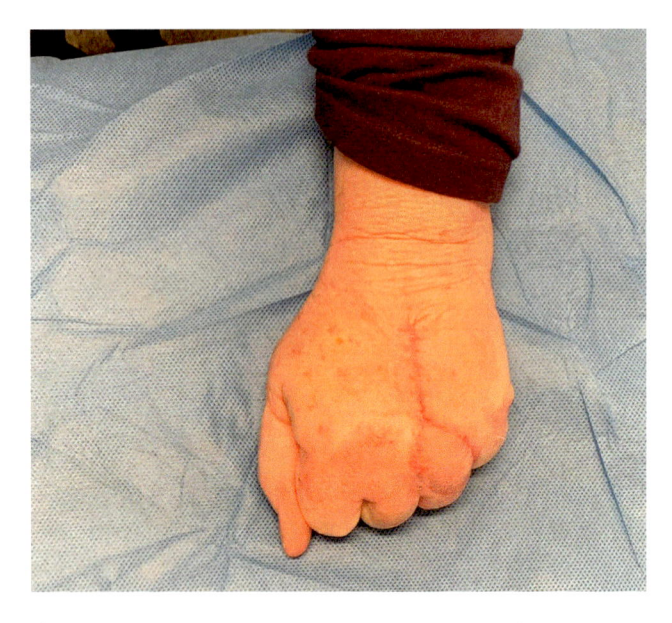

Fig. 26.15 Demonstration of full flexion after DMCA flap reconstruction over MCPJ

26.6 Core Surgical Techniques in Flap Dissection

The flaps are raised under tourniquet control but without exsanguination to allow direct visualization of the vessels.

26.7 FDMA Flap

1. The donor site is marked out: the dorsum of the proximal phalanx of the index finger, with the artery delineated using a pencil Doppler ultrasound.
2. The borders of the flap are incised – this is down to the paratenon laterally and distally, but at the proximal edge just through the dermis, down to the adipofascial layer. The skin flaps overlying the pedicle are raised thin, in the subdermal plane.
3. The FDMA flap is raised distal to proximal, with dissection initially superficial to the paratenon. Care must be taken when dissecting at the MCPJ not to injure the FDMA or cutaneous branches that supply the skin island.
4. At the level of the dorsal interosseous muscle, dissection becomes deeper, just above the muscle, to incorporate the FDMA (which runs in the epimysium). The width of the adipofascial tissue raised can extend to the second metacarpal and should incorporate dorsal veins to minimize venous congestion. This dissection is continued proximally to achieve as much length as is required. Branches running into the muscle can be ligated with microligaclips or coagulated. It is important to not skeletonize the vessel; it is often visualized at the end of dissection and can be transilluminated through the adipofascial tissues.
5. For dorsal defects, a subcutaneous tunnel is made, through which the flap is passed with the help of a silk suture. For volar defects, tunneling risks constriction of the pedicle so make an incision along the direction the flap must travel.
6. A neurotized FDMA flap, incorporating a branch of the SBRN, is particularly useful for sensate reconstruction of volar thumb defects. Two-point discrimination of 10 mm can be achieved.
7. A full-thickness skin graft is used to resurface the donor defect on the index finger (hence the importance of preserving paratenon). If any of the flap pedicle is exposed and cannot be covered without excessive compression, the pedicle can also be grafted. The skin flaps overlying the FDMA pedicle donor site are closed primarily.

26.7.1 Reverse Dorsal Metacarpal Artery Perforator (Quaba) Flap.

1. For the Quaba flap, a pivot point is planned in the distal third of the intermetacarpal space and the perforator iden-

tified with handheld Doppler. The defect is templated and used to design the flap, extending proximally over the intermetacarpal space and based around the pivot point.

2. The flap is raised proximal to distal, preserving paratenon of the extensor tendons, until the distal edge of the junctura is reached.

   Alternatively, the flap can also be raised retrograde as anatomical studies have shown that skin perforators arising from the palmar metacarpal artery are often consistent; therefore, the retrograde approach is based on the connection between the dorsal metacarpal artery (DMA) and the palmar arterial system at the level of the metacarpal head. A retrograde approach involves identifying the most distal perforator first from the palmar source vessel, starting the dissection in the webspace [6].

   The variable anatomy of the third to fifth dorsal metacarpal arteries sometimes prevents successful flap harvest [4].

3. The perforator is not skeletonized and a cuff of adipofascial tissue around it is preserved.
4. The flap is rotated into the defect and tourniquet released to assess perfusion and check there is no kinking or restriction at the rotation point. Further (cautious) dissection around the perforator may be needed to avoid tension.
5. The flap is inset, the flap often becomes hyperemic, and surgeons can dissect and include a dorsal vein which may help to avoid flap congestion.
6. The donor site can be closed directly.

26.8 Clinical Scenario

26.8.1 Case Scenario A: Figs. 26.2, 26.4, 26.5, 26.6, 26.7, and 26.8
Surgeon Dariush Nikkhah

- A 65-year-old carer developed a squamous cell carcinoma (SCC) of the dorsum of her thumb nail bed complex. Biopsy confirmed a poorly differentiated SCC, and after multidisciplinary team discussion, decision was made to perform a wider excision and post operative radiotherapy. The patient had excision of the SCC and entire nail bed complex down to bone, and a FDMA flap was raised to resurface the defect. At 1 year the patient remained disease-free and had full function of the hand with an excellent donor site outcome.

26.8.2 Case Scenario B: Figs. 26.3, 26.10, 26.12, 26.13, 26.14, and 26.15
Surgeon Dariush Nikkhah

- A 55-year-old patient suffered a traumatic loss of soft tissue above the extensor tendon of her ring finger with an exposed MCPJ. A reverse dorsal metacarpal artery flap was designed to reconstruct the defect. The patient made a full recovery and as demonstrated at 3 months had no flexion or extension deficit in the hand.

26.9 Pearls and Pitfalls

Pearls

Tips for FDMA Flaps

- Raising thin skin flaps over the FDMA allows preservation of veins within the adipofascial tissue of the pedicle.
- Taking all the first dorsal interosseous fascia and dorsal epimysium, and not skeletonizing the pedicle, allows safe flap elevation. It also protects the venae comitantes from unnecessary trauma.
- A distal dorsal branch of the radial nerve can be incorporated to neurotize the flap.
- Dorsal defects may not need a subcutaneous tunnel for the flap, but palmar defects may necessitate one.
- A cutaneous tail can be incorporated, extending proximally from the flap over the FDMA pedicle. This can maintain small cutaneous vessels and reduce tension when closing skin over the pedicle, in cases where the flap is not tunneled (or if the tunnel will be too tight).

Tips for Reverse DMCA Flaps

- Be careful in the vicinity of the perforator – careful dissection is needed to release tethering fibrous bands without skeletonizing the vessels. This allows rotation without constriction of the perforator and veins.
- More radial Quaba flaps are more reliable.
- It is possible to incorporate tendon with DMCA flaps.
- The Quaba flap is a good option for webspace defects where retrograde dissection can identify vessels on which to base the Quaba or extended Quaba flap (Fig. 26.16).
- The flap can be based on a more distal perforator to increase the flap reach – the perforator is level with the distal webspace, and the perfusion is via the first dorsal branch of the palmar digital artery. Extended flaps can reach palmar defects and even to the level of the DIPJ.

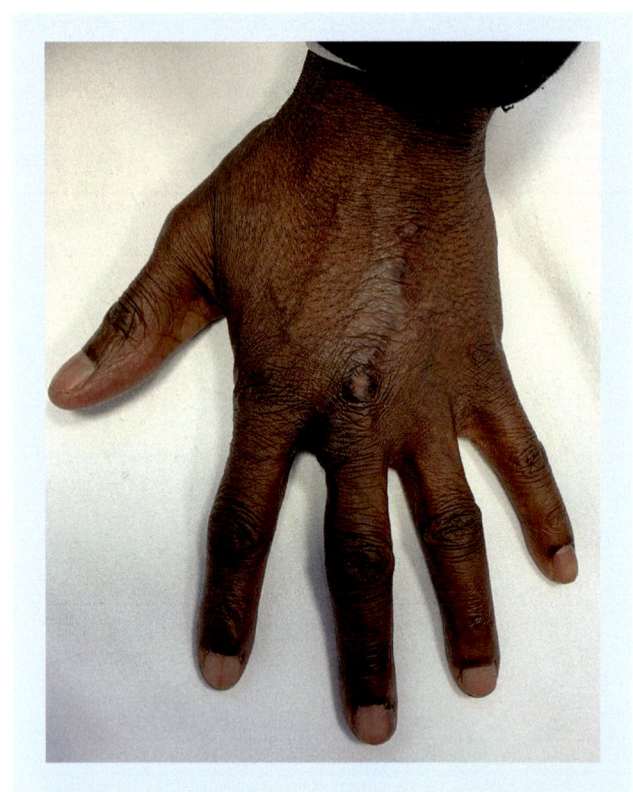

Fig. 26.16 1- month follow up if webspace reconstruction after SCC excision with reverse DMCA flap

Pitfalls
- Take care when dissecting around the pedicle just proximal to the MCPJ; taking a cuff of surrounding tissue and a cutaneous tail can help to avoid injury at this zone.
- The Foucher flap is not ideal for volar thumb resurfacing as it does not provide glabrous tissue (free pulp transfer is the gold standard).
- The Foucher flap may struggle to reach the very tip of the thumb and may require IPJ flexion to achieve closure.
- Donor sites can be stiff or require skin grafts; utilize hand therapy services to minimize stiffness.
- Care must be taken to use bipolar cautery on a low setting; making use of micro ligaclips for any small branches may help avoid thermal injury.

26.10 Selected Readings

- Maruyama Y. The reverse dorsal metacarpal flap. British journal of plastic surgery, 1990; 43:24–27.
- *Maruyama described the reverse dorsal metacarpal flap, reporting a consistent vascular basis and a role in covering small soft tissue defects of the hand. Eight cases were included in the study, and the reverse dorsal metacarpal flap was utilized to reconstruct wide range of defects, a result of acute trauma, burn ulcerations, tumors, syndactyly, and contractures. The flaps were raised to include the fascia over the dorsal interosseous muscles, the proximal DMA was divided, and the arch of rotation was the distal metacarpal, at connections between the terminal branches and the palmar metacarpal and digital arteries. The constancy of second dorsal metacarpal artery was demonstrated as the artery most frequently used. The author reports good outcomes in seven of the eight cases, reporting distal partial necrosis of one case based on the fifth dorsal metacarpal artery* [3].
- Foucher G, Braun J. A New Island Flap Transfer from the Dorsum of the Index to the Thumb. Plast Reconstruct Surg J. 1979: 63;344–349.
- *Foucher et al. describe an island "Kite" flap from the dorsum of the index finger, raised on the first dorsal metacarpal artery with one or two veins and innervated by terminal branches of the radial nerve. From 30 cadaveric specimens, the anatomy of the FDMA was delineated and the operative technique described. The vascular bundle is reported to be reliable; in 12 cases the authors report no flap necrosis. This flap can be used for reconstruction of thumb defects* [1].
- Quaba A, Davison PM. The distally based dorsal hand flap. Br J Plast Surg. 1990: 43;28–39.
- *The authors describe a distally based dorsal hand flap raised on a direct cutaneous branch of the second, third, and fourth dorsal metacarpal artery. Anatomical studies are supplemented with a clinical series of 21 patients. This flap was used to reconstruct defects (post-excisional for skin lesions, burns, and contractures) on the dorsum of the metacarpals, phalanges, distal palm, and web spaces. In 21 cases, they report one flap failure and one partial flap loss, both intended to reconstruct distal palmar defects. Most donor sites were amendable to direct closure; others required split- thickness or full- thickness skin grafts* [4].
- Omokawa S, Tanaka Y, Ryu J, Kish V. The anatomical basis for reverse first to fifth dorsal metacarpal arterial flaps. J Hand Surg(British and European Volume). 2004: 30B;40–44.
- *Omokawa et al. studied the cutaneous vascularity arising from the first to the fifth dorsal metacarpal arteries in order to understand the anatomical basis of reverse dorsal metacarpal arterial flaps. This cadaveric specimen study demonstrated that the first to the third metacarpal arteries consistently anastomose with the palmar arterial system. Each artery gave off four to eight skin perforators along the length of the metacarpal. The diameter of the perforators was larger at the distal third of the metacarpal; therefore it may contrib-*

ute most of the dorsal cutaneous vascularity of the hand. Fourth and fifth dorsal metacarpal arteries passed palmary into the interosseous muscles at the mid-level of the metacarpal. Anatomy of the fifth metacarpal was found to be more variable and seldom reached the metacarpophalangeal joint (MCPJ); thus it can only be used in cases where it does extend to the MCPJ [7].

- Yoon T, Carrera A, Benito-Ruiz J, Ferreres A, Serra-Renom J. The anatomical basis of the fourth dorsal metacarpal flap: a cadaveric dissection. J Hand surg. 2006: 31A;711–716.

- *Yoon et al. studied the vascularization of the fourth dorsal intercarpal space demonstrating consistency of the distal recurrent branch of the dorsal metacarpal artery. These findings suggest that flaps may be reliably raised based solely on the distal recurrent branch. Excluding the fourth dorsal metacarpal artery increases efficiency of dissection with a proposed reduction in donor site morbidity [8].*

References

1. Foucher G, Braun JB. A new island flap transfer from the dorsum of the index to the thumb. Plast Reconstr Surg. 1979;63(3):344–9.
2. Holevich J. A new method of restoring sensibility to the thumb. J Bone Joint Surg Br. 1963;45:496–502.
3. Maruyama Y. The reverse dorsal metacarpal flap. Br J Plast Surg. 1990;43(1):24–7.
4. Quaba AA, Davison PM. The distally-based dorsal hand flap. Br J Plast Surg. 1990;43(1):28–39.
5. Sherif MM. First dorsal metacarpal artery flap in hand reconstruction. I. Anatomical study. J Hand Surg Am. 1994;19(1):26–31.
6. Unluer Z, Ruston J, Nikkhah D. The retrograde approach to the reverse dorsal metacarpal artery flap. J Plast Reconstr Aesthet Surg. 2020;
7. Omokawa S, Tanaka Y, Ryu J, Kish VL. The anatomical basis for reverse first to fifth dorsal metacarpal arterial flaps. J Hand Surg Br. 2005;30(1):40–4.
8. Yoon TS, Carrera A, Benito-Ruiz J, Ferreres A, Serra-Renom JM. The anatomic basis of the fourth dorsal metacarpal flap: a cadaveric dissection. J Hand Surg Am. 2006;31(5):711–6.

27

Digital Artery Flaps: Homodigital and Heterodigital Island Flaps

Sirke Rinkoff, Julia Ruston, and Dariush Nikkhah

27.1 Introduction

Homodigital island flaps relocate tissue from a nonessential area of the digit to an area needing robust coverage or a nongraftable wound bed [1]. They are based on one of the two digital arteries to each finger and rely on the knowledge that sacrifice of one artery does not (usually) compromise perfusion to the digit. Weeks and Wray first described the homodigital island flap based on the digital artery in 1973 to cover soft tissue defects on the proximal digit. Homodigital island flaps can be anterograde and advanced distally for pulp defects (such as the oblique triangular neurovascular flap of Venkataswami and Subramanian [2]). This is commonly indicated for volar oblique amputations of the digit.

Reverse-flow flaps have facilitated pulp reconstruction further, based on retrograde flow through the digital artery, via anastomosis from the contralateral side (Lai et al. [3] and Kojima et al. [4]). These are indicated for fingertip and nailbed reconstruction, but can also be used to cover defects on the dorsum over the distal interphalangeal joint. Lai describes how the flap is outlined over the lateral donor proximal phalanx according to the site and shape of the defect; this is then raised with the distal digital artery acting as a pedicle. An extended flap incorporating dorsal skin over the metacarpophalangeal joint is also described for major finger defects in which the standard flap does not provide sufficient cover.

Koshima et al. [5] described the digital artery perforator (DAP) flap, and there are numerous subsequent "freestyle" perforator flap variations. The digital artery perforator flap is used for resurfacing the fingertip; the flap is based on the medial or lateral aspect of the finger proximal to the defect. During flap elevation the digital artery perforator and the subcutaneous venular system near the defect are preserved, and the flap is then rotated 180° into the defect.

The concept of elevating an islanded flap based on antegrade digital artery flow is credited to Moberg and Littler, although Esser may have been the first person to describe an "island flap" in 1917. In 1961, Tubiana and Duparc described further principles of a neurovascular heterodigital skin island flap, such as selecting donor site and how to elevate the flap.

The heterodigital island flap has the advantage of importing (potentially neurotized) glabrous skin into another digit which may be too extensively injured for a homodigital flap or where the defect is too proximal for a reverse flap (e.g., over the middle phalanx). It can be useful for large volar defects where return of sensation is critical, e.g., thumb pulp. The donor site is usually the ulnar side of the middle or radial side of the ring finger. The disadvantage of the heterodigital flap is that it requires morbidity to another digit, and there have been problems with cross-localization of sensation to the donor digit, cold intolerance, and hyperesthesia or paresthesia of the donor digit.

27.2 Anatomy of Homo- and Heterodigital Island Flaps

The digital artery runs along the ulnar and radial aspects of the finger, dorsal to the digital nerve, within a fatty-areolar channel between Cleland's and Grayson's ligaments. Each finger has two palmar digital arteries, the larger and most dominant of which is usually the closest toward the midline (e.g., ulnar digital artery of the index and radial digital artery of the little finger) (as described by Haerle et al. [6]). The middle and ring fingers often demonstrate codominant digital vessels, and therefore homodigital flaps are especially suited to these fingers, with least risk of inadequate perfusion or cold intolerance, after dividing one artery for the flap. Digital artery diameter varies in size from approximately

S. Rinkoff · J. Ruston · D. Nikkhah (✉)
Royal Free Hospital, London, UK
e-mail: s.rinkoff@nhs.net; julia.ruston@nhs.net; d.nikkhah@nhs.net

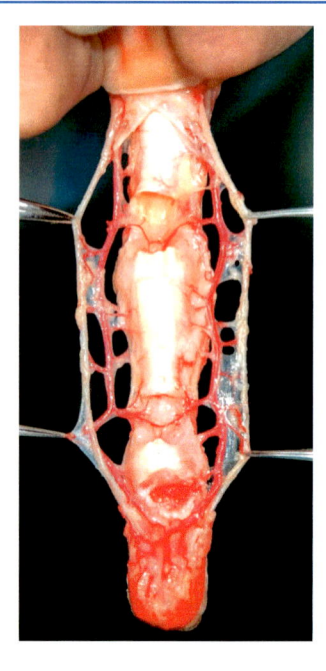

Fig. 27.1 Latex infused picture demonstrating the anatomy of the blood supply and arches of the finger and hand. (Picture courtesy of G Pafitanis, D Song, Z Yumao, see chapter 51 Cadaveric Flap Anatomy section)

1 mm proximally to 0.5 mm at the level of the distal interphalangeal joint (DIPJ). Lai's line (which is the junction of the darker dorsal skin and the volar lighter skin on the digit) is a useful surface landmark for the digital artery.

Interconnections between the radial and ulnar digital arteries form the anatomic basis and feasibility of many digital flaps (as seen in Fig. 27.1). Transverse palmar arches connect the digital arteries at relatively constant locations, deep to the flexor tendons:

1. Proximal arch: C1 pulley
2. Middle arch: C3 pulley
3. Distal arch: just distal to the FDP insertion

The middle and distal arches are larger in caliber than the proximal and facilitate retrograde vascular flow into distally based flaps. Multiple small palmar branches arise from each digital artery, usually laterally, and run in the subcutaneous tissue. These provide the perfusion to the palmar skin islands mobilized in some homodigital flaps. Three dorsal branches arise from each digital artery to supply the dorsal digital skin and anastomose with their contralateral counterparts to form arcades on the dorsum of the finger. There is also a rich network of vessels arising from the distal transverse arch at the fingertip.

The superficial palmar arch gives rise to three common digital arteries, which anastomose with corresponding palmar metacarpal branches from the deep palmar arch. Around the level of the metacarpophalangeal joint, each common digital artery bifurcates into the proper digital arteries, which run into adjacent digits (from the ulnar aspect of the index to the radial aspect of the little finger). The border digits have more variable vascular anatomy, but usually the radial digital artery of the index finger (radialis indicis) arises from the radial artery as it becomes the deep palmar arch. The ulnar digital artery to the little finger usually arises from the superficial palmar arch directly. The heterodigital island flap can be mobilized as proximally as the origin of the supplying vessel from the superficial palmar arch, and this enables their transposition to defects that may lie further than just an adjacent digit.

Venous drainage of the finger is via dorsal and palmar systems. The dorsal system is dominant, with a more constant arrangement of longitudinal subcutaneous veins and numerous interconnections. The palmar longitudinal veins are venae comitantes accompanying the digital arteries; these form the venous drainage of most homodigital island flaps.

The digital nerve can be differentiated from the artery by its pearly white consistency and the presence of Pacinian corpuscles. A dorsal branch arises which may run either deep or superficial to the digital artery and in most cases arises proximal to the proximal digital flexion crease Lai et al. [7]. It courses obliquely to innervate the lateral skin over the proximal phalanx (from which the reverse homodigital island flap is fashioned) and the dorsal skin over the middle phalanx. The skin overlying the metacarpophalangeal joint (MCPJ) which is included in an extended reverse homodigital flap is supplied by the superficial sensory branch from the corresponding radial or ulnar nerve.

In Littler's original description of the heterodigital island flap, the digital nerve on the donor finger was transected and incorporated into pedicle of the flap. Modifications of this have been described. Rose et al. [8] recommended preserving the nerve in the donor digit. To eliminate double sensibility, coapting the transected nerve has been suggested; however, the problem of the loss of the digital nerve in the donor digit remains. To avoid this, Lee et al. [1] described a lateral middle phalangeal finger flap where the proper digital nerve (PDN) for the donor digit was left intact. They dissected fascicles from branches of the PDN and the dorsal branch of the PDN (DBPDN) and coapted these to the nerve stumps of PDNs at the recipient finger. This can be visualized in Fig. 27.2; in image c the heterodigital island flap is raised on the digital artery with the DBPDN, and in image d this has been coapted to the ulnar digital nerve stump of the thumb. More recently, Wang et al. [9] suggested including the PDN and DBPDN in the flap and bridging the donor nerve defect with a nerve graft taken from the remaining proximal portion of the DBPDN.

Fig. 27.2 (a–d) Illustrate a heterodigital island flap neurotized with the DBPDN for thumb reconstuction (illustration by Julia Ruston)

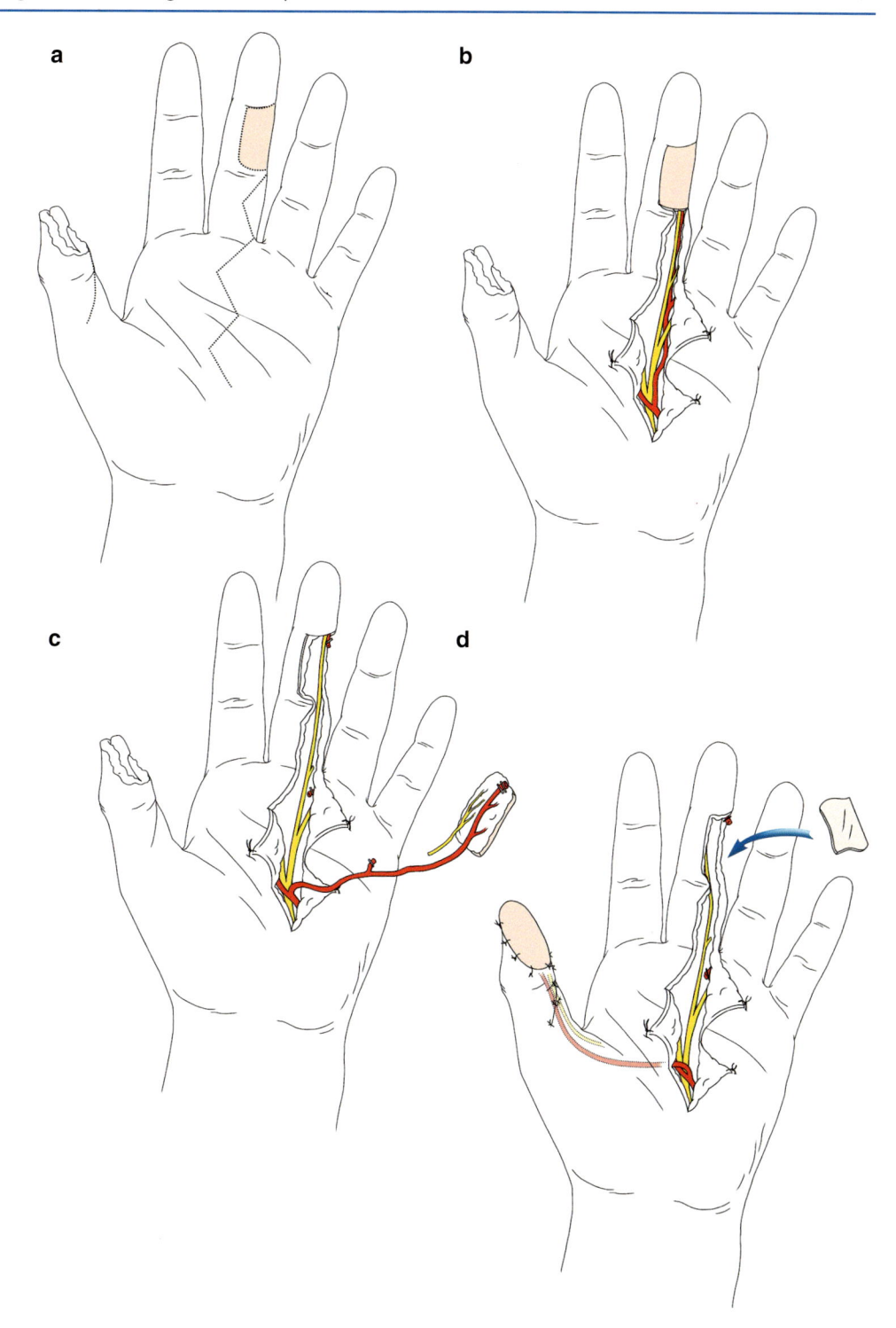

27.3 Preoperative Investigation

The digital artery can be identified through palpation or the aid of a fine Doppler probe. As this flap requires you to sacrifice one of the digital arteries, it is important to check there has been no injury to the digital artery on the contralateral side of the digit. The patency of both digital vessels can be confirmed with a digital Allen's test. For a heterodigital island flap, the adjacent digit should also be assessed, as the donor digital artery may need to be dissected proximally to its origin from the superficial palmar arch, and this necessitates ligation of the digital artery to the adjacent finger (at the bifurcation of the common digital artery). To perform a digital Allen's test, ask the patient to flex and extend their finger repeatedly while the digital arteries are compressed to achieve blanching of the finger; blanching of the finger will persist while compression is maintained on the digital arteries. Testing both ulnar and radial digital arteries separately, release of compression on one digital artery should cause the finger to become pink if the artery is patent; however if it is occluded, the finger will remain blanched.

27.4 Flap Design and Markings

27.4.1 Reverse Homodigital Island Flap

Lai's line can be used to mark the location of the digital artery preoperatively. The defect is templated and mapped on to the lateral aspect (radial or ulnar) of the proximal phalanx of the affected digit. Either a zigzag or a midaxial skin incision over the lateral border of the finger can be used, and this is marked preoperatively, between the flap and the defect (as in Fig. 27.3).

For the middle and ring fingers, the flap is usually elevated from the same side as the defect of the involved digit. This allows less stretching of the pedicle during transposition. For the index and little finger, the preference is the ulnar side and radial side of the proximal phalanx, respectively.

27.4.2 Heterodigital Island Flap

Lee et al. described a heterodigital island flap known as the mid-lateral phalangeal flap. They suggested basing the flap on the lateral ulnar side of the middle phalanx of the middle finger for a thumb defect and on the lateral ulnar side of the ring finger for a little finger defect, according to the size and shape of the pulp defect. The flap is centered on the mid-lateral line of the donor finger and extends from the mid-dorsal line to the mid-palmar line and from the proximal interphalangeal joint to the distal interphalangeal joint.

A palmar zigzag incision is drawn, to allow dissection of the pedicle to the level of the common digital artery or to the superficial palmar arch (as in this case).

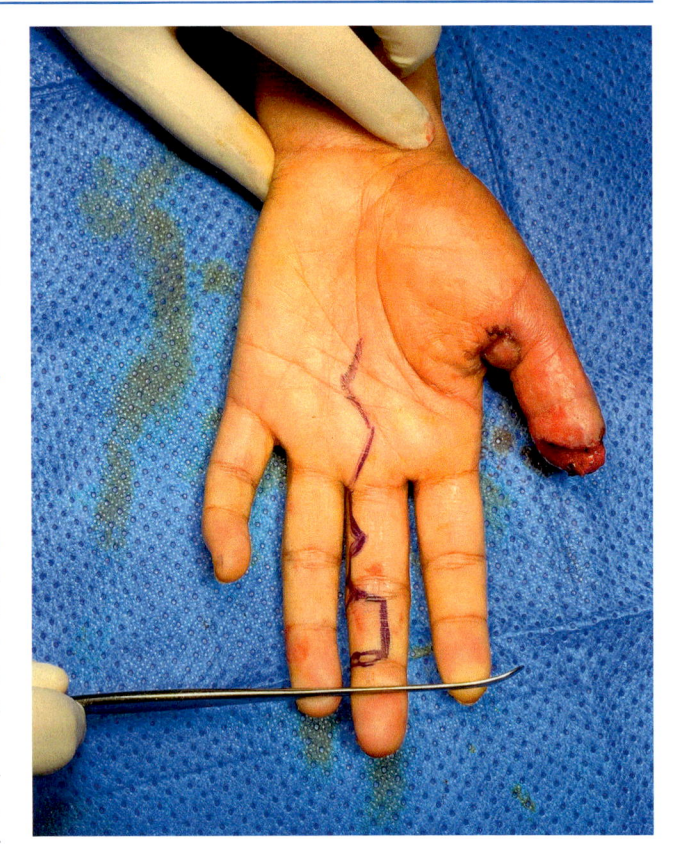

Figure 27.4 shows the skin markings for a heterodigital island flap to thumb defect. The flap is marked on the lateral ulnar aspect of the middle phalanx, and a zigzag excision extends on the lateral border of the digit to meet the palmar incision.

Fig. 27.4 Skin markings for a heterodigital island flap to thumb defect

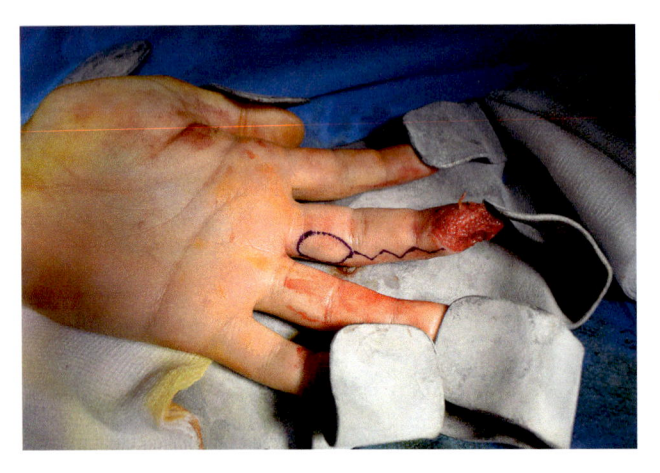

Fig. 27.3 Demonstrates a volar oblique amputation of the RMF pulp

27.5 Flap Raise/Elevation: A Step-by-Step Guide

27.5.1 Reverse Homodigital Island Flap

Dissection of reverse homodigital island flap (Fig. 27.5)
1. Skin is incised along the markings and skin flaps raised in the subcutaneous plane, to facilitate exposure of the neurovascular bundle. The flap, overlying the lateral border of the proximal phalanx, is incised and the neurovascular bundle is identified first proximally.

Fig. 27.5 Dissection of a reverse homodigital island flap

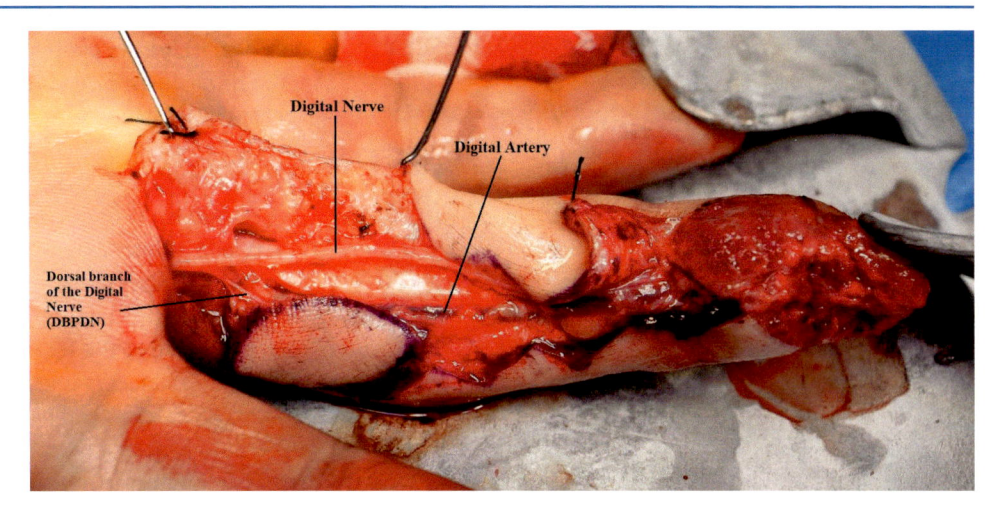

2. The nerve and artery are carefully separated, and the nerve is retracted in the palmar direction Fig 27.5, to preserve it. The dorsal branch of the digital nerve can be preserved, but may also be raised with the flap and subsequently coapted with a digital nerve distally in the defect using 9.0 Nylon (a neurotized homodigital island flap).
3. The digital artery is ligated proximally and divided.
4. Dissection deep to the artery allows gradual elevation and mobilization of the flap and the pedicle. As dissection progresses distally, deep and dorsal branches of the artery are divided, and a cuff of adipofascial tissue is maintained around the pedicle to preserve venous drainage. The artery itself is not well visualized in the dissection (rather just tethering branches as they are encountered) to avoid skeletonizing the vessel.
5. Caution should be taken in the vicinity of the transverse arches, as these form the pivot point for the flap and must not be injured. The middle or distal can be used depending on the length of pedicle required for the flap to reach the defect—dissection to the most distal arch results in a longer pedicle.
6. Once pedicle length is adequate to rotate 180° into the defect without tension, stop dissection (there is no need to dissect all the way to the distal arch if the pedicle length is adequate; this minimizes risk of inadvertent damage).

Flap inset and closure (Fig. 27.6)
7. The flap is inset at the fingertip with loose sutures to minimize compromise from postoperative swelling of the skin paddle.
8. A full-thickness skin graft is inset to the donor defect proximally, and the skin incision is closed.
9. The pedicle can be covered with remaining skin graft or left open (closure of the skin is usually not possible over the pedicle, without compression). As healing occurs, this contracts with time. In Fig. 27.6 a jelonet tie-over dressing is used to bolster the graft and Kaltostat covers the graft donor site.

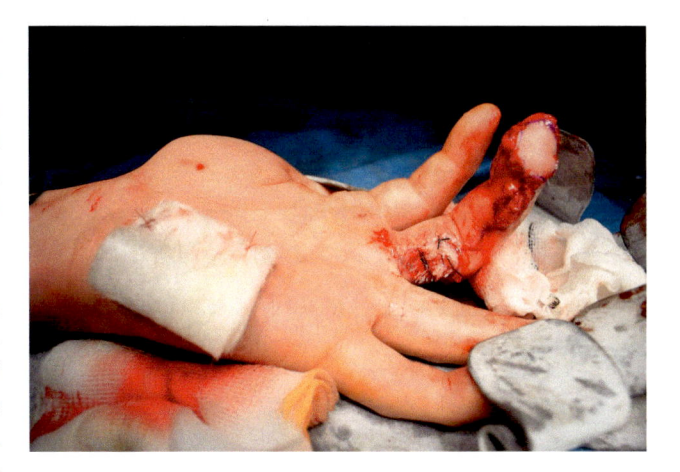

Fig. 27.6 Reverse homodigital island flap inset and closure

27.5.2 Heterodigital Island Flap

Dissection of the flap (Fig. 27.7)
1. The flap is dissected from the flexor sheath/periosteum of the middle phalanx and the digital artery is divided distally. Care is taken to preserve the proper digital nerve (as pictured).

Dissection of the DBPDN and the pedicle (Fig. 27.8)
2. The dorsal branch of the proper digital nerve is taken with the flap; this allows it to be coapted to the digital nerve at the recipient site. The digital artery is dissected to the superficial palmar arch – with ligation of the radial digital artery to the ring finger in this case, at its origin from the common digital artery.

Length of the pedicle is tested (Fig. 27.9)
3. The length of the pedicle is tested to check it can reach the recipient site without tension at the thumb tip.

The flap is passed under a tunnel of skin to the thumb tip (Fig. 27.10)
4. A silk suture is used to aid the passage of the flap through a subcutaneous tunnel to the thumb

Perfusion of the flap is checked (Fig. 27.11)
5. The tourniquet is released so that perfusion of the flap can be checked and haemostasis performed.

The flap is secured in place and a FTSG sutured to donor site (Fig. 27.12)
6. The flap is secured in place, a full-thickness skin graft inset into the donor site and the remaining skin incisions sutured.

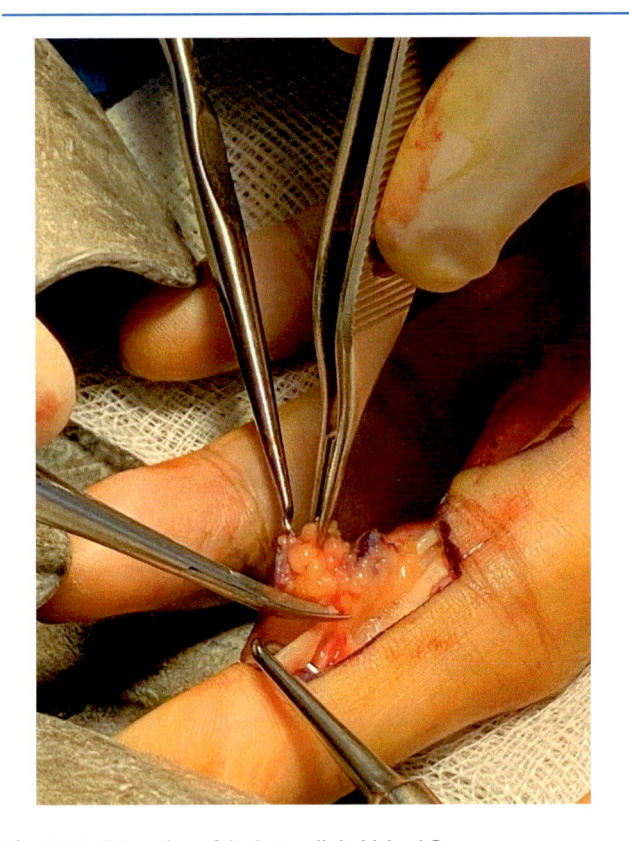

Fig. 27.7 Dissection of the heterodigital island flap

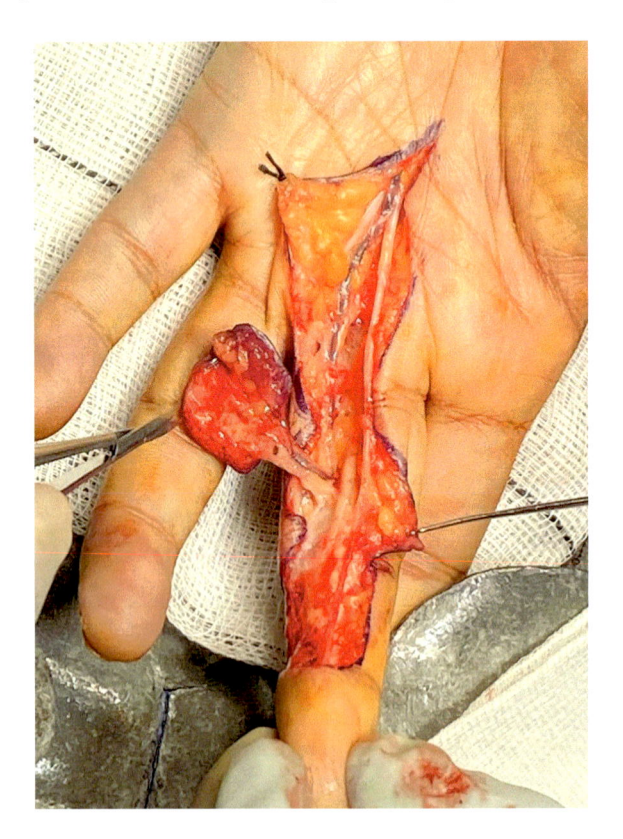

Fig. 27.8 Dissection of the DBPDN and the pedicle for heterodigital island flap

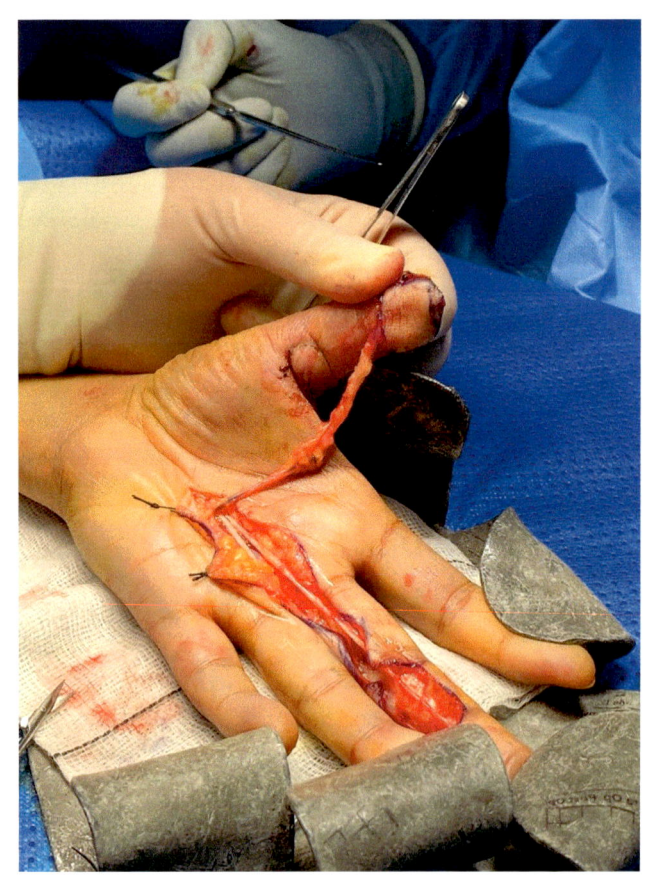

Fig. 27.9 Pedicle length is tested for a heterodigital island flap

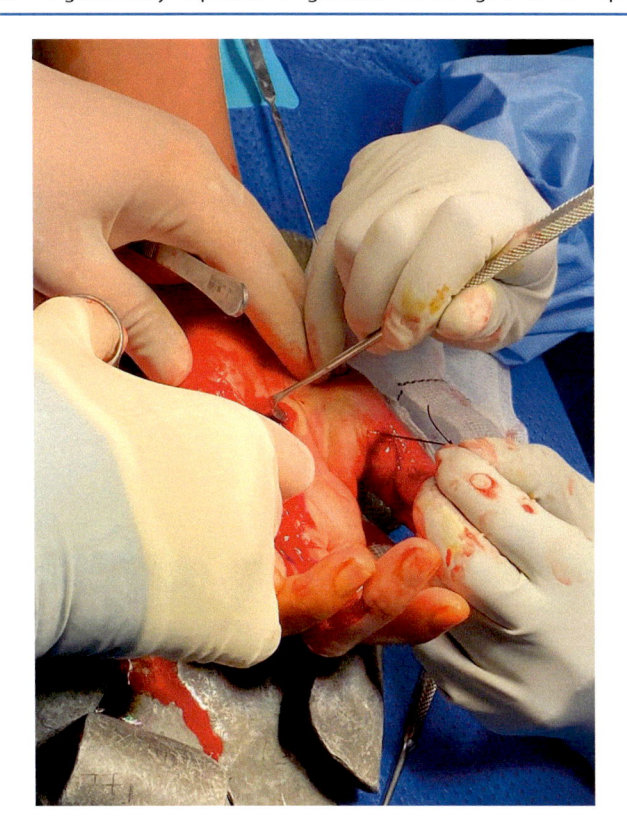

Fig. 27.10 The heterodigital island flap is passed under a tunnel of skin to the thumb tip

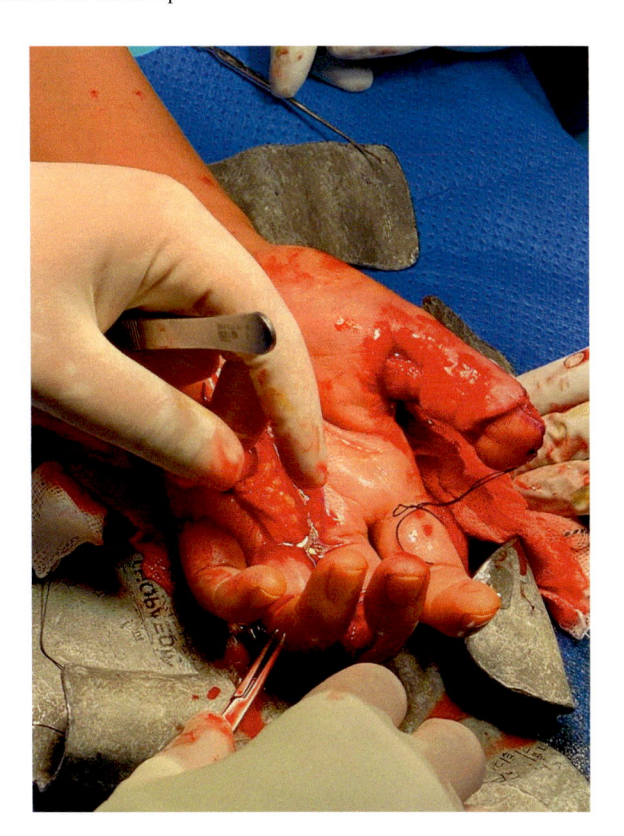

Fig. 27.11 Perfusion of the heterodigital island flap is checked

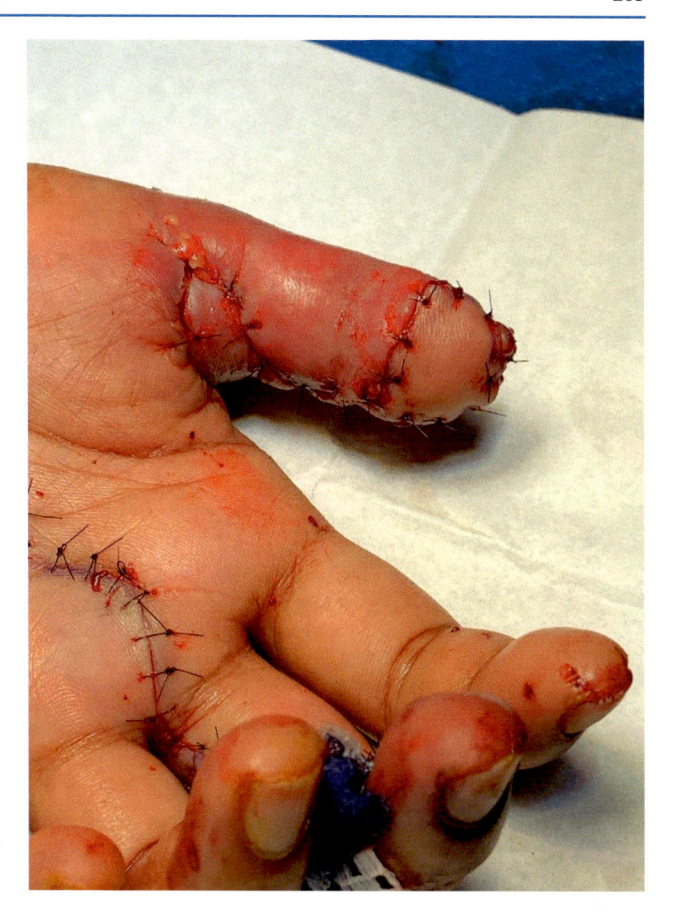

Fig. 27.12 Heterodigital island flap is secured in place

27.6 Core Surgical Techniques

27.6.1 Reverse Homodigital Island Flap : Surgeon Dariush Nikkhah

This flap is most easily raised using an arm tourniquet and loupe magnification under regional or general anesthesia. The wound is thoroughly cleaned and debrided. The skin markings are incised. Firstly, the flap over the lateral border of the proximal phalanx and the skin incisions on the lateral border of the digit are extended distally to the defect.

The main digital nerve is identified as can be seen in Fig. 27.5 and preserved. The flap is dissected free preserving a cuff of soft tissue around the artery, preserving venous drainage of the flap. The senior author uses fine microsurgical instrumentation for dissection of the nerve away from the digital artery, including microscissors and fine-handled tenotomies. For vessel side branches, one can use bipolar with heat sinking technique or microligaclips to avoid thermal injury to the main digital artery. Once the flap is dissected, the digital artery is ligated and divided proximally. The flap can then be raised on the pedicle and inset into the defect.

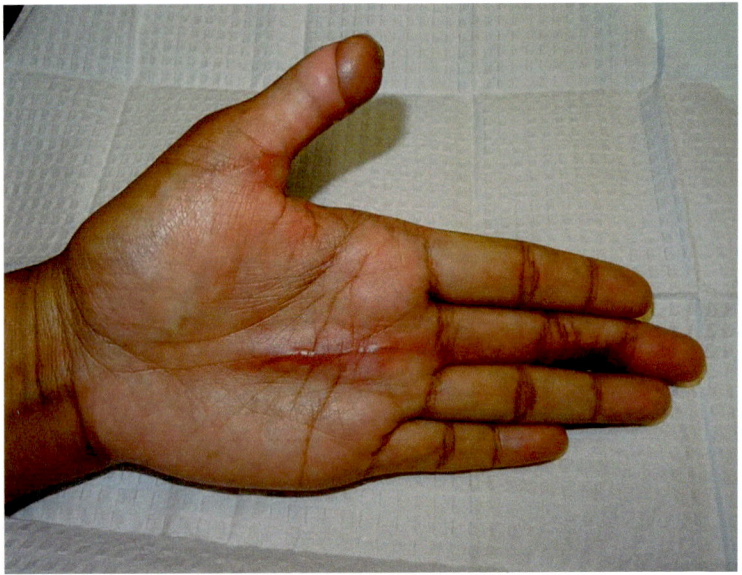

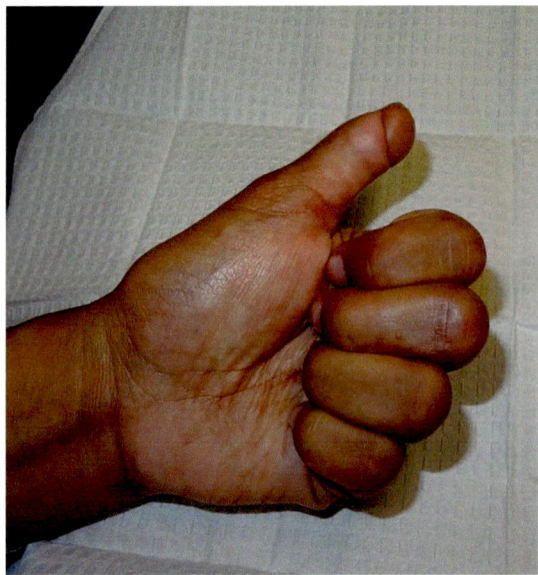

Fig. 27.13 Six-month post-op outcome for a heterodigital island flap

The arc of rotation is centered on the distal transverse palmar arch at the distal interphalangeal joint, giving the flap a wide reach in a variety of clinical situations. The flap can be sensate if the dorsal sensory branch is included in the skin paddle. In Fig. 27.6 you can see the flap inset at the fingertip; a skin graft has been harvested from over the hypothenar eminence and has been inset over the flap donor site. The skin graft can be harvested from other sites but if using the groin, avoid taking hair-bearing skin.

27.6.2 Heterodigital Island Flap : Surgeon Dariush Nikkhah

This procedure should be done under general or regional anesthesia with tourniquet control. In this example which demonstrates a mid-lateral phalangeal flap, the flap is raised from the ulnar side of the middle finger (donor) over the middle phalanx.

A zigzag incision is made from the distal margin of the flexor retinaculum in the palm to the finger web, and then a lateral zigzag incision extends up the digit. The pedicle is raised carefully in a retrograde fashion, protecting a 5 mm cuff of adipofascial tissue around the artery. This is important (as with homodigital artery flaps) for venous drainage of the flap. Gentle traction on the pedicle allows visualization of nerve and vessel branches to the flexor tendon and joints which are divided. The branch of the common digital artery to the ring finger is ligated, and the common digital artery is dissected as far proximally as the superficial palmar arch. This is the pivot point. As with the reverse homodigital island flap, side branches of the artery can be clipped with microligaclips, or bipolar with heat sink technique can be used.

A stitch secured to the flap is used to aid its passage through the subcutaneous tunnel from the donor site to the recipient site (thumb tip). Once the flap is in place, the pedicle is checked for any evidence of tension or kinking. The tourniquet is released to check perfusion and perform hemostasis prior to closure. A FTSG from the forearm was sutured to the defect on the donor finger. A jelonet bolster has been used to secure the FTSG.

Figure 27.13 shows the outcome at 6 months post-op for this patient. The patient had protective sensation.

27.7 Clinical Scenario

27.7.1 Reverse Homodigital Island Flap : Surgeon Dariush Nikkhah

An 18-year-old woman sustained a burn to the right index finger, while cooking. After debridement she was left with a full-thickness defect over the distal interphalangeal joint (Fig. 27.14).

This was an isolated injury and the patient was otherwise well and a nonsmoker. A reverse homodigital island flap from the ulnar border of the proximal index provided robust and padded soft tissue cover (Fig. 27.15).

The wound had healed at 2 weeks and the patient had an uneventful recovery (Fig. 27.16).

27.7.2 Heterodigital Island Flap : Surgeon Dariush Nikkhah

A 50-year-old man required multiple washouts for a flexor sheath infection of his index finger, with resultant skin loss

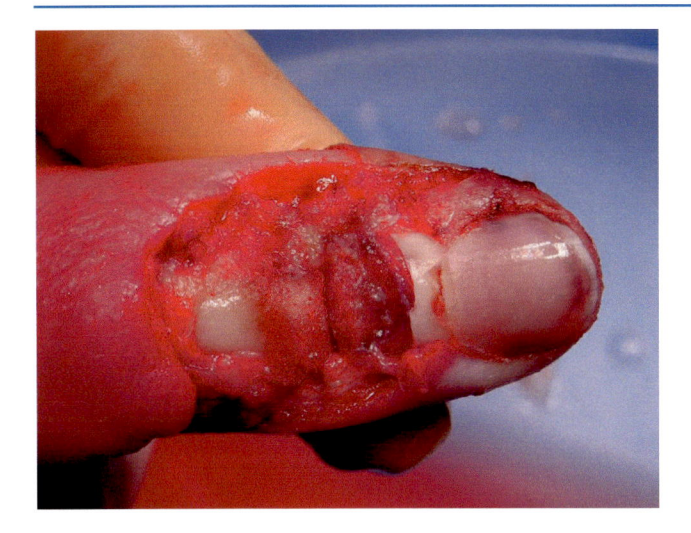

Fig. 27.14 Injury to the finger with defect over DIPJ

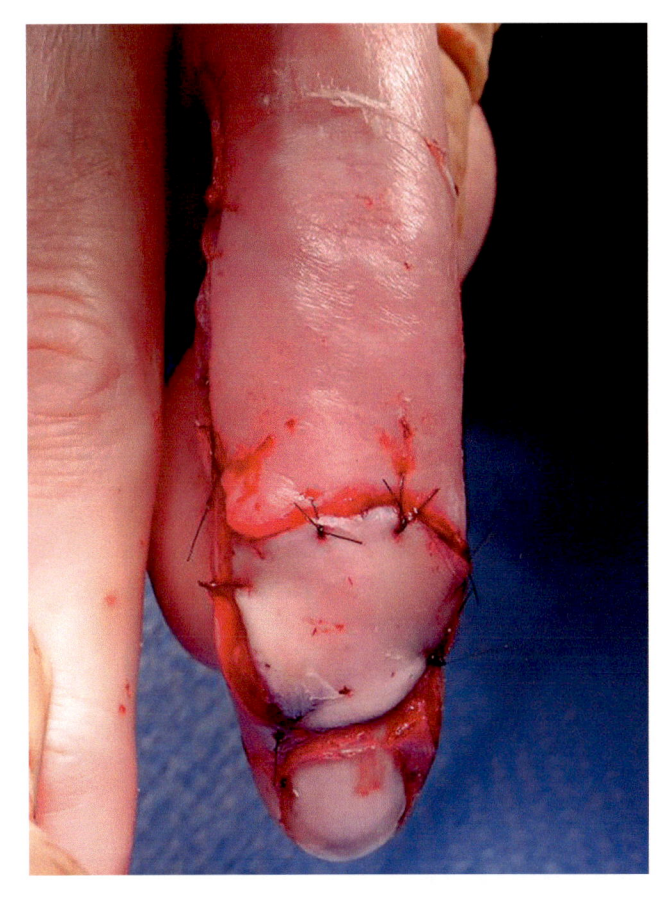

Fig. 27.15 Intraoperative view showing reverse homodigital island flap to defect

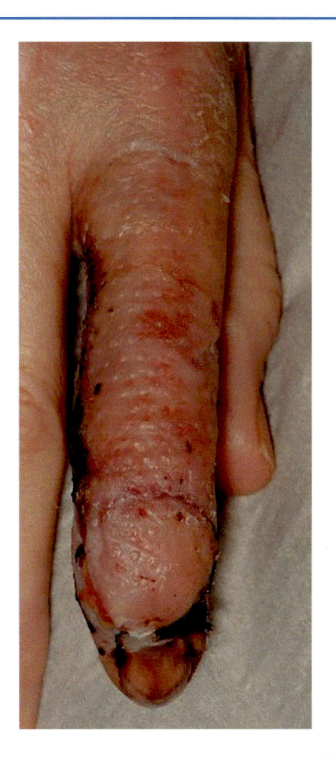

Fig. 27.16 Two-week postoperative outcome for reverse homodigital island flap

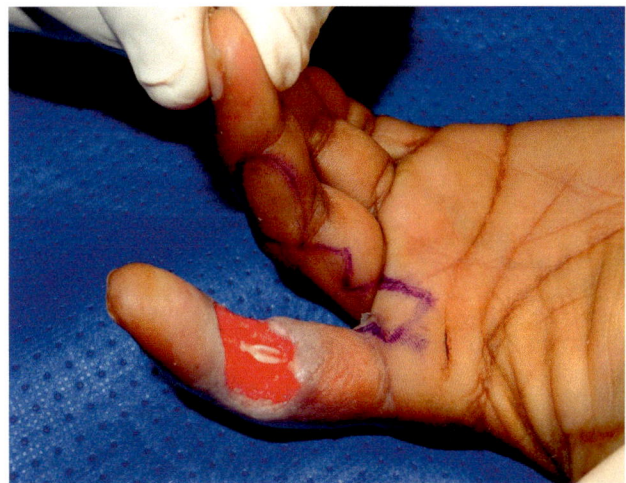

Fig. 27.17 Skin markings for heterodigital island flap

over the volar aspect of the middle phalanx. Following resolution of the infection, he had a defect with flexor tendon exposed. Using the principles described previously, a heterodigital island flap was designed based on the radial digital artery of the middle finger, to cover the defect on the index finger. The donor site in this case was closed primarily due to skin laxity.

Figure 27.17 shows the index finger defect, with exposed tendon and skin markings for a heterodigital island flap.

Figure 27.18 shows how the flap is raised on the radial digital artery of the middle finger and is ready to be inset into the defect (Fig. 27.19). The digital nerve from donor finger is still intact (seen retracted with skin flap).

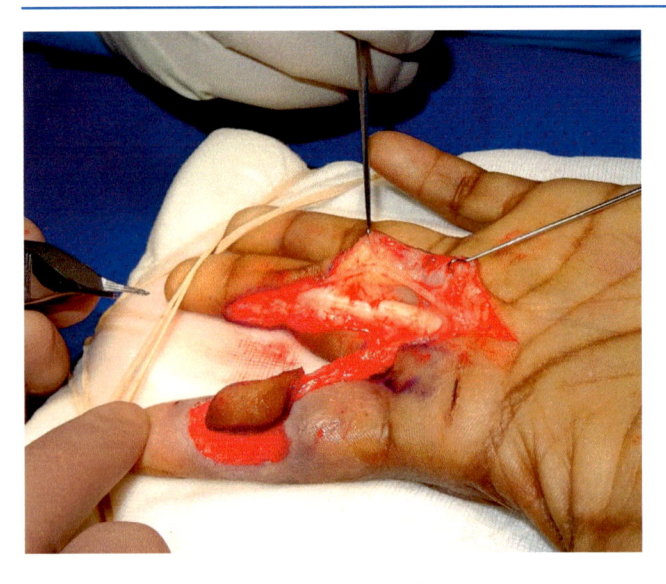

Fig. 27.18 Heterodigital island flap is raised and ready to be inset

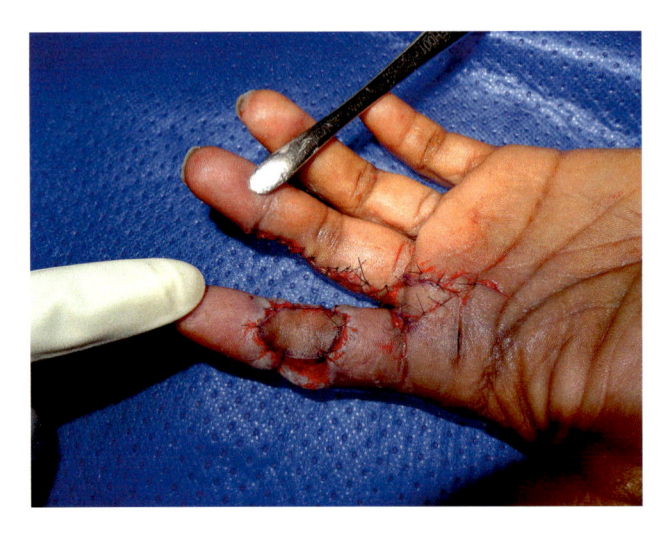

Fig. 27.19 Final flap inset to cover index finger, donor site closed primarily

27.8 Pearls and Pitfalls [10–18]

Pearls

- For a reverse homodigital island flap, identify the digital nerve rather than the artery first, and start proximal to the flap. It is then dissected free from the adipofascial tissue that surrounds the artery. The flap can then be raised quicker and without the need to hunt for the digital artery.
- Elevating the hand postoperatively can help reduce venous congestion.
- If there is concern about the blood supply from the contralateral digital artery, the ipsilateral digital artery can be initially clamped to check the blood supply to the digit before it is ligated and divided.
- When performing a mid-lateral phalangeal flap, make the subcutaneous tunnel wide, and use a silk suture to aid passing the flap through the tunnel.
- For a heterodigital island flap, avoid the need for sensory reeducation and donor numbness by preserving the main digital nerve on the donor finger and taking just the dorsal branch.
- Use a thick FTSG skin graft to close the donor site.

Pitfalls

- Avoid skeletonizing the pedicle as this may result in damage of the venous drainage or vascular supply of the flap.
- A reverse homodigital island flap needs to be inset loosely to avoid compression of the pedicle, which usually leads to venous compromise of the flap. Leaving the area of the pedicle open or applying a small split-thickness graft will avoid flap loss.
- If reconstructing the fingertip with a retrograde homodigital island flap, make sure the distal arch is intact, and if there is any question that it is compromised, a homodigital flap should not be performed.
- Avoid performing antegrade and retrograde homodigital flaps on infected or vascularly compromised digits as this may compromise the digit further.
- Make sure the patient understands the donor site from a heterodigital island flap is unsightly, and offer them microsurgical alternatives (hand or foot).

27.9 Selected Readings

- Lai et al. The Reverse Digital Artery Flap for Fingertip Reconstruction. Ann Plast Surg. 1989 Jun;22(6):495–500. doi: 10.1097/00000637-198906000-00005.
- *This is the original paper describing the reverse homodigital island flap. It describes the anatomy and relationship of the digital artery and nerve. It describes how to raise*

- Lai et al. A Versatile Method for Reconstruction of Finger Defects: Reverse Digital Artery Flap. Br J Plast Surg. Aug-Sep 1992;45(6):443–53. doi: 10.1016/0007-1226(92)90208-f.
- *This paper describes in more detail the reverse homodigital island flap. It includes a cadaveric dissection examining the anatomy of the dorsal sensory nerve. It also describes an extended flap and an innervated flap.*
- Kojima et al. Reverse Vascular Pedicle Digital Island Flap. Br J Plast Surg. 1990 May;43(3):290–5. doi: 10.1016/0007-1226(90)90074-a.
- *This paper also describes a reverse homodigital island flap. It describes eight fingers in which this flap was used.*
- Tan R E S & Lahiri A. Vascular Anatomy of the Hand in Relation to Flaps. Hand Clin 2020 (36) 1–8.
- *Detailed review of anatomical studies of vasculature of the whole hand.*
- Littler JW. Neurovascular pedicle transfers of tissue in reconstructive surgery of the hand. J Bone Joint Surg. 1956, 38A: 917.
- *This is Littler's original description of elevating an island flap.*
- Lee et al. Innervated Lateral Middle Phalangeal Finger Flap for a Large Pulp Defect by Bilateral Neurorrhaphy. Plast Reconstr Surg 2006 Oct;118(5):1185–93; doi: 10.1097/01.prs.0000221002.75057.a4.
- *This describes the mid-lateral phalangeal flap demonstrated in the step-by-step guide in this chapter.*
- Wang et al. Modified Heterodigital Neurovascular Island Flap for Sensory Reconstruction of Pulp or Volar Soft Tissue Defect of Digits. J Hand Surg Am 2020 Jan;45(1):67.e1–67.e8. doi: 10.1016/j.jhsa.2019.04.014. Epub 2019 Jun 22.
- *This describes the techni\que of using the proximal DBPDN as a nerve graft for the transected donor PDN.*

References

1. Lee YH, Baek GH, Gong HS, Lee SM, Chung MS. Innervated lateral middle phalangeal finger flap for a large pulp defect by bilateral neurorrhaphy. Plast Reconstr Surg. 2006;118(5):1185–93.; discussion 1194. https://doi.org/10.1097/01.prs.0000221002.75057.a4.
2. Venkataswami R, Subramanian N. Oblique triangular flap: a new method of repair for oblique amputations of the fingertip and thumb. Plast Reconstrue Surg. 1980;66(2):296–300.
3. Lai CS, Lin SD, Yang CC. The reverse digital artery flap for fingertip reconstruction. Ann Plast Surg. 1989 Jun;22(6):495–500. https://doi.org/10.1097/00000637-198906000-00005.
4. Kojima T, Tsuchida Y, Hirasé Y, Endo T. Reverse vascular pedicle digital island flap. Br J Plast Surg. 1990;43(3):290–5. https://doi.org/10.1016/0007-1226(90)90074-a.
5. Koshima I, Urushibara K, Fukuda N, Ohkochi M, Nagase T, Gonda K, Asato H, Yoshimura K. Digital artery perforator flaps for fingertip reconstructions. Plast Reconstr Surg. 2006;118(7):1579–84. https://doi.org/10.1097/01.prs.0000232987.54881.a7.
6. Haerle M, Häfner HM, Schaller HE, Brunelli F. Dominances in finger arteries. J Hand Surg Br. 2002;27(6):526–9. https://doi.org/10.1054/jhsb.2002.0856.
7. Lai CS, Lin SD, Chou CK, Tsai CW. A versatile method for reconstruction of finger defects: reverse digital artery flap. Br J Plast Surg. 1992;45(6):443–53. https://doi.org/10.1016/0007-1226(92)90208-f.
8. Rose EH. Small flap coverage of hand and digit defects. Clin Plast Surg. 1989;16(3):427–42.
9. Wang H, Yang X, Chen C, Huo Y, Wang B, Wang W. Modified Heterodigital Neurovascular Island flap for sensory reconstruction of pulp or volar soft tissue defect of digits. J Hand Surg Am. 2020;45(1):67.e1–8. https://doi.org/10.1016/j.jhsa.2019.04.014.
10. Ashbell TS, Kutz JE, Kleinert HE. The digital Allen test. Plast Reconstr Surg. 1967;39(3):311–2. https://doi.org/10.1097/00006534-196703000-00013.
11. Littler JW. Neurovascular pedicle transfers of tissue in reconstructive surgery of the hand. J Bone Joint Surg. 1956;38A:917.
12. Moberg E. Aspects of sensation in reconstructive surgery of the upper extremity. J Bone Joint Surg Am. 1964;46:817–25.
13. Moledina J, Reissis D, Nikkhah D. Maneuvers to aid raising and survival of the Homodigital Island flap. Plast Reconstr Surg Glob Open. 2016;4(9):e1056. https://doi.org/10.1097/GOX.0000000000001056.
14. Niranjan NS, Armstrong JR. A homodigital reverse pedicle island flap in soft tissue reconstruction of the finger and the thumb. J Hand Surg Br. 1994;19(2):135–41. https://doi.org/10.1016/0266-7681(94)90149-x.
15. Tan RES, Lahiri A. Vascular anatomy of the hand in relation to flaps. Hand Clin. 2020;36(1):1–8. https://doi.org/10.1016/j.hcl.2019.08.001.
16. Tubiana R, Duparc J. Restoration of sensibility in the hand by neurovascular skin island transfer. J Bone Joint Surg. 1961;43B:474.
17. Weeks PM, Wray RC. Management of acute hand injuries. St. Louis: Mosby; 1973. p. 140.
18. Xarchas KC, Tilkeridis KE, Pelekas SI, Kazakos KJ, Kakagia DD, Verettas DA. Littler's flap revisited: an anatomic study, literature review, and clinical experience in the reconstruction of large thumb-pulp defects. Med Sci Monit. 2008;14(11):CR568–73.

Radial Forearm Flap

Shahriar Raj Zaman, Qadir Khan, Jeremy M. Rawlins, Allan Ponniah, and Dariush Nikkhah

28.1 Introduction

The radial forearm free flap (RFFF) was first described in 1978 in China at the Shenyang Military Hospital and then subsequently in a 1981 case series of 60 patients for resurfacing predominantly the neck for burn contractures [1, 2]. It has been described as a Mathes and Nahai type B fasciocutaneous flap [3]. Traditionally it has been utilized as a fasciocutaneous flap that includes volar forearm skin, fascia and the radial artery; however the flap may also include bone, cutaneous nerves, flexor tendons and even the brachioradialis muscle. As such, it has become known for its versatility, reliability and its ease of harvest. The flap can also be pedicled to cover elbow defects or applied as a reverse radial forearm flap for hand/thumb defects [3]. Perforator-based and adipofascial flaps have also been described for dorsal hand injuries [4]. For a period of time following its development, it became the workhorse fasciocutaneous flap for those defects requiring soft, thin and pliable reconstructions with long pedicles. Its use now is predominantly, but not limited to, in head and neck cancer reconstruction for intra-oral lining and glossectomy defects [5]. The less than optimal aesthetic donor site morbidity has led to other fasciocutaneous flaps such as the anterolateral thigh (ALT) or the medial sural artery perforator (MSAP) flap being utilized now more frequently [6]. Nevertheless, the RFFF represents a reliable choice in situations where others are not feasible.

28.2 Anatomy

The RFFF can be designed off the whole volar forearm, but traditionally the distal radial forearm is harvested due to its slender composition at this level. The arterial supply is based on the septocutaneous branches of the radial artery, which traverses proximally in the septum between the brachioradialis (BR) and pronator teres (PT) and distally between the BR and flexor carpi radialis (FCR). In the proximal third, there is a constellation of perforators (4, range 0–10) that are large and well-spaced, whereas in the distal third, they are more numerous and smaller in size (9, range 4–14) [1]. The radial artery is accompanied by venae comitantes throughout its course in a ladder-like configuration whereby the valves can be bypassed by the frequent interconnections and thus permitting retrograde drainage [1, 3]. Superficial venous drainage is traditionally provided by the nearby large cephalic vein which ascends on the radial volar forearm and can be dissected as far proximally as the deltopectoral groove. A sensate flap can be raised based on the lateral cutaneous nerve of the forearm which supplies the radial volar forearm, and if ulnar enough, the medial cutaneous nerve of the forearm could also be harvested. For an osteocutaneous flap, a segment of radius up to 10–12 cm in length and 40% in cross section is able to be harvested through periosteal branches that filter down from deep fascia in the intermuscular septum [1, 3]. The concept of subfascial and suprafascial flaps has also been explored and will be discussed further below.

With regard to anatomical variations, McCormack found both the radial and ulnar arteries to be present 100% of the time in their 750 dissections [7]. Subsequent work by Coleman and Anson found an absence of branches from the superficial palmar arch to the thumb and index finger in over 10% of dissections [8]. In 50% of dissections, the deep arch from the radial artery did not communicate with the ulnar artery [8]. In such a combination, the thumb would completely be dependent on the radial artery, and so a RFFF would necessitate a vein graft to ensure thumb vascularity.

S. R. Zaman · J. M. Rawlins
Royal Perth Hospital, Perth, WA, Australia

Q. Khan
Fiona Stanley Hospital, Murdoch, WA, Australia

A. Ponniah · D. Nikkhah (✉)
Royal Free Hospital, London, UK
e-mail: allan.ponniah@nhs.net; d.nikkhah@nhs.net

28.3 Preoperative Investigation

Preoperatively, an Allen's test must be performed to ensure adequate vascularity to the hand if the radial artery were to be ligated. In the Allen's test, both the radial and ulnar arteries are occluded through finger pressure at the wrist whilst asking the patient to make a fist a few times to allow venous exsanguination of the hand. The patient then opens their hand, and pressure off the ulnar artery is released whilst maintaining occlusion of the radial artery. A hand colour that returns to pink within several seconds is one where the RFFF will be safe to use. A thorough surgical history is paramount to ascertain any previous injuries including fractures (especially if an osteocutaneous flap is planned) or vascular injuries. If harvesting an osteocutaneous flap, an x-ray aids in planning and assessing for previous fractures. Caution also must be taken particularly in the elderly or vasculopaths whereby unknown atheroma may increase the risk of failure or complications. In such cases, a CT angiogram would be recommended. Once a side is chosen for harvest, the radial artery can be palpated at the level of the volar wrist and traced proximally with a handheld Doppler up to the level of cubital fossa depending on the length of pedicle needed.

28.4 Flap Design and Markings

Begin by marking the course of the radial artery and cephalic vein from the wrist to the cubital fossa. Coarsely this is represented by a line 1 cm inferior to the centre of the antecubital fossa to the scaphoid tubercle but can be more accurately traced with a handheld Doppler. Mark the BR and FCR tendons by palpating them distally on the wrist. The axis of the flap will be slightly ulnar to this line in order to avoid the hairier dorsal wrist. The dimensions of the flap for marking are determined by the defect for reconstruction and generally are made over the distal third of the forearm (Fig. 28.1).

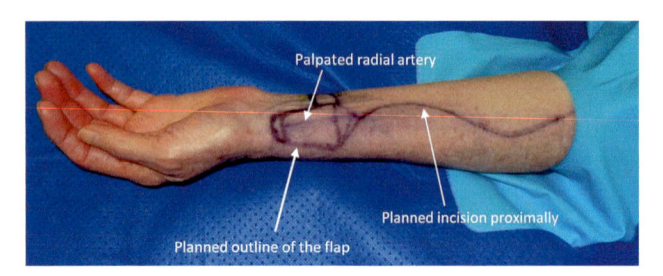

Fig. 28.1 Flap design and markings

28.5 Flap Raise/Elevation: A Step-by-Step Guide

Step 1 Position and Incision
With the patient supine, the arm is on an arm table extended to 90 degrees. The arm is elevated for exsanguination, tourniquet applied and the forearm supinated. Make an incision on the ulnar border of the flap down through subcutaneous tissue until forearm fascia is reached. The fascia is incised proximally over the muscle and down to the paratenon of the flexor carpi ulnaris (FCU) tendon distally.

Step 2 Ulnar to Radial Subfascial Raise: Standard Method
Elevation at this subfascial level proceeds ulnar to radially superficial to the underlying muscles/tendons with haemostasis along the way. It's important to preserve the paratenon of all the tendons. As the dissection is subfascial, the volar forearm veins and the lateral and medial cutaneous nerves (depending on how ulnar the flap is) will be already within the flap (Fig. 28.2). The nerves and veins will be encountered at the proximal edge of the flap, and so prepare whatever is necessary for the reconstruction. Proceed radially till edge of previously marked FCR.

Step 3 Pedicle Dissection Proximally
Whilst waiting for recipient site preparation, dissection of the radial artery and its venae proximally can be performed (Fig. 28.3). This can be aided with a self-retainer retractor in the septum between FCR and BR to expose the vascular pedicle (Fig. 28.4). Take care to apply micro-haemostatic clips to the small muscle branches off the radial artery. Free the pedicle circumferentially proximally to the skin paddle (Fig. 28.5). If the cephalic vein is also going to be included in the flap, then its dissection can also be performed at this point.

Step 4 Radial Incision
The radial border of the flap is then incised 1 cm radial to the artery. Care must be taken to identify and protect the superficial radial nerve and its branches (Fig. 28.6). Clip and divide the cephalic vein at the distal edge of the flap if it is to be included. The free border of BR muscle and its tendon is seen and retracted radially. The radial artery and its venae will be seen along the ulnar side of the BR tendon and the radial border of FCR tendon. Dissect along BR muscle edge, ensuring the intermuscular fascia is not breached as the vascular pedicle is within.

28 Radial Forearm Flap

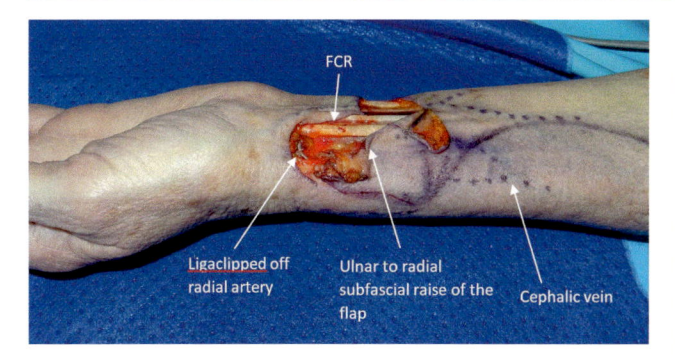

Fig. 28.2 Subfascial ulnar to radial raise with the distal radial neurovascular bundle ligaclipped

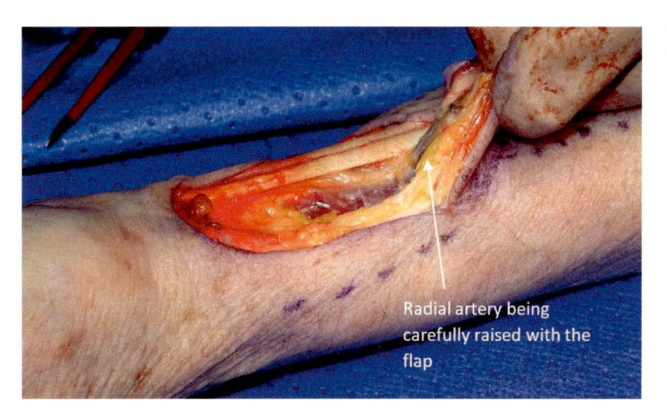

Fig. 28.3 Distal to proximal raise of the RFFF

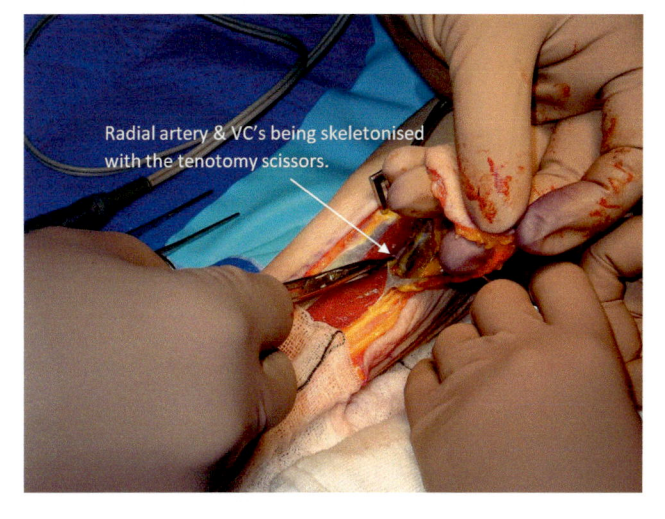

Fig. 28.4 Careful dissection of the pedicle between BR and FCR

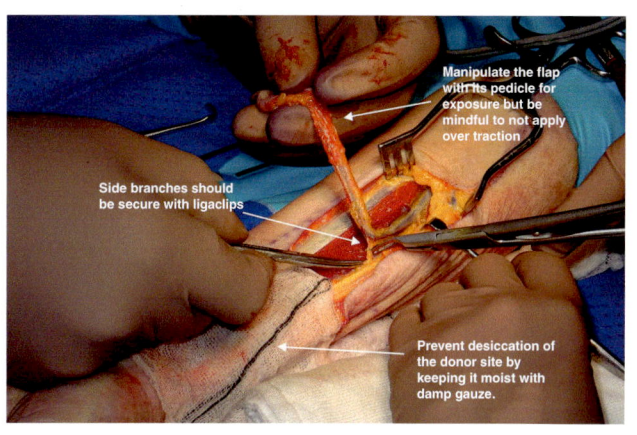

Fig. 28.5 Meticulous ligaclipping of the side branches with gentle traction

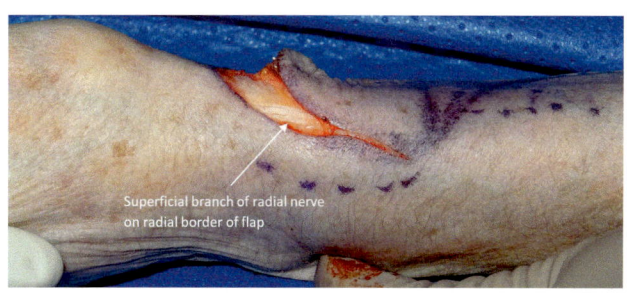

Fig. 28.6 Care must be taken around the radial border of the flap to avoid injury to the superficial branch of the radial nerve

Step 5 Divide Radial Artery and Venae Distally

At the distal edge of the flap, isolate and divide the radial artery and its venae. At this point the vascular pedicle of the flap should be the only attachment remaining to the underlying tissues as the rest of the flap has been raised already. Proceed then to create a plane under the pedicle from distal to proximal along its length ensuring haemostasis of any small branches. Once free of all its attachments, release the tourniquet and assess circulation of the flap.

Step 6 Division of Pedicle for Transfer

Once the recipient site is ready for transfer, the pedicle is prepared for division (Fig. 28.7). At the proximal pedicle end, carefully separate the venae from the radial artery to allow adequate length for anastomoses. Beginning with the venae, double clip the side that will remain and divide distal to this. Do the same for the artery. This will now render the flap ischaemic.

Step 7 Donor Site Closure

For a sizeable RFFF that isn't amenable for a hatchet flap, a skin graft is used. The FCR and BR muscle bellies are approximated with absorbable sutures, ensuring the paratenon isn't injured. Apply a skin graft, a bulky dressing and a resting volar plaster of Paris.

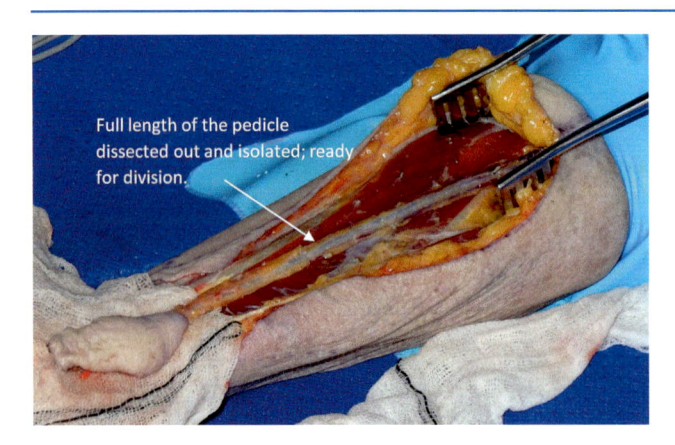

Fig. 28.7 Flap islanded and pedicle dissected out as far proximally as required

28.6 Core Surgical Techniques in Flap Dissection

28.6.1 Skin Paddle Design

The cutaneous design is open to great variation depending on what is required. The standard RFFF is designed over the distal volar third of the forearm. The design for the reverse RFF is with the skin paddle in the proximal forearm, and the pivot point is the palpable radial pulse at the level of the wrist. The skin island is designed centrally along the radial artery axis (illustrated in case scenario B). The flap can also be split into several skin islands based on the septocutaneous perforators.

28.6.2 Ulnar to Radial Approach

The subfascial flap elevation technique is the standard method; however a suprafascial flap harvest can also be performed. It was hypothesized that the subfascial flap improved flap vascularity by way of preserving the subfascial vascular plexus. The suprafascial flap on the other hand was thought to leave a more suitable donor site for graft take and tendon excursion which was subsequently confirmed by Chang et al. [9]. A decade later, a definitive anatomical study found that the deep fascia did not contribute to the perfusion of the RFFF as was initially thought [10].

28.6.3 Osteocutaneous Flap

RFFF as an osteocutaneous flap has fallen out of favour due to better donor sites such as the free fibula flap and thus its use is rare. Available bone is from distal to pronator teres insertion to the distal styloid which gives approximately 10–12 cm length of boat-shaped bone segment in an adult [1]. The wrist and forearm is then placed into a plaster of Paris for 3–4 weeks to prevent a radius fracture; some surgeons plate the donor site for further rigid stability [1, 3].

28.6.4 Flap Dissection and Instrumentation

Dissection with a blade is generally the standard but can also be done with fine bipolar cautery at low settings especially near the pedicle. DeBakey forceps are used when handling vessels, and micro-ligaclips for clipping off the numerous side branches of the radial artery are recommended.

28.6.5 Tendon Inclusion

Depending on what the requirements of the reconstruction are, vascularized tendon can be transferred with the flap. The palmaris longus can be used if a fascial sling is required in cases of angle of mouth or lower lip reconstruction [1]. The BR tendon can also be utilized in pedicled reverse RFF for extensor defects.

28.6.6 Vein Harvest

For the free flap, harvesting a superficial vein (usually cephalic vein) is always worthwhile, even though the flap will generally be fine with venous drainage via the deep venae system. This applies also for the reverse pedicled flap for the hand defects [11].

28.6.7 Donor Site

The donor site morbidity represents the most unappealing feature of this flap, particularly if grafting is required. Full-thickness grafts from lateral groin (hairless) are preferred to split-thickness grafts for cosmesis, and suprafascial flaps have been found to improve graft take [9]. The ulnar transposition flap ("hatchet flap") was popularized by the Canniesburn group in the late 1980s and is applicable for the small donor site defects [12]. Acellular dermal matrices such as Integra or Matriderm have also shown promising results as staged constructions of the donor site.

28.7 Clinical Scenario

28.7.1 Clinical Scenario A: Surgeons Jeremy Rawlins and Qadir Khan

A 58-year-old female patient with a left nasal alar invasive BCC (Fig. 28.8). Staged excision and reconstruction was planned due to the extent and inconspicuous clinical borders of the tumour. Anatomical subunits were marked using the contralateral side as the template. A subfascial RFFF from the non-dominant forearm was raised (Figs. 28.9 and 28.10). The RFFF was folded for nasal lining and along with a cheek advancement flap for the medial cheek defect (Fig. 28.11). The fascial side of the flap was temporarily split skin grafted whilst awaiting the next stage (Figs. 28.12 and 28.13). The donor was closed with a full-thickness skin graft.

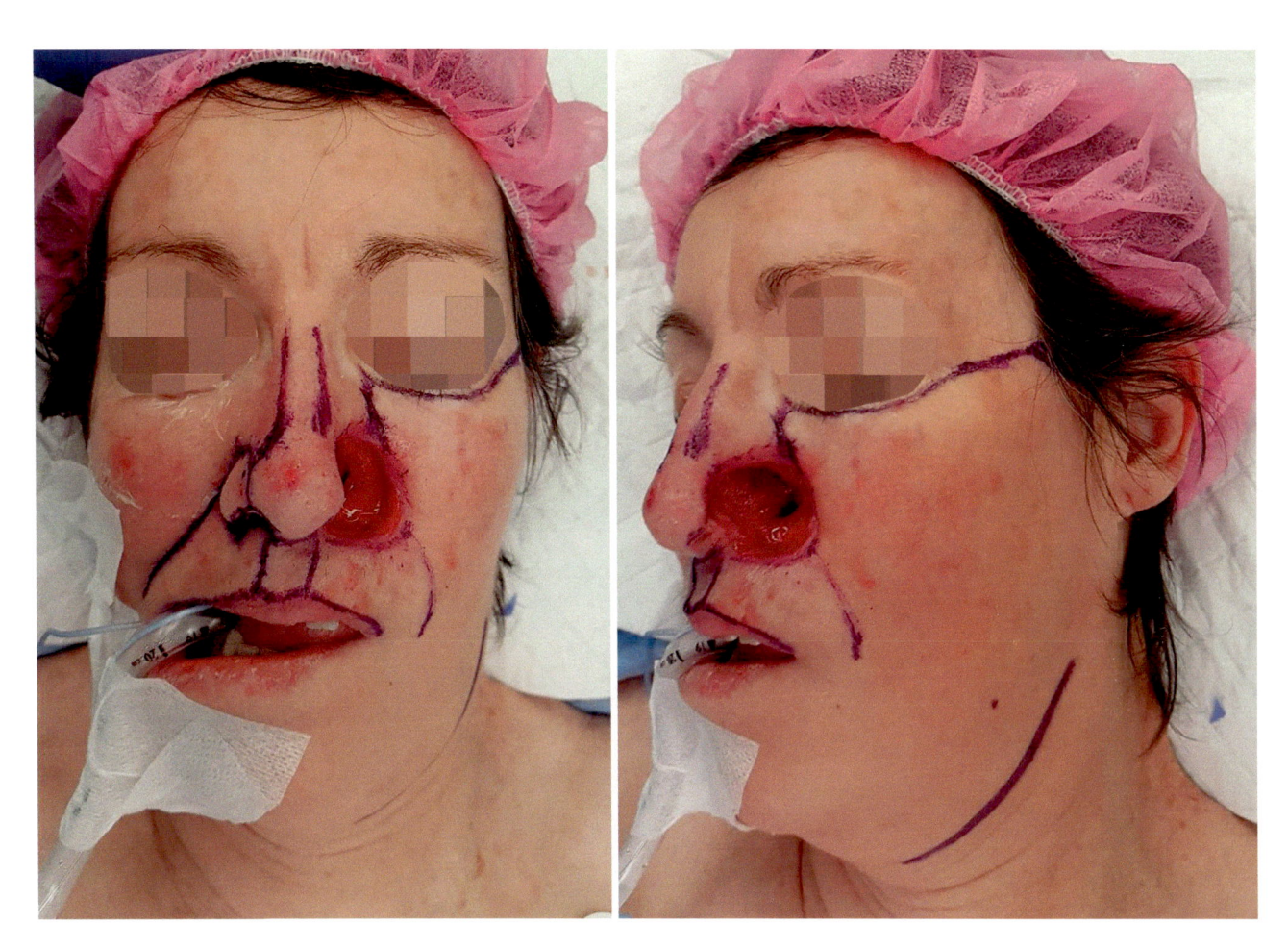

Fig. 28.8 Left alar/nasal and medial cheek defect with the anatomical subunits marked out

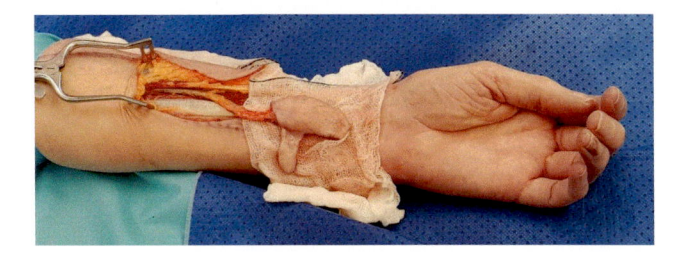

Fig. 28.9 Subfascial radial forearm flap raise. The cephalic vein was not included due to the small size of the flap

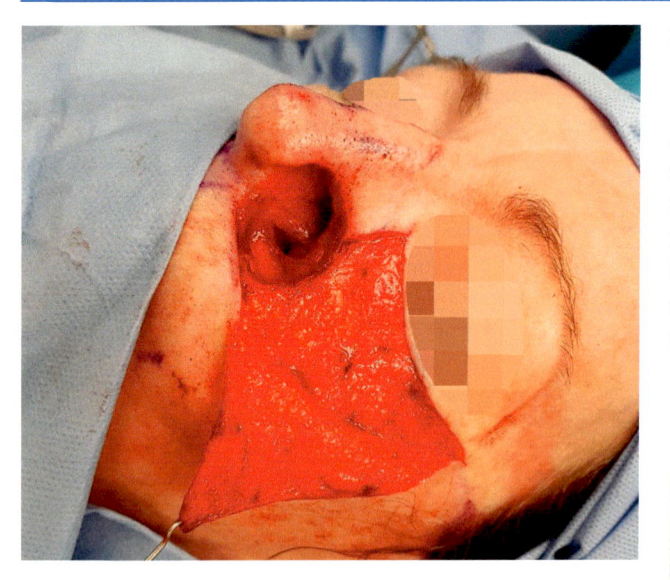

Fig. 28.10 The flap divided and placed in the plastic sleeve, ready for tunnelling to the neck vessels for microanastomoses

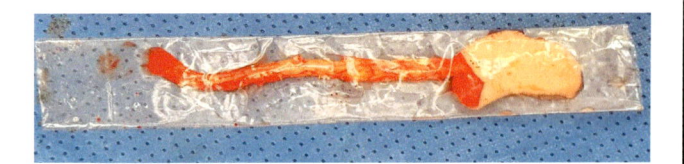

Fig. 28.11 Cheek advancement flap raised for the medial cheek defect

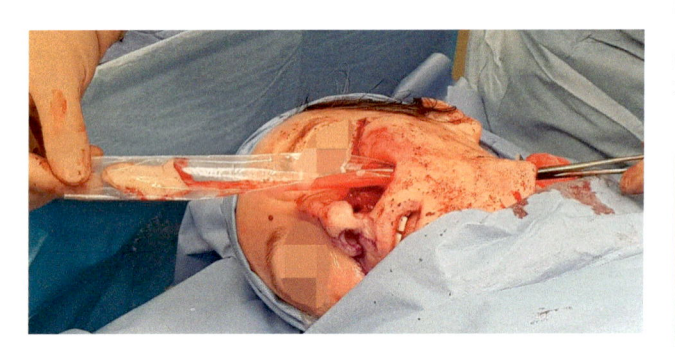

Fig. 28.12 The flap pedicle being tunnelled safely to the neck vessels. The plastic sleeve safeguards the pedicle from any untoward injury during the tunnelling

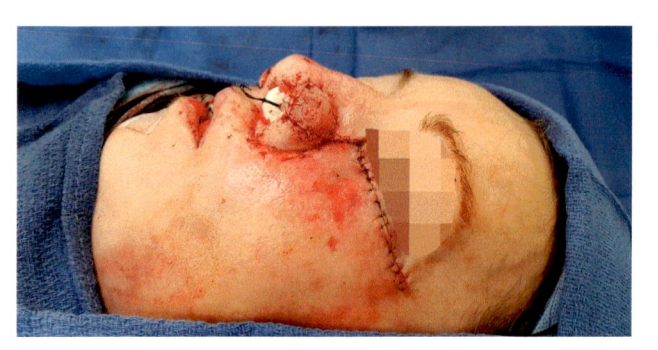

Fig. 28.13 Stage 1 complete. Nasal packs have been inserted to stent the nostrils open temporarily

28.7.2 Clinical Scenario B: Surgeons Dariush Nikkhah and Norbert Kang

A 60-year-old manual worker crushed his hand under heavy machinery. He had an exposed third metacarpal with a unicortical fracture, with tendon and periosteum stripped off the metacarpal (Fig. 28.14). A reverse radial forearm flap was performed after debridement (Fig. 28.15). He had an uneventful recovery, and at 6 months postoperatively, he had full range of movement and declined further debulking surgery (Fig. 28.16).

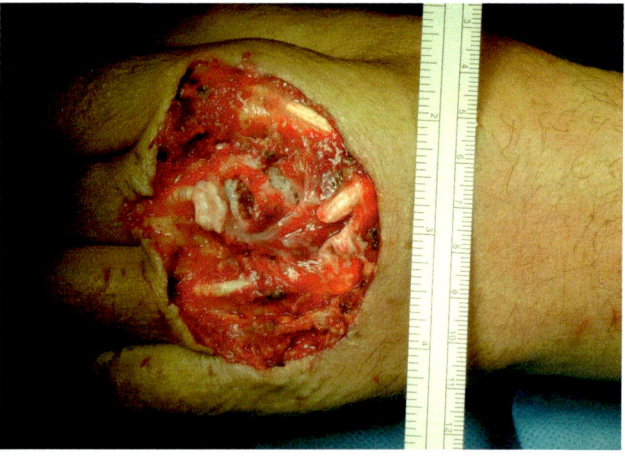

Fig. 28.14 Size of dorsal hand defect post definitive debridement and ready for reconstruction

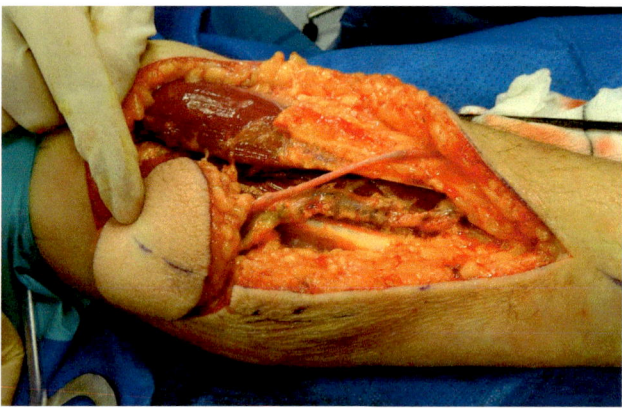

Fig. 28.15 Reverse radial forearm flap raised and islanded

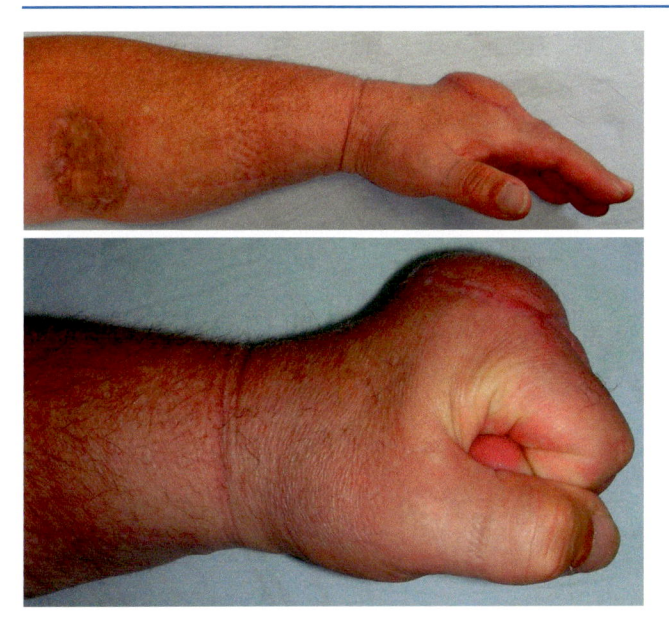

Fig. 28.16 Postoperatively, he had full range of movement with no restrictions

28.7.3 Clinical Scenario C: Surgeons Dariush Nikkhah and Allan Ponniah

A 69-year-old woman presented with aggressive recurrent poorly differentiated cutaneous squamous cell carcinoma of the nose. The lesion was fixed to the nasal bone, and CT imaging demonstrated extension of the tumour into the upper lateral cartilages and nasal bone—without evidence of lymphadenopathy. A partial rhinectomy was performed, and the upper septum, upper and lower lateral cartilage, nasal bone and nasal side wall were removed en bloc (Fig. 28.17). The lesion was narrowly excised at the deep margin, and after MDT discussion due to its aggressive and locally invasive nature, it was felt that immunotherapy with cemiplimab should be given over radiotherapy as this would allow for a better chance for later nasal reconstruction. After assessment at the craniofacial MDT, decision was made to perform a trilaminar reconstruction with internal lining imported as a free tissue transplant. The most suitable donor site was the forearm which was templated intraoperatively; the flap was taken as a suprafascial flap to reduce bulk (Figs. 28.18 and 28.19). The advantage of this approach would allow more accurate tailoring of the inner lining, which is not possible with locoregional flaps. Free flap reconstruction of the inner lining provides a customised and templated solution which allows for a robust blood supply for cartilage constructs. The radial forearm flap was raised on the nondominant hand, and the donor site was closed primarily with a hatchet flap. Superficial veins were harvested, and an 11 cm pedicle was taken for a tensionless anastomosis with the facial artery and facial vein in the neck with 9.0

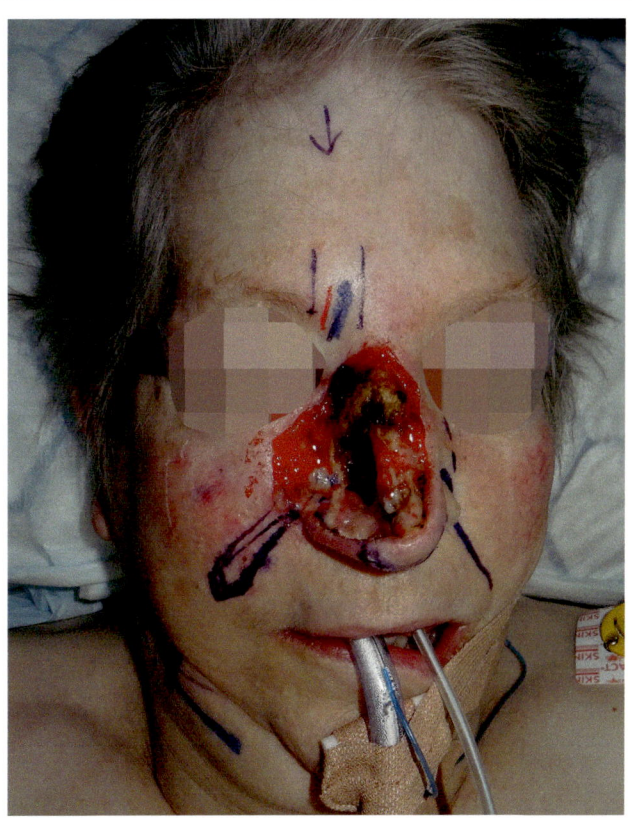

Fig. 28.17 Nasal defect post SCC cancer resection

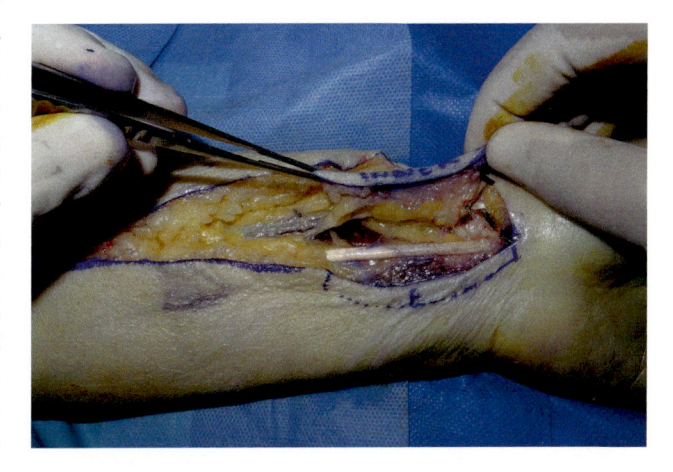

Fig. 28.18 Intraoperative picture demonstrating harvest of a suprafascial radial forearm flap for inner lining

ST. An alar batten graft was taken from the right conchal bowl to recreate the external valve. A full-thickness forehead flap was used to cover the cartilage and inner lining radial forearm flap in the same operation. Two subsequent revision operations which involved forehead flap debulking and pedicle division were performed. The patient had an excellent cosmetic outcome and remains cancer-free at 12 months (Fig. 28.20).

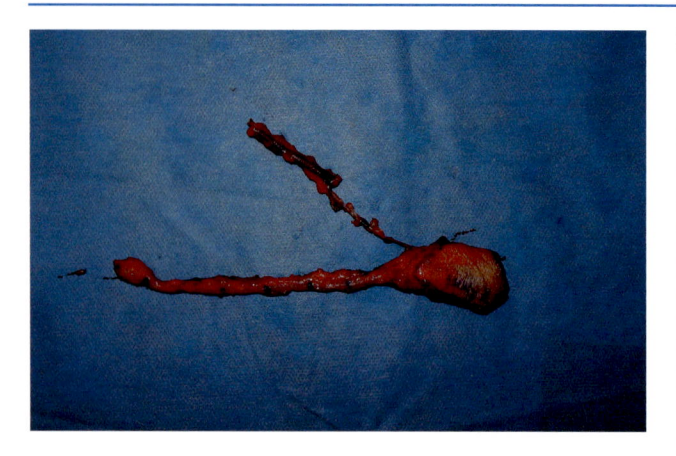

Fig. 28.19 Postage stamp size radial forearm flap with cephalic vein and radial artery demonstrated before transplantation

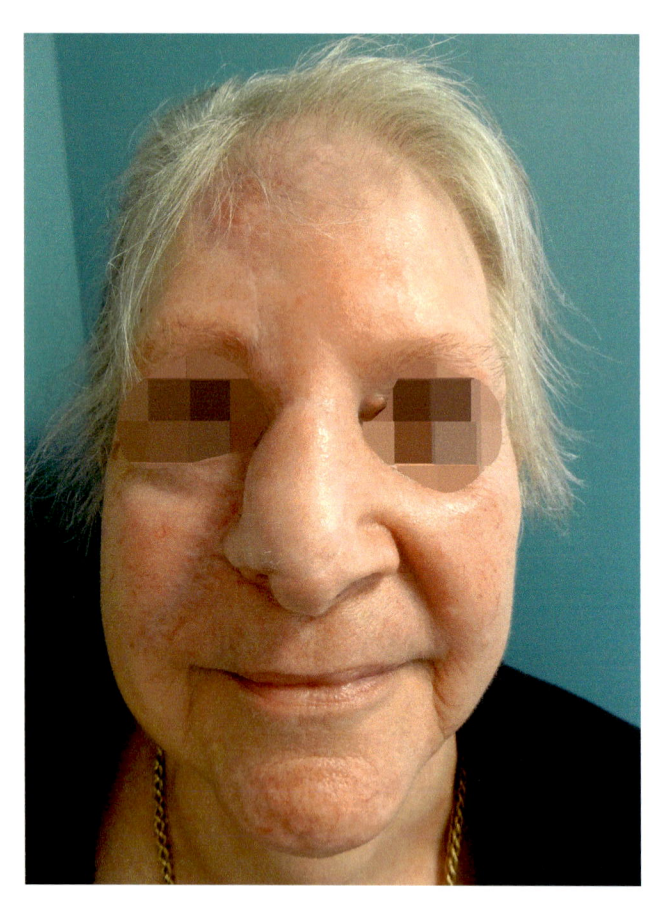

Fig. 28.20 12-month result after reconstruction

28.8 Pearls and Pitfalls [13]

Pearls
1. Proximal pressure above the elbow provides a degree of venous occlusion and thus can help identify more clearly the superficial veins.
2. Avoid the distal most 2 cm of the volar wrist to reduce the risk of tendon exposure from flap elevation.
3. Proximal incision to flap should be designed with the closure of the resultant defect in mind. If an ulnar transposition (hatchet) flap is planned, then plan design with the backcut. Otherwise a "lazy S" incision can be made if a split skin graft is planned for the donor site.
4. To ensure a true subfascial dissection, incise the fascia until the underlying muscle can be clearly seen.
5. To avoid injury to the paratenon and subsequent wound healing and tendon glide problems, utilize a sharp scalpel to dissect above the paratenon.

Pitfalls
1. Care must be taken to avoid an iatrogenic injury to the superficial branch of the radial nerve with the radial flap incision.
2. Following the radial incision, retract the BR muscle radially to avoid injuring the vascular pedicle.
3. Injuring the paratenon during subfascial dissection can lead to donor site healing issues.
4. A common pitfall with not taking a superficial vein as a lifeboat (usually cephalic) could place the flap at risk of venous congestion.
5. Misplacement of the flap not over the radial artery perforators in reverse pedicled flaps can result in flap necrosis.

28.9 Selected Readings

- Wei FC, Mardini, S. Chapter 25 Radial Forearm Flap. In: Flaps and Reconstructive Surgery. Pp 320–338. In: *Flaps and Reconstructive surgery.*
- *A modern encyclopaedia on reconstructive plastic surgery. The chapter is an excellent source on all aspects on the radial forearm flap.*
- Manktelow RT. Forearm Flap. In: *Microvascular Reconstruction.* 1986. pp 25–30.
- *Foreworded by Professor Ian Taylor himself, this book was a definitive landmark on flaps in reconstructive surgery during a time when reconstructive microsurgery was in its teens.*
- Mathes S, Nahai F. Radial Forearm Flap. 1997. pp. 775–802.
- *A succinct summary of the key aspects of a radial forearm flap raise with good cadaveric pictures. One of the pioneering volumes on reconstructive flap surgery.*
- Soutar DS, Mc Gregor IA. The radial forearm flap in intraoral reconstruction: The experience of 60 consecutive cases. Plast Reconstr Surg. 1986; 78(1). pp. 1–8.
- *From Canniesburn, Scotland, a 60-case review of the utility of the RFFF in intraoral reconstruction at a time when a reliable flap did not appear to be available.*
- Timmons MJ, Missotten FEM, Poole MD, Davies DM. Complications of radial forearm flap donor sites. Br J Plast Surg. 1986;39(2):176–8.
- *An important paper examining the complications of radial forearm free flaps including skin graft failure, swelling of the hand, stiffness, reduced strength and sensation, cold-induced symptoms and fractures of the radius. Their paper was on 15 patients from across 2 centres.*
- Jones NF, Jarrahy R, Kaufman MR. Pedicled and Free Radial Forearm Flaps for Reconstruction of the Elbow, Wrist and Hand. Plast Reconstr Surg. 2008; 121(3). pp. 887–898.
- *A single surgeon's experience from California with 67 pedicled and free RFF for reconstruction of the elbow, wrist and hand. The authors recommend the anterograde pedicled flap for elbow coverage and the reverse RFF as the optimal choice for moderate-sized defects of the wrist and hand.*
- Chang SCN, Miller G, Halbert CF, Yang KH, Chao WC, Wei FC. Limiting Donor Site Morbidity by Suprafascial Dissection of the Radial Forearm Flap. Microsurgery. 1996. 17: pp. 136–140.
- *In response to problems with donor site complications with subfascial raises, this paper examined the technique of suprafascial flap elevation to prevent donor site problems with considerable value.*
- Schaverien M, Saint-Cyr M. Suprafascial Compared With Subfascial Harvest of the Radial Forearm Flap: An Anatomic Study. J Hand Surg Am. 2008; 33(1): pp. 97–101.
- *An anatomical study examining the difference between suprafascial and subfascial RFFF raises. Based on radiology, the draining patterns were assessed and deemed that the deep fascia doesn't contribute to the perfusion of the RFFF for viability.*

References

1. Wei FC, Mardini S. Flaps and reconstructive surgery. Flaps and reconstructive. Surgery. 2009
2. Manktelow RT, Manktelow RT. Forearm flap. In: Microvascular reconstruction; 1986.
3. Mathes S, Nahai F. 8J - Radial Forearm Flap. 1997. pp. 775–802.
4. Taghinia AH, Carty M, Upton J. Fascial flaps for hand reconstruction. J Hand Surg Am [Internet]. 2010;35(8):1351–5. https://doi.org/10.1016/j.jhsa.2010.05.015.
5. Soutar DS, Mc Gregor IA. The radial forearm flap in intraoral reconstruction: the experience of 60 consecutive cases. Plast Reconstr Surg. 1986;78:1.
6. Timmons MJ, Missotten FEM, Poole MD, Davies DM. Complications of radial forearm flap donor sites. Br J Plast Surg. 1986;39(2):176–8.
7. Mccormack LJ, Cauldwell EW, Anson BJ. Brachial and antebrachial arterial patterns; a study of 750 extremities. Surg Gynecol Obstet. 1953;96:43.
8. Coleman SS, Anson BJ. Arterial patterns in the hand based upon a study of 650 specimens. Surg Gynecol Obstet. 1961;113:409.
9. Chang SCN, Miller G, Halbert CF, Yang KH, Chao WC, Wei FC. Limiting donor site morbidity by suprafascial dissection of the radial forearm flap. Microsurgery. 1996;17(3):136–40.
10. Schaverien M, Saint-Cyr M. Suprafascial compared with subfascial harvest of the radial forearm flap: an anatomic study. J Hand Surg Am. 2008;33(1):97–101.
11. Jones NF, Jarrahy R, Kaufman MR. Pedicled and free radial forearm flaps for reconstruction of the elbow, wrist, and hand. Plast Reconstr Surg. 2008;121(3):887–98.
12. Elliot D, Bardsley AF, Batchetor AG, Soutar DS. Direct closure of the radial forearm flap donor defect. Br J Plast Surg. 1988;41(4):358–60.
13. Wolff K-D, Hölzle F. Raising of microvascular flaps. Springer; 2011.

Posterior Interosseous Artery Flap

Douglas Copson, Dariush Nikkhah, and Mark Pickford

29.1 Introduction

The PIA flap is a regional fasciocutaneous flap, which can be used to cover small- to medium-sized defects. The anterograde PIA variant is suitable for coverage of elbow defects, and the more common distally based PIA flap for cover of the dorsal hand and first webspace. Its main benefits include its thin pliable nature and avoiding disrupting the two major arteries within the forearm. We the authors see its utility in small non-graftable defects where the donor site may be closed directly or a small skin graft used with minimal morbidity. Large defects may be better served by thin fasciocutaneous free flaps, or alternatively the PIA flap may be raised without skin, i.e. as an adipofascial or pure fascial flap, with a view to grafting the flap and directly closing the donor site.

The PIA flap was described around the same time by Zancolli and Angrigiani as well as Penteado and Masquelet.

At the sixth European Hand Surgery Course in Umea (Sweden) in 1985, Zancolli and Angrigiani described the reverse posterior interosseous artery flap. The flap was published in Spanish literature by Zancolli and Angrigiani 1986 and in the English literature in the *Journal of Hand Surgery* in 1988 [1]. In this paper the PIA flap was described as an option for coverage of the dorsum of the hand and first webspace; 25 cases were performed between 1984 and 1987, 21 for first webspace release, 3 for reconstruction of dorsal hand defects and 1 for a volar wrist defect. In this paper the vascular anatomy and surgical technique are described.

The flap was also described by Penteado and Masquelet in 1986 in French literature as well as by Penteado, Masquelet and Chevrel in English literature in 1986 [2]. The latter paper is an early anatomical study/original description of the PIA flap; dissection of 70 cadaveric forearms and the anatomical findings underlying the flap were described. The authors reported two cases of anterograde PIA flaps and ten distally based variants.

Since its first description, multiple variations of the PIA flap have been described, which include the distally based PIA flap, anterograde PIA flap, extended PIA flap and adipofascial and pure fascia variants.

29.1.1 Characteristics (Types)

29.1.1.1 Distally Based PIA Flap

The distally based PIA flap is the most common variant used today and the original form as it was described. It is based on the distal communication between the anterior interosseous artery and the posterior interosseous artery and allows for coverage of defects of the dorsal hand and first webspace up to the level of the MCPJ.

29.1.1.2 Anterograde PIA Flap

The posterior interosseous artery flap can be designed in an anterograde fashion with a pivot point where the PIA enters the extensor compartment. In this fashion it can be used to cover defects of the elbow and proximal forearm.

Supplementary Information The online version contains supplementary material available at [https://doi.org/10.1007/978-3-031-07678-7_29].

D. Copson (✉)
Royal Perth Hospital, Perth, WA, Australia

D. Nikkhah
Royal Free Hospital, London, UK

M. Pickford
Queen Victoria Hospital East Grinstead, East Grinstead, UK

© Springer Nature Switzerland AG 2023
D. Nikkhah et al. (eds.), *Core Techniques in Flap Reconstructive Microsurgery*, https://doi.org/10.1007/978-3-031-07678-7_29

29.1.1.3 Fascia-Only Reverse PIA Flap

Fascia-only variant of the reverse PIA flap. The original article highlights an improved cosmesis of the donor site as no graft is required; it is a super-thin and very pliable fascial flap, well suited to dorsal hand coverage. The flap is raised in much the same manner at the reverse PIA flap [3].

29.1.1.4 Extended PIA Flap

The extended PIA flap is a variant described to extend the reach of the reverse PIA flap to reach the fingertips. Instead of using the PIA's communication with the AIA to perfuse the reverse-flow flap, the dorsal intercarpal arch, originating from the radial artery, is used and the AIA communication divided. The dorsal intercarpal arch communicates with the PIA via the fifth extensor compartment artery. This moves the pivot point of the flap to the level of the carpus, rather than 2 cm proximal to the DRUJ, greatly extending the reach of the flap [4].

29.2 Anatomy

The PIA flap is a fasciocutaneous flap, based on the septocutaneous perforators coming off the posterior interosseous artery; a detailed knowledge of the arterial anatomy is important.

The common interosseous artery arises from the ulnar artery and branches into the anterior and posterior interosseous arteries in the proximal volar forearm. The PIA passes dorsally between the radius and ulna at a point just distal to the chorda obliqua ligament, through the proximal aspect of the interosseous membrane; this point lies approximately 6 cm distal to the lateral epicondyle.

When viewed from the extensor aspect, the PIA enters into the extensor compartment between the distal edge of supinator and the proximal origin of APL; this point is at the junction of the upper and middle thirds of the forearm. Just after entering the extensor compartment, the interosseous recurrent artery is given off, from which a large proximal cutaneous perforator may arise; the PIA lies on the septum between ECU and EDM and passes distally in the forearm. It reduces in size and becomes more superficial in the middle third of the forearm, lying just under the deep fascia rather than near the interosseous membrane. At a point 2 cm proximal to the DRUJ, a communication exists between the PIA and AIA; this communication is the basis of the distally based posterior interosseous artery flap. Distal to the PIA-AIA communicating branch, the PIA also has a communication with the dorsal carpal arch, which is the basis of the extended PIA flap [2, 5].

Along its course the PIA gives off muscular, osseous and fasciocutaneous perforators. These fasciocutaneous perforators provide the cutaneous supply on which the flap relies.

The PIA perforators are divided into proximal, middle and distal third perforators. The most common perforator relied upon in a classic PIA flap is in the middle third of the forearm, just distal to the mid-axial point.

Use of the proximal perforators for reverse PIA flaps has been described to extend the reach of the flap, but this comes with the added risk to the posterior interosseous nerve (PIN) as there exists a closer relationship between the PIA and branches of the PIN in the proximal third of the forearm.

The posterior interosseous nerve is of utmost importance as the sole motor innervation to the extensor compartment of the forearm and must, therefore, be preserved. The PIN enters the dorsal compartment between the two heads of supinator and lies on the radial side of the artery giving off multiple branches. The nerve branch of the PIN to ECU commonly passes just proximal to the large proximal perforator but can pass between the proximal perforator and the remainder of the perforators in the septum, necessitating division of this perforator.

29.2.1 Anatomical Variations

- Origin of the PIA may be from the ulnar artery directly instead of the common interosseous branch in up to 10% of cases. This does not affect the reliability of the PIA flap.
- There is a large proximal perforator which has a degree of anatomical variability as its source vessel may be the posterior interosseous artery or the posterior interosseous recurrent artery.
- The motor branch of the PIN to ECU may cross the recurrent PIA or the PIA proper in the proximal third of the dorsal forearm. In these cases care must be taken to preserve the nerve branch. This may limit which proximal perforators may be harvested with the flap.

29.3 Preoperative Investigation

Preoperative assessment begins with a thorough history of prior injury or surgical intervention to the dorsal forearm and wrist. The current mechanism of injury must also be taken into account and zone of injury assessed as to whether it encroaches on the territory of the flap.

Preoperative imaging is not strictly necessary although CT angio and Doppler investigations can offer additional information. Handheld Doppler assessment can be used to localise septocutaneous perforators as well as localise the communication between the PIA and the AIA [6].

With a good-quality, high-resolution CT angiogram, it is possible to visualise the posterior interosseous artery.

29.4 Flap Design and Markings

1. With the forearm in a pronated position, mark a line between the lateral epicondyle of the humerus and DRUJ. (This is the axis of intermuscular septum between ECU and EDM.)
2. Mark a point 2 cm proximal to the DRUJ (this is the location of the communication between the AIA and PIA which acts as the vascular supply and pivot point when performing a reverse PIA flap).

3. Template the defect and plan the flap in reverse based around the pivot point:
   – In our practice the proximal extent of the flap should not extend above a point 6 cm below the lateral epicondyle of the humerus. More proximal skin paddle locations have been described up to the level of the elbow but in our view come with increased risk of distal flap complications.
   – For dorsal hand defects, template the defect after debridement and with the hand in flexion as not to underestimate the size of the defect.
   – Flaps with a width greater than 4 cm will likely require grafting of the donor site which should be taken into consideration.
   – The size and shape of the skin paddle may be varied to include only the skin required to reconstruct the defect or, in addition, a thin strip of skin over the septum as advocated by some authors in a racquet-shaped skin paddle [7]. In our view the latter is unnecessary, because the septum, which is always raised with the flap, is both slender and robust.

29.5 Flap Raise/Elevation: A Step-by-Step Guide

Step 1: Markings
(See Previous Section and Fig. 29.1)

Step 2: Patient Positioning
Surgery is performed under general or regional anaesthetic with the patient supine. A padded hand table and arm tourniquet are used as well as loupe magnification, typically 2.5x or similar. The arm is not exsanguinated before inflation of the tourniquet to aid identification of the vessels.

Step 3: Locating the Septum (Fig. 29.2 and 29.3)
Dissection commences in the distal third of the forearm; the little finger may be flexed and extended to identify EDM muscle belly and tendon through the translucent deep fascia (Video 29.1). The forearm fascia is incised radial to the 5/6 septum and EDM muscle retracted to visualise the septum and PIA that lies against it. Once the septum and PIA are clearly identified, a second parallel incision is made on the ulnar side of the septum, which continues proximally to the level of the flap itself.

Step 4: Centring the Flap on the Septum
(Fig. 29.4 and 29.5)
Provisional flap markings are then checked to ensure that the flap/skin paddle is actually centred over 5/6 septum; this is particularly important when raising narrow flaps, where there is little margin for error. An incision around the ulnar border of the flap is then made, and fascia over ECU is harvested with the flap.

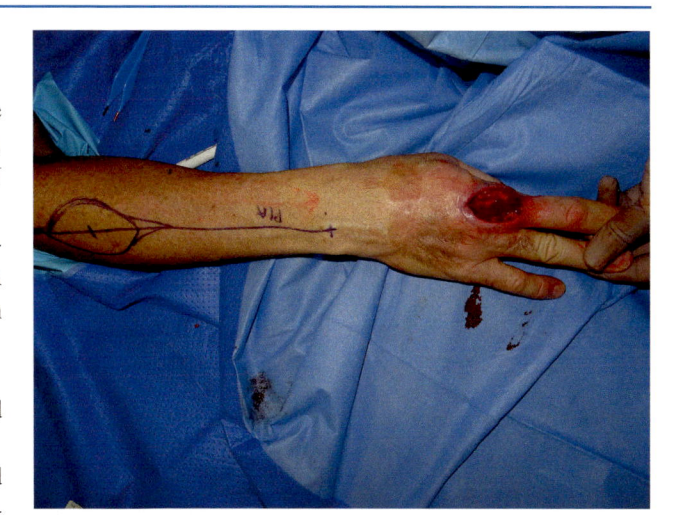

Fig. 29.1 Markings for PIA flap to cover MCPJ. With the forearm in a pronated position, mark a line between the lateral epicondyle of the humerus and DRUJ. (This is the axis of intermuscular septum between ECU and EDM)

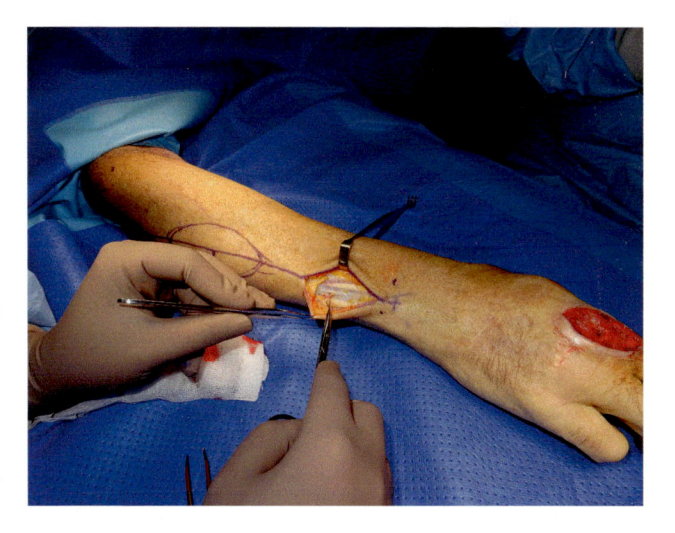

Fig. 29.2 Dissection starts in the distal third of the forearm – note a perforator emerging between the ECU and EDM septum

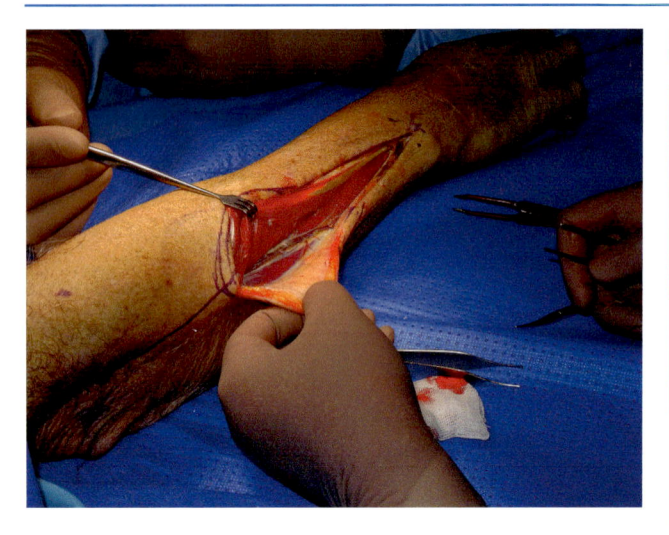

Fig. 29.3 The forearm fascia is incised radial to the 5/6 septum and EDM muscle retracted to visualise the septum and PIA that lies against it. Note the perforators going into the skin paddle of the PIA flap

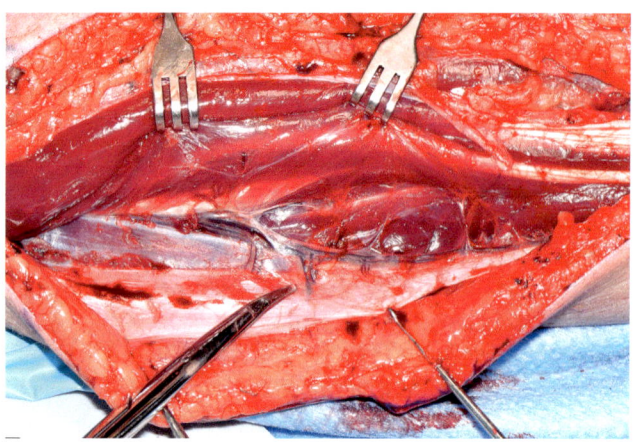

Fig. 29.5 Location of multiple perforators going into PIA skin paddle – the flap axis is centred on the basis of these perforators

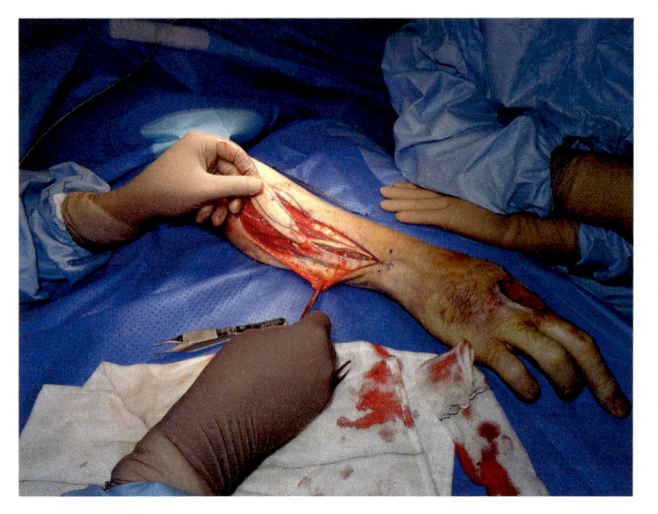

Fig. 29.4 Flap is centred over the 5/6 septum and the fascial strip over ECU is harvested to protect the PIA pedicle

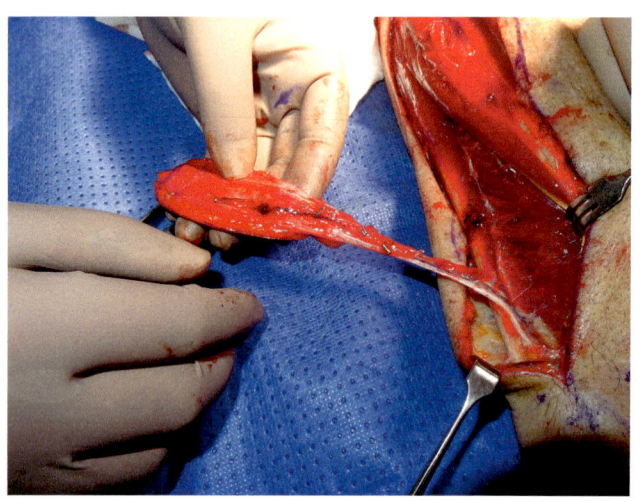

Fig. 29.6 The PIA is divided proximally with the use of ligaclips and islanded for skin coverage of the hand

Step 5: Pedicle/Septum Dissection (Fig. 29.6)
The flap is raised in a proximal to distal fashion once the septum has been identified. The PIA is divided proximally with the use of ligaclips. Muscle perforators are similarly clipped or divided after cautery with fine bipolar forceps, and the PIA and venae comitantes are harvested with the intermuscular septum preserving branches of the PIN.

Step 6: Flap Inset (Fig. 29.7a, b)
A superficial tunnel is created to allow for compression-free delivery of the flap to the primary defect; any tunnel wide enough to allow easy passage of the skin paddle will easily accommodate the narrow vascular pedicle. The flap is inset, and the donor site closed either primarily or by split thickness skin graft.

Note
If raising an anterograde PIA flap, the dissection is carried out in a similar fashion, with the location of the septum being initially identified distally, by incising the fascia over EDM. The dissection in an anterograde PIA flap progresses from distal to proximal, ligating the PIA at the level of the communication with the AIA [8].

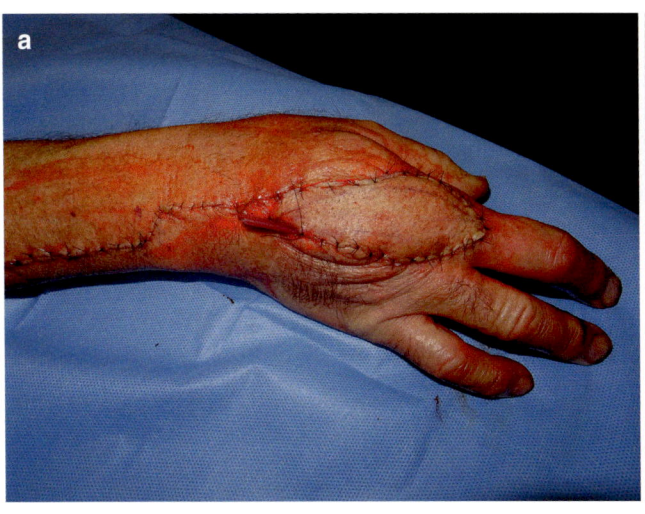

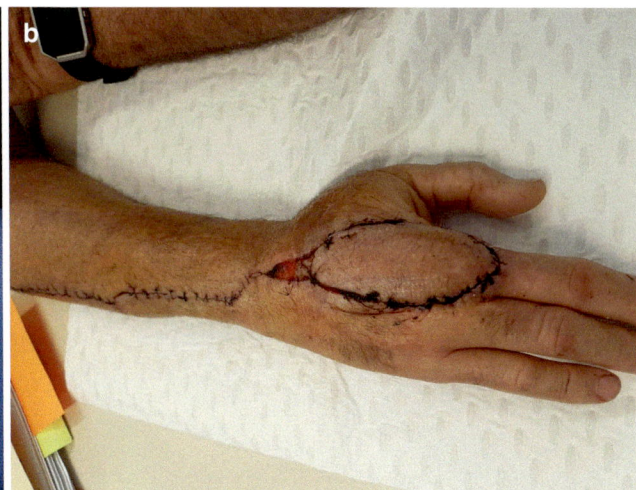

Fig. 29.7 (**a**) PIA flap inset. (**b**) Outcome at 2 weeks

29.6 Core Surgical Techniques in Flap Dissection

Step 1: Markings (See Previous Section and Fig. 29.1)
The markings act as a guide but may need to be adjusted based on the location of the intermuscular septum. It is important to not commit to the flap borders until the septum is identified.

Steps 3 and 4: Locating the Septum and Centring the Flap on the Septum (Figs. 29.2, 29.3, 29.4, and 29.5)
As mentioned in the previous section, moving the little finger through its range of motion can aid in the identification of EDM tendon and muscle belly as demonstrated in Video 29.1.

Step 5: Pedicle/Septum Dissection (Fig. 29.6)
Pedicle dissection is relatively straightforward once the septum is identified. We find retraction of the muscle best performed by an assistant rather than a self-retainer. Care must be taken at the proximal extent of the dissection, where the PIA and PIN are in close proximity, and the proximal nerve branch to ECU is most at risk as it may cross the artery.

Step 6: Flap Inset (Fig. 29.7a, b)
As with all pedicled flaps, it is important to avoid venous compression. The best technique to avoid compression will depend on the specific case but may, occasionally, involve dividing the overlying skin.

29.7 Clinical Scenario

29.7.1 Scenario A (Dorsum of the Hand/MCPJ): Surgeon Dariush Nikkhah

The most common scenario which lends itself to the PIA flap is a dorsal hand defect with exposed tendon or bone in an otherwise uninjured upper limb.

29.7.1.1 Case 1: Video 29.1: Surgeon Dariush Nikkhah

The associated images 1–7 and Video 29.1 show the right hand of a gentleman with an exposed right middle finger MCPJ. Tendon and an open joint were at the base of the wound after debridement of an infected wound and septic MCPJ. In this scenario a reverse PIA flap is used to cover the defect.

29.7.1.2 Case 2: Video 29.2: Surgeon Mark Pickford

A gentleman presented with a large SCC of the right thumb necessitating amputation. Video 29.1 demonstrates a reverse PIA flap being used to cover the defect.

29.7.2 Scenario B (Dorsum of the Hand Free PIA Flap): Surgeon Petr Vondra

A 57-year-old man sustained a circular saw injury to his left hand which resulted in open fractures and significant soft tissue loss over the dorsum of the hand (Fig. 29.8). Under axillary block we performed osteosynthesis first and second

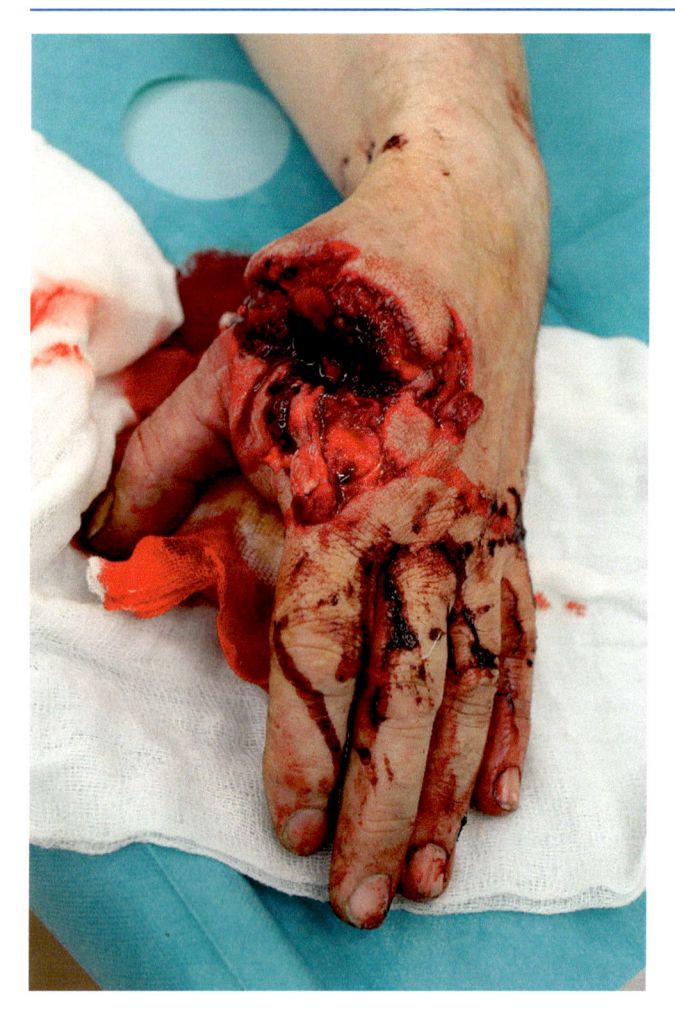

Fig. 29.8 Circular saw injury to his left hand which resulted in open fractures and significant soft tissue loss over the dorsum of the hand

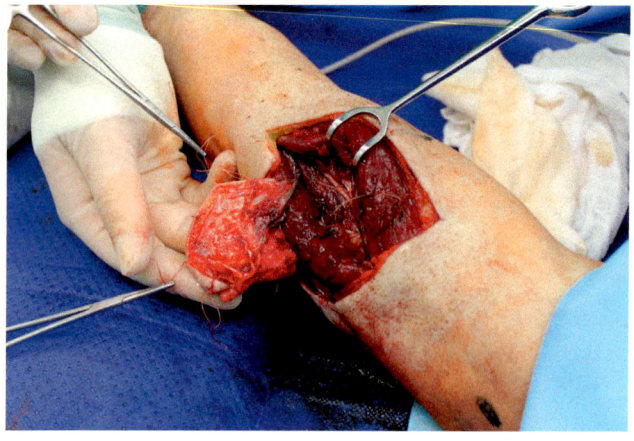

Fig. 29.9 Harvest of a free PIA flap under regional anaesthetic

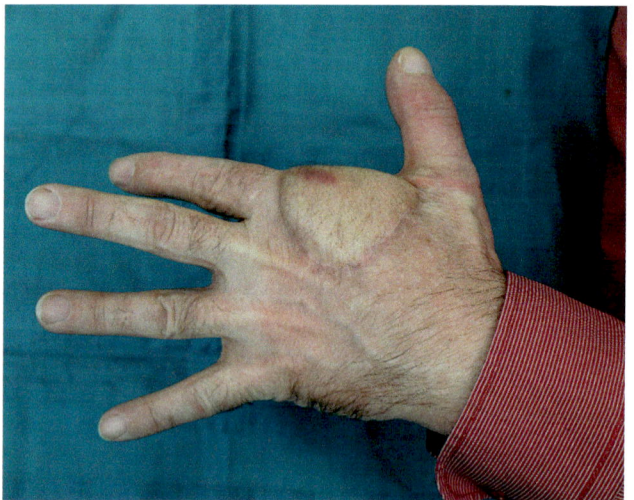

Fig. 29.10 Long-term result

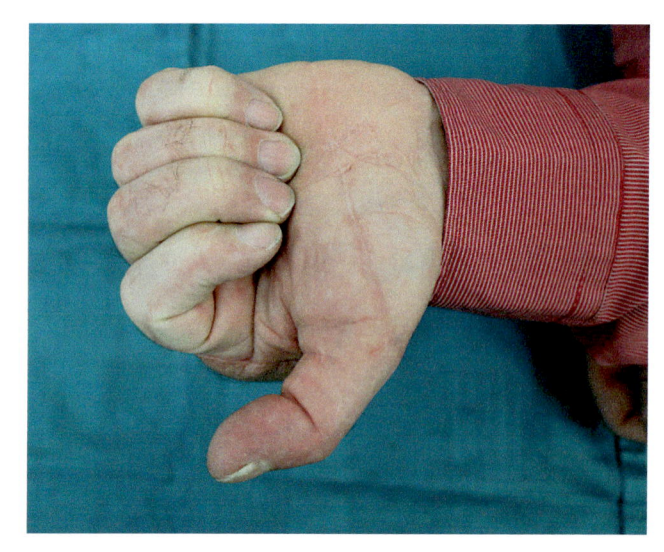

Fig. 29.11 Patient able to achieve near full flexion

metacarpal bones with plate fixation. A vein graft was used to repair a segmental defect in the radial artery.

At second stage we performed a free ipsilateral PIA flap, anastomosed end to side to the vein graft and local veins (Fig. 29.9). The secondary defect was partially sutured under tension and skin grafted. Final result on photo is after 6 (Fig. 29.10) months from injury, the patient regained good two-point sensation and excellent range of motion (Fig. 29.11).

29.8 Pearls and Pitfalls

Pearls
- When identifying the septum between EDM and ECU, moving the little finger and visualising the tendons through the translucent deep fascia can aid accurate identification of EDM. Looking for arterial branches travelling in the fascia can also help locate the septum [9].
- Harvest a strip of fascia over EDM and ECU, as well as the 5/6 septum. This protects the underlying flap pedicle and avoids unnecessary and risky dissection of the vessels off the septum.
- Do not attempt to skeletonise the pedicle or dissect out the perforating vessel between the AIA and the PIA. Both manoeuvres risk damage to the pedicle.

Pitfalls
- **Unnecessary Proximal Dissection:** Dissection of the most proximal perforator is possible but increases risk to the PIN. If the defect can be closed using a middle third septocutaneous perforator, then base the flap on this perforator.
- **Underestimating the Size of the Defect:** The defect should be debrided before the defect size is measured and the final skin paddle designed. Dorsal hand defects should also be measured with the hand flexed into a fist as to not underestimate the size of the defect [10].

29.9 Selected Readings

- Posterior Interosseous Island Forearm Flap. J Hand Surg. 2 May 1988; 13-B.
- *This paper is the original description, in the English language, of the reverse posterior interosseous artery flap, as described by Zancolli and Argrigiani in 1988. The same authors published a description of the flap in Spanish medical literature 2 years previously (1986). It should be the starting point for anyone considering performing this flap as it provides a good description of the anatomy and surgical technique and gives case examples.*
- Penteado CV, Masquelet AC, Chevrel JP. The anatomic basis of the fascio-cutaneous flap of the posterior interosseous artery. Surg Radiol Anat. 1986;8(4):209–15. doi: 10.1007/BF02425069. PMID: 3107143.
- *This paper is an early anatomical and clinical study of the PIA flap. In this paper two anterograde and ten reverse PIA flaps are described.*
- Zaidenberg EE, Zancolli P, Farias Cisneros E, Miller AG, Moreno R. Antegrade Posterior Interosseous Flap for Nonhealing Wounds of the Elbow: Anatomical and Clinical Study. Plast Reconstr Surg Glob Open. 2018 Nov 7;6(11):e1959. doi: 10.1097/GOX.0000000000001959. PMID: 30881783; PMCID: PMC6414117.
- *This paper published in 2018 provides detail on the vascular anatomy pertinent to the less frequently used anterograde posterior interosseous artery flap.*
- Zaidenberg EE, Farias-Cisneros E, Pastrana MJ, Zaidenberg CR. Extended Posterior Interosseous Artery Flap: Anatomical and Clinical Study. J Hand Surg Am. 2017 Mar;42(3):182–189. doi: 10.1016/j.jhsa.2017.01.004. PMID: 28259275.
- *This CME style article published in the Journal of Hand Surgery outlines the anatomical basis and surgical technique for the extended PIA flap and provides a more detailed description of this less common variant than can be entered into in this chapter.*
- Techniques to enable identification and safe elevation of the posterior interosseous artery flap: Part 1 and 2. Nikkhah D, Pickford M. J Plast Reconstr Aesthet Surg. 2019 Jun;72 [4]:1030–1048. doi: 10.1016/j.bjps.2019.02.006. Epub 2019 Mar 5. PMID: 30871942 No abstract available.
- *Short communication detailing technical steps in safe elevation of this flap and identifying the pedicle.*

References

1. Zancolli EA, Angrigiani C. Posterior interosseous island forearm flap. J Hand Surg. 1988;13B:130–5.
2. Penteado CV, Masquelet AC, Chevrel JP. The anatomic basis of the fascio-cutaneous flap of the posterior interosseous artery. Surg Radiol Anat. 1986;8(4):209–15. https://doi.org/10.1007/BF02425069. Original French publication: Masquelet AC, Penteado CV. Le Lambeau interosseux postérieur. Ann Chir Main (sous presse). 1986
3. Jakubietz RG, Bernuth S, Schmidt K, Meffert RH, Jakubietz MG. The fascia-only reverse posterior interosseous artery flap. J Hand Surg Am. 2019;44(3):249.e1–5. https://doi.org/10.1016/j.jhsa.2018.06.012. Epub 2018 Jul 19
4. Zaidenberg EE, Farias-Cisneros E, Pastrana MJ, Zaidenberg CR. Extended posterior interosseous artery flap: anatomical and clinical study. J Hand Surg Am. 2017;42(3):182–9. https://doi.org/10.1016/j.jhsa.2017.01.004.
5. Costa H, Soutar DS. The distally based island posterior interosseous flap. Br J Plast Surg. 1988;41(3):221–7. https://doi.org/10.1016/0007-1226(88)90104-x.
6. Puri V, Mahendru S, Rana R. Posterior interosseous artery flap, fasciosubcutaneous pedicle technique: a study of 25 cases. J

Plast Reconstr Aesthet Surg. 2007;60(12):1331–7. https://doi.org/10.1016/j.bjps.2007.07.003. Epub 2007 Aug 23

7. Acharya FNB, Bhat MS, Bhaskarand MS. The posterior interosseous artery flap technical considerations in raising an easier and more reliable flap. J Hand Surg. 2012;37A:575–82.

8. Zaidenberg EE, Zancolli P, Farias Cisneros E, Miller AG, Moreno R. Antegrade posterior interosseous flap for nonhealing wounds of the elbow: anatomical and clinical study. Plast Reconstr Surg Glob Open. 2018;6(11):e1959. https://doi.org/10.1097/GOX.0000000000001959. PMID: 30881783; PMCID: PMC6414117.

9. Nikkhah D, Pickford M. Techniques to enable identification and safe elevation of the posterior interosseous artery flap: part 1 and 2. J Plast Reconstr Aesthet Surg 2019 Jun;72(6):1030–1048. doi: https://doi.org/10.1016/j.bjps.2019.02.006. Epub 2019 Mar 5. PMID: 30871942.

10. Shibata M, Iwabuchi Y, Kubota S, Matsuzaki H. Comparison of free and reversed pedicled posterior interosseous cutaneous flaps. Plast Reconstr Surg. 1997;99:791–802.

Venous Flaps

Christopher Deutsch and Jamil Moledina

30.1 Introduction

Venous flaps—cutaneous free flaps raised on a venous plexus alone—are a unique subset of free flaps, which have specific characteristics ideally suiting them to reconstruction of the upper limb and, in particular, the hand and digits.

The technique was originally described in animal models by Nakayama [1] and subsequently translated into clinical practice for reconstruction of skin defects in digital replantation [2, 3]. The early flaps in humans were based solely on venous inflow, through the venous flap, with blood then returned to the venous system as a true "flow-through" flap. Anastomosis of an artery to the inflow of the venous flap has been used to enhance oxygen delivery to the transposed tissue, to increase the size and versatility of these flaps [4]. As such, venous flaps can be classified according to both their recipient inflow and outflow:

- V-V-V (vein-to-vein-to-vein). Venous inflow passes through the veins of the flap into an outflow vein as a true flow-through flap. This is most commonly useful on the dorsum of the hand where recipient veins are readily accessible and metabolic demands are relatively low.
- A-V-A (artery-to-vein-to-artery). As another flow-through flap, arterial inflow passes into the flap and is drained back into a distal artery. This technique is particularly useful in reconstructing a segmental arterial defect, thus perfusing both flap and tissue beyond, in addition to providing soft tissue cover, as may be required in complex digital revascularization.
- A-V-V (artery-to-vein-to-vein). Arterialized venous flaps are more similar to conventional free flaps, where the flap is designed in such a way as to restore vascular anatomy approximating a normal artery-to-venous system through a capillary bed. They are a useful option where reconstruction of the artery in continuity is not required for distal digital reperfusion, such as at the fingertip or elsewhere on the hand. The authors recommend the use of arterialized, as opposed to flow-through, flaps wherever possible, given the flap survival benefits of restoring a capillary bed.

30.2 Anatomy

Venous flaps are not defined by an anatomical donor site, but rather are united by the absence of an anatomical arterial-capillary-venous flow pattern. The flap can be raised on any subcutaneous venous network where an inflow and outflow vein can be selected and where the network is closely associated with the overlying skin; this is most commonly the dorsum of the foot, the volar forearm, and the medial leg.

The physiological mechanism for survival of these flaps is debated. It is certainly true that non-arterialized venous flaps will be required to survive on a lower PaO_2 than is normal and that for such flaps in particular, neovascularization is likely to be key to their long-term survival. The low PaO_2 may indeed be a significant driver in neovascularization. Even in the case of arterialized venous flaps, flow studies have shown that where blood flow passes through the flap in a straightforward anterograde manner (i.e., in the natural direction of flow-through venous valves), the peripheral flap is largely bypassed. A solution to this problem of shunting has been to divert the flow around the flap in a retrograde manner [5], so that resistance provided by the valves pushes blood out to the peripheries. More recently, this has been superseded by in-flap ligation of vessels, known as shunt restriction, to encourage one vessel to act as an afferent "artery" and one as an efferent "vein," rather than relying on one vein to do both and thus forcing blood into the peripheries of the flap [6]. This technique drives blood through a capillary system between the main afferent and efferent vessels and significantly improves the survival of these flaps.

C. Deutsch (✉) · J. Moledina
Department of Plastic Surgery, St George's University Hospitals NHS Foundation Trust, London, UK

30.3 Preoperative Investigation

The venous flap donor site is usually planned to be readily expendable, and as such no specific preoperative investigation is required beyond standard preoperative planning for any microsurgical procedure. As these flaps are usually very thin, the superficial venous plexus can be easily assessed clinically, and indeed this is the most appropriate way to design the flap accurately. Handheld vein visualization devices may have a role when superficial veins are hard to see.

30.4 Flap Design and Markings

1. The venous networks of the volar forearm and dorsal foot make excellent donors for venous flaps (Fig. 30.1).
2. Numerous tributaries to the basilic and cephalic veins of the forearm are readily identified under the pliable skin of the volar forearm; compression of the forearm or upper arm may improve their visibility (Fig. 30.2).
3. The defect can be templated and superimposed over visible veins, with a note made of the position of the recipient artery and veins (Fig. 30.3).
4. The inflow vessel needs to be positioned in the flap to allow for anastomosis to the recipient vessel.
5. For an arterialized flow-through flap (A-V-A), a suitable vein should be selected to act as the inflow to the flap, paying attention to ensure an anterograde direction of flow. The vessel should run through the flap and then anastomosed to a distal artery in the defect.
6. For an arterialized venous flap (A-V-V), the inflow artery should enter the flap, ideally centrally, and run only for a short distance in the flap before being terminated by ligation or distally anastomosed to an outflow artery if an arterial defect needs to be bridged. The authors suggest that approximately one quarter to one third, but certainly less than half, of the surface of the flap overlies the arterialized vein, with the rest of the flap dedicated to outflow vein(s) (Fig. 30.4).
7. Outflow veins must also be selected in an appropriate position for anastomosis to the outflow recipient vessels (Fig. 30.5).
8. In arterialized venous flaps, in-flap ligations should be planned to be prevent all large connections between inflow and outflow vessels; this shunt restriction recreates a capillary bed and reduces the problem of direct shunt between the inflow and outflow systems.
9. The flap design can be adjusted to fit a wide range of defects. Design features such as concatenation of two skin paddles (to resurface adjacent digits), or the inclusion of additional structures such as the tendon of the palmaris longus, allow reconstruction of complex defects (Fig. 30.6).
10. The donor venous plexus must fit with the recipient vessels, and if it does not, then a different donor site must be explored.

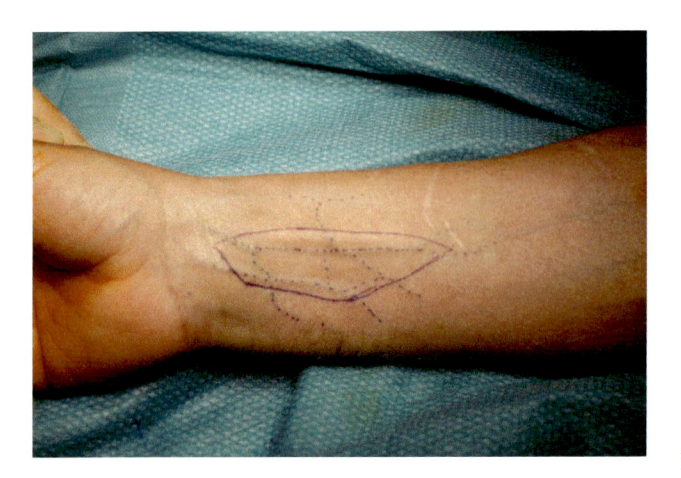

Fig. 30.1 The venous plexus comprising tributaries to the cephalic and basilic veins of the forearm

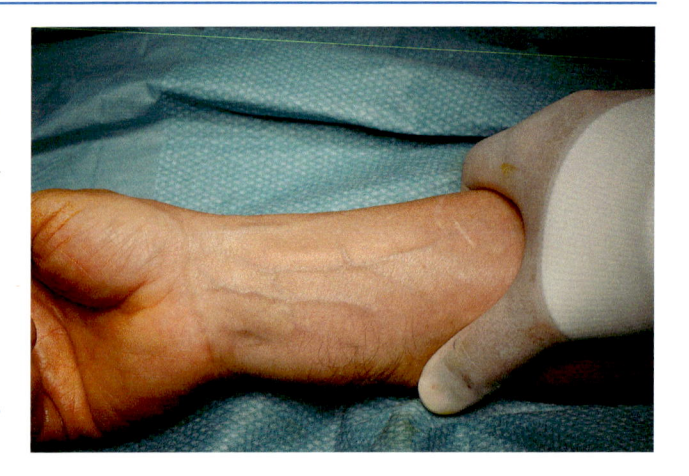

Fig. 30.2 Manual compression of the forearm distends the veins and makes them easily visible for flap planning

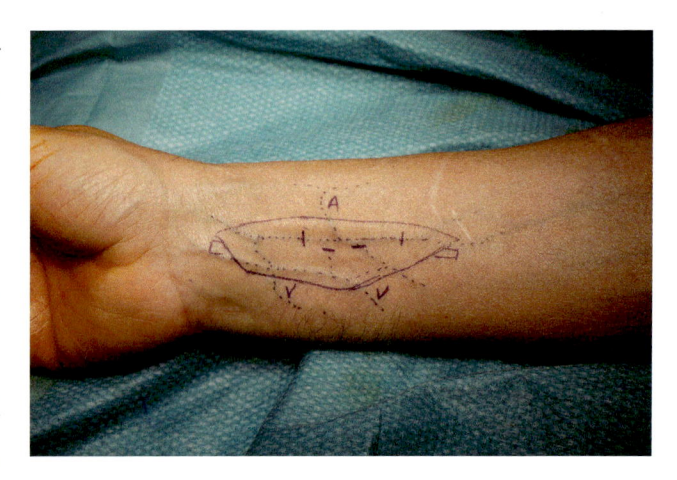

Fig. 30.3 The defect can be templated and superimposed over the venous network for flap design

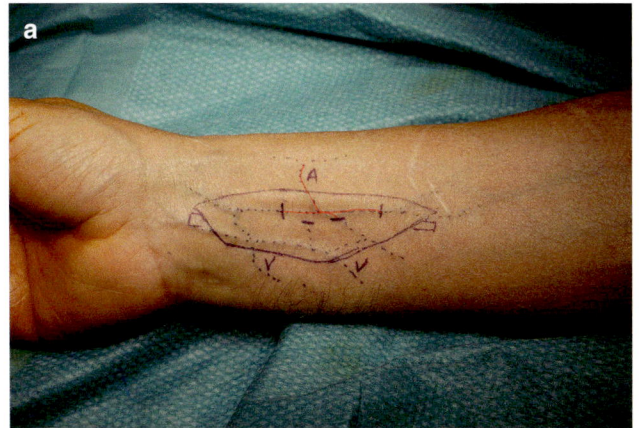

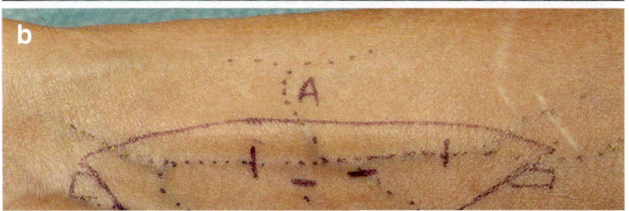

Fig. 30.4 (**a**, **b**) The arterialized inflow to the flap should be ideally positioned centrally, and terminated by ligation after running for a short distance within the flap (marked in red)

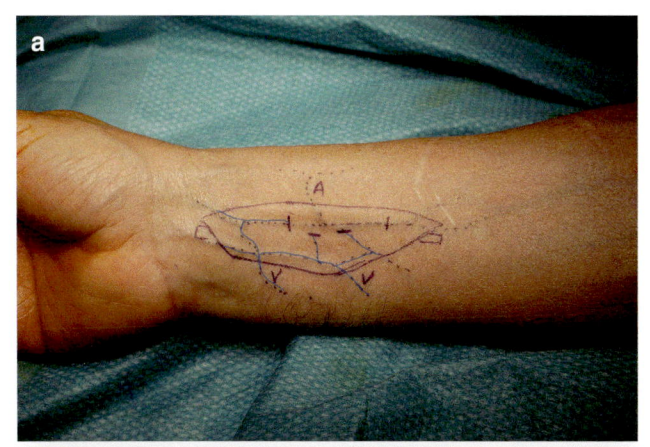

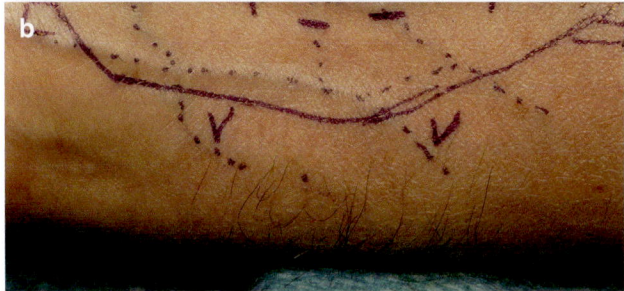

Fig. 30.5 (**a**, **b**) The outflow veins (marked in blue) are positioned to match the position of recipient veins. [**Alternative Figure**—The outflow venous network (*highlighted*) is positioned to match the position of the recipient veins.]

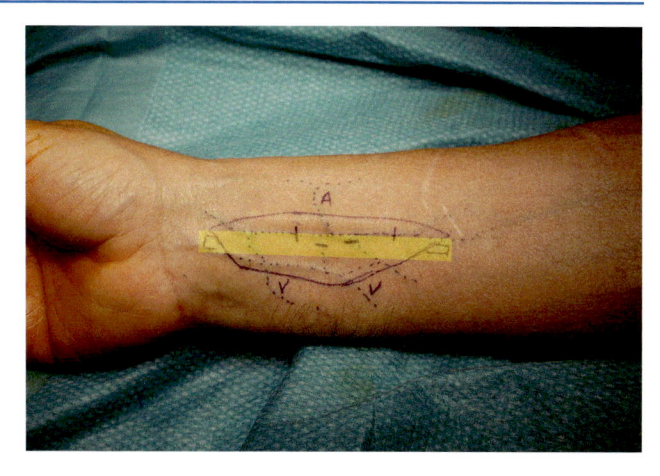

Fig. 30.6 Tendon (*highlighted*), such as palmaris longus, can be included within the flap for reconstruction of composite defects

30.5 Flap Raise/Elevation: A Step-by-Step Guide

1. Design
   In venous flaps, design is a critical phase. The inflow and outflow vessels must be carefully selected to match up to the intended recipient vessels (Fig. 30.7).
2. Tourniquet inflation
   Inflate an upper arm tourniquet.
3. Ulnar skin incision
   Begin on the ulnar border of the flap, closest to the operating surgeon. Incise carefully just through the dermis as the veins are very superficial and can easily be damaged. Once the veins are identified, they can be followed away from the flap to obtain an adequate pedicle length, usually up to 2 cm, and then ligated and divided (Fig. 30.8).
4. Radial skin incision
   Repeat the process for the radial border of the flap, again taking care not to injure the superficial venous network. Preserve some length even on veins that have not been identified for anastomosis as backup vessels (Fig. 30.9).
5. Complete sub-flap dissection
   Once the vessels have been dissected and ligated circumferentially around the flap, the flap can be raised relatively easily, by simply freeing it from the underlying forearm fascia with sharp dissection (Fig. 30.10).
6. Raise completed
   The flap is ready for inset after performing in-flap ligation on the underside using microvascular ligation clips or suture ties. Here the flap has been raised with paratenon and tendon for vascularized tendon reconstruction (Fig. 30.11).

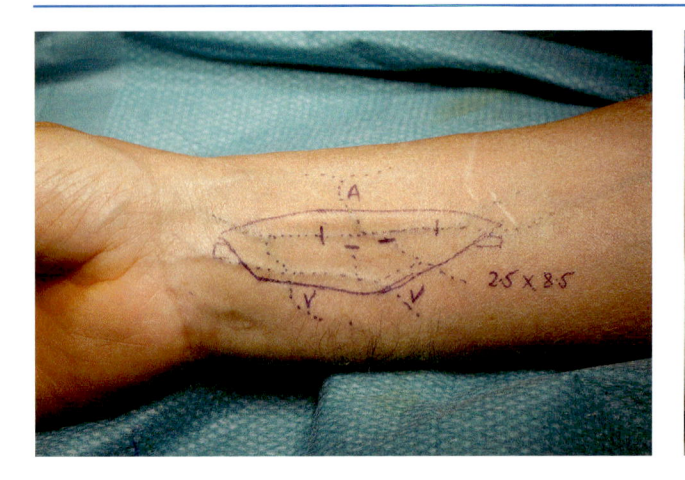

Fig. 30.7 The flap design completed, prior to raising

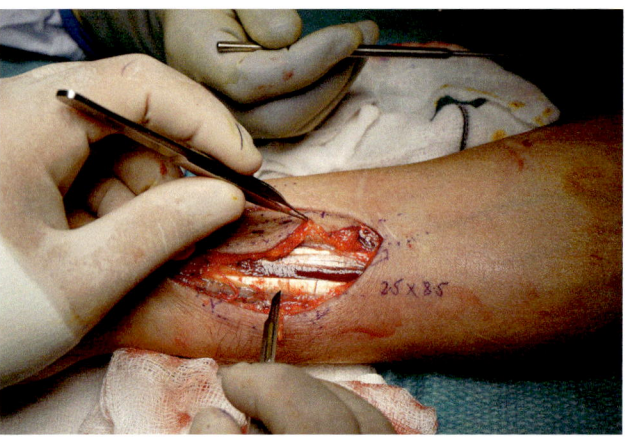

Fig. 30.10 Sharp dissection is used to raise the flap from the underlying forearm fascia

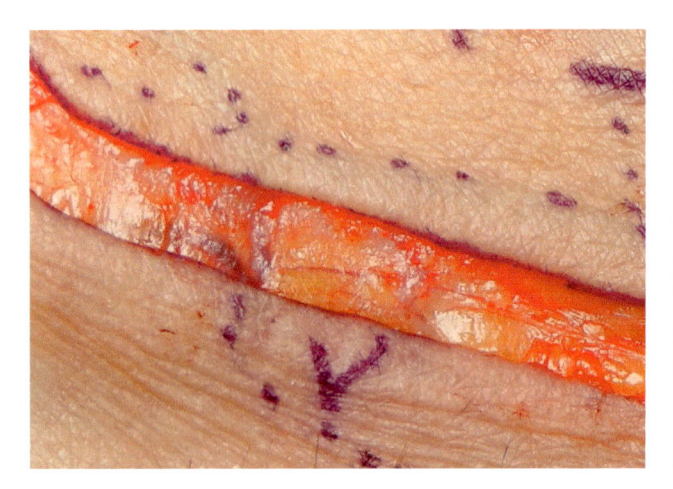

Fig. 30.8 The veins are very superficial and easily injured

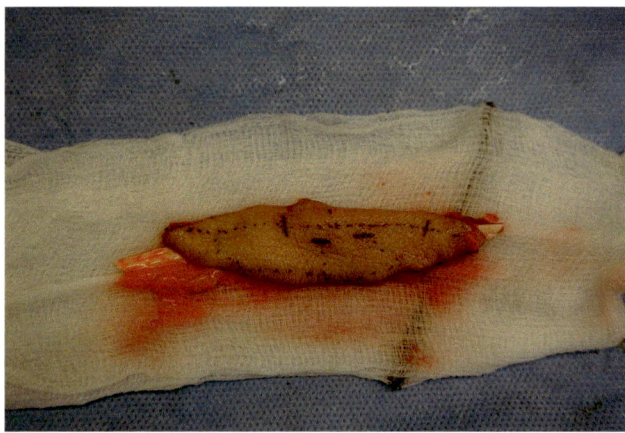

Fig. 30.11 The flap is raised, here including a vascularized section of tendon

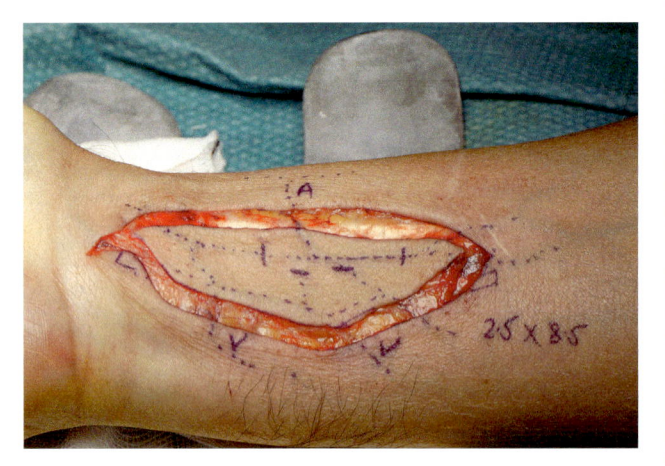

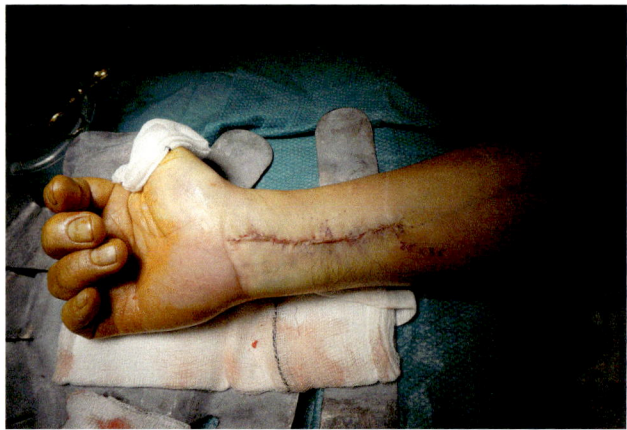

Fig. 30.9 Circumferential incision is completed with all veins having been identified

Fig. 30.12 The donor site is closed primarily using an absorbable monofilament suture

7. Donor site closure

   The donor site can usually be primarily closed if the width of the flap is less than 2.5 centimeters using an absorbable monofilament suture. If a larger flap is raised or the skin closure is very tight, a full-thickness skin graft from the medial upper arm or a split-thickness skin graft is required (Fig. 30.12).

30.6 Core Surgical Techniques in Flap Dissection

1. Tourniquet
   An upper arm tourniquet is inflated to 250 mmHg, and exsanguination is by arm elevation and gentle manual compression only, so that the veins remain partly filled.
2. Vessel Dissection
   Sharp dissection using a 15 blade is preferred, with dissection along the vessels using the blade, fine tenotomy scissors, or microsurgery scissors. The first incision should be only just through the dermis until the veins are identified as the vessels may be immediately subdermal.
3. Sub-Flap Dissection
   Dissection just above the fascia of the forearm is a clear and safe plane, in which the flap can be readily raised. If required, tendon can be raised within its paratenon, in continuity with the skin component of the flap, for reconstruction of segmental tendon defects (see Case 1).
4. In-Flap Ligation
   Shunt restriction substantially improves the intra-flap blood flow. Ligation of shunting vessels using microvascular ligation clips or suture ties is strongly advised in arterialized venous flaps. This is performed on the underside of the flap after it has been raised, according to pre-planned design of the intended vascular pattern.
5. Hemostasis
   All free ends of the venous plexus must either be anastomosed to recipient vessels or ligated, and this should be checked before final inset as otherwise a hematoma may result once the vasospasm settles fully after inset is completed.

30.7 Clinical Scenario: Surgeon Jamil Moledina

A 45-year-old man presented to the emergency department following an injury with an electric router while working. Assessment revealed a complex, grossly contaminated wound to the dorsum of the left thumb, spanning from the head of the first metacarpal to the base of the distal phalanx. The dorsal cortex of the proximal phalanx and EPL from Zones 1 to 3 was lost with the overlying skin. The IPJ and MCPJ were exposed with loss of their ulnar collateral ligaments. The wound was thoroughly debrided surgically, and a venous flap from the contralateral forearm raised with a section of flexor tendon to simultaneously reconstruct tendon and skin (Figs. 30.13, 30.14, 30.15, 30.16, 30.17, 30.18, and 30.19).

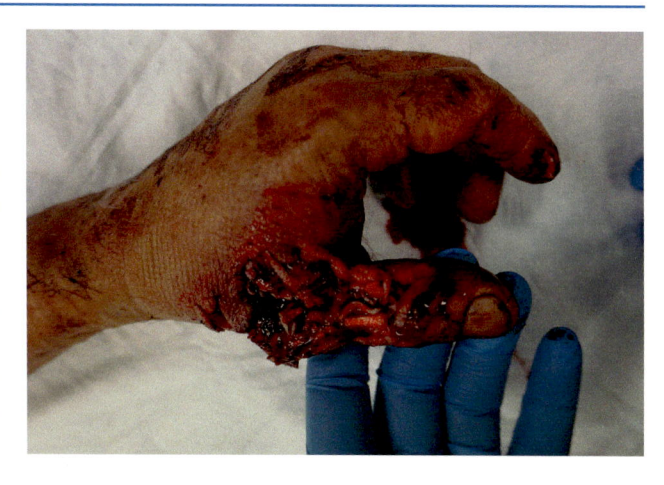

Fig. 30.13 The complex wound to the thumb, caused by an electric router

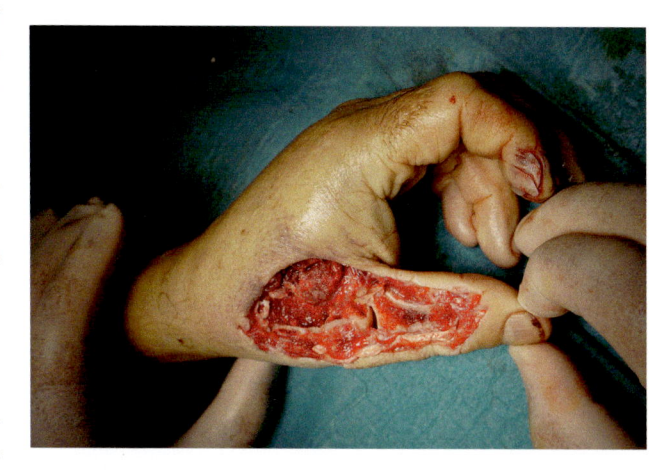

Fig. 30.14 The surgically debrided wound with open interphalangeal- and metacarpophalangeal joints, ulnar collateral ligaments, unicortical injuries to the metacarpal and proximal phalanx, and loss of skin and extensor pollicis longus

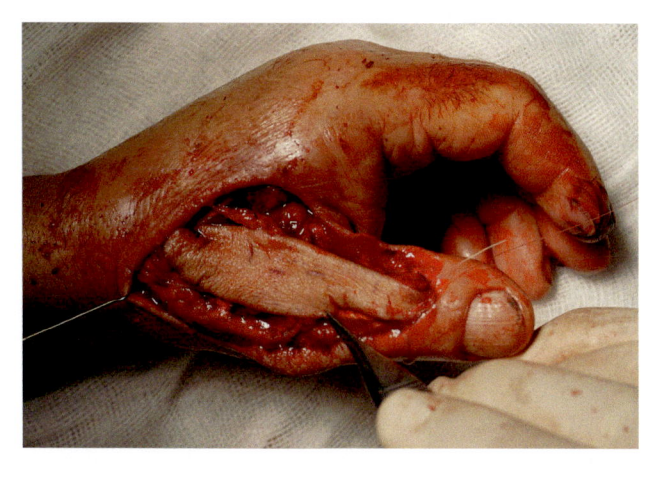

Fig. 30.15 The flap during inset; the microvascular anastomoses have been completed and the flap is perfused

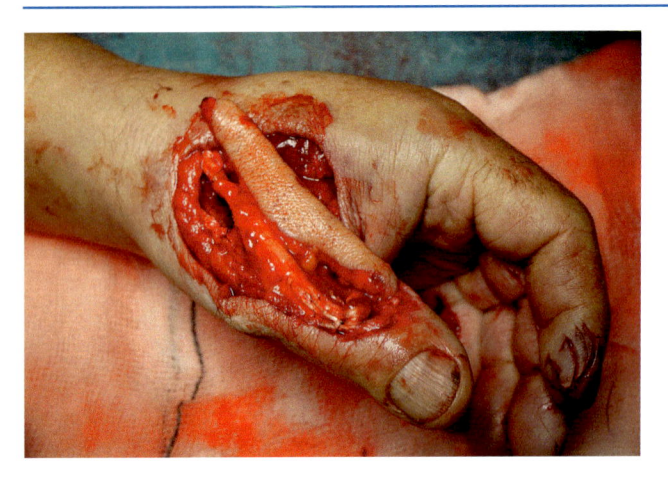

Fig. 30.16 The flap during inset; the vascularized tendon has been interposed

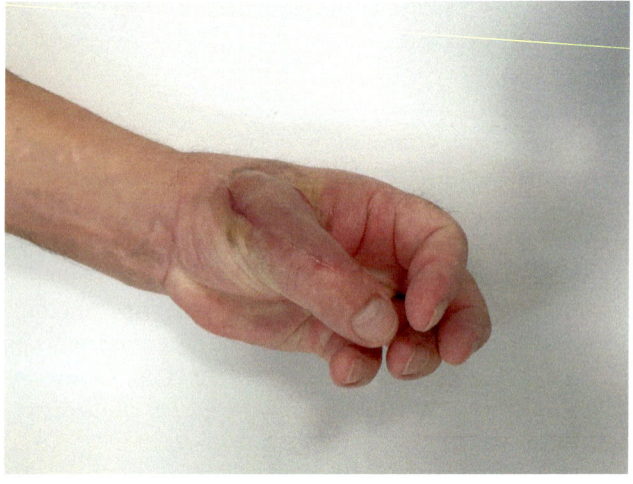

Fig. 30.19 Demonstration of thumb opposition

30.8 Pearls and Pitfalls

Pearls

- Use multiple outflow veins (at least two), ideally each with separate flow pathways.
- Ensure no more than a quarter to a third of the flap area is directly supplied by the arterialized vessel.
- Plan all flow anterograde to avoid potential complications with venous valves.
- Perform shunt-restricting ligations before reperfusing flap.
- Perform all anastomoses before releasing clamps and allowing inflow to the flap.

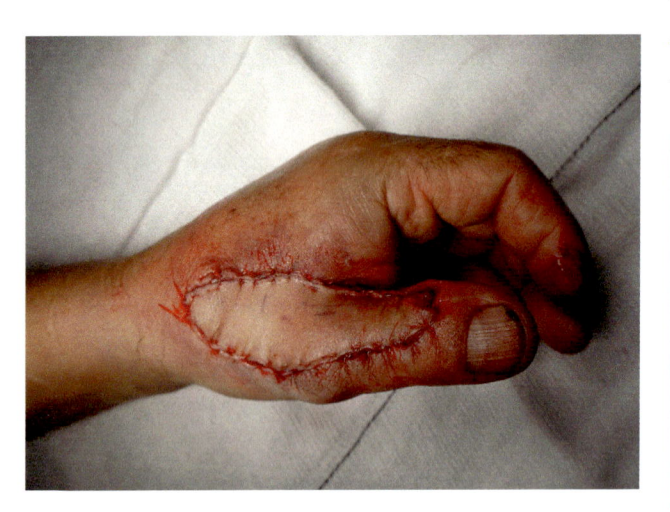

Fig. 30.17 The flap immediately postoperatively

Pitfalls

- Hematoma. Ensure all open or reserved vessels are anastomosed or ligated before inset to reduce the risk of postoperative bleeding.
- Damage to vessels. Veins are thin walled and very superficial, so take extreme care when incising the skin.
- Redundancy of arterialized vein. The donor vessel will expand substantially after anastomosis when the pressure increases. Trim the vessel to an appropriate length or allow a gentle curve without kinking.

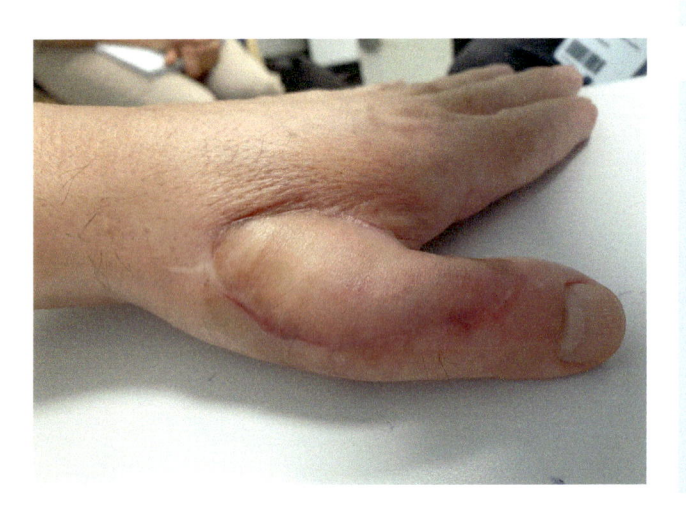

Fig. 30.18 The flap result at 3 months

- Incorrect pedicle length. Plan the position of the recipient and donor veins carefully before raising the flap, to ensure the pedicles are appropriately placed.
- Incorrect skin paddle size. Allow for substantial postoperative swelling of flap by taking this into account in skin paddle design.

30.9 Selected Readings

- Nakayama Y, Soeda S, Kasai Y. Flaps nourished by arterial inflow through the venous system: an experimental investigation. Plast Reconstr Surg. 1981;67 (3):328–334.

  This paper is an early description of the arterialized venous flap, in rat models, to prove the concept of arterio-venous anastomosis in free flap survival. Comparison between types of flaps, initially pedicled with supporting microvascular anastomoses and later islanded on just microvascular anastomoses, demonstrated good flap survival, compared to composite grafts which predictably fully necrosed.

- Lin, YT, Henry SL, Lin CH, Lee HY, Lin WN, Lin CH, Wei FC. The Shunt-Restricted Arterialized Venous Flap for Hand/Digit Reconstruction: Enhanced Perfusion, Decreased Congestion, and Improved Reliability. The Journal of Trauma: Injury, Infection, and Critical Care 2010;69 (2), 399–404.

  This work provides a comprehensive description of a core principle in venous flaps – shunt restriction. The techniques of restriction are described in terms of four vascular arrangements, and the subsequent improvement in peripheral perfusion of the flaps, as well as reduced venous congestion, as demonstrated by laser Doppler flowmetry.

- Inoue G, Maeda N, Suzuki K. Resurfacing of skin defects of the hand using the arterialised venous flap. Br J Plast Surg 1990;43: 135–139.

  Inoue provides a good description of indications for the use of the venous flap in the hand in a case series of 22 patients. Of these, 12 were reconstructed in an A-V-A manner, and 10 in an A-V-V manner. Many flaps covered bone or tendon and as such provided good evidence of their vascularized nature. They report an overall survival of 95%.

- Woo SH, Kim KC, Lee GJ, Ha SH, Kim KH, Dhawan V, Lee KS. A retrospective analysis of 154 arterialised venous flaps for hand reconstruction: an 11 year experience. PRS 2007;119 (6):1823–1838.

  This paper showcases a wide range of applications of venous free flaps in a large retrospective case series. Interesting modifications are also presented, including simultaneous cover of adjacent digits, the use of vascularized tendon, and innervated flaps. They report flaps as large as 14x9cm in the hand, with complete survival.

- Brooks D, Buntic RF, Taylor C. Use of the venous free flap for salvage of difficult ring avulsion injuries. Microsurgery 2008;28:397–402.

  A typical indication for A-V-A venous flaps is in ring avulsion injuries, where the venous flap is used to both reconstruct segmental arterial injury and soft tissue. Here Brooks presents eight cases, reporting good, supple skin quality and good range of movement in the reconstructed digits.

References

1. Nakayama Y, Soeda S, Kasai Y. Flaps nourished by arterial inflow through the venous system: an experimental investigation. Plast Reconstr Surg. 1981;67(3):328–34.
2. Honda T, Nomura S, Yamauchi S, Shimamura K, Yoshimura M. The possible applications of a composite skin and subcutaneous vein graft in the replantation of amputated digits. Br J Plast Surg. 1984;37(4):607–12.
3. Tsai SM, Matiko JD, Breidenbach W, et al. Venous flaps in digital revascularization and replantation. J Reconstr Microsurg. 1987;3:113.
4. Yoshimura M, Shimada T, Imura S, Shimamura K, Yamauchi S. The venous skin graft method for repairing skin defects of the fingers. Plast Reconstr Surg. 1987;79(2):243–50.
5. Moshammer HET, Schwarzl FX, Haas FM, et al. Retrograde arterialized venous flap: an experimental study. Microsurgery. 2003;23:130–4.
6. Lin YT, Henry SL, Lin CH, Lee HY, Lin WN, Lin CH, Wei FC. The shunt-restricted arterialized venous flap for hand/digit reconstruction: enhanced perfusion, decreased congestion, and improved reliability. J Trauma Injury Infect Crit Care. 2010;69(2):399–404.

Free Thenar Flap

Dimitris Reissis, Petr Vondra, and Zheng Yumao

31.1 Introduction

The free thenar flap was first described by Tsai in 1991 [1], based on the radial digital artery of the thumb. Following this, the arterial supply of the thenar region has been further studied and the free thenar flap redefined, initially by Kamei et al. in 1993 [2] and then Omokawa et al. in 1997 [3], with its arterial supply optimized to come from the superficial palmar branch of the radial artery (SUPBRA) [4].

It is a fasciocutaneous flap, primarily used as a free flap to reconstruct medium-large (up to 2 × 10 cm) defects of the volar surface of the digits, in circumstances where local or island homodigital and heterodigital flaps, such as the cross-finger flap, are of insufficient size or precluded due to injury to the adjacent finger. It is useful for volar defects with exposed bone or tendon [5] and is preferable for patients who would rather not sacrifice any soft tissue component from the foot or for whom the defect is too large for a partial second toe pulp flap, for example.

It has many advantages, approaching ideal replacement for the volar tissues of the fingers [6], with excellent tissue match providing thick, glabrous skin with ample soft tissue to restore sufficient bulk and contour of pulp and volar aspect of digits, while enabling maintained length of the injured finger. It also has minimal donor site morbidity, provided the flap width is kept to 2 cm or less to allow primary closure, with an inconspicuous scar that can be hidden in the mid-palmar crease [1, 2, 6, 7].

It also has a role as a pedicled thenar flap, to reconstruct volar defects of the adjacent thumb. In all cases it allows for limiting the patients' morbidity to one hand, with preservation of all major vessels to the digits [3, 4] within a single operative field (in contrast to harvesting a free partial toe flap), and therefore offers a single site for early rehabilitation with no need for postoperative immobilization, as opposed to use of cross-finger flaps or traditional pedicled island thenar flaps.

The flap is often raised and inset without neurorrhaphy, but still has a tendency to neurotize well and become sensate [6]. It can also be raised as a sensory flap by the inclusion of a named nerve. Options for this include the palmar cutaneous branch of the median nerve (PCBMN) [6, 8], lateral antebrachial cutaneous nerve (LABCN) [2], or superficial branch of the radial nerve (SBRN) [3, 9]. Yang et al. (2010) [8] have proposed the PCBMN as the most constant and useful nerve to provide innervation to the flap, in view of anatomical variations related to the LABCN and SBRN (Yang and Mckinnon) [10], allowing for the flap to be constantly innervated.

31.2 Anatomy

The free thenar flap is a fasciocutaneous flap based on the superficial palmar branch of the radial artery (SUPBRA), which has a constant anatomy and reliable direct cutaneous perforators to a constant skin area of roughly 3 × 4 cm over the thenar eminence.

The SUPBRA originates from the radial artery at the level of the styloid process of the radius, approximately 2.5 cm proximal to the scaphoid tubercle [2, 4]. It then runs distally under the flexor retinaculum and branches to give superficial and main (deep) branches. The superficial branch provides cutaneous branches to the skin of the thenar eminence and distal wrist skin. The main branch then enters the base of the thenar musculature and passes deep between abductor pollicis brevis and opponens pollicis muscles to form the superficial volar arch together with the branch from the ulnar artery. It can also supply arterial perforators to the first web space.

The SUPBRA should not be confused with the dorsal terminal continuation of the radial artery, which passes dorsally

---

D. Reissis (✉) · P. Vondra
Royal Free Hospital, London, UK
e-mail: dreissis@nhs.net

Z. Yumao
Department of Hand and Foot Surgery, Taizhou Hospital, Wenzhou Medical University and The Third Affiliated Hospital of Southern Medical University, Taizhou, Zhejiang Province, China

© Springer Nature Switzerland AG 2023
D. Nikkhah et al. (eds.), *Core Techniques in Flap Reconstructive Microsurgery*, https://doi.org/10.1007/978-3-031-07678-7_31

toward and beneath the extensor pollicis longus through the anatomical snuff box.

Once fully dissected, the pedicle is about 2 cm in length, with an average diameter of 1.4 mm (range 0.8–3 mm) [6], which provides an accurate size match to the digital vessels for anastomosis.

The flap can also be based on the independent branch of the radial artery; however this has been found to be present in only 13.3% of the cases [8].

Venous drainage is via the venae comitantes of the SUPBRA or superficial palmar veins continuing as distal forearm veins, of which either or both can be harvested reliably and effectively.

The nerve supply can be provided from segments of the PCBMN, which is present in 100% of the cases. Additionally, the LABCN (present in 43% of the cases) or the SBRN (present in 46% of the cases) can be used if one is present, although these can both be absent in 33% of the cases [8].

31.3 Preoperative Investigation

In view of the consistent arterial supply, which is universally present in all patients, routine preoperative imaging is not required for free thenar flap harvest. However, CT angiography may be useful in patients with previous hand/upper limb injury or surgery or patients with diabetes and atherosclerotic disease.

A standard handheld Doppler ultrasound (8–10 Hz) is routinely used to map the path of the SUPBRA preoperatively on the operating table [6]. This is identified by tracing the pulse of the radial artery distally across the radio-carpal joint radial to the flexor carpi radialis tendon.

Before the tourniquet is inflated, superficial volar veins located between the thenar eminence and distal forearm are also marked.

31.4 Flap Design and Markings

The arterial supply is first mapped out and marked using a handheld Doppler ultrasound probe as above. In some patients the vessel can be seen as a pulsation at the point that it crosses the distal wrist crease. It is usually palpable as a pulse just distal to the scaphoid, as it passes the radio-carpal joint along a line radial to the flexor carpi radialis tendon. Dorsiflexing the wrist can help to palpate the artery if difficult to feel in the neutral position.

On inspection, the superficial volar veins that drain the flap can be marked in the region starting radial to the mid-palmar crease and passing proximally across the wrist and into the distal forearm as they pass in an ulnar direction. If these are not easily visible, one may dangle the hand and forearm to increase venous filling to aid this.

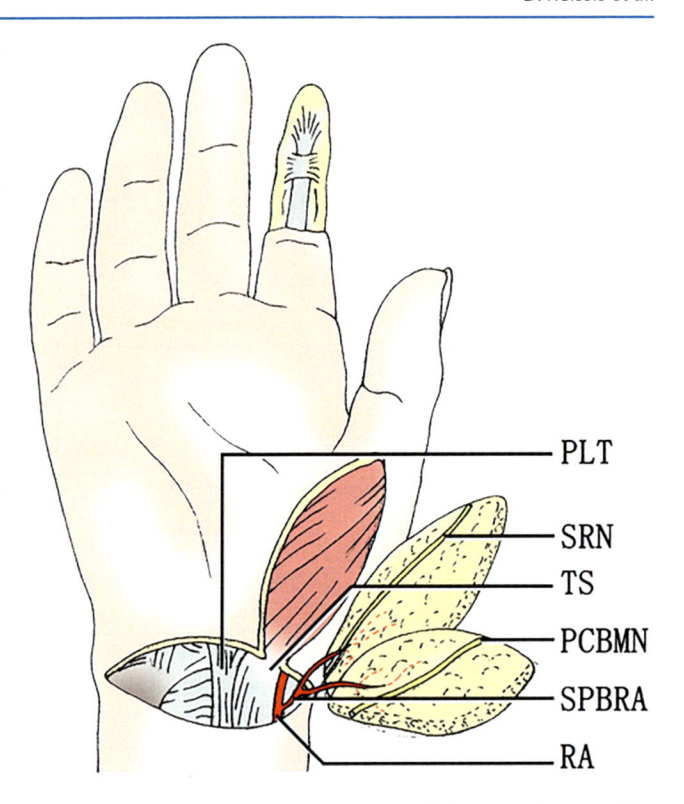

Fig. 31.1 RA, radial artery. SUPBRA, superficial palmar branch of the radial artery. PCBMN, palmar cutaneous branch of the median nerve. SBRN, superficial branch of the radial nerve. TS, tubercle of the scaphoid. PLT, palmaris longus tendon

The free thenar flap is then designed as a curvilinear ellipse, as templated to the defect, with the long axis in the direction of the mid-palmar crease (Fig. 31.1). While the length can be extended up to 10 cm, one should maintain a maximum width of 2 cm to enable direct closure of the donor site without tension [6, 8, 11].

Key landmarks for design of the flap skin paddle are the scaphoid tubercle and a line coming down from radial border of the ring finger. The longitudinal axis of the flap should lie on the line connecting both points. This corresponds to the course of the arterial and neural pedicles longitudinally and includes the skin destinations of the PCBMN [8].

The wrist flap based on the cutaneous perforators of the SUPBRA can be designed with the skin paddle orientated transversely across the wrist/distal volar forearm [12] (Fig. 31.1). This does not provide glabrous skin, but also provides hairless skin with a relatively inconspicuous donor site scar that can be closed directly as long as the flap width is kept less than 2–3 cm depending on skin laxity.

31.5 Flap Raise/Elevation

Positioning
- Position the patient supine with their hand out on an arm table. Dissection is carried out under tourniquet control,

which is inflated after 1-minute elevation of the arm rather than exsanguination with an Esmarch.

Incision
- Make the first skin incision in a longitudinal curvilinear orientation, starting at the volar wrist crease and extending 2–3 cm proximally along the distal forearm [2].

Dissection: Arterial Pedicle
- Carefully dissect toward the radial artery, and identify the origin of the SUPBRA at the point that it bifurcates from the radial artery – usually 2.5 cm proximal to the scaphoid tubercle and 1 cm proximal to the wrist crease (Fig. 31.2).
- (If basing the flap on the independent branch of the radial artery, its origin is more proximal, roughly 3 cm proximal to the wrist crease.)
- The SUPBRA is differentiated from the main branch of the radial artery by its superficial and medial course, whereas the latter deviates dorsally and laterally into the anatomical snuffbox.
- Follow the SUPBRA distally.
- Throughout the dissection maintain clear visualization of both the superficial and main (deep) branches of the SUPBRA, by keeping in a plane deep to the main branch—care is required as this crosses the level of the distal wrist crease into the palm, and you may need to incise the most superficial fibers of the thenar muscles in order to include and not damage this main branch of the SUPBRA [6].
- Identify the superficial branch of the SUPBRA as it provides cutaneous branches to skin of the thenar eminence.
- Carefully ligate the main branch of the SUPBRA as it passes deep into the thenar muscles (Fig. 31.3).

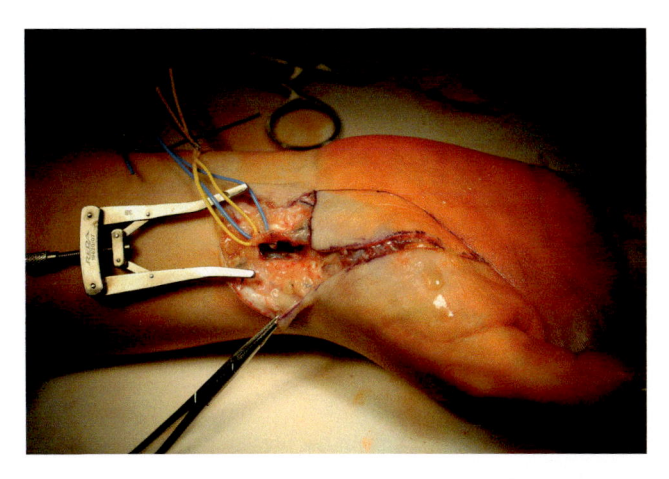

Fig. 31.2 Identification of the SUPBRA during dissection of the proximal arterial pedicle

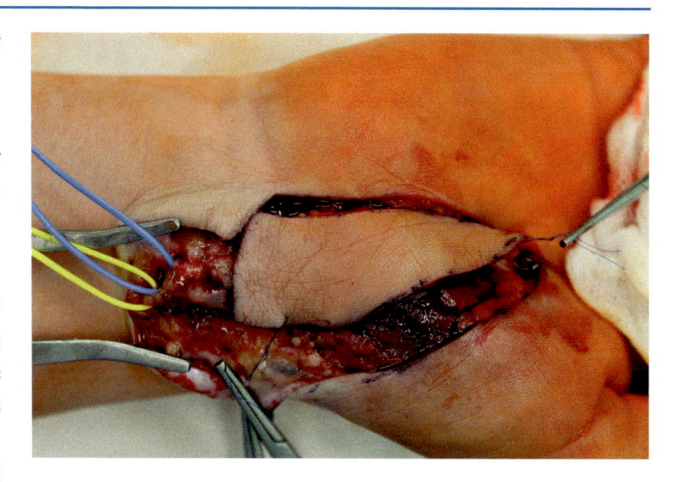

Fig. 31.3 Complete dissection of the SUPBRA following ligation of the distal branch as it passes deep into the thenar muscles

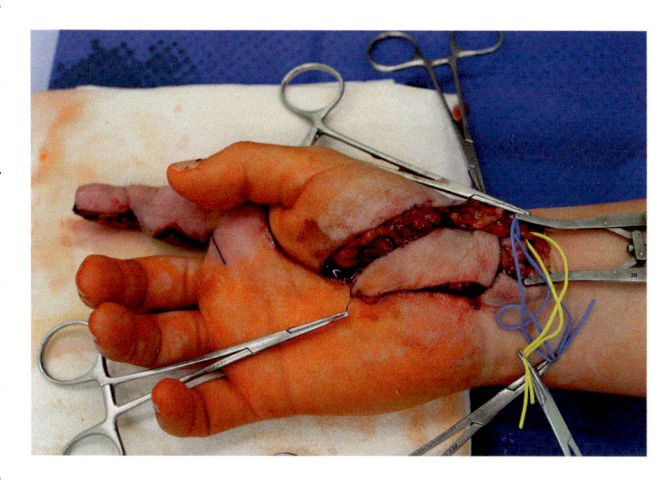

Fig. 31.4 Raising of a fasciocutaneous free SUPBRA flap, with dissection following a radial-ulnar direction over the thenar muscles underlying the flap

Dissection: Flap
- Incise the radial-distal border of the flap skin paddle first.
- Ligate the distal end of the subcutaneous veins in this region of the thenar eminence.
- Deepen this incision to the fascia over the thenar muscles, and then lift as a fasciocutaneous flap in an ulnar direction (Fig. 31.4).
- On the ulnar-proximal half of the flap, make only a superficial incision into the upper dermis taking care to identify and preserve the subcutaneous palmar veins leading into the subcutaneous distal forearm.
- If including a sensory supply, identify and preserve the PCBMN, which passes medially from the proximal aspect of the flap skin paddle.
- Alternatively, if using either the LABCN or SBRN as the sensory supply, these course laterally from the proximal aspect of the flap skin paddle.

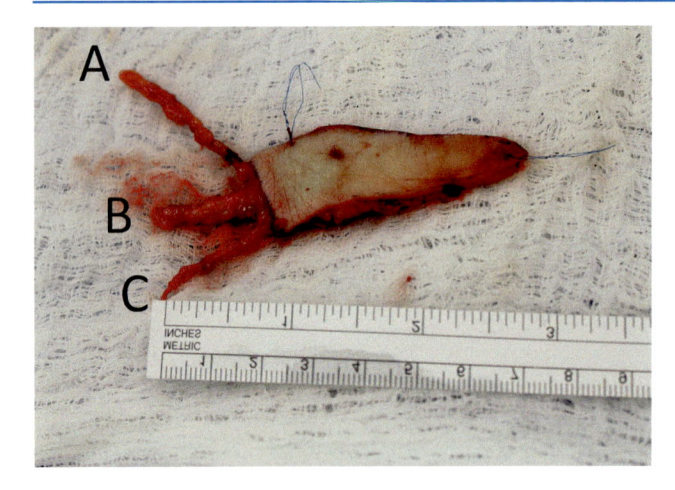

Fig. 31.5 Raised free SUPBRA flap. (**a**) superficial vein. (**b**) SUPBRA. (**c**) SBRN

- Once all key structures are identified, complete the incision of the skin paddle proximally.

Flap Raise
- Before disconnecting the flap, let the tourniquet down to assess flap circulation – if the distal connection of the pedicle to the superficial palmar arch or other vessels in the first web space is still intact, this can be clamped with a microclamp and the tourniquet released to check perfusion.
- Ligate the SUPBRA at the point that it arises from the radial artery to maximize pedicle length.
- Complete dissection of the vein(s) and nerve proximally slightly longer than required (Fig. 31.5).

Flap Inset
- Inset the flap into the defect with loose skin sutures.
- Anastomose the SUPBRA to the digital artery – usually performed in an end-to-end fashion using 10–0 nylon.
- Anastomose the vein to a dorsal digital vein again using handsewn anastomosis, usually in an end-to-end fashion using 10–0 nylon.
- Anastomose the nerve to a digital nerve in end-to-end fashion using 8–0 or 9–0 nylon perineural sutures (Fig. 31.6).

Donor Site Closure
- Close donor site primarily – if a flap width of up to 2 cm has been used.
- The thumb may need to be flexed to facilitate closure.

Dressing
- Apply a plaster of Paris dressing to immobilize the recipient site/digit and wrist, and elevate to reduce postoperative edema and pain.
- Ensure a window in the dressing to monitor the flap postoperatively.

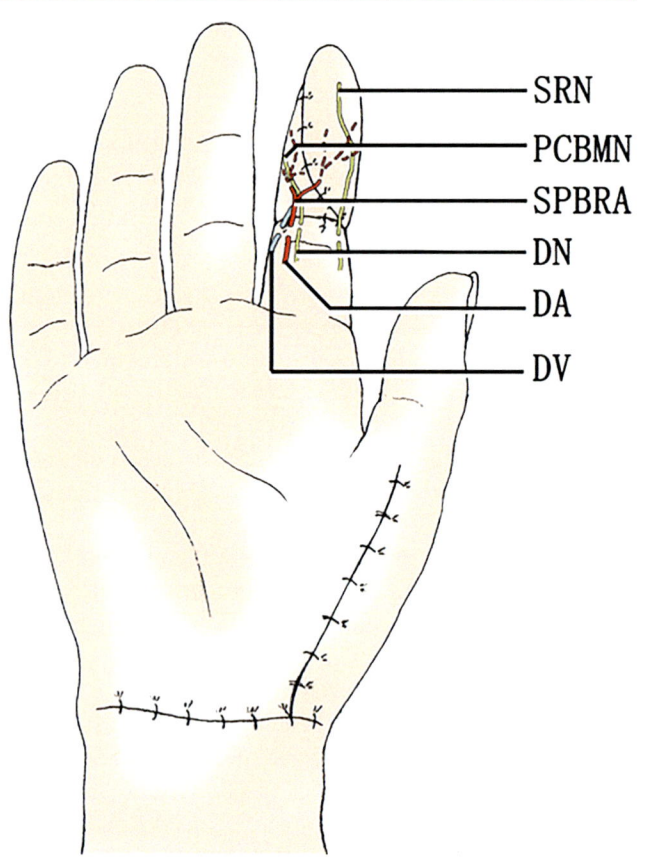

Fig. 31.6 Schematic demonstrating the anastomoses of a free SUPBRA flap for reconstruction of a volar digital defect. The SRN and PCBMN can be anastomosed to either available DN. The SUPBRA is anastomosed to the DA. The vein is anastomosed to a DV. SUPBRA, superficial palmar branch of the radial artery. PCBMN, palmar cutaneous branch of the median nerve. SBRN, superficial branch of the radial nerve. DA, digital artery. DV, digital vein. DN, digital nerve

31.6 Core Surgical Techniques in Flap Dissection

- Ligate the SUPBRA flush with its origin from the radial artery to maximize pedicle length.
- Dissect extra length of the vein into the distal forearm to enable an easier anastomosis to a more proximal and therefore larger vein in the digit close to the web space.
- Inclusion of a sensory nerve and neurorrhaphy to a digital nerve is not always required. Significant functional sensory recovery can occur as a result of neurotization from the relatively high density of nerve receptors in the skin of the thenar eminence, similarly to outcomes from pedicled thenar island flaps [13–15].
- For thumb reconstruction, a reverse pedicled thenar flap can be used – this relies on the presence of distal connections of the superficial radial artery, which are present in only 60% of the cases [16].

- The deep branch of the SUPBRA can also be used as the vascular pedicle of the flap [6], as opposed to the superficial branch. The deep branch gives branches along its course to the overlying skin and allows a longer length of pedicle (up to 6.5 cm) to be used, compared with a maximum length of 2.5 cm with the superficial branch.

31.7 Clinical Scenarios

Case 1: Surgeon Petr Vondra

A 47-year-old woman sustained a crush injury resulting in a full-thickness defect of the volar-ulnar aspect of her right index finger. She was keen to restore a more natural shape of her fingertip while maintaining her nail. She was treated with a free thenar SUPBRA flap from the same hand. The flap was raised based on the SUPBRA, superficial vein, and SRN proximally. These were anastomosed to the ulnar digital artery, an ulnar-dorsal digital vein, and the ulnar digital nerve, respectively. She has a satisfactory outcome at 9 months with restoration of protective sensation and maintained nail appearance (Fig .31.7).

Case 2: Surgeon Dr Yumao

A 41-year-old gentleman sustained traumatic tip and pulp amputations of his left middle and ring fingers. The resultant defects were reconstructed using bilateral free wrist SUPBRA flaps. Both flaps were raised based on the SUPBRA, venae comitantes, and the PCBMN. These were anastomosed to the radial digital artery, volar digital veins, and the radial digital nerve, for both flaps/digits. Both flaps survived with satisfactory healing and contour of the pulp of each digit. He recovered 8 mm two-point discrimination in each digit and good functional range of motion at the DIPJ with satisfactory donor site scars at both wrists (Fig. 31.8).

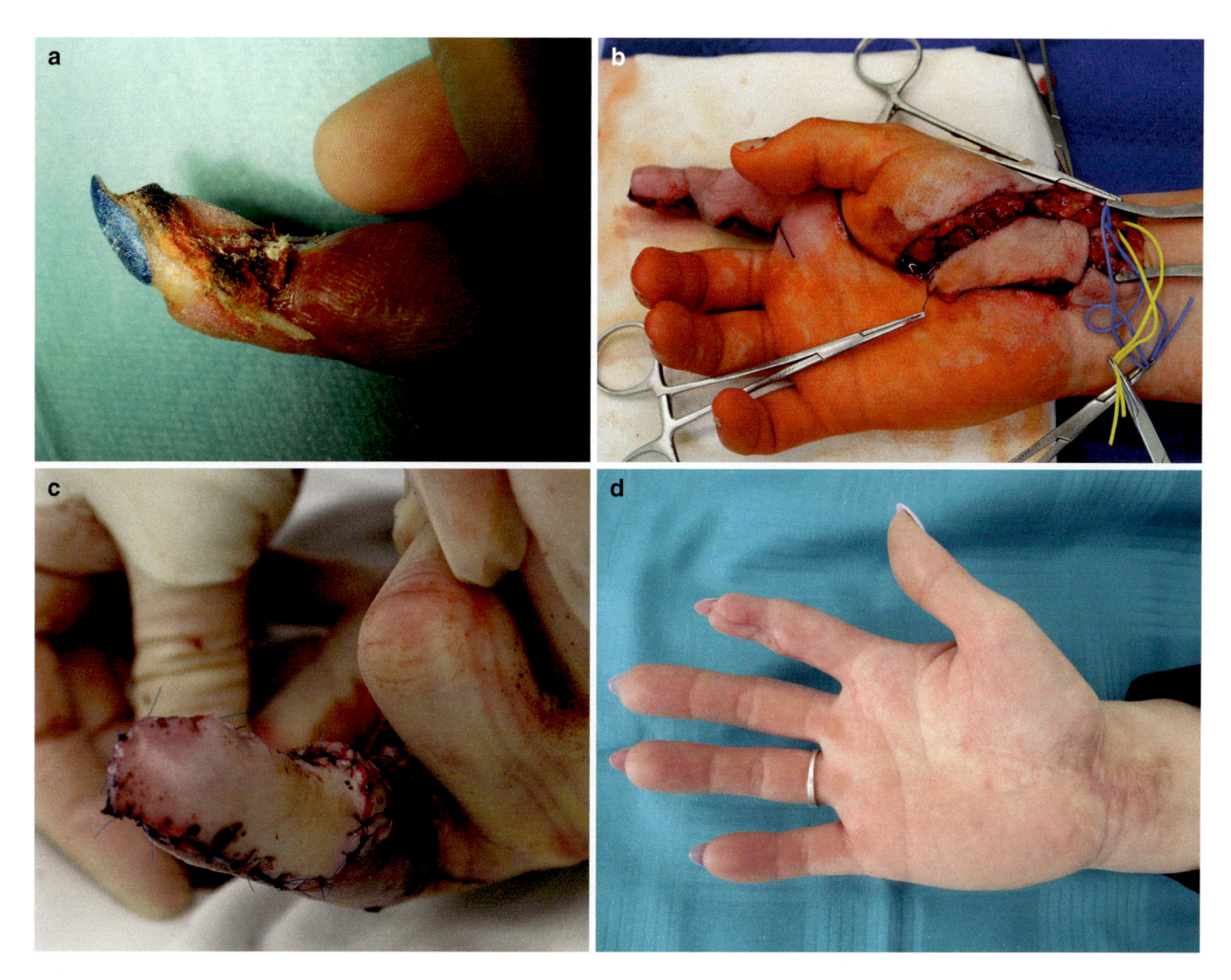

Fig. 31.7 Case 1. (**a**) Full-thickness burn defect on the volar-ulnar aspect of her right index finger. (**b**) Free thenar SUPBRA flap raised based on the SUPBRA, superficial vein, and SRN. (**c**) Flap inset on table. (**d**) Outcome of the flap and donor site scars at 1 year postoperatively

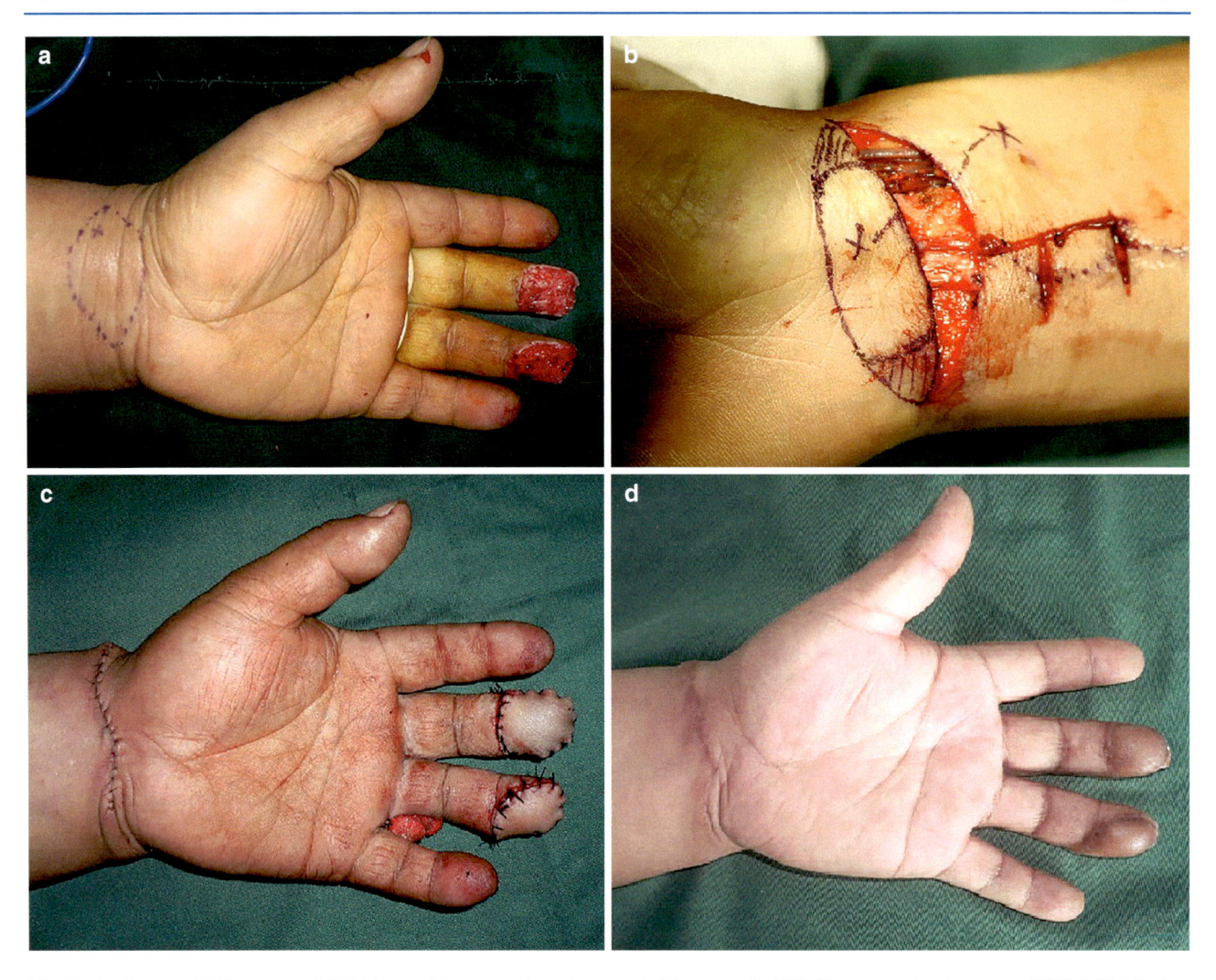

Fig. 31.8 Case 2. (**a**) Traumatic full-thickness defects on the volar aspect of the patient's left middle and ring fingers. (**b**) Free wrist SUPBRA flaps were raised bilaterally (shown on the contralateral right wrist) based on the SUPBRA, venae comitantes, and PCBMN. (**c**) Flaps inset on table. (**d**) Outcome of the flaps and left donor site scar at 18 months

Case 3: Surgeon D Nikkhah

A 49 year old gentleman sustained a traumatic volar oblique amputation of his right thumb. After debridement and osteosynthesis of a P2 fracture with a single Kirschner wire a free thenar flap was raised to reconstruct the defect. The flap encorporated a long superficial vein and the superficial palmar branch of the radial artery as marked in Fig. 31.9a. The flap was anastomosed to the ulnar digital artery with 9.0 ST end to end and the long superficial vein was anastomosed to a dorsal vein with 10.0ST. A small skin graft was placed over the pedicle to avoid compression and the flap was loosely inset to provide glabrous support to the thumb. The patient made an uneventful outcome and early results demonstrated at 2 months Fig. 31.9b with the patient resuming work as a labourer.

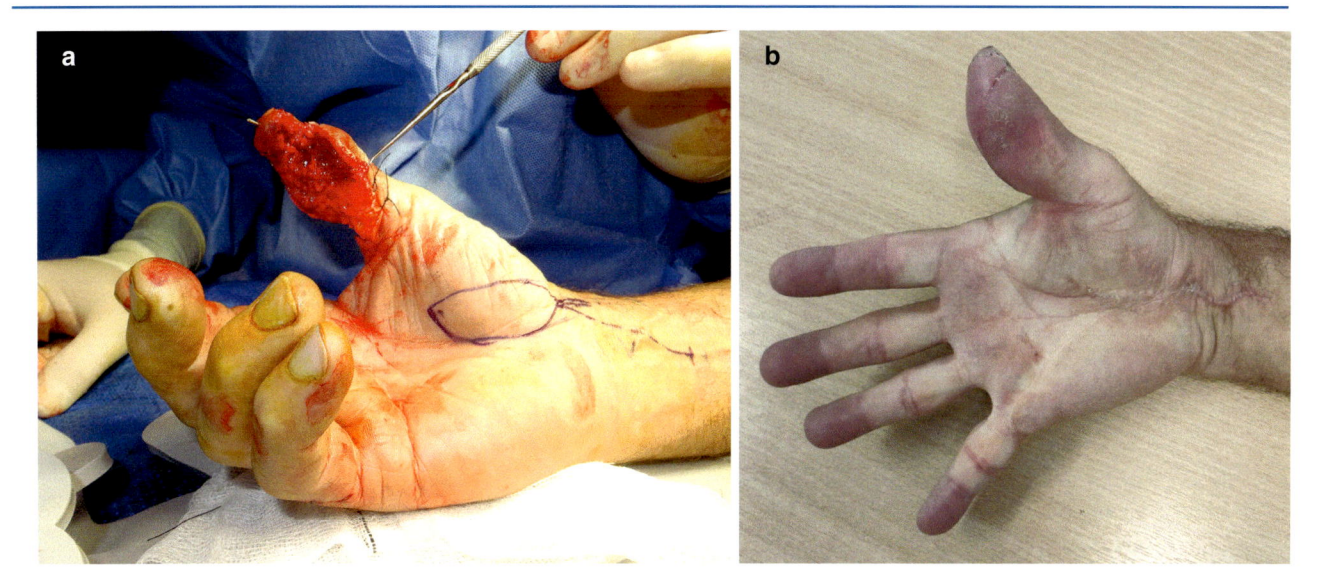

Fig. 31.9 (**a**) Volar oblique amputation of thumb, with free thenar flap marked to resurface thumb pulp (**b**) early result at 2 months with minimal donor site morbidity and a well padded glabrous reconstruction of the thumb

31.8 Pearls and Pitfalls

Pearls

- Perform the arterial anastomosis first, so that the vein can fill with prominent backflow to assist the handsewn venous anastomosis [6].
- Perform the venous anastomosis to the proximal dorsal digital or distal dorsal hand veins in order to improve the size match and flow [6].
- Inset the flap loosely – use a split skin graft from the hypothenar eminence over the loose fatty areolar tissue covering the pedicle if required to avoid potential compression from direct closure [6].
- Design the flap obliquely and centrally located over the mid-palmar crease [6].
- It is possible to base the flap on a subcutaneous vein only and used as an arterialized venous flow-through flap, with arterial inflow and outflow to revascularize the digit and also provide skin coverage of the digit [1].
- Avoid long-term pain at the site of nerve division, by carefully dissecting and burying the nerve ends to avoid neuroma formation [5].
- The free thenar flap may also be used for reconstruction of intraoral defects following excision of oral SCC or other small-medium-sized defects in the hard palate, for example [17].

Pitfalls

- If a flap of width larger than 2 cm is raised, this may require the use of a skin graft for donor site closure, which will significantly compromise donor site morbidity [2, 6].
- Avoid injury to the recurrent motor branch of the median nerve, which may pass through or distal to the transverse carpal ligament (Types I–III) [18].
- Avoid the pedicle being too short by measuring the length required and ensuring this is less than 2 cm.
- If the flap appears too bulky after inset, allow this to settle before performing a debulking procedure several months postoperatively [6].
- Avoid poor postoperative outcome, but ensuring the patient attends for adequate hand therapy and complies with this [6].

31.9 Selected Readings

- Tsai TM, Sabapathy SR, Martin D. Revascularisation of a finger with a thenar mini-free flap. J Hand Surg Am 1991;16 (4):604e6.
  Summary: This is the first case report of the use of a free flap from the thenar region. This was performed for a patient with a devascularized left index finger with a soft tissue defect on the volar side. The thenar mini-free flap

was raised at the level of the MCPJ of the thumb, based on the radial digital artery of the thumb that was anastomosed to the ulnar digital artery of the index finger. A volar vein was also harvested with the flap and anastomosed to a dorsal vein. The arterial anastomosis clotted off postoperatively, but flow was restored with revision of the anastomosis, and no further complications were encountered. The donor site was noted to be minimal with good range of motion of the thumb.

- Kamei K, Ide Y, Kimura T, A new free thenar flap. Plast Reconstr Surg 1993;92 (7):1380e4.

  Summary: This was the first description of the free thenar flap based on the superficial palmar branch of the radial artery. The authors report two cases of traumatic volar defects of the fingers, for which local/pedicled flaps would not have been large enough and cross-finger flaps were deemed unsatisfactory due to stiffness caused postoperatively. Both flaps survived uneventfully and successfully reconstructed the defects with some sensory recovery. The anatomy of the SUPBRA is described clearly along with the main advantages of the flap, including requiring only one operative field, providing a sensory flap with good tissue match and minimal donor site morbidity, compared with other options such as a cross-finger flap or a partial toe transfer.

- Omokawa S, Ryu J, Tang JB, Han J. Vascular and neural anatomy of the thenar area of the hand: its surgical applications. Plast Reconstr Surg. 1997;99 (1):116–121. doi:10.1097/00006534-199701000-00018

  Summary: This anatomical study investigated the vascular and neural supplies of the thenar region in 30 fresh cadavers. The superficial palmar branch of the radial artery was found in all hands. It had an average diameter of 1.4 mm (0.8–3.0 mm). The constant area supplied by the SUPBRA was 4x3cm over the proximal part of the abductor pollicis brevis and opponens pollicis muscles. This supported the fact that a fasciocutaneous flap could be reliably harvested from the thenar region, based on the SUPBRA. In 63% of the hands dissected, the SUPBRA was connected to other arteries in the palm, suggesting that the flap can also be transferred as a reverse-pedicled island flap in these cases. The predominant sensory innervation of the flap was found to be from a branch of the superficial radial nerve.

- Iwuagwu, F.C., Orkar, S.K. and Siddiqui, A. Reconstruction of volar skin and soft tissue defects of the digits including the pulp: experience with the free SUPBRA flap. Journal of Plastic, Reconstructive & Aesthetic Surgery, 2015, 68 (1), pp.26–34.

  Summary: Following an initial publication in 2011 by the same authors, in which the term "SUPBRA" flap was first coined, this article presents a case series of 13 patients for whom a range of traumatic digital defects were reconstructed using a free SUPBRA flap. Flap dimensions ranged from 2x5cm to 2x10cm. They reported no flap failures and good functional outcomes with ideal tissue match, minimal donor site morbidity, and return of protective sensation despite no neurorrhaphy performed except in one patient. They conclude that the free SUPBRA flap has many advantages, approaching the ideal replacement for the volar tissue of the fingers.

References

1. Tsai TM, Sabapathy SR, Martin D. Revascularisation of a finger with a thenar mini-free flap. J Hand Surg Am. 1991;16(4):604c6.
2. Kamei K, Ide Y, Kimura T. A new free thenar flap. Plast Reconstr Surg. 1993;92(7):1380e4.
3. Omokawa S, Ryu J, Tang JB, Han J. Vascular and neural anatomy of the thenar area of the hand: its surgical applications. Plast Reconstr Surg. 1997;99(1):116–21. https://doi.org/10.1097/00006534-199701000-00018.
4. Iwuagwu Fortune C, Orkar Sam K, Aftab S. Free superficial palmar branch of the radial artery flap for the reconstruction of defects of the volar surface of the digits, including the pulp. Plast Reconstr Surg. 2013;131(2):308ee9e.
5. Garg R, Fung BK, Chow SP, Yuk Ip W. A free thenar flap–a case report. J Orthop Surg Res. 2007;2(1):1–3.
6. Iwuagwu FC, Orkar SK, Siddiqui A. Reconstruction of volar skin and soft tissue defects of the digits including the pulp: experience with the free SUPBRA flap. J Plast Reconstr Aesthet Surg. 2015;68(1):26–34.
7. Mabvuure NT, Pinto-Lopes R, Iwuagwu FC, Sierakowski A. A systematic review of outcomes following hand reconstruction using flaps from the superficial palmar branch of the radial artery (SUPBRA) system. J Plast Reconstr Aesthet Surg. 2020;
8. Yang JW, Kim JS, Lee DC, Ki SH, Roh SY, Abdullah S, Tien HY. The radial artery superficial palmar branch flap: a modified free thenar flap with constant innervation. J Reconstr Microsurg. 2010;26(08):529–38.
9. Omokawa S, Mizumoto S, Iwai M, et al. Innervated radial thenar flap for sensory reconstruction of the fingers. J Hand Surg Am 1996;21:373e80, 373.
10. Mackinnon SE, Dellon AL. The overlap pattern of the lateral antebrachial cutaneous nerve and the superficial branch of the radial nerve. J Hand Surg [Am]. 1985;10:522–6.
11. Sassu P, Lin CH, Lin YT, Lin CH. Fourteen cases of free thenar flap: a rare indication in digital reconstruction. Ann Plast Surg. 2008;60(3):260–6. https://doi.org/10.1097/SAP.0b013e31806ab39f.
12. Sakai S. Free flap from the flexor aspect of the wrist for resurfacing defects of the hand and fingers. Plast Reconstr Surg. 2003;111:1412–20. discussion 1421–1422
13. Melone CP Jr, Beasely RW, Carstens JH Jr. The thenar flap: an analysis of its use in 150 cases. J Hand Surg. 1982;7:291e7.
14. Kim KS, Kim ES, Hwang JH, Lee SY. Thumb reconstruction using the radial midpalmar (perforator based) island flap (distal thenar perforator based island flap). Plast Reconstr Surg. 2010;125:601e8.
15. Iwuagwu F, Siddiqui A. Pedicled (antegrade) SUPBRA flap for wound cover on volar aspect of thumb. J Plast Reconstr Aesthet Surg. 2012;65(5):678e80.
16. Omokawa S, Takaoka T, Shigematsu K, et al. Reverse-flow island flap from the thenar area of the hand. J Reconstr Microsurg. 2002;18:659–63.
17. Gaggl A, Bürger H, Brandtner C, Singh D, Hachleitner J. The microvascular thenar flap as a new possibility for super-thin soft tissue reconstruction in the oral cavity—initial clinical results. Br J Oral Maxillofac Surg. 2012;50(8):721–5.
18. Kozin SH. The anatomy of the recurrent branch of the median nerve. J Hand Surg Am. 1998;23(5):852–8. https://doi.org/10.1016/S0363-5023(98)80162-7.

Medial and Lateral Arm Fasciocutaneous Flaps

32

Katerina Kyprianou, Georgios Pafitanis, Dajiang Song, and Youmao Zhen

32.1 Introduction

32.1.1 First Description, Origin and Evolution of Medial Arm Flap Vascularity

The medial arm flap was first described by Tagliacozzi in 1597. In 1975, Daniel et al. described the medial arm with its associated medial brachial cutaneous nerve, where the arterial supply was thought to be a cutaneous branch arising from the superior ulnar collateral artery (SUCA). Similarly, Kaplan and Pearl (1980) described an axial pattern flap supplied by SUCA and vein. Subsequently, Dolmans et al. (1979) dissected the medial arm flap and reported the SUCA was absent in 20% of the dissections, with Matoub et al. (1981) reporting five arterial variations supplying the flap. In 1982, Song et al. indicated that the medial arm was supplied by a branch from the SUCA and described variations in terms of the SUCA being absent and sometimes too small for free flap transfer.

32.1.2 Medial Arm Flap Characteristics

The medial arm flap is a fasciocutaneous flap with a Type B pattern of circulation according to Mathes and Nahai classification. The standard flap is based on the upper segmental subcutaneous perforator and the flap can reach and cover up to the axilla. Reverse or distally based flaps are designed on the lower segmental perforators. Those are useful for staged transfer such as in nasal reconstruction (Tagliacozzi flap). Additionally, a flap based on the posterior ulnar collateral vessels can be elevated as a distally based flap.

32.1.3 Common Indications

The medial arm flap can be used both as a pedicled and free flap. As a pedicled flap, it can be used for coverage for the nose, axilla, antecubital fossa and breast reconstruction. As a free flap, it can be used for distant coverage for the head and neck area, as well as both upper and lower extremities.

The following flap modifications of the medial arm flap exist:

1. Segmental transposition: Achievable due to the segmental nature of blood supply to this flap. Distally based transposition is also feasible by basing the flap on the subcutaneous vessels, particularly useful for staged distant transfer as in nasal reconstruction.
2. Innervated flap: Microvascular transplantation of a neural sensory flap based on intercostobrachial or medial cutaneous nerve of the arm can be performed.
3. Reverse flap: A reverse island flap based on the ulnar recurrent vessel can be used for coverage of the antecubital fossa. This is the reverse medial arm flap or the ulnar recurrent fasciocutaneous flap.

K. Kyprianou
Department of Plastic Surgery and Burns, Chelsea and Westminster Hospital, London, UK

G. Pafitanis (✉)
London Reconstructive Microsurgery Unit (LRMU), Department of Plastic Surgery, Emergency Care and Trauma Division (ECAT). The Royal London Hospital, Barts Health NHS Trust & University College Hospital London (UCLH), London, UK
e-mail: g.pafitanis@qmul.ac.uk

D. Song
Department of Oncology Plastic Surgery, Hunan Province Cancer Hospital, Changsha, Hunan, China

Y. Zhen
Department of Hand and Foot Surgery, Enze Hospital of Taizhou, Enze Medical Center, Taizhou, Zhejiang, China

32.2 Anatomy

The vascular supply of the medial arm flap has been described as variable septocutaneous blood supply, and perhaps this is one of the major reasons why this flap has not been widely popularised. It's primarily characterised by a dominant pedicle, the SUCA, and a minor pedicle that mostly originates from the brachial artery, with their interconnected collateral anastomotic cutaneous networks.

32.2.1 Vascular Supply: Superior Ulnar Collateral Artery (SUCA)

The vascular anatomy of the arm originates from the axial artery, renamed as brachial artery as it enters the proximal arm region. The brachial artery crosses through the septum between triceps and biceps and gives off the profunda brachii artery that supplies the triceps muscle and the posterior fasciocutaneous region of the arm via multiple small branches.

The SUCA is considered the main supply to the medial arm, with 1–2 cm length and calibre of up to 2 mm. Direct cutaneous branches of the brachial artery, septocutaneous perforators provide significant blood supply to the medial arm skin. It is an axial cutaneous artery approximately 5 cm below the pectoralis major muscle and coursing in the subcutaneous planes approximately 10 cm beyond. The nomenclature of the SUCA is characterised by three anatomical variations: (1) originating from the profunda (~60%), (2) originating directly from the brachial artery (~20%) and (3) originating from both profunda and brachial arterial branches (~20%). The calibre of the SUCA is adequate for dissection of free flap in the case of (1) or (2); however, in the case of (3), the arterial pedicle calibre requires the ability for submillimetre microvascular anastomosis or could be utilised as a pedicled flap. Extra care should be taken as the biceps musculocutaneous blood supply also arises in very close proximity (~7 cm) below the pectoralis major muscle and through the muscle supplies the anterior arm skin via more than two musculocutaneous perforators.

Posteriorly, the ulnar collateral artery which is an axial cutaneous vessel can be found 7cm from the elbow and occasionally forms branches that connect the SUCA cutaneous network to the elbow. Posteriorly, the ulnar collateral artery, a larger in calibre vessel, travels between the proximal heads of the flexor carpi ulnaris to gives its muscle branches and courses us and posterior to the medial condyle along with the ulnar nerve, to be anastomosed with the SUCA.

32.2.2 Nerve Supply

The medial cutaneous nerve of the arm offers sensory innervation to the skin paddle of the medial arm flap. The superior region is primarily innervated by the intercostobrachial nerve and the inferior region by the medial cutaneous nerve of the arm (C8-T1).

32.2.2.1 Anatomical Studies (Vasculature or Angiosomes)

In the medial flap territory, the major blood supply is provided by the septocutaneous perforators, which arise from the brachial artery, SUCA, inferior ulnar collateral artery or superficial brachial artery if present. Hwang et al. found that a constant perforator could be found within a circle of diameter 2.89 cm, centred 8.9 cm above and 1.2 cm medial to the medial epicondyle. Perignon et al. reported the same but for a circle of radius 2.4 cm, centred at 7.5 cm above and 0.5 cm medial to the medial epicondyle. Finally, Tinhofer et al. reported the same but for a circle of radius 3 cm, centred at 8 cm above and 1 cm medial to the medial epicondyle. Xue et al. reported that an average of 4.5 perforators can be found along the medial intermuscular septum of the arm, which is consistent with previous observations. According to the angiosome theory, elevating a medial arm flap with full length should be based on at least 1.5 perforator angiosomes connected by true anastomoses, as medial arm flaps based on a single perforator have less favourable survival.

32.3 Preoperative Investigation

Preoperative planning of the flap includes identification of the SUCA using the handheld Doppler and marking of the large subcutaneous veins, to include at least one large superficial vein. The dominant SUCA could be also identified in a computerised tomography as usually has larger calibre than 2 mm, along the course of the brachial artery.

32.4 Flap Design and Markings

The patient is positioned supine, and a line drawn from the anterior axillary fold or coracoid process to the medial epicondyle of the humerus, which is the main landmark. The skin island lies along the medial inner aspect of the arm and can be centred along the distal third of the line drawn above. The size of skin island can be up to 20x8cm. The anterior border of the flap is incised first to identify the biceps and dissection continues to the intermuscular septum. The pedicle (SUCA) enters the flap on the deep surface through the medial intermuscular septum of the arm. The point where the pedicle enters the flap is at the midpoint of the key landmark line from the coracoid process to the medial epicondyle. Proximally, the SUCA is closely involved with the ulnar nerve.

32.5 Flap Raise/Elevation: A Step-by-Step Guide

1. Anterior incision from the flap design required is made and the deep fascia is divided (Fig. 32.1).
2. Flap is elevated carefully at subfascial plane until the medial intermuscular septum is seen and the brachial artery and median nerve are identified and dissected (Fig. 32.2).

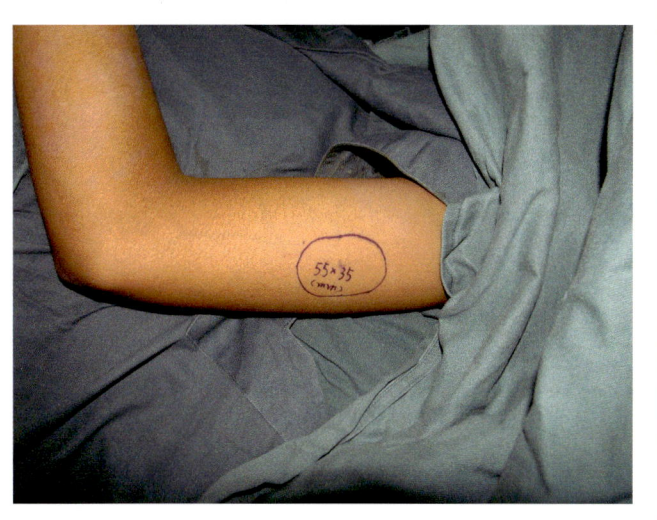

Fig. 32.1 Flap design

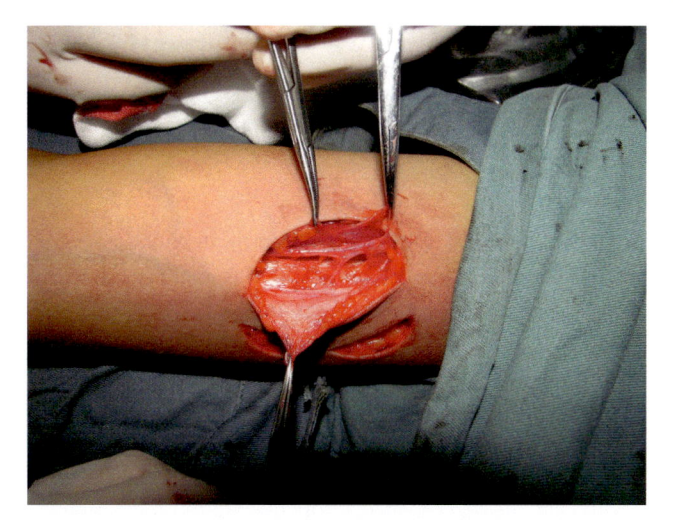

Fig. 32.2 Flap is elevated at the subfascial plane until the medial intermuscular septum is seen

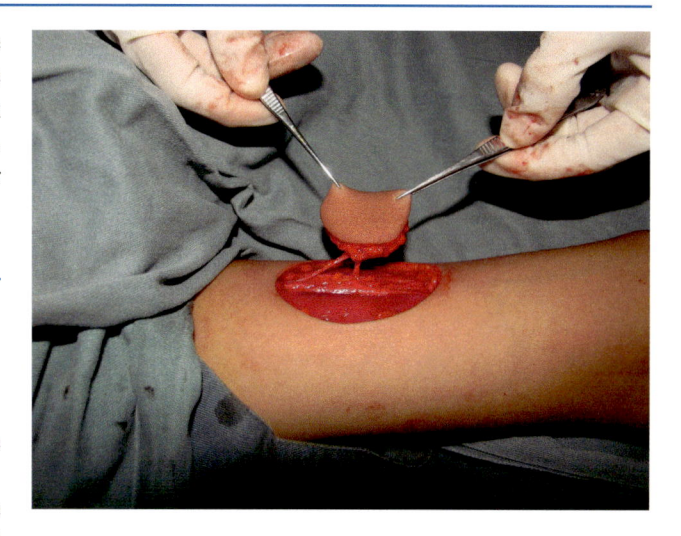

Fig. 32.3 Flap is islanded on its pedicle

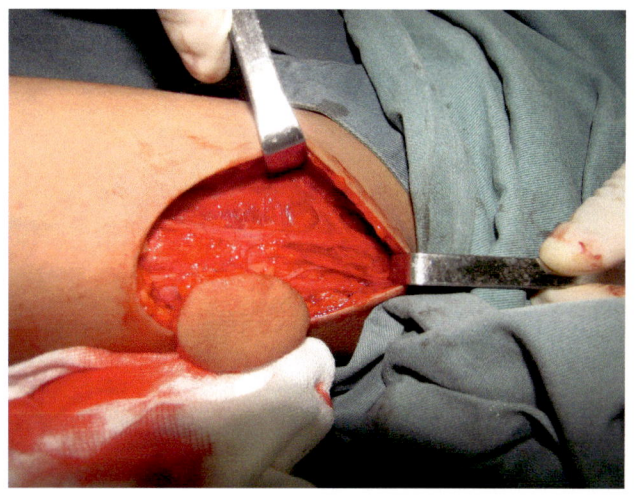

Fig. 32.4 The anterior and posterior incisions are undermined and dissected to allow identification of a subcutaneous vein in proximity or overlying the muscular fascia and SUCA pedicle

3. The posterior incision is made at the fascia over the triceps and the flap can be islanded on its pedicle (Fig. 32.3).
4. If the flap is elevated up to the mid- to distal third of the inner arm at the subfascial level, the ulnar nerve must be identified and separated from the intermuscular septum (Fig. 32.4).
5. The anterior and posterior incisions are undermined and dissected to allow identification of a subcutaneous vein in proximity or overlying the muscular fascia and SUCA pedicle (Fig. 32.4).
6. The flap could be harvested for free tissue transfer (Fig. 32.5).
7. If the reverse flap has been chosen, the collateral distal arm connections should be identified to allow safe rotation to cover the defect around the elbow joint.

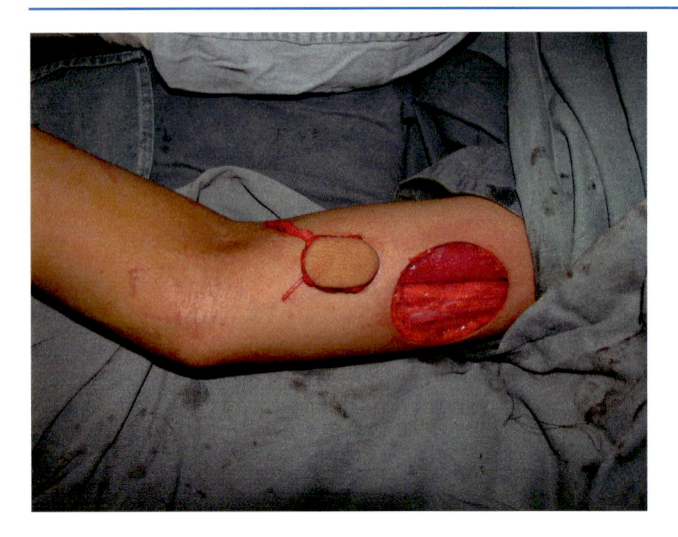

Fig. 32.5 The flap harvested for free tissue transfer

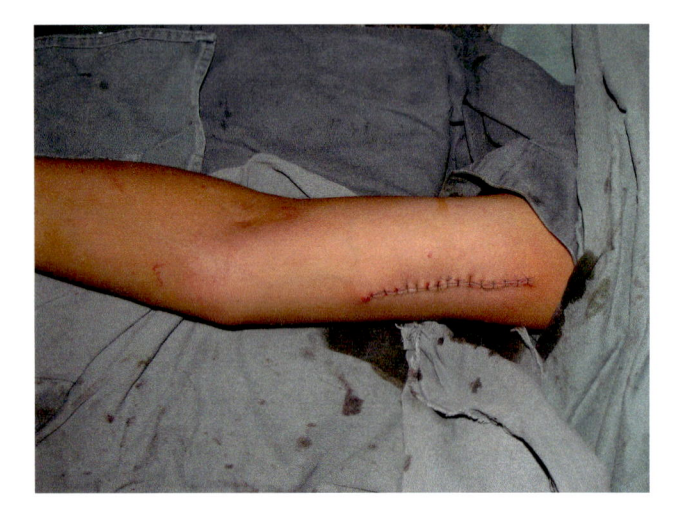

Fig. 32.6 The donor site can be closed primarily

8. For the small flaps, the donor site can be closed primarily. Larger flaps may require split thickness skin graft of the donor site; however, that is not advisable since there are other numerous alternative flaps that can be used for larger fasciocutaneous skin paddles (Fig. 32.6).

32.6 Core Surgical Techniques in Flap Dissection

32.6.1 Standard Flap

The standard flap is based proximally on the SUCA and is elevated either for free tissue transfer or local transposition. Technical considerations for its dissection are detailed:

1. The flap is designed as an ellipse centred along the middle to distal third of the key line drawn from the coracoid process to the medial epicondyle of the humerus. The distal extent of the flap is 3 cm above the medial epicondyle.
2. The anterior incision is made first and dissection is continued through the skin and subcutaneous tissues to the deep fascia.
3. The deep fascia is elevated off the biceps muscle, and dissection continues from lateral to medial towards the medial intermuscular septum.
4. As the medial intermuscular septum is approached, the septocutaneous branches are easily identified. These are usually branches of the SUCA.
5. At this stage the posteromedial half of the incision is made, and the posteromedial half of the flap is elevated from medial to lateral. The dissection starts over the triceps muscle, continues over the exposed ulnar nerve and extends across the brachialis to the medial intermuscular septum.
6. The deep plane of elevation includes the areolar fascia to protect the superior brachial collateral artery. Care is taken to avoid the intermuscular septum that contains the ulnar and median nerves and the brachia/artery. Protection is facilitated by marking the brachial artery course between the biceps and triceps. Proximal to the point where the superior ulnar collateral artery penetrates the skin, the dissection requires more care, so as not to transect this direct cutaneous artery as it exits the intermuscular septum.
7. The medial cutaneous nerve of the arm and the basilic vein or a branch are divided and included in the flap.
8. Once the medial and lateral halves of the dissection meet the intermuscular septum, the SUCA is traced proximally to its origin from the brachial artery. In its proximal course, the ulnar nerve is intimately involved with the SUCA.
9. Proximal dissection of the SUCA to its origin will yield a pedicle length of up to 3 cm.
10. At this stage the flap is ready for transfer as a free flap or transposition.

32.6.2 Reverse Flap

The reverse medial arm flap is based on the posterior ulnar collateral vessels. The design of the flap is the same as the standard flap. The vascular bases of the flap, the posterior ulnar collateral vessels, run deep to the ulnar nerve along the anterior border of the triceps muscle coursing diagonally from the medial epicondyle to the midline of the upper arm:

1. Dissection of the flap is initiated through the medial incision and the flap elevated across the intermuscular septum.
2. The SUCA and its septocutaneous branches are identified and isolated and the SUCA ligated at its origin.
3. The lateral incision is then made.

4. The flap is elevated across to the ulnar nerve.
5. At this stage the posterior ulnar recurrent vessels are identified, dissected off the ulnar nerve included within the flap, and the flap dissected from above down towards the medial epicondyle.
6. The flap is now ready for transposition superiorly into the antecubital area.
7. The flap is placed in the defect without tension and sutured.

32.6.3 Free Flap

For free tissue transfer, the flap is based on its dominant SUCA:

1. The anterior incision is made and the dissection continued down to biceps and the medial intermuscular septum.
2. The SUCA is identified and the septocutaneous branch is traced to the flap.
3. Once it has been established that the SUCA is the dominant supply and the vessel is suitable for microvascular transfer, flap elevation proceeds as described for the standard flap.

32.7 Clinical Scenarios

32.7.1 Medial Arm Flap

A 45-year-old gentleman underwent right foot first webspace reconstruction with a thin and pliable fasciocutaneous medial arm flap. The medial arm flap was raised in the exact dimensions of the defect (3.5 × 5.5 cm). The superior ulnar collateral artery and the basilic vein were used as the dominant pedicles (Fig. 32.7). Microvascular anastomosis was achieved with a dorsal incision to identify branch of the dorsalis pedis artery and a cutaneous vein on the medial dorsum of the foot, overlying the first webspace. The flap inset along with primary closure of the dorsal extension incision for the microvascular arterial and venous anastomosis achieved excellent webspace reconstruction and coverage of the big toe lateral wound defect (Figs. 32.8 and 32.9).

32.7.2 Lateral Arm Flap

The lateral arm flap, a flap with consistent vascular pedicle, similar to the medial arm flap can also be used for similar indications. It is based on the radial collateral artery, a branch of the brachial artery. The flap is designed in the humerus axis, posterior to the biceps, brachialis and brachioradialis sarcomeres. During flap elevation, the pedicle is seen within the septum between triceps and biceps muscles, along with

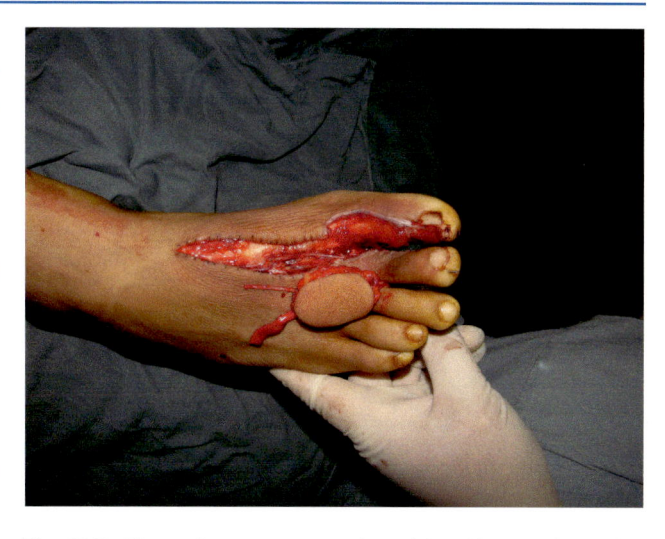

Fig. 32.7 First webspace reconstruction with a thin and pliable free fasciocutaneous medial arm flap

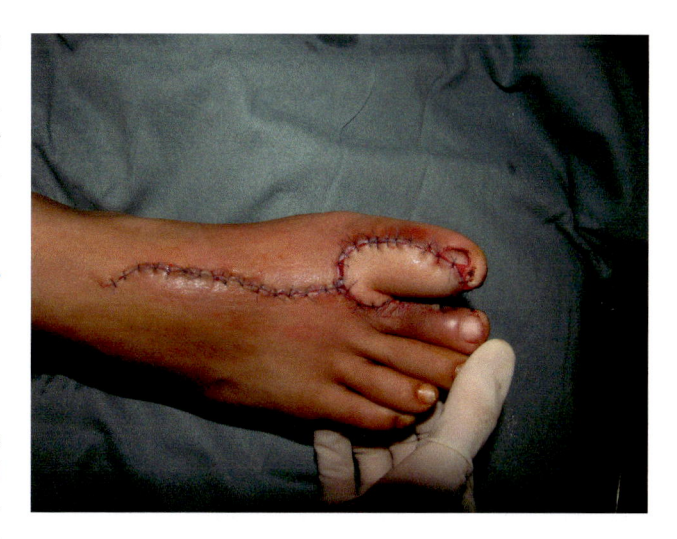

Fig. 32.8 Microvascular anastomosis was achieved with a dorsal incision to identify branch of the dorsalis pedis artery and a cutaneous vein

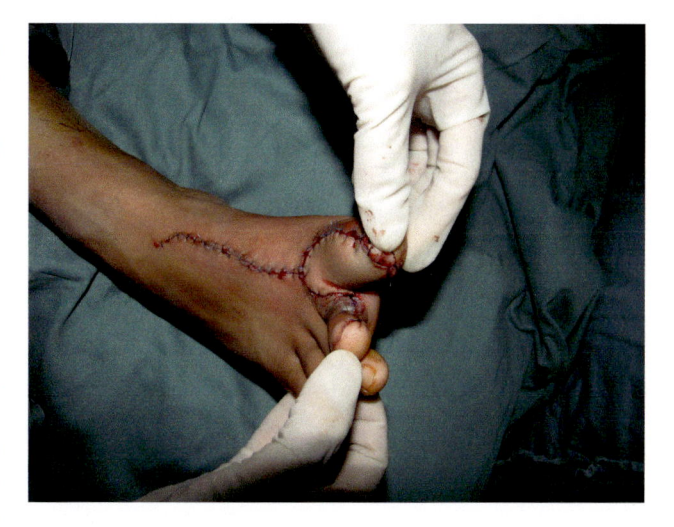

Fig. 32.9 The flap inset achieved primary closure of the foot dorsum and like-to-like webspace reconstruction of the big toe lateral wound defect

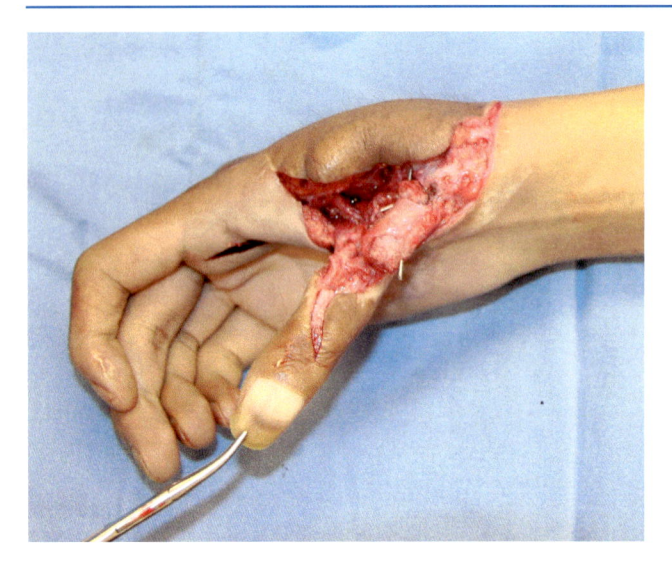

Fig. 32.10 Right hand thenar eminence skin, muscle and first metacarpal bone defect

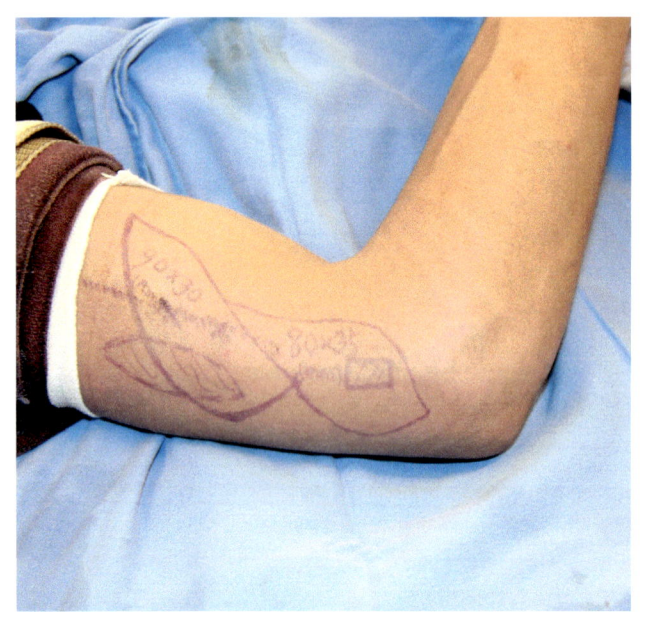

Fig. 32.11 A chimeric bi-paddle lateral arm flap, along with a small segment of the triceps sarcomere to obliterate the thenar muscle defect and a small distal humerus bone component, was designed

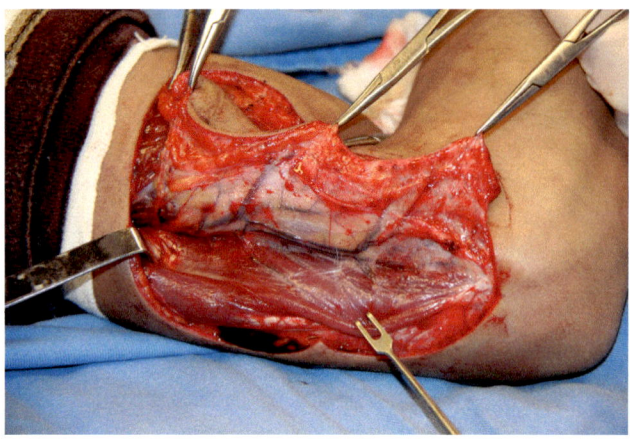

Fig. 32.12 The chimeric paddles raised en-bloc of two perforators of the lateral arm flap, along with a small segment of the triceps sarcomere on the distal pedicle

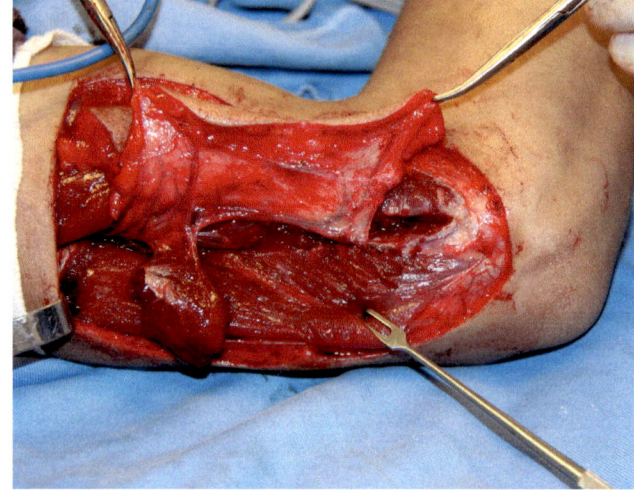

Fig. 32.13 The small segment of the triceps sarcomere to obliterate the thenar muscle defect is demonstrated along with the distal humerus bone segment

multiple small musculocutaneous perforators, that could be used to harvest small chimeric muscle components for composite reconstructions, i.e. thenar eminence and first webspace reconstruction.

A 35-year-old gentleman required a composite reconstruction of his right hand thenar eminence skin, muscle and first metacarpal bone defect (Fig. 32.10). A chimeric bi-paddle lateral arm flap, along with a small segment of the triceps sarcomere to obliterate the thenar muscle defect and a small distal humerus bone component, was raised (Fig. 32.11). Figure 32.12 demonstrates the radial collateral artery within the septum with the multiple muscular branches and the distal humeral branch. The chimeric configuration of the flap dissected allowed the composite reconstruction of all defect characteristics of the right thenar eminence along with the small $1 \times 1 \times 1$ cm defect of the first metacarpal (Figs. 32.13 and 32.14). Figure 32.15 shows the complementary pattern of the chimeric free flap components with the composite defect after the microvascular anastomosis to the radial artery and branch of the cephalic vein.

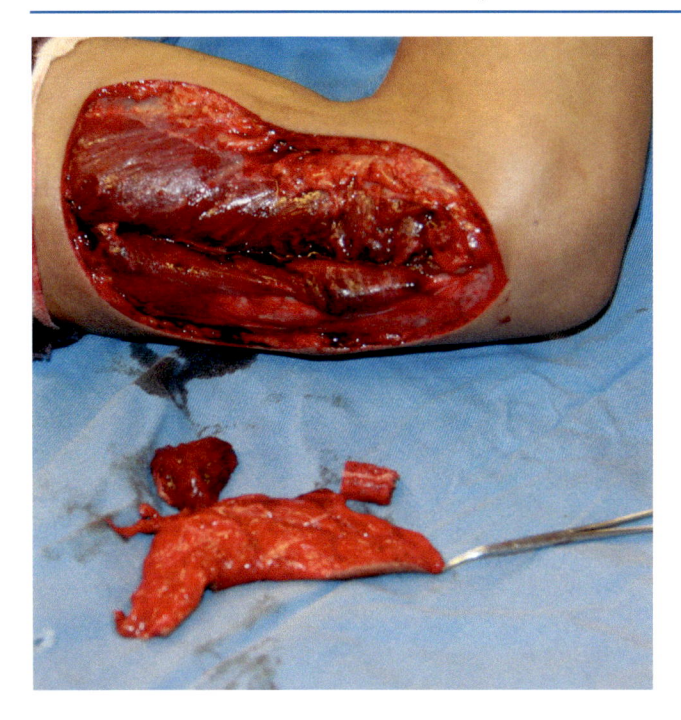

Fig. 32.14 The chimeric flap raised

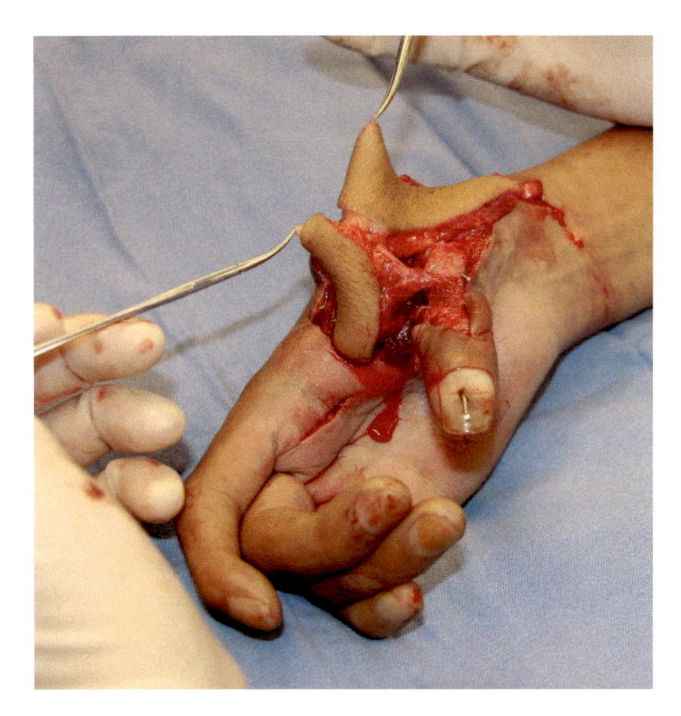

Fig. 32.15 The chimeric configuration of the flap dissected allowed the composite reconstruction of all defect characteristics of the right thenar eminence along with the small defect of the first metacarpal

32.8 Pearls and Pitfalls

Pearls
- The basilic vein or a major branch is crucial to be identified and included within the anterior incision during flap elevation.
- The arc of rotation in cases when the reverse configuration is chosen must take into consideration the joint movement to reduce the risks of scar contracture.
- It is ideal to use the medial arm free flap when requiring thin pliable fasciocutaneous flap that could be also innervated via the medial cutaneous nerve of the arm.

Pitfalls
- Larger-size flaps that will require skin graft closure of the donor site are not advisable since numerous other alternatives are available.
- This is not a flap of first choice; however, it offers a pliable and good-quality skin especially in elderly.
- The septocutaneous perforators are usually branches of the superior ulnar collateral artery. However, on occasion these branches may arise directly from the brachial artery or may not course through the intermuscular septum but through the posteromedial aspect of the biceps muscle.

32.9 Selected Readings

- Kaplan EN, Pearl RM. An arterial medial flap – vascular anatomy and clinical applications. Ann Plast Surg. 1980;4(3):205–15.
- *A comprehensive vascular anatomical reference from the early stages of reconstructive microsurgery, demonstrating the arterial blood supply of the medial arm flap. Detailed nomenclature, vascular branches and clinical applications are also revealed.*
- Xue B, Zang M, Chen B, Tang M, Zhu S, Li S, Han T, Liu Y. Septocutaneous perforator mapping and clinical appli-

cations of the medial arm flap. J Plast Reconstr Aesthet Surg. 2019;72(4):600–8. doi: 10.1016/j.bjps.2019.01.025. Epub 2019 Feb 10. PMID: 30808600.
- *A retrospective study of 36 patients who underwent reconstructive surgery using a medial arm flap, aiming to clarify the distribution of septocutaneous perforators and its relationship with pedicled flap design. Given its rich septocutaneous perforator distribution, the medial arm flap can be harvested reliably with versatile design and minimal donor site morbidity, thus deserving more attention in reconstructive surgery.*
- Matloub HS, Ye Z, Yousif NJ, Sanger JR. The medial arm flap. Ann Plastic surg. 1992 Dec 1;29(6):517–22.
- *A cadaveric study of 40 fresh cadaver arms, looking at the vascular supply to the medial side of the arm after latex injection. This study demonstrated that the superior ulnar collateral artery was present in 39 of 40 dissections and was the most consistent prominent blood supply to this area.*
- Gong X, Cui JL, Lu LJ. The medial arm pedicled perforator flap: application of phenomenon of one perforator perfusing multiple perforator angiosomes. Injury. 2014 Dec;45(12):2025–8. doi: 10.1016/j.injury.2014.09.005. Epub 2014 Sep 21. PMID: 25294118.
- *A study of eight flaps using the medial arm pedicled perforator flaps to treat skin defects around the elbow with seven flaps surviving uneventfully. This study confirmed the phenomenon of one perforator perfusing multiple perforator angiosomes in the medial arm and showed that it is a useful tool for skin defects around the elbow.*
- Hou C, Chang S, Lin J, Song D. Medial arm perforator flap. In: Surgical Atlas of Perforator Flaps. Dordrecht: Springer; 2015. https://doi.org/10.1007/978-94-017-9834-1_9.
- *A detailed published literature regarding the medial arm island flap in a reverse configuration. Special considerations regarding the local fasciocutaneous flap based on the recurrent ulnar arterial branches are demonstrated and discussed.*

The Groin Flap: The Workhorse Flap for Upper Limb Reconstruction

Hari Venkatramani, David Zargaran, Dariush Nikkhah, Julia Ruston, and S. Raja Sabapathy

33.1 Introduction

The groin flap was first described by Ian A McGregor and Ian T Jackson in 1972. They assessed the role of the superficial circumflex iliac vessels in supplying a self-contained vascular territory and raised the groin flap based on these vessels [1]. They described the design of the flap and its excellent usage as a pedicled flap in 35 patients. Taylor et al. in 1973 described the clinical application of detaching the vascular pedicle from the groin to use it as a free flap to cover a post traumatic wound in the lower limb claiming it to be the first described free flap [2].

The ease of harvest and reliable vascular anatomy made the pedicled groin flap a workhorse flap for coverage of soft tissue defects distal to the elbow. The robust lymphatics at the base of the flap are responsible for lack of oedema both in the flap as well as the part of the hand distal to the flap. Furthermore, venous drainage through a superficial set into the saphenous system and the cosmetically advantageous location of the scar make the pedicled groin flap a strong potential candidate for upper extremity reconstruction. Its use as a pedicled flap has been well established by the group at Ganga Hospital who perform the case over 200 times a year despite being a centre of microsurgical excellence [3].

Modifications have been made for its use as a tubed flap [4] for reconstructing degloved digits, islanded flap [5], osteocutaneous flap [6] and a vascularised groin lymph node flap [6, 7] alongside its already established role as a free flap. The free flap has been successfully described as an effective solution for soft tissue coverage in the paediatric population with good outcomes in congenital, trauma and neoplastic reconstructions [8].

The free groin flap has been criticised for its variable vessel origin, limited length of vascular pedicle, inconsistent calibre [9] and, when inclusive of tissue medially, the presence of donor pubic hair. However, its many proponents have demonstrated that it can be an effective solution with appropriate planning and vessel selection.

33.2 Anatomy

The groin flap is an axial pattern, type A, fasciocutaneous flap based on the Cormack and Lamberty classification [10]. The arterial supply of the flap is based on superficial circumflex iliac artery (SCIA) a branch of the femoral artery. The venous drainage is through a network of superficial veins superficial circumflex iliac veins (SCIV) which are 1.5 mm in diameter and ultimately drain into saphenous venous network (Fig. 33.1).

The superficial circumflex iliac artery is 1.92 ± 0.6 mm in diameter [11] and arises deep to deep fascia, approximately 2.8 ± 1 cm below the inguinal ligament [12]. It gives a superficial branch which travels towards the anterior superior iliac spine (ASIS), and the artery then traverses deep to the fascia over the sartorius and sometimes piercing the muscle and emerging superficially along the lateral border of the muscle. It gives many skin branches at this stage. The following variations in arterial anatomy (Fig. 33.2) should be kept in mind when raising as a free flap:

- Direct origin from the femoral artery—42–45%.

H. Venkatramani (✉) · S. R. Sabapathy
Department of Plastic, Hand and Reconstructive Microsurgery, Ganga Hospital, Coimbatore, Tamil Nadu, India

D. Zargaran
Royal Free Hospital, London, UK

D. Nikkhah
Department of Plastic, Reconstructive and Aesthetic Surgery, Royal Free Hospital, London, UK

J. Ruston
Department of Plastic Surgery, The Royal Free Hospital, London, UK

© Springer Nature Switzerland AG 2023
D. Nikkhah et al. (eds.), *Core Techniques in Flap Reconstructive Microsurgery*, https://doi.org/10.1007/978-3-031-07678-7_33

- Common origin along with superficial inferior epigastric artery (SIEA)—48%.
- Large SCIA with absent SIEA—10–15%.

There are two key venous drainage systems in the area with the dominant system being the superficial cutaneous veins which involve the SCIV and SIEV which join into a common trunk before draining into the saphenous vein. The venae comitantes along the SCIA are small at approximately 1 mm in diameter and form the deep system of venous drainage. The sensation to the lateral aspect of the groin flap is provided and supplied by the lateral cutaneous branches of the 12th thoracic subcostal nerve with further supply from the lateral femoral cutaneous nerve (Fig. 33.3).

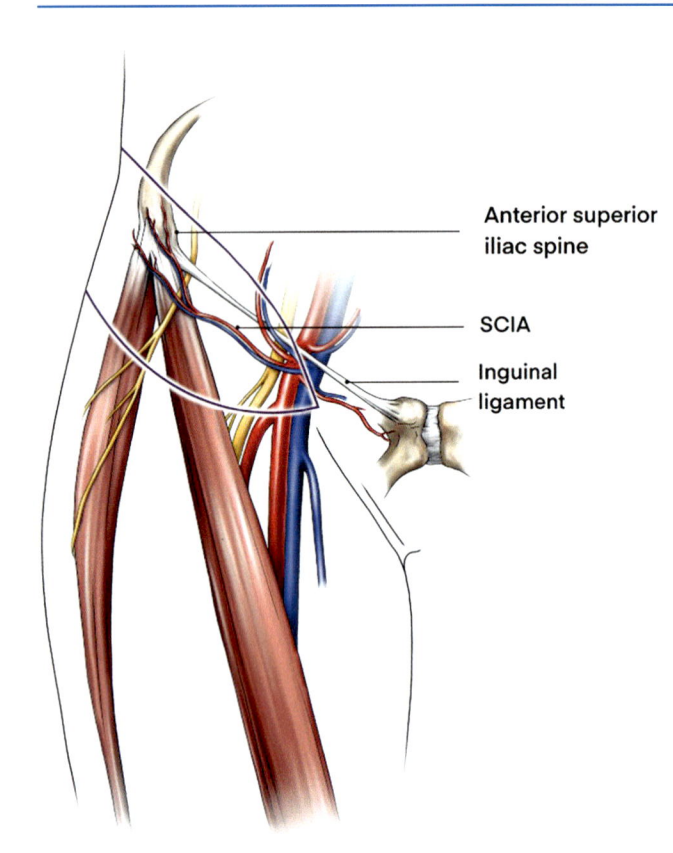

Fig. 33.1 Markings for standard pedicled groin flap

a) 42–45%
Direct from femoral artery

b) 48%
Common origin with SIEA

c) 10–15%
Large SCIA with absent SIEA

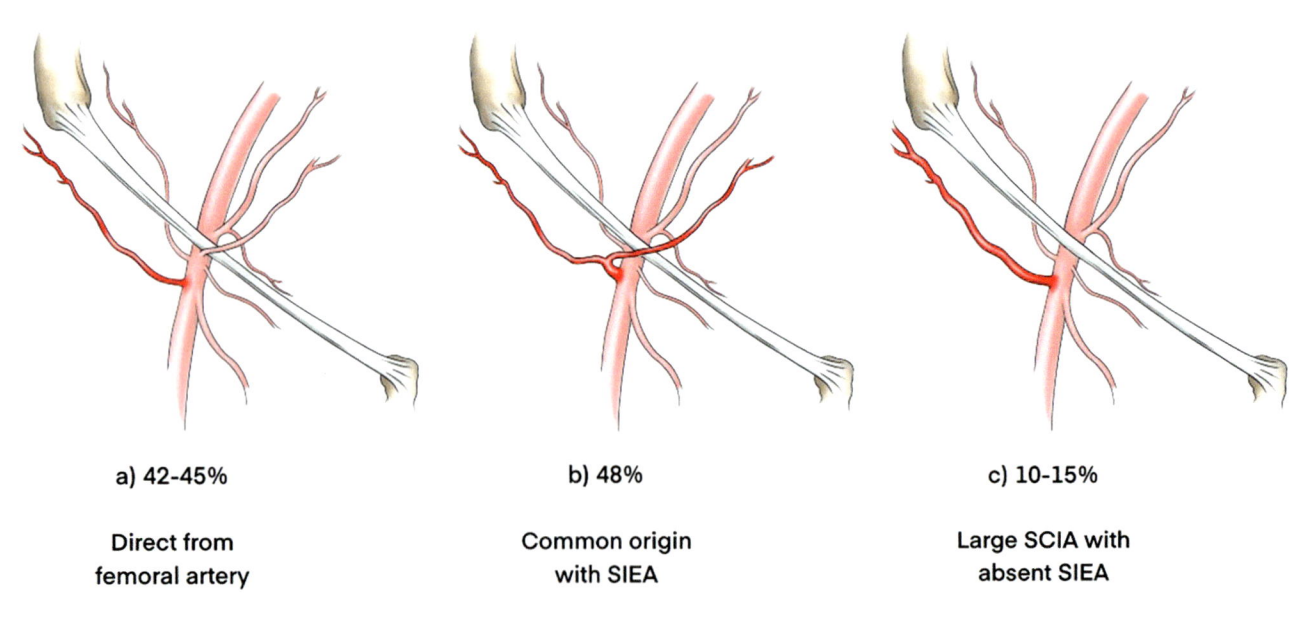

Fig. 33.2 Variations in vessel anatomy of the groin flap

Fig. 33.3 Incorporation of the lateral cutaneous branches providing a sensory groin flap

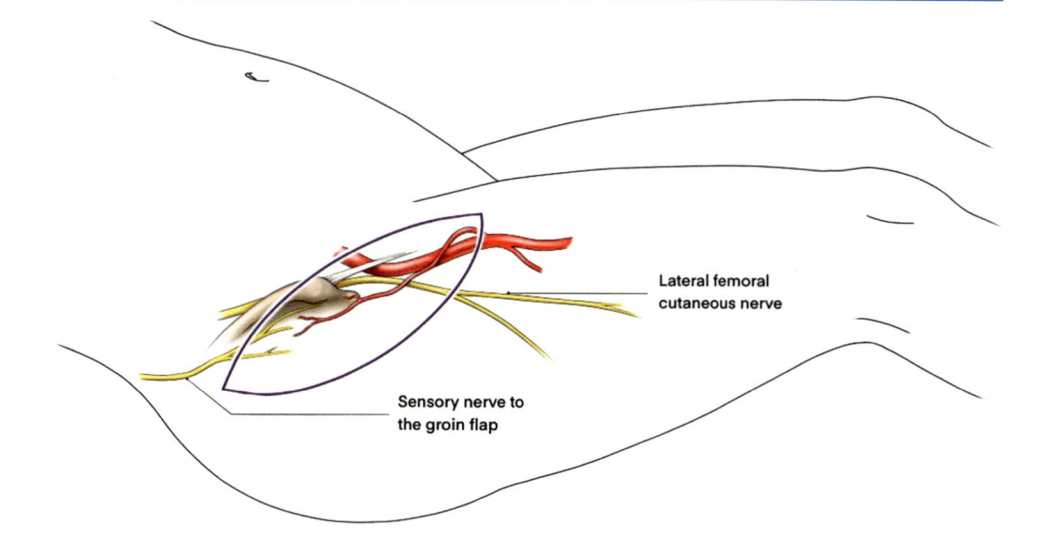

33.3 Preoperative Investigation

The high incidence of anatomical variation makes preoperative marking of vessels and preparation essential. Handheld Doppler is used to identify the femoral artery first. The origin of SCIA can be marked by a handheld Doppler, but we find the use of ultrasound colour Doppler scan more useful in identifying and marking the artery and accompanying veins [13]. The size and direction of the vessels also can be identified with ultrasound colour Doppler scan. The more superficial and thin groin flap harvested needs a higher frequency ultrasound probe. The standard probes of 13–20 Mhz are enough for the main vessels. CT angiograms are not used for this purpose. We prefer to trim the pubic hair in all cases of groin flaps, and it is very important to keep in mind the outline of hair and not to raise any part of it while transferring the flap.

33.4 Flap Design and Markings

First mark the midline, and then trace your hand to identify the most prominent point along the hip which is the ASIS. Now draw a line from midline to ASIS which is the inguinal ligament. Along the ASIS draw the outline of the sartorius muscle.

The next step is to palpate the femoral artery and mark it. Two finger breadths below and parallel (3 cm) to the inguinal ligament the SCIA is given off, and it goes towards the ASIS. At the lateral border of the sartorius, the pedicle becomes superficial (Fig. 33.4).

The flap is marked 5 cm below and above the inguinal ligament and the length on an average between 10 and 20 cm is marked. Primary closure is possible if the width of the flap is up to 10 cm.

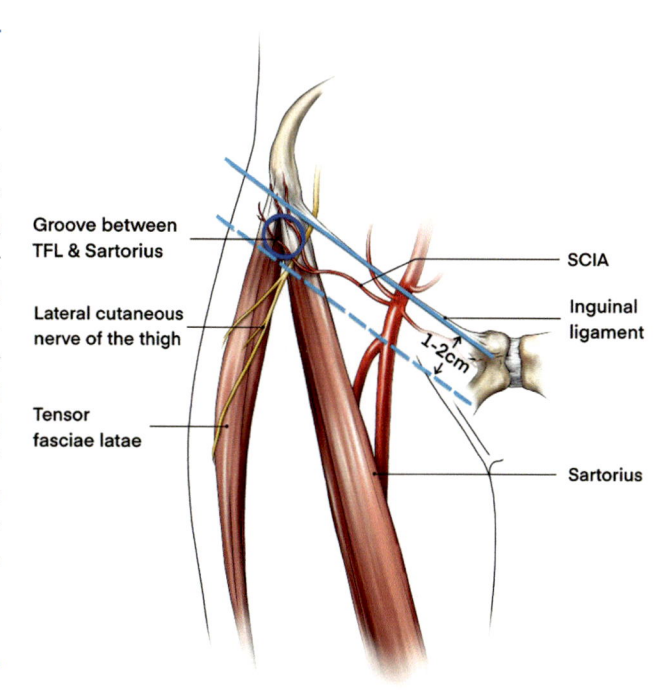

Fig. 33.4 Illustration of anatomical landmarks determining the location of the SCIA

33.5 Flap Raise/Elevation: A Step-by-Step Guide

Setup

- Position of patient: Supine with a folded sheet under the hip to raise the side of harvest. Good access to the lateral aspect of groin is important.
- Anaesthesia: The surgery can either be done under regional anaesthesia or general. If regional is preferred, an upper limb block and spinal or combined spinal with epidural anaesthesia is advised.

Fig. 33.5 Illustration demonstrating the plane of dissection incorporating the fascia over the sartorius so that the SCIA is included in a pedicled or free groin flap

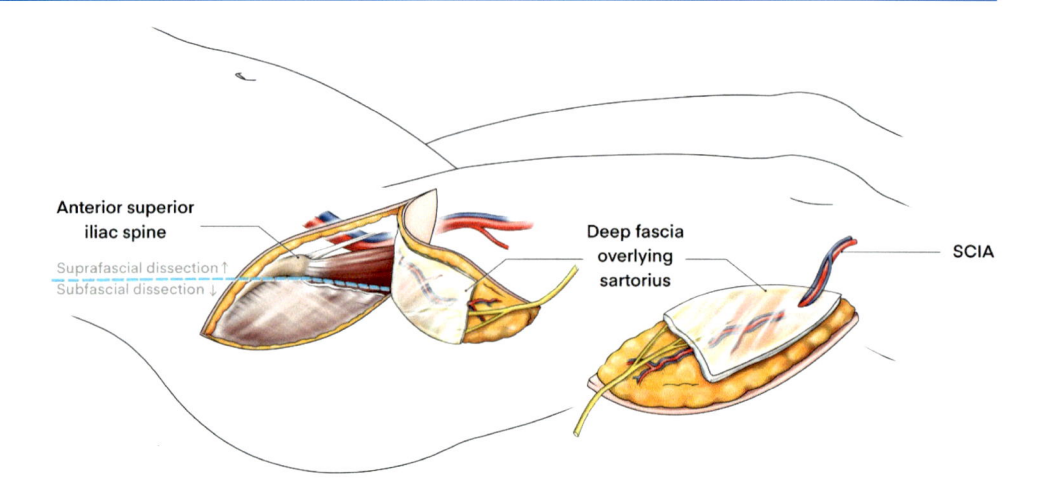

Pedicled Groin Flap

- **Incision** made on superior margin followed by lateral margin using a number 10 or number 15 blade.
- **Flap raise:** The flap is raised suprafascially till we reach the lateral margin of the sartorius. Once the lateral border of the sartorius is reached, the dissection proceeds subfascially (Fig. 33.5).
- **Pedicle identification**: Once the fascia over the sartorius is raised, along the medial margin, the SCIA can be seen and raised along with the flap. There may be small muscular branches entering the sartorius which need to be carefully cauterised with bipolar cautery.
- **Pedicle dissection**: The lateral femoral cutaneous nerve is seen 1 cm inferior and medial to ASIS and should be safeguarded. It could be sacrificed if coming between the pedicles. The flap is raised up to its origin from the femoral artery. As mentioned before in more than half of the patients, we will encounter common trunk of SCIA and SIEA. The dissection proceeds up to the femoral artery in case of free groin flap, whereas in pedicle flap we can stop the dissection up to medial border of the sartorius.
- **Closure of donor site:** Up to 10 cm width of flap can be closed primarily in most cases; wider flaps would need skin grafting of donor site. Flexing the hip and knee facilitates donor site closure.
- **Flap division:** The flap is divided at 3 weeks and inset is completed. In case of tubed groin flap as done for thumb loss or degloving, a delay at the base of flap is done at 3 weeks, and then final division and inset are given at 4 weeks. The delay is carried out under local anaesthesia, a handheld Doppler is used to mark the axial vessel and then the incision is kept, and the vessels are divided and cauterised. The skin closed and at the time of division, the incision passes through the delay site.

Free Groin Flap Identification of the SCIA pedicle should ideally be performed preoperatively with a colour/pencil Doppler. If the location of SCIA is not clear and if there is a combined SCIA and SIEA take-off from the femoral artery, it is better we visualise their origin from the femoral artery first.

- **Incision**: A medial incision is first made and overlying the femoral vessels and the origin if SCIA is seen. The origin also gives us an idea on the size of the pedicle. Once visualised the incision is kept lower and parallel to inguinal ligament. If on medial access incision we find that the vessel size is too small, a pedicled flap can still be raised for extremity reconstruction.
- **Alternative incision**: An alternative approach which some authors advocate is making the incision in the same fashion as the pedicled approach; however, a medial approach enables tailoring of the length of the pedicle and the skin paddle. This was the initial description as per Taylor et al.
- **Flap dissection** is carried out subfascially till the sartorius, and upon reaching the sartorius, the pedicle previously identified is kept in full view on the medial aspect of the flap. Further, dissection should continue right to the origin of the femoral artery to ensure maximal pedicle length. The incision of fascia is then performed with both the pedicle in view medially and the medial aspect of the sartorius identified laterally. *Note*: Inclusion of the deep branch of SCIA is paramount, which runs beneath the fascia of the sartorius.
- **Venous selection for anastomosis:** In addition to the venae comitantes, we advocate incorporation of another superficial vein.

33.6 Core Surgical Techniques in Flap Dissection

- **Pedicle appraisal.** Upon identification of the pedicle for the free groin flap, if the pedicle is too small or insufficient, the superficial inferior epigastric artery could offer

an alternative or consideration given to the contralateral side.
- **Skin flap raising.** When determining how thin the flap is to be upon initial inset, holding the distal edges of the flap under tension with skin hooks and the use of toothed forceps with McIndoe scissors has been found to be effective.
- **Donor site closure.** Flexion of the hip can help facilitate donor site closure.
- **Skin island placement**. Lateral placement of the skin island provides both an increase in pedicle length and reduction of the thickness of the medial portion of the flap and helps avoid the presence of hair-bearing tissue.
- **Dissection over the sartorius muscle** (critical step).
- **Adjustment of flap markings**. Once the pedicle has been identified through dissection, the markings can be adjusted to centralise the pedicle on the flap.

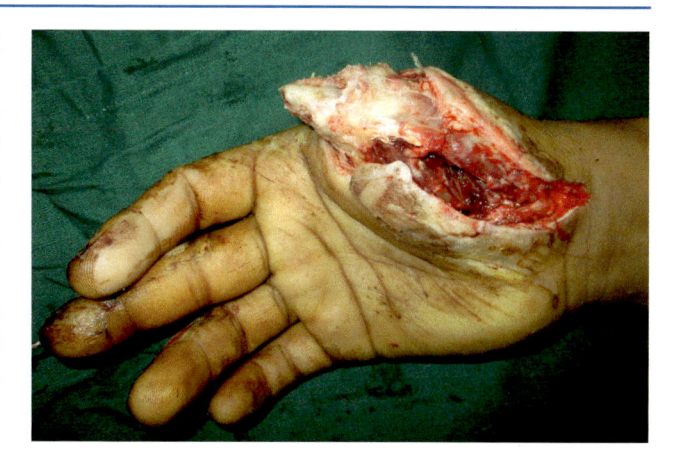

Fig. 33.7 Status after debridement

33.7 Clinical Scenario

33.7.1 Clinical Scenario A: Dr. Sabapathy and Dr. Venkatrami: Loss of Thumb Following Trauma (Figs. 33.6, 33.7, 33.8, 33.9, 33.10, 33.11, 33.12, and 33.13)

The first stage is surgical debridement and pedicled groin flap cover. The key steps are marking the flap and keeping the flap base along the medial border of the sartorius. The opposite thumb girth is measured and the flap designed keeping the width of the flap equal on both sides of the line marking the course of SCIA. The flap is inset into the dorsal side first, and then tubing starts, and the seam of the flap is kept along the medial inner aspect of the new thumb. This way we have both options once the flap has settled, namely, osteoplastic reconstruction using an iliac crest bone graft and a Littler's island flap for sensation. The other option is second toe transfer with part of metatarsal. This patient had the former.

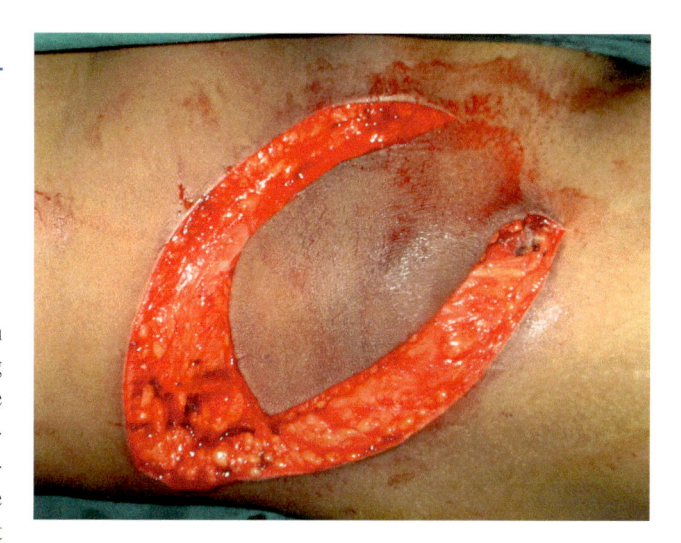

Fig. 33.8 A groin flap has been raised to cover the defect and provide soft tissue for further reconstruction

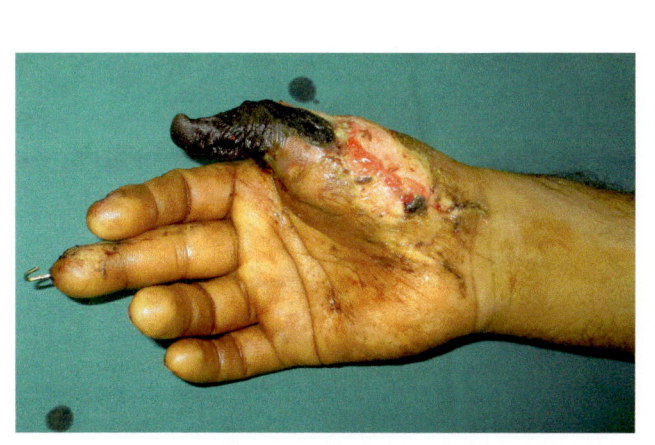

Fig. 33.6 Crush injury right hand which has resulted in gangrene of the thumb referred for further reconstruction

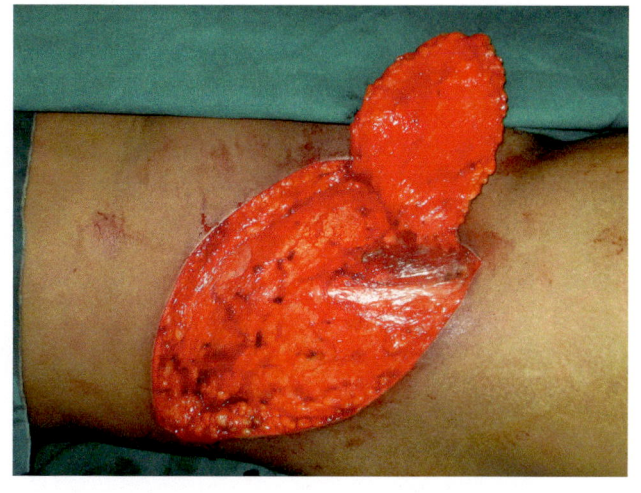

Fig. 33.9 Groin flap raised up to anti-superior iliac spine

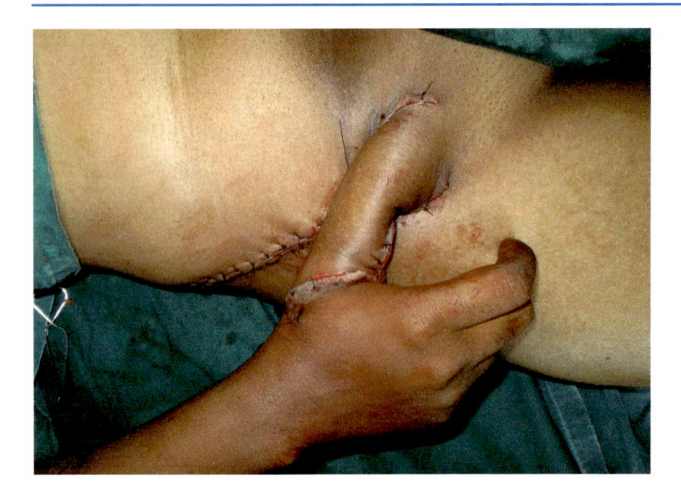

Fig. 33.10 The flap is attached in the direction of the thumb. (Note: Suture line comes from inner side which could be opened up for further reconstruction. The donor area primarily closed)

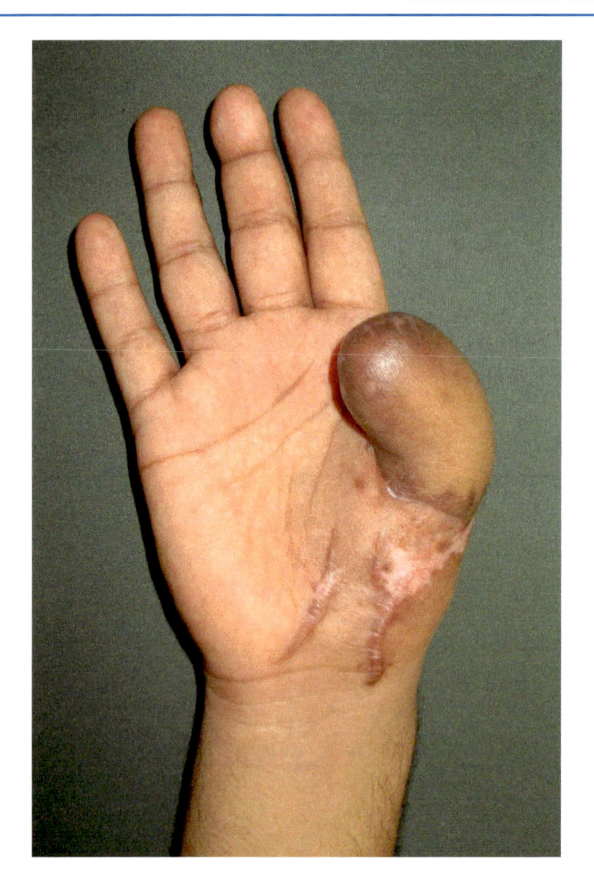

Fig. 33.11 The flap after division before further reconstruction. The flap length is adequate for both osteoplastic reconstruction and toe transfer

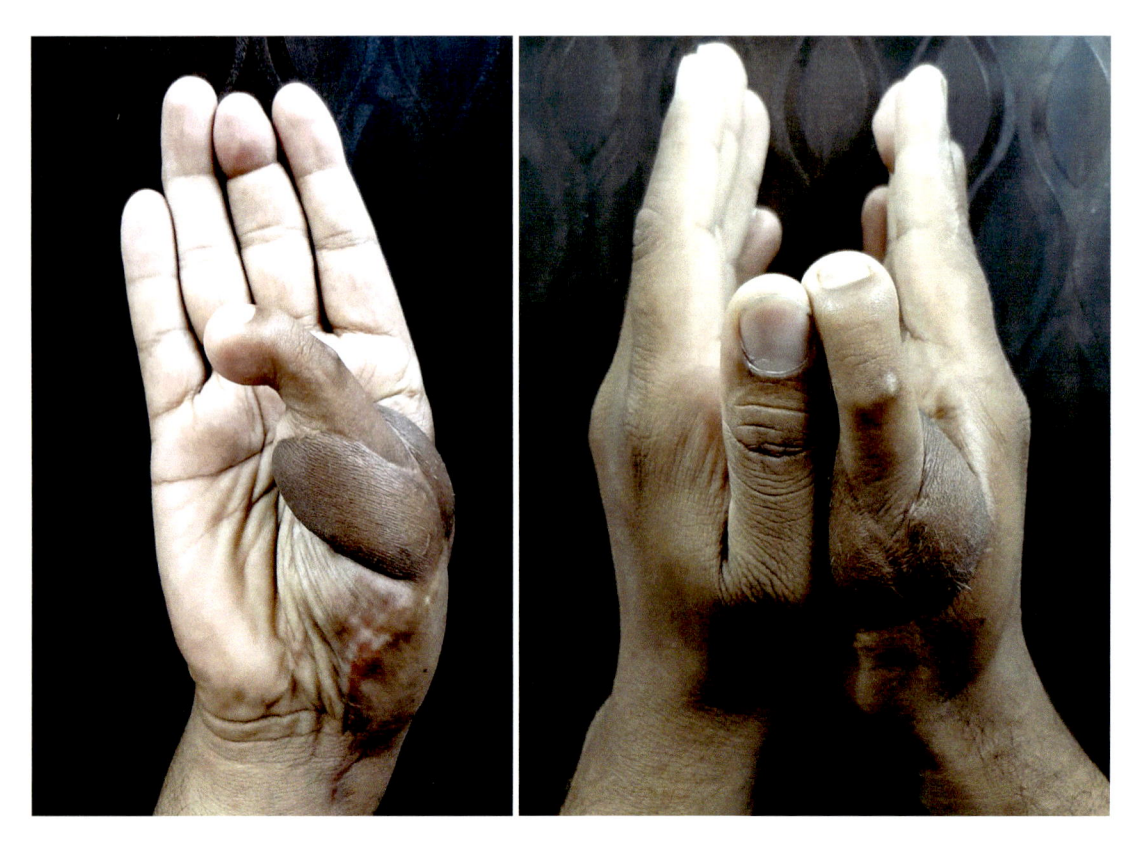

Figs. 33.12 and 33.13 Second toe transfer done using flap skin on the side and flap excised

33.7.2 Clinical Scenario B: Dr Dariush Nikkhah and Dr Jeremy Rawlins Elbow Resurfacing with Free Groin Flap

A 56-year-old man sustained a motor vehicle accident (Fig. 33.14). He had an elbow defect with exposed olecranon

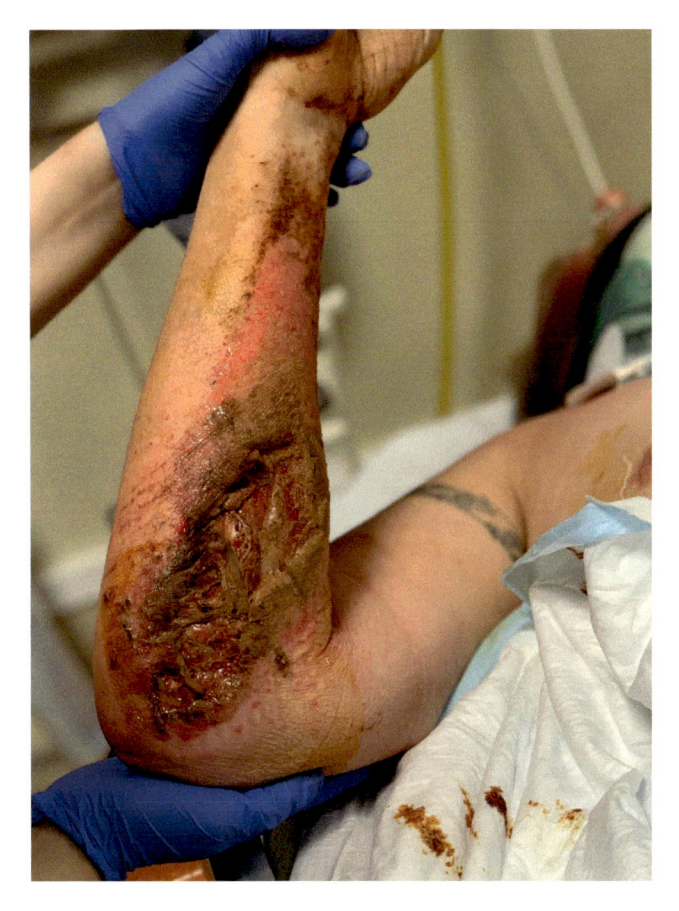

Fig. 33.14 Elbow defect pre-debridement

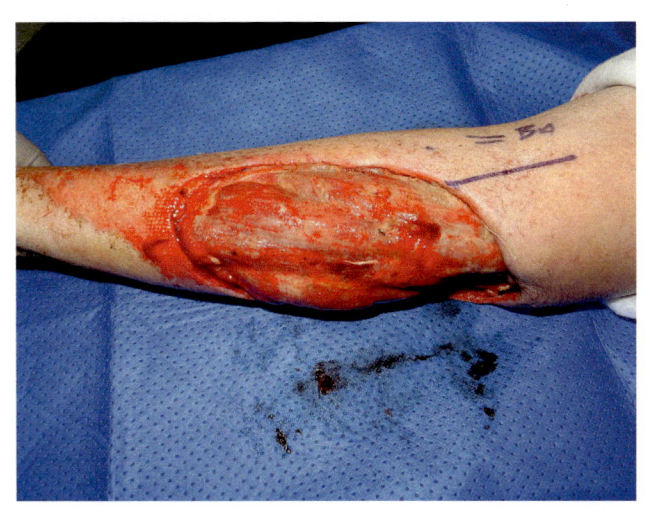

Fig. 33.15 Post-debridement of the elbow showing exposed olecranon

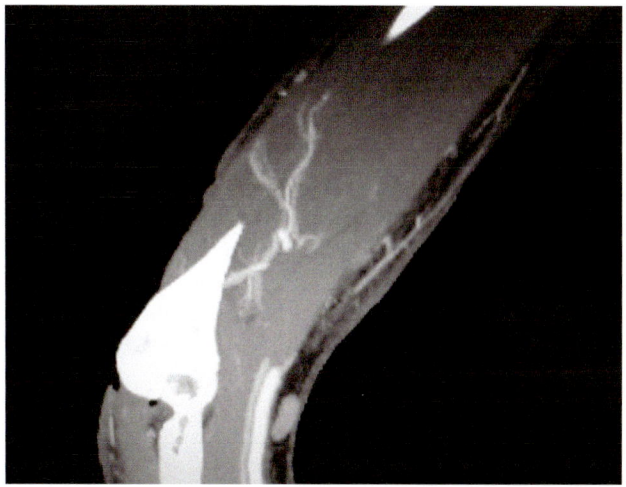

Fig. 33.16 Radial artery perforator chosen as recipient vessels for free groin flap

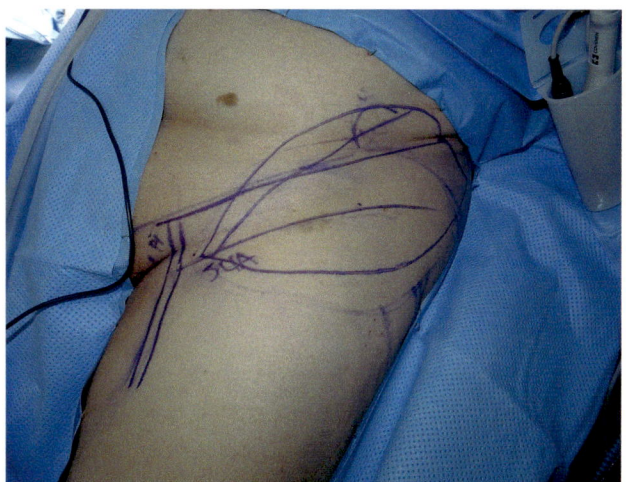

Fig. 33.17 Markings for a modified free groin flap

after initial debridement (Fig. 33.15). A CT angiogram demonstrated good recipient vessels with a perforator emerging from the radial artery (Fig. 33.16). A modified free groin flap was harvested through a medial approach. The SCIA/V vessels were anastomosed to a perforator originating from the radial artery, and a secondary superficial vein was anastomosed for additional venous drainage (Figs. 33.17, 33.18, and 33.19). The patient had an uneventful outcome (Fig. 33.20).

33.7.3 Case Scenario C: Dr Sabapathy and Dr Venkatrami

This case demonstrates a staged pedicled groin flap for volar skin loss of the right middle ring and little fingers (Figs. 33.21, 33.22, 33.23, 33.24, 33.25 and 33.26).

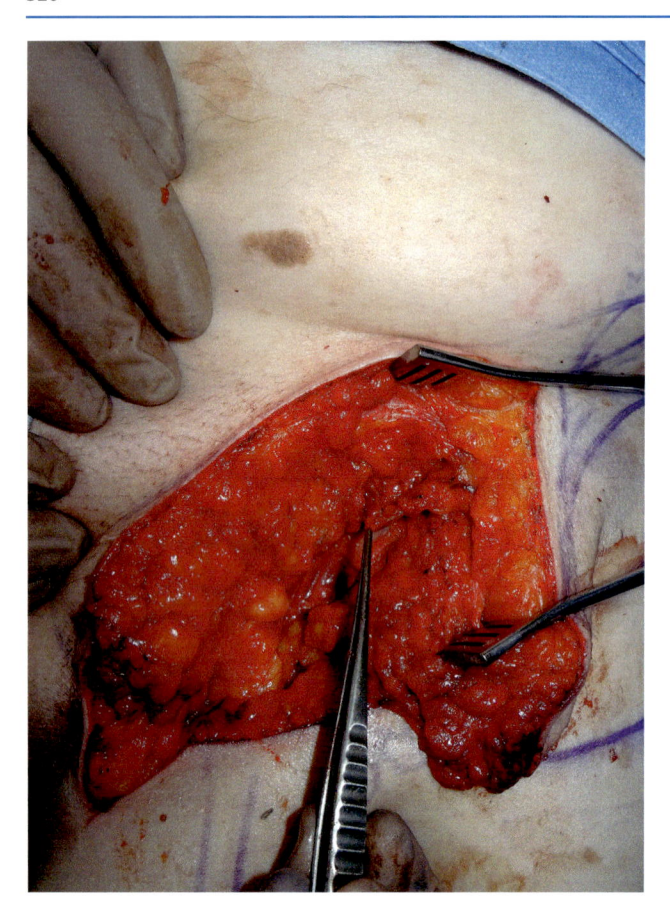

Fig. 33.18 Medial approach demonstrating SCIA/V vessels

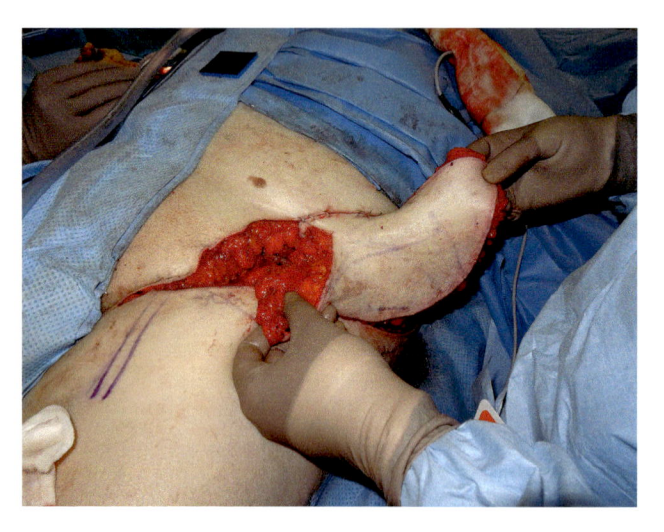

Fig. 33.19 Free groin flap raised demonstrating short pedicle

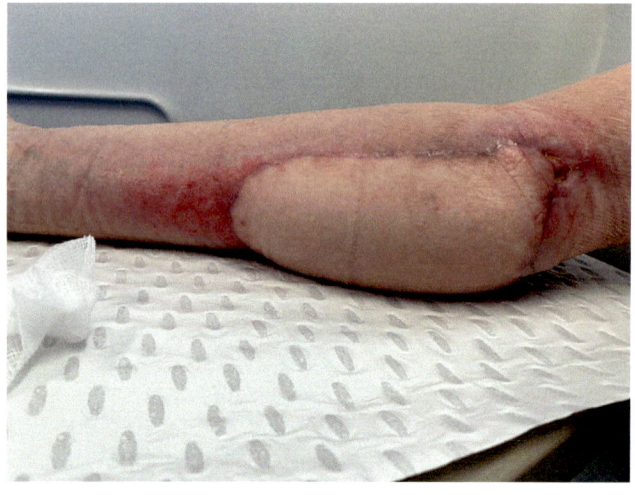

Fig. 33.20 Early result demonstrating robust wound coverage in a single stage

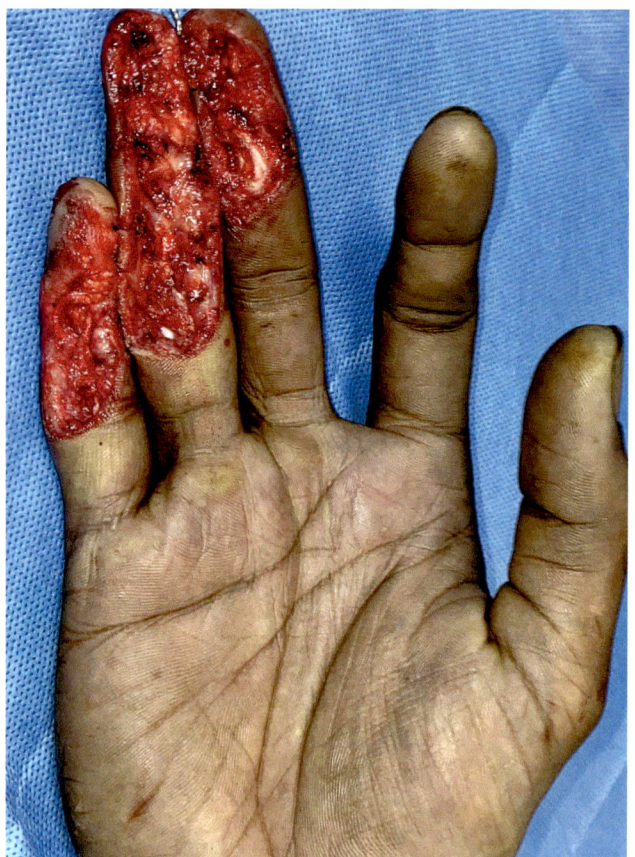

Fig. 33.21 Composite tissue loss on volar aspect of the right, middle, ring and little fingers with exposure of the flexor tendons after debridement and loss of FDP in the ring finger

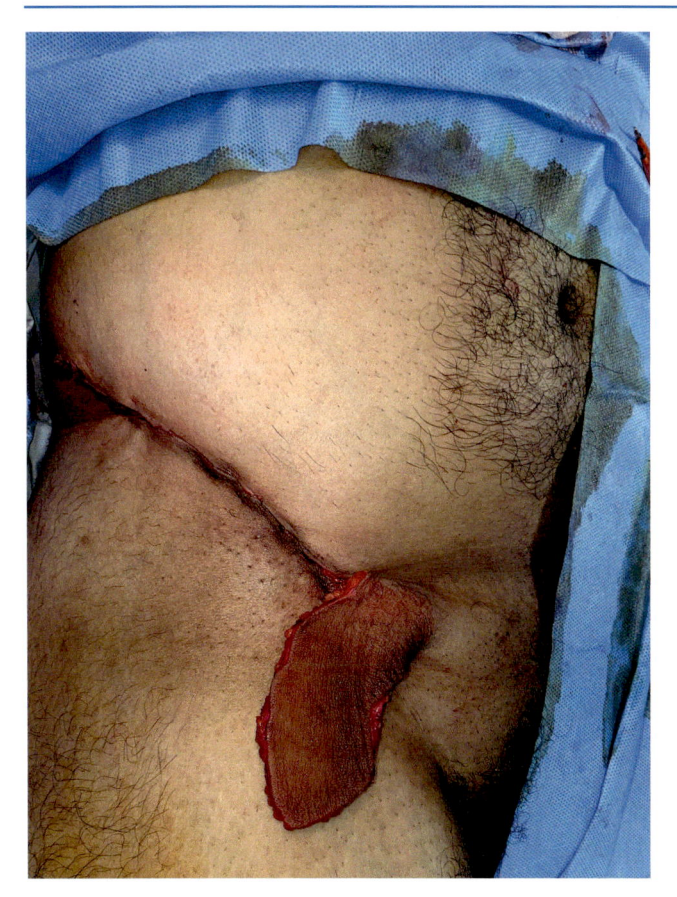

Fig. 33.22 Pedicled groin flap raised and the donor area closed

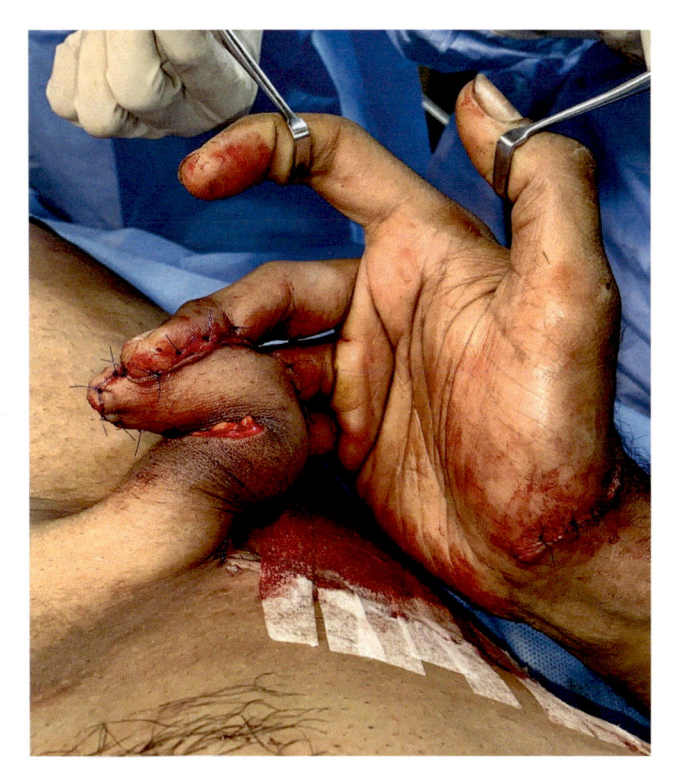

Fig. 33.23 Groin flap inset into the defect

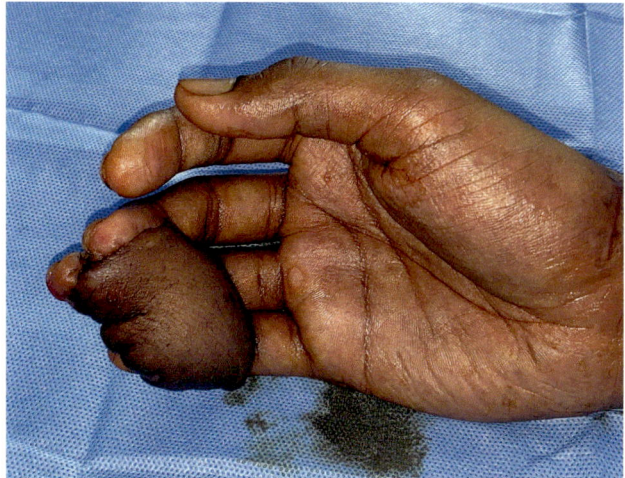

Fig. 33.24 Picture after division

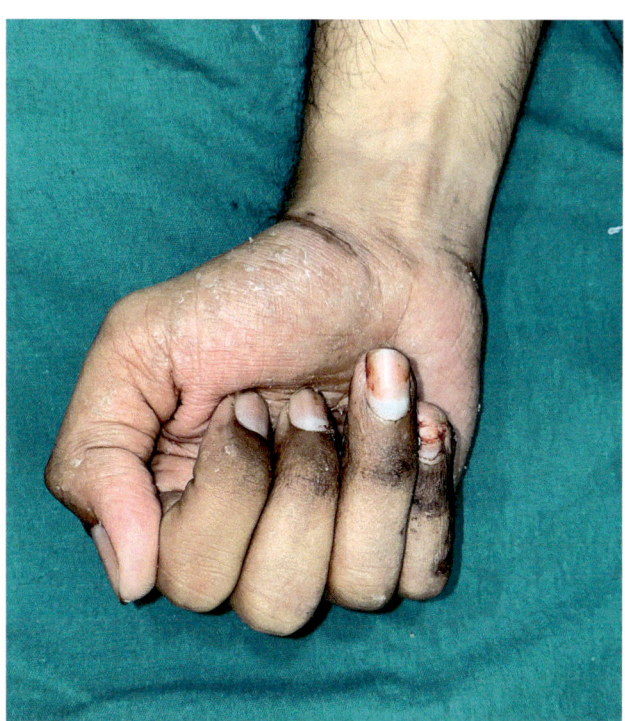

Fig. 33.25 Functional outcome after syndactyly separation and thinning of flaps

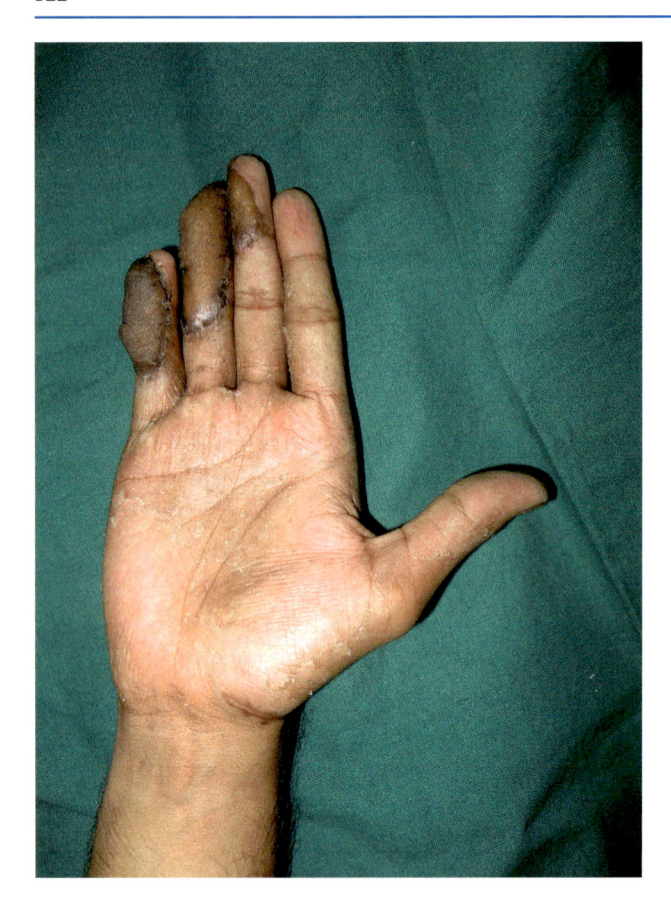

Fig. 33.26 Final result after flap inset and digits separated

33.8 Pearls and Pitfalls

> **Pearls**
> Hairless skin lies along the groin crease laterally and the skin island should be centred over this region.
> - Primary closure possible in majority of cases if the width of the flap is less than 10 cm. One can also undermine the upper abdominal flap to facilitate closure.
> - The inclusion of lymphatic tissue in the flap helps mitigate distal oedema.
> - Secondary thinning is safe [14].
> - Can take really long flap going along the trunk.

> **Pitfalls**
> - In patients with a high BMI, there is difficulty in harvest and it may not be an appropriate choice of flap.
> - Pedicle size and length can be short and small when used as free flap. The pedicle length can range from 2 cm – 6 cm however placing the skin island more lateral can help provide a longer pedicle when performing a free flap.
> - Joint stiffness in crush injury of the hand (particularly in pedicled flap).
> - Edge necrosis if a very long flap is raised.
> - Need for delay in tubed flaps.

33.9 Selected Readings

- McGregor IA, Jackson IT. The groin flap. Br J Plast Surg. 1972 Jan;25(1):3–16. https://doi.org/10.1016/s0007-1226(72)80003-1.
  First paper to describe the groin flap [1].
- Smith PJ, Foley B, McGregor IA, Jackson IT. The anatomical basis of the groin flap. Plast Reconstr Surg. 1972 Jan;49(1):41–7. https://doi.org/10.1097/00006534-197, 201,000-00008.
  Anatomical paper identifying that the superficial circumflex iliac artery was consistently present [15].
- Knutson GH. The groin flap: a new technique to repair traumatic tissue defects. Can Med Assoc J. 1977 Mar 19;116(6):623–5.
  Seminal paper which popularised the groin flap [16].
- Cobb ARM, Koudstaal MJ, Bulstrode NW, Lloyd TW, Dunaway DJ. Free groin flap in hemifacial volume reconstruction. Br J Oral Maxillofac Surg. 2013 Jun;51(4):301–6. https://doi.org/10.1016/j.bjoms.2012.09.004.
  Consecutive case series of 14 patients who had hemifacial augmentation with a free groin flap [5].
- Hough M, Fenn C, Kay SP. The use of free groin flaps in children. Plast Reconstr Surg. 2004 Apr 1;113(4):1161–6. https://doi.org/10.1097/01.prs.0000110329.68009.4c.
  Consecutive case series of 33 patients who had reconstructions with a free groin flap for a variety of aetiologies including trauma, congenital and tumour based [8].

- Sabapathy SR, Bajantri B. Indications, Selection and use of distant pedicled flaps in upper limb reconstryction. Hand Clin 2014;30(2):185–199.

  An article which provides all the important technical tips to obtain good outcomes with the pedicled groin and abdominal flaps.

References

1. McGregor IA, Jackson IT. The groin flap. Br J Plast Surg. 1972 Jan;25(1):3–16.
2. Taylor GI, Daniel RK. The free flap: composite tissue transfer by vascular anastomosis. Aust N Z J Surg. 1973 Jul;43(1):1–3.
3. Bajantri B, Latheef L, Sabapathy SR. Tips to orient pedicled groin flap for hand defects. Tech Hand Up Extrem Surg. 2013 Jun;17(2):68–71.
4. Jokuszies A, Niederbichler AD, Hirsch N, Kahlmann D, Herold C, Vogt PM. The pedicled groin flap for defect closure of the hand. Oper Orthop Traumatol. 2010 Oct;22(4):440–51.
5. Cobb ARM, Koudstaal MJ, Bulstrode NW, Lloyd TW, Dunaway DJ. Free groin flap in hemifacial volume reconstruction. Br J Oral Maxillofac Surg. 2013 Jun;51(4):301–6.
6. Aydin T, Feyzi K, Tayfun T, Berna T. Reconstruction of wide scrotal defect using groin fasciocutaneous island flap combined with a strip of deep fascia. J Plast Reconstr Aesthet Surg. 2010 Aug;63(8):1394–5.
7. Zeltzer AA, Anzarut A, Braeckmans D, Seidenstuecker K, Hendrickx B, Van Hedent E, et al. The vascularized groin lymph node flap (VGLN): anatomical study and flap planning using multidetector CT scanner. The golden triangle for flap harvesting. J Surg Oncol. 2017 Sep;116(3):378–83.
8. Hough M, Fenn C, Kay SP. The use of free groin flaps in children. Plast Reconstr Surg. 2004 Apr 1;113(4):1161–6.
9. Chuang DC, Jeng SF, Chen HT, Chen HC, Wei FC. Experience of 73 free groin flaps. Br J Plast Surg. 1992 Mar;45(2):81–5.
10. Cormack GC, Lamberty BG. A classification of fascio-cutaneous flaps according to their patterns of vascularisation. Br J Plast Surg. 1984 Jan;37(1):80–7.
11. Sinna R, Hajji H, Qassemyar Q, Perignon D, Benhaim T, Havet E. Anatomical background of the perforator flap based on the deep branch of the superficial circumflex iliac artery (SCIP flap): a cadaveric study. Eplasty. 2010 Jan 18;10:e11.
12. Gentileschi S, Servillo M, De Bonis F, Albanese R, Pino V, Mangialardi ML, et al. Radioanatomical study of the pedicle of the superficial circumflex iliac perforator flap. J Reconstr Microsurg. 2019 Nov;35(9):669–76.
13. Tashiro K, Harima M, Kato M, Yamamoto T, Yamashita S, Narushima M, et al. Preoperative color Doppler ultrasound assessment in planning of SCIP flaps. J Plast Reconstr Aesthet Surg. 2015 Jul;68(7):979–83.
14. Kimura N, Saitoh M, Hasumi T, Sumiya N, Itoh Y. Clinical application and refinement of the microdissected thin groin flap transfer operation. J Plast Reconstr Aesthet Surg. 2009 Nov;62(11):1510–6.
15. Smith PJ, Foley B, McGregor IA, Jackson IT. The anatomical basis of the groin flap. Plast Reconstr Surg. 1972 Jan;49(1):41–7.
16. Knutson GH. 7. The groin flap: a new technique to repair traumatic tissue defects. Can Med Assoc J. 1977 Mar 19;116(6):623–5.

Superficial Circumflex Iliac Artery Perforator Flap: A Thin and Versatile Option for Limb and Head and Neck Reconstruction

Juan Enrique Berner, Dariush Nikkhah, and Tiew Chong Teo

34.1 Introduction

The superficial circumflex iliac artery perforator (SCIP) flap was first described by Koshima et al. in 2004 [1], as the evolution of the free groin flap popularised by McGregor and Jackson [2]. The SCIP flap can be a thin reconstructive option for most patients, by harvesting skin superior and lateral to the inguinal ligament.

The donor site can be easily closed primarily even when large flaps are designed, leaving a well concealed oblique scar on the iliac fossa. Dissection of the flap and its pedicle is relatively superficial, avoiding tedious raising in difficult anatomical planes. The vascular anatomy of the SCIP flap allows the raising of multiple skin paddles, lymph nodes [3] and even small segments of iliac crest bone [4]. This versatility has been the reason for its recent popularity for lower limb [5], hand [6] and head and neck reconstruction [7].

We have recently proposed a classification system for SCIP flaps based on the contents transferred [6]:

- Type 1: Standard SCIP flap.
- Type 2: Adipofascial SCIP flap.
- Type 3: SCIP flap with multiple skin paddles.
- Type 4: Osteocutaneous SCIP flap.
- Type 5: SCIP flap with vascularised lymph node transfer.
- Type 6: Neurotised SCIP flap.

Supplementary Information The online version contains supplementary material available at [https://doi.org/10.1007/978-3-031-07678-7_34].

J. E. Berner (✉)
Royal Victoria Infirmary, Newcastle upon Tyne, UK

D. Nikkhah
Royal Free Hospital, London, UK
e-mail: d.nikkhah@nhs.net

T. C. Teo
Queen Victoria Hospital, East Grinstead, UK

It has been criticised that its small calibre and short pedicle limit the applications of this flap. However, adequate planning and recipient vessel selection can facilitate its execution.

34.2 Anatomy

The superficial circumflex iliac artery (SCIA) is a cutaneous branch arising from the femoral artery close to the origin of the superficial inferior epigastric artery. The SCIA supplies skin, tegumentum and superficial lymph nodes in the groin area. It follows a supero-lateral course branching into a superficial/medial and a deep/lateral branch [8]. The deep branch runs in the deep fascia, providing muscular perforators to the sartorius muscle, and the skin and iliac bone lateral to this muscle. The superficial branch, instead, follows a superior course crossing the level of the inguinal ligament. It pierces the superficial fascia to then supply the skin superior and laterally heading towards the anterior superior iliac spine (ASIS).

The SCIP flap can be harvested based on perforators arising from the deep/lateral or superficial/medial branches, or even both to obtain a chimeric flap [9]. However, if a single skin paddle is needed, the superficial/medial perforator is more amenable for dissection. This can be found in the great majority of patients around a point 4.5 cm lateral to the pubic tubercle and 1.5 cm superior to it [10].

The length of the pedicle of the SCIP flap will depend on the design of its skin paddle. A more laterally placed flap will therefore have a longer pedicle. The average length of the SCIP pedicle is 6 cm, but can be as long as 8 cm, including vessels of around 1 mm calibre [6].

Compared to the traditional groin flap, the SCIP presents multiple advantages. Its pedicle length can be adjusted as it can be directly incised along its course. The SCIP is a thinner flap, as it can be safely raised at the level of Scarpa's fascia until the pedicle is reached, compared to the groin flap which has to include the deep fascia over sartorius. Furthermore, due to its location inferior to the inguinal ligament, the groin flap is more likely to include hair bearing skin.

© Springer Nature Switzerland AG 2023
D. Nikkhah et al. (eds.), *Core Techniques in Flap Reconstructive Microsurgery*, https://doi.org/10.1007/978-3-031-07678-7_34

34.3 Pre-Operative Investigation

In some centres, the use of computed tomography angiography (CTA) has been advocated to facilitate the planning of the SCIP flap [11]. However, in our experience this is not routinely required. With the patient lying supine in the operative table, the location of the superficial/medial SCIA perforator can be confirmed using a hand-held Doppler device.

More recently, Pereira et al. have proposed the use of augmented reality for planning SCIP flaps. If a CTA has been performed, smartphone-based technology can combine the vascular anatomy with the superficial landmarks in order to ease raising [12]

34.4 Flap Design and Markings

Considering the dimensions of the defect, the SCIP skin paddle can be designed as an ellipse, including the non-hair-bearing skin above the inguinal ligament (Fig. 34.1).

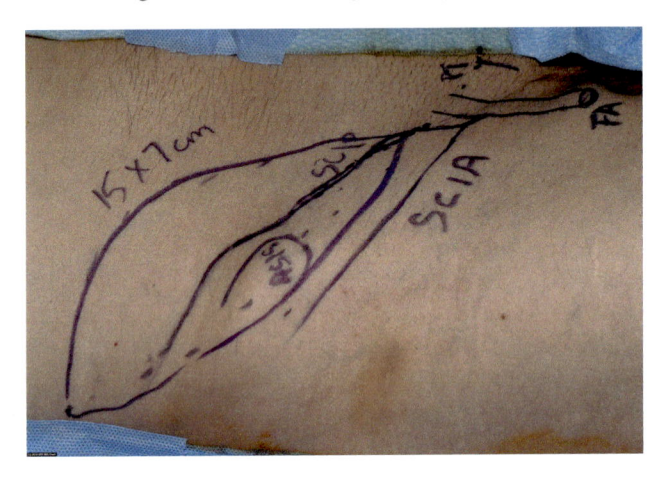

Fig. 34.1 Landmarks drawn before SCIP flap transfer. The ASIS is marked and a line drawn to the pubic tubercle; this illustrates the inguinal ligament. 2 cm below this is the SCIA emerging from the femoral artery. The SCIP perforator is marked emerging superolaterally above the inguinal ligament

We tend to orientate this ellipse parallel to the supero-lateral course of the latter. This particular location allows harvesting a thin flap, while allowing a tensionless closure by mobilising abdominal tissues. As we prefer to raise this flap in an anterograde manner, we also mark an incision line over the course of the SCIP pedicle [6]. This is not required if the flap is raised retrogradely, in other words, from lateral to medial.

34.5 Flap Raise/Elevation: A Step-by-Step Guide

1. *Incision over SCIP pedicle.* An incision over the course of the previously identified SCIP pedicle is performed using a number 15 or 10 blade. We routinely prefer using perforators arising from the medial/superficial branch of the SCIA. Sharp dissection is continued through the superficial flap until the pedicle is visualized (Fig. 34.2a, b). We prefer using the medial to lateral approach as demonstrated here.
2. *Pedicle dissection.* Using a combination of blunt, sharp and bipolar dissection the SCIP pedicle is dissected along its course. Debakey forces are used carefully handling the vessels. The pedicle is traced to its origin on the SCIA (Fig. 34.3a, b).
3. *Pedicle appraisal and flap design adjustment.* Once the pedicle has been exposed it can be appraised before committing to the raising of the skin paddle. If necessary its design can be adjusted to obtain a longer pedicle (Fig. 34.4).
4. *Skin flap raising and incorporation of extra superficial vein.* While protecting the previously dissected pedicle, the margins of the flap can be incised using a cold blade. Raising can be done either at the level of the external oblique muscle fascia, or through Scarpa's fascia using finger-switch diathermy [13] (Fig. 34.5a). We

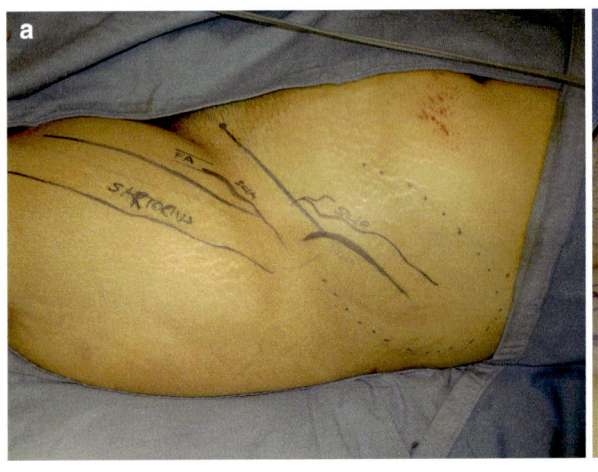

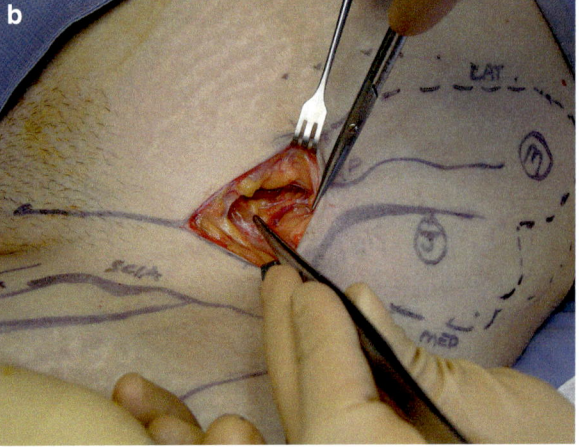

Fig. 34.2 (a) Landmarks of the SCIP flap before elevation. (b) Medial approach to SCIP flap, showing identification of the superficial perforator

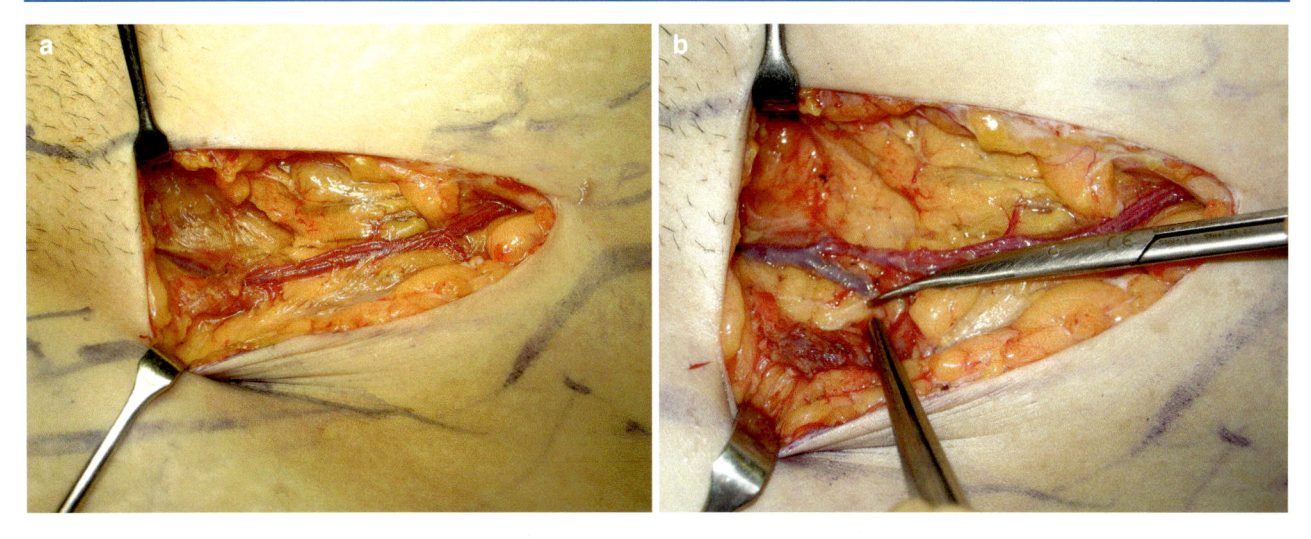

Fig. 34.3 (**a**) Dissection of SCIP pedicle adjusting desired pedicle length and dissection down to its origin at the SCIA (**b**)

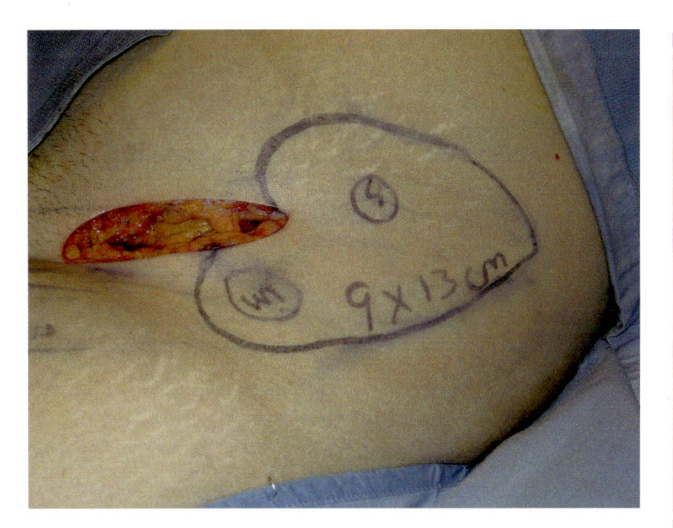

Fig. 34.4 The skin paddle is finalised after templating the defect to be reconstructed

also routinely include an extra superficial vein. (Fig. 34.5b).

5. *Pedicle division and transfer.* The pedicle can be then clipped in its origin and divided for transfer. By this stage the recipient vessels should be prepared. If anastomosing to a perforator on the recipient site, this can be done end-to-end. If anastomosing to a named vessel is preferred, usually it is done end-to-side due to vessel discrepancy (Fig. 34.6).

6. *Donor site closure.* Abdominal laxity allows tensionless closure of large flaps in the groin area. It is important not to undermine the abdomen to avoid contour deformities. Closure is obtained by using 2–0 PDS dermal sutures and 3–0 monocryl subcuticular suture (Fig. 34.7).

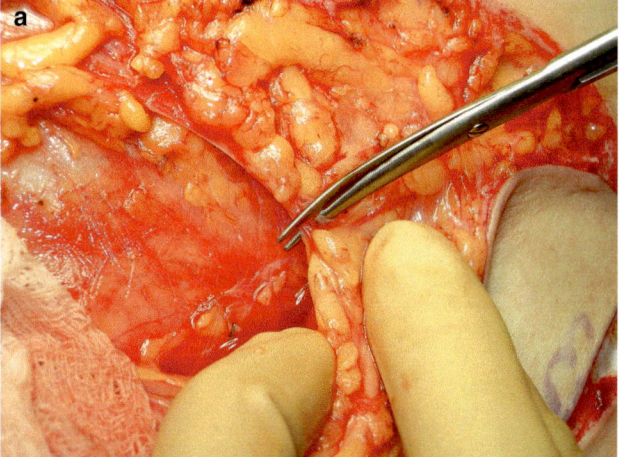

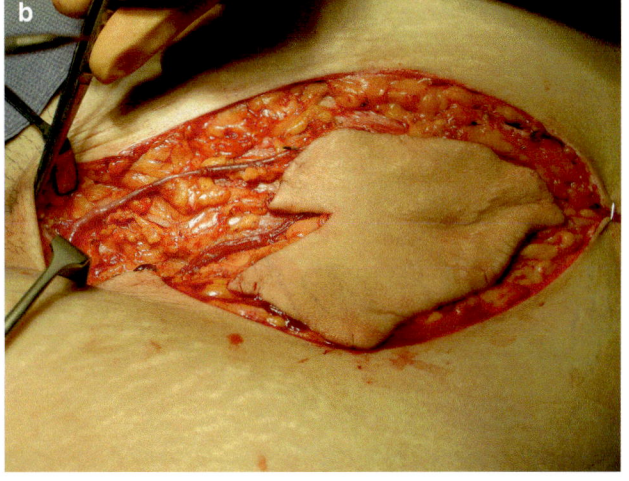

Fig. 34.5 (**a**) The flap is raised off the external oblique fascia superiorly and (**b**) an extra superficial vein is incorporated into the skin flap

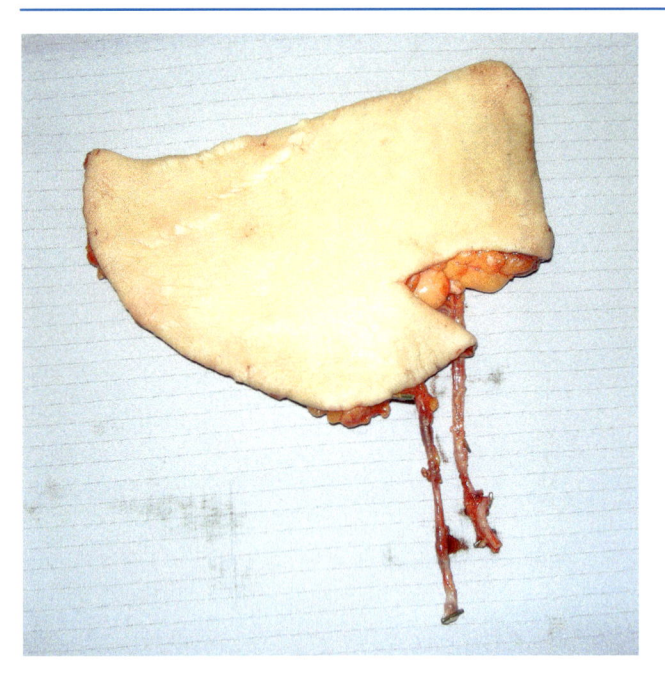

Fig. 34.6 The pedicle is divided before SCIP transfer. The vein is marked with blue ink. A pedicle length of 6 cm was taken in this case

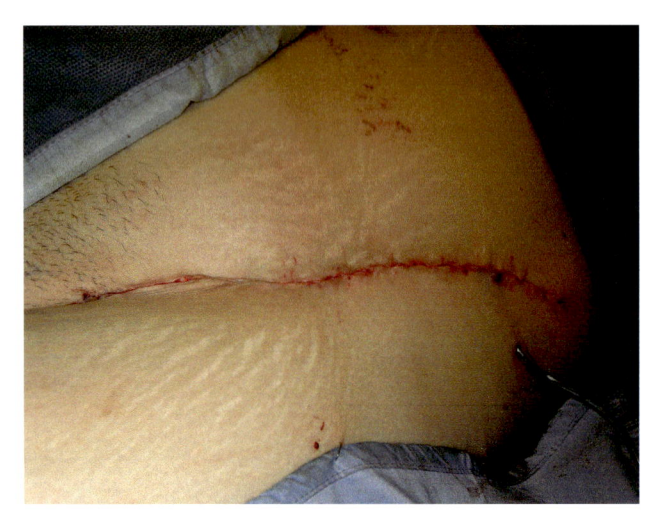

Fig. 34.7 The donor site is closed in layers and a suction drain is placed

34.6 Core Surgical Techniques in Flap Dissection

1. *Incision over SCIP pedicle.* The use of a West self-retaining retractor provides adequate retraction, easing sharp dissection. No assistant is needed for raising this flap.
2. *Pedicle dissection.* Debakey forceps and tenotomy scissors are our preferred instruments for pedicle dissection, along with bipolar diathermy. Vessel Loops can be used to carefully retract vessels as the pedicle is freed up from neighbouring tissues.
3. *Pedicle appraisal and flap design adjustment.* It is advantageous to adjust the flap design to include any superficial veins in its vicinity. This can be later used as a lifeboat if drainage via the SCIP venae comitans is inadequate.
4. *Skin flap raising.* At this point it is convenient to have an assistant holding Senn-Mueller retractors, especially if dissection through Scarpa's fascia is decided.
5. *Pedicle division and transfer.* If the calibre of the SCIP artery is too small for a safe anastomosis in the hand of the operating surgeon, the main trunk of the SCIA can be taken at its origin from the femoral artery. By doing this the pedicle can be lengthened to a limited extent.
6. *Donor site closure.* We do not tend to insert drains on the donor site for this flap unless a very large flap has been taken with significant undermining of the abdominal wall.

34.7 Clinical Scenario

Case Scenario 1 Surgeon TC Teo A 46-year-old female underwent an excision of a painful leiomyoma on her left upper arm. A 14 × 25 cm defect was created that required reconstruction with a large superficial circumflex iliac artery perforator (SCIP) flap. The anterograde raising of this flap is shown, first incising over its pedicle to identify the SCIP vessels to then subsequently complete the whole raising of the skin paddle. The flap was then inset in the defect while and the donor site was closed directly. Patient presented an uneventful recovery. (Figs. 34.8, 34.9, 34.10, and 34.11).

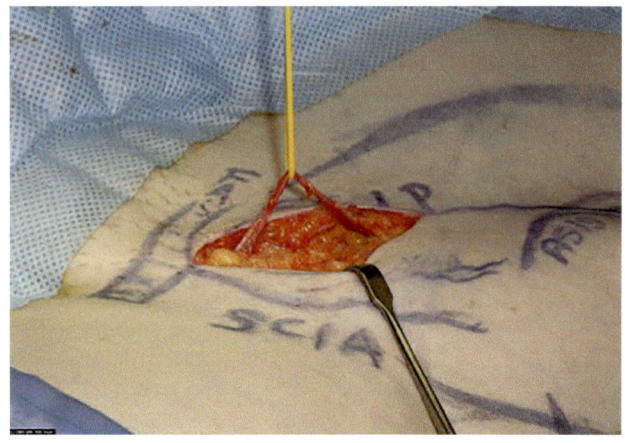

Fig. 34.8 Medial approach to the pedicle of SCIP

Fig. 34.9 Large 19 by 25 cm SCIP flap raised to reconstruct Leiomyoma defect

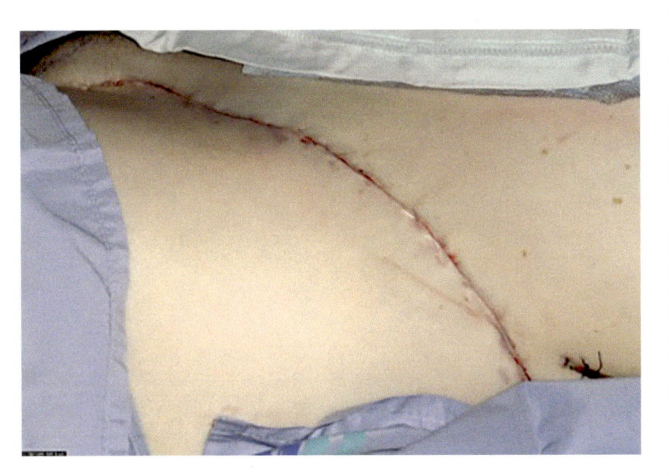

Fig. 34.10 Tensionless donor site closure after large SCIP flap

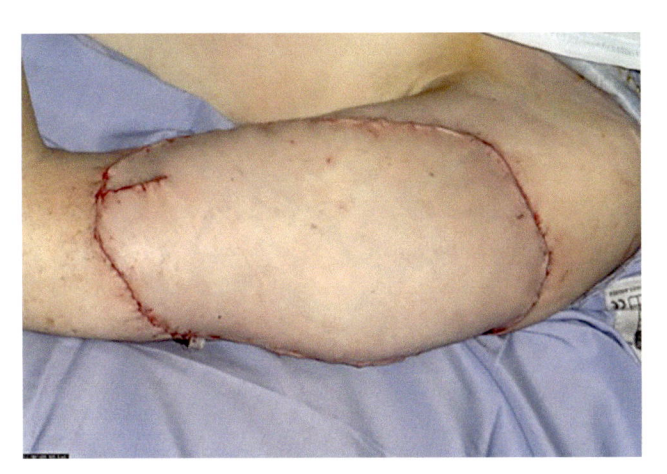

Fig. 34.11 Leiomyoma defect closed with SCIP flap

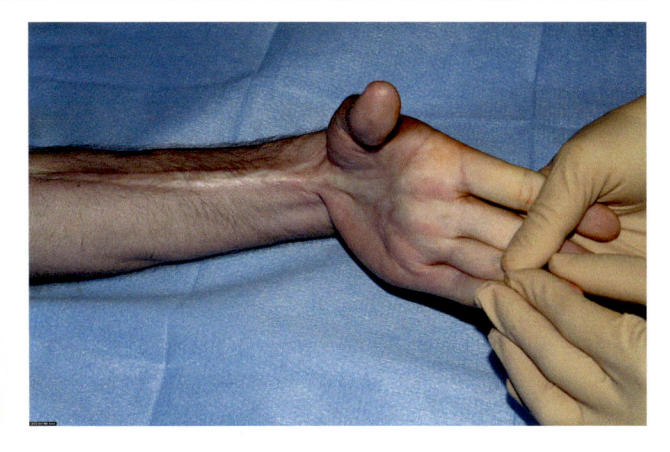

Fig. 34.12 Patient with significant wrist flexion contracture secondary to Volkmann's contracture

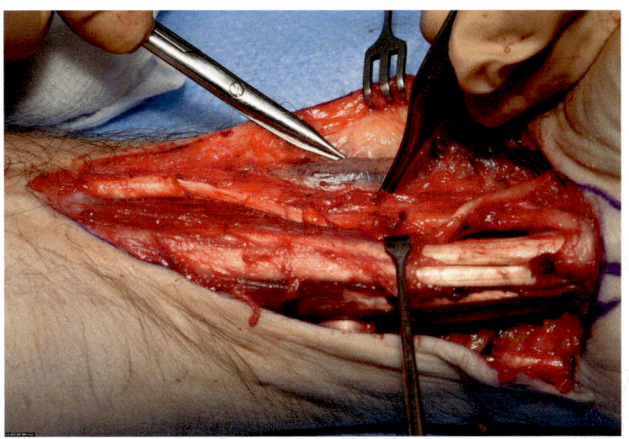

Fig. 34.13 Wrist contracture released with resultant defect with exposed flexor tendons. Radial vessels dissected as recipient vessels for SCIP flap

Case Scenario 2 Surgeon TC Teo and D Nikkhah A 37-year-old man was referred to our unit for a long-standing left forearm and hand Volksmann contracture, following a missed compartment syndrome years ago. In order to get his wrist in to a more functional position, an extensive scar release was performed, including flexor tendon lengthening and a proximal row carpectomy. The resulting defect was resurfaced with a 15 × 7 SCIP flap anastomosed end to side to the radial artery and end to end to the Venae Comitans. The intraoperative photographs showing the preparation of the radial vessels, raising of the SCIP pedicle, inset and postoperative results are shown (Figs. 34.12, 34.13, 34.14, 34.15, and 34.16).

Case Scenario 3 Surgeon TC Teo A 49-year-old man sustained a Gustilo 3B open tibial fracture after a motor vehicle accident, an external fixator frame was placed after initial debridement by the orthopaedic team. An SCIP flap was designed to reconstruct the defect. The flap resurfaced the defect, and anastomosis was made end to side to the posterior tibial artery and end to end to the associated venae comitans. The patient made a full recovery, with bony union and a healed reconstruction without any long-term sequelae (Figs. 34.17, 34.18, 34.19, and 34.20).

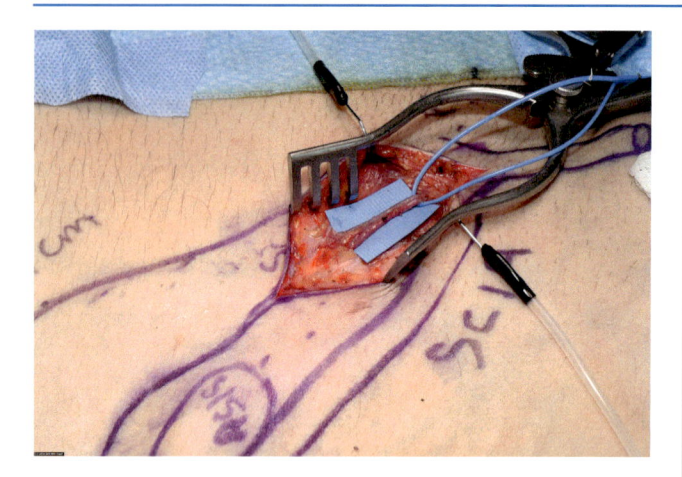

Fig. 34.14 Medial approach to SCIP with vessels identified under Scarpa's fascia

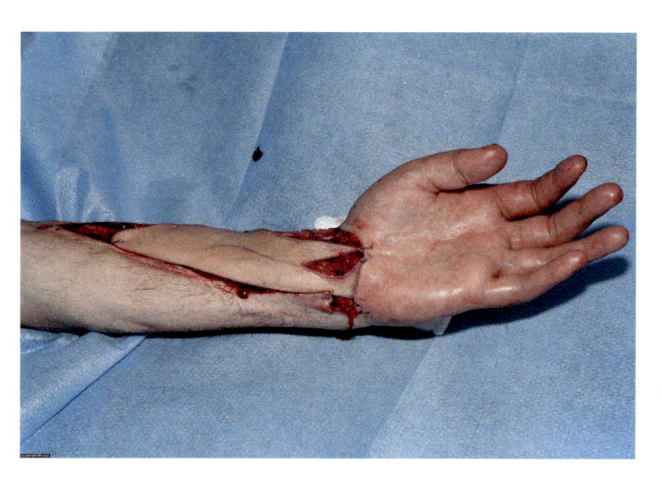

Fig. 34.15 SCIP inset over soft tissue defect at wrist at end of case

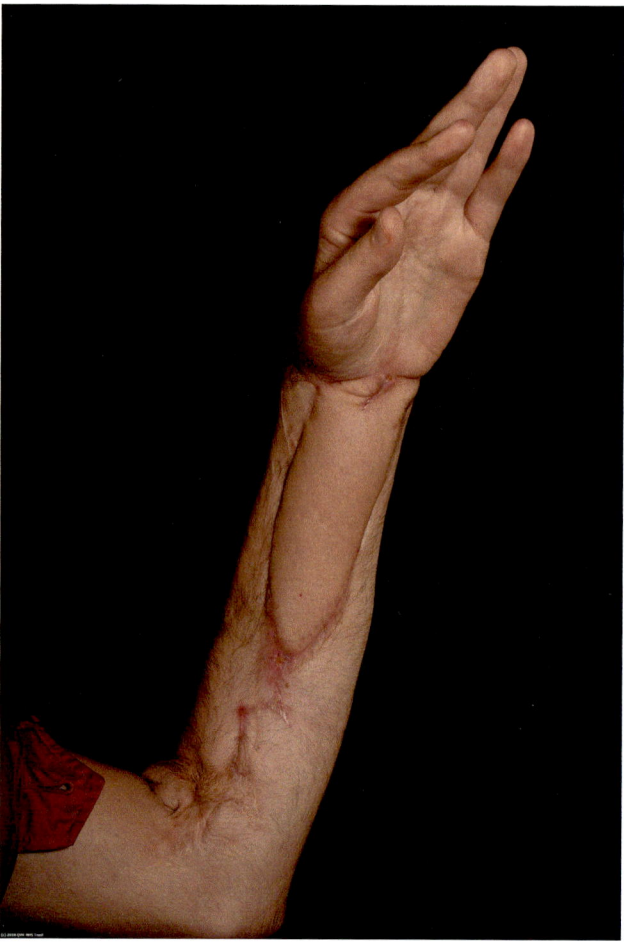

Fig. 34.16 Result at 6 months

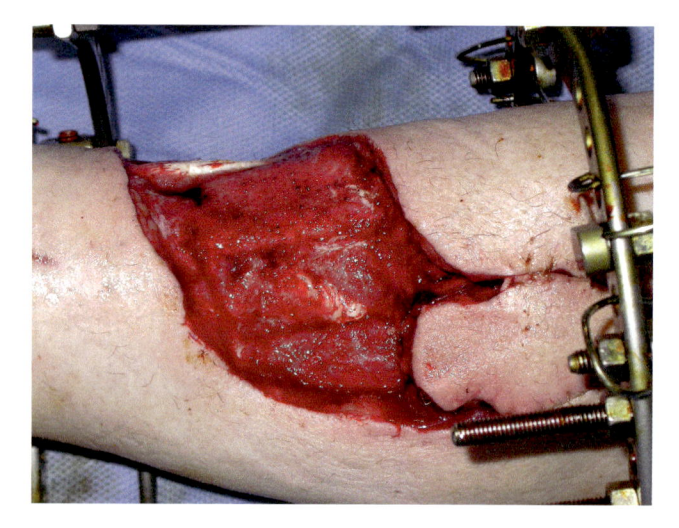

Fig. 34.17 Open tibial fracture in middle third of lower extremity

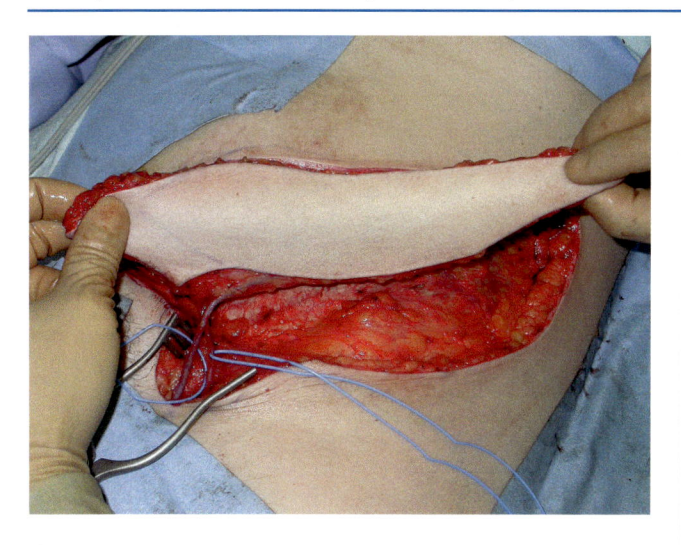

Fig. 34.18 SCIP flap raised and templated for lower limb defect

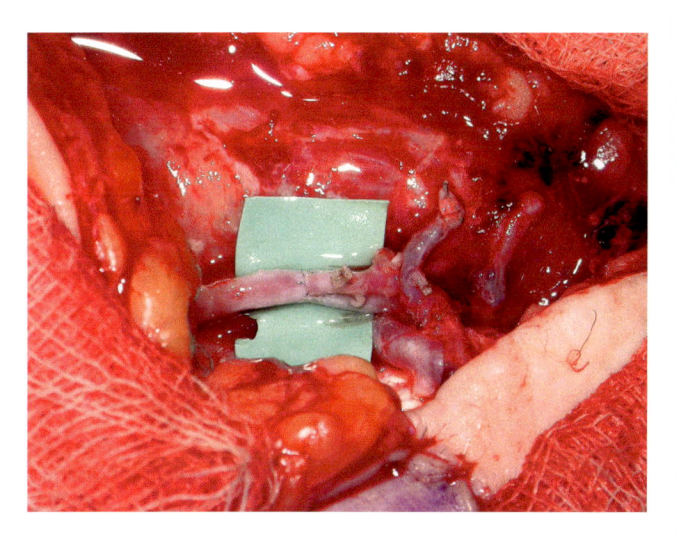

Fig. 34.19 End to side anastomosis onto the PTA and end to end anastomosis onto venae comitans

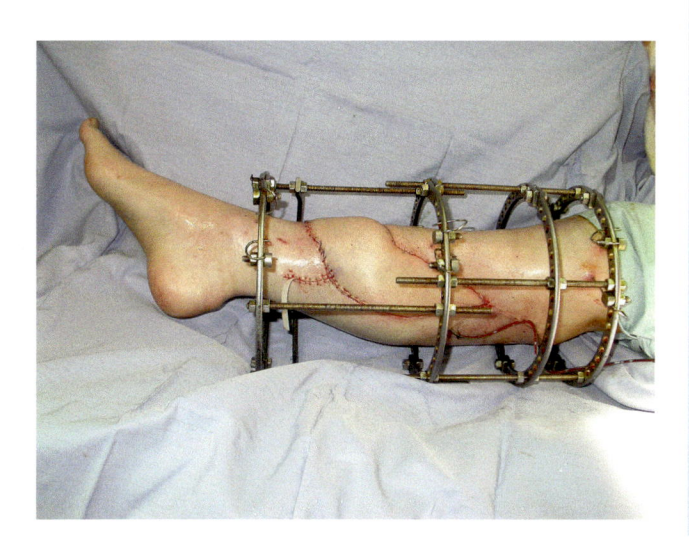

Fig. 34.20 Final result at end of case

34.8 Pearls and Pitfalls

> **Pearls**
> - Place skin paddle over inguinal ligament, incorporating non- hair-bearing skin if possible.
> - An incision over the SCIP pedicle allows visualising its calibre and length before committing to raising the whole flap. In rare occasions, raising can be abandoned and a contralateral SCIP or SIEA flap raised.
> - There are multiple superficial veins running in the groin region. This should always be included in the flap if possible. These superficial veins tend to have a larger calibre than the SCIP vena comitans and are particularly useful in small flaps to reduce the chances of venous congestion.
> - If the calibre of the SCIP artery is inadequate for safe anastomosis, a segment of the larger SCIA can be harvested.
> - Avoid undermining of the abdomen prior to closure to avoid contour deformities or pulling on the umbilicus.

> **Pitfalls**
> - SCIP flap dissection is mostly superficial and therefore raising can be quick in experienced hands. It is an excellent choice when there are recipient vessels in the wound or just next to it. If a longer pedicle is required, another alternative should be sought.
> - Small flaps are prone to venous congestion. Incorporating a superficial vein with the flap can solve this problem.
> - It is important to have in mind that the SCIP pedicle runs through superficial groin lymph nodes. Careful dissection is key to minimise the risk of seroma and lymphoedema.
> - Surgeons raising this flap should be prepared to work with vessels of 0.8–1 mm calibre. Often it is necessary to perform an end to side anastomosis in extremity reconstruction due to the significant vessel mismatch.
> - The artery in the SCIP flap is often smaller than the vein, it can be simple to confuse the two, and it is best to mark the vein with blue ink or place a microsurgical clamp over it to help distinguish the two structures.

34.9 Selected Readings

- Pereira N, Parada L, Kufeke M, Troncoso E, Roa R. A new planning method to easily harvest the superficial circumflex iliac artery perforator flap. J Reconstruct Microsurg. 2020 Mar;36(03):165–70.
- *This recent article presents an anatomy-based planning strategy using CT-angiography which can be useful for surgeons familiarising with the SCIP flap*
- Koshima I, Nanba Y, Tsutsui T, Takahashi Y, Urushibara K, Inagawa K, Hamasaki T, Moriguchi T. Superficial circumflex iliac artery perforator flap for reconstruction of limb defects. Plastic and reconstructive surgery. 2004 Jan 1;113(1):233–40.
- *Inceptional article by Prof. Koshima, being the first publication to present the use of this flap in the literature.*
- Goh TL, Park SW, Cho JY, Choi JW, Hong JP. The search for the ideal thin skin flap: superficial circumflex iliac artery perforator flap—a review of 210 cases. Plastic and reconstructive surgery. 2015 Feb 1;135(2):592–601.
- *Largest case series of SCIP flaps to date, demonstrating its reliability for limb reconstruction as super-thin flap. The authors describe the lateral to medial approach of SCIP flap elevation.*
- Berner JE, Nikkhah D, Zhao J, Prousskaia E, Teo TC. The versatility of the superficial circumflex iliac artery perforator flap: a single surgeon's 16-year experience for limb reconstruction and a systematic review. J Reconstruct Microsurg. 2020 Feb;36(02):093–103.
- *Largest case series in Western population. The SCIP classification based on the included tissues is presented along with a description of the anterograde raising technique.*

References

1. Koshima I, Nanba Y, Tsutsui T, Takahashi Y, Urushibara K, Inagawa K, Hamasaki T, Moriguchi T. Superficial circumflex iliac artery perforator flap for reconstruction of limb defects. Plast Reconstr Surg. 2004;113:233. https://doi.org/10.1097/01.PRS.0000095948.03605.20.
2. McGregor IA, Jackson IT. The Groin Flap. Br J Plast Surg. 1972; https://doi.org/10.1016/s0007-1226(72)80003-1.
3. Pereira N, Cámbara Á, Kufeke M, Roa R. Post-traumatic lymphedema treatment with superficial circumflex iliac artery perforator lymphatic free flap: a case report. Microsurgery. 2019;39:354. https://doi.org/10.1002/micr.30437.
4. Pan ZH, Jiang PP, Zhao YX, Wang JL. Treatment of complex metacarpal defects with free chimeric iliac Osteocutaneous flaps. J Plast Surg Hand Surg. 2017;51:143. https://doi.org/10.1080/2000656X.2016.1205502.
5. Goh TL, Park SW, Cho JY, Choi JW, Hong JP. The search for the ideal thin skin flap: superficial circumflex iliac artery perforator flap--a review of 210 cases. Plast Reconstr Surg. 2015; https://doi.org/10.1097/PRS.0000000000000951.
6. Berner JE, Nikkhah D, Zhao J, Prousskaia E, Teo TC. The versatility of the superficial circumflex iliac artery perforator flap: a single Surgeon's 16-year experience for limb reconstruction and a systematic review. J Reconstr Microsurg. 2020;36:93. https://doi.org/10.1055/s-0039-1695051.
7. Green R, Rahman KM, Owen S, Paleri V, Adams J, Ahmed OA, Ragbir M. The superficial circumflex iliac artery perforator flap in intra-Oral reconstruction. J Plast Reconstr Aesthet Surg. 2013;66:1683. https://doi.org/10.1016/j.bjps.2013.07.011.
8. Yoshimatsu H, Steinbacher J, Meng S, Hamscha UM, Weninger WJ, Tinhofer IE, Harima M, Fuse Y, Yamamoto T, Tzou CHJ. Superficial circumflex iliac artery perforator flap: an anatomical study of the correlation of the superficial and the deep branches of the artery and evaluation of perfusion from the deep branch to the Sartorius muscle and the iliac bone. Plast Reconstr Surg. 2019;143:589.
9. Gentileschi S, Servillo M, De Bonis F, et al. Radioanatomical study of the pedicle of the superficial circumflex iliac perforator flap. J Reconstr Microsurg. 2019;35:669. https://doi.org/10.1055/s-0039-1693144.
10. Suh HS, Jeong HH, Choi DH, Hong JP. Study of the medial superficial perforator of the superficial circumflex iliac artery perforator flap using computed tomographic angiography and surgical anatomy in 142 patients. Plast Reconstr Surg. 2017;139:738. https://doi.org/10.1097/PRS.0000000000003147.
11. Pereira N, Parada L, Kufeke M, Troncoso E, Roa R. A new planning method to easily harvest the superficial circumflex iliac artery perforator flap. J Reconstr Microsurg. 2020;36:165. https://doi.org/10.1055/s-0039-1698444.
12. Pereira N, Kufeke M, Parada L, Troncoso E, Bahamondes J, Sanchez L, Roa R. Augmented reality microsurgical planning with a smartphone (ARM-PS): a dissection route map in your pocket. J Plast Reconstr Aesthet Surg. 2019;72:759. https://doi.org/10.1016/j.bjps.2018.12.023.
13. Hong JP, Choi DH, Suh H, Mukarramah DA, Tashti T, Lee K, Yoon C. A new plane of elevation: the superficial fascial plane for perforator flap elevation. J Reconstr Microsurg. 2014; https://doi.org/10.1055/s-0034-1369807.

Lateral Circumflex Femoral Artery—Anterolateral Thigh Flap: Anterolateral Thigh Flap

Robert Miller, Dariush Nikkhah, Edmund Fitzgerald O'Connor, and Jeremy Rawlins

35.1 Introduction

First published by Song in 1984, the anterolateral thigh (ALT) flap is one of the key perforator-based workhorse flaps for regional or free tissue transfer reconstruction [1, 2]. Since its inception, it has been extensively described for reconstruction of defects across the body. Together with consistently high flap success, minimal donor site morbidity and the ability to use a two-team approach, this is a key flap in the reconstructive surgeon's armament.

Based on work in the late twentieth century on septocutaneous vessels, Song's original paper described three thigh flaps (anteriolateral, anteriomedial and posterior). They described a flap thickness between 1 and 3 cm, with a total area of 800 cm [2] that could be neurotised [1]. Since then, the ALT flap has evolved to provide muscle, fascia and skin tissue components in various combinations, as well as use as a flow-through or chimeric flap. Furthermore, by limiting the flap width dimension, primary closure of the donor site can be achieved, reducing the donor site morbidity and improving cosmesis.

Most commonly, the ALT is raised as a free flap for head and neck and lower limb reconstruction. However, it can also be used as a pedicled flap, most commonly for lower abdominal wall, groin and perineal reconstruction.

Supplementary Information The online version contains supplementary material available at [https://doi.org/10.1007/978-3-031-07678-7_35].

R. Miller
Department of Plastic and Reconstructive Surgery, St George's Hospital, London, UK

D. Nikkhah (✉)
Department of Plastic, Reconstructive and Aesthetic Surgery, Royal Free Hospital, London, UK
e-mail: d.nikkhah@nhs.net

E. F. O'Connor
Department of Plastic and Reconstructive Surgery, St. Thomas' Hospital, London, UK

J. Rawlins
Department of Plastic Surgery, Royal Perth Hospital, Perth, WA, Australia

35.2 Anatomy

The ALT flap is centred at the mid-point of a line drawn between the anterior superior iliac spine (ASIS) superiorly and the superior lateral aspect of the patella inferiorly. The arterial supply is derived from the lateral circumflex femoral artery (LCFA) which arises proximally from the profunda femoris artery and runs deep to the rectus femoris (RF) and sartorius. The LCFA divides into the ascending, transverse and descending branches, which most commonly follow an intramuscular course (87% musculocutaneous vs. 13% septocutaneous [3]) to supply the subcutaneous tissue and skin of the thigh. This is contrary to Song's original description of predominantly septocutaneous vessels [1].

The ALT flap is most commonly based on perforators from the *descending* branch. However, other perforator patterns have been described [4]. The descending branch travels along the medial edge of the vastus lateralis (VL) in the intra-muscular septum between VL and RF, giving off perforators within a 3 cm radius of the mid-point between the ASIS – superior lateral patella. In a minority of patients, the descending branch divides into medial and lateral branches at this mid-point, with the lateral branch providing perforators to the lateral thigh. Septocutaneous perforators travel between the RF and VL, traversing the fascia to supply the skin, while musculocutaneous perforators course through the VL for approximately 3–5 cm, before exiting the fascia to supply the overlying skin [2]. Studies examining the vascular territories of the thigh flaps have demonstrated that linking vessels and recurrent flow from the subdermal plexus facilitate perfusion between perforator zones. This allows an unthinned extended ALT to be raised on a single perforator [5]. Venous drainage most commonly comes from two venae comitantes running with the arterial pedicle, which go onto drain into the femoral vein.

Sensory innervation comes from the lateral femoral cutaneous nerve, which passes under the inguinal ligament just medial to the ASIS and travels under the tensor fascia lata, before piercing it. Motor innervation to the VL is derived from a branch of the femoral nerve which travels with the descending branch of the LFCA in the intramuscular septum.

Variations may occur in different ethnic groups. However, this has not been widely reported or confirmed. One difference is the thickness of the adipose thigh layer, which is typically greater in western population and less in Asian populations. Koshima also reports finding aberrant anatomy with loss of the RF-VL septum more commonly in Caucasians [6].

35.3 Pre-Operative Investigation

Routine pre-operative imaging is not indicated for ALT flap harvest. However, CT angiography may be pertinent in patients with prior upper thigh/ pelvic injury or surgery or patients with severe arterial atherosclerotic disease.

A standard hand-held doppler is used routinely to map perforators pre-operatively, most commonly found in a 3 cm radius around the mid-point between the ASIS – superior lateral patella. Although these devices are cheap and accessible, their accuracy has been questioned [5] and will often not allow the surgeon to determine the pedicle course or the site of fascial perforation. For more accurate perforator mapping, CTA can be used [7, 8].

More recently, colour-coded duplex sonography has gained popularity. This can be used by the operating surgeon both pre- and intra-operatively providing both anatomic and haemodynamic information and has high sensitivity and specificity values. It has been advocated to facilitate accurate pre-operative planning and perforator selection, subsequently decreasing flap raise time and allowing potential complications due to variations in anatomy to be identified prior to surgery commencing [9].

35.4 Flap Design and Markings

Flap marking (Fig. 35.1):

- Mark the ASIS and superior lateral aspect of the patella.
- Draw a longitudinal line connecting the two landmarks. This should lie over the groove (septum) between RF and VL, which can be palpated in thin patients.

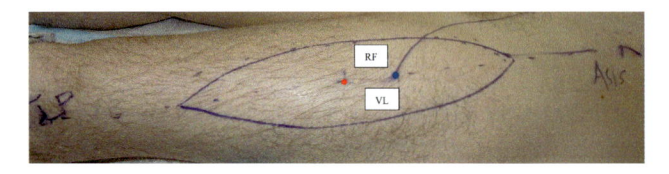

Fig. 35.1 Pre-op markings. *ASIS* Anterior Superior Iliac Spine, *LP* lateral patella, *RF* rectus femoris, *VL* Vastus lateralis, *Red dot and circle* Mid-point of line around which a 3 cm radius circle can be drawn, *Blue dot* perforator

- Draw a 3 cm circle around the mid-point to define the likely exit of perforators (commonly in inferior lateral quadrant) [2].
- Mark skin perforators with a hand-held Doppler.

Flap design key points:

- Template or measure the defect to design the flap on the longitudinal axis of the thigh.
- Although, the flap can be successfully raised on one perforator, where possible, incorporate two perforators. Marking a second backup perforator is helpful in case the primary perforator is of insufficient size/ calibre.
- Limit the flap width to approximately 8 cm to facilitate primary closure [2].
- Limit the flap length to approximately 22 cm for a single pedicle [2].

35.5 Flap Raise/Elevation: A Step-by-Step Guide

1. Incise the medial marking of the flap.
2. Incise the subcutaneous tissue down to thigh fascia.
3. At this point:
   a. Either stop at the muscle fascia and dissect laterally in a **supra-fascial** plane until the skin perforator(s) is identified and chosen. Isolate the perforator(s) and dissect through the fascia. Supra-fascial flaps offer the advantage of a thinner flap, better suited for dorsal hand or foot defects.
   b. Or *incise* the fascia over the RF (preserving the epimysium) and dissect laterally in a sub-fascial plane to the RF-VL septum.
4. Identify the RF-VL septum. Note the yellow fat between the two muscles to help identify the septum. Additionally, the VL and RF muscle fibres contract in different directions. Stimulating the muscles can help differentiate them and identify the septum. Figure 35.2.

5. Retract the RF medially to expose the RF-VL septum and inspect for the presence of septocutaneous perforators Fig. 35.3.

If septocutaneous perforators are not present, continue sub-fascial dissection until the perforator is identified passing through the muscle (Fig. 35.4). If the perforator is of a good caliber, there is no need to take a second perforator.

Once the chosen perforator(s) are identified, dissect the pedicle retrogradely either through a septocutaneous course

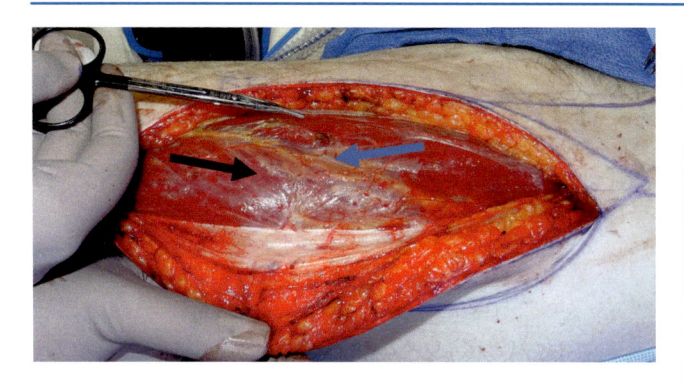

Fig. 35.2 Tenotomy scissors = RF; black arrow = VL; blue arrow = RF-VL septum (note the yellow fat)

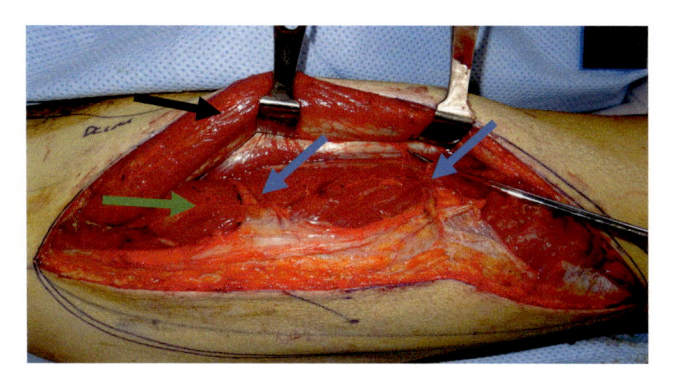

Fig. 35.3 Medial retraction of the RF (black arrow) demonstrates clearly the RF-VL septum. Green arrow = VL. In this case there are septocutaneous perforators visible arising from the septum (blue arrow)

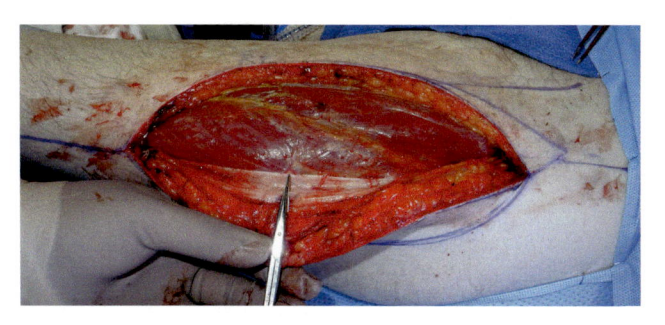

Fig. 35.4 Tenotomy scissors highlighting musculocutaneous perforators perforating the fascia

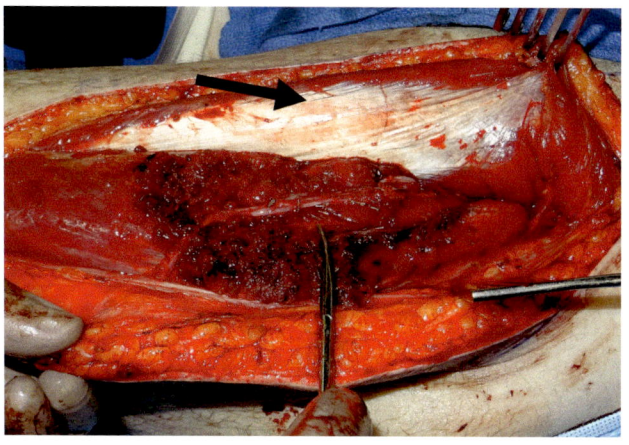

Fig. 35.5 Black arrow = Retracted RF; tenotomy scissor tips = perforator after VL intramuscular dissection

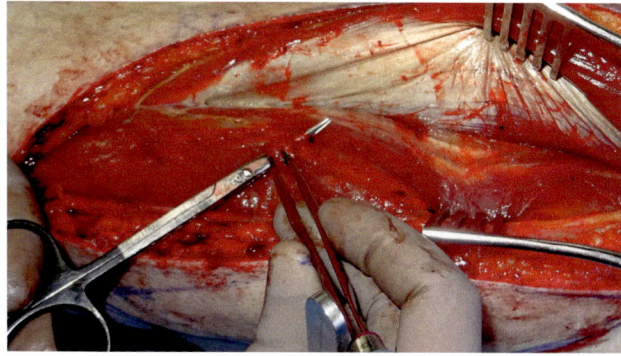

Fig. 35.6 Tenotomy scissors placed on top of the perforator with bipolar used to dissect the muscle off above

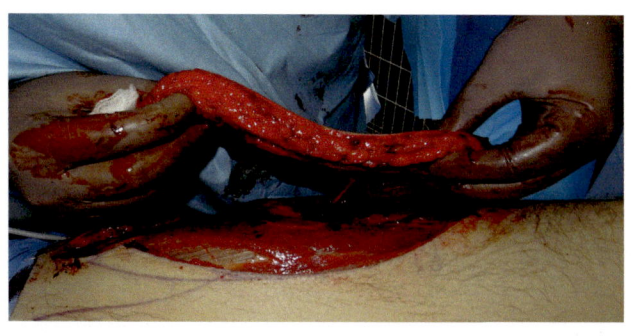

Fig. 35.7 Subfascial ALT raised on a single perforator prior to perforator division

through the RF – VL septum (Fig. 35.3) or through the VL (Fig. 35.5) using the deroofing technique (fig. 35.6) (Video 35.1), heat-sink bipolar technique or ligaclips can be used for side branches coming off the pedicle

- Dissect the pedicle retrogradely to the descending branch of the LFCA or until adequate pedicle length is achieved, at which point the pedicle can be divided. Up to 10–11 cm of pedicle length can be achieved if dissected to rectus femoris branch [2].
- Incise the lateral marking of the flap down through fascia to isolate, and then divide, the pedicle (Fig. 35.7).

35.6 Core Surgical Techniques in Flap Dissection

General techniques:

- The final flap design should be reassessed, and modified if necessary, after identification of the skin perforators.

- For retrograde musculocutaneous perforator dissection, the anterior muscle fibres can be lifted with toothed forceps, the tenotomy scissors spread in a transverse plane over the vessel and the muscle fibres divided [2]. Alternatively, the tenotomy scissors can be passed in a longitudinal direction over the vessel, creating a tunnel. Monopolar or Bipolar cautery can then be used to cut onto the scissors, effectively deroofing the vessel [3]. See Fig. 35.6. Video 35.1.
- Intra-muscular branches commonly arise laterally and posteriorly. Tenotomy scissors can be used to make a window around them, after which they can be ligated. Alternatively, bi-polar cautery can be used; however, this increases the risk of thermal damage to the pedicle unless a heat sink bipolar technique is used [10].
- A cuff of VL muscle can be taken around the pedicle. This both increases speed of elevation and provides muscle to fill dead-space if necessary.
- For septocutaneous perforators, dissection is simpler. The pedicle should again be dissected retrogradely but can simply be separated from the surrounding tissue until the desired length is reached. See Fig. 35.3.
- The motor nerve to the RF and VL should be protected during pedicle dissection.

Problem solving:

- If a perforator is absent or of insufficient size, the same medial incision can be used with proximal extension to look for the transverse (Fig. 35.8) or ascending branch of the branch of the LFCA. In these cases, it may be necessary to convert to a tensor fascia lata flap or anteromedial thigh flap. Failing this, it may be necessary to swap to the contralateral thigh.
- If donor site closure is not possible, a skin graft might be needed, although this is cosmetically unsatisfactory. Alternatively, a modified key-stone flap [10] or V-Y advancement flaps can be used [2].

Considerations for use as a pedicle flap:

- Design and harvest should follow the same steps as outlined above. For a proximally based pedicle flap the pivot point is approximately 2 cm below the inguinal ligament. The flap can then be rotated medially over the RF or tunneled subcutaneously laterally [2].

Modifications:

- Up to the entire length of the VL can be included in the flap (Fig. 35.9), providing sufficient muscle branches from the descending branch of the LFCA are preserved. The VL can also be raised as a stand-alone muscle flap, based on the descending branch of the LFCA, without the ALT skin.

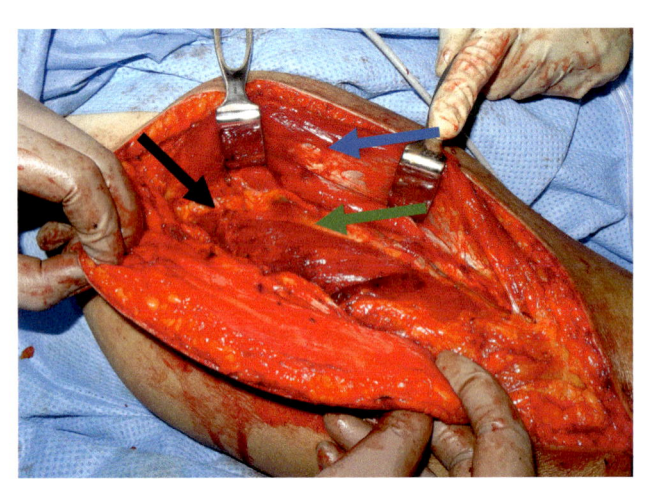

Fig. 35.8 Medial retraction of the RF (blue arrow) demonstrating the RF-VL septum (green arrow) with no distal perforator. However, a proximal transverse LCFA branch perforator supplying the partially raised ALT flap is demonstrated (black arrow)

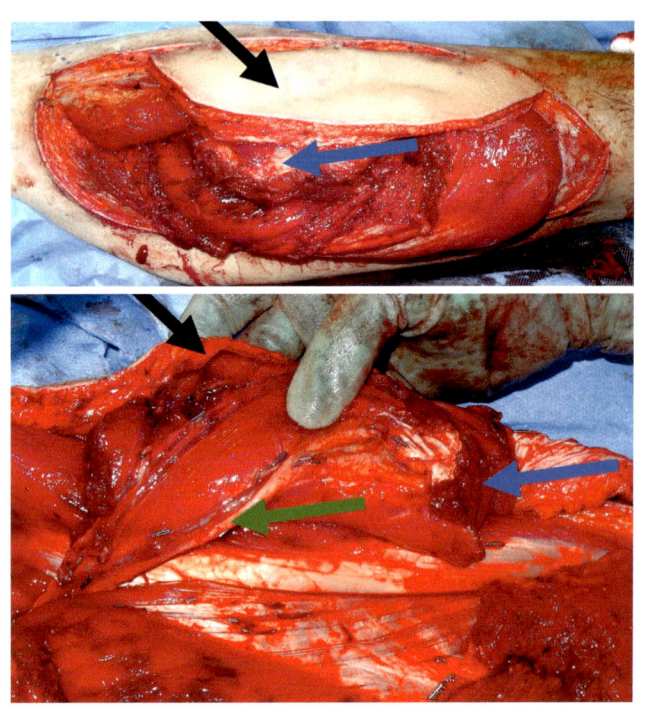

Fig. 35.9 ALT flap (black arrow) taken with a segment of VL (blue arrow). The pedicle is demonstrated in the lower image (green arrow)

- The RF muscle can be incorporated in a chimeric ALT flap, provided the branches from the descending branch of the LFCA are preserved.
- The TFL can be raised in conjunction with the ALT if the ascending branch of the LFCA is included. The TFL can be used for simultaneous reconstruction of other soft tissue components (such as tendon).
- The ALT flap can be thinned up to a thickness of 3 mm. However, it is advised to keep a 2 cm radius around the skin pedicle [2]. Alternatively, thigh fat can be included to add bulk to the flap. Placing the skin paddle distally on the thigh facilitates a thinner flap [4] (almost 50% thinner) as demonstrated in the two images within Fig. 35.10.
- A fasciocutaneous flap, without the overlying skin, can also be raised based on the same pedicle. The approach for raising is the same as for a subfascial flap but without the need to preserve the skin perforators.
- The flap can be innervated with the lateral femoral cutaneous nerve to provide sensation or the motor branch to the VL to provide animation. A nerve stimulator can be used to check whether the nerve branch is sensory or motor.
- The ALT flap can also be raised with multiple skin paddles if more than one perforator is identified. This can be useful in head and neck reconstruction where bipaddle ALT flaps can be used to reconstruct pharyngooesophageal defects and at the same time to resurface the neck.

35.7 Clinical Scenario

Case 1 Marine injury propeller injury

Dariush Nikkhah & Jeremy Rawlins

A 35-year-old male was struck by the propeller of a boat whilst in the sea. He suffered unicortical metatarsal fractures with associated soft tissue defect. He was managed in line with British Orthopaedic Association / British Association of Plastic, Reconstructive and Aesthetic Surgery guidelines. The wound was debrided within 24 hours and reconstructed on day three with a joint ortho-plastics team approach. A thin subfascial ALT was used and anastomosed onto the dorsalis pedis vessels. Bony fixation was not required (Fig. 35.11).

Case 2 Upper limb flexor tenolysis, neurolysis and forearm defect reconstruction

Dariush Nikkhah & Jeremy Rawlins

A 26-year-old male suffered a forearm crush injury which had originally been managed by split thickness skin grafting. He required excision of the skin graft, tenolysis, neurolysis of the ulnar and median nerves and resurfacing with a flow through ALT flap (Fig. 35.12). He had an excellent outcome with full range of motion achieved at 1 year follow-up (Video 35.2).

Case 3 Orbital exenteration and medical maxillectomy reconstruction

Graeme Glass & Dariush Nikkhah

A 46-year-old lady presented with an aggressive squamous cell carcinoma of the maxilla and orbit. She underwent orbital exenteration and medial maxillectomy. A right sided ALT flap was raised with a cuff of vastus lateralis to fill the dead space in the right cheek. The ALT was anastomosed to the facial artery and vein after de-epitheliasing the skin paddle. She had an uneventful post-operative recovery (Fig. 35.13).

The final video in this chapter provides a summary and overview of the ALT flap raise (Video 35.3).

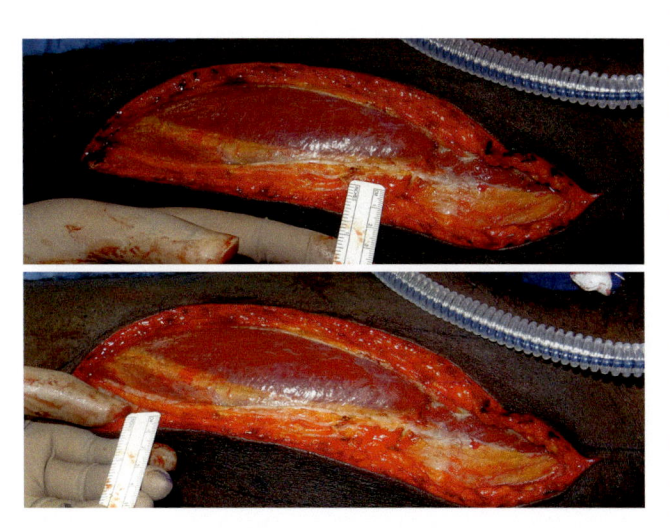

Fig. 35.10 Demonstration of the difference in ALT flap thickness along the thigh. Upper image = proximal; Lower image = distal

Fig. 35.11 Upper images demonstrate pre-operative defect (left) vs. post-operative reconstruction (right). The lower image demonstrates a subfascial ALT with a single isolated intra-muscular perforator

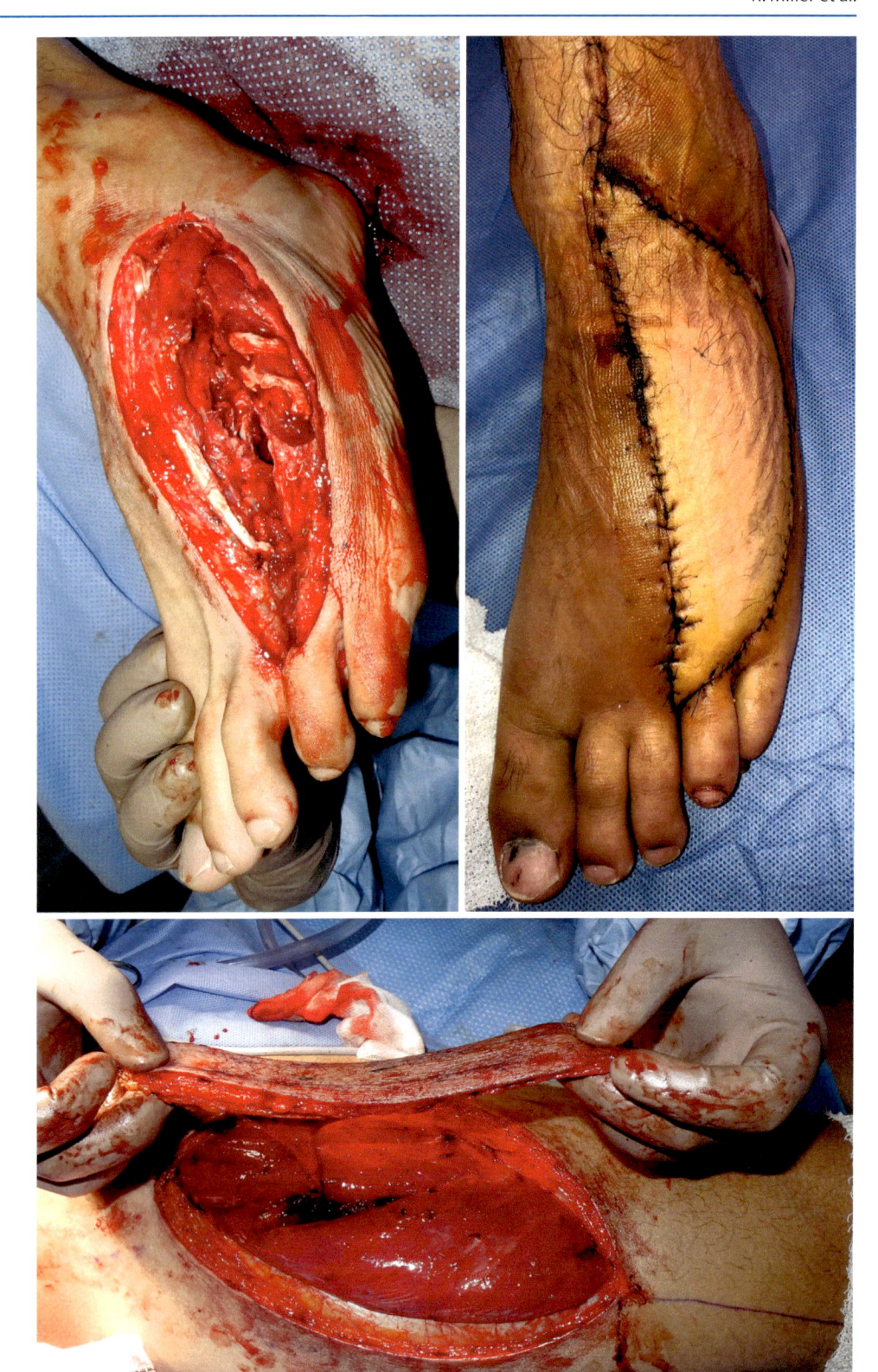

35 Lateral Circumflex Femoral Artery—Anterolateral Thigh Flap: Anterolateral Thigh Flap

Fig. 35.12 Images demonstrating pre-op deformity (upper left), intra-op defect post tenolysis and neurolysis (upper right), post-op defect reconstruction with thin subfascial ATL (lower left) and follow-up image (lower right)

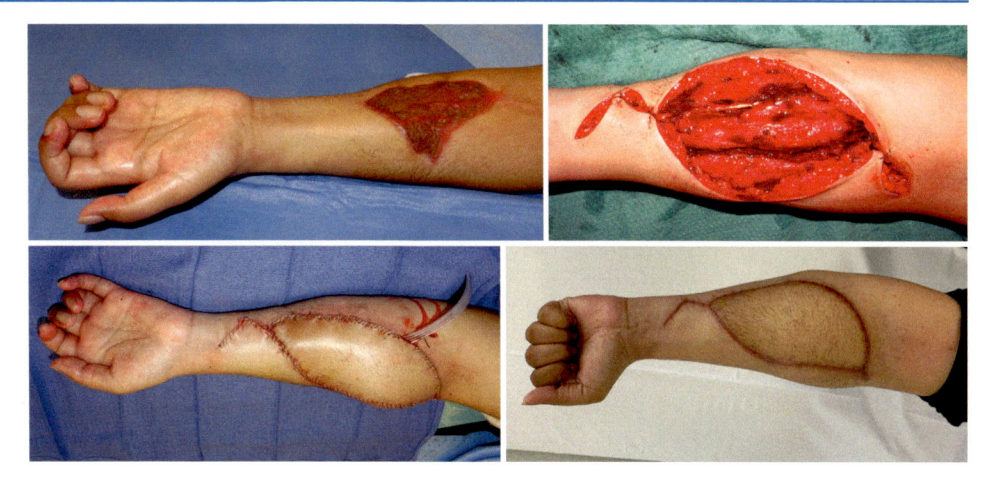

Fig. 35.13 Upper images show post orbital exenteration (left) and post flap inset (right). The lower image demonstrates ALT skin paddle in place within the orbit with the pedicle tunneled to allow anastomosis onto the facial artery. The cuff of VL is fulling the dead-space of the maxilla

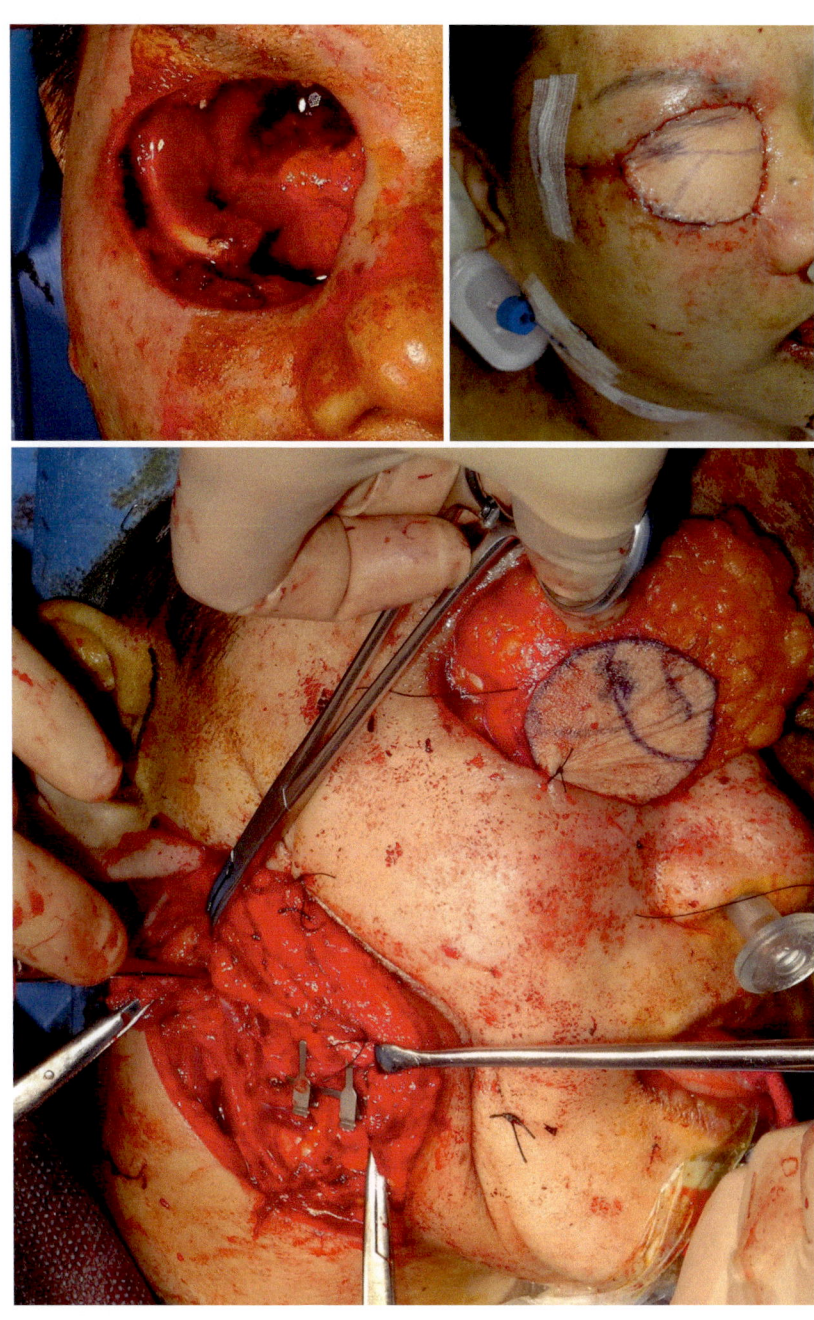

35.8 Pearls and Pitfalls

Pearls

- Flap design does not need to be centred over the identified skin vessel. An eccentric design is acceptable and can provide additional pedicle length (particularly for pedicle flaps) [2]. Furthermore, using a distal skin paddle can provide a thinner flap, if required, as shown in Fig. 35.10.
- Distal incision extension can help visualise and identify the RF/VL septum to prevent confusion with the septum between the two heads of the RF.
- Proximal extension as a lazy 'S' can provide additional exposure to maximise pedicle length [10].
- Identification of the most proximal perforator may be helpful as this will often have the shortest intramuscular course [11].
- Include a cuff of fascia around the pedicle during supra-fascial flap harvest.
- After flap raise use a large nylon suture to take the tension off the donor site and aid subsequent closure (if not being done immediately). See Fig. 35.14.

Pitfalls

- Skin colour mismatch between ALT and recipient site. The thigh may be significantly paler and provide a poor cosmetic outcome.
- Similar attention should be given to hair growth, particularly when used for intra-oral reconstruction.
- Twisting of the pedicle during inset. Lifting the flap once raised to see the natural lie of the pedicle will aid placement.
- Not supporting the flap during the raise may cause tension or traction on the pedicle, which in turn may cause the vessels to spasm. This is more pertinent in the supra-fascial raise when both medial and lateral incision are made prior to pedicle dissection.
- Loss of sensation to the ALT. Patients should be counselled pre-operatively. This can be reduced by preserving cutaneous nerves in a supra-fascial elevation.

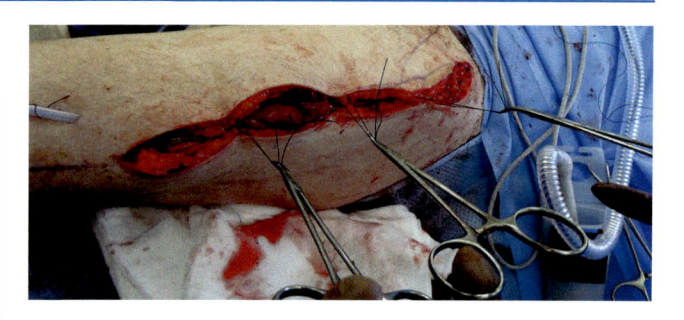

Fig. 35.14 Temporary donor site closure using a large dermal silk suture. This will facilitate subsequent closure

35.9 Selected Readings

- Song YG, Chen GZ, Song YL. The free thigh flap: a new free flap concept based on the septocutaneous artery. British journal of plastic surgery. 1984 Apr 1;37(2):149–59.
- *The original paper describing the three thigh flaps is a must read for its historic value and the impact it has had on microsurgical reconstruction. Song et al., describe the anteromedial, anterolateral and posterior thigh flaps based on their work on septocutaneous perforators* [1].
- Wei FC, Jain V, Celik N, Chen HC, Chuang DC, Lin CH. Have we found an ideal soft-tissue flap? An experience with 672 anterolateral thigh flaps. Plast Reconstr Surg. 2002;109(7):2219–26.
- *Published in 2002, this was a seminal paper highlighting the versatility and reliability of the ALT flap in microsurgical reconstruction. It also solidified the consensus that ALT perforators are predominantly musculocutaneous, in contrast to Song's original description* [3].
- Kehrer A, Sachanadani NS, da Silva NP, Lonic D, Heidekrueger P, Taeger C, Klein S, Jung EM, Prantl L, Hong JP. Step by Step Guide to Ultrasound-Based Design of Alt Flaps by the Microsurgeon–Basic and Advanced Applications and Device Settings. Journal of Plastic, Reconstructive & Aesthetic Surgery. 2019; 73(6)1081–1090.
- *The use of ultrasound in flap design is gaining popularity worldwide. This recent publication offers a step-*

wise guide for the use of colour-coded duplex sonography in identifying and mapping ALT perforators based on the authors experience of 125 ALT flaps over two centres. Although perforator mapping using ultrasound technology is not routinely necessary for ALT flap harvest, it offers an excellent opportunity to learn these skills [9].

- Yu P. Characteristics of the anterolateral thigh flap in a Western population and its application in head and neck reconstruction. Head & Neck: Journal for the Sciences and Specialties of the Head and Neck. 2004 Sep;26(9):759–69.
- *This paper balances the experience of the ALT flap from Asian cohorts with the experience of 72 ALT flaps in a Western population (Texas, USA). It offers excellent illustrations demonstrating the anatomical variations of the ALT pedicle (Fig. 35.3) and the likelihood of encountering these perforators (Fig. 35.1). Familiarising oneself with these anatomical variations will aid efficient and effect flap raise* [4].
- Saint-Cyr M, Oni G, Lee M, Yi C, Colohon SM. Simple approach to harvest of the antierloateral thigh flap. Plastic and reconstructive surgery. 2012; 129 (1):207–11.
- *This concise paper from Saint-Cry offers a stepwise approach to ALT perforator identification, choice and ALT raise. It highlights the authors' preference for selecting a proximal perforator to reduce the need for perforator dissection with* Fig. 35.6 *offering an easy-to-follow algorithm* [11].

References

1. Song YG, Chen GZ, Song YL. The free thigh flap: a new free flap concept based on the septocutaneous artery. Br J Plast Surg. 1984;37(2):149–59.
2. Wei F-C, Mardini S. Flaps and reconstructive surgery. Elsevier; 2009.
3. Wei FC, Jain V, Celik N, Chen HC, Chuang DC, Lin CH. Have we found an ideal soft-tissue flap? An experience with 672 anterolateral thigh flaps. Plast Reconstr Surg. 2002;109(7):2219–26. discussion 2227-2230
4. Yu P. Characteristics of the anterolateral thigh flap in a Western population and its application in head and neck reconstruction. Head Neck. 2004;26(9):759–69.
5. Saint-Cyr M, Schaverien M, Wong C, et al. The extended anterolateral thigh flap: anatomical basis and clinical experience. Plast Reconstr Surg. 2009;123(4):1245–55.
6. Koshima I. Free anterolateral thigh flap for reconstruction of head and neck defects following cancer ablation. Plast Reconstr Surg. 2000;105(7):2358–60.
7. Smit JM, Klein S, Werker PM. An overview of methods for vascular mapping in the planning of free flaps. J Plast Reconstr Aesthet Surg. 2010;63(9):e674–82.
8. Rozen WM, Ashton MW, Pan WR, et al. Anatomical variations in the harvest of anterolateral thigh flap perforators: a cadaveric and clinical study. Microsurgery. 2009;29(1):16–23.
9. Kehrer A, Sachanadani NS, da Silva NPB, et al. Step-by-step guide to ultrasound-based design of alt flaps by the microsurgeon - basic and advanced applications and device settings. J Plast Reconstr Aesthet Surg. 2019;73(6):1081–90.
10. Nikkhah D, Miller R, Pafitanis G, Vijayan R, Sadigh P. Five simple techniques to enable rapid elevation and donor site closure of the anterolateral thigh flap. J Hand Microsurg. 2019;11(1):54–6.
11. Saint-Cyr M, Oni G, Lee M, Yi C, Colohan SM, Colohon SM. Simple approach to harvest of the anterolateral thigh flap. Plast Reconstr Surg. 2012;129(1):207–11.

Transverse Upper Gracilis (TUG) Flap: A Reliable Alternative for Breast Reconstruction

36

Juan Enrique Berner and Adam Blackburn

36.1 Introduction

The gracilis muscle has been a common donor site for free tissue transfer since the 1970s [1]. This expendable muscle in the adductor compartment of the thigh has demonstrated to be a reliable alternative, easy to raise and a constant vascular pedicle [2]. Even though its musculocutaneous variant had been described previously, it was Yousif et al. who introduced the transverse upper gracilis (TUG) flap in 1992 [3]. His anatomical studies demonstrated that musculocutaneous perforators arising in the proximal portion of the gracilis muscle follow a transverse course anteriorly and posteriorly. This is the basis for the transverse design of the TUG skin paddle, which results in a well concealed donor site scar in the groin crease [4].

It was a decade after its inception, that Arnez et al. would popularise the use of this flap for breast reconstruction, as an alternative to abdominal free flaps [5]. In many microsurgical centres, the TUG flap has become the second-best option for patients undergoing autologous breast reconstruction [6]. This can be particularly useful as a single or stacked flap, particularly in slim patients [7]. More recently, modifications to the TUG have been proposed, intending to avoid scars in the gluteal crease while optimising volume harvest. This has been achieved by modifying the orientation of the skin paddle [8].

36.2 Anatomy

The gracilis is the most superficial muscle in the adductor compartment of the thigh. It originates in the ischiopubic ramus and inserts in the anteromedial proximal tibia, via the pes anserinus conjoint tendon. It acts primarily as a hip adductor even though it also plays a role in hip flexion and knee extension.

It is perfused by a branch of the medial circumflex femoral artery, running between adductor longus and magnus, entering the gracilis muscle approximately 10 cm inferior to the pubic tubercle [3]. A motor branch of the obturator nerve pierces into the gracilis muscle close to the entry of its vascular pedicle, usually at a 45° angle. Harvesting the nerve to gracilis allows transferring this muscle as a functional flap [9], though this is not indicated for breast reconstruction.

Two anatomical landmarks are important for raising the skin paddle of the TUG flap. Anteriorly, the long saphenous vein runs in the femoral triangle towards the saphenofemoral junction. The TUG flap spares this vein and care should be taken not to harvest tissues that are deep and lateral to it, which can disrupt lymphatic drainage to the lower extremity. Posteriorly, the posterior cutaneous nerve of the thigh arises from the great sciatic foramen under the piriformis muscle. It pierces the deep fascia in the posterior midline of the thigh, from where it travels inferiorly providing sensation to the skin in the posterior thigh. This structure should be avoided during the raising of the TUG flap, preserving sensation and avoiding neuroma formation in a pressure-bearing area [10].

36.3 Pre-Operative Investigation

Given its constant vascular anatomy, no routine preoperative investigations are used to plan the raising of a TUG flap. However, for breast reconstruction, careful analysis should be performed, especially for delayed cases.

The profunda artery perforator (PAP) arises posterior to the gracilis muscle, approximately 8 cm inferior to the gluteal crease [11]. Locating this perforator using computed tomography angiography in conjunction with hand-held Doppler can be useful as a lifeboat if the skin paddle over the gracilis is inadvertently undermined [12].

J. E. Berner (✉)
Royal Victoria Infirmary, Newcastle upon Tyne, UK

A. Blackburn
Queen Victoria Hospital, East Grinstead, UK

© Springer Nature Switzerland AG 2023
D. Nikkhah et al. (eds.), *Core Techniques in Flap Reconstructive Microsurgery*, https://doi.org/10.1007/978-3-031-07678-7_36

36.4 Flap Design and Markings

Marking of this flap starts with the patient standing, facing away from the surgeon. The posterior midline of the thigh is marked first, as this will be the posterior most point of the skin ellipse. It is convenient at this stage to mark the posterior portion of the superior margin of the flap on the gluteal crease. The patient is then asked to lie down with the hip abducted and the knee flexed. In this position the adductor longus tendon can be seen and felt and the gracilis muscle lies in "the hollow" posterior to it (Fig. 36.1). The anterior marking of the apex of the flap is approximately 2 finger breadths lateral to the lateral border of adductor longus, at the point where the thin groin skin becomes thicker thigh skin. The width of the skin paddle over the gracilis tends to range from 7 to 10 cm; however, this should be routinely checked by means of a "pinch-test" (Fig. 36.2). On the operative table markings are templated and re-checked for symmetry in bilateral cases. (Figs. 36.3 and 36.4).

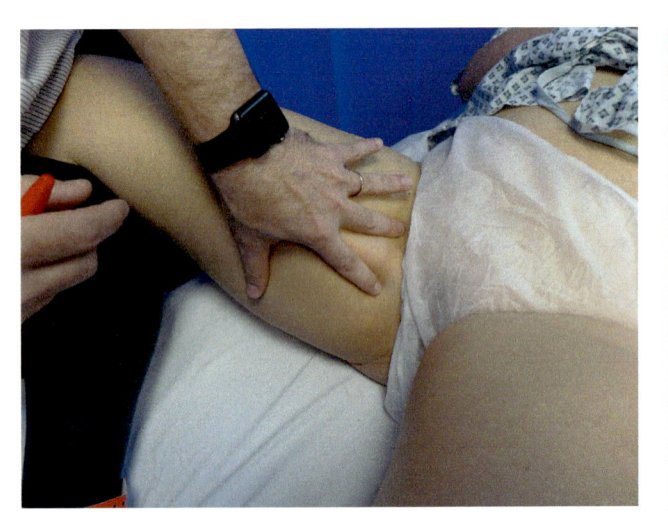

Fig. 36.1 Palpation of the adductor longus muscle. The gracilis muscle is posterior to the adductor longus

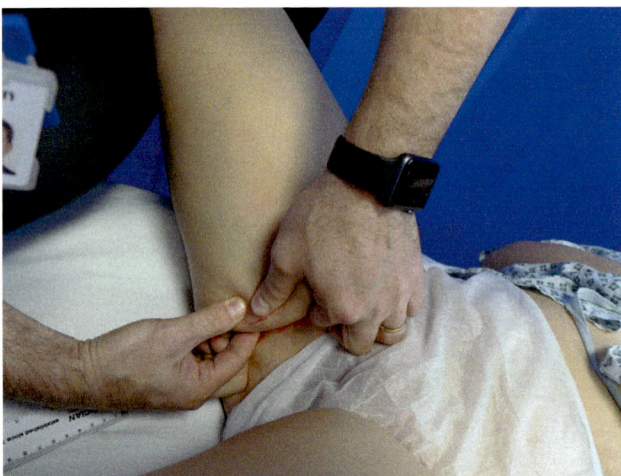

Fig. 36.2 Pinch test to determine the width of skin paddle to be included with flap

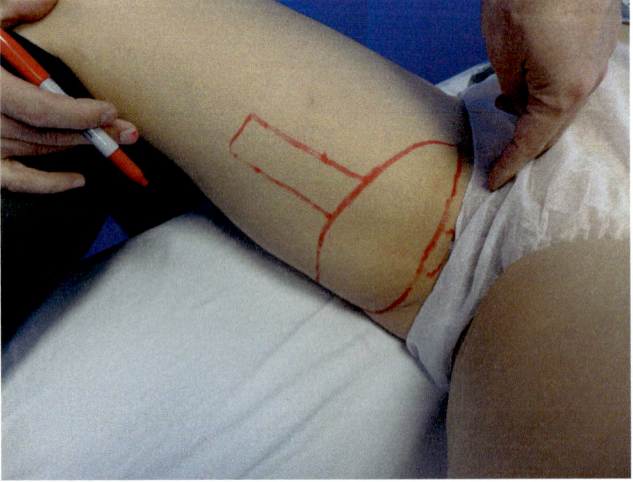

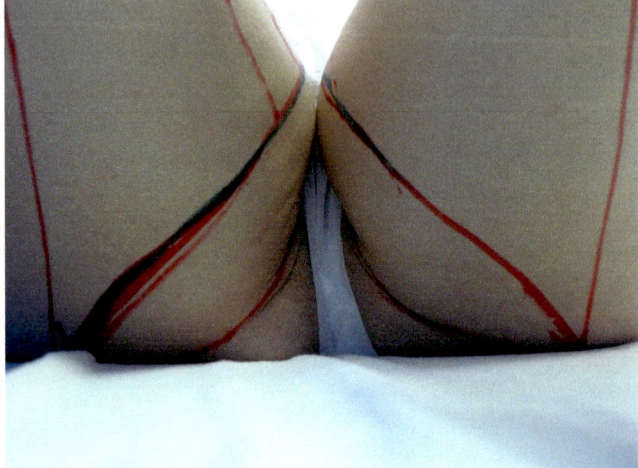

Figs. 36.3 and 36.4 Marking of the flap, which should be checked for symmetry if bilateral flaps are being harvested

36.5 Flap Raise/Elevation: A Step-by-Step Guide

1. **Patient Positioning and Skin Incision.** With the patient lying supine on the operating table, the thigh is abducted and the knee flexed, while paying attention to pressure areas around the ankle. Pressure sores and sciatica have been reported as possible complications. Pneumatic calf compression is used routinely for deep venous thrombosis prophylaxis (Figs. 36.5 and 36.6). Staples can be used to mark opposing margins of the skin paddle. A cold blade is used to incise around the skin paddle markings.

2. **Anterior Raising of the Flap.** Flap raising is started on the anterior aspect of the flap keeping the plane of dissection on the superficial fascia to avoid inadvertent harvest of lymphatic tissues until the great saphenous vein comes into view. Medial to the great saphenous vein the plane of dissection changes (Fig. 36.7). A deeper incision allows visualising the adductor longus fascia, which is incised and included in the flap. If a tributary of the great saphenous vein is seen crossing the skin paddle, this is divided near the great vein and included with the harvest.

3. **Superior Margin Dissection.** While the fascia over the adductor longus can be incised to be included of the flap care must be taken to preserve the fascia over the gracilis muscle for a 2–3 cm superiorly to prevent the muscle contracting and skin perforators being damaged (Fig. 36.8). The plane can get deeper once again posterior to this muscle. 2–3 cm from the posterior midline care must be taken not to divide the deep fascia to avoid injury to the posterior cutaneous nerve of the thigh.

4. **Inferior Margin Dissection.** The thigh skin just inferior to the incision can be undermined to augment the amount of tissue harvested with the flap. Once more it is preferable to respect the gracilis fascia when visualised (Fig. 36.9).

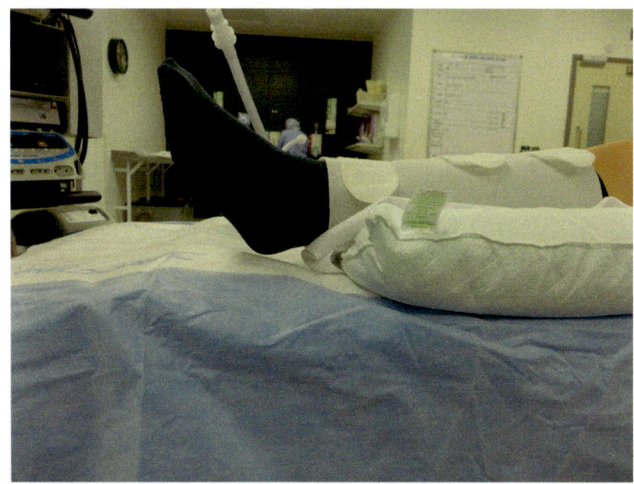

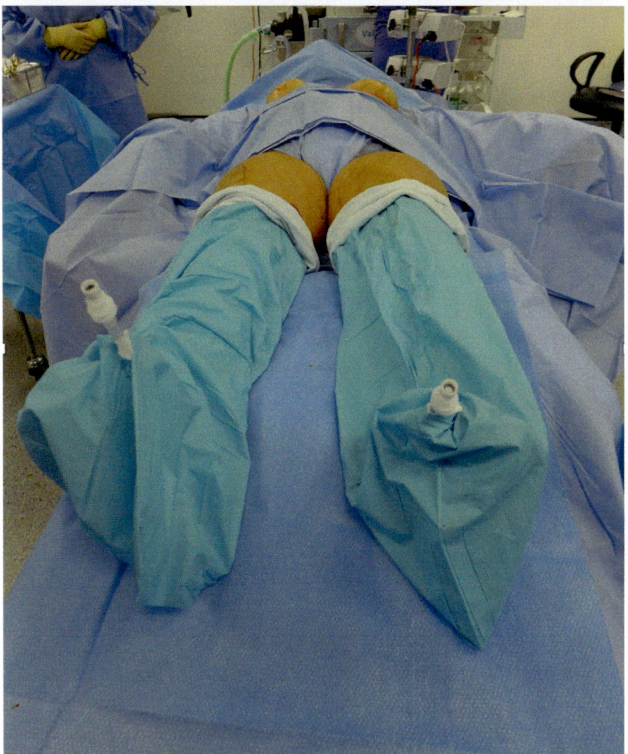

Figs. 36.5 and 36.6 Positioning of patient with pillow under legs and intermittent pneumatic compression devices on legs

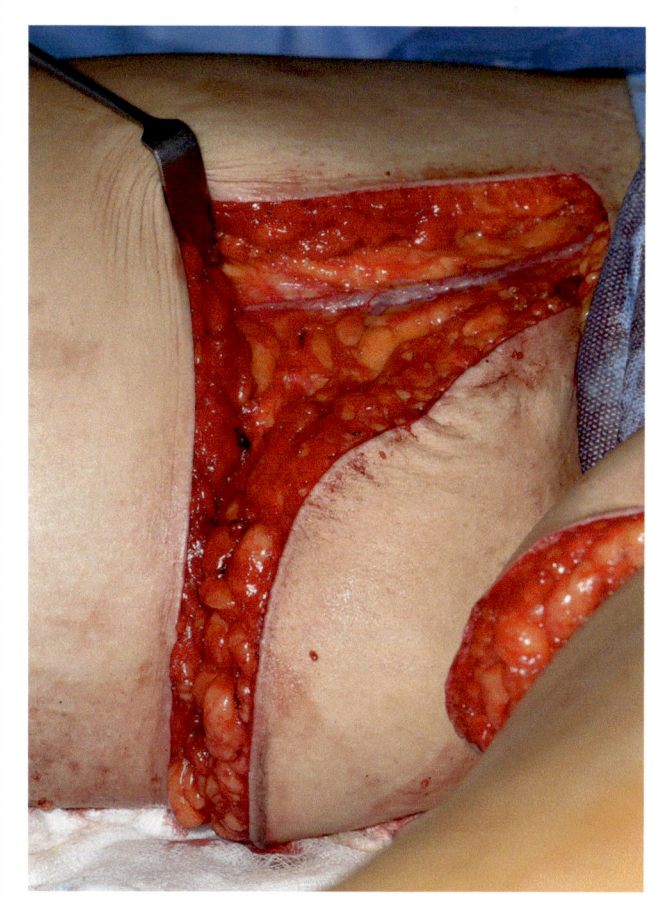

Fig. 36.7 Anterior raising of skin paddle. A tributary to the great saphenous vein can be taken with the flap

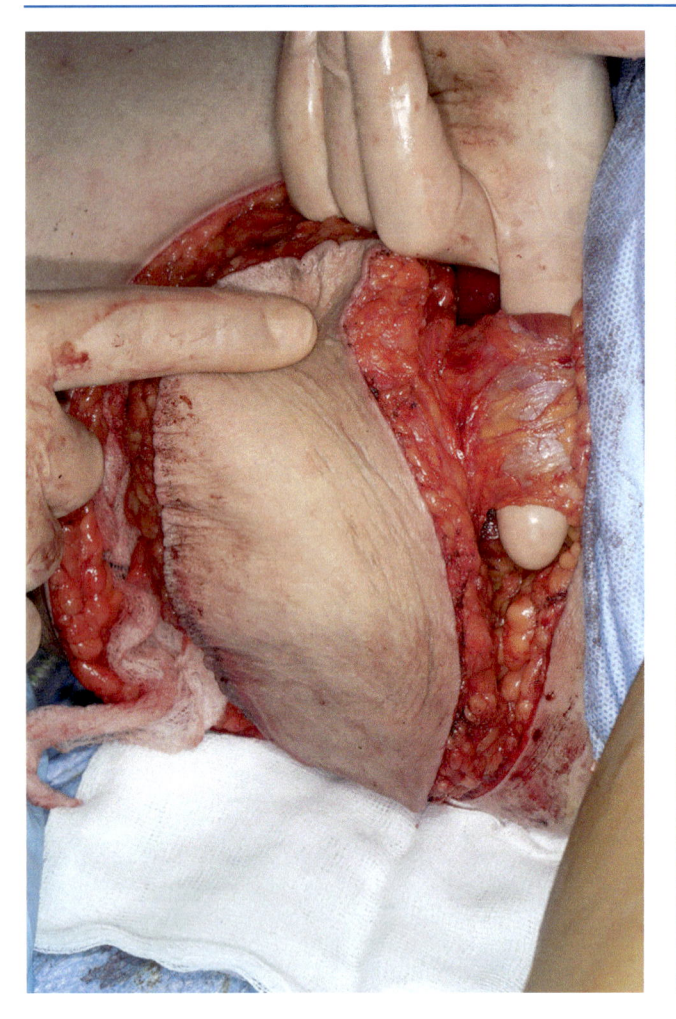

Fig. 36.8 The gracilis muscle is identified

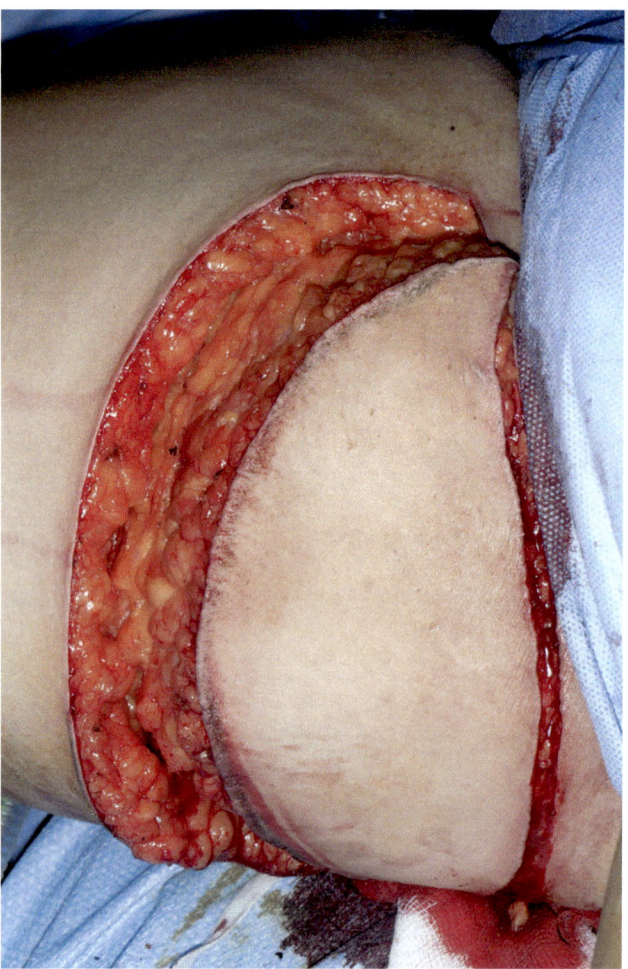

Fig. 36.9 The flap can then be islanded by committing with the inferior and posterior incisions

5. **Identification of the Gracilis Pedicle.** The loose areolar tissue between the gracilis and adductor longus can be released until the pedicle is visualised. It is advisable not to discard any vessels until the gracilis pedicle is confirmed as other muscle branches run in its vicinity (Fig. 36.10).
6. **Dissection around Gracilis Muscle.** Once the position of the pedicle has been confirmed, dissection through the loose areolar tissue around the gracilis muscle can be performed superior and inferior to the vessels. (Fig. 36.11).
7. **Pedicle Dissection.** The gracilis pedicle can be then dissected following its course in between adductor longus and magnus with the help of a Travers self-retaining retractor. Obturator nerve branches to adductor longus and should be spared as they run over the pedicle to avoid untoward morbidity. Dissection is finished when the medial circumflex femoral artery is seen. Large branches coming from the pedicle to adductor longus and magnus need to be controlled using ligaclips (Fig. 36.12).
8. **Completion of Raising and Detachment.** A mobile pedicle eases the rest of the gracilis muscle dissection. Perfusion of the skin paddle can then be confirmed. The gracilis muscle is then divided as proximal as possible while protecting the pedicle. The process is repeated inferiorly. Even though muscle tends to atrophy, it can still add volume to the flap and it is a suitable bed for future fat grafting. Once ready for transfer, the artery and vein to gracilis can be clipped and divided.
9. **Closure of the Donor Site.** A size 16 drain is placed in the defect left by the gracilis harvest, exiting anteriorly in the groin. Meticulous closure is key for donor site complication avoidance. We prefer to use skin staples as provisional closure, paying attention to address any potential posterior dog ear deformity (Fig. 36.13). Layered closure from posterior to anterior, with interrupted 2–0 Vicryl and 3–0 Monocryl, is adequate.

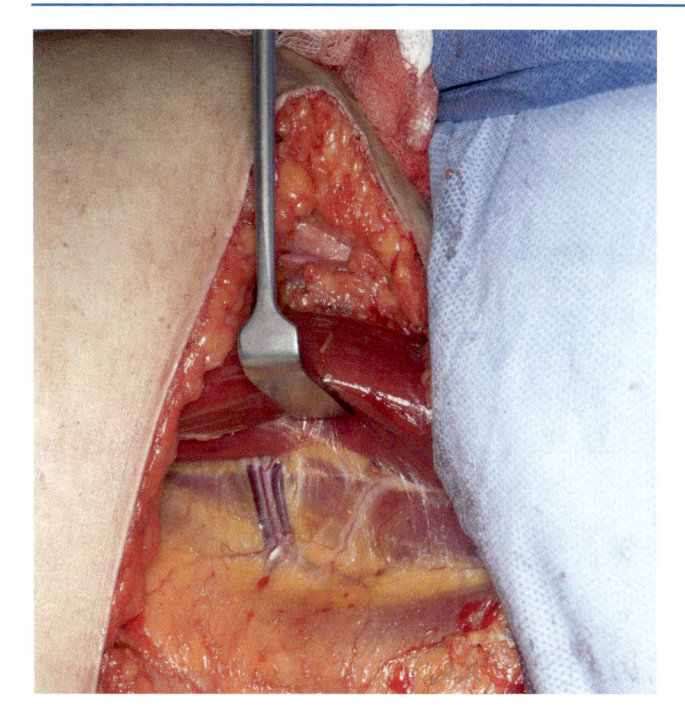

Fig. 36.10 Retraction of the adductor longus muscle reveals the pedicle to the gracilis nerve along with the branch to gracilis from the obturator nerve

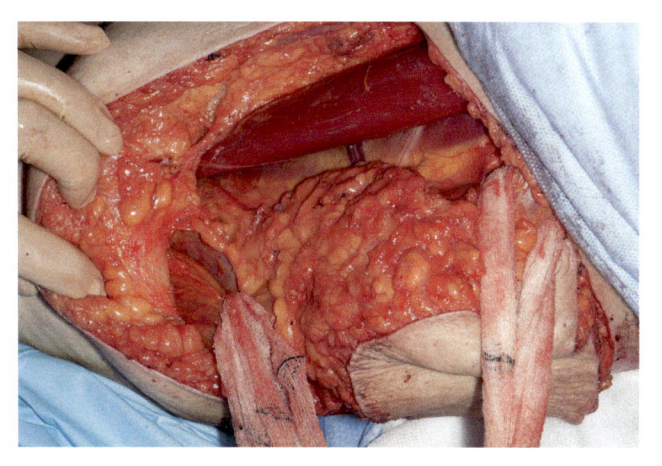

Fig. 36.11 The gracilis muscle can be retracted using two gauzes which facilitates dissection through the areolar plain between adductor longus and magnus muscles

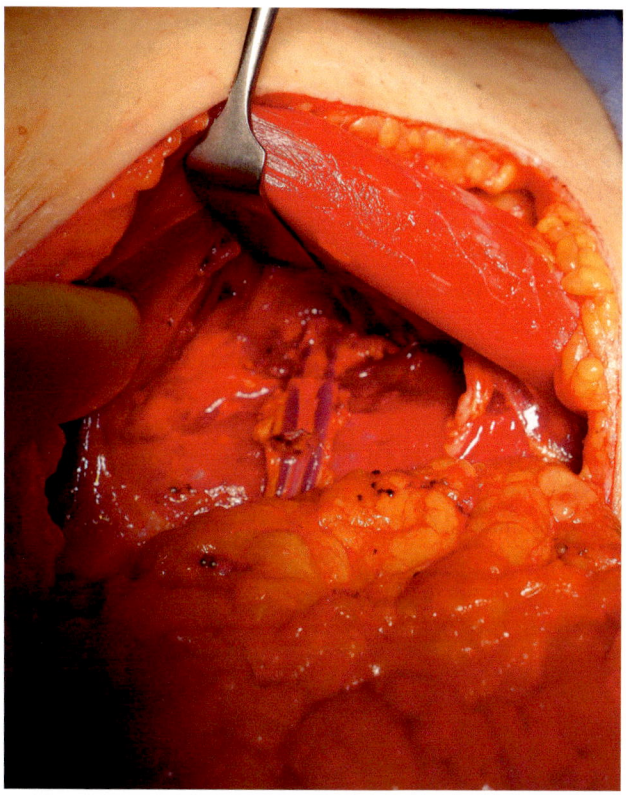

Fig. 36.12 Dissection of the pedicle is complete when the source vessel is reached

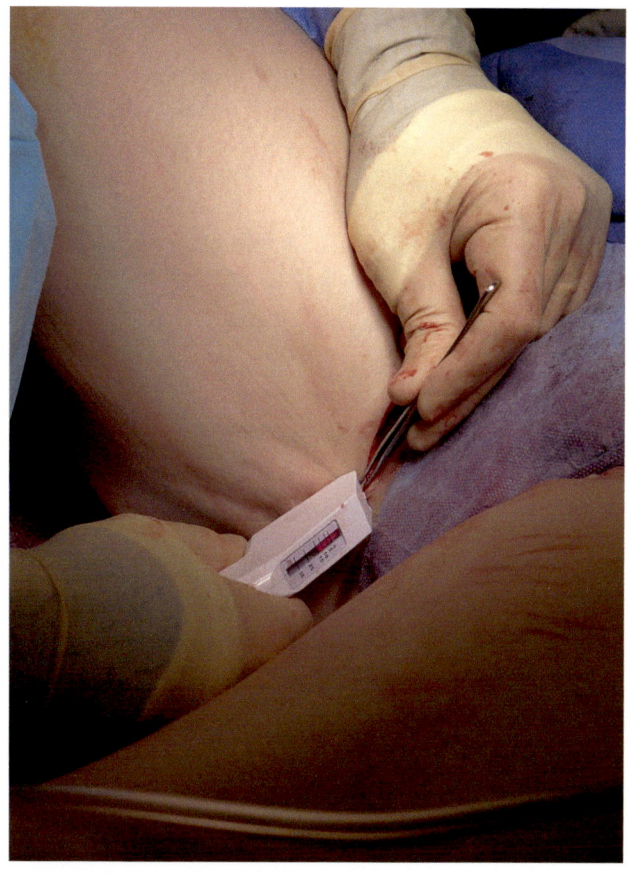

Fig. 36.13 Temporary closure using staples allows avoiding a posterior dog ear deformity when suturing the donor site

36.6 Core Surgical Techniques in Flap Dissection

1. **Patient Positioning and Skin Incision.** Even though raising does not take long for this flap, hyperabduction of the hip and pressure sores in the lateral ankle area should be avoided. An assistant holding the abducted thigh can help avoid this issue.
2. **Anterior Raising of the Flap.** We perform most of the skin paddle dissection using finger-switch diathermy in coagulation mode. Dissection around the great saphenous vein can be performed using Debakey forceps and tenotomy scissors.
3. **Superior Margin Dissection:** Trying to incorporate tissues superior to this incision is usually pointless, as there is minimal subcutaneous fat on the groin and gluteal creases. As previously mentioned, injury to the posterior cutaneous nerve of the thigh should be avoided.
4. **Identification of the Gracilis Pedicle.** The artery and vein to gracilis enter the flap with its nerve, classically described as forming a 45 degree angle.
5. **Dissection around Gracilis Muscle.** Finger dissection superior and inferior to the pedicle allows freeing the muscle circumferentially. A moist gauze can be used to wrap around the gracilis muscle as a visual aid assisting in the later dissection.
6. **Pedicle Dissection.** After identifying the vessels to gracilis, these can be dissected out using bipolar diathermy and Debakey forceps. We reserve the use of ligaclips for large branches only. Even though these provide adequate control, they can also easily get in the way while dissecting under adductor longus. The heat-sinking technique protecting the pedicle with the Debakey forces avoids heat damaging it.
7. **Completion of Raising and Detachment.** We do not routinely harvest the whole muscle, but some length can be useful to fill the upper breast pole. It is advisable if bilateral TUG flaps are raised, that the surgeon detaching the muscle does so at both sides. This allows harvesting similar muscle length.
8. **Closure of the Donor Site.** We have recently adopted the use of barbed sutures to accelerate donor site closure. This is technically more difficult to get right compared with interrupted stitching. We advise putting a few deep 2–0 vicryl stitches to preserve tissue alignment before using the barbed suture.

36.7 Clinical Scenario

36.7.1 Bilateral TUG

A 56-year-old female patient previously treated for breast cancer with bilateral skin-sparing mastectomies and implant-based reconstructions, presenting worsening capsular contracture (Fig. 36.14a). She was referred to our service for consideration of salvage with bilateral autologous reconstruction. CT-angiography demonstrated lack of suitable abdominal perforators, therefore decided to proceed with bilateral TUG flaps. A first stage free flap surgery was performed, including monitoring skin paddles (Fig. 36.14b) was later followed by excision of the skin paddles under local anaesthetic, nipple reconstruction with local flap and tattooing of the areola (Fig. 36.14c).

36.7.2 Unilateral TUG

A 45-year-old female patient that underwent a skin sparing mastectomy and immediate breast and nipple reconstruction with a TUG flap (Fig. 36.15a, b).

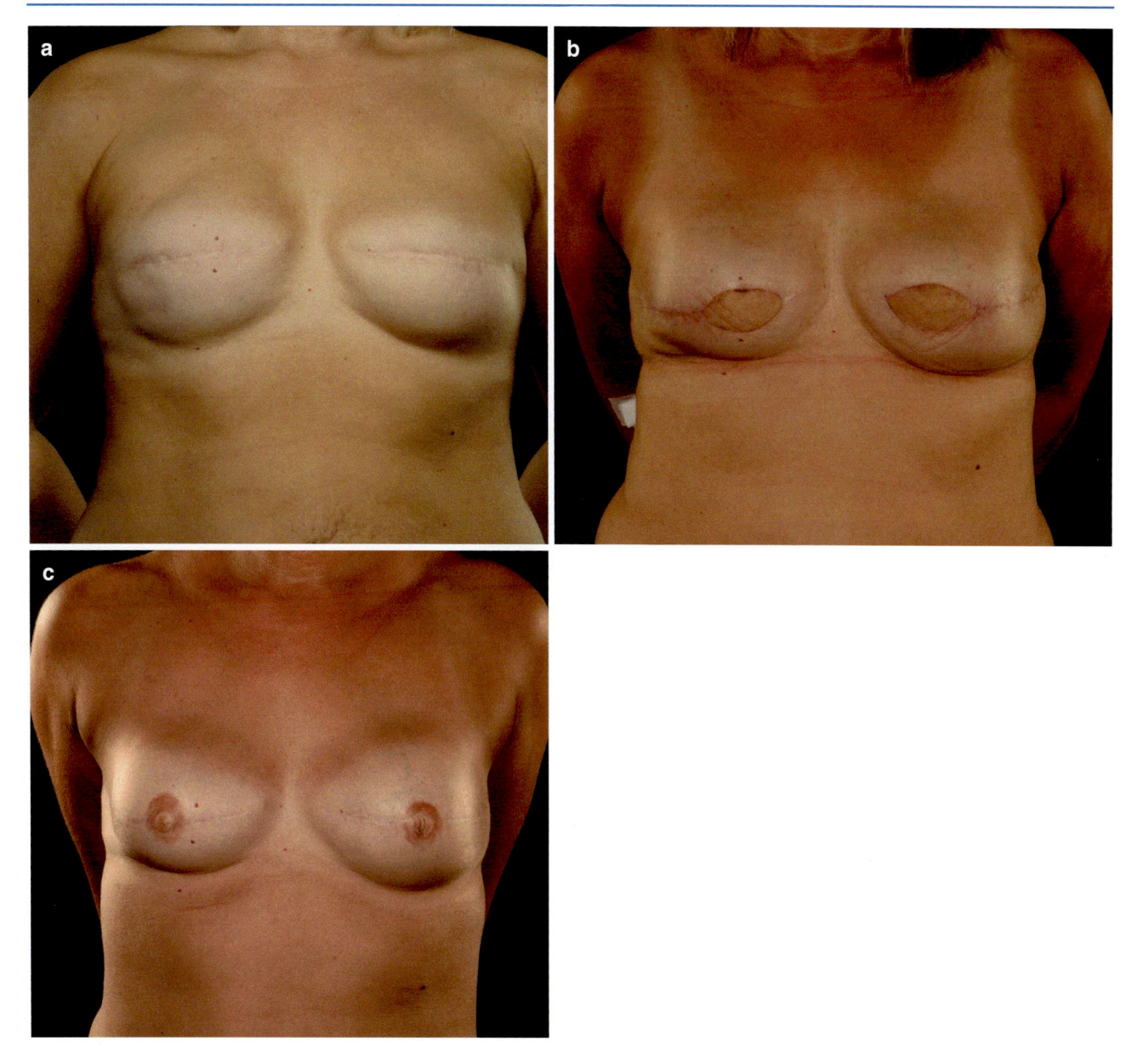

Fig. 36.14 (a–c) Case of bilateral breast reconstruction with TUG flaps

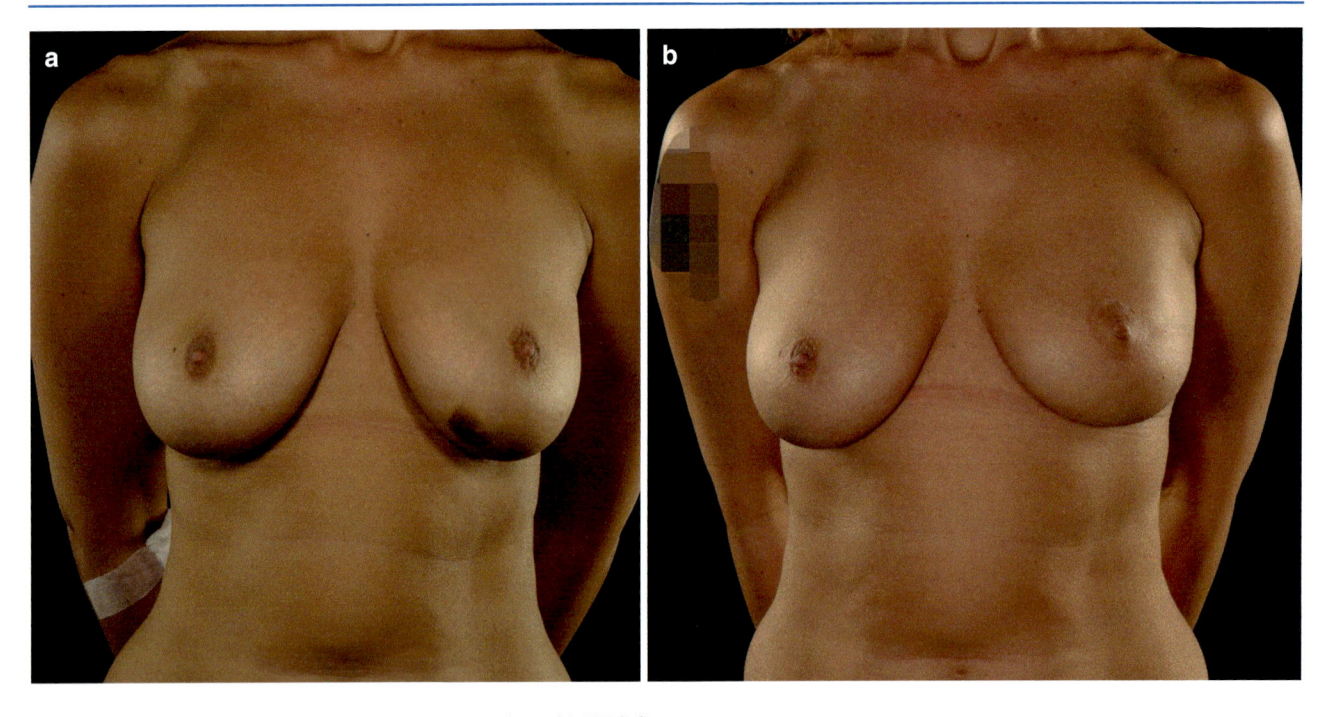

Fig. 36.15 (**a**, **b**) Case of unilateral breast reconstruction with TUG flaps

36.8 Pearls and Pitfalls

Pearls
- The transverse skin paddle of the TUG flap can be modified to a more diagonal direction to avoid placing a posterior scar in a pressure area [13]. We have used an L-shaped modification to increase the volume of this flap (approximately 30–40%) with good results [14].
- The dissection of the pedicle as it reaches the medial circumflex femoral artery can be difficult as the adductor longus needs to be retracted. If this step is problematic the lateral septum of the adductor longus can be opened up, allowing direct visualisation of the gracilis pedicle as it reaches its source vessel [15].
- For immediate breast reconstruction cases, we prefer accessing the internal mammary vessels under the fourth costal cartilage, as at this level there is less calibre mismatch with the gracilis pedicle.
- For insetting this flap in immediate breast reconstruction cases, we prefer to place the anterior limb of the flap medially and the skin paddle along the bottom to recreate the medial, inferior and lateral poles. The inferior gracilis muscle stump can be secured in the upper pole, which usually requires subsequent fat grafting.
- Immediate nipple reconstruction can be achieved with a TUG flap [10] (Fig. 36.16).

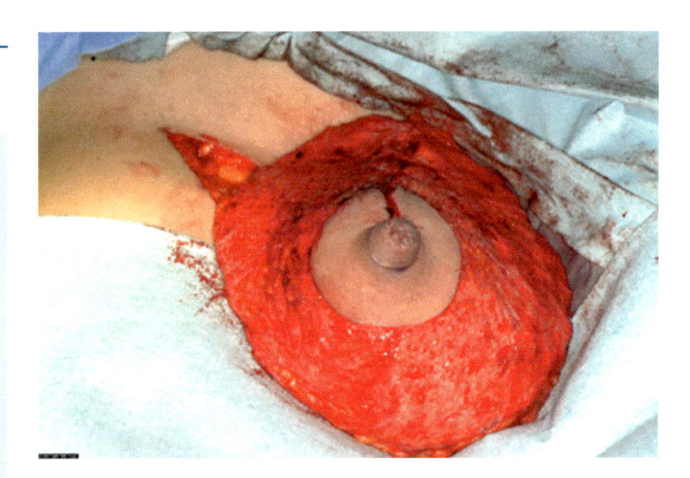

Fig. 36.16 Immediate nipple–areola complex reconstruction coning a TUG flap

Pitfalls
- As previously mentioned, the muscle division is best if performed by the same surgeon, so similar volumes can be harvested.
- For delayed breast reconstruction, excessive coning of the flap to increase projection can result in an unnatural narrow breast.
- The operating microsurgeon should be prepared to perform end-to-side arterial anastomosis if the vessel calibre mismatch is close to 3:1.

36.9 Selected Readings

1. ZM Arnez, D Pogorelec, F Planinsek, U Ahcan. Breast Reconstruction by the Free Transverse Gracilis (TUG) Flap. Br J Plast Surg. 2004 Jan;57(1):20-6.

   Inceptional paper that later popularised the use of this flap as a second option for breast reconstruction, demonstrating its safety and applications

2. Russe E, Kholosy H, Weitgasser L, Brandstetter M, Traintinger H, Neureiter J, Wechselberger G, Schoeller T. Autologous fat grafting for enhancement of breast reconstruction with a transverse myocutaneous gracilis flap: a cohort study. J Plast Reconstr Aesthet Surg. 2018 Nov;71(11):1557–62.

   This outcomes study demonstrates the utility of adjunct fat transfer to optimise results after TUG flaps for breast reconstruction

3. Saour S, Libondi G, Ramakrishnan V. Microsurgical Refinements With the Use of Internal Mammary (IM) Perforators as Recipient Vessels in Transverse Upper Gracilis (TUG) Autologous Breast Reconstruction. Gland Surg. 2017 Aug;6(4):375–9.

   The internal mammary vessels are the recipient of preference. The TUG fap has a shorter pedicle than the DIEP flap. Therefore, it is helpful to have recipient in the wound

4. Fattah A, Figus A, Mathur B, Ramakrishnan VV. The transverse Myocutaneous Gracilis flap: technical refinements. J Plast Reconstr Aesthet Surg. 2010 Feb;63(2):305–13.

   This article contains an excellent description of the TUG flap raising technique

5. Park JE, Alkureishi LWT, Song DH. TUGs Into VUGs and Friendly BUGs: Transforming the Gracilis Territory Into the Best Secondary Breast Reconstructive Option. Plast Reconstr Surg. 2015 Sep;136(3):447–54.

   This paper describes some of the skin paddle modifications for the TUG flap.

References

1. Heckler FR. Gracilis Myocutaneous and muscle flaps. Surg: Clin Plast; 1980. p. 7.
2. Zukowski M, Lord J, Ash K, Shouse B, Getz S, Robb G. The Gracilis free flap revisited: a review of 25 cases of transfer to traumatic extremity wounds. Ann Plast Surg. 1998;40:141. https://doi.org/10.1097/00000637-199802000-00006.
3. Yousif NJ, Matloub HS, Kolachalam R, Grunert BK, Sanger JR. The transverse Gracilis musculocutaneous flap. Ann Plast Surg. 1992;29:482. https://doi.org/10.1097/00000637-199212000-00002.
4. Schoeller T, Wechselberger G. Breast reconstruction by the free transverse Gracilis (TUG) flap. Br J Plast Surg. 2004;57:481. https://doi.org/10.1016/j.bjps.2004.02.016.
5. Arnez ZM, Pogorelec D, Planinsek F, Ahcan U. Breast reconstruction by the free transverse Gracilis (TUG) flap. Br J Plast Surg. 2004;57:20. https://doi.org/10.1016/j.bjps.2003.10.007.
6. Moller L, Berner JE, Dheansa B. The reconstructive journey: description of the breast reconstruction pathway in a high-volume UK-based microsurgical Centre. J Plast Reconstr Aesthet Surg. 2019;72:1930. https://doi.org/10.1016/j.bjps.2019.07.017.
7. Rozen WM, Patel NG, Ramakrishnan VV. Increasing options in autologous microsurgical breast reconstruction: four free flaps for "stacked" bilateral breast reconstruction. Gland Surg. 2016;5:255.
8. Dayan JH, Allen RJ. Lower extremity free flaps for breast reconstruction. Plast Reconstr Surg. 2017;140:77S. https://doi.org/10.1097/PRS.0000000000003944.
9. Sacak B, Gurunluoglu R. The innervated Gracilis muscle for microsurgical functional lip reconstruction: review of the literature. Ann Plast Surg. 2015;74:204. https://doi.org/10.1097/SAP.0b013e3182920c99.
10. Fattah A, Figus A, Mathur B, Ramakrishnan VV. The transverse Myocutaneous Gracilis flap: technical refinements. J Plast Reconstr Aesthet Surg. 2010;63:305. https://doi.org/10.1016/j.bjps.2008.10.015.
11. Allen RJ, Haddock NT, Ahn CY, Sadeghi A. Breast reconstruction with the Profunda artery perforator flap. Plast Reconstr Surg. 2012;129:16e. https://doi.org/10.1097/PRS.0b013e3182363d9f.
12. Nicholas T, Haddock SST. Consecutive 265 Profunda artery perforator flaps: refinements, satisfaction, and functional outcomes. Plast Reconstr Surg Glob Open. 2020;8 https://doi.org/10.1097/GOX.0000000000002682.
13. Dayan E, Smith ML, Sultan M, Samson W, Dayan JH. The diagonal upper Gracilis (DUG) flap: a safe and improved alternative to the TUG flap. Plast Reconstr Surg. 2013;132:33–4.
14. Berner JE, Henton JMD, Blackburn A. The L-shaped modification of the transverse upper gracilis (TUG) flap. Eur J Plast Surg. 2020;43:1–6.
15. King ICC, Obeid N, Woollard AC, Jones ME. Maximizing length and safety in gracilis free flap dissection. J Plast Reconstr Aesthet Surg. 2016;69:1452–3.

37. Medial Circumflex Femoral Artery: Gracilis Muscle Flap

Robert Miller, Dariush Nikkhah, and Graeme Glass

37.1 Introduction

The gracilis flap is a versatile option for regional and free flap reconstruction. First published in 1952 by Pickrell as a pedicle muscle flap for anal reconstruction [1] it was thereafter described as a pedicled musculocutaneous flap [2, 3] and finally as a free flap in 1976 [4]. In the form of a free flap it has become a well-established reconstructive option for small extremity wounds, functional limb reconstruction and facial reanimation. As a pedicle flap, it is used in groin, perineal and vaginal reconstruction. With a single dominant vascular pedicle supplemented by additional segmental minor pedicles, it is a type II flap according the to the classification of Mathes and Nahai [5].

The flexibility of the gracilis flap lies with the fact that a variable length of muscle may be harvested, from a short segment centred on the dominant pedicle to the entire length of the muscle including tendon. Further modifications include the addition of a portion of adductor longus muscle as a chimeric flap [6] or the inclusion of a perforator-based fasciocutaneous component based on a cutaneous perforator from the main pedicle. Moreover, with a single motor nerve branch it may be utilized as a functional muscle flap. As it can be raised either as a muscle flap or a musculocutaneous flap, there is versatility in both volume and texture. Moreover, the muscle will atrophy with time and is thus useful when contour adaptation is important [7]. Importantly, with an excellent donor site scar hidden in the medial thigh and almost no power deficit in thigh adduction post-harvest, the use of this flap is without appreciable donor site morbidity.

37.2 Anatomy

The gracilis has a broad origin from the inferior portion of the pubic symphysis and inferior ramus of the pubis with both muscular and tendinous components. It then tapers into a slender, flat and thin muscle running superficially down the medial thigh. In the proximal thigh, the gracilis is found medial and posterior to the adductor longus (AL), of which the proximal tendon can be easily palpated in the medial thigh with the patient lying supine in a frog leg position. The distal third of the muscle then runs posteriorly to the sartorius, and anteriorly to the adductor magnus, as it passes posteriorly to the medial femoral condyle along with the sartorius. The gracilis inserts between the sartorius (anterior) and semitendinosus (posterior) tendons on the anteromedial aspect of the proximal tibia, together forming the pes anserinus.

The gracilis is based on a single dominant vascular pedicle. Most commonly this is the terminal branch of the medial femoral circumflex artery, in turn arising from the profunda femoris artery. However, the dominant pedicle may also arise from the profunda femoris artery directly. On entering the muscle, the artery divides, most commonly into three branches [8] before ultimately forming anastomoses with the minor pedicles. Additional minor pedicles are present with the most common configuration consisting of two minor pedicles [9] usually from the superficial femoral artery, although the distal minor pedicle may arise from the popliteal artery [9]. Usually the arterial pedicle is accompanied by two venae comitantes which join prior to draining into the profunda femoris vein. The length of the venous pedicle is therefore 1–2 cm shorter than the arterial pedicle, which is approximately 7 cm in length [6].

The presence of at least one skin perforator measuring over 0.5 mm has been reported in the majority of cases [8, 10]. Skin perforators are most consistently found over the proximal third of the muscle, loosely associated with the position of the dominant pedicle [8, 9, 11]. Predominantly, the skin perforators pursue a musculocutaneous course but septocutaneous (between gracilis and AL) skin perforators have also been described.

Motor innervation to the gracilis is from a single anterior branch of the obturator nerve (L2–4), which runs between the gracilis and AL supplying both. The nerve can be found deep to the vessels, entering the muscle approximately 1–1.5 cm proximal (superior) to the pedicle [6, 12]. It may be dissected under adductor longus [8] to its bifurcaton with the posterior branch which supplies adductor magnus and (usually) adductor brevis. The posterior branch must be preserved. Typically, the distance from the point of entry into gracilis and the bifurcation with the posterior branch is 4-5 cm, in our experience, or 2–4 cm from the obturator foramen. A sensory branch of the anterior obturator nerve supplying the medial thigh skin (medial cutaneous nerve of the thigh) runs as a separate branch in tandem to the motor branch [6].

An appreciation of the above anatomy is particularly important when considering flap thinning in cases of facial reanimation, for example. The muscle can be thinned but great care must be taken when doing so to avoid compromising the vascular supply and/or nerve input to the portion of the muscle designated to the flap.

37.3 Pre-Operative Investigations

Routine pre-operative imaging is not indicated. However, angiography studies may be pertinent in patients with prior upper thigh/ pelvic injury or surgery. It has been suggested that pre-operative non-invasive angiography may be used to predict the territory supplied by different pedicle arrangements, facilitating a safer approach to the design of composite tissue flaps [13]. Similarly, while hand held-Doppler is not used routinely pre- or intra-operatively for gracilis muscle harvest alone, it may be used to identify perforators when incorporating a cutaneous component into gracilis flap design [10].

37.4 Flap Design and Markings

37.4.1 Marking

With the patient supine in a frog leg position (hip abducted and the knee flexed), the adductor longus tendon is clearly palpated and marked. The gracilis can be palpated posterior/inferiorly (approximately two finger breadths) to this in the medial thigh. Its origin should be identified and marked from the inferior portion of the pubic symphysis and inferior ramus of the pubis. Finally, the medial tibial condyle should be palpated and marked to indicate its insertion (Fig. 37.1). A line connecting the midpoint of the origin to the insertion should be marked. The proximal two-thirds represent the muscle component and the distal third the tendon. Approximately 10 cm distal to the inferior pubic symphysis is marked as the most likely site of the pedicle and skin perforators, which enter the flap from the superior lateral aspect.

37.4.2 Flap Design

Flap design will depend on the indication. There are no significant differences to flap design for a pedicle or free flap. If the gracilis muscle alone is needed, an incision should be marked approximately 2 cm posterior to the main portion of the muscle body, with or without a secondary incision marked over the insertion. The length of the proximal incision and need for a secondary incision at the insertion will depend on the length of muscle and tendon required, and should be adapted accordingly.

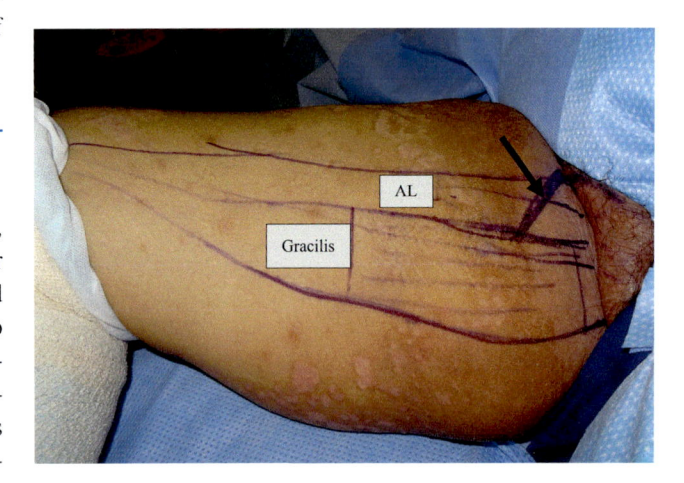

Fig. 37.1 The adductor longus (AL) is palpated and then marked. Approximately 2 cm posterior to this the gracilis is palpated and marked. The course of the pedicle is also marked (black arrow)

If a musculocutaneous flap is needed, an oval-shaped skin paddle should be designed over the gracilis muscle. If a short paddle is needed, this should be centred over the muscle pedicle. If a longer paddle is required, this should be designed as an extension of the short paddle to incorporate the most reliable perforators. It should be remembered that the distal skin paddle may be unreliable and careful evaluation of the perforator arrangement is necessary as part of the approach considered here [14]. The width of the flap should not exceed the ability to close the skin directly without tension. This is typically up to 5 cm but the 'finger grasp' test to evaluate the feasibility of primary closure is essential before committing [6]. A transverse skin paddle design has also been described [13, 15] which can be harvested as a musculocutaneous flap or fasciocutaneous flap based on a mapped perforator [16].

37.5 Flap Raise/Elevation – A Step-by-Step Guide

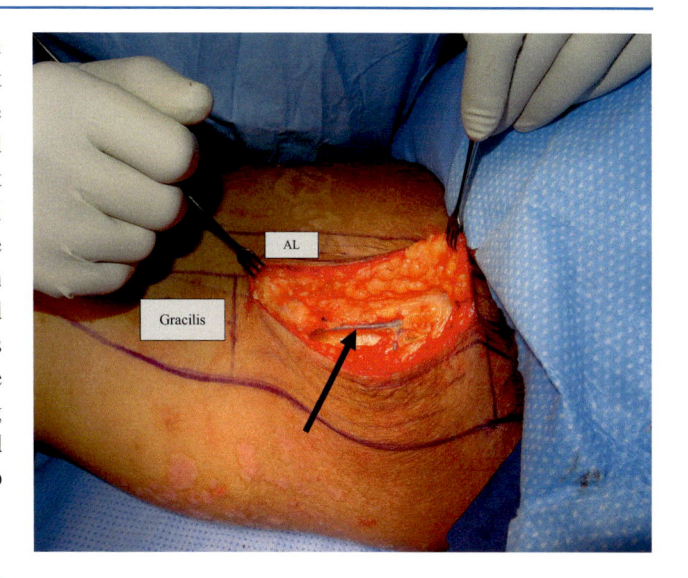

Fig. 37.3 Identification of the great saphenous vein (black arrow) superficially

The patient should be positioned supine, with the knee flexed and the hip flexed and abducted (externally rotated). In this position the hip, knee and foot must be supported to stabilize the position (Fig. 37.2).

- **Step 1.** Incise the skin based on the above discussed markings. If raising a musculocutaneous flap, incise just the distal aspect or at the tendon insertion if harvesting tendon.
- **Step 2.** Identify and preserve the great saphenous vein (GSV) running obliquely over the AL and gracilis (Fig. 37.3).
- **Step 3.** Incise down to the gracilis muscle fascia (Fig. 37.4).
  (a) If raising a musculocutaneous flap, incise down to the gracilis tendon. Identify the gracilis as it runs distally to insert between the sartorius and semitendinosus. Identify the muscle and confirm that the designed skin paddle is orientated over the muscle. Continue the incision proximally and along the anterior border of the skin paddle. Alternatively, a new proximal incision can be made on the anterior aspect of the skin paddle.
- **Step 4.** Incise the fascia exposing the AL superiorly and the anterior border of the gracilis inferiorly. Continue the fascial incision exposing the required gracilis muscle length (Fig. 37.5).
- **Step 5.** Isolate the muscle from the surrounding tissue using blunt dissection.
- **Step 6.** Gently retract the gracilis medially and superiorly to help identify and protect the pedicle.
- **Step 7.** Separate the fascial connections between the gracilis and AL anterior medially, adductor magnus posterior and sartorius distally until the pes anserinus.
- **Step 8.** Retract the AL laterally and superiorly/ anteriorly to facilitate dissection of the neurovascular pedicle entering the muscle posteriorly (Fig. 37.6).
  (a) For the musculocutaneous flap, identify the AL-gracilis septum and include this in the pedicle dissection (to include septocutaneous perforators. However, also remember, the main pedicle may run a septocutaneous course).
- **Step 9.** Dissect the pedicle proximally as it runs between the adductor longus and magnus, ligating branches to the adductor longus (Fig. 37.7).
- **Step 10.** Identify the motor nerve deep and separate to the vessels (Fig. 37.8). Dissect the nerve to the required length, if needed.

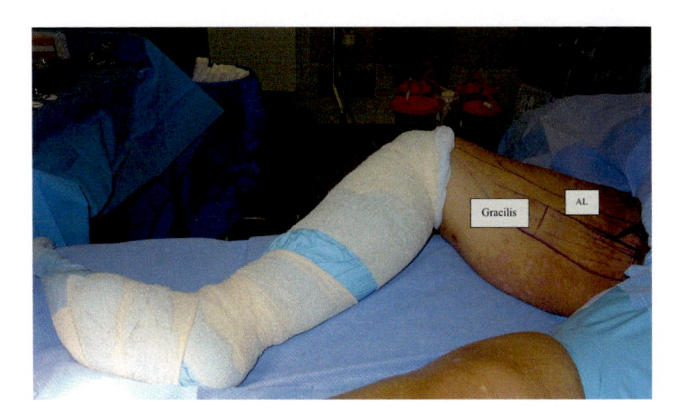

Fig. 37.2 Patient positioned in frog leg position

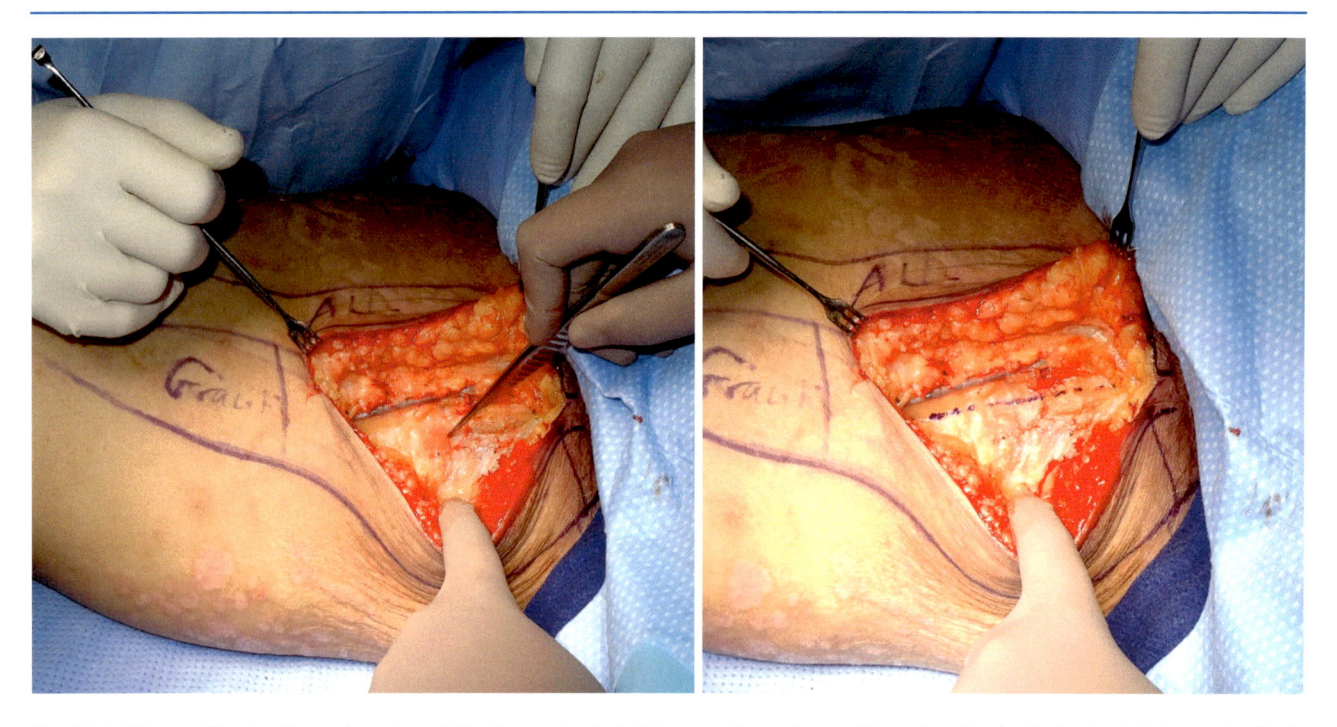

Fig. 37.4 The gracilis should now be palpated. The forceps in the left image point to the gracilis enclosed in fascia. In the right image the fascia between adductor longus and gracilis is marked for incision

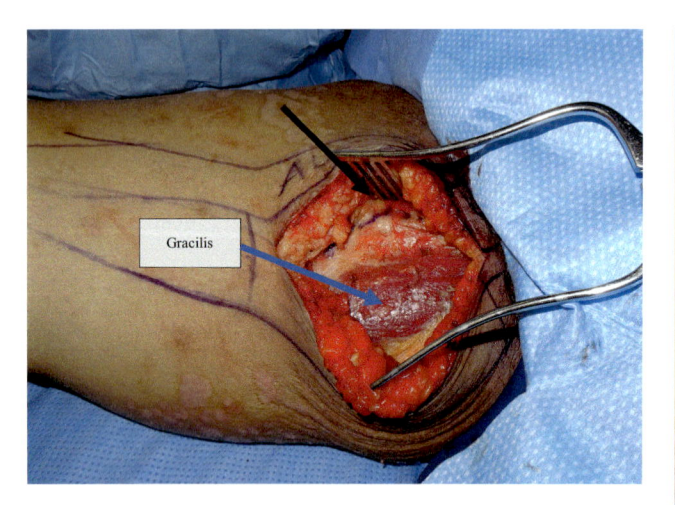

Fig. 37.5 Dissection to expose the gracilis muscle (blue arrow) with the GSV retracted superiorly (black arrow)

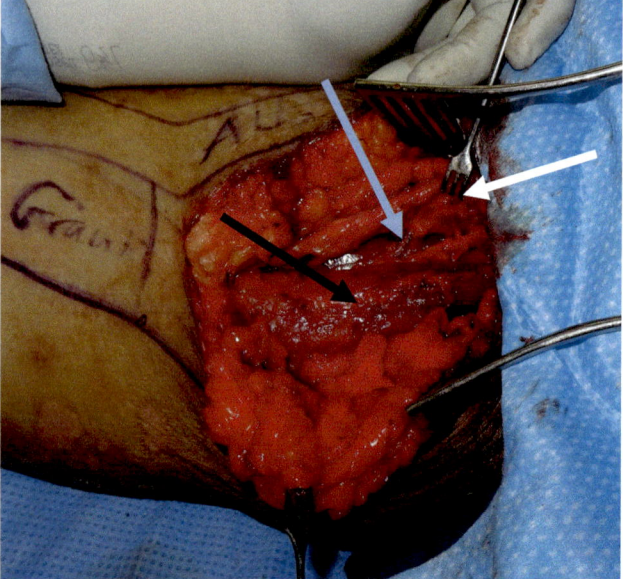

Fig. 37.6 Retraction of the AL superiorly (white arrow) aids identification of the neurovascular pedicle (blue arrow) entering the gracilis (black arrow)

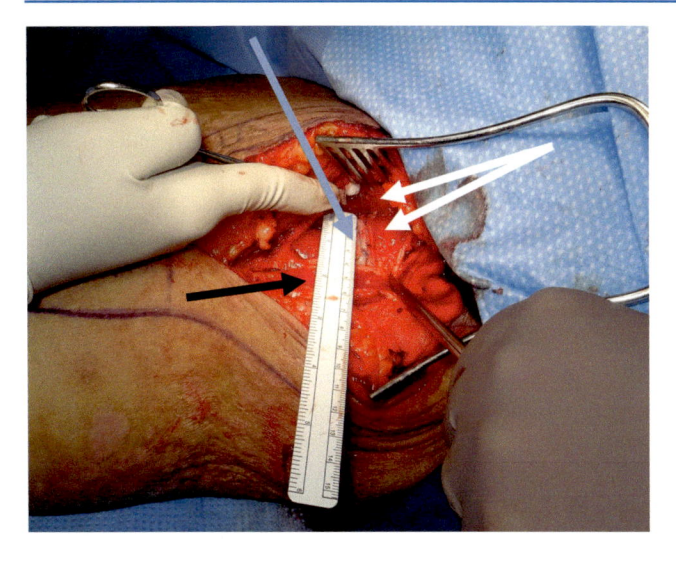

Fig. 37.7 The pedicle (blue arrow) is dissected proximally between the AL and adductor magnus (white arrows). The gracilis is indicated by the black arrow

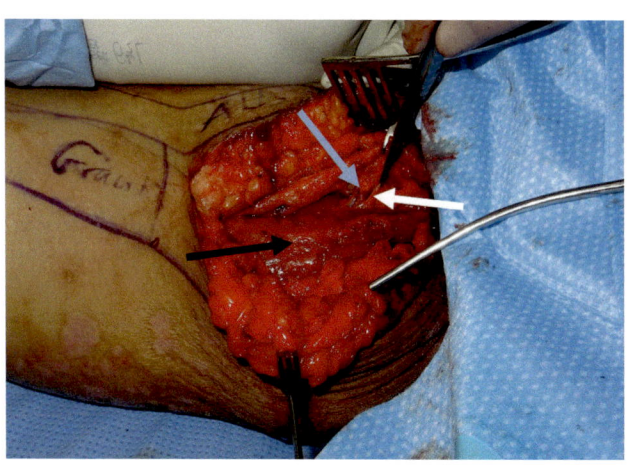

Fig. 37.8 Black arrow = gracilis. Blue arrow = pedicle. White arrow = motor nerve

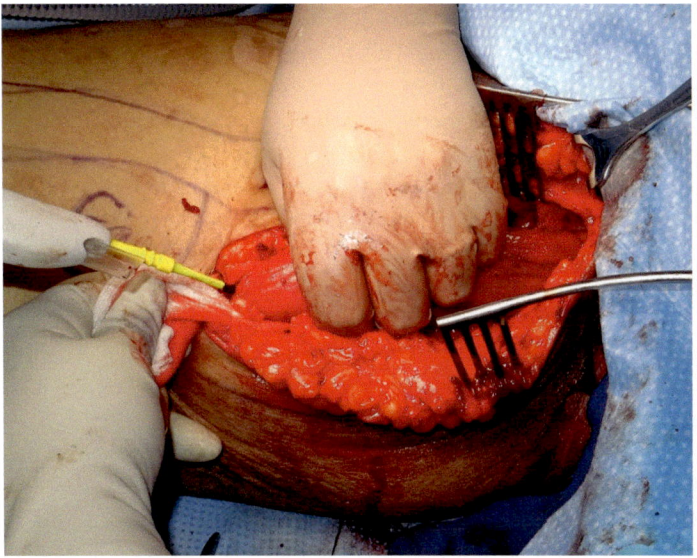

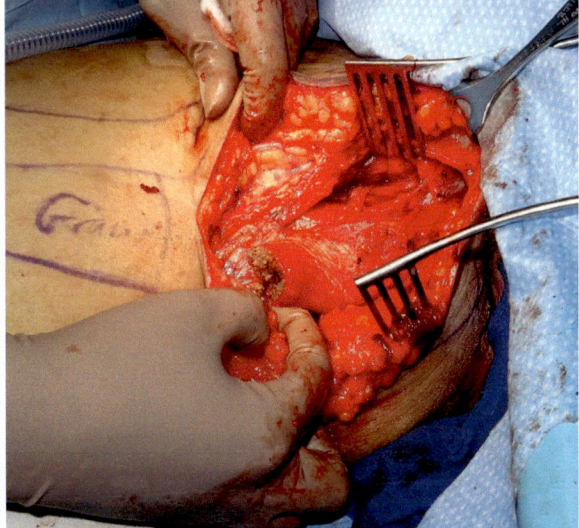

Fig. 37.9 A swab is placed around the proximal gracilis and monopolar cautery used to divide it

- **Step 11.** Free the flap distally. During this you may encounter further pedicles, which can either be preserved or ligated.
- **Step 12.** Place the gracilis at resting tension and mark the muscle at set intervals (every 1 cm, for example. See clinical case 1). This step is necessary for reanimation procedures to facilitate tensioning at inset. It may be omitted when muscle tensioning is not necessary (for example, in lower limb trauma).
- **Step 13.** Divide the flap distally. Options:
  (a) Split the muscle distally at the required length. Place a swab around the muscle and slow division with monopolar cautery can be used to reduce bleeding (Fig. 37.9).
  (b) Split the gracilis tendon approximately 5 cm distal to the musculotendinous junction.
  (c) Make a separate distal incision over the insertion, trace the tendon down to the tibia (between the sartorius and semitendinosus) and harvest at its insertion (Fig. 37.10).
- **Step 14.** Divide the flap proximally, either through the muscle or through the proximal tendinous origin, depending on the length required.
  (a) Remember for the musculocutaneous flap you will also need to incise the posterior border of the skin paddle.

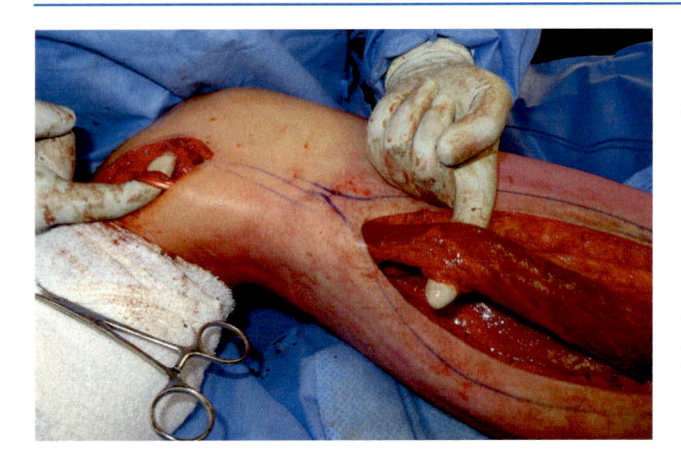

Fig. 37.10 This demonstrates a distal incision at the tendinous insertion which will be divided for harvest

37.6 Core Surgical Techniques in Flap Dissection

There are several modifications and techniques to the gracilis flap raise. This is predominantly regarding the flap dimensions and components raised as outlined in step 13 above.

For muscle-only flaps (step 13a), the muscle and proximal tendinous portion can be trimmed to the appropriate size and shape. Unless inclusion of one or both musculotendinous junctions is essential, trimming of the muscle to length is dependent on adequate positioning of the pedicle.

If the distal gracilis tendon is needed (step 13 b and c), the flap may be raised with or without a skin paddle. Most commonly this is used in limb reconstruction and may only require a small skin paddle for flap monitoring, if so desired. However, these should be used with caution as the skin paddles can be unreliable, appearing unhealthy when the underlying muscle is healthy. If a long length of tendon is required it should be remembered that there are two slips of the distal tendon (see Fig. 37.11 lower image). The first, inserting to the medial tibial condyle, can be divided. The main terminal slip can be raised with tibial periosteum to achieve approximately 1 cm more length [6]. Whether using muscle alone or a musculocutaneous flap for functional free flap reconstruction, the muscle should be marked prior to division. This can be under functional or resting tension. Whichever is used, the same should be used at inset (Figs. 37.12 and 37.13b).

For musculocutaneous flaps, the surgeon should ensure the paddle is appropriately designed over the gracilis muscle and it may be necessary to redesign the skin paddle once the gracilis muscle is identified. If a large skin paddle is needed, from step 6 above you should aim to include septa between the gracilis – adductor magnus and gracilis – sartorius to increase the septocutaneous supply and improve skin paddle survival. If independent movement between muscle and skin is desired this can be achieved by separating the skin flap and muscle. This can be done with ligation/ cautery of musculocutaneous perforators until the proximal AL-Gracilis septum is reached, at which point septal perforators to the skin can be identified and preserved. The skin paddle can then be rotated and placed at inset [6].

Similarly, the gracilis flap can be raised with an independent skin flap from a medial circumflex perforator artery as a conjoint flap [6, 16]. This requires identification of musculocutaneous perforators pre-op using a hand-held Doppler and the skin paddle should be designed centred longitudinally on the selected perforator and elevated as a perforator flap with intra-muscular dissection of the perforators to the main vessel. Elevation of the gracilis muscle flap is then carried out as described above. Similarly, a transversely orientated skin paddle [15] can be designed for a musculocutaneous flap in breast reconstruction. In this case it is not necessary to isolate the transverse skin paddle as a perforator flap. The flap raise should follow the steps for musculocutaneous flap raise above with an adapted skin paddle design.

When using the gracilis muscle or musculocutaneous flap as a pedicled flap in reconstruction of the lower abdomen, groin, vagina or perineum the steps outlined above for flap raise can be followed without division of the pedicle. Patient positioning depends on access to the recipient site, with supine, lithotomy and even prone positioning described as necessary [17].

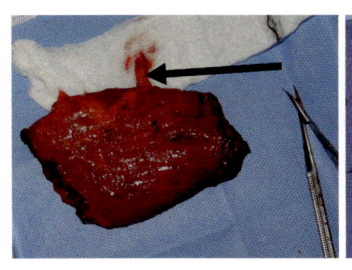

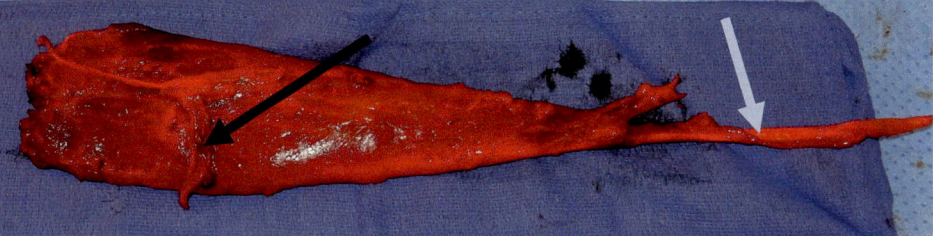

Fig. 37.11 Different flap harvest designs. The top image demonstrating muscle alone for a lower limb reconstruction and the lower image demonstrating the full muscle length with distal tendon (blue arrow) for free functional muscle transfer. Black arrow = pedicle

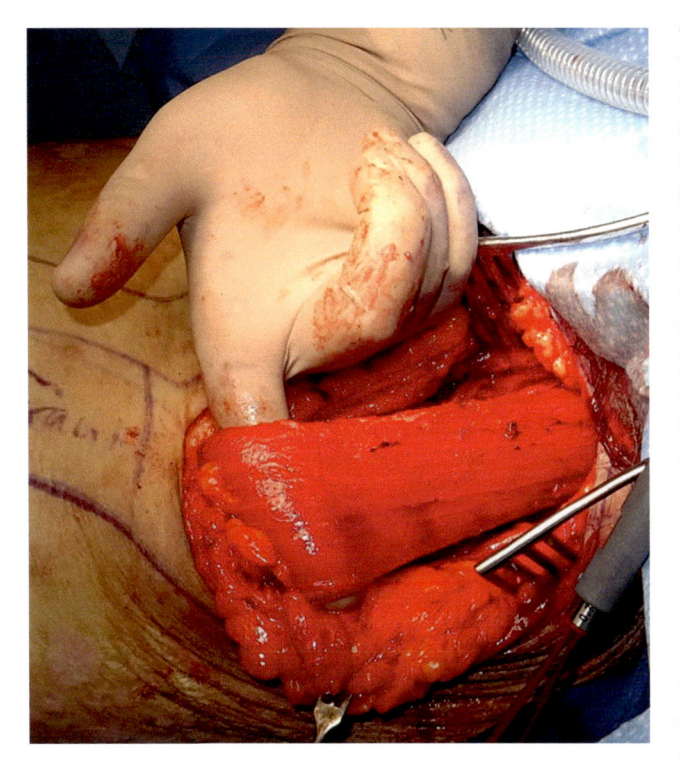

Fig. 37.12 The muscle can be placed under functional tension and marked at 1 cm intervals prior to division

37.7 Clinical Scenario

37.7.1 Case 1: Facial Reanimation: Surgeon Graeme Glass

This case demonstrates an innervated free gracilis flap for left-sided facial reanimation in a child. Pre-operative examination revealed significant facial asymmetry at rest and on dynamic facial movement. The flap was harvested with the vascular pedicle and motor nerve clearly demonstrated in Fig. 37.13a. The gracilis muscle was marked (Fig. 37.13b) to ensure correct tensioning on transfer and inset as discussed above. Figure 37.13c demonstrates the flap inset and tensioning. The vascular pedicle and motor branch can be clearly seen at inset. The flap was thinned to approximately 10 g in situ. The facelift type access was closed and the buried flap was monitored by hourly Doppler signals for the first 24 h followed by 2 hourly to 36 h. A Penrose drain secured in the post-auricular region was removed at 24 h as was a suction drain to the thigh. Post-op recovery was uneventful and facial therapy commenced at 2 weeks. Dynamic facial movement was reestablished at week 7.

37.7.2 Case 2: Upper Limb Reanimation: Surgeons Dariush Nikkhah and Jeremy Rawlins

The gentleman in this case suffered a pan plexus injury to his brachial plexus after a high-speed motorbike road traffic accident. Previous nerve transfers had been unsuccessful. In this case a free functional gracilis muscle transfer was performed to reanimate elbow flexion. The gracilis flap was harvested with gracilis tendon using a two-team approach. The arterial flap pedicle was anastomosed onto the thoracoacromial artery and the flap obturator nerve was anastomosed to the spinal accessory nerve. The proximal end of the gracilis was anchored onto the clavicle and the distal end inserted with a Krakow repair onto the biceps tendon. A small window was kept to monitor the muscle and a Doppler signal was recorded (Fig. 37.14). The patient had an uneventful post-operative recovery and achieved an MRC 4 as demonstrated in the video (Video 37.1).

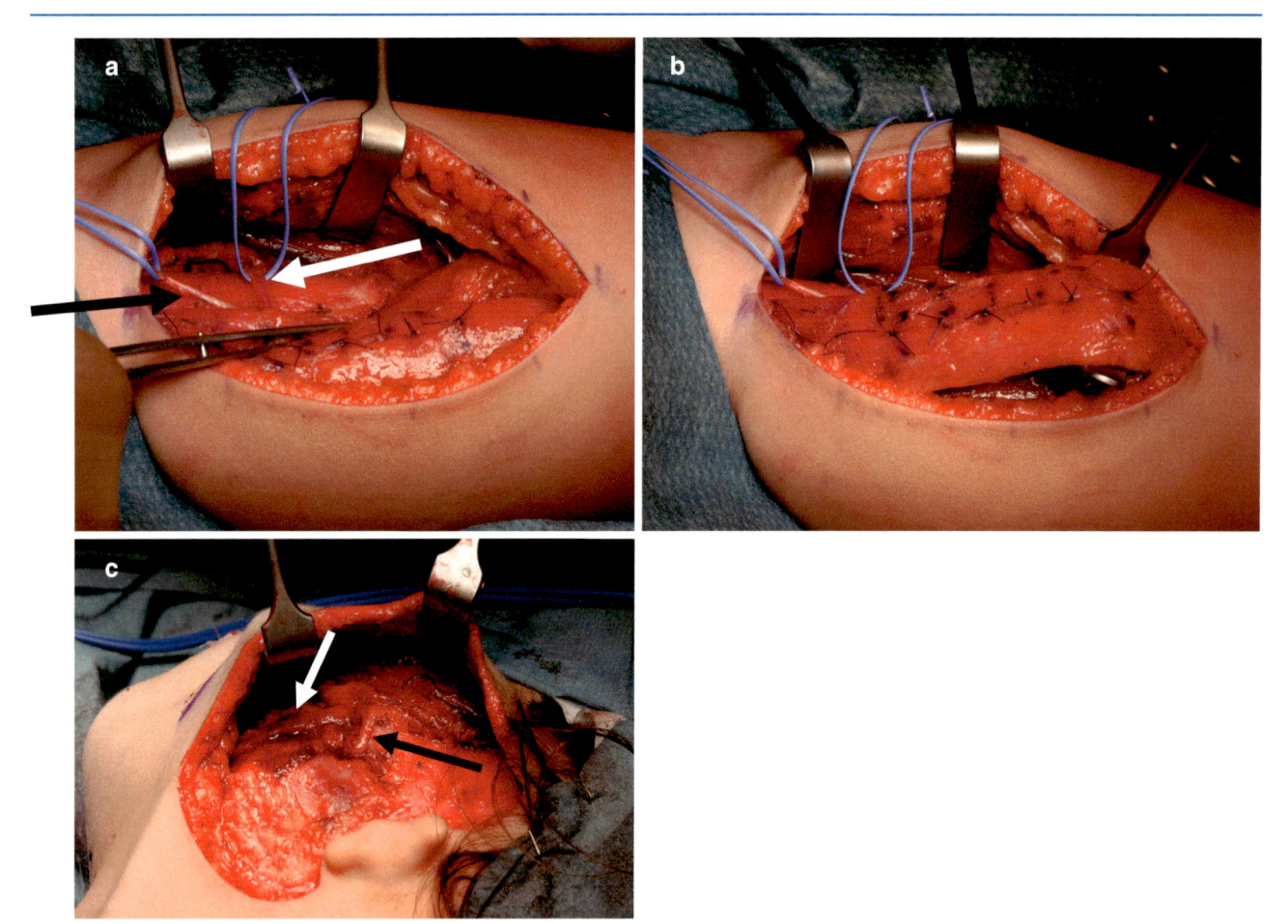

Fig. 37.13 (**a**) This demonstrated the gracilis muscle flap prior to division of the pedicle and muscle. The motor nerve is seen on the left (black arrow) and the pedicle superiorly (white arrow). (**b**) This demonstrated the marking of the muscle to facilitate tensioning on inset. (**c**) This demonstrates the flap after inset and after thinning with the motor nerve (black arrow) and vascular pedicle (white arrow) again highlighted

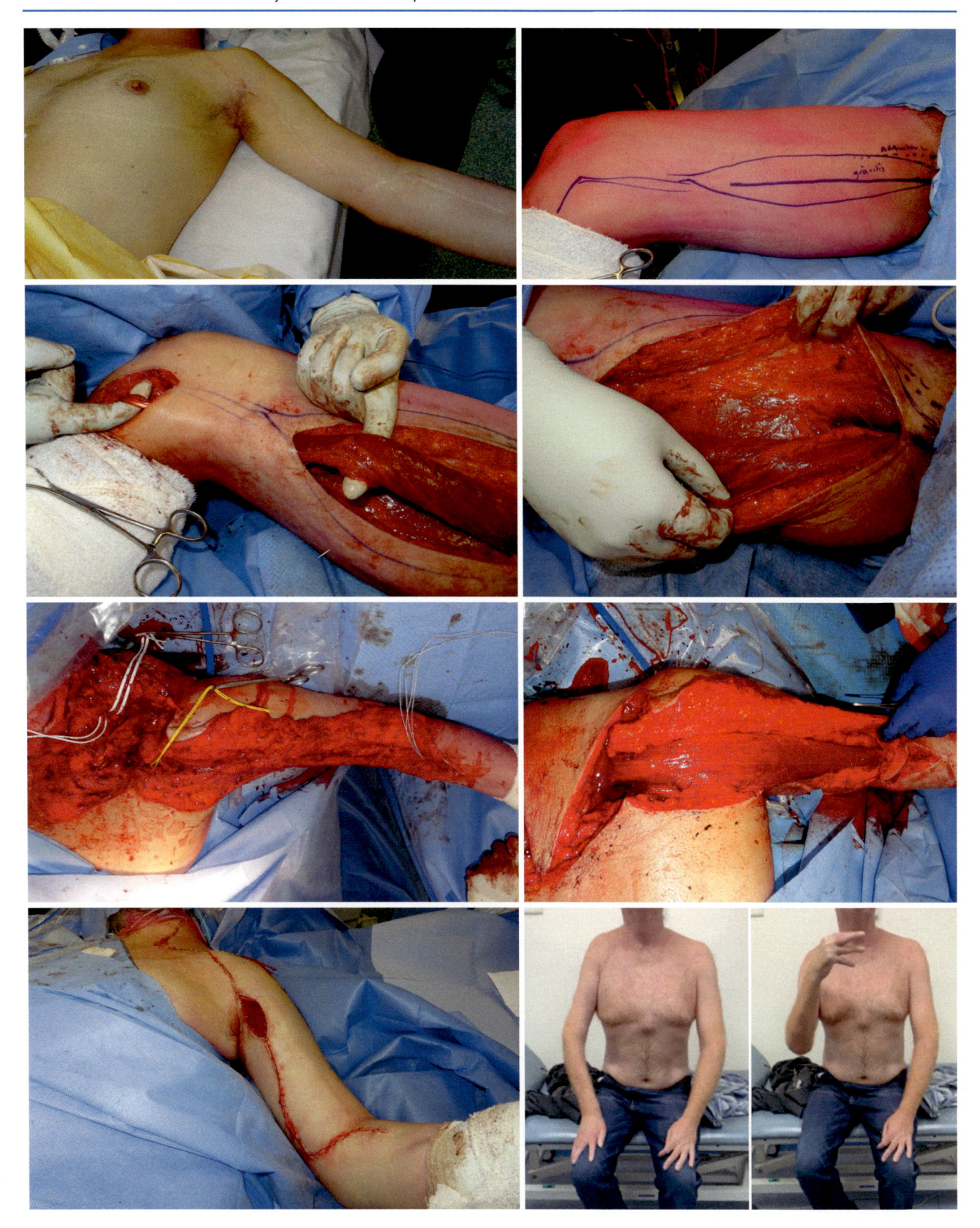

Fig. 37.14 These images demonstrate the patient journey from pre-op, intra-op flap raise and inset and post-operative outcome. Note the window left post-operatively to allow flap monitoring. The post-operative images demonstrating 4/5 elbow flexion power at 6 months

37.8 Pearls and Pitfalls

Pearls

- Suturing the skin paddle to the muscle fascia is advised during the harvest of musculocutaneous flaps to prevent shearing of the musculocutaneous perforators.
- When using a skin paddle, starting flap elevation with the anterior incision allows the adductor longus to be easily identified by its prominent proximal tendon (which is also easily palpated). This gracilis is readily identified posteriorly to this in the upper thigh and allows the step of a distal incision to identify the gracilis tendon and check skin paddle placement to be omitted.
- When using a free gracilis muscle flap, a small window can be left to allow flap monitoring instead of using a skin paddle which may not correlate to the underlying muscle (Fig. 37.14).
- Alternatively, a buried free gracilis flap may be monitored using Doppler ultrasound only. In the absence of peer-reviewed evidence a reasonable protocol is hourly monitoring for the first 24 h and 2 hourly overnight for the next 12 h. At this point, the senior author discontinues protocolled monitoring.
- If using the gracilis as a functional muscle, the resting tension of the inset must equal the resting tension of the muscle in situ. To help get this right, measure and mark (with absorbable sutures) 1 cm intervals along the muscle in situ. Measure again during flap inset to ensure the tension is right.
- When using a free gracilis flap for facial reanimation, it is advisable to use the gracilis muscle from the same side as the side of the face to be reanimated, as, during inset, the orientation of the nerve and vessels better corresponds to the position of the facial vessels and the likely nerve donors. (If performing the procedure in two teams, the flap harvest surgeon may sit on the opposite side while the facial preparation is done on the ipsilateral side).
- Measure the distance between the junction of the tragus and zygomatic arch and the oral commissure and add 2–3 cm for the muscle split. This provides the length of the muscle flap harvest. Next measure the distance between the palpable facial artery as it curves around the body of the mandible and the oral commissure. This provides an estimate for the length of the pedicle needed.
- Inset the distal flap prior to the arterial and venous anastomosis. Then do the nerve coaptation followed be the proximal flap insertion. This provides flap stability while maintaining flexibility of inset and minimizes ischaemic time.

Pitfalls

- Do not confuse the adductors for the gracilis. This may happen if the incision is not marked approximately 2 cm posterior to the main portion of the muscle body. When the patient is supine with the knee flexed (as positioned on the operating table) the gracilis is not under tension and will fall posteriorly. If the incision markings have not been placed as described, the gracilis may be posterior to the incision, causing confusion.
- Insufficient pedicle length. Dissect the pedicle right to its insertion from profunda femoris. This can be facilitated by a window above the adductor longus to help take as much pedicle as needed [18].
- Muscle flaps are more sensitive to ischaemia and therefore one should limit the ischaemic time of the muscle. Ensure the microsurgical setup is well prepared to facilitate this. Aim for an ischaemic time of less than 2 h.
- Pedicle mismatch. Be prepared to do end to side anastomosis or perforator to perforator in lower limb.
- It can be more challenging to elevate muscle flaps versus fasciocutaneous flaps down the line if the flap needs to be elevated to facilitate removal of metal work in the lower limb, for example. Muscle flaps can die if the pedicle is divided down the line and therefore careful case selection is advised when used in lower limb trauma.

37.9 A Note on Monitoring Muscle Flaps for Vascular Compromise

Studies indicate that irreversible ischaemic changes occur within 2 h of compromised skeletal muscle [19]. We must therefore assume that we have a window of no more than 2 h from the onset of flap compromise to the re-establishment of tissue perfusion. In practical terms, the likelihood of successful surgical salvage of a congested muscle flap is therefore low. Logically, the decision about whether to commence a protocol of post-operative flap monitoring must therefore consider whether the resources and logistical infrastructure at the surgeons' disposal can facilitate a rapid return to the operating room if necessary. This must be balanced against the fact that flap monitoring is demanding on clinical time and exhausting for the patient. Thus, given that most flap problems occur within the first 36 h, a rigorous protocol of flap monitoring during this critical period seems reasonable. By contrast, there is little logical merit in prolonged, tapered protocols. Ultimately, the time to make these decisions is not in the lull of mental exhaustion that follows a successful free flap surgery. Protocols should be agreed in advance based on the resources available and deviations from agreed protocols must have a basis in logic.

37.10 Selected Readings

- Giordano PA, Abbes M, Pequignot JP. Gracilis blood supply: anatomical and clinical re-evaluation. Br J Plast Surg. 1990;43 (3):266–272.

  This classic paper provides the groundwork for anatomical investigations and studies of the gracilis flap vasculature, following on from the work by Mathes and Nahai [9].

- Hattori Y1, Doi K, Abe Y, Ikeda K, Dhawan V. Surgical approach to the vascular pedicle of the gracilis muscle flap. J Hand Surg Am. 2002 May;27 (3):534–6.

  This paper describes an easy and safe approach to the vascular pedicle of the gracilis muscle flap. With this technique the vascular pedicle can be harvested with maximum length and the largest possible calibre for functioning free muscle transfer [20].

- Tremp M, Oranges CM, Wang WJ, Wettstein R, Zhang YX, Schaefer DJ, Kalbermatten DF. The "nugget design": A modified segmental gracilis free flap for small-sized defect reconstruction on the lower extremity. J Plast Reconstr Aesthet Surg. 2017.

  The paper introduces a technical refinement for small-sized three-dimensional defect reconstruction on the foot using a segmental free gracilis muscle flap supplied but secondary proximal pedicles. Although in the majority of cases the gracilis is based on it is dominant pedicle, it should be remembered that this is a versatile flap that can be adapted to a wide range of reconstructions [21].

- Franco MJ, Nicolson MC, Parikh RP, Tung TH. Lower Extremity Reconstruction with Free Gracilis Flaps. J Reconstr Microsurg. 2017 Mar;33 (3):218–224.

  This paper discusses the use of the gracilis flap in lower limb reconstruction. It supports its use for small- and medium-sized defects and highlights the benefit of a denervated muscle flap for this reconstruction with good long-term outcomes [7].

- Coelho JAJ, McDermott FD, Cameron O, Smart NJ, Watts AM, Daniels IR. Single centre experience of bilateral gracilis flap perineal reconstruction following extra-levator abdominoperineal excision. Colorectal Dis. 2019;21 (8):910–91.

  This recent paper reports the authors use of the gracilis flap for perineal reconstruction. They have found success in positioning the patient prone, as discussed above, and is worth reviewing if this is to be attempted [17].

- Doi K, Sakai K, Kuwata N, Ihara K, Kawai S. Double free-muscle transfer to restore prehension following complete brachial plexus avulsion. The Journal of Hand Surgery. 1995 May 1;20 (3):408–14.

  A fantastic paper from Doi et al. on the use of double functional free muscle transfers in brachial plexus injury. Although in this series the gracilis is not used in isolation, it is the favoured flap and highlights its importance in the function of reconstructing the upper limb [22].

References

1. Pickrell KL, Broadbent TR, Masters FW, Metzger JT. Construction of a rectal sphincter and restoration of anal continence by transplanting the gracilis muscle; a report of four cases in children. Ann Surg. 1952;135(6):853–62.
2. Orticochea M. The musculo-cutaneous flap method: an immediate and heroic substitute for the method of delay. Br J Plast Surg. 1972;25(2):106–10.
3. McCraw JB, Massey FM, Shanklin KD, Horton CE. Vaginal reconstruction with gracilis myocutaneous flaps. Plast Reconstr Surg. 1976;58(2):176–83.
4. Harii K, Ohmori K, Sekiguchi J. The free musculocutaneous flap. Plast Reconstr Surg. 1976;57(3):294–303.
5. Mathes SJ, Nahai F. Classification of the vascular anatomy of muscles: experimental and clinical correlation. Plast Reconstr Surg. 1981;67(2):177–87.
6. Wei F-C, Mardini S. Flaps and reconstructive surgery. Elsevier; 2009.
7. Franco MJ, Nicoson MC, Parikh RP, Tung TH. Lower extremity reconstruction with free Gracilis flaps. J Reconstr Microsurg. 2017;33(3):218–24.
8. Peek A, Müller M, Ackermann G, Exner K, Baumeister S. The free gracilis perforator flap: anatomical study and clinical refinements of a new perforator flap. Plast Reconstr Surg. 2009;123(2):578–88.
9. Giordano PA, Abbes M, Pequignot JP. Gracilis blood supply: anatomical and clinical re-evaluation. Br J Plast Surg. 1990;43(3):266–72.
10. Lykoudis EG, Spyropoulou GA, Vlastou CC. The anatomic basis of the gracilis perforator flap. Br J Plast Surg. 2005;58(8):1090–4.
11. Kappler UA, Constantinescu MA, Büchler U, Vögelin E. Anatomy of the proximal cutaneous perforator vessels of the gracilis muscle. Br J Plast Surg. 2005;58(4):445–8.
12. Magden O, Tayfur V, Edizer M, Atabey A. Anatomy of gracilis muscle flap. J Craniofac Surg. 2010;21(6):1948–50.
13. Whitaker IS, Karavias M, Shayan R, et al. The gracilis myocutaneous free flap: a quantitative analysis of the fasciocutaneous blood supply and implications for autologous breast reconstruction. PLoS One. 2012;7(5):e36367.
14. Krishnan K. An illustrated handbook of flap-raising techniques. New York: Thieme; 2008. p. 24–8.
15. Yousif NJ, Matloub HS, Kolachalam R, Grunert BK, Sanger JR. The transverse gracilis musculocutaneous flap. Ann Plast Surg. 1992;29(6):482–90.
16. Hallock GG. The medial circumflex femoral (gracilis) local perforator flap--a local medial groin perforator flap. Ann Plast Surg. 2003;51(5):460–4.
17. Coelho JAJ, McDermott FD, Cameron O, Smart NJ, Watts AM, Daniels IR. Single Centre experience of bilateral gracilis flap perineal reconstruction following extra-levator abdominoperineal excision. Color Dis. 2019;21(8):910–6.

18. King IC, Obeid N, Woollard AC, Jones ME. Maximizing length and safety in gracilis free flap dissection. J Plast Reconstr Aesthet Surg. 2016;69(10):1452–3.
19. Labbe R, Lindsay T, Walker PM. The extent and distribution of skeletal muscle necrosis after graded periods of complete ischemia. J Vasc Surg. 1987;6(2):152–7.
20. Hattori Y, Doi K, Abe Y, Ikeda K, Dhawan V. Surgical approach to the vascular pedicle of the gracilis muscle flap. J Hand Surg Am. 2002;27(3):534–6.
21. Tremp M, Oranges CM, Wang WJ, et al. The "nugget design": a modified segmental gracilis free flap for small-sized defect reconstruction on the lower extremity. J Plast Reconstr Aesthet Surg. 2017;70(9):1261–6.
22. Doi K, Sakai K, Kuwata N, Ihara K, Kawai S. Double free-muscle transfer to restore prehension following complete brachial plexus avulsion. J Hand Surg Am. 1995;20(3):408–14.

Profunda Artery Perforator Flap

38

Tomoyuki Yano

38.1 Introduction

The profunda artery perforator (PAP) flap was first introduced as a free flap for soft tissue defects by Angrigiani et al. (2001). Allen et al. (2012) applied this technique in the field of breast reconstruction in 2012. Since then, various studies on PAP flap breast reconstruction have been conducted, and the PAP flap has become one of the alternative flap options for autologous breast reconstruction. Nowadays, the PAP flap is a thin and pliable flap option for head and neck reconstruction and soft tissue defect in the extremity as well.

An advantage of the PAP flap is it has less anatomical variation and it has a straightforward pedicle dissection. A skin paddle can harvest adequate adipose tissue volume without any damage to surrounding muscles, which leads to less donor site morbidity after surgery. Moreover, the donor site wound will be nicely hidden in the posterior medial side of the thigh or inguinal crease. A disadvantage of the PAP flap is that only a limited width of the skin paddle can be harvested to achieve primary safe donor site closure. A small- to moderate-sized defect, which needs a certain amount of adipose tissue, will be a good indication for the PAP flap.

38.2 Anatomy

The profunda femoris artery gives off three perforators in the posterior compartment of the thigh. The first perforator of the profunda femoris artery supplies the adductor magnus and gracilis muscles. This perforator penetrates these muscles, takes an intra-muscular course, or a septal course, and branches to the posterior medial thigh skin (Fig. 38.1). Usually, the first perforator is approximately 8–10 cm from the groin crease and 2–3 cm below the gracilis muscle.

Finally, this perforator gives off two or three cutaneous branches to the posterior medial thigh region. The location of perforators are consistent, and there is little anatomical variation. Actually, in our experience with 38 cases of the PAP flap, there was no case that did not have any single perforator in the posterior medial region. You can always find at least one adequate perforator of the PAP flap in the posterior medial region, and this might be a distinct difference between the PAP flap and ALT flap. On the other hand, the second and third perforators of the profunda femoris artery supply the semi-membranosus, biceps femoris and vastus lateralis muscles.

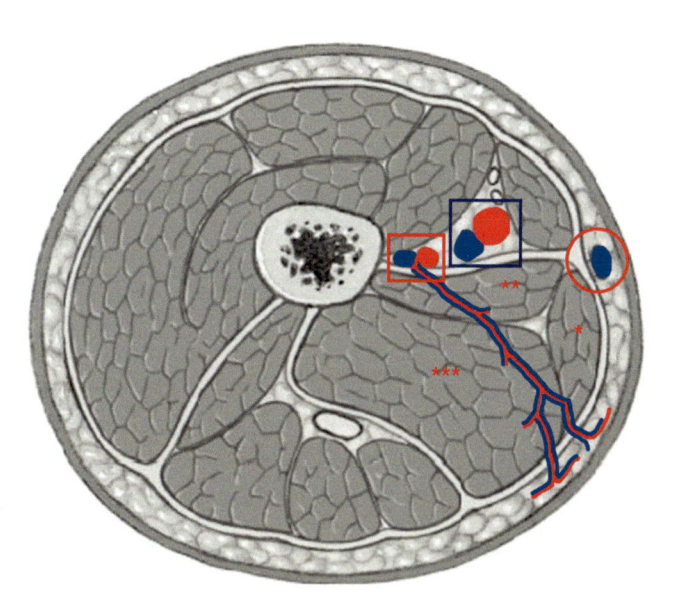

Fig. 38.1 A schema of the anatomy of the PAP flap. The red and blue boxes indicate the profunda artery and vein, the femoral artery and vein. The red circle shows the great saphenous vein. The single, double and triple asterisks indicate the gracilis muscle, adductor longus muscle and adductor magnus muscle, respectively. The red line with accompanying double blue line represents the perforator of the PAP flap

T. Yano (✉)
Cancer Institute hospital for JFCR, Tokyo, Japan

38.3 Pre-Operative Investigation

PAP flap perforators from the profunda femoris artery usually tend not to have anatomical variations or anomalies, a hand-held Doppler will be enough for pre-operative investigation. After identifying the adductor longus and gracilis muscles, two or three perforators will be found with a hand-held Doppler below these two muscles. However, if CT angiography is available, a CT image will provide more specific information to identify the dominant perforators in each patient.

Nowadays, a duplex ultrasound is another useful tool to perform pre-operative investigation for free flap planning. Duplex ultrasound images provide the exact raising point of perforators from the adductor magnus muscle, and show the size and quality of the perforators. Kehrer et al. (2018) reported that they could map almost the exact emergence point of the PAP flap perforators with no false-negative sign. This information will help to determine which perforator to include in the flap.

38.4 Flap Design and Markings

The perforators are marked and the flap design is drawn as the patient is positioned in the frog-leg position (Fig. 38.2a, b). The adductor longus muscle can be palpated between the pubic tubercle and medial knee joint, when you ask the patient to adduct the thigh. Just below the adductor longus muscle, the gracilis muscle can be palpated, and these two muscles are marked on the surface of the medial thigh. One to three perforators will be marked during the pre-operative investigation with a hand-held Doppler, CT angiography or duplex ultrasound. A red circle with an asterisk indicates a dominant perforator in this case. Because the donor site exists close to the hip joint, and the donor site wound tends to have relatively strong tension according to the patient's body movement post-operatively, it recommends designing the width of the PAP flap less than 8 cm for a safe donor site closure.

There are two types of flap incision markings, the transverse and vertical designs (Fig. 38.2a, b). The design can be selected according to patient demands, the amount of subcutaneous fat and perforator locations.

If indocyanine green (ICG) angiography is available, it is recommended to evaluate the lymphatic flow of the medial thigh in order to avoid damaging the lymphatic system, as reported by Karakawa et al. (2020). White arrows show the medial lymphatic flow in this patient.

38.5 Flap Raise/Elevation: A Step-by-Step Guide

Step 1. Make a Skin Incision. Find the Great Saphenous Vein If Necessary

Start by making a skin incision to the anterior incision line of the flap. In the subdermal tissue, the great saphenous vein (short white arrows) and its branch, named the posterior

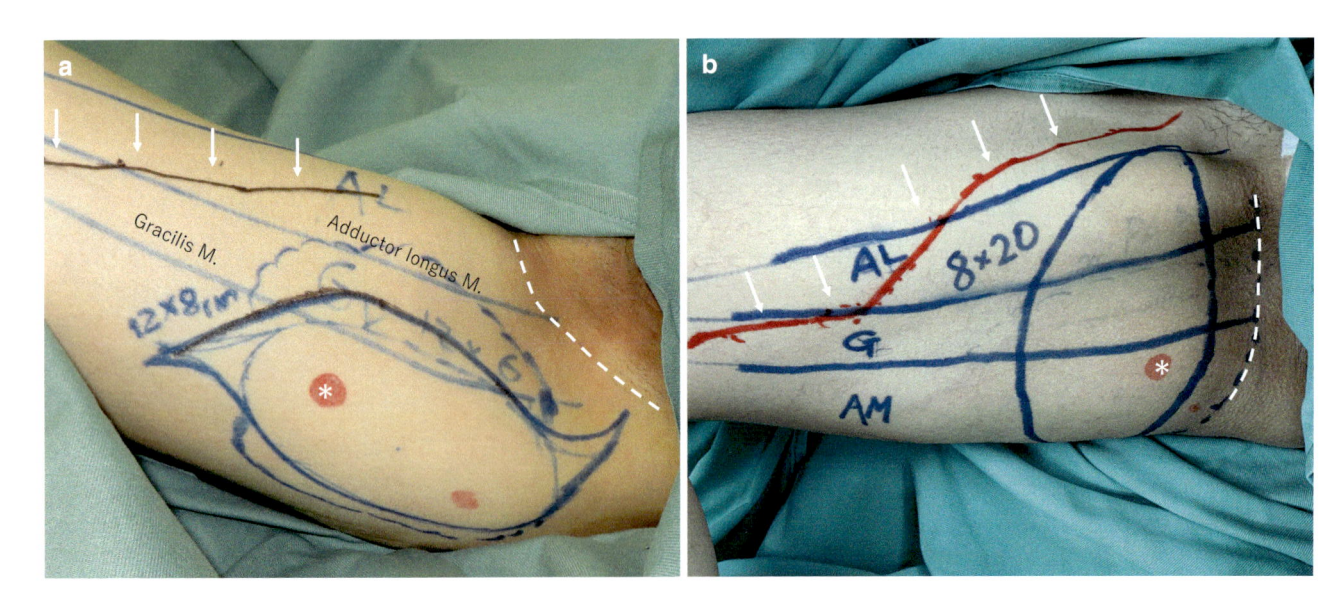

Fig. 38.2 (**a**) (left): Vertical design of the PAP flap (left), (**b**) (right): transverse design of the PAP flap. White arrows indicate lymphatic vessel identified with ICG lymphography. White asterisk shows a dominant perforator. White dotted line represents inguinal crease

accessory saphenous vein (long white arrows), can be identified (Fig. 38.3). Karakawa et al. (2019) reported the usability of including the accessory saphenous vein in the PAP flap. If the recipient vein has a rather large calibre size, and the flap needs a large drainage vein, including the accessory saphenous vein in the flap will be another option for flap venous drainage.

Step 2. Find the Landmark Muscle, The Adductor Longus Muscle

After making the skin incision, it is easy to dissect the skin paddle from the anterior border to the posterior border. Dissection of the skin paddle continues under the deep fascia, which will help you to identify both the adductor longus and gracilis muscles. You can identify the adductor longus muscle first, just after making an incision into the deep fascia (Fig. 38.4a).

Step 3. Find the Second Landmark Muscle, the Gracilis Muscle

Next to the adductor longus muscle, the gracilis muscle will appear 2–3 cm posterior to the adductor longus muscle. The adductor longus and gracilis muscles are key muscles to tell you that your dissection is in the right layer, and you will find the adductor magnus muscle next to these two muscles (Fig. 38.4b).

Step 4. Identify the Adductor Magnus Muscle

The adductor magnus muscle is next to the gracilis muscle (Fig. 38.5a). To start dissecting the adductor muscle means that you have stepped into the "Hot zone" to find the perforators from the profunda femoris artery penetrating the adductor magnus muscle. Therefore, dissection should be meticulous once you have found the adductor magnus muscle.

Step 5. Identify the Dominant Perforator of the PAP Flap

Usually, the perforators from the profunda femoris artery give off several skin perforators. You can choose one or two perforators that will be suitable for a flap setting. The white arrows show the dominant perforator (Fig. 38.5b). Sometimes two skin perforators are found to be joined during muscular dissection. Therefore, if you can find two close skin perforators, it is recommended to dissect both perforators expecting both perforators to be joined together, and the flap can have a stable vascular supply.

Step 6. Dissection of the Flap Pedicle to Obtain Enough Length for Flap Setting

Once the perforator is identified, skeletonizing the perforator is relatively straightforward. Unlike the DIEP flap or ALT flap pedicle, the PAP flap pedicle usually runs straight into the profunda femoris artery. This route makes skeletonizing the PAP flap pedicle rather simple. But the perforator gives off several small muscle branches (Fig. 38.6a), so careful ligation and separation are necessary. The muscle branch of the PAP flap becomes relatively larger in the proximal side, and the calibre size of the side branch vessels become large enough for micro-anastomosis (Fig. 38.6a). This side branch will be a recipient vessel if the stacked PAP flap is considered for use.

In the end, the PAP flap with adequate bulk can be harvested (Fig. 38.6b). The PAP flap can include the posterior saphenous vein as a lifeboat vessel for an extra drainage.

38.6 Core Surgical Techniques in Flap Dissection

First, after making the skin incision to the anterior incision line, you have to perform careful dissection of subcutaneous tissue so as not to damage the saphenous vein (Step 1). When you try to identify the landmark muscles, the adductor lon-

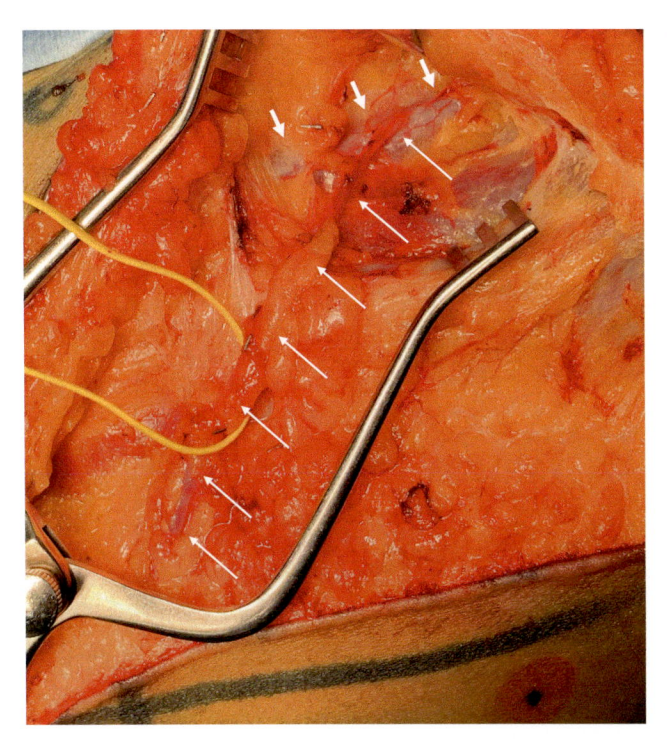

Fig. 38.3 Short white arrows indicate the great saphenous vein, and long white arrows show the posterior accessory saphenous vein branched off from the great saphenous vein

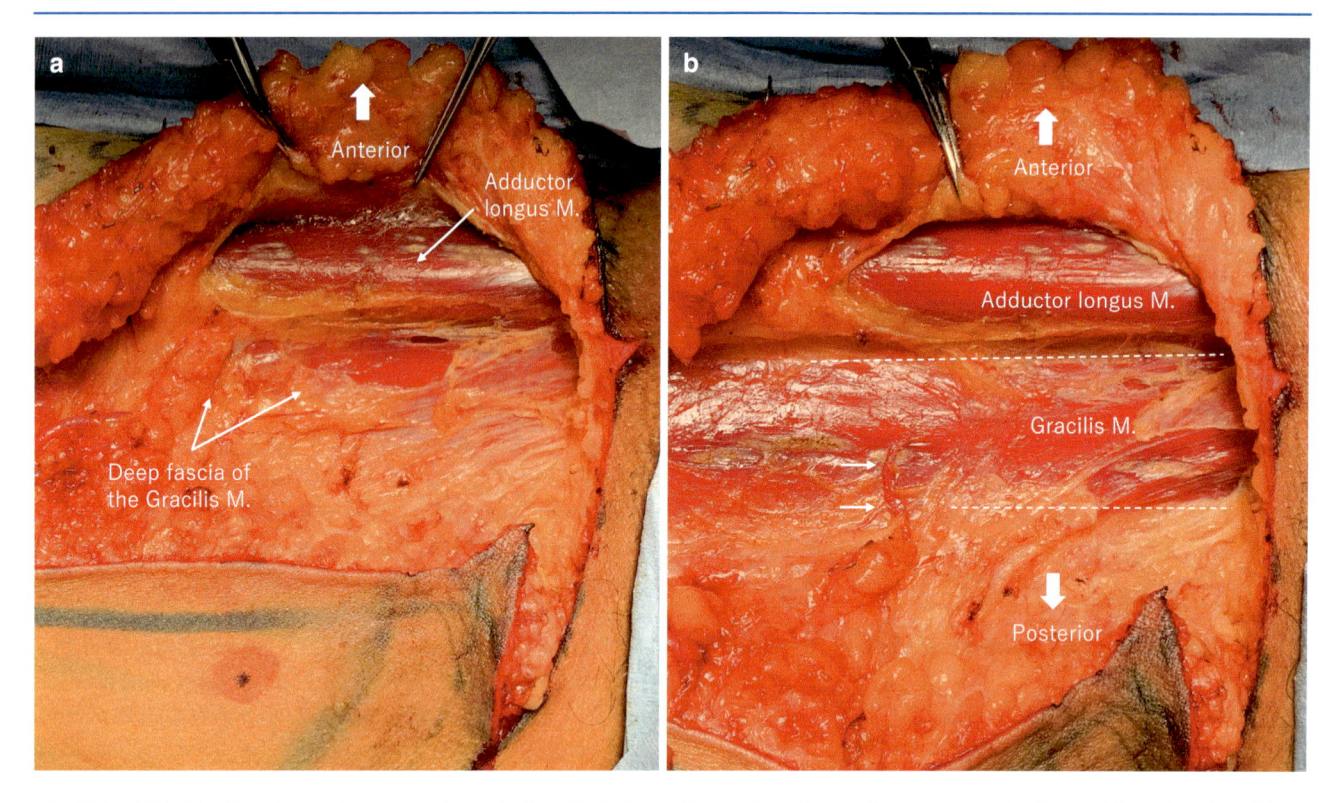

Fig. 38.4 (**a**) (left): The adductor longus muscle can be identified after opening the deep fascia, (**b**) (right): the gracilis muscle can be found posterior to the adductor longus muscle. Short arrows indicate the perforator from the gracilis muscle to the skin paddle. White dotted lines show the anterior and posterior border of the gracilis muscle

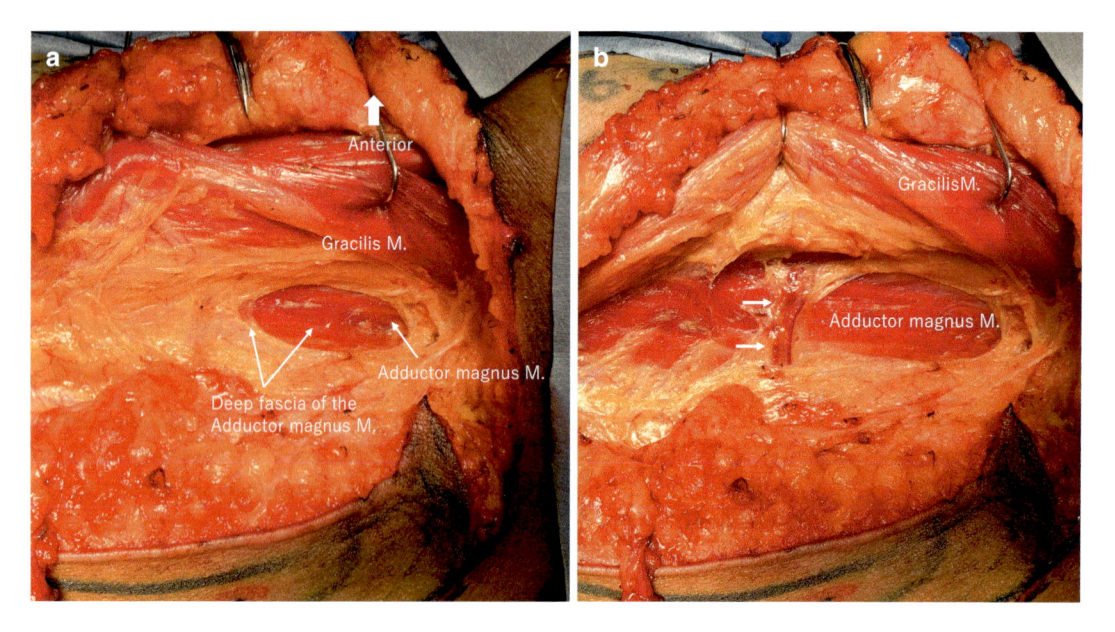

Fig. 38.5 (**a**) (left): The adductor magnus muscle can be identified after dissecting the deep fascia next to the gracilis muscle, (**b**) (right): white arrows indicate the perforator from the adductor magnus muscle to the skin paddle

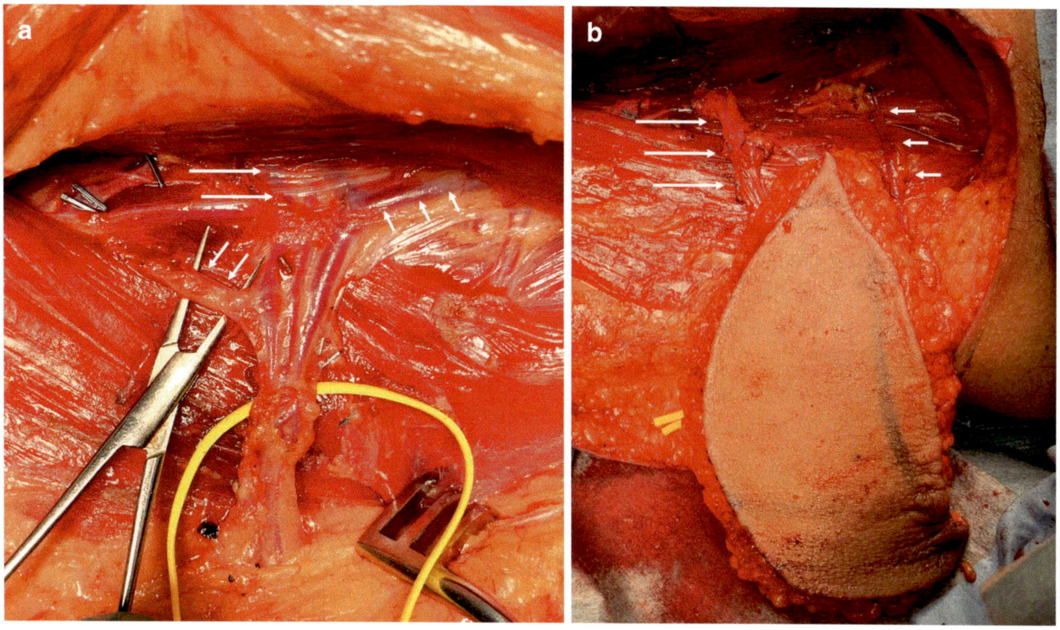

Fig. 38.6 (**a**) (left): Both white arrows indicate side branches of the PAP flap pedicle, which can use as a recipient vessel for the stacked PAP flap, (**b**) (right): white short and long arrows indicate the posterior saphenous vein and the PAP flap pedicle, respectively

gus and gracilis muscles, subfascial dissection makes it easy for you to find these muscles. Therefore, you have to open the fascia of the adductor longus, gracilis and adductor magnus one by one as shown in steps 2–4 (Figs. 38.4a and 38.6a). If you are confused about which muscle you are dissecting, the gracilis muscle will be a guide for you. The gracilis muscle has a distinctive shape (step 3). It looks like a muscle belt, and it is easily separated from the surrounding tissues. Once you can recognize the gracilis muscle, you can identify the adductor magnus muscle posterior to the gracilis muscle.

Usually, you can find two or three perforators penetrating the adductor magnus muscle. You can choose which one to dissect according to the size or location of the perforator. Sometimes, there is one dominant perforator, which is the largest of the vessels. Because the PAP flap has a limited number of perforators in the medial posterior thigh area, it is not difficult to decide which perforator to include compared to the DIEP flap, which has multiple choices of perforators (step 5). During the pedicle skeletonization, two Weitlaner retractors or similar retractors will help you to provide a stable dissection window. Start with deroofing the perforator, and the surrounding muscles are divided with a fine mosquito or dissecting scissors. Several muscular branches from the PAP flap pedicle can be observed during intra-muscular dissection. Careful separation of these branch vessels with a surgical ligation clip and a Bipolar should be continued until you can obtain enough length of the flap pedicle for the flap setting. Even though the flap pedicle seems to have enough length for your plan, it is recommended to dissect further to provide an extra 1 or 2 cm length. Because the PAP flap pedicle tends to become shorter after a flap harvesting, this extra dissection will prevent you having trouble with flap setting. When you have skeletonized approximately 8 to 10 cm of the flap pedicle, the calibre size of the perforator becomes large enough up to about 2 mm to anastomose to any kind of recipient vessels, such as the internal mammary artery or superior thyroid artery (step 6).

38.7 Clinical Scenario

38.7.1 Scenario 1

The PAP flap could be an alternative option of breast reconstruction for a patient with small- to medium-sized breast. Moreover, the PAP flap is another option for breast reconstruction if a patient has multiple scars in the abdomen, does not have enough fat for breast reconstruction in the abdomen and lumbar region, or plans a future pregnancy. The PAP flap can be placed in the defect with a cone shape or transverse settings according to the shape of the patient breast.

38.7.2 Scenario 2

The PAP flap is available for a simple small to the medium size of head and neck defect such as hemi-glossectomy or parotidectomy defect. Using the PAP flap, pliable skin with adequate volume of adipose tissue can be transferred to the defect. In this scenario, the skin paddle is better to design in the vertical fashion by including the distal perforator of the PAP flap. Sometimes, the PAP flap pedicle becomes shorter than expected, and which makes the flap setting difficult for head and neck defect. Vertical design with the distal perforator enables the flap to extend its pedicle length with de-epithelializing part of the skin paddle as a part of the flap pedicle.

38.8 Pearls and Pitfalls

Pearls
- Find and identify the adductor longus and gracilis muscles first. These key muscles tell you that you are in the right plane to dissect.
- Continue to dissect under the deep fascia until you can identify the adductor magnus muscle.
Sometimes during a skin paddle elevation, a relatively robust perforator from the gracilis originating from the medial femoral circumflex system can be found. In this scenario, you can switch to harvesting the flap as a transverse upper gracilis (TUG) flap.
- In the case of head and neck reconstruction, often the defect needs a rather long flap pedicle. In this scenario, you can de-epithelialize part of the flap, and use this part as an extension of the pedicle.
- There is a possibility of harvesting the innervated PAP flap including the cutaneous branch of the obturator nerve.

Pitfalls
- Do not take too large a skin paddle. The width of the PAP flap is recommended to harvest within 8 cm for a safe donor site primary closure. Donor site wound problems can be more serious after harvesting the PAP flap if you harvest too much material for the skin paddle.
- It is recommended to create a flap pedicle that is as long as possible. The PAP flap pedicle tends to be shorter than you expect after detaching the flap from the donor site. Usually, one single perforator will be enough for nourishing small- to medium-sized PAP flap. On the other hand, ICG angiographies such as SPY system or PDE neo will always help you to reduce the risk of fat necrosis or wound healing post-operatively.
- In some cases, the donor site scar is little bit lower than a patient has expected due to the location of the perforator.
- When you perform flap dissection of the posterior part of the flap, you should take care not to damage the posterior femoral cutaneous nerve.
- In some cases, a hemi-lateral PAP flap might provide only limited volume for breast reconstruction. For instance, sometimes the PAP flap cannot provide enough volume in the breast upper pole area. In that case, you can consider using both sides of the PAP flap as a stacked PAP flap. It is a very rare scenario for the PAP flap, but if you cannot find any single adequate perforator to raise the PAP flap, you can switch to use the medial circumflex artery perforator as TUG flap or to harvest the PAP flap from the contralateral side of the thigh.

38.9 Selected Readings

- Angrigiani C, Grilli D, Thorne CH. The adductor flap: a new method for transferring posterior and medial thigh skin. Plast Reconstr Surg 2001;107:1725–1731.
- *The first article about the application of the PAP flap as a free flap for soft tissue defects.*
- Allen RJ, Haddock NT, Ahn C, Sadeghi A. Breast reconstruction with the profunda artery perforator flap. Plast Reconstr Surg 2012;129:16–23.
- *The first report to describe the usability of the PAP flap for breast reconstruction.*
- Haddock NT, Gassman A, Cho MJ, Teotia SS. 101 consecutive profunda artery perforator flaps in breast reconstruction: lessons learned with our early experience. Plast Reconstr Surg 2017; 140: 229–239.
- *A report on the experiences of using a large number of PAP flaps for breast reconstruction*
- Qian B, Xiong L, Li J, Sun Y, Sun J, Guo N, Wang Z. A systematic review and meta-analysis on microsurgical safety and efficacy of profunda artery perforator flap in breast reconstruction. J Oncol 2019;29:1–12.
- *A systematic review and meta-analysis on the PAP flap in breast reconstruction.*
- Ito R, Huang JJ, Wu JCW, Lin MCY, Cheng MH. The versatility of profunda femoral artery perforator flap for oncological reconstruction after cancer resection-clinical cases and review of literature. J Surg Oncol 2016; 114:193–201.
- *A report on the usability of the PAP flap for various kinds of defects.*
- Heredero S, Sanjuan A, Falguera M, Dean A, Ogledzki M. The thin profunda femoral artery perforator flap for tongue reconstruction. Microsurgery 2020; 40:117–124.
- *Report on experiences of the usage of the PAP flap for head and neck reconstruction.*
- Largo RD, Chu CK, Chang EI, Liu J, Abu-Ghname A, Wang H, Schaverien MV, Mericli AF, Hanasono MM, Yu P. Perforator Mapping of the Profunda Artery Perforator Flap: Anatomy and Clinical Experience. Plast Reconstr Surg 2020; 146: 1135–1145.
- *PAP flap perforator mapping in the medial thigh area for flap design and planning.*
- Algan S, Tan O. Profunda femoris artery perforator flaps: a detailed anatomical study. J Plast Surg Hand Surg 2020; 54: 377–381.
- *Anatomical study on the detailed information of perforators of the PAP flap using fresh cadavers.*
- Kehrer A, Hsu MY, Chen YT, Sachanandani N, Tsao CK. Simplified profunda artery perforator (PAP) flap design using power Doppler ultrasonography (PDU): a prospective study. Microsurgery 2018;38: 512–523.
- *Clinical evaluation and description of the perforator of the PAP flap using power Doppler ultrasonography.*
- Karakawa R, Yoshimatsu H, Tanakura K, Miyashita H, Shibata T, Kuramoto Y, Yano T. An anatomical study of the lymph-collecting vessels of the medial thigh and clinical applications of lymphatic vessels preserving profunda femoris artery perforator (LpPAP) flap using pre- and intraoperative indocyanine green (ICG) lymphography. J Plast Reconstr Aesthet Surg 2020;73:1768–1774.
- *Clinical and anatomical study of the relation between lymphatic vessels and the profunda femoris artery perforator.*
- Karakawa R, Yoshimatsu H, Fuse Y, Hayashi A, Tanakura K, Heber UM, Weninger WJ, Tzou CHJ, Meng SM, Yano T. The correlation of the perforators and the accessory saphenous vein in a profunda femoris artery perforator flap for additional venous anastomosis: a cadaveric study and clinical application. Microsurgery 2019;40:200–206.
- *Cadaveric and clinical evaluation of usage of the posterior saphenous vein for the PAP flap.*
- Ciudad P, Maruccia M, Orfaniotis G, Weng HC, Constantinescu T, Nicoli F, Cigna E, Socas J, Sirimahachaiyakul P, Sapountzis S, Kiranantawat K, Lin SP, Wang GJ, Chen HC. The combined transverse upper gracilis and profunda artery perforator (TUGPAP) flap for breast reconstruction. Microsurgery 2016; 36: 359–366.
- *Explaining the idea of conjoined TUG flap and PAP flap for breast reconstruction.*

Medial Femoral Condyle Flap

Anthony L. Logli and Alexander Y. Shin

39.1 Introduction

The medial aspect of the knee, and specifically the descending genicular artery (DGA), was first recognized as a potential donor site for a vascularized flap in 1981 [1]. In 1985, the osteoarticular branch (OAB) of the DGA was realized as a flap supply source in harvesting the adductor magnus tendon and tubercle [2].

The contemporary medial femoral condyle (MFC) flap was first described in 1988 as a free corticoperiosteal flap to address pseudoarthrosis of the upper limb [3]. The innovative feature of this flap was inclusion of cortical bone, thereby preventing disruption of the highly osteogenic cambrium layer of periosteum violated with vascularized periosteal flaps [4].

The MFC flap can be raised as a pedicled or free corticoperiosteal, corticocancellous, or osteochondral graft with or without a neurotized skin island. The flap is extremely versatile and can be shaped according to donor site needs without compromising blood supply. Use of the MFC graft has been described in the clavicle [5–7], manubrium [8], humerus [4, 5, 9, 10], metacarpal [4, 11], scaphoid [12–15], capitate [16, 17], lunate [16, 18], forearm [4, 5], tibia [19, 20], femur [21], talus [5], calcaneus [22], as well as head and neck reconstruction [23–27] with indications encompassing radiation-induced pathologic fractures, primary or recalcitrant nonunions, or sites with known or anticipated poor vascularity or healing potential [6, 28]. When inclusive of cartilage from the trochlea, the graft is instead given the moniker of medial femoral trochlea (MFT) graft [29, 30].

39.2 Anatomy

The vascular anatomy of the medial knee in the context of vascularized grafts was first explored by Hertel and Masquelet in 1989, simultaneously marking the appearance of the MFC flap in the American literature [19]. The MFC flap is supplied by the descending (or supreme) genicular artery (DGA) (present intraoperatively in 93% of knees) and venae comitantes [13, 19, 31]. The DGA originates off the medial aspect of the superficial femoral artery (SFA) approximately 14 cm above the joint line (11–18 cm) just before the SFA passes through the adductor magnus hiatus [4, 13, 19]. Mean diameter and length is sufficient for microvascular anastomosis at 1.5–2.1 mm and 1.2 cm, respectively [19, 31]. It consistently branches into an osteoarticular branch (OAB) (90% from the DGA; 6% directly from the SFA), the predominant supply for the MFC graft, a saphenous artery branch (SAB) (79% present), which can simultaneously supply a skin flap for transfer, and a muscular branch (MB) [13, 19]. The mean distance of the OAB origination is 11.3 cm above the joint line [13]. The vessel runs on the posterior surface of the medial intermuscular septum with a mean diameter of 1.2 mm at its origin [19]. Proximal branching near the origin (40%) and distal branching near the adductor tubercle (60%) then occurs, where the OAB splits into medial and lateral branches, some of which supply the posterior border of the vastus medialis. Just proximal to the knee joint capsule and MCL origin, the OAB joins with the sMGA to create a rich, almost circular, anastomosis supplying the overlying periosteum. Recent mappings and in-depth reexamination of the microvascular anatomy of this region suggest there to be an average of 30 osteoarticular perforators extending to a depth of 13 mm with highest concentration of these located in the posterior-distal quadrant of the condylar surface [31].

Independently perfused or dual-supply MFC grafts based off the superomedial genicular artery (sMGA) were described early-on to further enhance flap vascularity [4]. While dual

A. L. Logli
Orthopaedic Surgery, Mayo Clinic, Rochester, MN, USA

A. Y. Shin (✉)
Division of Hand Surgery, Department of Orthopaedic Surgery, Mayo Clinic, Rochester, MN, USA
e-mail: shin.alexander@mayo.edu

vascularity remains an option, incorporation is not essential. The sMGA is present 98% of the time and originates from the medial aspect of the popliteal artery at a mean distance of 5.2 cm above the joint line [13, 32]. These vessels are typically shorter, smaller, harder to dissect, and have no cutaneous vascular supply to support skin if needed for transfer, however, they are the dominant supply to the MFC region in 23% of intraoperative exposures and the only vessel in 7% of cases [32]. In the native knee, both the DGA and sMGA serve as the principal nourishment to the periosteum of the MFC, while playing a relatively minor role in corticomedullary perfusion [5]. Thus, destruction of residual perfusion to the donor site bed is not a concern.

39.3 Preoperative Investigation

The anatomy of the medial knee is highly consistent, thereby obviating the need for preoperative vascular mapping in most instances. If desired, Doppler ultrasonography can be used. This may be most useful to identify and mark the SAB if a skin island is planned. This vessel is located distally in the medial thigh just posterior to the midlateral line [21]. It perfuses an area of skin approximately 361 cm^2 [33]. Smaller skin islands, measuring up to 70 cm^2, may also be raised solely on cutaneous perforators of the DGA [33]. Prior incisions should be recognized and incorporated if possible. Use of the ipsilateral knee is preferred for recipient sites of the upper extremity. This allows two surgical teams in the room to operate simultaneously. In upper extremity recipients, use of the ipsilateral knee also allows the patient to use a cane in the contralateral hand if necessary. Otherwise, either knee may be used.

The patient is placed supine with the hip and knee flexed and externally rotated. The recipient site should be exposed first if not done simultaneously by a second operating team. A sterile tourniquet is applied to the proximal thigh and raised (usually to 300 mmHg) just prior to medial thigh incision and exposure.

39.4 Flap Design and Markings

A bulk section of distal medial femoral metaphyseal bone 6–8 cm in length may be harvested in most instances, as well as 5–7 cm corticoperiosteal flaps. The proximal extent of periosteal perfusion of the DGA is much greater (up to 13.7 cm or 29% of total femur length in cadaveric specimens) [34]. Despite this, it is important not to extend the harvest past the metaphyseal-diaphyseal junction as it creates a stress riser that may result in a delayed supracondylar femur fracture. This is a well-known complication in the total knee replacement literature when femoral condyle bone cuts extend past the metaphyseal diaphyseal junction [35]. Thin corticoperiosteal grafts with large dimensions (8 × 13 cm^2) have been successfully raised for humeral non-unions in the past with no known incident of perioperative fracture [36].

The portion of the MFC used for flap harvest is that which has the greatest density of perforating vessels. This has been previously defined as the posterior-distal quadrant of the femoral condyle and has the following borders: (1) the hamstring insertion and medial collateral ligament (MCL) origin posteriorly, (2) the anterior horn of the medial meniscus anteriorly, (3) the hamstring insertion proximally, and (4) the proximal pole of the patella distally.

39.5 Flap Raise/Elevation: A Step-by-Step Guide

1. Incision
    Incision is dependent on indication. A straight 18–20 cm medial thigh incision starting at the joint line and extending proximally along the posterior border of the vastus medialis is used for non-articular grafts (Fig. 39.1), while a 15 cm curvilinear incision with the apex at the proximal pole of the patella is used when inclusion of articular cartilage into the graft is desired.
2. Exposure
    (a) Vastus medialis muscle fascia is divided at its posterior border along the entire length of the incision and the muscle belly is retracted anteriorly to fully appreciate the MFC and overlying vascularity in the bed of the wound (Fig. 39.2).
3. Graft Planning
    (a) Once the supply vessel has been chosen (DGA or sMGA), the pedicle should be isolated by suture ligation of the unused vessel. The planned graft is then outlined on the MFC periosteum using bipolar electrocautery at posterior-distal aspect of the MFC for non-articular grafts, anterior-proximal MFC for articular grafts, and broadly across the condylar surface for corticoperiosteal grafts in order to maximize perfusion potential (Fig. 39.3—structural (a), corticoperiosteal (b), and MFT (c) graft plans are shown).
4. Graft Separation
    (a) A small very sharp curved osteotome or microsagittal saw is used to vertically divide the borders of the graft to the desired depth. The proximal border is the last cut made for non-articular grafts while division

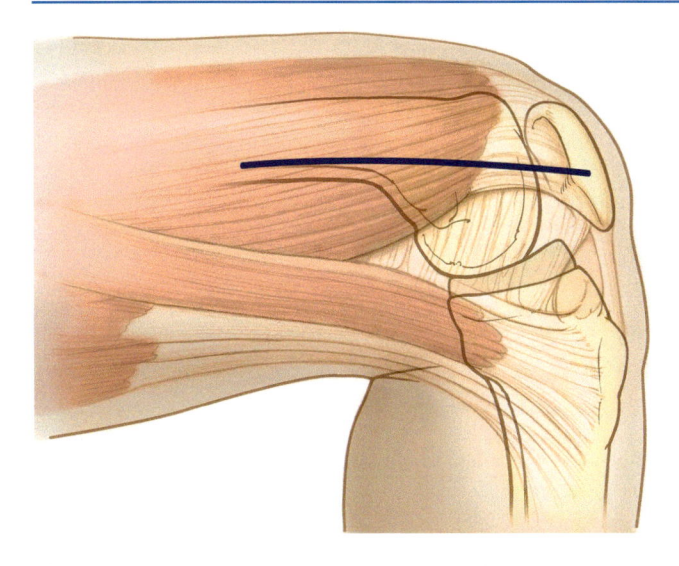

Fig. 39.1 Illustration of the medial knee incision for obtaining a nonarticular graft starting at the joint line and extending proximally 18–20 cm. For an articular graft, the incision would curve distally starting at the proximal pole of the patella. (Reproduced with permission of the Mayo Foundation)

through the cartilage is the final cut made in articular grafts (Fig. 39.4—structural (a) and corticoperiosteal (b) graft separation is shown).

5. Graft Elevation
   (a) One critical step unique to raising a structural graft to prevent graft fragmentation or fracture is to raise an adjacent small wedge of bone 1–2 cm large. This permits undercutting the graft with a curved osteotome at the desired depth and elevation of the graft en-bloc. Otherwise, nonstructural grafts may be elevated after the final cut is carefully made (Fig. 39.5—structural (a) and corticoperiosteal (b) graft elevation is shown with the additional technical feature recommended when raising a structural graft highlighted (c)).

6. Graft Preparation and Division
   (a) The graft pedicle is clipped and divided. Once, harvested, it is customized according to recipient site geometry (Fig. 39.6—structural (a) and corticoperiosteal (b) grafts shown after graft division).

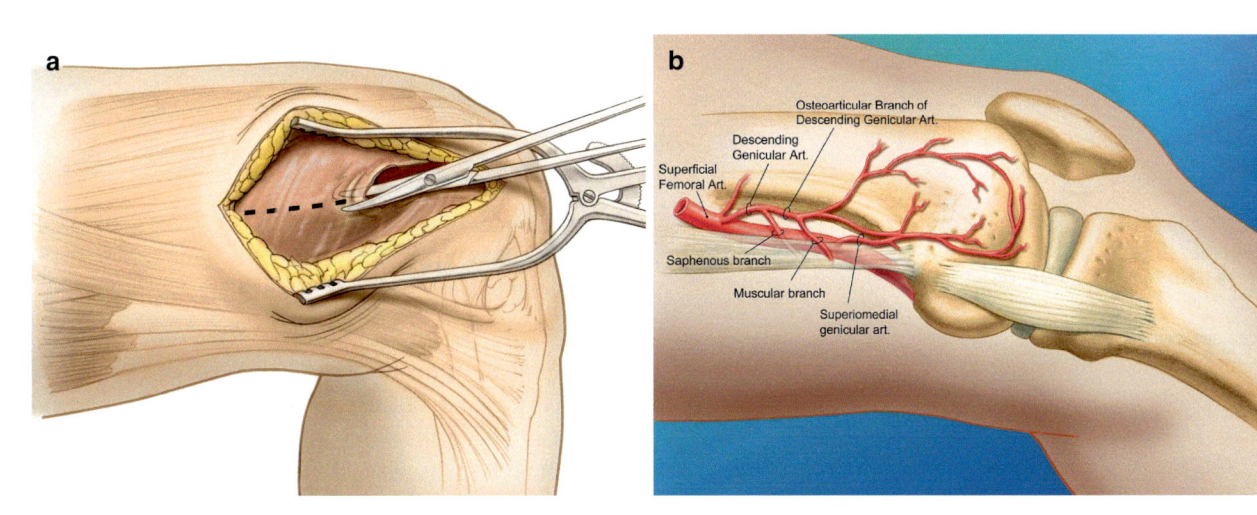

Fig. 39.2 Illustration showing release of the fascia overlying the vastus medialis in-line with the skin incision (**a**). Once the vastus medialis is retracted anteriorly, the medial femoral condyle and overlying vasculature will be visualized in the bed of the wound (**b**). (Reproduced with permission of the Mayo Foundation)

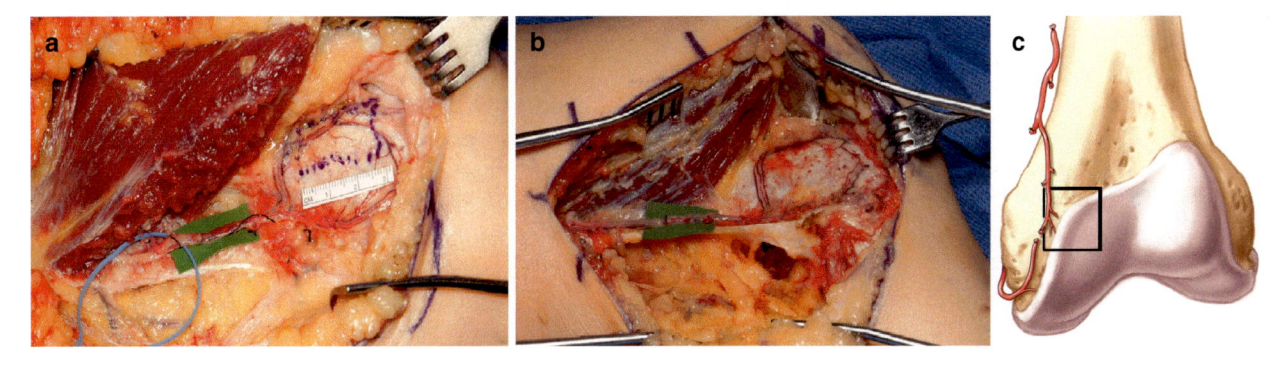

Fig. 39.3 The chosen pedicle (DGA or sMGA) is isolated and clearly visualized using a green background (**a**, **b**). Bipolar cautery or a surgical marker can be used to outline the planned dimensions of the graft. Shown is a planned structural (**a**), corticoperisoteal (**b**), and articular (**c**) graft. (Reproduced with permission of the Mayo Foundation)

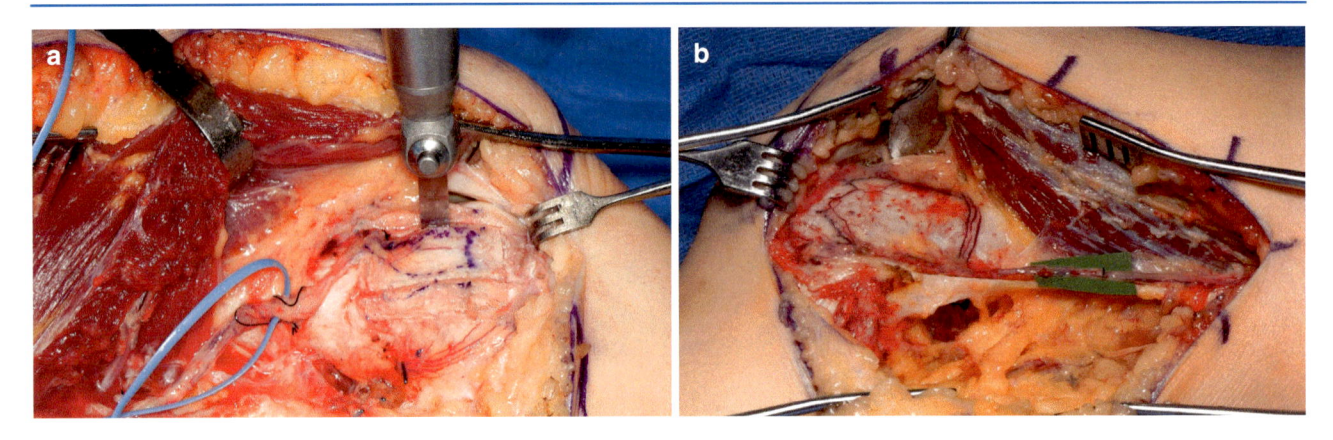

Fig. 39.4 A microsagittal saw (**a**) or sharp, curved osteotome (**b**) may be used to permit graft separation. Shown is a structural (**a**) and corticoperiosteal graft (**b**) being carefully separated from the medial femoral condyle donor site

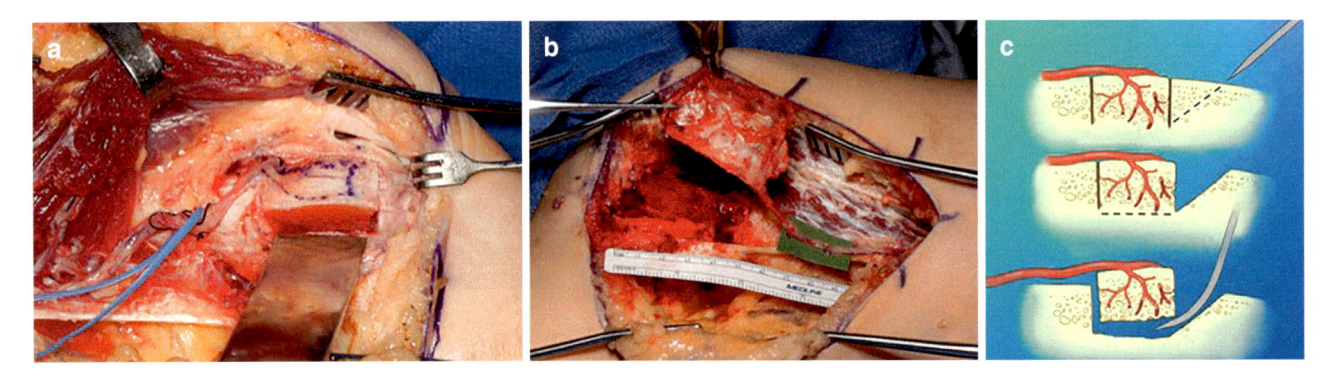

Fig. 39.5 A small block or wedge of bone is removed adjacent to a planned structural graft so that it can be elevated en-bloc using a curved osteotome. An example of this critical step is shown clinically (**a**) and in an illustrated form (**b**). This is not necessary for raising a corticoperiosteal graft (**c**). (Reproduced with permission of the Mayo Foundation)

7. Donor Site Closure
    (a) The donor site defect is filled with synthetic hydroxyapatite bone filler (for non-articular grafts) and the wound is irrigated and closed in a layered fashion with absorbable sutures over suction drains.
8. Graft Inset and Anastomosis
    (a) Non-articular grafts should be inset and fixed into the donor bed while corticoperiosteal grafts are wrapped around bone and fixed with sutures. Both press-fit and supplemented fixation options may be used for articular grafts. Microvascular anastomosis is then performed using an operative microscope and adequacy of perfusion confirmed (Fig. 39.7—structural graft for scaphoid osteonecrosis (a), MFT graft for proximal pole scaphoid nonunion with fragmentation (b) and corticoperiosteal graft for clavicle nonunion (c) are shown).

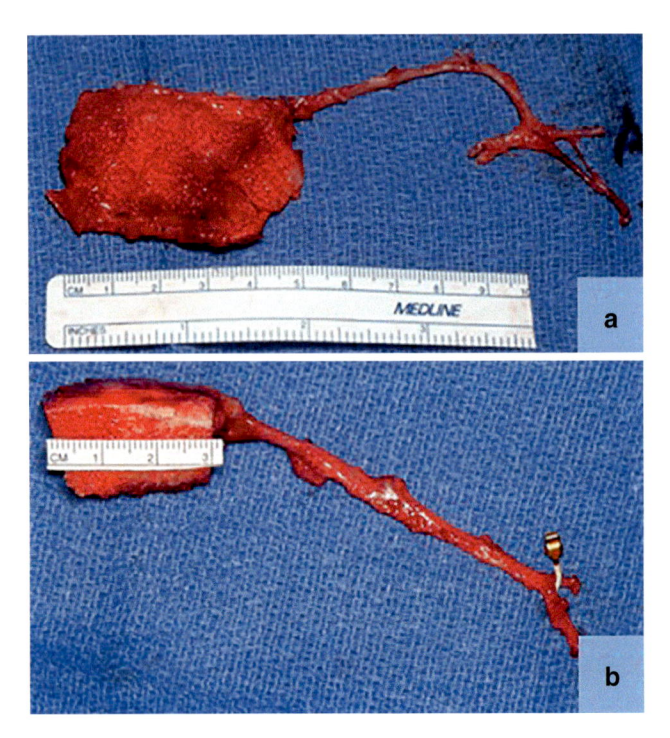

Fig. 39.6 A divided and custom-trimmed corticoperiosteal (**a**) and structural (**b**) medial femoral condyle vascularized bone graft and associated pedicle is shown

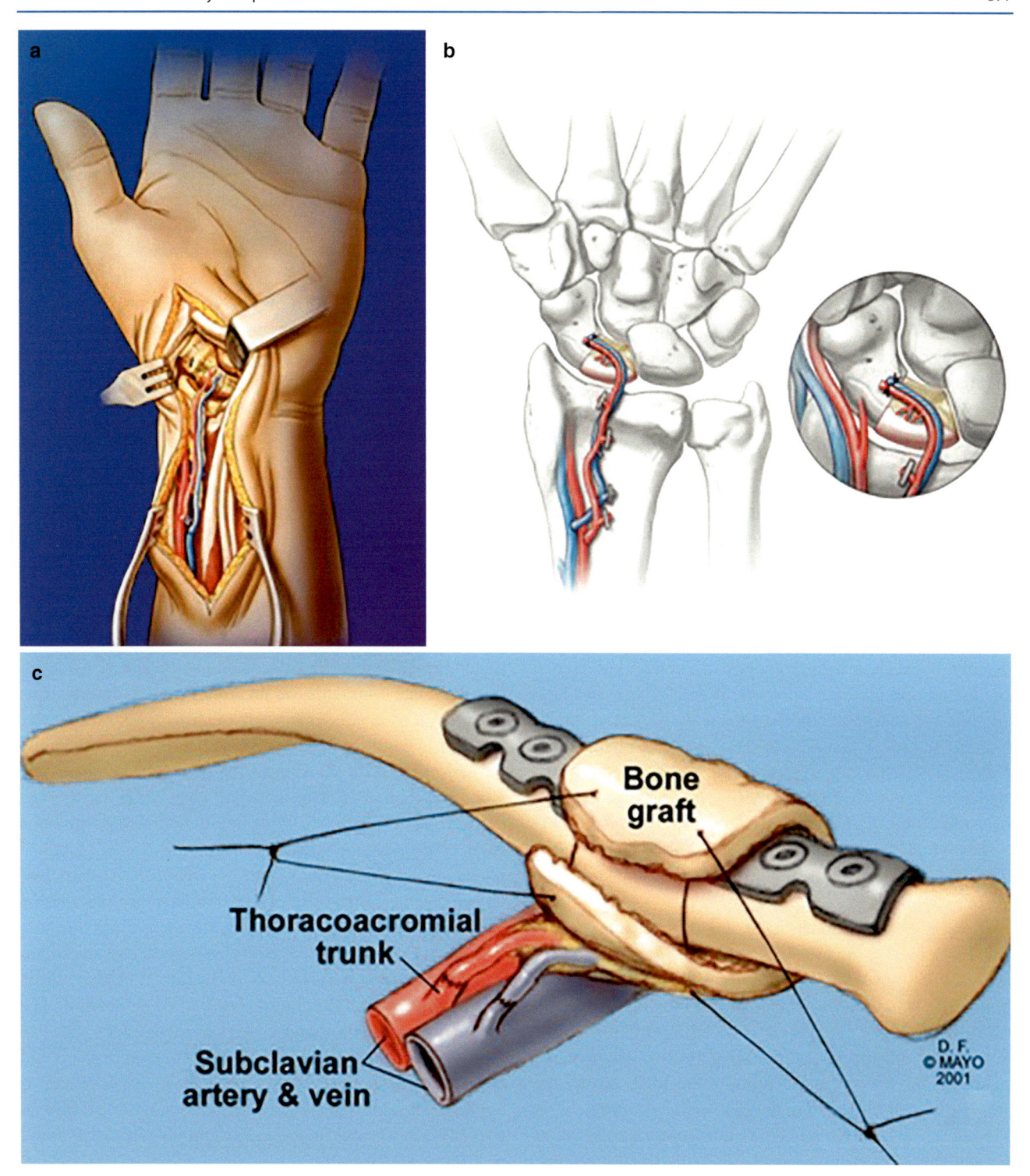

Fig. 39.7 Illustrations of a medial femoral condyle structural bone graft (**a**) and medial femoral trochlear graft (**b**) used for scaphoid reconstruction after insetting and microvascular anastomosis is shown. Conversely, corticoperisoteal grafts are typically wrapped around the recipient site, such as a clavicular nonunion undergoing revision open reduction and internal fixation (**c**). (Reproduced with permission of the Mayo Foundation)

39.6 Core Surgical Techniques in Flap Dissection

Under tourniquet control, a medial thigh incision starting at the most palpable, distal edge of the femur and extending proximally along the posterior border of the vastus medialis is used (Step 1—Incision). A curved incision is used instead when a component of articular cartilage is desired for the graft. The incision should be extended as necessary, which may be the case with more muscular patients. This should be anterior to the SAB signal if a skin island is planned. In all cases, the SAB is protected if identified during exposure. Electrocautery and self-retaining retractors are used to dissect through subcutaneous tissue down to fascia and then to make a small distal rent at the posterior border of the vastus medialis fascia. Metzenbaum scissors are used to complete the fascial divide proximally along the entire length of the incision, and the vastus medialis is lifted from its compartment anteriorly. The MFC and overlying vascularity can then be fully appreciated in the bed of the wound (Step 2—Exposure). Posterior retraction of the sartorius muscle may be needed for improved visualization. The DGA may be visualized on the floor of the wound just anterior to the adductor magnus tendon proximally and overlying the MFC distally. If the DGA is large enough, the sMGA branch may be ligated and divided. However, if the DGA is not large enough, the sMGA should be used and DGA contribution ligated instead. A green background is placed beneath the chosen pedicle for ease of recognition. Once the supply vessel has been chosen (DGA or sMGA), the planned graft can be outlined on the MFC periosteum using bipolar electrocautery (Step 3—Graft Planning). Planning a slightly larger flap than measured is important to allow for later customization.

Next, graft separation is dependent on graft composition. For a structural graft, a small curved osteotome or microsagittal saw (9 mm wide blade) is used perpendicular to the bone surface to vertically divide all but the proximal border of the graft where the pedicle is travelling (Step 4—Graft Separation). Identifying and avoiding the medial epicondyle of the femur will prevent disturbing the MCL during this step. Proximally, removal of the graft is done in three stages. First, a vessel loupe should be used to gently lift the vascular pedicle out of harm's way. Second, the small osteotome is similarly used perpendicular to the bony surface to make a vertical, proximal divide. Finally, the small osteotome is used 1–2 cm proximally to the proximal border of the planned graft at a 45° angle to undercut the graft (Step 5—Graft Elevation). This prevents levering out an incomplete or fragmented graft. The floor of the graft can then be lifted out of the donor site without damage or tension to the vascular pedicle. Viability of the graft can be ascertained by assessing for punctate bleeding from the periosteum. The tourniquet may be deflated if necessary, to visualize this. Graft separation and elevation is performed similarly for articular grafts, with exceptions being that the knee capsule needs to be entered first and that the last cut is made through the cartilage to ensure an adequate amount is incorporated (Step 5—Graft Separation and Step 6—Graft Elevation). The process of graft separation differs in corticoperiosteal grafts, where a curved osteotome is instead used running almost parallel to the cortical surface and where gradual separation occurs from the margins toward the center (Step 5—Graft Separation). Elevation is completed from distal to proximal by prying the graft away from the underlying cancellous bone beneath the vascular pedicle (Step 6—Graft Elevation).

The size and dimensions of the graft are then carefully scrutinized. Additional cancellous bone can be harvested from the donor site at this time. The pedicle is followed proximally and dissected free to maximize pedicle length before being clipped and sharply divided. The pedicle is usually at least 6 cm in length and close to the origin of the donor vessel. One clip is placed on the artery and two clips on any venae comitantes to facilitate ease of identification during anastomosis (Step 6—Graft Preparation and Division). Trimming and customization of the graft should be performed after division of the pedicle. The donor site wound is then copiously irrigated with sterile saline. The bony defect is grafted with synthetic hydroxyapatite bone filler of the surgeon's choice. The donor site is closed in layers using absorbable sutures (Step 7—Donor Site Closure). Deep fascia and patellar retinacular tissues using interrupted 0-Vicryl sutures in a figure-of-eight fashion. Buried, interrupted 2–0 Monocryl is used to close subcutaneous tissue over a 10-French supra-fascial channel drain set to bulb suction. A running 3–0 barbed suture followed by an occlusive mesh and 2-octyl cyanoacrylate adhesive dressing are used for skin. The knee is dressed in a soft and bulky compressive dressing and a knee immobilizer is applied. The drain is typically discontinued on postoperative day 1 for non-articular grafts and postoperative day 2 or 3 for articular grafts.

Structural grafts should be inset into the donor bed as an interposition graft, while corticoperiosteal grafts are wrapped around the recipient bone. In most instances, further stabilization is then necessary and is dependent on the anatomic region of the donor site. Once satisfied with graft security, end-to-side arterial anastomosis followed by an end-to-end microvenous repair is performed using an operative microscope and 8–0 or 9–0 nylon suture in an interrupted fashion (Step 8—Graft Inset and Anastomosis). Patency of the vessels and perfusion of the graft are visually confirmed prior to closure. Recipient site closure is performed in a layered fashion and is dependent on the anatomic site.

Postoperatively, the knee immobilizer is to be worn over the first few days for patient comfort as knee flexion may be uncomfortable. Immediate weight-bearing and range of motion is permitted and is usually tolerated well. A cane is supplied and may be used in the contralateral hand for support in the first few days after surgery.

39.7 Clinical Scenario

A healthy, 19-year-old, right-hand-dominant college freshman injured his left wrist during a fall while playing soccer. It initially was treated as a sprain. Due to ongoing pain, medical evaluation was sought 1 year after injury, and he was diagnosed with a scaphoid nonunion. Physical examination revealed pain in the anatomic snuffbox and diminished active wrist range of motion in all planes. Imaging demonstrated a nonunion of the scaphoid waist with a large cystic area and sclerosis of the proximal pole concerning for potential avascular necrosis (Fig. 39.8). A MFC vascularized bone graft from the ipsilateral leg was recommended and performed. The graft measured 10 × 10 × 10 mm and was taken from the posterior-distal aspect of the MFC off the DGA. Once inset, the graft was pre-drilled and fixed with a 24 mm cannulated, scaphoid-specific screw under fluoroscopic guidance. Standard reanastomosis and closure followed. Patient was placed in a bulky, long-arm thumb spica splint and returned for suture removal 2 weeks later. He was transitioned into a short arm cast for a period of 3 months at which time plain films and a CT scan were obtained demonstrating healing at the bone graft site (Fig. 39.9). He was given a custom-fabricated splint to be weaned out of in 4–6 weeks and initiated gentle range of motion with a skilled hand therapist. He was seen back 6 months and 1 year from surgery with excellent pain-free range of motion of the wrist and knee with no complication (Fig. 39.10).

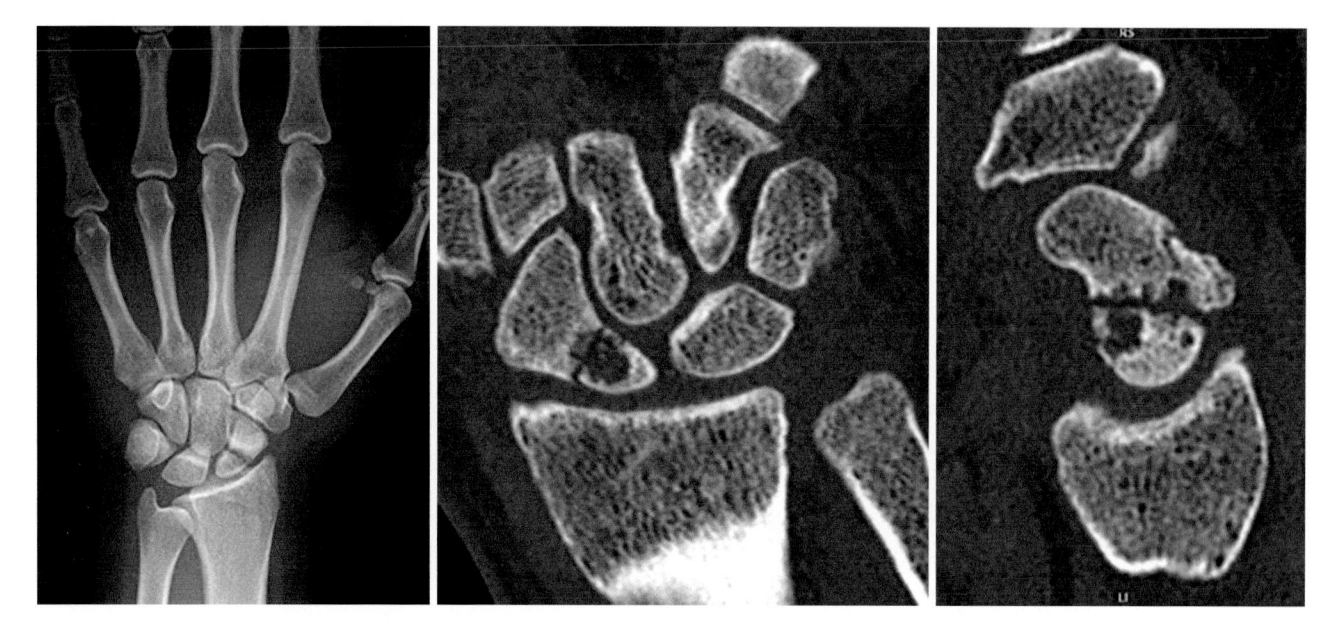

Fig. 39.8 Left wrist demonstrating a scaphoid waist nonunion with cystic resorption and sclerosis of the proximal pole without fragmentation or deformity (left—PA wrist; middle—coronal CT; right—scaphoid-axis, sagittal CT)

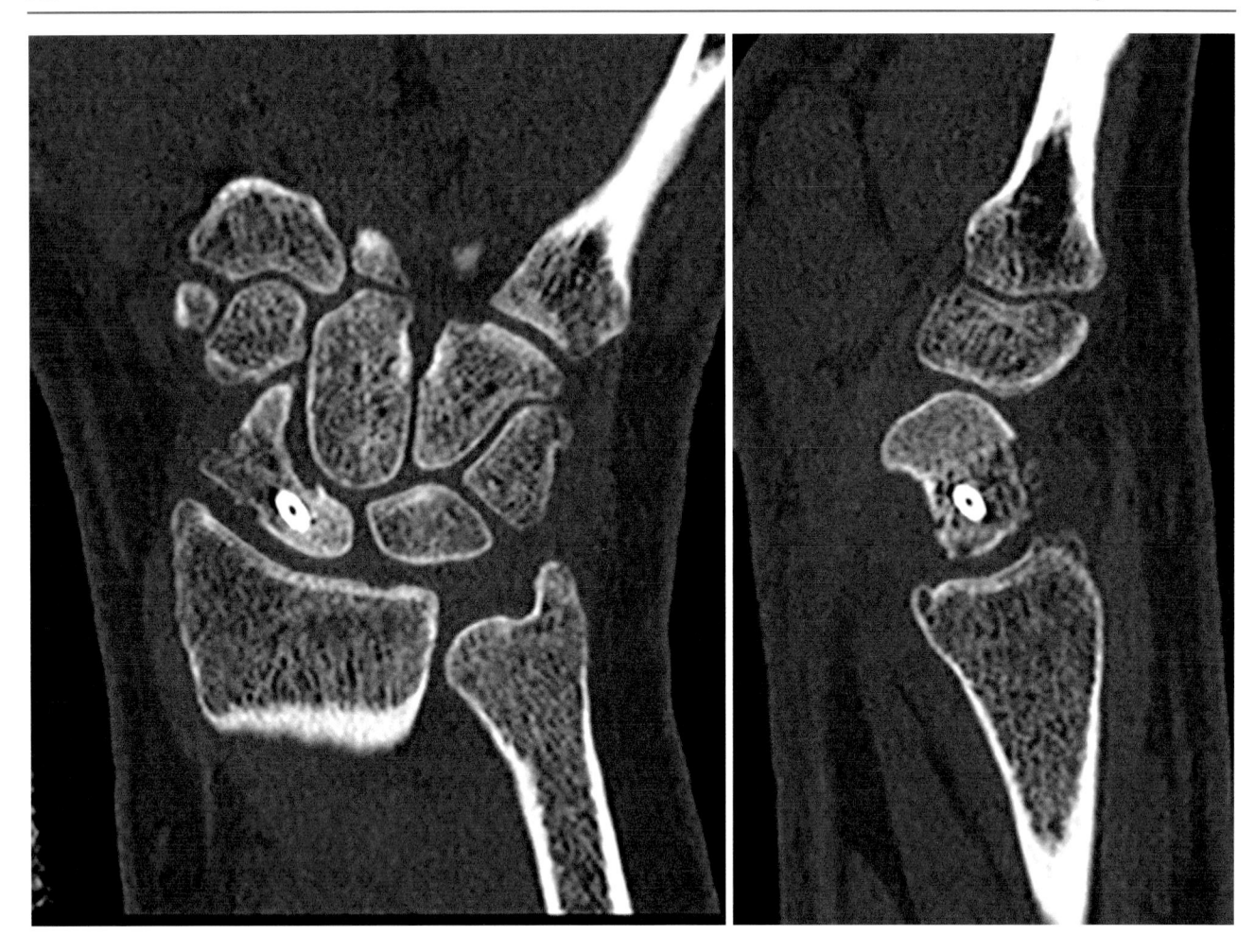

Fig. 39.9 Left wrist demonstrating proximal and distal incorporation of the vascularized MFC graft approximately 3 months after surgery (left—coronal CT; right—sagittal CT)

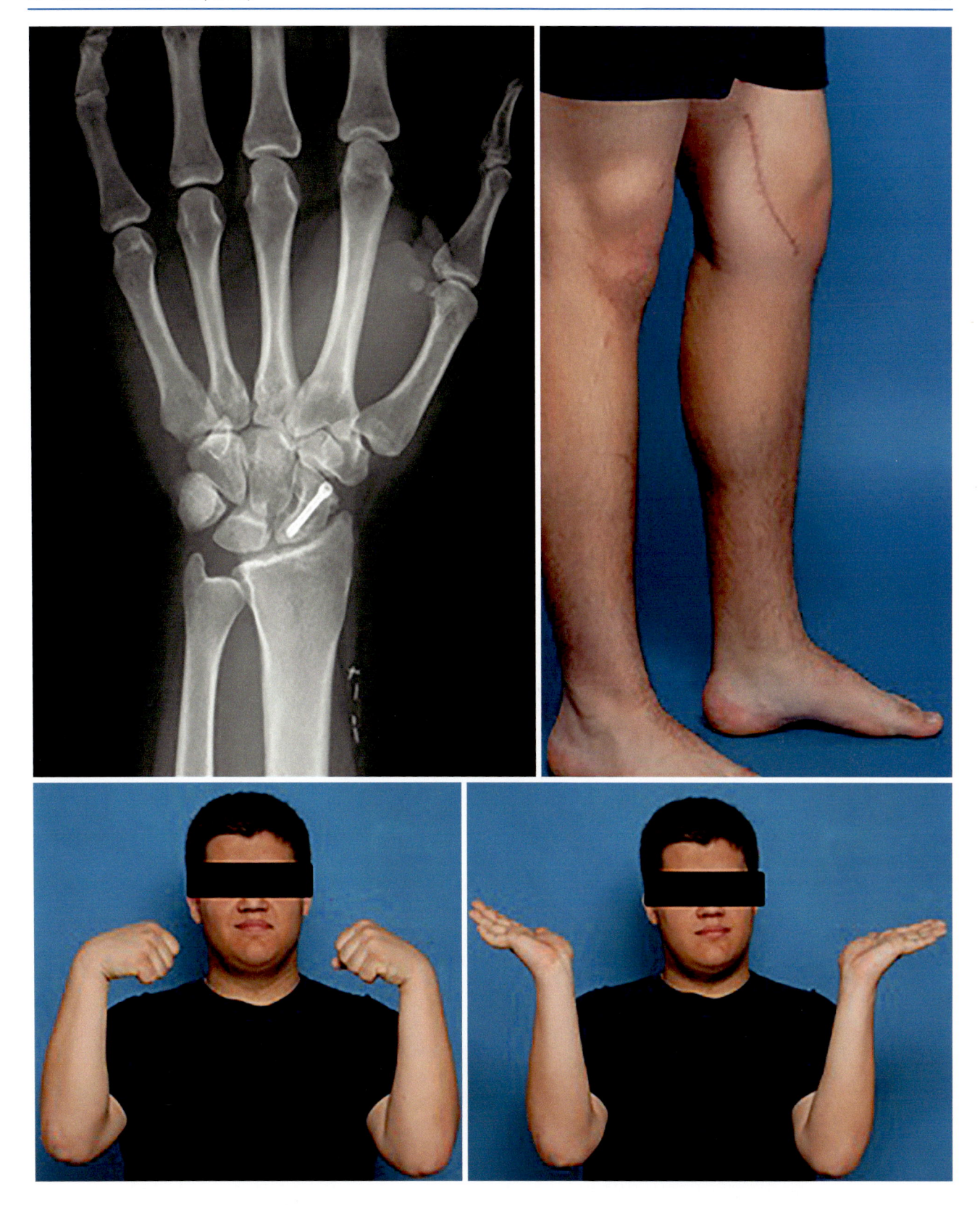

Fig. 39.10 Patient returns 6 months after surgery with a healed scaphoid, pain-free wrist, excellent motion, and no complication (top left—PA wrist; top right—healed medial knee incision; bottom left—final wrist flexion; bottom right—final wrist extension)

39.8 Pearls and Pitfalls

Pearls
- It is important to identify both the DGA and the sMGA and choose the largest caliber vessel to serve as the graft's primary vascular supply. This is usually, but not always, the DGA.
- Thin corticoperiosteal grafts are much easier to shape while large corticocancellous grafts will serve more of a structural role. Functional expectations of the graft should be pre-determined to maximize its potential.
- To ensure graft viability after being raised, check for bleeding edges of the periosteum, cortical, and cancellous bone.

Pitfalls
- In addition to raising the graft according to pre-planned dimensions, making an additional cut at a 45° angle just distal to the graft and elevating an extra wedge of bone allows for easier removal of the graft and decreases the risk of graft fracture or corticoperisoteal separation.
- Particularly when considering large grafts, it is critical to identify and avoid important surrounding anatomy. The adductor magnus tendon, superficial femoral artery proper, superficial medial collateral ligament and knee joint capsule are such structures.
- While large, viable grafts can be obtained from the MFC region [34], we recommend the proximal extent of the graft not pass the metaphyseal flare due to the risk of iatrogenic femur fracture as has been observed before with femoral notching [35].
- For interposition scaphoid reconstruction, insetting of the graft is the most difficult part. Correction of DISI deformity and minimal bone resection of the proximal and distal poles is necessary. Overstuffing has been suggested but is exceedingly difficult to accomplish. Normal anatomy is restored, and the length of the scaphoid rarely is "overstuffed" [37].

39.9 Selected Readings

- Sakai K, Doi K, Kawai S. Free vascularized thin corticoperiosteal graft. Plastic and reconstructive surgery. 1991;87(2):290–8.
- *Sakai et al. provide us with the first description in the American literature of the MFC graft used in a free fashion. All 6 patients had upper extremity nonunions that previously failed one or more operations and went on to union 2–3.5 months after being treated with a free corticoperiosteal MFC graft.*
- Larson AN, Bishop AT, Shin AY. Free medial femoral condyle bone grafting for scaphoid nonunions with humpback deformity and proximal pole avascular necrosis. Tech Hand Up Extrem Surg. 2007;11(4): 246–58.
- *One of the most common applications for a free MFC graft has been scaphoid nonunions, particularly when osteonecrosis of the proximal pole and/or deformity is present. This article presents our original surgical technique, which has not changed considerably since.*
- Hertel R, Masquelet AC. The reverse flow medial knee osteoperiosteal flap for skeletal reconstruction of the leg. Description and anatomical basis. Surg Radiol Anat. 1989;11(4):257–62.
- *This article presents the first description of the contemporary MFC graft in the American literature. It was described as a pedicled graft for treatment of local nonunions and osteonecrosis. More importantly, it describes the vascular basis for the MFC graft in the context of relevant surrounding anatomy through the cadaveric prosection of 50 specimens.*
- Hugon S, Koninckx A, Barbier O. Vascularized osteochondral graft from the medial femoral trochlea: anatomical study and clinical perspectives. Surg Radiol Anat. 2010;32(9):817–25.
- *The MFC graft can be modified into an osteochondral flap using cartilage from the medial femoral trochlea. In these instances, it is typically referred to as an MFT graft. This article offers the first anatomic evaluation of the MFT graft and suggests its feasibility for the treatment of defects often seen in Kienböck's disease or proximal pole of the scaphoid pathology.*
- Yamamoto H, Jones D Jr, Moran SL, Bishop AT, Shin A. The arterial anatomy of the medial femoral condyle and its clinical implications. J Hand Surg (European Volume). 2010;35(7):569–74.
- *These authors define the microvascular anatomy of the MFC graft while also reexploring the macrovascular*

anatomy some 20 years after its initial description. This work significantly contributed to our understanding of the posterior-distal quadrant of the MFC to be the optimal location for flap elevation as it reliably has the highest density of perforating vessels.

- Oh C, Pulos N, Bishop AT, Shin AY. Intraoperative anatomy of the vascular supply to the medial femoral condyle. J Plast Reconstr Aesthet Surg. 2019;72(9):1503–8.
- *This work explores the intraoperative macrovascular anatomy of the MFC graft in 113 patients. The major limitation of all prior anatomic descriptions was a reliance on information gained from a limited number of cadaveric specimens. It found the DGA to be present in 93% of patients and dominant 77% of the time with the sMGA absent in 2% of cases.*
- Mehio G, Morsy M, Cayci C, Sabbagh MD, Shin AY, Bishop AT, et al. Donor-site morbidity and functional status following medial femoral condyle flap harvest. Plast Reconstr Surg. 2018;142(5):734e–41e.
- *This article thoroughly explores knee donor site morbidity related to MFC graft harvest in 75 patients. These authors found an overall complication rate of 18.6% with the majority being saphenous nerve paresthesias with increasing flap size as a significant risk factor. Fifty-one percent of patients had functional outcomes comparable to a normal knee at 13 months.*

References

1. Acland R, Schusterman M, Godina M, Eder E, Taylor G, Carlisle I. The saphenous neurovascular free flap. Plast Reconstr Surg. 1981;67(6):763–74.
2. Masquelet A, Nordin J, Guinot A. Vascularized transfer of the adductor magnus tendon and its osseous insertion: a preliminary report. J Reconstr Microsurg. 1985;1(3):169–74.
3. Sakai K. Free vascularized bone and periosteal graft for pseudarthrosis in the upper limb. J Jpn Soc Surg Hand. 1988;5:698–704.
4. Sakai K, Doi K, Kawai S. Free vascularized thin corticoperiosteal graft. Plast Reconstr Surg. 1991;87(2):290–8.
5. Doi K, Sakai K. Vascularized periosteal bone graft from the supracondylar region of the femur. Microsurgery. 1994;15(5):305–15.
6. Fuchs B, Steinmann SP, Bishop AT. Free vascularized corticoperiosteal bone graft for the treatment of persistent nonunion of the clavicle. J Shoulder Elb Surg. 2005;14(3):264–8.
7. Huang TC-T, Sabbagh MD, Lu C-K, Steinmann SP, Moran SL. The vascularized medial femoral condyle free flap for reconstruction of segmental recalcitrant nonunion of the clavicle. J Shoulder Elb Surg. 2019;28(12):2364–70.
8. Aibinder W, Torchia M, Bishop A, Shin A. Vascularized medial femoral condyle graft for manubrium nonunion: case report and review of the literature. J Surg Orthop Adv. 2017;26(3):173–9.
9. Muramatsu K, Doi K, Ihara K, Shigetomi M, Kawai S. Recalcitrant posttraumatic nonunion of the humerus: 23 patients reconstructed with vascularized bone graft: 23 patients reconstructed with vascularized bone graft. Acta Orthop Scand. 2003;74(1):95–7.
10. Yajima H, Maegawa N, Ota H, Kisanuki O, Kawate K, Takakura Y. Treatment of persistent non-union of the humerus using a vascularized bone graft from the supracondylar region of the femur. J Reconstr Microsurg. 2007;23(2):107–13.
11. Sammer DM, Bishop AT, Shin AY. Vascularized medial femoral condyle graft for thumb metacarpal reconstruction: case report. J Hand Surg Am. 2009;34(4):715–8.
12. Doi K, Oda T, Soo-Heong T, Nanda V. Free vascularized bone graft for nonunion of the scaphoid. J Hand Surg Am. 2000;25(3):507–19.
13. Larson AN, Bishop AT, Shin AY. Free medial femoral condyle bone grafting for scaphoid nonunions with humpback deformity and proximal pole avascular necrosis. Tech Hand Up Extrem Surg. 2007;11(4):246–58.
14. Jones DB Jr, Bürger H, Bishop AT, Shin AY. Treatment of scaphoid waist nonunions with an avascular proximal pole and carpal collapse. A comparison of two vascularized bone grafts. J Bone Joint Surg Am. 2008;90(12):2616–25.
15. Choudry UH, Bakri K, Moran SL, Karacor Z, Shin AY. The vascularized medial femoral condyle periosteal bone flap for the treatment of recalcitrant bony nonunions. Ann Plast Surg. 2008;60(2):174–80.
16. Higgins JP, Bürger HK. Osteochondral flaps from the distal femur: expanding applications, harvest sites, and indications. J Reconstr Microsurg. 2014;30(7):483–90.
17. Kazmers NH, Rozell JC, Rumball KM, Kozin SH, Zlotolow DA, Levin LS. Medial femoral condyle microvascular bone transfer as a treatment for capitate avascular necrosis: surgical technique and case report. J Hand Surg Am. 2017;42(10):841.e1–6.
18. Hachisuka H, Sunagawa T, Ochi M, Morrison WA. A vascularized medial femoral condyle cortico-periosteal graft for total lunate reconstruction. J Orthop Sci. 2020;25(2):354–8.
19. Hertel R, Masquelet AC. The reverse flow medial knee osteoperiosteal flap for skeletal reconstruction of the leg. Description and anatomical basis. Surg Radiol Anat. 1989;11(4):257–62.
20. Cavadas PC, Landín L. Treatment of recalcitrant distal tibial nonunion using the descending genicular corticoperiosteal free flap. J Trauma Acute Care Surg. 2008;64(1):144–50.
21. Doi K, Hattori Y. Vascularized bone graft from the supracondylar region of the femur. Microsurgery. 2009;29(5):379–84.
22. Hsu C-C, Loh CYY, Lin C-H, Lin Y-T, Lin C-H, Wong J. The medial femoral condyle flap to re-vitalise the femoral head for calcaneal reconstruction. J Plast Reconstr Aesthet Surg. 2017;70(7):974–6.
23. Choi JW, Jeong WS, Kwon SM, Koh KS. Medial femoral condyle free flap for premaxillary reconstruction in median facial dysplasia. J Craniofac Surg. 2017;28(1):e57–60.
24. Taylor EM, Wu WW, Kamali P, Ferraro N, Upton J, Lin SJ, et al. Medial femoral condyle flap reconstruction of a maxillary defect with a 3D printing template. J Reconstr Microsurg Open. 2017;2(01):e63–8.
25. Banaszewski J, Gaggl A, Andruszko A. Medial femoral condyle free flap for head and neck reconstruction. Curr Opin Otolaryngol Head Neck Surg. 2019;27(2):130–5.
26. Martin D, Bitonti-Grillo C, De Biscop J, Schott H, Mondle J, Baudet J, et al. Mandibular reconstruction using a free vascularised osteocutaneous flap from the internal condyle of the femur. Br J Plast Surg. 1991;44(6):397–402.
27. Pulikkottil BJ, Pezeshk RA, Ramanadham SR, Haddock NT. The medial femoral condyle corticoperiosteal free flap for frontal sinus reconstruction. J Craniofac Surg. 2017;28(3):813–6.
28. Kollitz KM, Pulos N, Bishop AT, Shin AY. Primary medial femoral condyle vascularized bone graft for scaphoid nonunions with carpal collapse and proximal pole avascular necrosis. J Hand Surg (European Volume). 2019;44(6):600–6.
29. Hugon S, Koninckx A, Barbier O. Vascularized osteochondral graft from the medial femoral trochlea: anatomical study and clinical perspectives. Surg Radiol Anat. 2010;32(9):817–25.
30. Houdek MT, Matsumoto JM, Morris JM, Bishop AT, Shin AY. Technique for 3-Dimesnion (3D) modeling of osteoarticu-

lar medial femoral condyle vascularized grafting to replace the proximal pole of unsalvagable scaphoid nonunions. Tech Hand Up Extrem Surg. 2016;20(3):117–24.
31. Yamamoto H, Jones D Jr, Moran SL, Bishop AT, Shin A. The arterial anatomy of the medial femoral condyle and its clinical implications. J Hand Surg (European Volume). 2010;35(7):569–74.
32. Oh C, Pulos N, Bishop AT, Shin AY. Intraoperative anatomy of the vascular supply to the medial femoral condyle. J Plast Reconstr Aesthet Surg. 2019;72(9):1503–8.
33. Iorio ML, Masden DL, Higgins JP. Cutaneous angiosome territory of the medial femoral condyle osteocutaneous flap. J Hand Surg Am. 2012;37(5):1033–41.
34. Iorio ML, Masden DL, Higgins JP. The limits of medial femoral condyle corticoperiosteal flaps. J Hand Surg Am. 2011;36(10):1592–6.
35. Lesh ML, Schneider DJ, Deol G, Davis B, Jacobs CR, Pelligrini VD Jr. The consequences of anterior femoral notching in total knee arthroplasty: a biomechanical study. JBJS. 2000;82(8):1096.
36. Kakar S, Duymaz A, Steinmann S, Shin AY, Moran SL. Vascularized medial femoral condyle corticoperiosteal flaps for the treatment of recalcitrant humeral nonunions. Microsurgery. 2011;31(2):85–92.
37. Giusti G, Bishop AT, Shin AY. Overstuffing of unstable scaphoid nonunions: a radiographic analysis of carpal parameters. J Hand Surg Am. 2019;44(5):423.e1–6.

Medial Sural Artery Perforator Flap

40

Dimitris Reissis, Dariush Nikkhah, Bernard Luczak, and Georgios Orfaniotis

40.1 Introduction

First described by Pedro Cavadas in 2001 [1], the Medial Sural Artery Perforator (MSAP) flap has quickly become a workhorse flap for reconstruction of both the head and neck and distal extremities [2, 3]. It is an evolution of the gastrocnemius muscle flap (Fig. 40.1), based on the musculocutaneous perforators arising through the medial gastrocnemius muscle.

Most commonly harvested as a free flap, the MSAP is primarily used to reconstruct small- to medium-sized defects where thin pliable tissue is required [4–6]. It is particularly useful for intra-oral reconstruction [7–14], for example after partial glossectomy. It is also used in reconstruction of lower leg, foot and ankle defects [4, 15–17], as well as full thickness defects of the hand [18–21], where other traditional flaps such as the ALT may be too bulky.

It also has a role as a pedicled flap [22, 23], for defects around the knee and upper leg, and can include a muscle component if required to fill dead space. It is a particularly versatile flap, with potential to tailor the flap design with multiple skin paddles each based on their own musculocutaneous perforators. It can also be harvested as a chimeric flap [24–26] including sections of plantaris tendon [18], sural [27] or saphenous nerve [19] for composite reconstruction tailored to the defect.

In view of its inconspicuous donor site and reduced donor morbidity with preservation of major vessels, the MSAP has notable advantages over other free flaps such as the radial forearm free flap [28–31], for similar reconstructive indications.

40.2 Anatomy

The MSAP flap is located along an axis drawn from the midpoint of the popliteal crease to the medial malleolus of the ankle. Thus the skin paddle overlies the medial gastrocnemius muscle.

The arterial supply is based on musculocutaneous perforators originating from the superficial branch of the medial sural artery, which itself is a branch of the popliteal artery at the level of the knee joint [32–34].

The distribution of these musculocutaneous perforators are variable, but almost universally present in all patients. Cavadas originally described an average of 2.2 perforators that can sustain the MSAP flap [1]. Further anatomical studies demonstrate a range of 2–8 perforators supplying the medial sural artery perforator territory, usually with a dominant perforator present [11, 34]. The intra-muscular branching patterns of the medial sural artery perforators has been classified as having single vessel perforators in 31%, two in 59% and three or more in 10% cases [32].

The perforators are most commonly located 12–17 cm below the popliteal crease along the line drawn from the midpoint of the popliteal crease to the prominence of the medial malleolus [32]. A dominant perforator is most often found 13 (±2) cm inferior and 2.5 (±1) cm lateral to the midpoint of the popliteal crease [32]. No perforator is found either less than 6 cm or more than 18 cm below the popliteal crease [11, 34].

The course of the perforator is intra-muscular through the medial head of gastrocnemius. The pedicle initially runs proximally towards the popliteal crease in the superficial muscle fibres of medial gastrocnemius muscle. After a short superficial course the vessel deepens down into the belly of gastrocnemius muscle giving multiple branches around

D. Reissis (✉) · D. Nikkhah
Royal Free Hospital, London, UK
e-mail: dreissis@nhs.net

B. Luczak
Royal Perth Hospital, Western Australia, Australia

G. Orfaniotis
Guy's and St Thomas' Hospital, London, UK

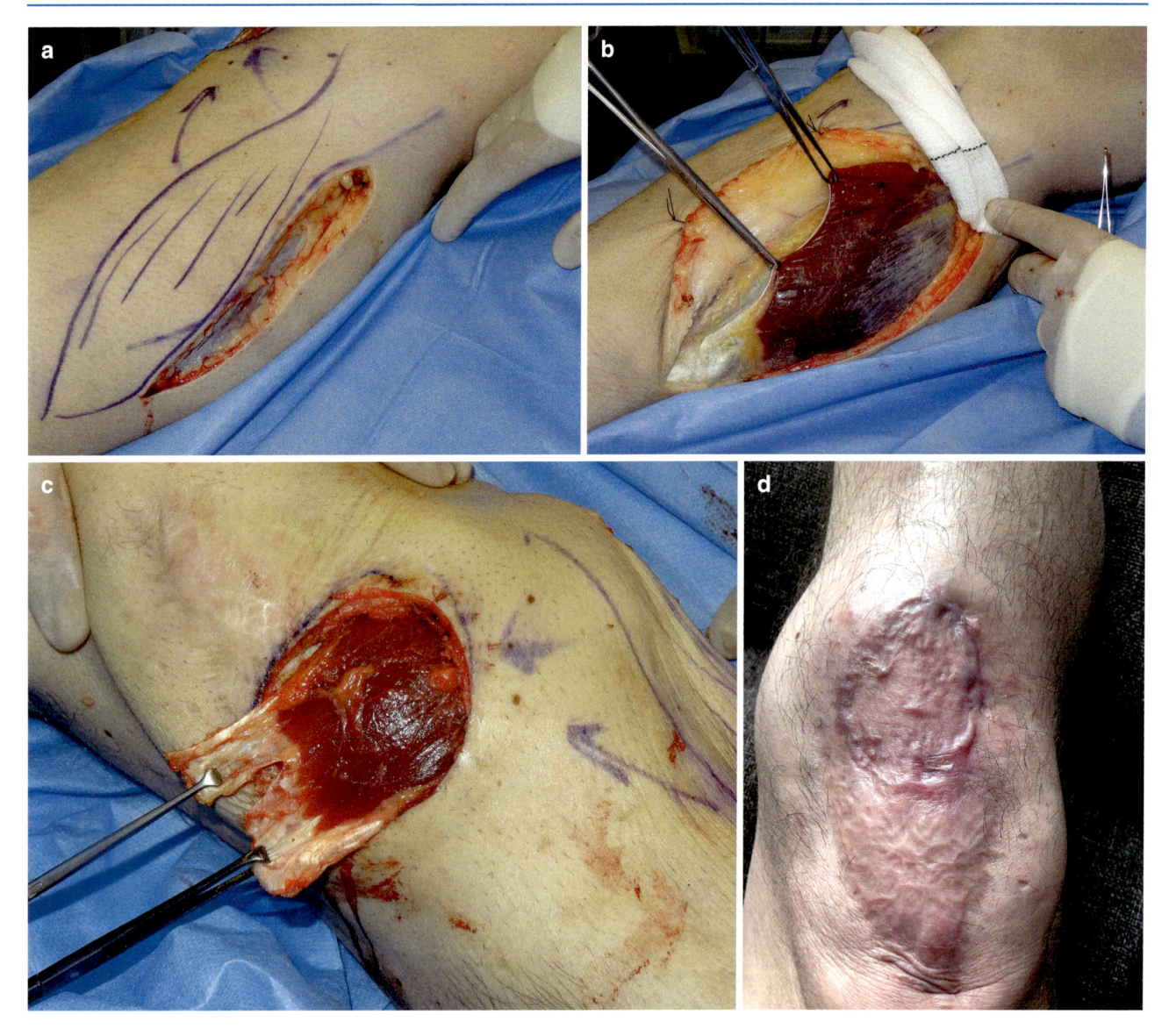

Fig. 40.1 (a) Pre-op markings of the pedicled Gastrocnemius muscle flap with the primary incision already made. The flap most often utilises the medial head of the gastrocnemius muscle, which in this case will be used to reconstruction a defect on the antero-lateral aspect of the knee. (b) Dissection of the medial head of gastrocnemius muscle, prior to division of the distal tendinous insertion. (c) Tension-free transfer of the pedicled gastrocnemius muscle flap into the recipient site defect on the antero-lateral knee. The muscle and distal tendon are secured in place and a skin graft placed over the muscle. (d) Healed gastrocnemius muscle flap with overlying skin graft at 6 months post-operatively. (Case Courtesy of D Nikkhah)

360°. Occasionally, the perforator may initially travel suprafascially along the muscle fascia for some distance prior to perforating through the superficial fascia, which must be identified early during dissection to avoid pedicle injury [4].

The length of the pedicle can range from 8 to 16 cm, depending on the location of the perforator and degree of dissection towards its origin from the medial sural artery [35, 36]. The arterial diameter of the vascular pedicle taken up to the medial sural artery is most commonly 1–2 mm [11]. This allows for tailoring of the pedicle length and vessel diameter to the defect being reconstructed and recipient vessels available. In the case of trauma or prior radiation to the recipient site, one can harvest a pedicle of adequate length to allow microvascular anastomosis outside the zone of trauma or radiation, with access to a choice of recipient vessels, for either end-to-end or end-to-side anastomosis.

Venous outflow is via the venae comitantes which parallel the course of the perforators and have a slightly larger diameter than the artery (3.5 mm). If required, an additional vein such as the short or long saphenous vein can be incorporated into the MSAP to improve venous drainage.

No nerve is usually included in the flap meaning it is insensate. However, harvesting the MSAP with a segment of the sural, saphenous or motor nerve to the gastrocnemius muscle as a nerve graft, may allow for functional reconstruction in the appropriate patient and setting [27].

The thickness of the flaps usually is as thin as 5 mm (range, 4–8 mm), allowing for a smooth profile where thin tissue is required at the recipient site, such as the foot and ankle and dorsum of hand [37]. Leahy et al. have shown than the medial calf is associated with 47% less supra-fascial adipose tissue than the ALT region in both men and women [38].

40.3 Pre-operative Investigation

Routine pre-operative imaging is not required for MSAP flap harvest. However, CT angiography may be useful in patients with previous lower limb injury or surgery or patients with diabetes and atherosclerotic disease.

A standard hand-held Doppler ultrasound (8–10 Hz) is routinely used to map perforators pre-operatively on the operating table [39]. These are most commonly found along the line marked from the midpoint of the popliteal fossa to the medial malleolus, in the region 6–18 cm below the popliteal crease and 1–3 cm lateral to the midline of the calf.

Colour duplex-Doppler has also been shown to be reliable for planning of sural artery perforator flaps due to high precision in detecting location of dominant perforators and ability to assess flow more accurately than standard Doppler ultrasound [40].

For more accurate perforator mapping with assessment of the intra-muscular pedicle course, branching pattern type [32] or the site of fascial perforation, CT angiogram [41], with or without 3D visualization reconstruction [42], can also be used. While these are more time- and resource-intensive, it has been shown that routine use of pre-operative CT angiogram may help determine which leg has the most favorable branching pattern type and intra-muscular course for flap harvest [32].

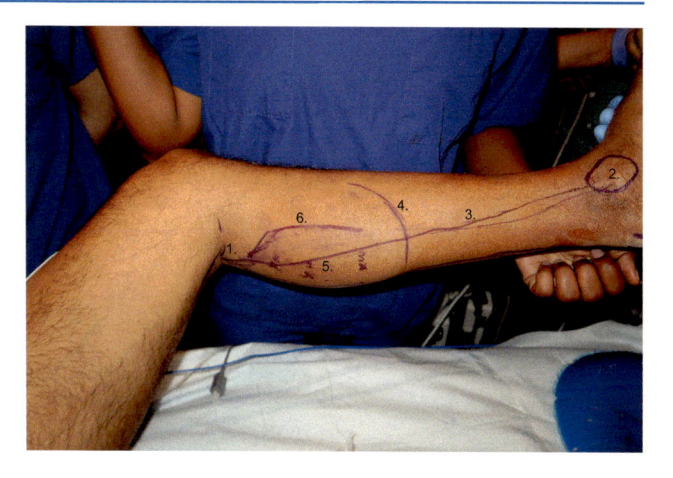

Fig. 40.2 Pre-op markings of the MSAP flap. (1) Midpoint of the popliteal fossa. (2) Medial malleolus. (3) Longitudinal line between the midpoint of the popliteal fossa and the medial malleolus. (4) Inferior border of the gastrocnemius. (5) Chosen perforators marked using an 'x' and number. (6) Anterior border of the flap

40.4 Flap Design and Markings

Flap Markings (Fig. 40.2)
- Mark the midpoint of the popliteal fossa and the medial malleolus.
  - Draw a longitudinal line connecting the two landmarks.
  - Starting at roughly 12 cm along and slightly posterior to this line, use a hand-held Doppler to identify the perforators. Ensure these are proximal to the inferior border of the gastrocnemius.
  - Mark the chosen perforator(s) using a clear 'x' and/or number.
  - Mark the anterior border of the flap.
  - Adjust the flap markings to ensure the perforator in the centre or upper edge of the flap depending on the laxity of skin and flap design [4]. If pedicle length is a priority, the perforator can also be located towards the distal aspect of the flap to lengthen the pedicle as much as possible.

Flap Design: Key Points
- Design the skin island of the MSAP free flap in a slightly oblique but predominantly longitudinal direction, to capture interconnecting choke vessels between the perforasomes of the lower limb [43].
- Limit the flap width to less than 6 cm width to enable primary closure [19].
  - Some series have suggested a flap width of up to 8 cm can also routinely enable direct closure with generally mild risk of donor site wound dehiscence [2, 5].
- Wherever possible use ipsilateral donor and recipient sites to restrict the dressings, scarring, pain and rehabilitation to a single limb.
  - This will still allow for a two-team approach if necessary, for shortened operative time and the use of a single tourniquet [4]. However, if there has been high energy trauma with diffuse soft tissue damage, the medial calf may be within the zone of trauma and preclude this, requiring harvest from the contralateral leg in these cases.

40.5 Flap Raise/Elevation: A Step-by-Step Guide

Positioning
- Position the patient supine with the thigh abducted, knee flexed and lower leg externally rotated, so the medial aspect of the calf is easily accessed.

Tourniquet

- Use of a mid-thigh tourniquet is recommended.
- If used, exsanguinate the lower leg only by elevation for 1 min, rather than using an eshmark, to maintain fill of venae comitantes and permit better visualization of the perforators.

Incision (Fig. 40.3)

- Make the anterior incision first.
- Be sure not to place this incision too posterior, as this would risk missing or injuring the perforators immediately.
- Incise down to fascia overlying the medial gastrocnemius muscle.

Identification of the Perforator(s)

- Identify and preserve any perforator passing through the subcutaneous tissue, however small initially, as this may be your main perforator.
- Take care to identify whether the perforator travels supra-fascially along the muscle fascia prior to perforating through the superficial fascia.
  - This can necessitate raising a wide skin paddle to keep the perforator central to the skin paddle, thus impacting donor site primary closure.
- Make an exploratory incision in the anterior aspect of the gastrocnemius fascia.
- Visualize and confirm perforator location and adequacy of size.
- Endoscope-assisted identification of the perforator(s) has been described but is not common practice [44].

Dissection

- Trace the course of the perforator through the medial gastrocnemius muscle by longitudinally splitting the superficial muscle fibres (Fig. 40.4).
- After a short superficial course, the vessel deepens down into the belly of gastrocnemius muscle giving multiple branches in all directions.
- Use careful bipolar dissection with a 'deroofing' technique with 'ligaclipping' and heat-sink diathermy of multiple side branches within the muscle.
  - Meticulous ligation/clipping of these tiny intra-muscular branches is mandatory to avoid intra-muscular haematoma in the immediate post-operative period.
- Dissect the pedicle retrogradely to the medial sural artery or until adequate pedicle length is achieved.
- Once the required length and calibre of pedicle vessel have been dissected, the posterior border of the flap is incised and the flap islanded on the pedicle(s).

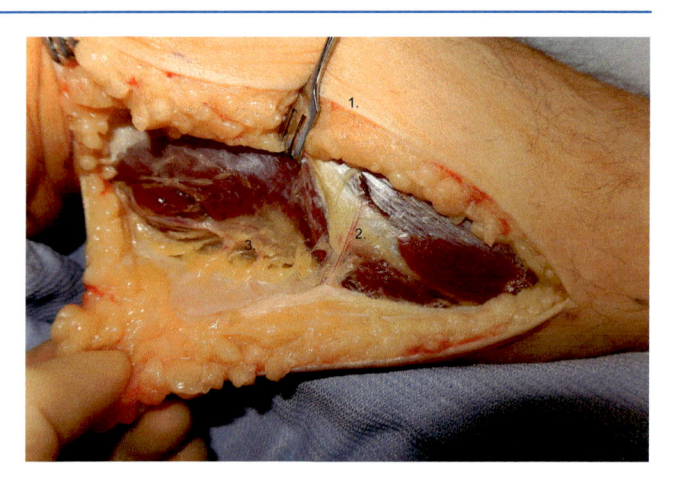

Fig. 40.3 Anterior incision and identification of perforators. (1) Anterior incision. (2) Main perforator arising from a larger deep musculocutaneous perforator. (3) Additional smaller and more proximal perforators, with predominantly supra-fascial course

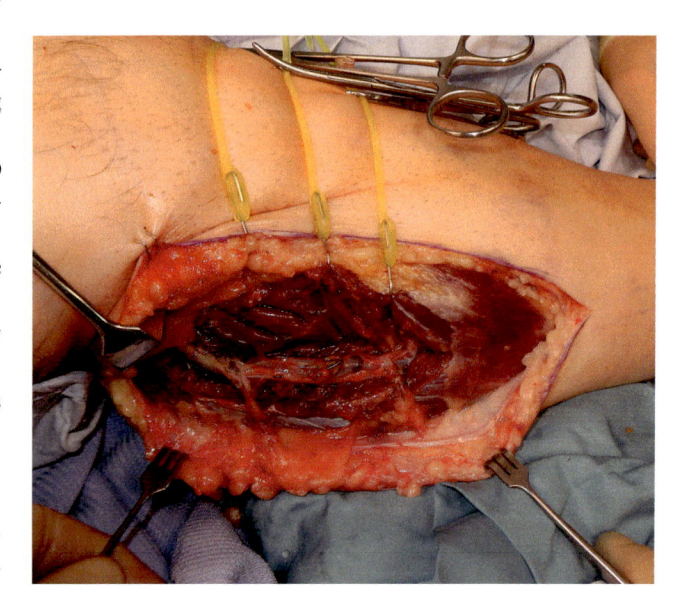

Fig. 40.4 Pedicle dissection. Main pedicle dissected free with longitudinal muscle-splitting dissection and ligaclipping of multiple side branches along its length. Two main perforators supply the skin paddle

- Once your pedicle dissection is complete and flap perfusion is confirmed, template the skin paddle to the defect and make the posterior incision, isolating the flap on the pedicle(s).
- Divide the pedicle proximally at the origin from the popliteal artery (Fig. 40.5).

Additional Flap Considerations

- If it is felt an additional vein will be required, ensure the small saphenous vein, which is normally located 3 cm from the dominant perforator [45], is protected throughout and included in the flap.

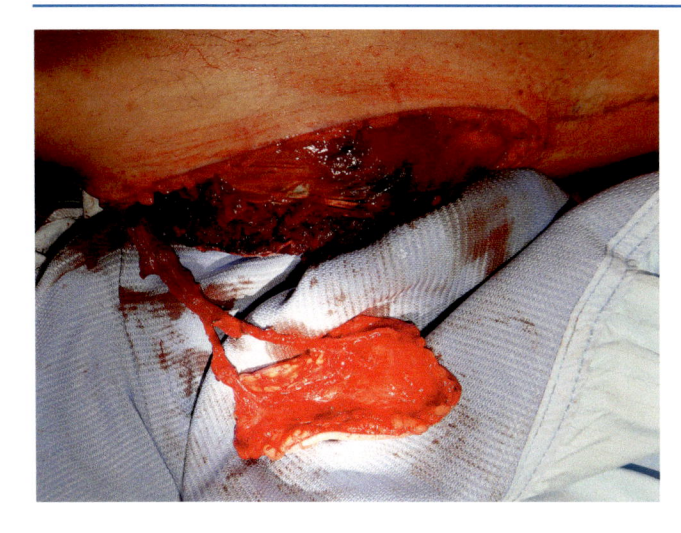

Fig. 40.5 Flap raised prior to division of the pedicle. The posterior skin incision has been made, after templating the flap to the recipient defect

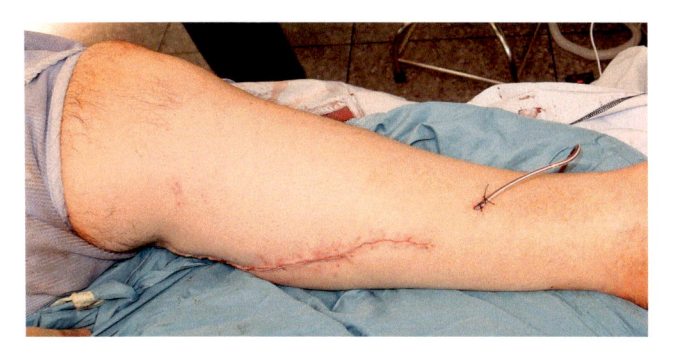

Fig. 40.6 Donor site closed primarily with a low vacuum suction drain in place

- Likewise, if a chimeric flap is required, an additional bulk of gastrocnemius muscle, plantaris tendon or sural nerve may be harvested as part of the flap too.

Closure
- Close the donor site primarily in layers (Fig. 40.6).
- Direct closure of the donor site is preferred as skin grafting to the calf compromises the aesthetics of the reconstruction.
- Place a low vacuum suction drain (to stay in place until draining <30 mL/24 h).

Post-operative Care
- Each department may have a different post-operative regime based on personal experience.
- The protocol must be flexible to the appearance and behaviour of the flap based on judicial clinical examination.
- An example of a post-operative regime for lower limb reconstruction may include:
  - Days 1–5: Elevation of the operated/recipient leg for 5 days.
  - Day 5: Begin dangling the limb for 5 min within a 1 h period. Increase the period dangling by 5 min each hour, 10 min in the second hour, 15 min in the third hour, until the leg is down for 30 min within the sixth hour.
- Laser Doppler perfusion imaging may be a valuable adjunct for post-operative flap monitoring if available, with the highest relative perfusion in the perforator zone of the flap between days 1 and 5 post-operatively [46].

40.6 Core Surgical Techniques in Flap Dissection

- Position the patient on the operating table before mapping the perforators with the Doppler ultrasound.
- Use safe dissection technique for deroofing the pedicle and using heatsink bipolar and ligaclipping of multiple muscular branches throughout.
- Reassess and modify the final flap design after the perforator(s) are identified and dissected fully, with release of the prior to disconnecting the flap.
- Harvest a segment of the short saphenous vein to provide the option for additional venous drainage, for use as both a free and pedicled flap [47].
- Avoid using the MSAP flap if it is required to be greater than 6 m width, to avoid the need for skin graft, which is unsightly and can result in tethered and poor quality scar [48].

40.7 Clinical Scenarios

40.7.1 Case 1

40.7.1.1 Partial Glossectomy Reconstruction
George Orfaniotis

A 46-year-old female underwent left partial glossectomy for a T2N0M0 SCC from her left tongue. The resultant defect was reconstructed with a free MSAP flap, which was based on a single perforator and anastomosed to superior thyroid artery and a branch of the internal jugular vein. The tumor resection and flap inset were performed transorally, with no requirement for a mandibular split. At 1 week post-operatively she was able to eat a soft diet and her speech was intelligible and easily understandable. At 4 months post-operatively the patient was back to her job as a motivational speaker and was also able to run 10 K (Fig. 40.7).

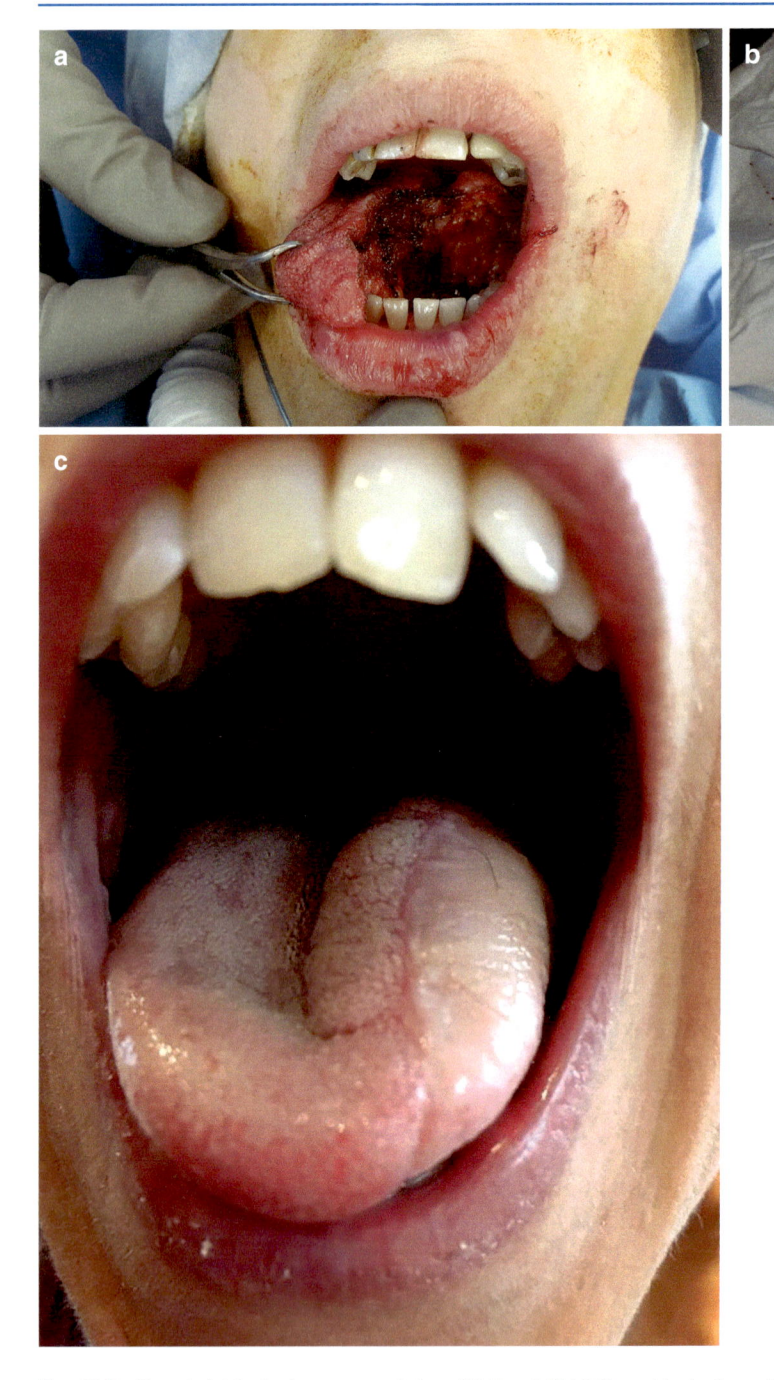

Fig. 40.7 Case 1. (**a**) Left glossectomy defect. (**b**) Free MSAP flap with single pedicle of sufficient length to anastomose to the ipsilateral transverse cervical vessels. (**c**) Result at 4 months post-operatively, with natural contour and mucosalisation of the flap epithelium on the tongue

40.7.2 Case 2

40.7.2.1 Pharyngeal Cancer Reconstruction
George Orfaniotis

A 62-year-old male with an invasive T4N1M0 pharyngeal SCC underwent total laryngo-pharyngectomy and bilateral neck dissection levels II–VI. Reconstruction was with a chimeric free MSAP flap with two skin paddles and a segment of gastrocnemius muscle, each based on their own individual musculocutaneous perforator. Pharyngeal reconstruction was achieved using an internal "patch" (6 × 5 cm) MSAP skin paddle, with the segment of the gastrocnemius muscle secured on top of this as extra waterproofing layer, also reducing the dead space. The second MSAP skin paddle was used to facilitate skin closure as well as to allow clinical flap monitoring. The flap was anastomosed to the right facial vessels, using a Cook-Schwartz Doppler probe to aid post-operative venous monitoring (Fig. 40.8).

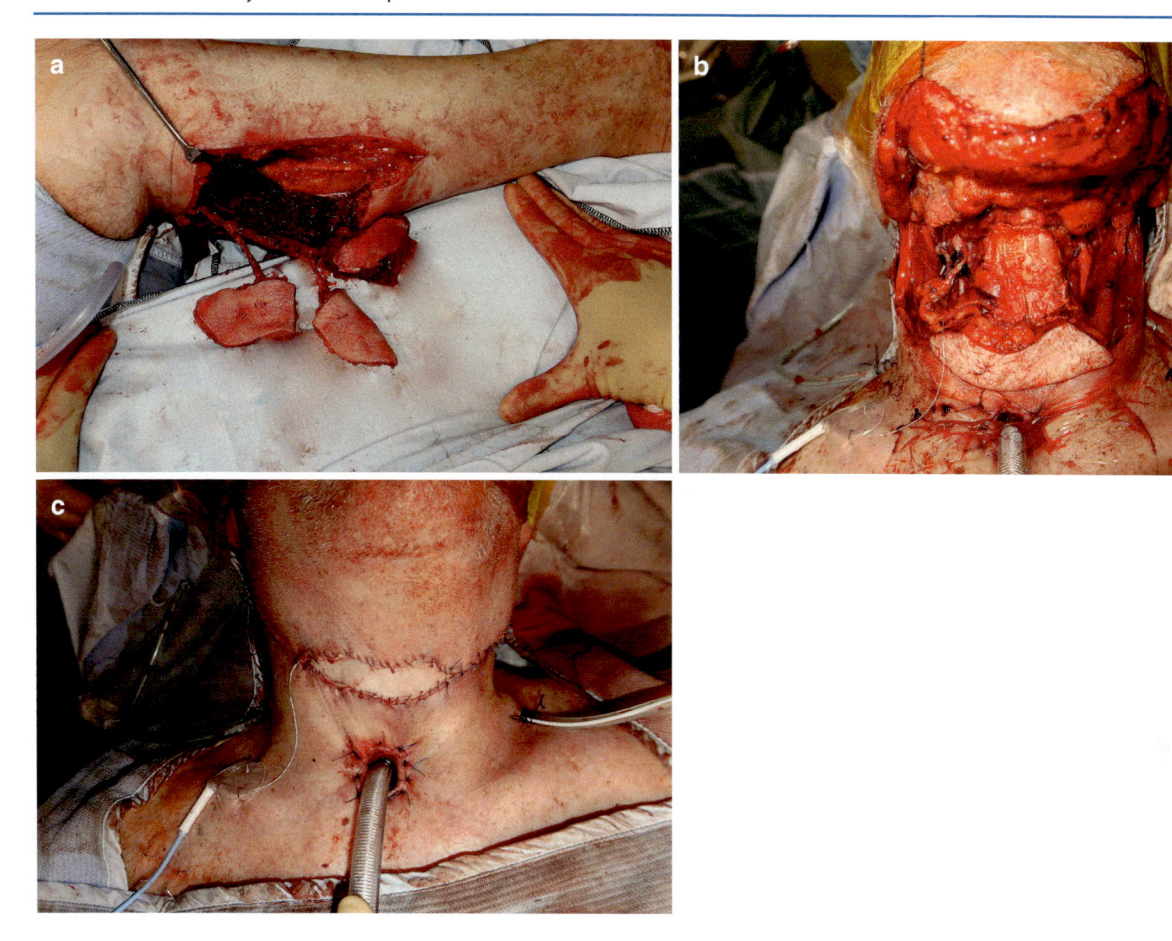

Fig. 40.8 Case 2. (**a**) Chimeric free MSAP flap being raised with two separate skin paddles and a segment of gastrocnemius muscle, each based on their own individual musculocutaneous perforator. (**b**) Defect following pharyngectomy and bilateral neck dissection with the free MSAP flap anastomosed to the right facial vessels and inset for simultaneous pharyngeal and soft tissue reconstruction. Note the Cook-Schwartz Doppler probe on one of the draining veins to aid post-operative venous monitoring. (**c**) Flap inset and closure, with tracheostomy, 2× low suction vacuum drains and the Doppler probe attached

40.7.3 Case 3

40.7.3.1 Open Ankle Wound Post-septic Arthritis

Dariush Nikkhah and Bernard Luczak

A 45-year-old man with diabetes developed septic arthritis of the ankle. After surgical debridement he had an exposed medial malleolus and associated soft tissue defect. An MSAP flap was raised from the contralateral calf to provide soft tissue coverage and tailored to the defect. This MSAP free flap was anastomosed to the anterior tibial artery and great saphenous vein, providing a stable reconstruction with minimal bulk and good contour to enable footwear. He had an uneventful post-operative recovery (Fig. 40.9).

Fig. 40.9 Case 3. (**a**) Left medial ankle soft tissue defect with exposed medial malleolus resulting from surgical debridement following septic arthritis of the ankle. (**b**) Free MSAP flap raised on two perforators (P1 and P2), with inclusion of the short saphenous vein (V) in addition to the venae commitantes. (**c**) Defect closure after MSAP flap inset with a low vacuum suction drain and separate Yates drain to reduce the risk of haematoma. Note the low profile of the flap to allow optimal contour of the medial malleolus and future footwear.

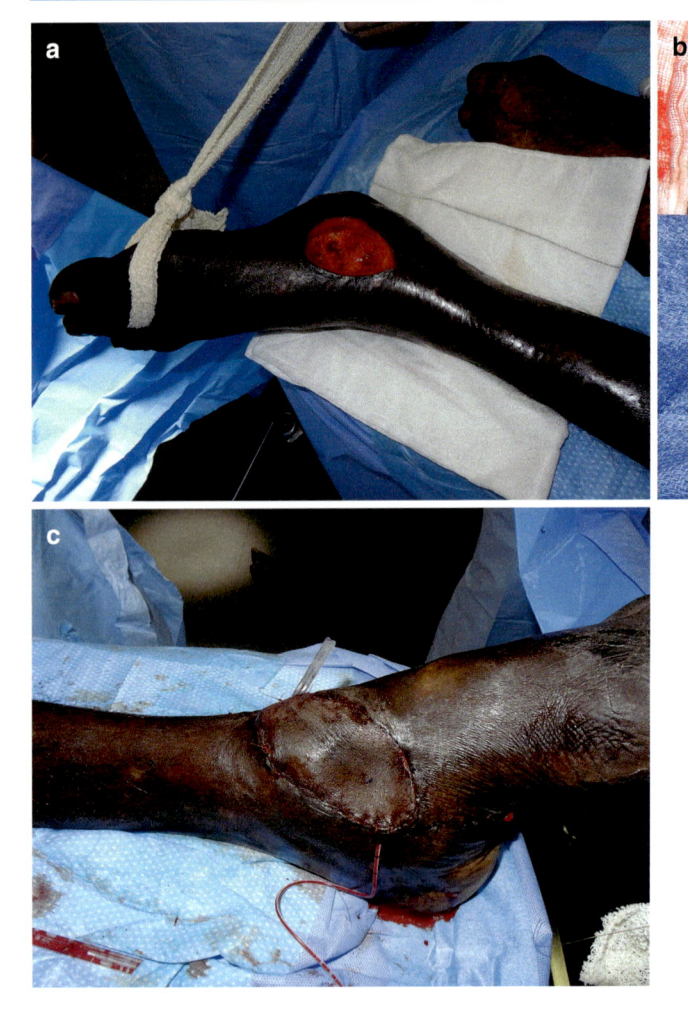

40.8 Pearls and Pitfalls

Pearls
- Incise the anterior border of the flap, with single incision in the fascia, to identify the perforator(s) before committing to your skin island.
- This flap can be raised with multiple very small size perforators, therefore preserve all options until the anatomy is revealed. If one is not comfortable with small size intra-muscular perforator dissection then an alternative flap option should be considered.
- The course of the perforator is always intramuscular and will require careful, often tedious, dissection using careful techniques described above.
- Flaps raised with a single small perforator may suffer from venous congestion. If the VCs are too small or damaged during dissection then the flap can be venous supercharged with the short saphenous vein (SSV). With careful dissection during the posterior incision, small branches of the SSV draining the flap can be preserved, and a good length of the SSV can be harvested proximally.
- Perform the dissection under tourniquet control without full exsanguination of the limb.
- Perform dissection under loupe magnification and preserve motor nerve branches to the gastrocnemius muscle. This can also be harvested as a nerve graft in a chimeric flap, if required.
- In cases of intra-oral reconstruction wait until the resection has finished before committing to the posterior incision. A template should be used with approximately the same thickness of the flap—such

as sterile blue sponge. The template should be measured accurately from the defect taking into consideration the three-dimensional configuration of intra-oral defects, as well as the extra tissue required to create the lingual sulcus.
- The template then is transferred to the calf and centred on the marked skin perforator. The skin flap should exactly match the template whilst still attached to its pedicle. Attempts to remove additional tissue once the flap is inset should be avoided as the perforator can be accidentally damaged or cause bleeding. If the flap was made larger than needed, then the reconstruction will be bulkier compromising the functional outcome.

Pitfalls
- Committing to your skin paddle before visualizing and confirming your perforator(s).
- Placing the first incision too posterior and missing or injuring the perforator from the outset.
- Damaging the pedicle during dissection of its long intramuscular course—good retraction, ligaclips, heat sink bipolar technique and deroofing technique are vital to avoid perforator damage.
- Closing the fascia over the muscle—this may increase the risk of compartment syndrome in the case of haematoma post-operatively.
- Attempting to close the donor site directly if the width of the flap is more than 6 cm—use an alternative flap if this is the case, to avoid an unacceptable donor site morbidity due to wound breakdown or use of a skin graft.

40.9 Selected Readings

- Cavadas PC, Sanz-Giménez-Rico JR, Gutierrez-de la Cámara A, Navarro-Monzonís A, Soler-Nomdedeu S, Martínez-Soriano F. The medial sural artery perforator free flap. Plast Reconstr Surg. 2001;108(6):1609–17.
- *Summary: This is the first description of the free MSAP flap in the literature, based on cadaveric studies and clinical case series and focused on its use for lower limb reconstruction. Based on 10 cadaveric leg dissections, a mean of 2.2 perforators (range, 1–4) from the medial sural artery were noted over the medial gastrocnemius muscle, clustered 9–18 cm from the popliteal crease. A series of six successful clinical cases, including five free flaps and one pedicled flap for ipsilateral lower-leg and foot reconstruction, demonstrated that while the dissection is somewhat tedious, the vascular pedicle can be considerably long and of suitable calibre with minimal donor-site morbidity.*
- Dusseldorp JR, Pham QJ, Ngo W, Gianoutsos M, Moradi, P. Vascular anatomy of the medial sural artery perforator flap: a new classification system of intra-muscular branching patterns. J Plast Reconstr Aesthet Surg. 2014;67:1267–75.
- *Summary: The objective of this study was to determine the pattern of intra-muscular course of the MSAP flap pedicle. Fourteen cadaveric specimens were dissected and CT angiograms of 84 legs were examined. Three types of arterial branching pattern were identified within the medial gastrocnemius, demonstrating one (31%), two (59%) or three or more (10%) main branches. A dominant perforator from the medial sural artery was present in 92% of anatomical specimens (13/14). Vertically, the location of the perforator from the popliteal crease was on average 13 cm (±2 cm). Transversely, the perforator originated 2.5 cm (±1 cm) from the posterior midline. Using CT angiography it was possible in ten consecutive patients to identify a more superficial intra-muscular branch and determine the leg with the optimal branching pattern type for flap harvest.*
- Mughal M, Gabuniya N, Zoccali G, Roblin P, Townley W. Functional outcomes of the medial sural artery perforator flap in oral cavity reconstruction. Ann Plast Surg. 2020;85(3):256–9.
- *Summary: This study assessed functional outcomes in patients with oral cavity tumors reconstructed with MSAP flaps, including speech and swallowing. Of the 38 patients included, 84.2% had intelligible speech at 6-month follow-up and further improvement at 1 year (92.1%). All patients resumed feeding on postoperative day 4, and only 7.8% (n = 3) of the patients required assistance with feeding at 1-year follow-up. Thus the authors conclude that the MSAP flap provides adequate small-volume replacement for oral cavity reconstructions, with most patients achieving a full diet with no restrictions by 1 year after reconstruction and excellent speech with little or no need for repetition in conversation.*
- Fitzgerald O'Connor E, Ruston J, Loh CYY, Tare M. Technical refinements of the free medial sural artery perforator (MSAP) flap in reconstruction of multifaceted ankle soft tissue defects. Foot Ankle Surg. 2020;26(2):233–8.
- *Summary: The authors present their retrospective review of 15 peri-ankle reconstructions using the MSAP flap—4 dorsal foot, 4 medial malleolar, 4 lateral malleolar and 3 tendo-achilles defects. All flaps in this series survived.*

There was one case of partial flap necrosis and no incidences of donor site dehiscence. All patients returned to full ambulation and none required subsequent flap revision. This study demonstrates the versatility of the free MSAP flap in reconstructing defects around the ankle area, by providing a thin, pliable, single stage and robust reconstruction, with a cosmetically ideal donor site.

References

1. Cavadas PC, Sanz-Giménez-Rico JR, Gutierrez-de la Cámara A, Navarro-Monzonís A, Soler-Nomdedeu S, Martínez-Soriano F. The medial sural artery perforator free flap. Plast Reconstr Surg. 2001;108(6):1609–17. https://doi.org/10.1097/00006534-200111000-00027.
2. Daar DA, Abdou SA, Cohen JM, Wilson SC, Levine JP. Is the medial sural artery perforator flap a new workhorse flap? A systematic review and meta-analysis. Plast Reconstr Surg. 2019;143(2):393e–403e. https://doi.org/10.1097/PRS.0000000000005204.
3. Xie XT, Chai YM. Medial sural artery perforator flap. Ann Plast Surg. 2012;68(1):105–10. https://doi.org/10.1097/SAP.0b013e31821190e6.
4. Fitzgerald O'Connor E, Ruston J, Loh CYY, Tare M. Technical refinements of the free medial sural artery perforator (MSAP) flap in reconstruction of multifaceted ankle soft tissue defects. Foot Ankle Surg. 2020;26(2):233–8. https://doi.org/10.1016/j.fas.2019.02.003.
5. Ives M, Mathur B. Varied uses of the medial sural artery perforator flap. J Plast Reconstr Aesthet Surg. 2015;68(6):853–8.
6. Sue GR, Kao HK, Borrelli MR, Cheng MH. The versatile free medial sural artery perforator flap: an institutional experience for reconstruction of the head and neck, upper and lower extremities. Microsurgery. 2020;40(4):427–33. https://doi.org/10.1002/micr.30543.
7. Mughal M, Gabuniya N, Zoccali G, Roblin P, Townley W. Functional outcomes of the medial sural artery perforator flap in oral cavity reconstruction. Ann Plast Surg. 2020;85(3):256–9. https://doi.org/10.1097/SAP.0000000000002352. PMID: 32205498.
8. Song X, Wu H, Zhang W, Chen J, Ding X, Ye J, et al. Medial sural artery perforator flap for postsurgical reconstruction of head and neck cancer. J Reconstr Microsurg. 2015;31(4):319–26.
9. Chen SL, Yu CC, Chang MC, Deng SC, Wu YS, Chen TM. Medial sural artery perforator flap for intraoral reconstruction following cancer ablation. Ann Plast Surg. 2008;61(3):274–9.
10. Chen SL, Chen TM, Dai NT, Hsia YJ, Lin YS. Medial sural artery perforator flap for tongue and floor of mouth reconstruction. Head Neck. 2008;30(3):351–7.
11. Kao HK, Chang KP, Chen YA, Wei FC, Cheng MH. Anatomical basis and versatile application of the free medial sural artery perforator flap for head and neck reconstruction. Plast Reconstr Surg. 2010;125(4):1135–45.
12. Choi JW, Nam SY, Choi SH, Roh JL, Kim SY, Hong JP. Applications of medial sural perforator free flap for head and neck reconstructions. J Reconstr Microsurg. 2013;29(7):437–42. https://doi.org/10.1055/s-0033-1343959.
13. Chalmers RL, Rahman KM, Young S, et al. The medial sural artery perforator flap in intra-oral reconstruction: a northeast experience. J Plast Reconstr Aesthet Surg. 2016;69(5):687–93. https://doi.org/10.1016/j.bjps.2016.01.005.
14. Sun QW, Gao PF, Wang CX, et al. Anatomical study and clinical application of medial sural artery perforator flap for oral cavity reconstruction. Ann Anat. 2020;227:151418. https://doi.org/10.1016/j.aanat.2019.151418.
15. Chen SL, Chen TM, Lee CH. Free medial sural artery perforator flap for resurfacing distal limb defects. J Trauma. 2005;58(2):323–7.
16. Chen SL, Chuang CJ, Chou TD, Chen TM, Wang HJ. Free medial sural artery perforator flap for ankle and foot reconstruction. Ann Plast Surg. 2005;54(1):39–43.
17. Kim ES, Hwang JH, Kim KS, Lee SY. Plantar reconstruction using the medial sural artery perforator free flap. Ann Plast Surg. 2009;62(6):679–84.
18. Jeevaratnam JA, Nikkhah D, Nugent NF, Blackburn AV. The medial sural artery perforator flap and its application in electrical injury to the hand. J Plast Reconstr Aesthet Surg. 2014;67(11):1591–4. https://doi.org/10.1016/j.bjps.2014.07.023.
19. Lin CH, Lin CH, Lin YT, Hsu CC, Ng TW, Wei F-C. The medial sural artery perforator flap: a versatile donor site for hand reconstruction. J Trauma. 2011;70(3):736–43.
20. Wang X, Mei J, Pan J, Chen H, Zhang W, Tang M. Reconstruction of distal limb defects with the free medial sural artery perforator flap. Plast Reconstr Surg. 2013;131(1):95–105.
21. Xie RG, Gu JH, Gong YP, Tang JB. Medial sural artery perforator flap for repair of the hand. J Hand Surg Eur. 2007;32(5):512–7. https://doi.org/10.1016/J.JHSE.2007.05.010.
22. Ling BM, Wettstein R, Staub D, Schaefer DJ, Kalbermatten DF. The medial sural artery perforator flap: the first choice for soft-tissue reconstruction about the knee. J Bone Joint Surg Am. 2018;100(3):211–7. https://doi.org/10.2106/JBJS.16.01401.
23. Tee R, Jeng SF, Chen CC, Shih HS. The medial sural artery perforator pedicled propeller flap for coverage of middle-third leg defects. J Plast Reconstr Aesthet Surg. 2019;72(12):1971–8. https://doi.org/10.1016/j.bjps.2019.08.006.
24. Zheng H, Liu J, Dai X, Schilling AF. Free conjoined or chimeric medial sural artery perforator flap for the reconstruction of multiple defects in hand. J Plast Reconstr Aesthet Surg. 2015;68(4):565–70. https://doi.org/10.1016/j.bjps.2014.12.031.
25. Sano K, Hallock GG, Hamazaki M, Daicyo Y. The perforator-based conjoint (chimeric) medial sural MEDIAL GASTROCNEMIUS free flap. Ann Plast Surg. 2004;53:588–92.
26. Hallock GG. Chimeric gastrocnemius muscle and sural artery perforator local flap. Ann Plast Surg. 2008;61(3):306–9.
27. Deek NFA, Hsiao JC, Do NT, et al. The medial sural artery perforator flap: lessons learned from 200 consecutive cases [published online ahead of print, 2020 Aug 19]. Plast Reconstr Surg. 2020;146:630e. https://doi.org/10.1097/PRS.0000000000007282.
28. Kao HK, Chang KP, Chen YA, Wei FC, Cheng MH. Comparison of the medial sural artery perforator flap with the radial forearm flap for head and neck reconstructions. Plast Reconstr Surg. 2009;124(4):1125–32.
29. Nugent M, Endersby S, Kennedy M, Burns A. Early experience with the medial sural artery perforator flap as an alternative to the radial forearm flap for reconstruction in the head and neck. Br J Oral Maxillofac Surg. 2015;53(5):461–3. https://doi.org/10.1016/j.bjoms.2015.02.023.
30. Taufique ZM, Daar DA, Cohen LE, Thanik VD, Levine JP, Jacobson AS. The medial sural artery perforator flap: a better option in complex head and neck reconstruction? Laryngoscope. 2019;129(6):1330–6. https://doi.org/10.1002/lary.27652.
31. Agrawal G, Gupta A, Chaudhary V, Qureshi F, Choraria A, Dubey H. Medial sural artery perforator flap for head and neck reconstruction. Ann Maxillofac Surg. 2018;8(1):61–5. https://doi.org/10.4103/ams.ams_137_17.
32. Dusseldorp JR, Pham QJ, Ngo Q, Gianoutsos M, Moradi P. Vascular anatomy of the medial sural artery perforator flap: a new classification system of intra-muscular branching patterns. J Plast Reconstr Aesthet Surg. 2014;67(9):1267–75. https://doi.org/10.1016/j.bjps.2014.05.016.

33. Hallock GG. Anatomic basis of the gastrocnemius perforator-based flap. Ann Plast Surg. 2001;47:517–22. https://doi.org/10.1097/00000637-200111000-00008.
34. Wong MZ, Wong CH, Tan BK, Chew KY, Tay SC. Surgical anatomy of the medial sural artery perforator flap. J Reconstr Microsurg. 2012;28:555–60.
35. Thione A, Valdatta L, Buoro M, Tuinder S, Mortarino C, Putz R. The medial sural artery perforators: anatomic basis for a surgical plan. Ann Plast Surg. 2004;53(3):250–5. https://doi.org/10.1097/01.sap.0000116242.26334.b5.
36. Altaf FM. The anatomical basis of the medial sural artery perforator flaps. West Indian Med J. 2011;60(6):622–7.
37. Akdeniz Doğan ZD, Çavuş Özkan M, Tuncer FB, Saçak B, Çelebiler Ö. A comparative clinical study of flap thickness: medial sural artery perforator flap versus anterolateral thigh flap. Ann Plast Surg. 2018;81(4):472–4. https://doi.org/10.1097/SAP.0000000000001488.
38. Leahy S, Toomey C, McCreesh K, O'Neill C, Jakeman P. Ultrasound measurement of subcutaneous adipose tissue thickness accurately predicts total and segmental body fat of young adults. Ultrasound Med Biol. 2012;38(1):28–34.
39. Zhao W, Li Z, Wu L, Zhu H, Liu J, Wang H. Medial sural artery perforator flap aided by ultrasonic perforator localization for reconstruction after oral carcinoma resection. J Oral Maxillofac Surg. 2016;74(5):1063–71. https://doi.org/10.1016/j.joms.2015.11.011.
40. Kosutic D, Pejkovic B, Anderhuber F, et al. Complete mapping of lateral and medial sural artery perforators: anatomical study with Duplex-Doppler ultrasound correlation. J Plast Reconstr Aesthet Surg. 2012;65(11):1530–6. https://doi.org/10.1016/j.bjps.2012.04.045.
41. He Y, Jin SF, Zhang ZY, Feng SQ, Zhang CP, Zhang YX. A prospective study of medial sural artery perforator flap with computed tomographic angiography-aided design in tongue reconstruction. J Oral Maxillofac Surg. 2014;72(11):2351–65. https://doi.org/10.1016/j.joms.2014.05.019.
42. Qing L, Hu Y, Tang J, Wu P, Yu F, Liang J. Three-dimensional visualization reconstruction of medial sural artery perforator flap based on digital technology. Zhongguo Xiu Fu Chong Jian Wai Ke Za Zhi. 2014;28(6):697–700.
43. Hallock GG. The medial sural artery perforator island flap as a simpler alternative for prophylactic skin augmentation prior to total knee arthroplasty. Int J Orthoplast Surg. 2019;2:1.
44. Shen XQ, Lv Y, Shen H, Lu H, Wu SC, Lin XJ. Endoscope-assisted medial sural artery perforator flap for head and neck reconstruction. J Plast Reconstr Aesthet Surg. 2016;69(8):1059–65. https://doi.org/10.1016/j.bjps.2016.01.029.
45. Al-Himdani S, Din A, Wright TC, Wheble G, Chapman TWL, Khan U. The medial sural artery perforator (MSAP) flap: a versatile flap for lower extremity reconstruction. Injury. 2020;51(4):1077–85. https://doi.org/10.1016/j.injury.2020.02.060.
46. Abdelrahman M, Jumabhoy I, Qiu SS, et al. Perfusion dynamics of the medial sural artery perforator (MSAP) flap in lower extremity reconstruction using laser Doppler perfusion imaging (LDPI): a clinical study. J Plast Surg Hand Surg. 2020;54(2):112–9. https://doi.org/10.1080/2000656X.2019.1703191.
47. Ranson J, Rosich-Medina A, Amin K, Kosutic D. Medial sural artery perforator flap: using the superficial venous system to minimize flap congestion. Arch Plast Surg. 2015;42(6):813–5. https://doi.org/10.5999/aps.2015.42.6.813.
48. Hallock GG. Medial sural artery perforator free flap: legitimate use as a solution for the ipsilateral distal lower extremity defect. J Reconstr Microsurg. 2014;30(3):187–92. https://doi.org/10.1055/s-0033-1357276.

Peroneal Artery Flaps: The Free Fibula Flap

Amitabh Thacoor, Daniel Butler, Dariush Nikkhah, and Jeremy Rawlins

41.1 Introduction

The fibula free flap (FFF) provides well-vascularised bone for the microsurgical reconstruction of defects following trauma or cancer. It was first described in 1975 by Taylor [1] for the reconstruction of two large traumatic tibial defects. Its first use in head and neck reconstruction occurred later in 1989 by Hidalgo [2] and it has since become the gold standard for the reconstruction of composite midface and oromandibular defects involving the intraoral mucosa (lining), mandibular bone and external skin (cover) [3].

Originally described as a purely osseous flap, the FFF can also be raised as an osteofasciocutaneous flap by including a skin paddle, which may also be sensate. It provides large calibre vessels with a long vascular pedicle and enough bone length (25 cm) to reconstruct near-total mandibular defects and withstand irradiation, with minimal long-term donor site morbidity [2]. Furthermore, the endosteal and periosteal blood supply safely permits multiple osteotomies, and the donor site is far away from the head and neck area to allow a two-team surgical approach.

Supplementary Information The online version contains supplementary material available at [https://doi.org/10.1007/978-3-031-07678-7_41].

A. Thacoor (✉)
Pan Thames Rotation, London, UK
e-mail: amitabh.thacoor@doctors.org.uk

D. Butler
Bay of Plenty District Health Board, Tauranga, New Zealand

D. Nikkhah
Department of Plastic, Reconstructive and Aesthetic Surgery, Royal Free Hospital, London, UK

J. Rawlins
Department of Plastic Surgery, Royal Perth Hospital, Perth, Australia

41.2 Anatomy

41.2.1 Bony

The lower extremity long bones include the principal weight-bearing tibia and the more slender fibula. Proximally, the fibular head articulates with the lateral condyle of the tibia while distally the fibula forms the lateral component of the ankle mortice. The syndesmosis between the distal fibula and tibia is essential in maintaining the stability of the ankle mortise and, thus, should be respected when planning flap harvest. At the fibular neck, the common peroneal nerve passes from the popliteal fossa, lateral to fibula and into the lateral compartment of the lower leg. Care should be taken when dissecting at this level.

41.2.2 Fascial

Four fascial compartments define the lower leg: anterior, lateral, superficial posterior and deep posterior compartments (Fig. 41.1). The anterior and deep posterior compartments are separated by the interosseous membrane, while the anterior and posterior crural intermuscular septa separate the lateral compartment from the anterior and posterior compartments respectively.

41.2.3 Vascular

The FFF is supplied by the peroneal artery (branching from the tibio-peroneal trunk) and its venae commitantes. The overlying skin is supplied by septocutaneous perforators, carried in the posterior crural intermuscular septum, which should be protected in osteofasciocutaneous flaps. Musculocutaneous perforators through the flexor hallucis longus and soleus muscles may also be additionally present. A skin paddle of 8 × 15 cm may be based on these perforators.

© Springer Nature Switzerland AG 2023
D. Nikkhah et al. (eds.), *Core Techniques in Flap Reconstructive Microsurgery*, https://doi.org/10.1007/978-3-031-07678-7_41

Fig. 41.1 Cross sectional anatomy of the lower leg. Muscles: *TA* tibialis anterior, *EDL* extensor digitorum longus, *EHL* extensor hallucis longus, *PL* peroneus longus, *PB* peroneus brevis, *TP* tibialis posterior, *FHL* flexor hallucis longus, *FDL* flexor digitorum longus, *S* soleus, *G* gastrocnemius, *P* plantaris. Fascial layers: *Anterior and posterior crural septa (green), Interosseous membrane (blue), Transverse crural septum (yellow).* Outline of the free fibula flap (black dotted) based on the peroneal artery and its venae commitantes and septocutaneous perforators through the posterior crural septum (green)

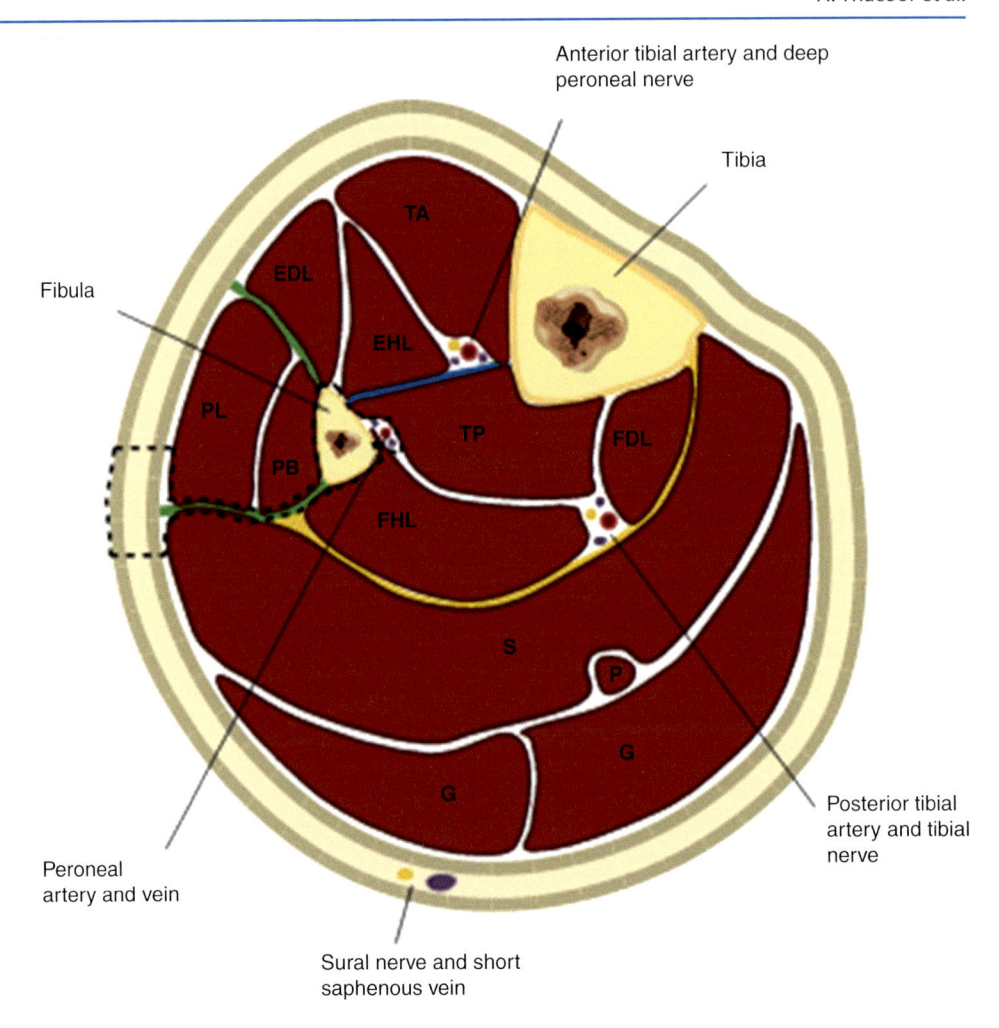

The fibula is supplied by an endosteal and periosteal blood supply, which allows multiple osteotomies to be performed safely. The peroneal vessels descend along the medial side of the fibula and lie posterior to the tibialis posterior muscle and anterior to the flexor hallucis longus muscle. Abnormal vascular branching patterns are known to exist, with a 0.1–4% incidence of peroneal artery absence and 0.2–7% incidence of arteria perona magna reported [4].

41.2.4 Nerves

The sural nerve, which lies superficially to the posterior border of the fibula and adjacent to the short saphenous vein is prone to iatrogenic injury and may be included for a sensate flap. In the lateral compartment of the leg, the superficial peroneal nerve passes from its position deep to the muscle proximally to passing through the investing fascia in the distal third of the lower leg. This nerve is often encountered when raising the skin island anteriorly and is easily damaged at this stage. The anterior neurovascular bundle (anterior tibial artery and deep peroneal nerve—anterior to the interosseous septum) and the posterior neurovascular bundle (posterior tibial artery and tibial nerve—medial to the flexor hallucis longus and deep to soleus muscle) are encountered during flap harvest and must be protected.

Thus the muscles encountered when raising an FFF include:

- Peroneus longus
- Peroneus brevis
- Extensor digitorum longus
- Extensor hallucis longus
- Tibialis posterior
- Soleus
- Flexor hallucis longus

41.3 Pre-operative Investigations

The role of routine pre-operative imaging prior to FFF harvest remains controversial. All patients planned for an FFF should undergo a physical examination to assess palpable pedal pulses and exclude varicosities [5]. However, a normal physical examination alone may not be sufficient in predicting vascular anomalies as it only identifies 28% of abnormalities present on imaging [4].

The purpose of preoperative imaging is to exclude large vessel branching anomalies, an absent peronal artery, ateria perona magna, peripheral vascular disease and identify the course and location of septocutaneous perforators [6]. Diagnostic modalities available include Doppler ultrasonography, conventional angiography, computed tomography angiography (CTA) and magnetic resonance angiography (MRA).

Doppler ultrasonography is a low-cost and readily available option but provides limited information on the vasculature. Conventional angiography, an invasive technique using arterial catheterization for contrast injection, has been associated with complications from arterial puncture and has largely been superseded by the less invasive CTA and MRA [4]. The additional capability afforded by CTA and MRA in mapping septocutaneous perforators as small as 0.3 mm as well as the relationship between the peroneal vessels and the fibula may facilitate surgical planning by guiding correct placement of the skin paddle to optimize perfusion and safer flap harvest [4, 7]. Current Level 1 evidence exists to support the use of angiography routinely to assess vascularity and reduce of risk of devastating leg ischaemia [5].

Furthermore, pre-operative CT images are also commonly used to aid three-dimensional modelling and virtual planning of osteotomies using a custom-made jig, particularly in mandibular reconstruction. This has been shown to help reduce operative time and increase accuracy in reconstruction [8].

41.4 Flap Design and Markings

The patient is positioned supine with the knee flexed and a sandbag under the ipsilateral hip. A tourniquet is applied. Surface markings include the head of the fibula proximally and the lateral malleolus distally. The axis of the bone is then drawn between these two surface landmarks. The proximal osteotomy is marked at least 7 cm below the head of the fibula to protect the common peroneal nerve. The distal osteotomy is marked at least 7 cm above the projection of the lateral malleolus to project the distal ankle syndesmosis (Fig. 41.2).

If a skin paddle is included, the location of the perforators are marked using Doppler ultrasound and the skin paddle is designed over the perforators. A skin paddle width of up to 4 cm can be closed primarily.

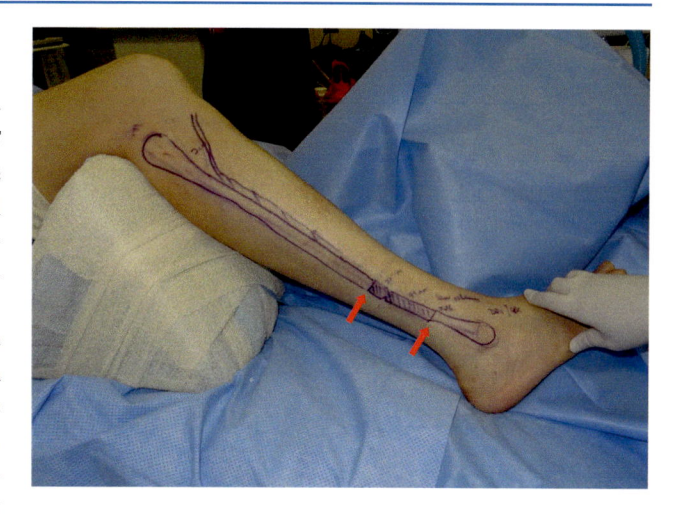

Fig. 41.2 Surface markings showing segment of fibula bone required (red arrows) for mandibular reconstruction in a case of osteoradionecrosis

41.5 Flap Raise/Elevation: A Step-by-Step Guide

- **Step 1: Incision and exposure of lateral compartment**
  A longitudinal incision is made through skin and subcutaneous fat down to muscle fascia to expose the lateral muscle compartment. The fascia is then incised longitudinally to expose the muscles of the lateral compartment—peroneus longus and peroneus brevis (Fig. 41.3). This dissection proceeds posteriorly in the subfascial plane until the posterior crural intermuscular septum is identified. To minimize the risk of iatrogenic damage to the septocutaneous perforators, this intermuscular septum can be identified more proximally on the lower leg first. Once the entire septum is exposed, suitable septocutaneous perforators to the skin can be identified.
- **Step 2: Dissection of lateral compartment muscles off fibula**
  A submuscular dissection then allows the lateral compartment muscles to be dissected off the lateral aspect of the fibula (Fig. 41.4), leaving a 2 mm cuff of muscle on to the fibula (Fig. 41.5). This thin cuff of muscle is essential to

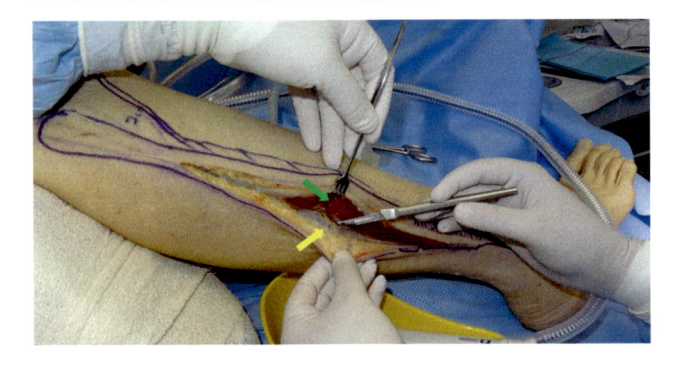

Fig. 41.3 Exposure of the lateral compartment muscles (green arrow). A perforator supplying the overlying skin is visible (yellow arrow), although not harvested in this case

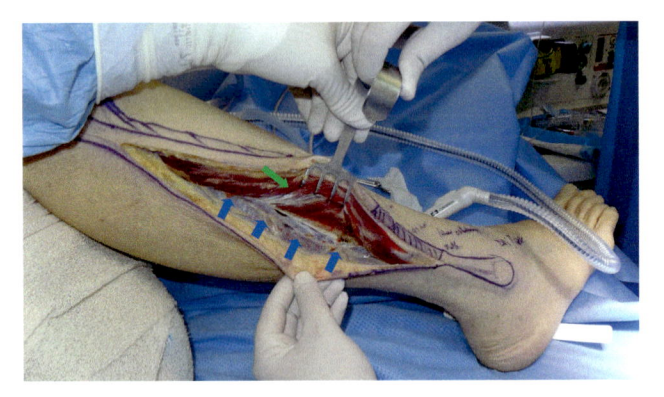

Fig. 41.4 Elevation of the muscles of the lateral compartment (green arrow). Septocutaneous Perforators going through the posterior crural septum are visualised (blue arrows)

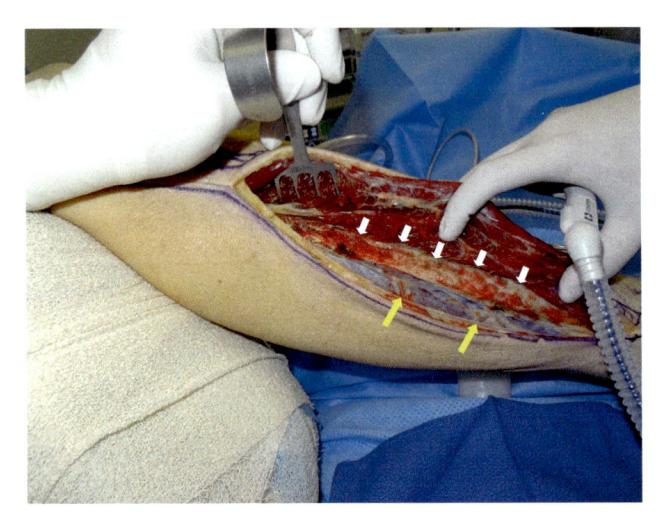

Fig. 41.5 A 2 mm cuff of muscle is left over the fibula to preserve periosteal blood supply (white arrows). Two perforators are also visible, which were not harvested in this case (yellow arrows)

avoid damage to the underlying periosteum. This continues up to the anterior crural septum. Anterior compartment muscle dissection then follows.

- **Step 3: Dissection of the anterior compartment muscles of fibula**
  After the anterior crural septum is divided, the muscles of the anterior compartment—extensor hallucis longus and extensor digitorum longus—are dissected off the anterior surface of the fibula, to expose the interosseous membrane (Fig. 41.6), which is incised longitudinally (Fig. 41.7). This reveals the tibialis posterior muscle. Attention is then focused to the posterior compartment.

- **Step 4: Dissection of the soleus muscle off the fibula**
  The posterior extent of the planned skin island is incised down through the fascia and dissection proceeds up to the

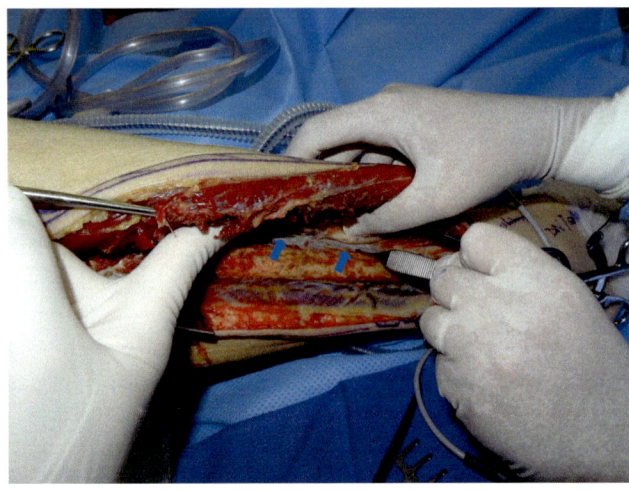

Fig. 41.6 The interosseous membrane becomes visible (blue arrows) following dissection of the anterior compartment muscles

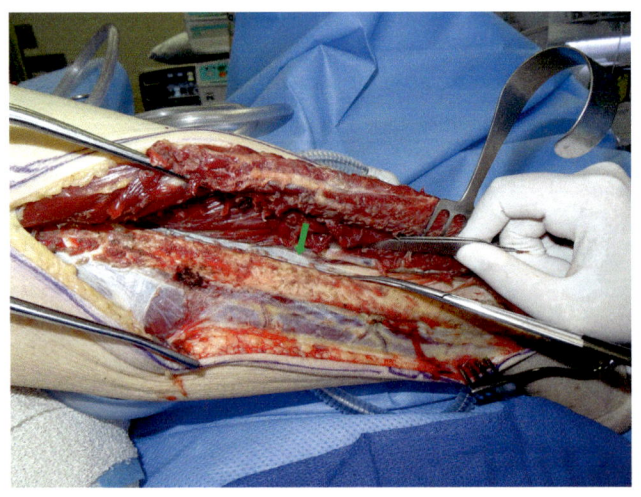

Fig. 41.7 The interosseous membrane becomes visible following dissection of the anterior compartment muscles (green arrow)

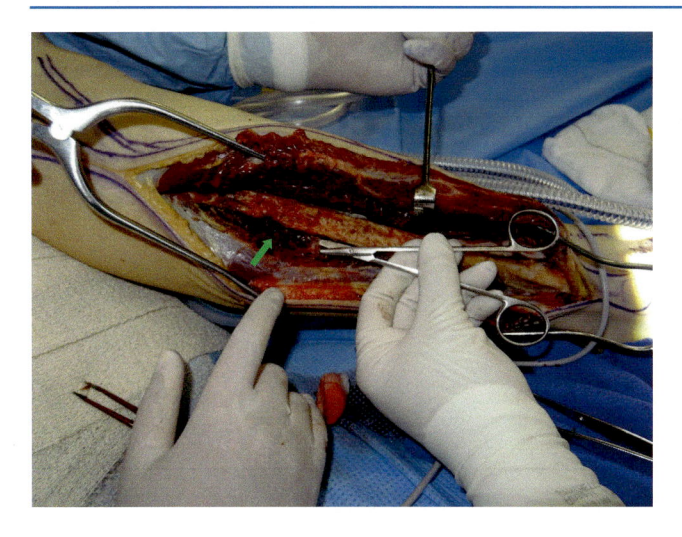

Fig. 41.8 Dissection of the muscles of the posterior compartment (green arrow)

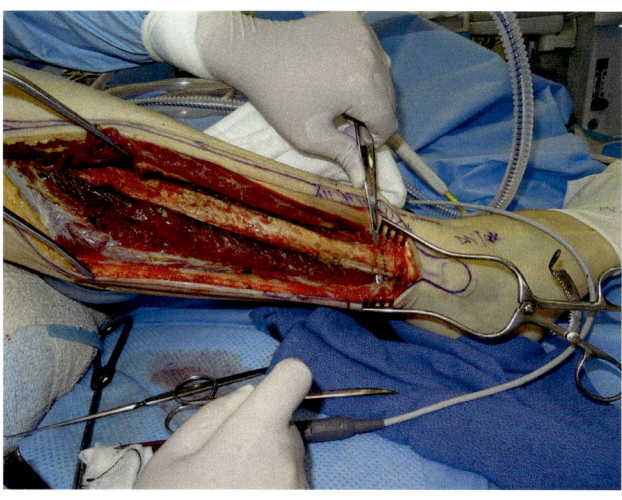

Fig. 41.10 Protection of the pedicle in preparation for the distal osteotomy

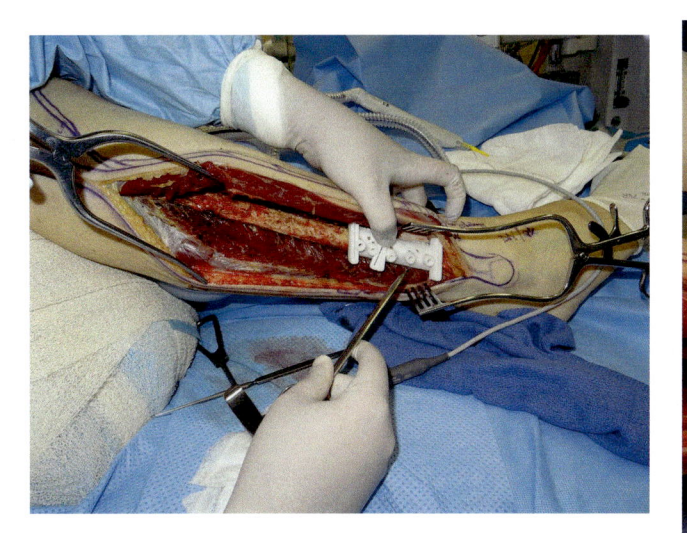

Fig. 41.9 Planning the distal osteotomy using a cutting jig

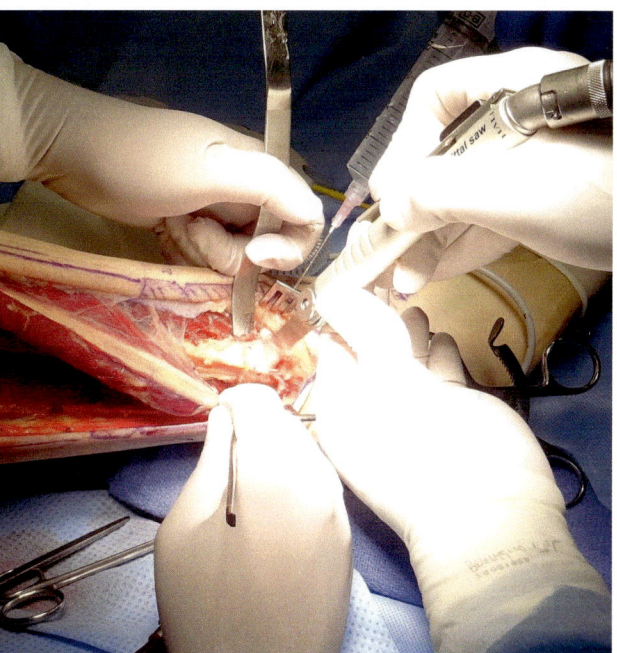

Fig. 41.11 Distal osteotomy with saline cooling

posterior crural intermuscular septum. The soleus muscle is dissected off the posterior crural septum (Fig. 41.8). As the flexor hallucis longus muscle is poorly visualized at this point, its dissection is best reserved for later (Step 7). There are branches that come off the septocutaneous perforators and pass posteriorly into the soleus muscle. These need to be divided after ensuring that the perforator continues proximally within the septum. Osteotomies can then be performed.

- **Step 5: Distal osteotomy**
  The distal osteotomy location is planned, ensuring it is at least 7 cm proximal to the lateral malleolus (a cutting jig can be used to aid planning—Fig. 41.9). A Howarth elevator (or malleable retractor) is used to get around the distal end of the fibula in a sub-periosteal plane (Fig. 41.10) and the distal osteotomy is performed using an oscillating saw, while the assistant uses saline irrigation to prevent thermal damage to the bone (Fig. 41.11).

- **Step 6: Proximal Osteotomy**
  The proximal osteotomy is performed, using a similar technique (Fig. 41.12). This osteotomy should be performed at 7 cm below the fibular head regardless of the length of bone required. This gives access to dissect the full length of vascular pedicle. Care should be taken to avoid injury to the deep peroneal nerve during this step. Following completion of the osteotomies, the fibula should be easily retractable laterally to expose the tibialis posterior muscle (Fig. 41.13).

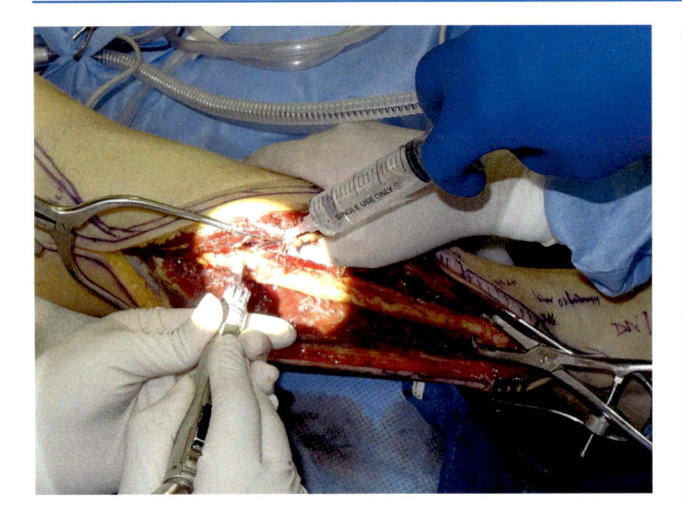

Fig. 41.12 Proximal osteotomy

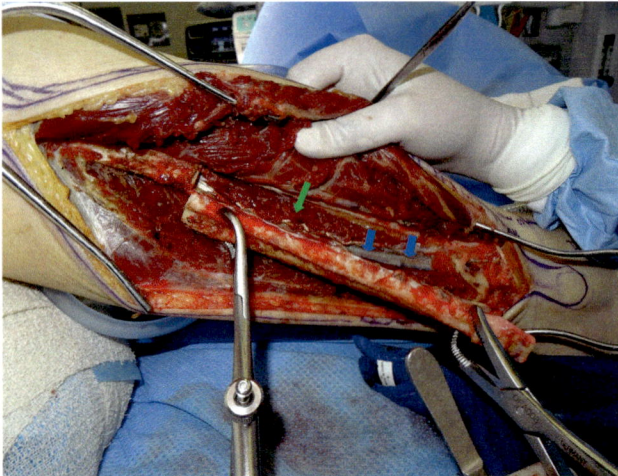

Fig. 41.14 Identification and dissection of the peroneal vessels (Blue arrows) through tibialis posterior (green arrow)

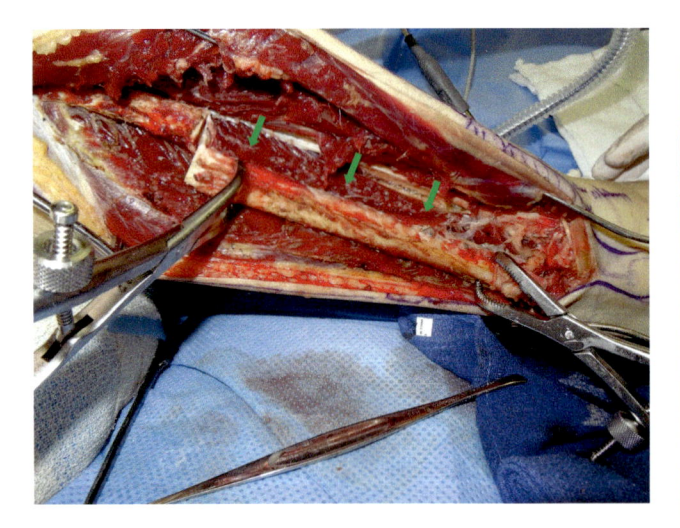

Fig. 41.13 Retraction of the fibula following osteotomies to expose the chevron-shaped tibialis posterior muscle (green arrows)

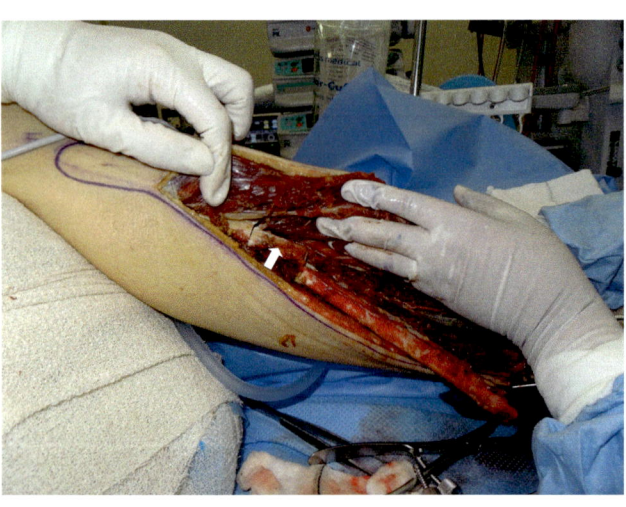

Fig. 41.15 Excision of proximal fibula before discarding to facilitate proximal dissection of pedicle (white arrow)

- **Step 7: Identification of the peroneal vessels**

  The distal end of the fibula is dissected underneath the interosseous membrane to identify the peroneal vessels. The distal end of the peroneal vessels are exposed and carefully clipped and divided. Tibialis posterior muscle is then dissected off the peroneal vessels from distal to proximal, and the flexor hallucis muscle (now better visualized) is dissected off the fibula, thereby islanding the flap (Fig. 41.14). Dissection should proceed until the origin of the pedicle from the tibioperoneal trunk. In order to facilitate proximal dissection of the pedicle, a window can be created by excising and discarding a portion of the proximal fibula (Figs. 41.15 and 41.16). Proximally, the tibial nerve and posterior tibial vascular bundles are encountered and should be carefully protected.

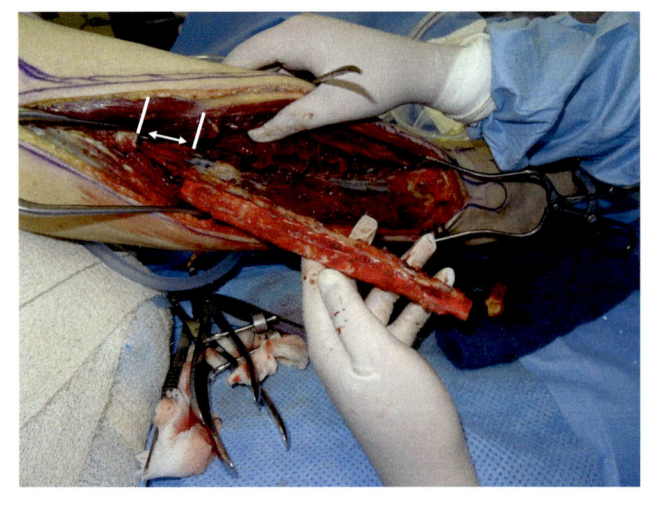

Fig. 41.16 Window created following discarding of proximal fibula

- **Step 8: Vessel clamping**

  The tourniquet is deflated and haemostasis performed. The peroneal artery and its associated venae commitantes can then be carefully inspected. The proximal end of the pedicle is clamped and transected and the flap safely detached.

- **Step 9: Wedge osteotomies**

  In cases of mandibular reconstruction, a cutting jig is placed over the fibula and secured with screws (Fig. 41.17). A Howarth elevator is used to protect the pedicle while wedge osteotomies can then be performed with an oscillating saw (Fig. 41.18) (Video 41.1).

- **Step 10: Closure**

  Following successful osteotomies (Fig. 41.19) and preparation of the recipient vessels (Fig. 41.20), the leg wound can be closed primarily or by split thickness skin grafting. A skin paddle of up to 4 cm wide can be closed primarily but split thickness skin grafting is required for larger defects. The leg is then immobilized in a posterior leg splint.

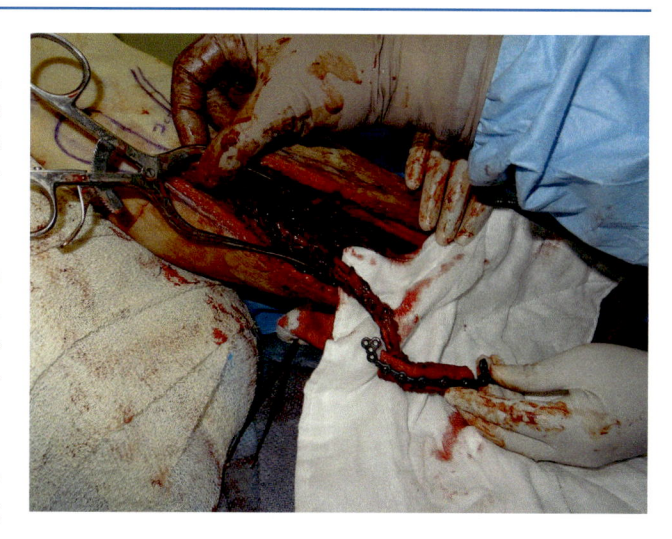

Fig. 41.19 Successful osteotomies and application of custom designed plates for bespoke mandibular reconstruction after osteoradionecrosis

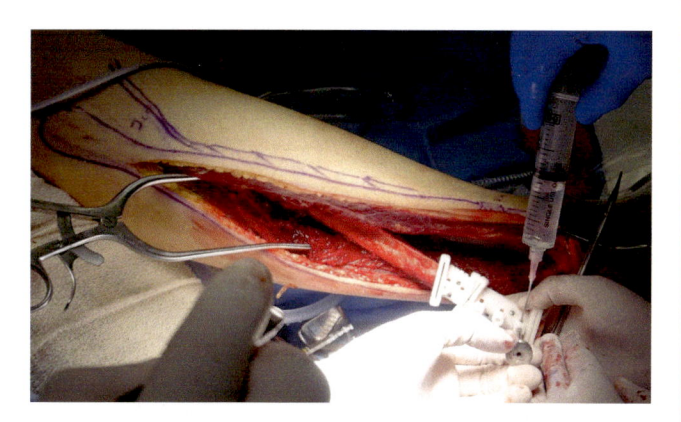

Fig. 41.17 Wedge osteotomies performed under warm ischaemia

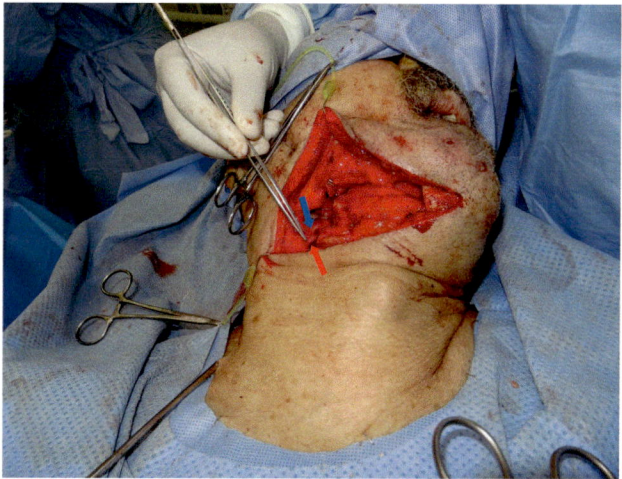

Fig. 41.20 Successful preparation of recipient vessels, in this case the facial artery (red arrow) and common facial vein (blue arrow) in the neck for mandibular reconstruction

41.6 Core Surgical Techniques in Flap Dissection

Markings The proximal osteotomy site should be at least 7 cm from the head of the fibula to prevent inadvertent damage to the deep peroneal nerve (Fig. 41.21). The distal osteotomy site should be at least 7 cm from the lateral malleolus to protect the integrity of the distal fibular ligaments and preserve ankle stability. The axis of the posterior border of the fibula is marked between the head of the fibula proximally and the lateral malleolus distally. This corresponds to the posterior crural septum, where the septocutaneous perforators are located. If an osteocutaneous FFF is

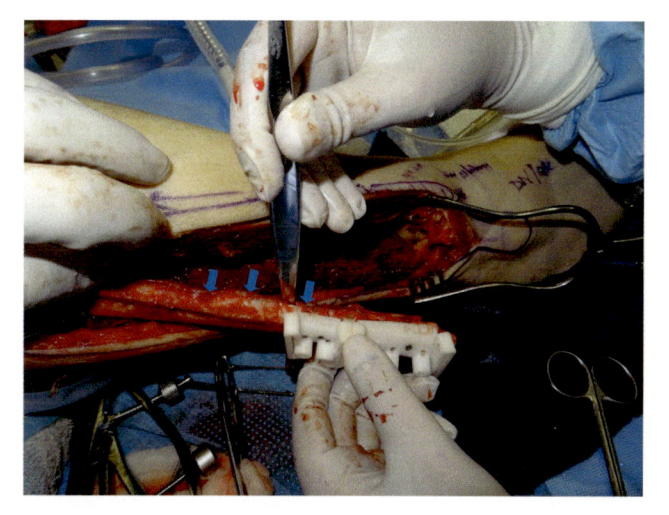

Fig. 41.18 Protection of the pedicle (blue arrows) using a Howarth elevator during wedge osteotomy

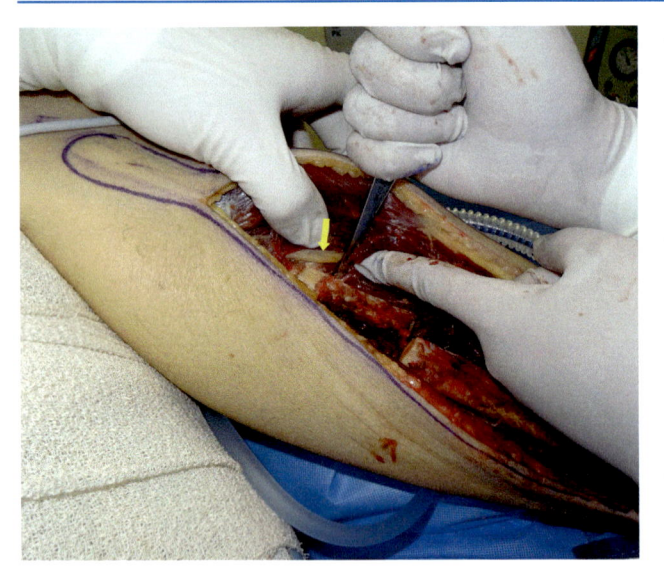

Fig. 41.21 Location of the deep peroneal nerve

raised, the skin paddle is centred over the posterior border of the fibula, to include skin perforators identified by Doppler ultrasound.

Elevation of lateral muscle compartment The anterior margin of the skin flap is incised first down to the muscles of the lateral compartment. Lateral traction is applied to the anterior skin flap while counter-traction is applied to the peroneal muscles anteriorly using cat's paw retractors. The peroneal muscles can be sharply dissected from the deep fascia up to the posterior crural septum. Septocutaneous perforators will become visible and must be carefully preserved, if a skin paddle is included. The lateral compartment muscles are dissected off the surface of the fibula, leaving a 2 mm cuff of muscle to preserve perosteal blood supply. This is continued up to the anterior crural septum, which is incised to access the anterior compartment.

Elevation of the anterior muscle compartment The anterior compartment muscles are dissected off the fibula. The surgeon's non-dominant thumb can be used to help retract the muscles and improve visibility of the interosseous membrane and also gauge the desired thickness of muscle retained on the surface of the fibula (Fig. 41.6). The interosseous membrane must be fully released to allow subsequent lateral retraction of the fibula to expose tibialis posterior muscle.

Elevation of the posterior muscle compartment The soleus muscle is bluntly separated from the flexor hallucis longus muscle, and is then dissected off the posterior aspect of the fibula. Large perforators through the gastrocnemius muscle emerge and need careful ligation.

Distal and proximal osteotomies Once the osteotomy sites have been marked, the overlying periosteum is incised and subperiosteal dissection using a Howarth elevator is performed. Following completion of the osteotomies, the fibula is retracted laterally using bone hooks (Fig. 41.13). This exposes the chevron-shaped tibialis posterior muscle.

Dissection of the peroneal vessels An avascular plane exists between tibialis posterior and the peroneal vessels. Tibialis posterior can therefore be dissected off the length of the peroneal vessels using a combination of bipolar cautery and ligation of side branches, which can be traced proximally to their junction with the posterior tibial vessels. Several side branches supplying tibialis posterior and soleus come into view, and must be ligated. Flexor hallucis longus muscle is now better visualized and can be dissected off the fibula. The vessels are clamped and ligated distally. In order to increase pedicle length and facilitate dissection proximally, a portion of fibula bone is excised and discarded to create a window for better visualization (Figs. 41.15 and 41.16). Once the desired pedicle length is obtained, the peroneal vessels are inspected, clamped and divided proximally. The flap can now be safely detached.

Wedge osteotomies In cases of mandibular reconstruction, a preoperative computer-generated plate contouring model and cutting jig may be designed to aid planning of osteotomies. Following complete elevation of the flap, the cutting jig is carefully placed over the fibula and secured in place with screws. Windows are made behind the planned osteotomy sites, where a malleable retractor is placed to protect the pedicle. Wedge osteotomies can then be safely performed under warm ischaemia (Figs. 41.17 and 41.18).

Closure The leg wound can be closed over a suction drain. A defect resulting from a skin paddle of up to 4 cm wide can be closed primarily, and split thickness skin grafting is required for larger defects. The leg is then immobilized in a posterior leg splint.

41.7 Clinical Scenario A: Surgeons Dariush Nikkhah, Qadir Khan, and Jeremy Rawlins

A 26-year-old fit and well male patient was diagnosed with a large mandibular odontogenic myxoma extending into the overlying soft tissue (Fig. 41.22). Following multidisciplinary assessment, surgical management by subtotal mandibulectomy and reconstruction with a free fibula osteocutaneous flap was recommended. The Pro Plan software was used preoperatively to aid surgical planning of intra-operative wedge osteotomies and bony plating. The peroneal artery was anastomosed to the recipient facial artery, a vena comitans was anastomosed to the recipient common facial vein and the skin paddle was used to reconstruct the floor of the mouth (Fig. 41.23). Complete resection was achieved and good chin projection and evidence of bony union was demonstrated on an early orthopantomogram (Fig. 41.24). The patient was also fitted with osseointegrated implants and has had an uneventful 12-month outcome (Videos 41.2 and 41.3).

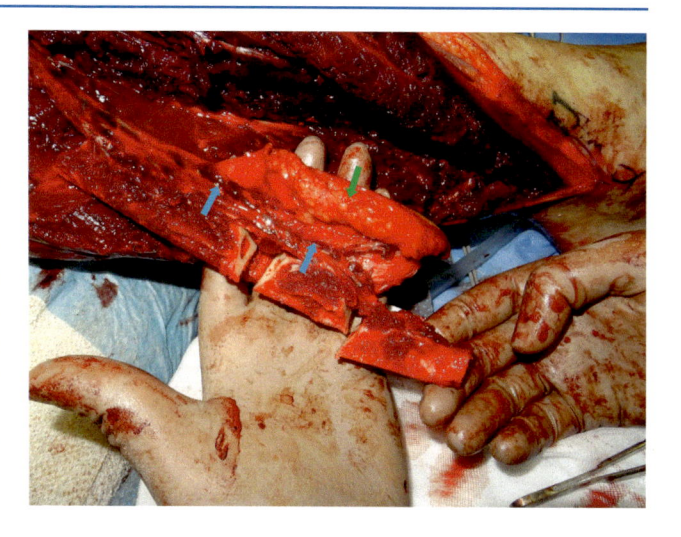

Fig. 41.23 Osteocutaneous fibula flap following osteotomies. Skin paddle (green arrow) peroneal pedicle (blue arrows)

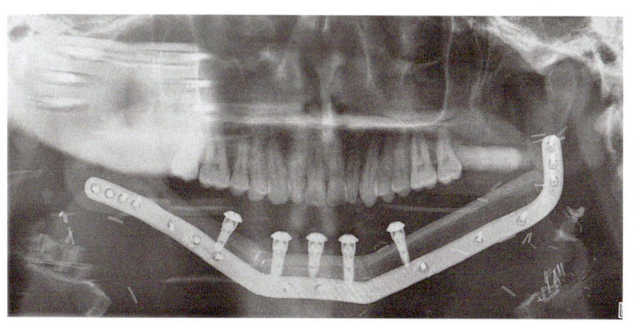

Fig. 41.24 Post-operative radiograph showing successful bony union and excellent symmetry

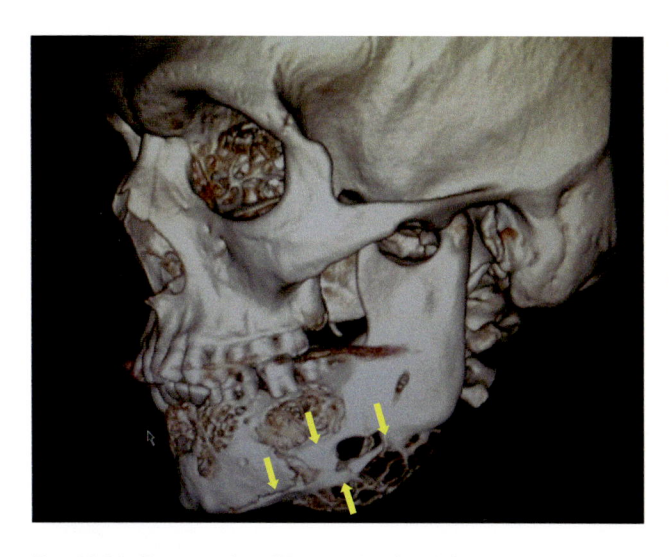

Fig. 41.22 Pre-operative CT scan showing left mandibular odontogenic myxoma (yellow arrows)

41.8 Clinical Scenario B: Surgeons Dariush Nikkhah, Qadir Khan, and Jeremy Rawlins

A 73-year-old male patient was diagnosed with osteoradionecrosis of the mandible following treatment for a previous SCC of the floor of the mouth. A decision was made to proceed with partial mandibulectomy and reconstruction with an osseous free fibula flap. The Pro Plan software was used preoperatively to aid surgical planning of intra-operative resection, wedge osteotomies and bony plating (Figs. 41.25 and 41.26). Following resection (Fig. 41.27), the peroneal artery was anastomosed to the recipient facial artery, a vena comitans was anastomosed to the recipient common facial vein. Complete resection was achieved and good post-operative mandibular contour was achieved (Fig. 41.28).

Fig. 41.25 ProPlan software for planning of osteotomies and bony plating

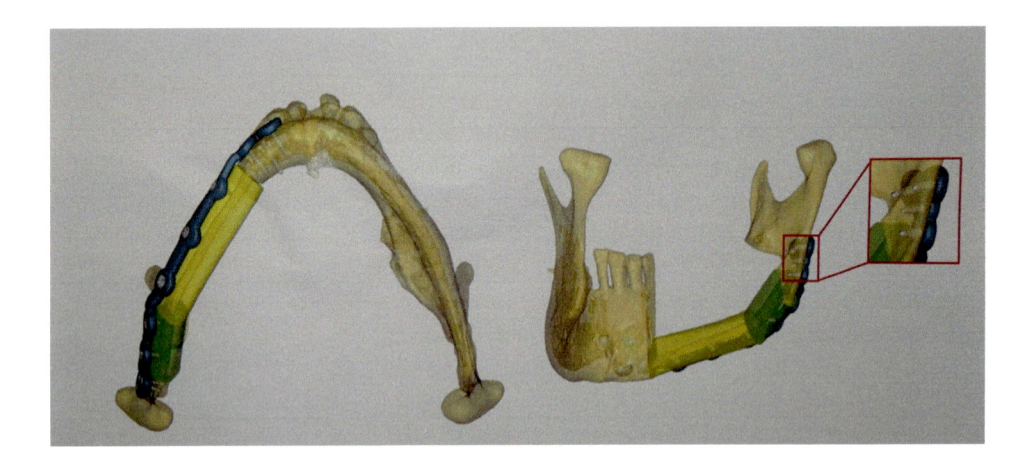

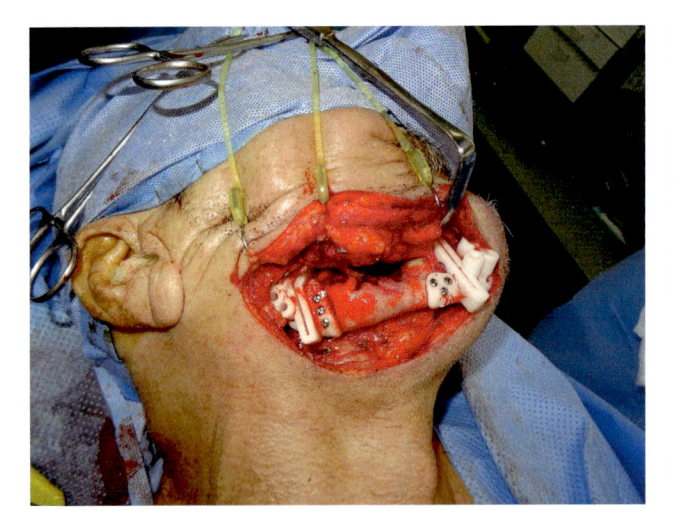

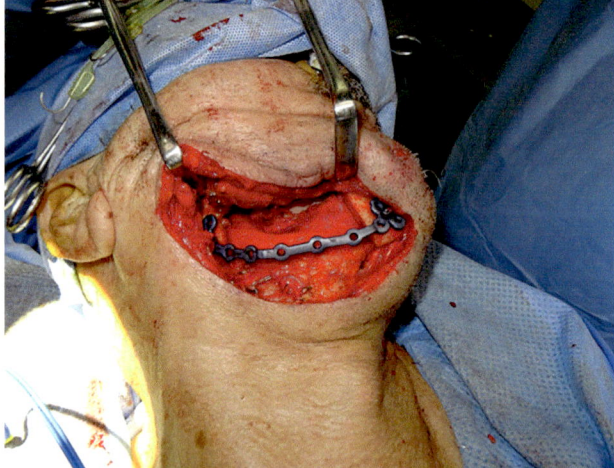

Fig. 41.26 Cutting jig used to aid surgical bony resection

Fig. 41.27 Resulting defect with mandibular plate visible

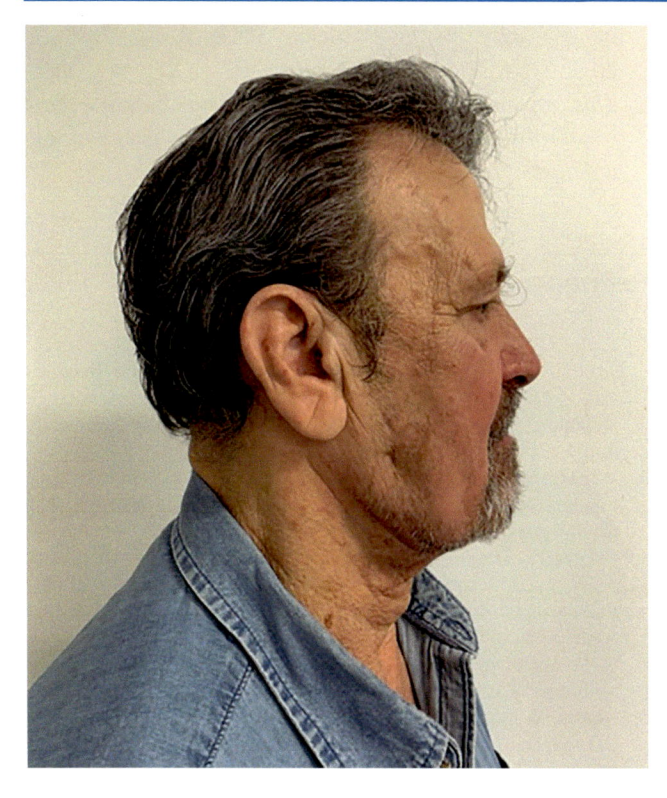

Fig. 41.28 Post-operative photograph demonstrating good mandibular contour

41.9 Pearls and Pitfalls

Pearls

- If an osteocutaneous flap is chosen, care must be taken not to damage the posterior crural septum, which carries most septocutaneous perforators to the skin paddle.
- Although septocutaneous perforators must be preserved in osteocutaneous flaps, musculocutaneous perforators may also be included to augment circulation where inadequate septocutaneous perforators are encountered.
- Always leave a thin cuff of muscle (at least 2 mm) over the fibula during flap elevation to preserve periosteal blood supply.
- In order to facilitate visualisation and dissection of the fibula pedicle proximally, a section of fibula (around 6 cm) may be removed and discarded.
- A thicker cuff of FHL can also be included in the flap to improve vascularity or to add bulk to obliterate dead space.

Pitfalls

- During dissection of the anterior compartment muscles, the anterior tibial vessels and deep peroneal nerve must be identified and protected by medial retraction using Langenbeck retractors.
- One should be mindful of the tibial nerve, which lies in very close proximity to the peroneal pedicle during dissection.
- If an osteocutaneous flap is raised, care must be taken not to damage the sural nerve and short saphenous vein during the posterior skin margin dissection by staying in a supra-fascial plane initially.
- The interosseous membrane should not be incised flush on to the fibula, but instead 5 mm away from it to avoid injury to the vascular pedicle and to aid in flexor hallucis longus repair.
- If less than 7 cm of fibula is left distally, a diastasis screw can be used to ensure ankle stability.

41.10 Selected Readings

- Taylor GI, Miller GDH, Ham FJ. The free vascularized bone graft. A clinical extension of microvascular techniques. Plast Reconstr Surg. 1975;55:533–44.
  This paper illustrates the first published description of the free fibula flap in the reconstruction of two cases involving extensive bone and soft tissue loss secondary to trauma.
- Hidalgo DA. Fibula free flap: a new method of mandible reconstruction. Plast Reconstr Surg 1989;84:71–9.
  This paper describes the first use of the free fibula flap in mandibular reconstruction. Twelve segmental mandibular defects were reconstructed using osseous and osteocutaneous free fibula flaps. Although all flaps survived, the author reported that the septocutaneous blood supply was generally inadequate to support the skin island for intraoral soft-tissue reconstruction.
- Wei FC, Chen HC, Chuang CC, Noordhoff MS. Fibular osteoseptocutaneous flap: anatomic study and clinical application. Plast Reconstr Surg. 1986;78(2):191–200.
  This anatomical study of 20 cadaver legs and 15 clinical cases demonstrates adequate circulation to the skin of the lateral aspect of the lower leg from the septocutaneous branches of the peroneal artery alone, and contrasts the original findings by Hidalgo (above).
- Alolabi N, Dickson L, Coroneos CJ, Farrokhyar F, Levis C. Preoperative angiography for free fibula flap

harvest: a meta-analysis. J Reconstr Microsurg. 2019;35(5):362–71.

This paper is the only published Level 1 evidence on the use of pre-operative angiography in free fibula harvest. It concludes that there is low-quality evidence to suggest a necessity for routine pre-operative angiography in all patients undergoing free fibula harvest.

- Roser SM, Ramachandra S, Blair H, et al. The accuracy of virtual surgical planning in free fibula mandibular reconstruction: comparison of planned and final results. J Oral Maxillofac Surg. 2010;68(11):2824–32.

This study evaluates the benefit of virtual surgery planning in free fibula flap reconstruction of mandibular defects. The authors conclude that a reasonably high level of accuracy was achieved in the mandibular and fibula osteotomies through use of the surgical cutting guides.

- Deek NF, Wei FC. Computer-assisted surgery for segmental mandibular reconstruction with the osteoseptocutaneous fibula flap: can we instigate ideological and technological reforms? Plast Reconstr Surg. 2016;137(3):963–70.

This review article draws comparisons between traditional and computer-aided techniques for mandibular reconstructions and highlights the important factors to be considered when planning soft tissue reconstruction.

- Al Deek NF, Kao HK, Wei FC. The fibula osteoseptocutaneous flap: concise review, goal-oriented surgical technique, and tips and tricks. Plast Reconstr Surg. 2018;142(6):913e–23e.

This review article describes challenges encountered when raising the free fibula flap and refined techniques to aid dissection and successful outcomes.

References

1. Taylor GI, Miller GDH, Ham FJ. The free vascularized bone graft. A clinical extension of microvascular techniques. Plast Reconstr Surg. 1975;55:533–44.
2. Hidalgo DA. Fibula free flap: a new method of mandible reconstruction. Plast Reconstr Surg. 1989;84:71–9.
3. Wei FC, Seah CS, Tsai YC, Liu SJ, Tsai MS. Plast Reconstr Surg. Fibula osteoseptocutaneous flap for reconstruction of composite mandibular defects 1994;93(2):294–304; discussion 305–6, 442.
4. Fukaya E, Grossman RF, Saloner D, Leon P, Nozaki M, Mathes SJ. Magnetic resonance angiography for free fibula flap transfer. J Reconstr Microsurg. 2007;23(4):205–11.
5. Alolabi N, Dickson L, Coroneos CJ, Farrokhyar F, Levis C. Preoperative angiography for free fibula flap harvest: a meta-analysis. J Reconstr Microsurg. 2019;35(5):362–71.
6. Akashi M, Nomura T, Sakakibara S, Sakakibara A, Hashikawa K. Preoperative MR angiography for free fibula osteocutaneous flap transfer. Microsurgery. 2013;33(6):454–9.
7. Rozen WM, Ashton MW, Stella DL, Phillips TJ, Taylor GI. Magnetic resonance angiography and computed tomographic angiography for free fibular flap transfer. J Reconstr Microsurg. 2008;24(6):457–8.
8. Zheng GS, Su YX, Liao GQ, et al. Mandible reconstruction assisted by preoperative virtual surgical simulation. Oral Surg Oral Med Oral Pathol Oral Radiol. 2012;113(5):604–11.

Posterior Tibial and Peroneal Perforators Flaps

Ahmed M. Yassin, Muholan Kanapathy, and Georgios Pafitanis

42.1 Introduction

Soft tissue reconstruction of the lower limb, especially the distal third is one the most challenging areas of reconstruction faced by plastic surgeons. The lack of excess soft tissue in this region limits the local flap option, hence making free tissue transfer as the preferred choice. However, the introduction of the concept of perforator flap by Kroll and Rosenfield in 1988 [1] and Koshima and Soeda in 1989 [2], followed by the introduction of propeller flaps by Hyakusosku in 1991 [3] transformed the design of local flaps, making them a more reliable option for the lower limb.

The most reliable perforators in the leg arise from the three main arteries: the posterior tibial (PTA), the peroneal (PA), and the anterior tibial (ATA). However, flaps based on the perforators arising from the first two arteries are the most commonly used. They can be used for reconstruction of defects in the distal third of the lower extremity, the foot, Achilles tendon, around the ankle joint including the medial and lateral malleolus, and down to the nonweight-bearing part of the heel [4]. They can also provide coverage for defects in the middle and upper third of the leg and around the knee joint.

Zhang and colleagues [5] in 1983 were the first to describe harvesting a medial leg cutaneous flap based on the PTA and its cutaneous branches. Venkataramakrishnan et al. [6] avoided sacrificing the PTA and reported raising posterior tibial artery perforator (PTAP) based V-Y advancement flaps. In a case report by Hallock in 1993 [7], he described the use of a PTAP flap to cover an exposed medial malleolus after rotating the flap 180° which is now known as a *propeller flap*.

A propeller flap can be defined as a fasciocutaneous flap, completely islanded on a single perforator and designed with two blades of unequal length. The perforator constitutes the pivot point of the flap, which allows it be rotated 90–180°. The long blade of the flap fits into the defect, while the short blade helps closure of part of the donor site [8].

On the other hand, peroneal artery perforator flap was first described by Donski and Fogdestam in 1983 [9], who raised a fasciocutaneous flap based on the distal cutaneous perforator originating from the peroneal artery about 5–7 cm superior to the lateral malleolus to cover the Achilles tendon.

42.2 Anatomy

42.2.1 Posterior Tibial Artery Perforator Flap

A cadaveric study done by Schaverien and Saint-Cyr [10] reported that perforators of PTA were the largest in the leg and were found in three clusters between the soleus and the flexor digitorum longus muscles, each being 4–9, 13–18, and 21–26 cm from the inter-malleolar line (Fig. 42.1a). Each cluster contains 23% of PTA perforators, and a perforator was found in each of them in 80% of the cadavers in the study. Multiple musculocutaneous perforators, usually passing through the soleus or gastrocnemius muscles, were also found in all zones of the leg, but were mainly located proximally. Two venae comitantes followed each perforator, and in the distal leg they are occasionally connected to the long saphenous vein [11].

The proximal two-thirds of the leg were found to have perforators with the largest caliber which pierce the deep fas-

Fig. 42.1 Diagram showing the territories of the PTA and PA perforator flaps. (**a**) Medial aspect of the leg showing the distribution of PTA perforators with the distance measures in centimeters proximal to the tip of the medial malleolus. (**b**) Lateral aspect of the leg showing the distribution of PA perforators with the distance measured in centimeters proximal to the lateral malleolus

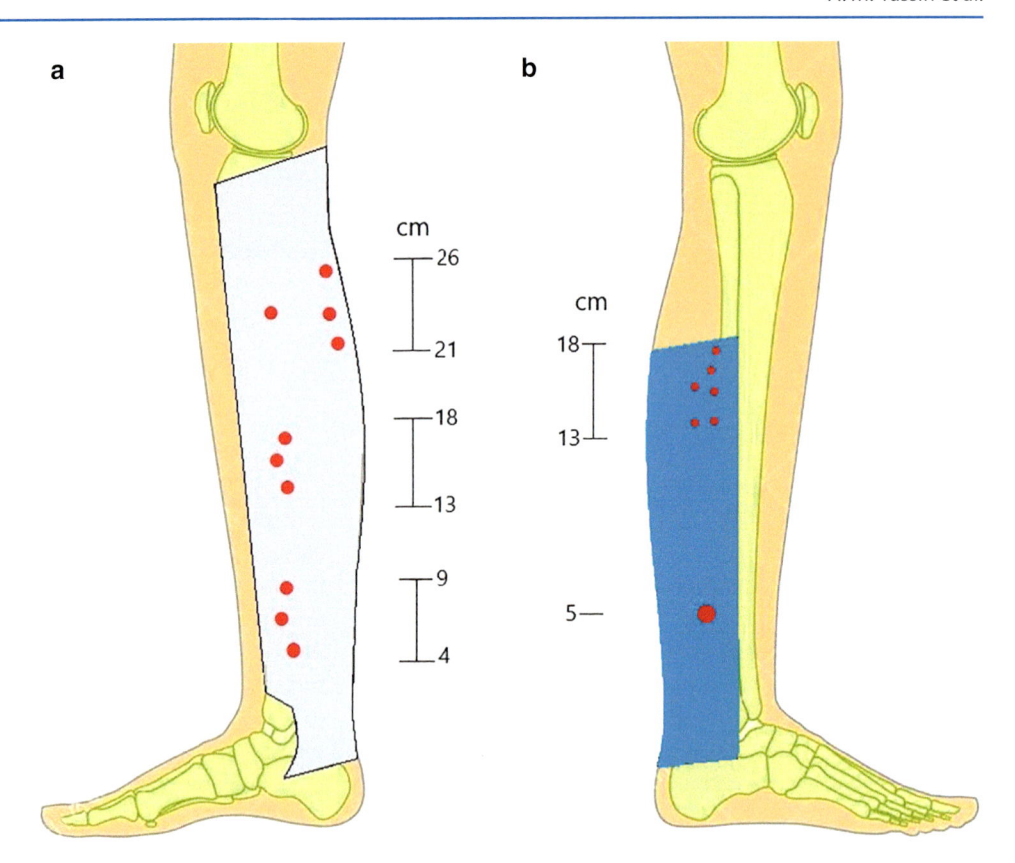

cia perpendicularly. This was found to be advantageous for the design of a propeller flap as it minimizes the chance of the perforators to kink if twisted [12].

When the PTAP flap is based on an appropriate perforator, its territory can extend from the anterior border of the tibia to the posterior midline, and about 2.5 times this width in terms of proximal to distal extension [13, 14].

42.2.2 Peroneal Artery Perforator Flap

PA supplies the posterolateral aspect of the leg through 5 ± 2 musculocutaneous and septocutaneous perforators, making the PA angiosome to extend from the posterior border of the fibula medially to the central raphe of Achilles tendon laterally [15]. These perforators are located at 3–5 cm interval, and most of them are found at about 13–18 cm superior to the lateral malleolus [10] (Fig. 42.1b). The musculocutaneous perforators predominate in the proximal leg and come through the soleus or peroneus longus muscles, while the septocutaneous perforators appear distally through the septum between the flexor hallucis longus and peroneus brevis [10]. About 5 cm above the lateral malleolus, a good-caliber perforator emerges from the PA, penetrates the interosseous membrane then divides into a superficial branch which supplies the skin of the lateral supramalleolar flap and a deep descending branch which anastomoses with the anterolateral branches of the anterior tibial artery [16].

The proportion of musculocutaneous to septocutaneous perforators widely varies between studies [17]. For example, Heitmann et al. [18] reported 34% of perforators to be musculocutaneous and 66% septocutaneous, while a study done by Yoshimura et al. reported these to be 71% musculocutaneous and 29% septocutaneous [19].

42.3 Preoperative Investigation

Perforators of the PTA and PA can be identified preoperatively using hand-held Doppler, color Doppler, Duplex ultrasound, thermal imaging, arteriography, high-resolution computed tomography, or magnetic resonance angiography [8, 20]. These modalities are useful in detecting the flap perforators, but they cannot provide information about the flap viability.

Hand-held Doppler is a simple useful tool for preoperative localization of adequate perforators; however, color Doppler is a more accurate method in terms of providing more data about the internal diameter of perforators [21]. Thermography has now also become an affordable and easy obtainable method for preoperative mapping, intraoperative decision-making and postoperative monitoring of propeller flaps using smartphone-compatible thermal imaging cameras [22]. On the other hand, computed tomography angiography (CTA) is now considered by many studies as the gold standard technique for mapping the cutaneous vasculature of the lower extremities. It can provide detailed information about the PTA and PA, and the anatomical data of their perforators including the diameter and course. Such data facilitated the preoperative mapping and the intraoperative dissection of the perforators [20, 23, 24].

It is also important to find a tool that can be used intraoperatively to detect the flap perfusion and the safe flap dimensions. Intravenous fluorescein administration is one of the methods used for prediction of flaps perfusion [25]. However, the indocyanine green near-infrared fluorescence angiography was found to be more accurate than the conventional fluorescein angiography in evaluating skin perfusion [26].

42.4 Flap Design and Markings

The most promising perforator near to the defect should be marked preoperatively using hand-held Doppler or any of the aforementioned modalities (Fig. 42.2). A pedicled perforator flap can be designed as a peninsular or islanded flap. In a peninsular flap, a skin bridge should be left intact during flap harvest in addition to the isolated perforator, and examples of this include the uni-bladed propeller, the transposition, and rotation flaps. On the other hand, an islanded flap, such as a twin-bladed propeller, keystone, and V-Y advancement, is only vascularized by the isolated perforator [15].

The most common design in the lower limb is the twin-bladed propeller flap (two blades of unequal sizes). For a proper design of this flap, the perforator should act as the pivot point of the flap. Then, the distance between the perforator and the distal end of the defect is measured and transferred proximally along the axis of the main source vessel. The distance between the perforator and the proximal border of the flap is equal to this measured distance plus 1 cm. The width of the proximal part of the flap, which should fill in the defect, equals to the width of the defect plus 0.5 cm. This compensates the expected flap contraction and allows for tensionless wound closure [27]. The short arm of the flap, which is the part between the perforator and the proximal tip of the defect, will be used to help closure of the secondary defect either completely or with a skin graft after complete flap dissection and rotation (Fig. 42.3).

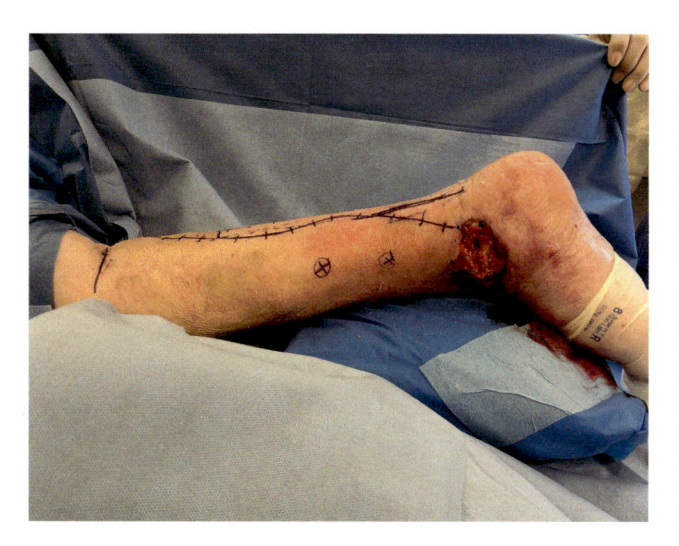

Fig. 42.2 Preoperative marking of the posterior tibial artery perforators

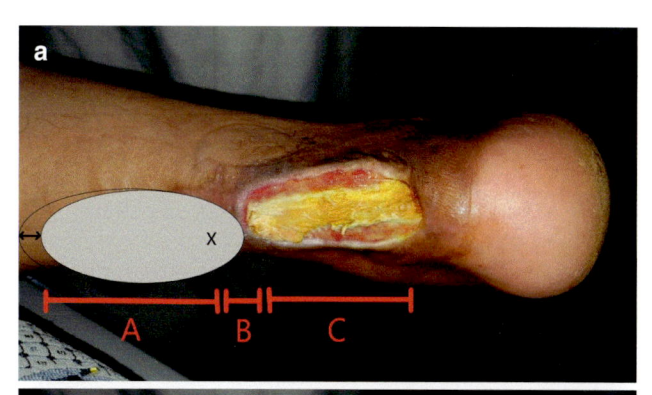

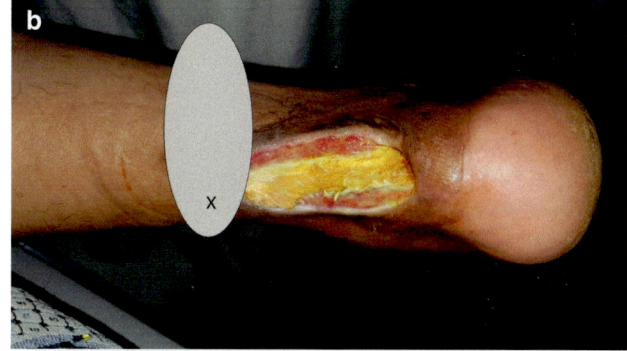

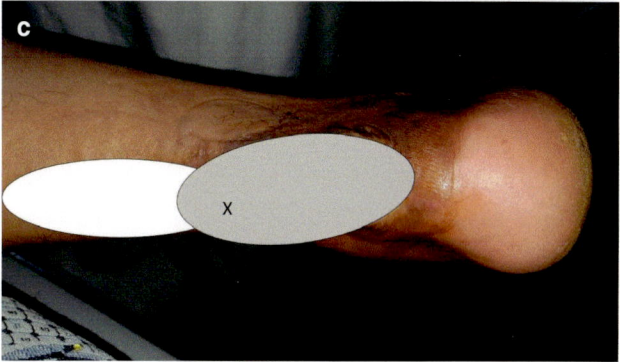

Fig. 42.3 The preoperative design for a twin-bladed propeller flap. (**a**) Marking of the flap. The distance between the perforator, marked as x, and the proximal tip of the flap (A) is equal to the length of the defect (C) plus the distance between the perforator and the proximal edge of the defect (B). Note that 1–2 cm should be added to (A) to compensate for the tissue retraction and help tension-free closure. (**b**) The flap will be rotated to cover the defect after complete dissection. (**c**) The defect will be completely covered with the long arm of the flap, while the short arm will help closure of part of the donor site. The remaining part can be covered with a split thickness skin graft or closed primarily if possible

42.5 Flap Raise/Elevation – A Step-By-Step guide

1. *Incision*

    The posterior border of the designed flap is incised as an exploratory incision down through the deep fascia (Fig. 42.4).

2. *Pedicle Dissection*

    The flap elevation is performed subfascially, identifying and preserving all potentially suitable perforators. Once all perforators are allocated, the best one should be selected based on the caliber, pulsatility, proximity to the defect, number and caliber of venae comitantes, orientation, and course (Fig. 42.5).

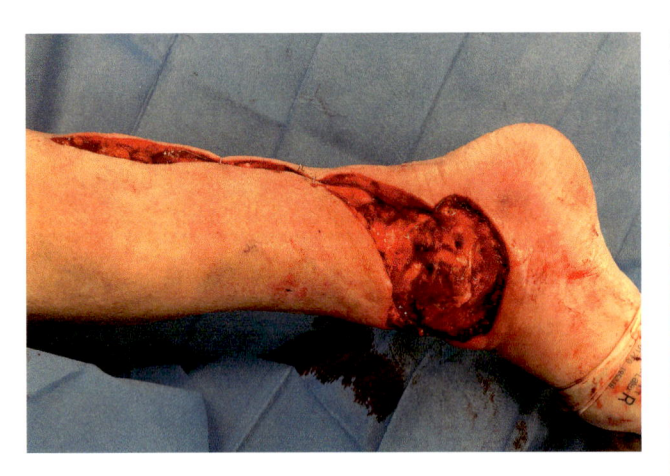

Fig. 42.4 Intraoperative photograph showing the incision of the posterior border of the flap down through the deep fascia

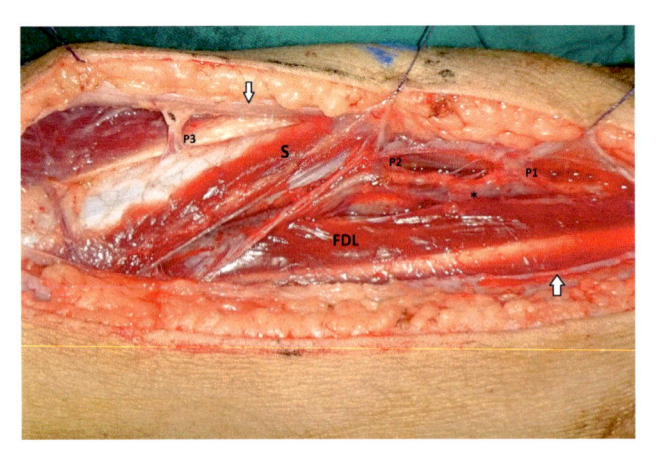

Fig. 42.5 Intraoperative photograph of a posterior tibial artery perforator flap. The incision was carried out down through the deep fascia (arrows). Three perforators were marked in this image; P1, P2, and P3 from distal to proximal. P1 and P2 were septocutaneous perforators passing through the septum between the soleus (S) and the flexor digitorum longus (FDL) and were traced down to the posterior tibial vessels (asterisk), while P3 was a musculocutaneous perforator piercing through the soleus muscle

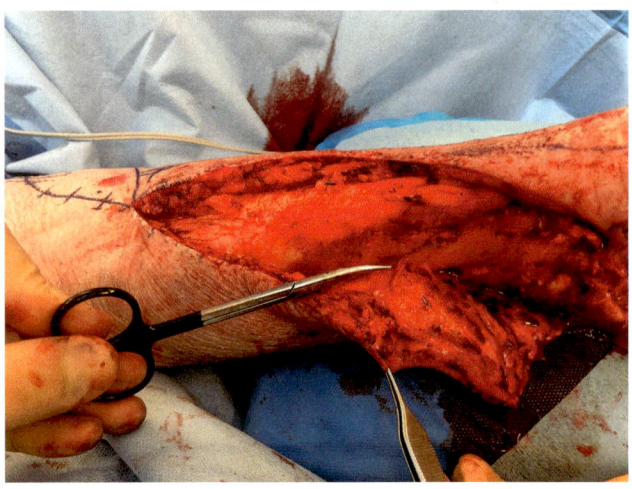

Fig. 42.6 Tenotomy scissor pointing to the most appropriate perforator of the flap

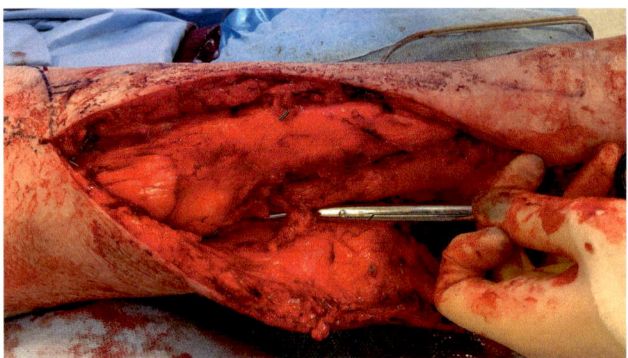

Fig. 42.7 The most appropriate perforator and its accompanying vein were dissected all around for a suitable length

3. *Pedicle Preparation*

    Once the most appropriate perforator is chosen, all other perforators must be ligated (Fig. 42.6). The perforator and its accompanying veins should then be dissected long enough to prevent kinking of the vessels when the flap is repositioned (Fig. 42.7). When high degree of rotation is required (more than 90–100°), perforator skeletonization or exposure of the source vessels will be necessary to minimize torsion (Fig. 42.8).

4. *Flap Adjustment*

    The flap can then be reevaluated and adjusted based on the chosen perforator (Fig. 42.9). The remaining outline of the flap is incised and dissected until completely islanded. The raised flap can now be transferred to the defect as a twin-bladed propeller, keystone, V-Y advancement, or even as a free perforator flap. The following steps should be undertaken to inset the flap as a twin-bladed propeller flap.

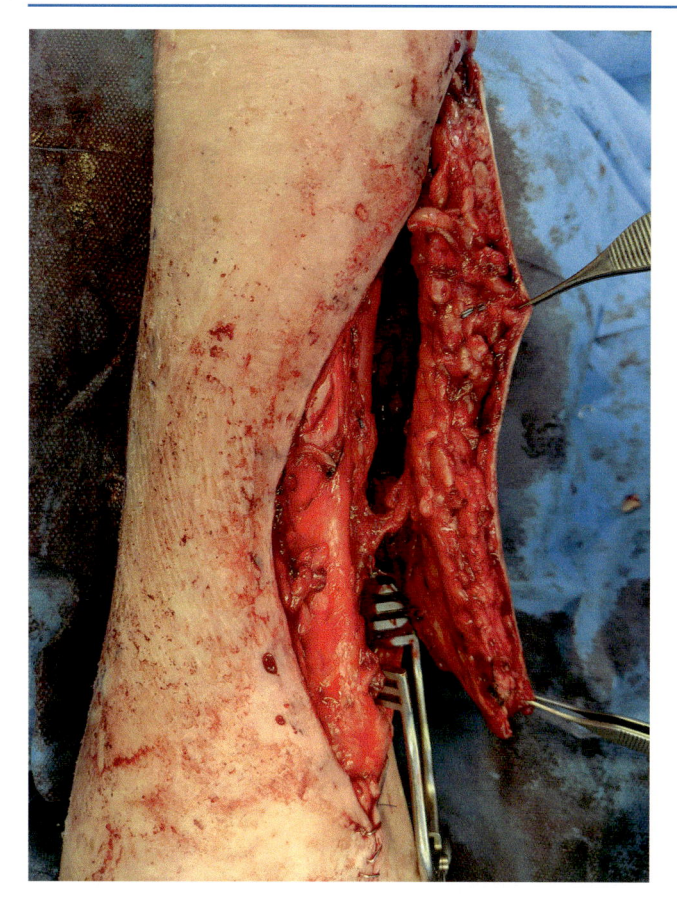

Fig. 42.8 Skeletonization of the perforator was carried out to minimize torsion of the pedicle

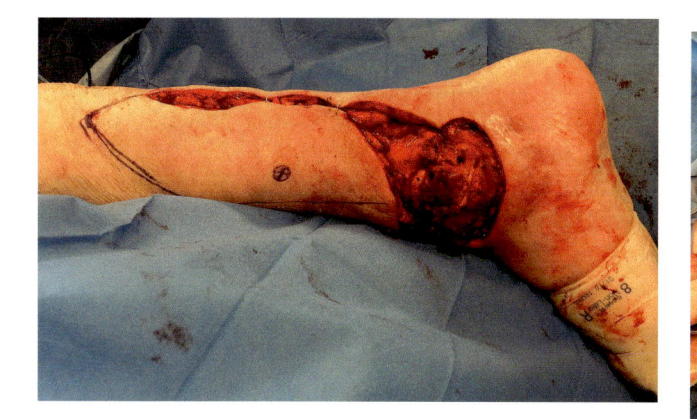

Fig. 42.9 The flap dimensions were adjusted based on the dissected perforator

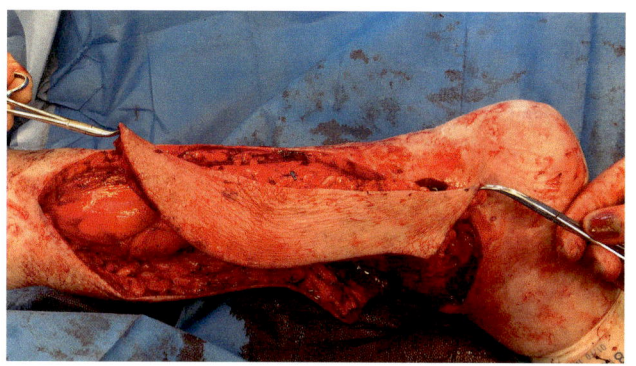

Fig. 42.10 The flap was rotated 180° to reach the recipient site

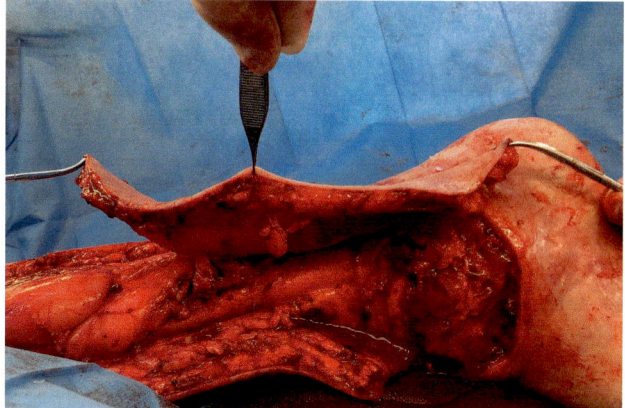

Fig. 42.11 Intraoperative photograph of the flap after being rotated 180° showing minimal torsion of the skeletonized perforator

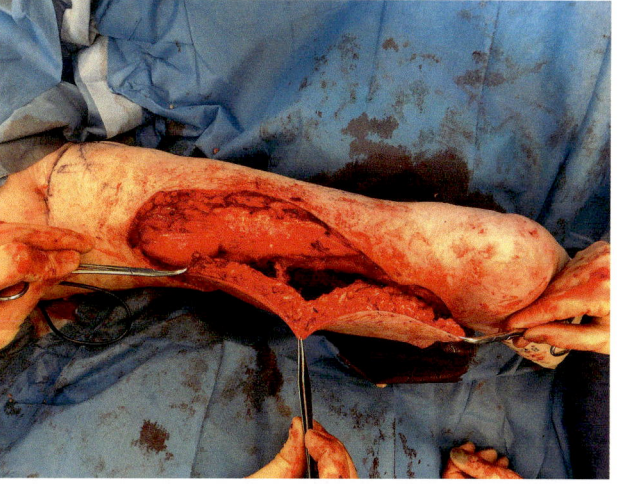

Fig. 42.12 After being rotated, the long blade of the flap filled the defect, while the short blade helped to cover part of the donor site

5. *Flap Transfer and Insetting*

The flap can be rotated up to 180° to reach the recipient site. The long blade of the propeller flap fills the defect, while the short blade is used to help closure of part of the donor site (Figs. 42.10, 42.11, and 42.12). This can be done using skin staples or 3–0 half-buried prolene sutures. Penrose or rubber drain can be used, but should be placed and secured well away from the perforator (Fig. 42.13).

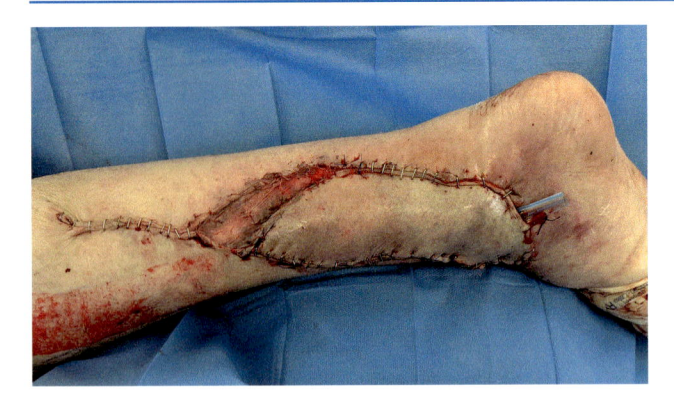

Fig. 42.13 Complete inset of the flap in its new position. A rubber drain was placed and secured away from the perforator. The donor site was partially closed primarily and the remaining part was skin grafted

6. *Donor Site Closure*

After complete inset of the flap in its new position, the donor site can be closed primarily if the flap area is small which enables tensionless closure and gives the best aesthetic result. In the case of a large donor site defect, a split-thickness skin graft can be used (Fig. 42.13).

42.6 Core Surgical Techniques in Flap Dissection (Propeller Flaps)

The use of a thigh tourniquet without exsanguination is advised to allow engorgement of the venae comitantes and optimize visualization of the perforators. An incision is first made along the posterior border of the planned flap down through the deep fascia using a blade (size 15 or 10), and then followed by subfascial dissection under loupe magnification by the means of sharp, blunt as well as bipolar dissection. Placing anchoring sutures at the flap edges helps to prevent the deep fascia from being separated from the skin and the subcutaneous fat with shearing forces during dissection and gives a better retraction and exposure.

At this stage, the flap dissection technique depends on the type of the flap harvested:

(a) Posterior tibial artery perforator flap:

Subfascial dissection is carried on over the flexor digitorum longus muscle, and the perforators can be identified and preserved on the undersurface of the fascia between the flexor digitorum longus and soleus muscles. PTA should be located and mobilized in the distal part of the initial incision to make dissection much easier, and then retracted towards the soleus muscle to make the intermuscular septum more defined. The identified perforators can then be followed down the septum until their origin from the PTA.

(b) Peroneal artery perforator flap:

Subfascial dissection is performed laterally until the musculocutaneous or septocutaneous perforators are identified, and then traced retrograde to the peroneal vessels. If the perforators are found piercing the soleus, peroneus longus or flexor hallucis longus muscles, they should be traced intramuscularly with ligation of any encountered muscular branches.

Multiple useful perforators are usually identified and the most appropriate one is selected based on its size, location, number of venae comitantes, subcutaneous course, and orientation. This chosen perforator might not be the one identified preoperatively using the hand-held Doppler or the CTA. If in doubt, an Acland clamp can be used to select between two similar-sized perforators.

Once this decision is made, the flap design is rechecked and modified accordingly to make sure that the proximal edge of the flap can be transferred to the distal edge of the defect without tension. The pedicle is then prepared by division of all fascial strands and muscular side branches associated with the perforator, especially those around the venae comitantes, for at least 2 cm to help the flap to rotate up to 180° without significant spiral twist of the pedicle. A long pedicle will result in a gentler twist, and therefore, less blood flow obstruction in this high degree of flap rotation.

Once the pedicle is prepared, the incision around the flap is completed and the rest of the flap is harvested. When the flap is totally islanded, it usually becomes hyperemic. The tourniquet is then released and the flap should not be rotated into the defect immediately after being completely islanded, but left in its original position for 10–15 min. This helps to relieve any vascular spasm involving the perforator, which usually happens following meticulous pedicle dissection, and the flap to reperfuse.

After confirming good perfusion of the flap, it can be rotated into the defect. At this stage, the flap is lifted from its position without applying too much tension on the pedicle, and then pivoted around the perforator. The flap can be rotated to fit into the defect in a clockwise or anticlockwise direction. This mainly depends on the angle between the longitudinal axis of the flap and the defect, and the perfect direction of rotation is one that causes the least tension and torsion of the pedicle.

The maximal angle of flap rotation is 180°, and it should not be rotated more than this angle as it can simply be rotated in the opposite direction. If the flap has to be rotated 180° to cover the defect, it should be rotated first in a clockwise direction. Then the degree of pedicle torsion is noted, any extra fascial strands causing compression on the venae comitantes are divided, and the flap perfusion is monitored. The same procedure should be repeated with the flap rotated in the anti-clockwise direction. The direction of rotation is then decided based on the angle which causes the least torsion to the perforator and maintains best flap perfusion. The results of a study done by Song et al. [28] emphasized the importance of this step and how the direction of flap rotation when a 180° of rotation is required can significantly affect the overall outcome of propeller flaps. They hypothesized that each perforator, and therefore each flap, might have a preferred direction of rotation over another. They also found out that the perforator flow can significantly be affected by the rotation direction, and the use of the preferred perforator direction may subsequently reduce the rate of the flap loss.

The first two skin sutures should be placed on the proximal and distal ends of the flap to guard against any further traction on the pedicle, then the rest of the flap is sutured in its new position. The donor site should not be closed under excess tension, as this will cause compression on the main vessel, affecting the blood supply of the flap, and causing edema of the distal leg. If complete primary closure of the donor site cannot be achieved, the remaining defect can be skin grafted.

42.7 Clinical Scenario

A 55-year-old hypertensive and diabetic male who works as a butcher presented with an exposed Achilles tendon of his right leg with superficial tendon necrosis. He sustained knife laceration to the back of his right lower leg 8 weeks before, followed by wound infection and skin necrosis which was surgically debrided, leaving the distal part of the Achilles tendon exposed. Superficial debridement of the necrotic part of the tendon was performed by the orthopedic team. Debridement of the wound edges was performed, resulting in a 11 × 6 cm defect. The defect was reconstructed using a posterior tibial artery perforator propeller flap. The flap was raised on a distal perforator closest to the defect, rotated about 160° and filled into the defect. Donor site was closed partially with the short blade of the flap and the remaining part was covered with a split-thickness skin graft. The flap survived completely and the patient had an uneventful postoperative recovery (Figs. 42.14, 42.15, 42.16, 42.17, 42.18, 42.19, and 42.20).

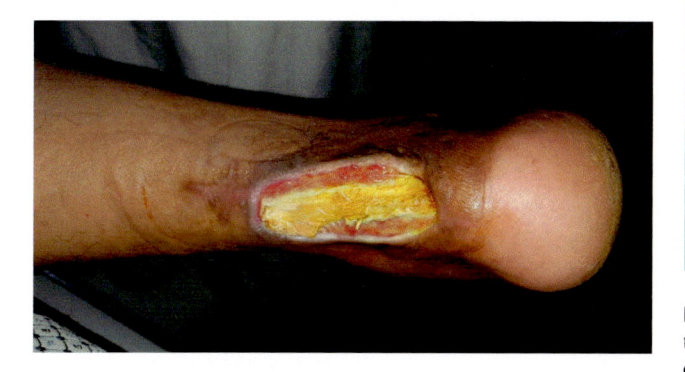

Fig. 42.14 Preoperative photo of right leg showing a skin loss and exposed Achilles tendon with superficial necrosis

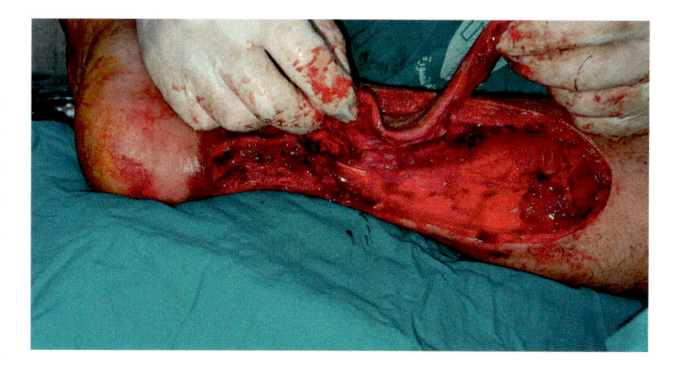

Fig. 42.15 Debridement of the recipient site was done. All the perforators were ligated except the most distal one on which the flap was harvested and the rest of the flap was then elevated

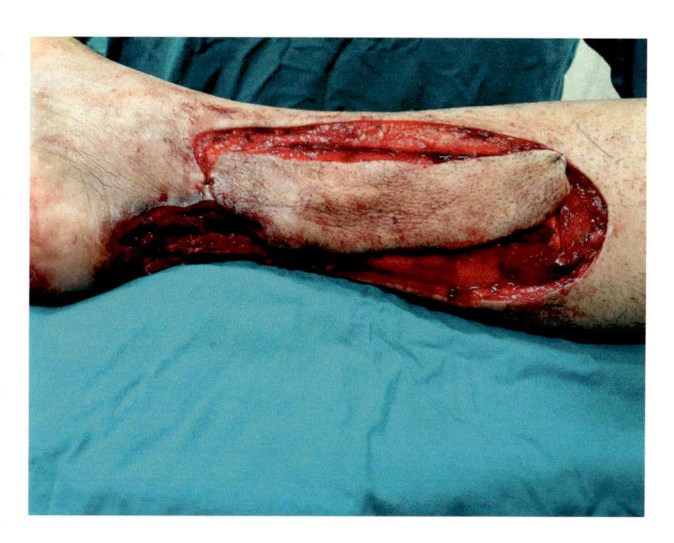

Fig. 42.16 The flap was not transferred immediately into the defect after being completely islanded, but sutured in its position for 10–15 min before rotation

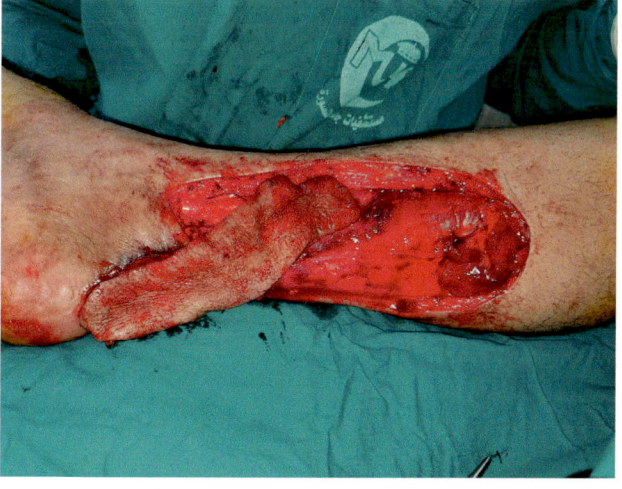

Fig. 42.17 The flap was then rotated into the defect. The long blade of the flap fitted into the defect, while the short blade covered part of the donor site

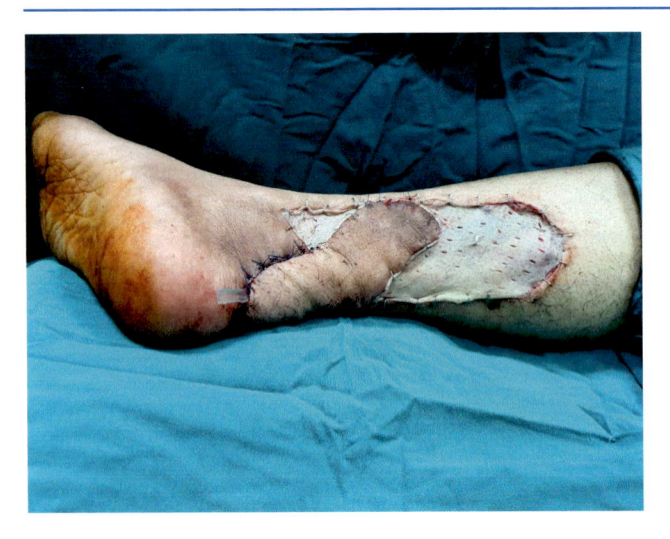

Fig. 42.18 The flap was sutured in its new position using 3–0 half-buried prolene sutures. A rubber drain was used and placed away from the pedicle. The remaining part of the donor site was covered with a split-thickness skin graft

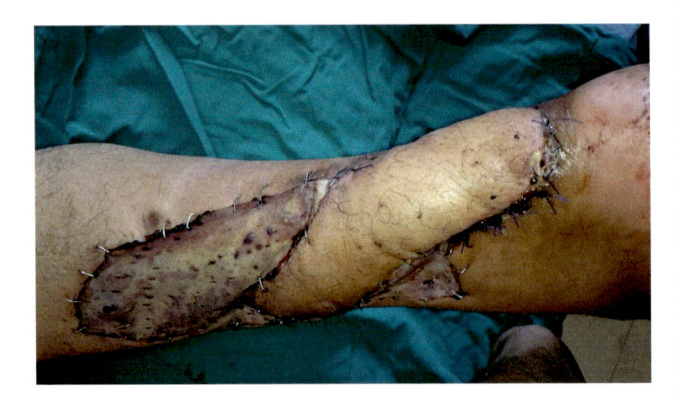

Fig. 42.19 5 days postoperative

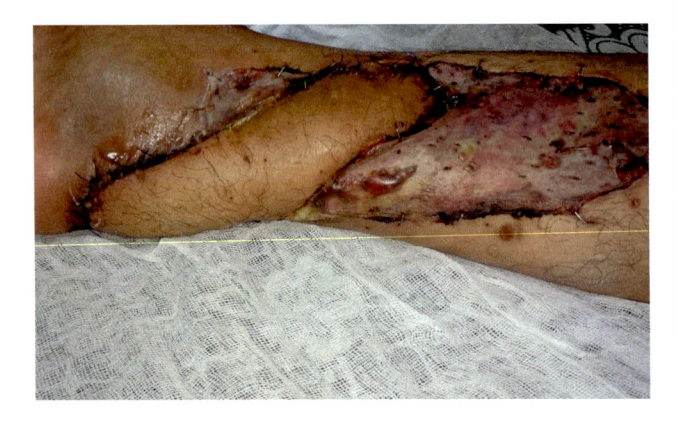

Fig. 42.20 Two weeks postoperative. The flap and the skin graft were both healing well

42.8 Pearls and Pitfalls

Pearls
- The initial incision over the flap should be designed with the possibility of becoming an edge for an alternative flap in case a suitable perforator is not detected intraoperatively.
- Avoid perforators that are too far from the defect, as they can cause the flap to be unnecessarily long.
- On the medial side of the leg, care should be taken not to include the long saphenous vein in the flap to avoid the vein becoming engorged with blood with nowhere to drain. Saphenous nerve should also be preserved to avoid postoperative distal numbness. On the lateral side of the leg, try to exclude the sural nerve to avoid loss of sensation of the lateral aspect of the distal leg and foot.
- When a perforator is chosen, it is best to make sure that the lateral dimensions of either sides of the pedicle are equidistant before cutting the other edge of the flap in order to avoid any excessive sideway traction on the pedicle after flap inset.
- If there is a reasonable cutaneous vein at the proximal border of the flap, it is recommended to dissect it for about 1–2 cm before ligating so it can be used as a lifeboat in case of flap congestion. In 2019, Kosutic [29] discussed the concept of hybrid perforator flaps. In this study, 25 perforator flaps were included, and in all of them, 1–2 superficial veins were dissected on the flap edge and used for prophylactic supercharging. After flap rotation, this prepared superficial flap vein was anastomosed microscopically with another vein on the edge of the defect. This additional step could enable the surgeon to harvest a larger flap more safely, use the entire raised flap more reliably, reduce the complications rate and improve the overall outcome of propeller flaps.
- Topical vasodilators as papaverine or verapamil can be applied around the perforator after completion of dissection and before flap rotation.

Pitfalls

- Perforators in an area of scar, granulation tissue, or zone of injury are more fragile and can be easily injured. According to the latest British Orthopaedic Association and British Association of Plastic, Reconstructive and Aesthetic Surgeons (BOA/BAPRAS) 2020 guidelines for the management of open fractures, the use of local perforator flaps should be limited to relatively low-energy injuries with a small-sized zone of injury. Free tissue transfer is recommended in cases of higher energy type of traumas and those associated with degloving injuries [30].
- A pedicle that is skeletonized more than required increases the risk of occlusive twist and hence affects the flap perfusion.
- Raising a propeller flap on two adjacent perforators can compromise its blood supply after inset, as they can be twisted around each other with flap rotation.
- Bulky dressing should be avoided as it can cause compression on the flap and vascular embarrassment. Bandaging should be soft and light, and a window should be made in the dressing to observe the flap.
- Venous congestion is the most common complication and the primary cause of flap necrosis. Flap salvage in that case should be commenced as soon as possible by removing some distal stitches to release excess tension, local heparinization of the flap or applying leeches. Negative pressure wound therapy will be valuable in such cases especially those that end with partial superficial flap necrosis.

42.9 Selected Readings

- Teo TC. The propeller flap concept. Clin Plast Surg. 2010;37(4):615–626, vi.
- *In this article, TC Teo describes the propeller flap concept as a versatile technique for reconstruction of defects in different parts of the body. He provides us with a very detailed description of the flap design and the surgical technique in harvesting propeller perforator flaps.*
- Low OW, Sebastin SJ, Cheah AEJ. A review of pedicled perforator flaps for reconstruction of the soft tissue defects of the leg and foot. Indian J Plast Surg. 2019;52(1):26–36.
- *This paper provides a historical review, the anatomical basis, the preoperative investigations and design of the common perforator-based flaps for reconstruction of leg and foot defects. It also focuses on the surgical technique and the postoperative follow-up of this kind of flaps.*
- Schaverien M, Saint-Cyr M. Perforators of the lower leg: analysis of perforator locations and clinical application for pedicled perforator flaps. Plast Reconstr Surg. 2008;122(1):161–70.
- *This cadaveric study provides a comprehensive anatomical illustration of the perforators arising from the main arteries of the leg (the anterior tibial, the posterior tibial, and the peroneal arteries), and how this can be applied clinically in the design of pedicled perforator flaps for reconstruction of the lower leg defects.*
- Georgescu AV. Propeller perforator flaps in distal lower leg: evolution and clinical applications. Arch Plast Surg. 2012;39(2):94–105.
- *The author highlighted some of the tips for the design and harvesting technique of propeller perforator flaps in the lower leg. He also addressed the most common complications that could happen postoperatively and the best way to deal with them.*
- Tajsic N, Winkel R, Husum H. Distally based perforator flaps for reconstruction of posttraumatic defects of the lower leg and foot. A review of the anatomy and clinical outcomes. Injury. 2014;45(3):469–77.
- *Tajsic et al. reviewed the surgical anatomy and techniques of the perforator flaps in the lower leg, analyzed the clinical outcomes in the included studies and illustrated some of the future trends that will be promising especially in terms of microvascular imaging for better monitoring of the healing capacity of perforator flaps.*
- Pignatti M, Pinto V, Docherty Skogh AC, Giorgini FA, Cipriani R, De Santis G, Hallock GG. How to design and harvest a propeller flap. Semin Plast Surg. 2020;34(3):152–60.
- *This article provided a good illustration for the preoperative investigation and planning for a propeller flap. Then the authors went through their standard step-by-step approach for the flap harvesting technique and a number of harvesting variations. They also discussed their postoperative flap monitoring protocol and their recommendations for the flap salvage in case of postoperative venous congestion.*

References

1. Kroll SS, Rosenfield L. Perforator-based flaps for low posterior midline defects. Plast Reconstr Surg. 1988;81(4):561–6.
2. Koshima I, Soeda S. Inferior epigastric artery skin flaps without rectus abdominis muscle. Br J Plast Surg. 1989;42(6):645–8.
3. Hyakusoku H, Yamamoto T, Fumiiri M. The propeller flap method. Br J Plast Surg. 1991;44(1):53–4.

4. Teo TC. Propeller flaps for reconstruction around the foot and ankle. J Reconstr Microsurg. 2021;37(1):22–31.
5. Zhang SC. [Clinical application of medial skin flap of leg—analysis of 9 cases]. Zhonghua Wai Ke Za Zhi [Chin J Surg]. 1983;21(12):743–5.
6. Venkataramakrishnan V, Mohan D, Villafane O. Perforator based V-Y advancement flaps in the leg. Br J Plast Surg. 1998;51(6):431–5.
7. Hallock GG. Evaluation of fasciocutaneous perforators using color duplex imaging. Plast Reconstr Surg. 1994;94(5):644–51.
8. Tajsic N, Winkel R, Husum H. Distally based perforator flaps for reconstruction of post-traumatic defects of the lower leg and foot. A review of the anatomy and clinical outcomes. Injury. 2014;45(3):469–77.
9. Donski PK, Fogdestam I. Distally based fasciocutaneous flap from the sural region. A preliminary report. Scand J Plast Reconstr Surg. 1983;17(3):191–6.
10. Schaverien M, Saint-Cyr M. Perforators of the lower leg: analysis of perforator locations and clinical application for pedicled perforator flaps. Plast Reconstr Surg. 2008;122(1):161–70.
11. Robotti E, Carminati M, Bonfirraro PP, et al. "On demand" posterior tibial artery perforator flaps: a versatile surgical procedure for reconstruction of soft tissue defects of the leg after tumor excision. Ann Plast Surg. 2010;64(2):202–9.
12. Jakubietz RG, Schmidt K, Zahn RK, et al. Subfascial directionality of perforators of the distal lower extremity: an anatomic study regarding selection of perforators for 180-degree propeller flaps. Ann Plast Surg. 2012;69(3):307–11.
13. Tang M, Mao Y, Almutairi K, Morris SF. Three-dimensional analysis of perforators of the posterior leg. Plast Reconstr Surg. 2009;123(6):1729–38.
14. Pontén B. The fasciocutaneous flap: its use in soft tissue defects of the lower leg. Br J Plast Surg. 1981;34(2):215–20.
15. Low OW, Sebastin SJ, Cheah AEJ. A review of pedicled perforator flaps for reconstruction of the soft tissue defects of the leg and foot. Indian J Plast Surg. 2019;52(1):26–36.
16. Masquelet AC, Beveridge J, Romana C, Gerber C. The lateral supramalleolar flap. Plast Reconstr Surg. 1988;81(1):74–81.
17. Georgescu AV. Propeller perforator flaps in distal lower leg: evolution and clinical applications. Arch Plast Surg. 2012;39(2):94–105.
18. Heitmann C, Khan FN, Levin LS. Vasculature of the peroneal artery: an anatomic study focused on the perforator vessels. J Reconstr Microsurg. 2003;19(3):157–62.
19. Yoshimura M, Shimada T, Hosokawa M. The vasculature of the peroneal tissue transfer. Plast Reconstr Surg. 1990;85(6):917–21.
20. Chen R, Huang ZQ, Chen WL, Ou ZP, Li SH, Wang JG. Value of a smartphone-compatible thermal imaging camera in the detection of peroneal artery perforators: comparative study with computed tomography angiography. Head Neck. 2019;41(5):1450–6.
21. Khan UD, Miller JG. Reliability of handheld Doppler in planning local perforator-based flaps for extremities. Aesthet Plast Surg. 2007;31(5):521–5.
22. Pignatti M, Pinto V, Docherty Skogh AC, et al. How to design and harvest a propeller flap. Semin Plast Surg. 2020;34(3):152–60.
23. Feng S, Min P, Grassetti L, et al. A prospective head-to-head comparison of color Doppler ultrasound and computed tomographic angiography in the preoperative planning of lower extremity perforator flaps. Plast Reconstr Surg. 2016;137(1):335–47.
24. Garvey PB, Chang EI, Selber JC, et al. A prospective study of preoperative computed tomographic angiographic mapping of free fibula osteocutaneous flaps for head and neck reconstruction. Plast Reconstr Surg. 2012;130(4):541e–9e.
25. Morykwas MJ, Hills H, Argenta LC. The safety of intravenous fluorescein administration. Ann Plast Surg. 1991;26(6):551–3.
26. Matsui A, Lee BT, Winer JH, Vooght CS, Laurence RG, Frangioni JV. Real-time intraoperative near-infrared fluorescence angiography for perforator identification and flap design. Plast Reconstr Surg. 2009;123(3):125e–7e.
27. Teo TC. The propeller flap concept. Clin Plast Surg. 2010;37(4):615–26, vi.
28. Song S, Jeong HH, Lee Y, et al. Direction of flap rotation in propeller flaps: does it really matter? J Reconstr Microsurg. 2019;35(8):549–56.
29. Kosutic D. Hybrid perforator flaps: introducing a new concept in perforator flap surgery. J Plast Reconstr Aesthet Surg. 2020;73(4):764–9.
30. Eccles S, Handley B, Khan U, McFadyen I, Nanchahal J, Nayagam S. Standards for the management of open fractures. Soft tissue reconstruction. Oxford: Oxford University Press; 2020.

Second Toe Free Flap

Dariush Nikkhah, Juan Enrique Berner, Petr Vondra, Bran Sivakumar, and Mark Pickford

43.1 Introduction

From a functional point of view, the thumb is the most important digit in the hand, able to effectively oppose with the remaining four ulnar fingers, which allows the gripping and manipulation of objects and tools. Congenital absence of a functioning thumb, or its loss due to acquired conditions, inevitably results in considerable loss of hand function. Even though attempts to reconstruct thumbs using tubed pedicled flaps were attempted in the nineteenth century, it was the Viennese surgeon Carl Nicoladoni who first described the use of a second toe for this purpose [1]. It was in 1898 that the first pedicled second toe to thumb transfer was performed for a 5-year-old patient, with its pedicle being divided 16 days later.

Thanks to the experimental work of Harry Buncke [2], the first successful microsurgical great toe-to-thumb transfer was performed in 1968 by the British surgeon John Cobbett in East Grinstead [3]. Even though the second toe tends to be smaller than the thumb, it offers two main advantages over the great toe donor site: (a) the second toe metatarso-phalangeal joint can be included, which is of use in proximal amputations and (b) the donor site is cosmetically favourable [4]. The second toe flap is preferred in digital reconstruction and also in children with congenital differences; it may be the preferred option for thumb reconstruction in children and female patients because of donor site considerations.

43.2 Anatomy

The second toe is perfused by its proper digital arteries, which emerge from the confluence of the dorsal and plantar metatarsal arteries in the area just proximal to the intermetatarsal ligament. The second toe free flap is raised with one or more dorsal subcutaneous veins, and the dominant metatarsal artery. The latter tends to be the dorsal system, derived from the dorsalis pedis artery in approximately 70% of the cases [5]; in these cases, the pedicle can be traced proximally on the dorsum of the foot to increase pedicle length. If the dorsal system is non-dominant, then a more tedious plantar dissection is required, which typically yields a shorter pedicle.

The second toe flap can be harvested with the metatarso-phalangeal joint and metatarsal if needed. The extensor digitorum longus and brevis tendons lie in a subcutaneous plane in the foot dorsum, while the flexor digitorum longus and brevis run inside a flexor sheath on the plantar aspect. Both proper digital nerves of the second toe derive from common digital nerve branches of the medial plantar nerve—intraneural dissection allows the principal digital nerves to be harvested with greater length if needed; dorsal cutaneous nerves should be harvested as well, to optimize sensibility in the transferred toe.

Supplementary Information The online version contains supplementary material available at [https://doi.org/10.1007/978-3-031-07678-7_43].

D. Nikkhah (✉)
Royal Free Hospital, London, UK

J. E. Berner
Barts and the Royal London Hospital, London, UK

P. Vondra
Hand and Plastic Surgery Institute, Vysoké nad Jizerou, Czech Republic

B. Sivakumar
Great Ormond Street Hospital, London, UK

Sidra Hospital Qatar, Doha, Qatar

M. Pickford
Queen Victoria Hospital, East Grinstead, UK

43.3 Pre-operative Investigation

Raising this flap for thumb reconstruction requires careful planning of the recipient site, considering the level of the amputation and surrounding soft tissues. An adequate first webspace is key to obtain an opposable reconstructed thumb, therefore this should be addressed before transferring a second toe.

The main benefit of pre-operative investigations concerning the donor site is to determine the dominant metatarsal artery. High definition computed tomography (CT) angiography is able to delineate the arterial perfusion of the foot, including its terminal branches; however, it involves radiation and use of contrast. Colour duplex ultrasound provides more information than a hand-held Doppler, being able to describe the subcutaneous vascular anatomy.

43.4 Flap Design and Markings

The second and third webspaces are marked at their mid points. From there a "V"-shaped incision is planned on both the plantar and dorsal surfaces, with the apex lying, approximately, over the metatarsophalangeal joint. The dorsal incision in extended proximally with Brunner flaps to allow adequate exposure of the neurovascular structures and extensors. The plantar incision can be extended proximally up to the metatarsal heads level with a straight line (Figs. 43.1 and 43.2), but is usually limited to avoid tender plantar scarring.

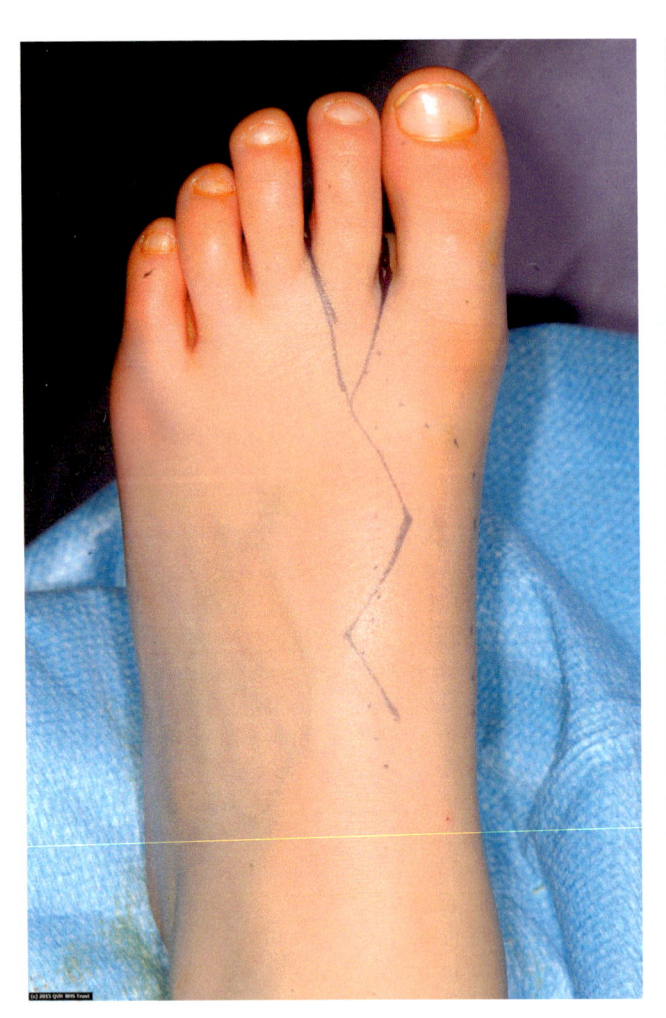

Fig. 43.1 Dorsal markings for second toe transfer

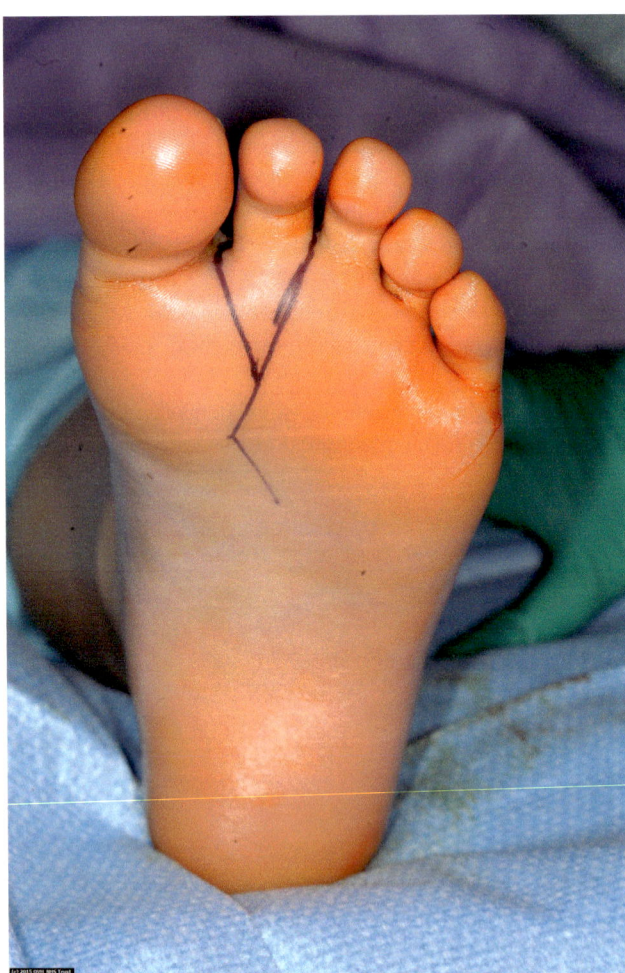

Fig. 43.2 Plantar markings for second toe transfer

43.5 Flap Raise/Elevation: A Step-by-Step

- **Step 1—Incision and Venous Dissection**: Under tourniquet control dorsal incisions are made and thin skin flaps are raised. Superficial veins draining the second toe are identified and protected, as these need to be included with the flap (Fig. 43.3).
- **Step 2—Retrograde Dissection**: Arterial dissection commences distally in the first web space; retrograde dissection determines whether the arterial supply to the second toe is dorsal dominant, or plantar dominant (Fig. 43.4). If there is a dorsal dominant circulation (70% cases) the first dorsal metatarsal artery can be traced proximally to its origin at the dorsal pedis. Debakey forceps and fine microsurgical instruments are used to handle the vessels; side branches are clipped with micro Ligaclips or cauterised with fine bipolar forceps. The dorsalis pedis is identified with its associated venae commitans by retracting the extensor hallucis brevis laterally. It is recommended to explore the arterial anatomy initially from the distal first web space, and simply follow the larger caliber vessels as they course dorsally or plantar wards i.e. to embark on toe elevation without preliminary imaging of the arterial supply. It is also recommended to dissect out the artery of the second web too, while preparing the nerve of that aspect, since this provides flexibility when selecting a suitable recipient vessel.
- **Step 3—Extensor Tendons:** The extensor digitorum brevis and longus can be easily identified and dissected for division and transfer. It is important to take sufficient length to allow a weave tenorrhaphy (Fig. 43.5).
- **Step 4—Cutaneous Nerves:** The deep peroneal nerve lies lateral to the dorsalis pedis, it should be marked with 6.0 nylon before division. Any sizeable dorsal cutaneous nerves supplying the second toe are harvested.
- **Step 5—Plantar Dissection and Flexor Tendons**: After raising and defatting the plantar skin flap, dissection proceeds into the first and second web spaces, where fascial bands must be divided to identify the proper digital arteries to the second toe; branches going to the great toe and middle toe are clipped and divided (Fig. 43.6). As the dissection proceeds, the plantar digital nerves and flexor tendons are also exposed (Fig. 43.6). Once adequate exposure is obtained, the dominant metatarsal artery of the first web is preserved and the secondary artery is divided and clipped. The senior author routinely harvests the second web artery as a back-up. If there is a plantar dominant circulation, pedicle length can be extended using an interposition vein graft (rather than an extended plantar dissection). The flexor digitorum longus and brevis are identified for division and transfer.

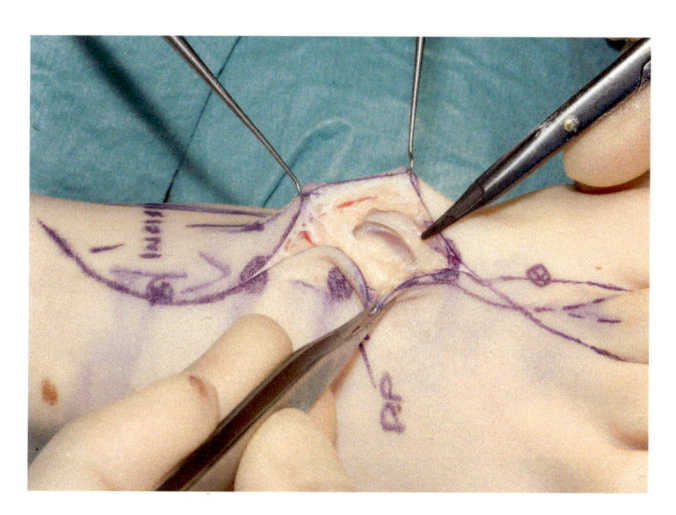

Fig. 43.3 Thin skin flaps raised over dorsal of foot demonstrating superficial dorsal veins

Fig. 43.4 Retrograde dissection in first webspace

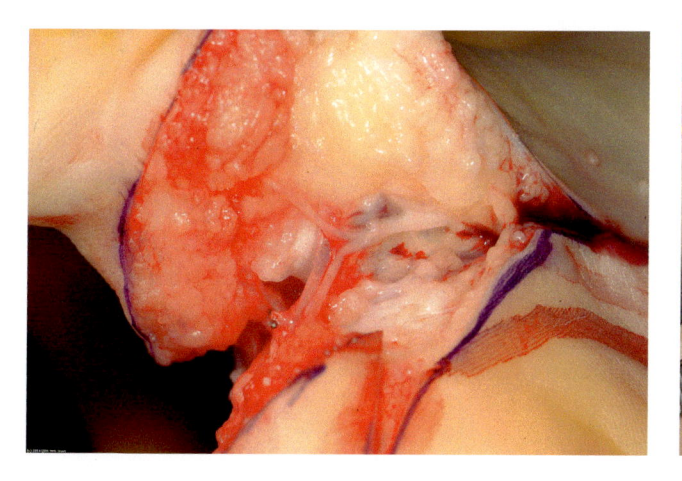

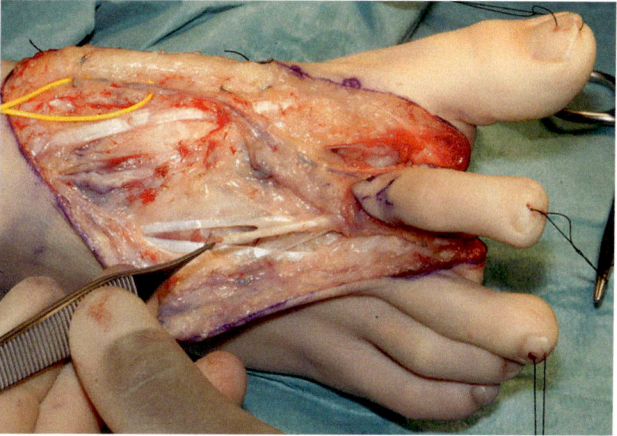

Fig. 43.5 Extensor tendons identified and divided

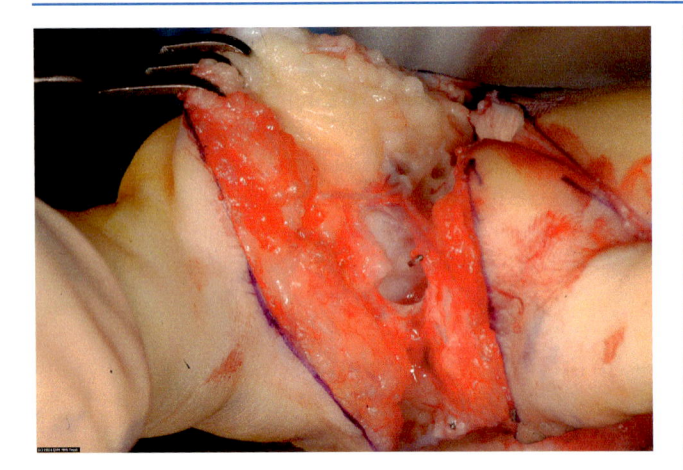

Fig. 43.6 Plantar dissection is demonstrated in this figure; the plantar digital nerves are identified, and here a plantar dominant arterial supply to the second toe is identified

- **Step 6—Metatarsophalangeal Joint Disarticulation:** Our preferred level for taking the second toe is at the metatarsophalangeal joint, but a segment of the metatarsal bone can also be harvested without significant morbidity. Disarticulation is performed by dividing the collateral ligaments, volar plate and capsule of the joint. The tourniquet is let down, after tenotomy of the extrinsic tendons but before division of the vascular supply, to assess perfusion (Fig. 43.7); if there is evidence of vasospasm warm saline or papaverine can be irrigated over the pedicle. Once the level of harvest is decided, the artery and vein are divided and the toe can then be removed and wrapped in a saline moistened gauze (Fig. 43.8).
- **Step 7—Recipient Preparation and Donor Site Closure:** At the recipient site a cruciate incision can be used to achieve wide exposure. Extensor and flexor tendons are tagged as well as recipient digital nerves; adequate tenolysis ensures good glide in recipient tendons. The recipient bone stump is usually prepared with an oscillating saw (Fig. 43.9). For thumb reconstruction the radial artery in the anatomical snuff box and associated venae commitans and dorsal veins are exposed and prepared; suitable side branches may be used for end-to-side anastomosis. The donor site is closed by approximating the soft tissues medial and lateral to the excision defect with strong PDS sutures. Skin is then closed with fine sutures.
- **Step 8—Osteosynthesis, Tendon Repair, Microsurgery:** Joint capsule is elevated off the base of the toe proximal phalanx to expose the proximal shaft; soft tissues are then protected by wrapping the toe in moist gauze, before care-

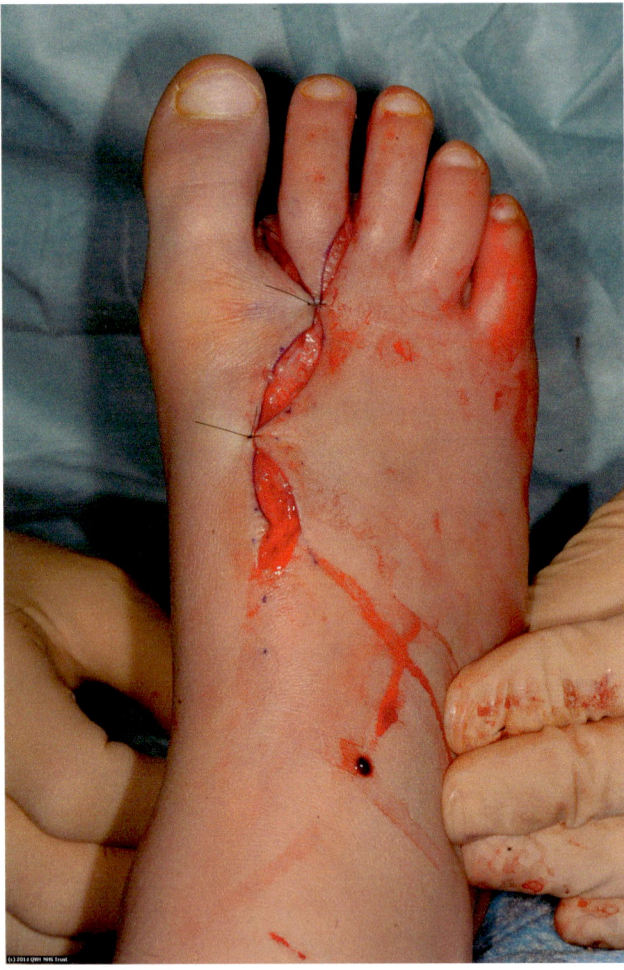

Fig. 43.7 Tourniquet is let down to assess second toe perfusion

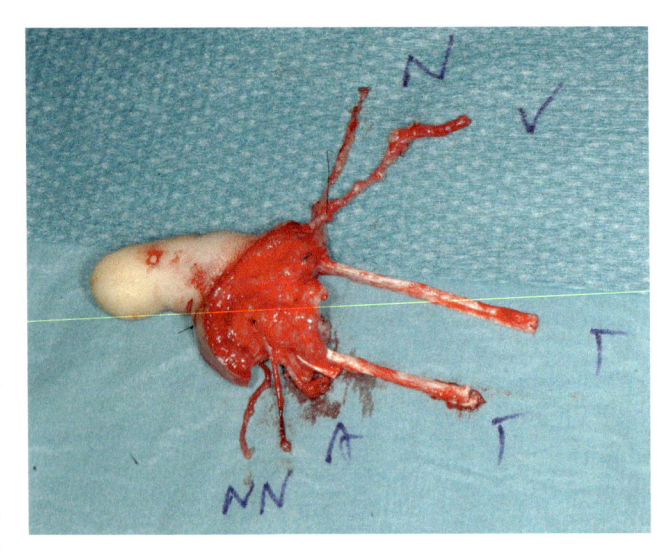

Fig. 43.8 Elevated second toe with structures marked

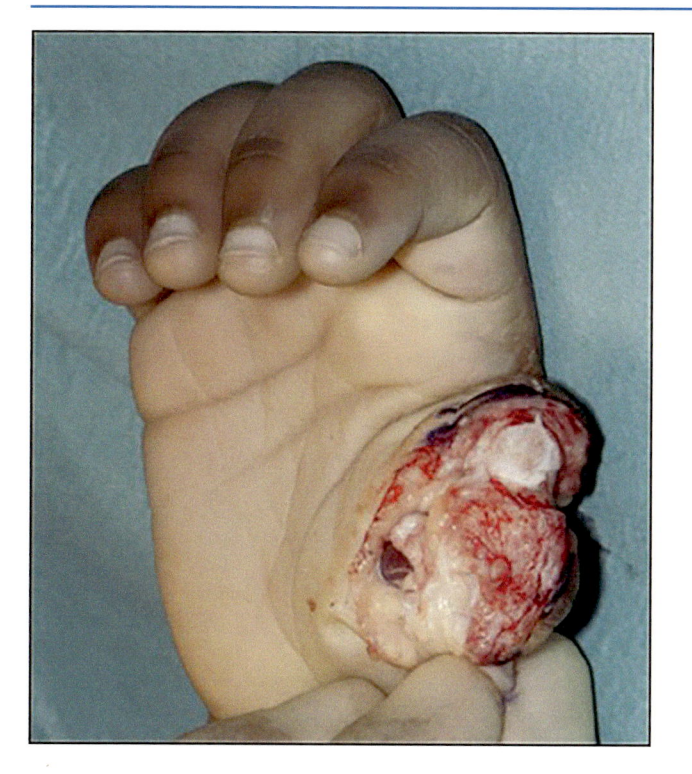

Fig. 43.9 Recipient bone prepared with oscillating saw for osteosynthesis

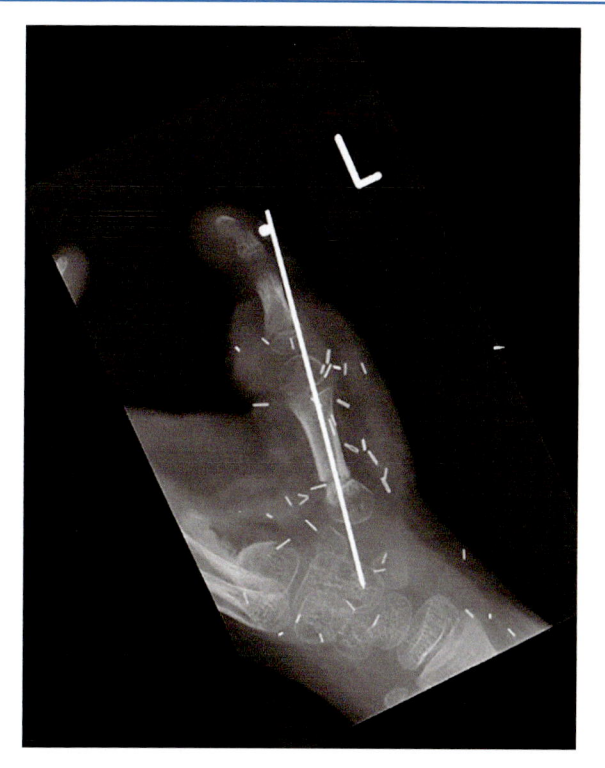

Fig. 43.10 Single axial Kirschner wire used for osteosynthesis of second toe transfer including metatarsal bone

fully removing the articular surface with an oscillating saw. Osteosynthesis is performed with two parallel interosseous wire loops, an interosseous wire and single Kirschner wire (Lister technique) or a single Kirschner wire (Fig. 43.10). It is important make sure that the thumb is in a good position for opposition. Tendons are repaired using a Pulvertaft weave. The digital nerves are repaired with 9.0 nylon. Arterial anastomosis is then performed, followed by two venous anastomoses if the veins are smaller than the artery.

- **Step 9—Skin Closure:** It is important to avoid harvesting excessive fat around the neurovascular structures of the donor toe, which can create unwanted tension during wound closure and also compromise the aesthetics of the reconstructed digit (Fig. 43.11). If skin closure without tension is not possible, we apply split thickness skin grafts over the base of the second toe and in some cases over the pedicle. This reduces the chance of pedicle compression and vascular compromise. A well-padded splint is applied so that no pressure is applied to the pedicle.

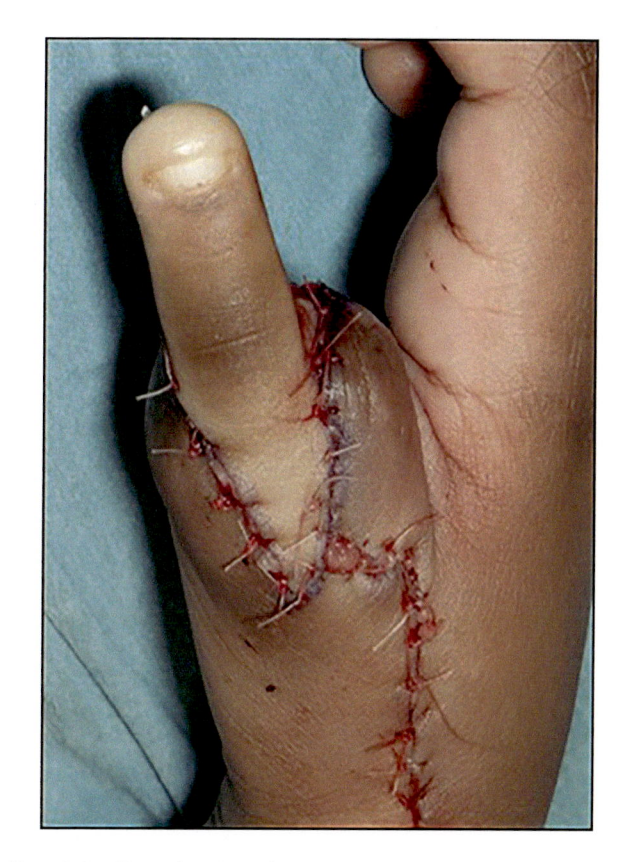

Fig. 43.11 Second toe inset for thumb reconstruction

43.6 Core Surgical Techniques in Flap Dissection

Retrograde Dissection Retrograde dissection from the distal first-web space quickly reveals whether the arterial supply is dorsal- or plantar-dominant. Needless dissection over the dorsum of the foot is avoided if a plantar dominant circulation is identified. The pedicle of a plantar dominant toe can be lengthened with an interposition vein graft.

Pedicle Dissection Care must be taken when dissecting the arterial and venous supply to the toe, we find handling with microsurgical instruments and use of microligaclips useful. Dissection should be performed with bipolar cautery on a low setting [6] and thermal damage can be avoided with heat sink bipolar technique.

Cutaneous Nerves As many cutaneous nerves as possible should be identified and repaired, since this improves the chances of good sensory recovery in the reconstructed digit.

Recipient Vessel In cases of symbrachydactyly there will be variations in anatomy and care must be taken to choose suitable veins and arteries for the toe transfer. It is preferred to go more proximal to larger vessels in the anatomical snuff box or wrist. Care must be taken to measure the required pedicle length before transfer and ascertain whether vein grafts are required.

Osteosynthesis We prefer intraosseous wire fixation or k-wires (particularly in children) over plate fixation. It allows for less dissection and preserves more periosteum. Rapid, simple and strong fixation can be achieved with two parallel box wires.

Donor Site Closure The morbidity with closure of the second toe donor site is minimal, we have noticed no long-term issues, apart from mild secondary clinodactyly of the remaining toes in the paediatric population (Figs. 43.12 and 43.13).

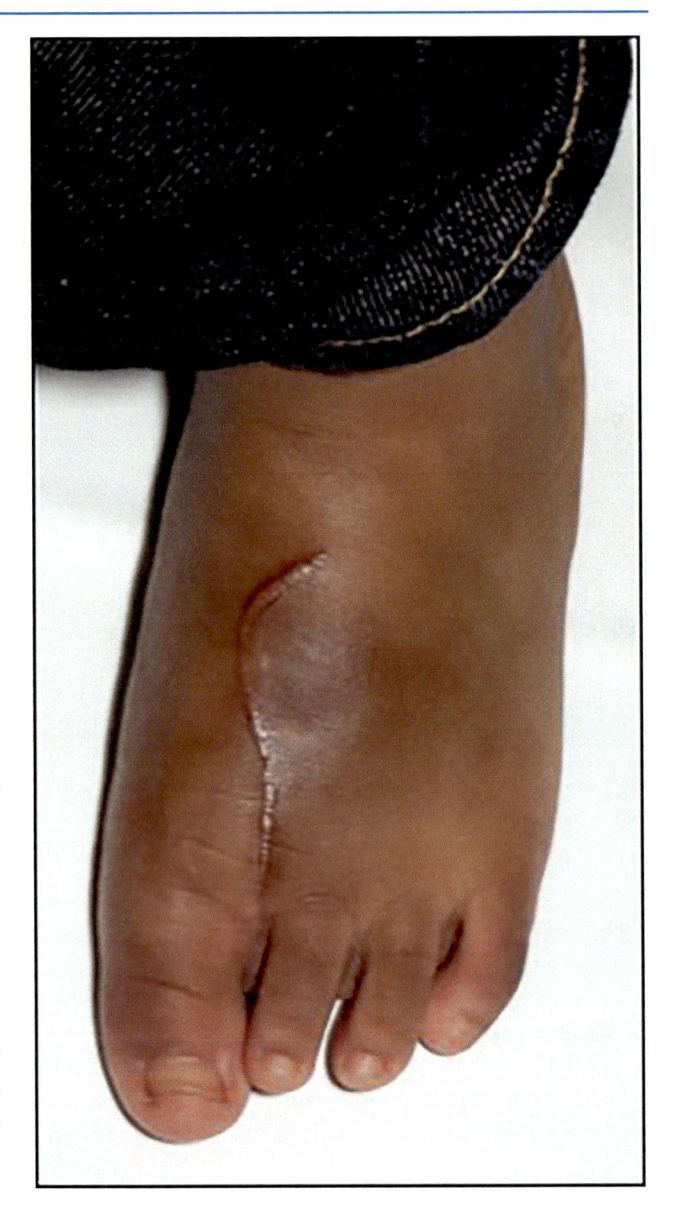

Fig. 43.12 Second toe donor site after unilateral second toe transfer—note the clinodactyly of remaining toes

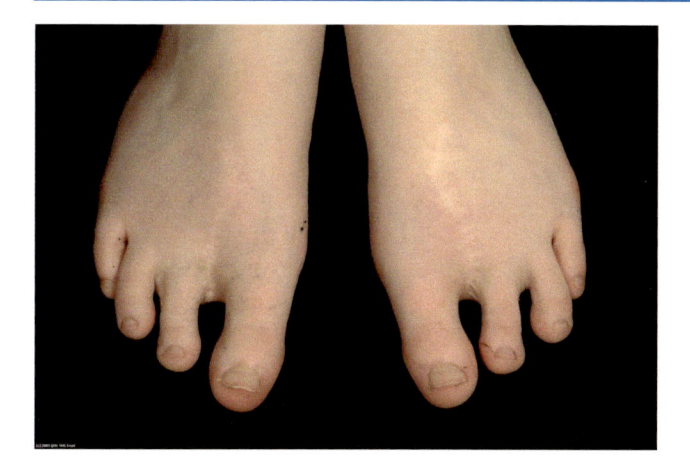

Fig. 43.13 Donor site after bilateral second toe transfer

43.7 Clinical Scenario

43.7.1 Case Scenario A: Congenital Hand—Symbrachydactyly—Surgeon Mark Pickford

A 4-year-old boy presented with monodactylous symbrachydactyly. After discussion with his parents they opted for a second toe transfer to provide large grasp and opposition. A second toe transfer was performed without complication. At 3-year follow-up the child was able to grasp and had a static 2 point discrimination of 5 mm (Figs. 43.14 and 43.15).

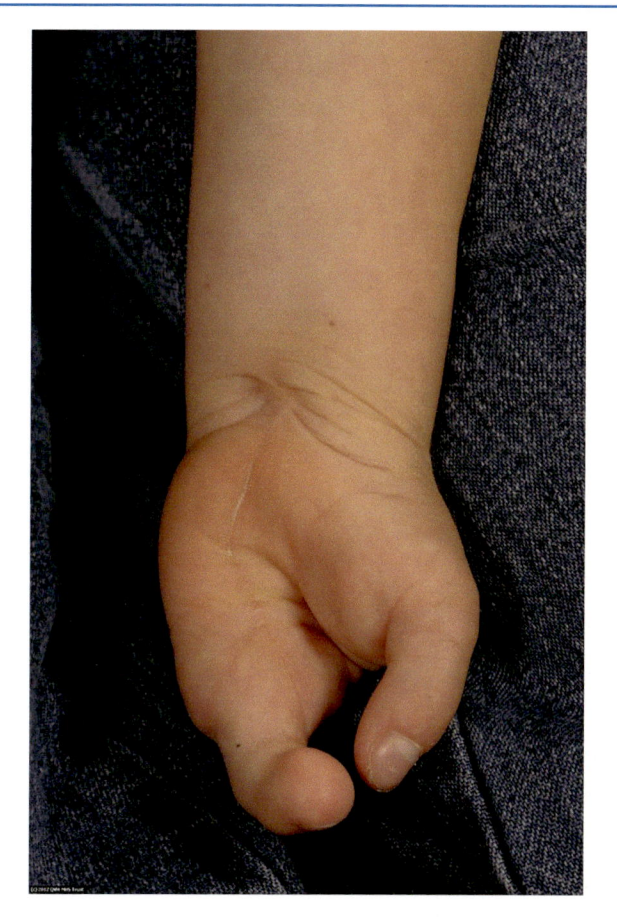

Fig. 43.14 Long-term outcome after second toe transfer for monodactylous symbrachydactyly

43.7.2 Case Scenario B: Traumatic Injury to the Hand—Surgeon Mark Pickford

A 45-year-old patient sustained a grenade injury to his left hand. He sustained a near total amputation of his non-dominant thumb, leaving part of his first metacarpal. In the first stage he had a pedicled posterior interosseous artery (PIA) flap imported into the first webspace. A second toe flap was raised and anastomosed to the anatomical snuff box with a bridging vein graft. He had an uneventful recovery (Figs. 43.16, 43.17, and 43.18).

43.7.3 Case Scenario C: Firework Injury to Hand—Surgeon Petr Vondra

A 15-year-old male sustained a devastating firework injury to his hand. The primary treatment was debridement and wound closure. The patient sustained complete loss of the first ray—only part of the trapezium remained, and only parts of the second to fourth metacarpal bones remained. From the fifth ray remained a well functional metacarpophalangeal joint and proximal phalanx of little finger (Fig. 43.19).

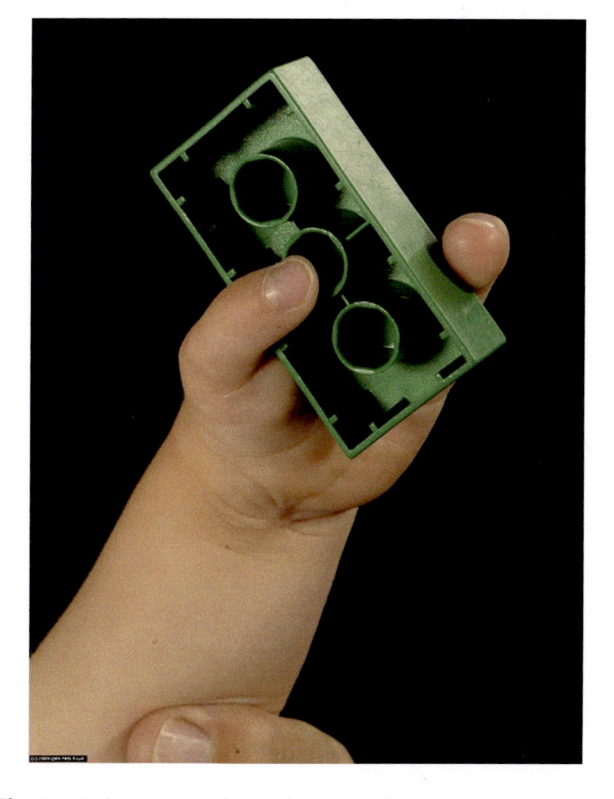

Fig. 43.15 Large grasp showed in same patient

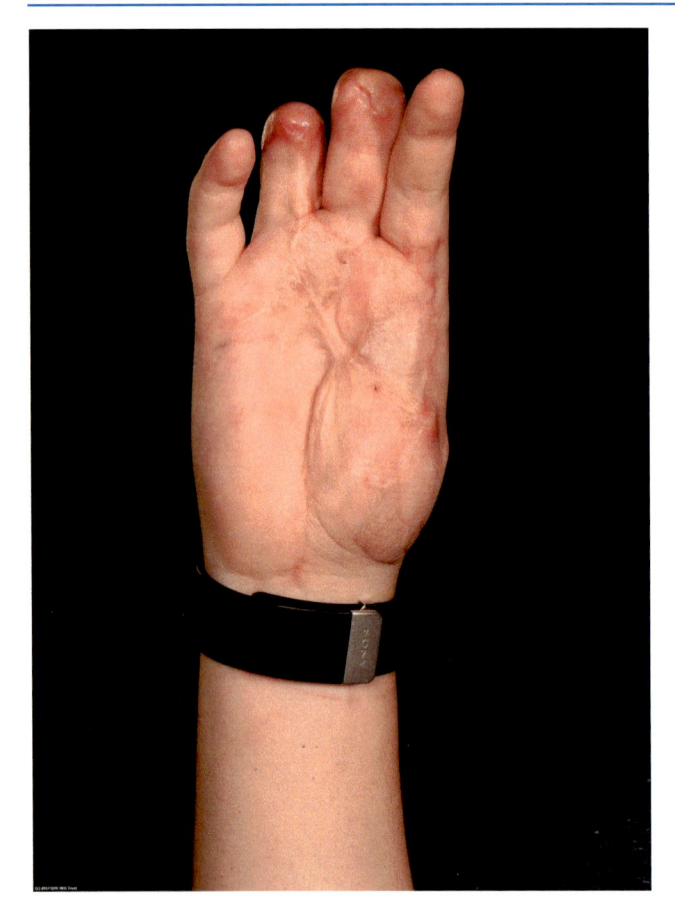

Fig. 43.16 Traumatic amputation of thumb secondary to a grenade blast

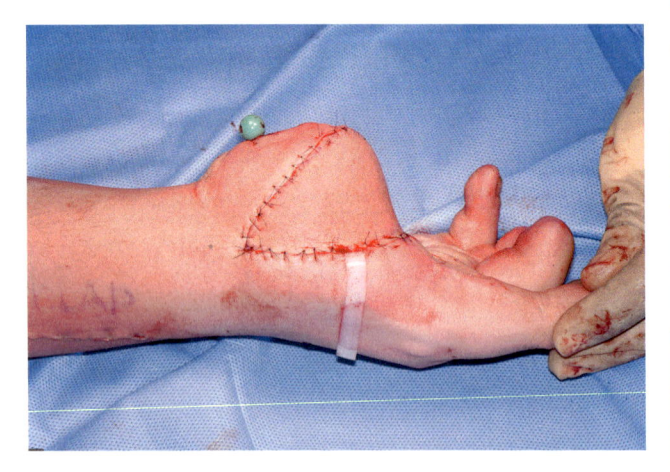

Fig. 43.17 First webspace in same patient is optimised with a PIA flap in anticipation for a second to transfer

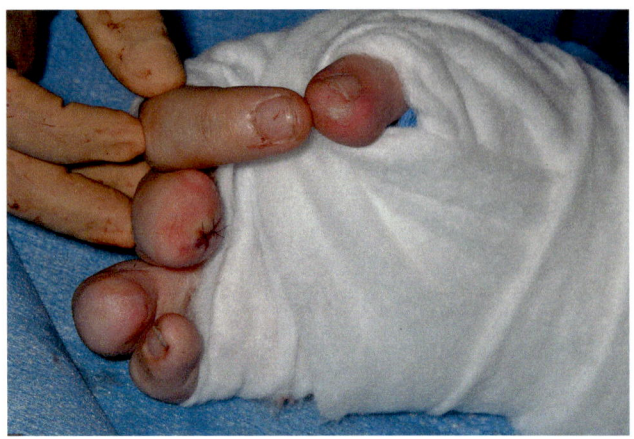

Fig. 43.18 On table result after second toe transfer to restore thumb opposition

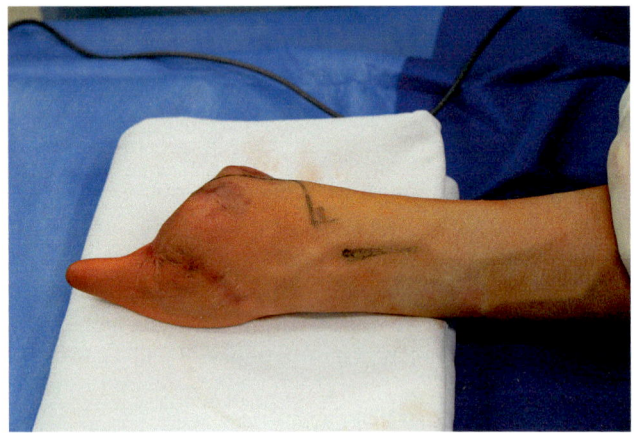

Fig. 43.19 Pre-op demonstrating intact fifth ray

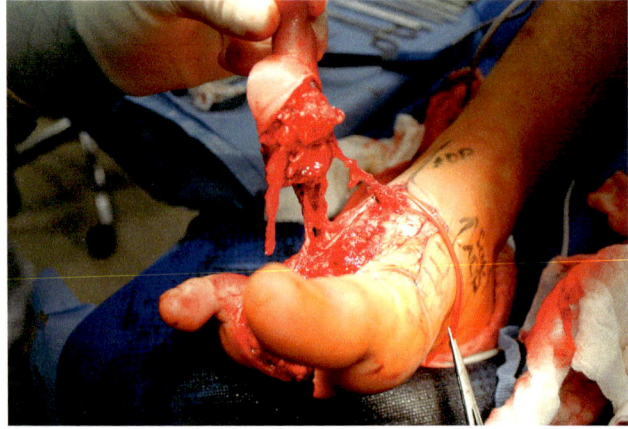

Fig. 43.20 Elevation of second toe

The patient underwent second toe to "thumb" microvascular reconstruction (Fig. 43.20). He regained sensation and movement and had an excellent donor site outcome (Fig. 43.21), but his webspace was too tight and he subsequently underwent a pedicled PIA flap for widening 6 months from toe to hand reconstruction. The final photos demonstrate good pinch at 1-year follow-up. (Fig. 43.22).

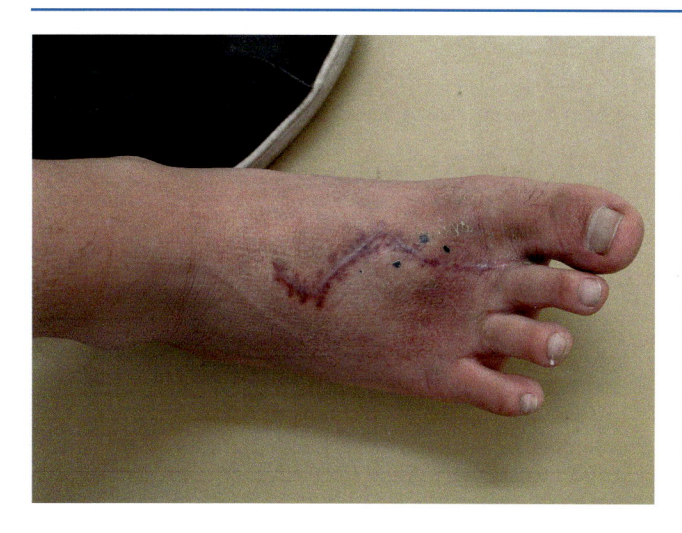

Fig. 43.21 Donor site outcome

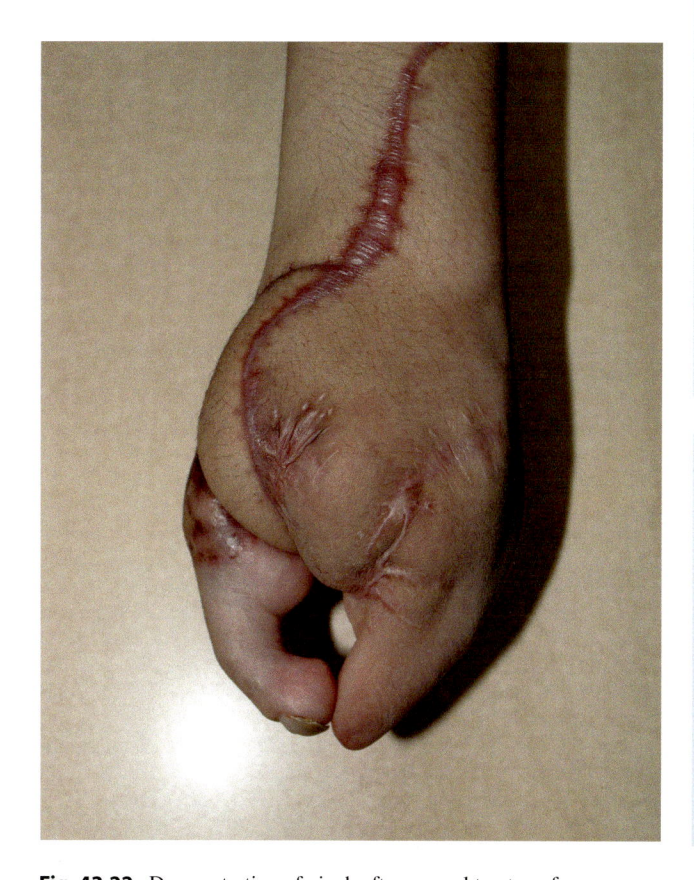

Fig. 43.22 Demonstration of pinch after second toe transfer

43.8 Pearls and Pitfalls

Pearls

- When incising the plantar triangle of skin one must leave most of the plantar fat on the foot, transferring the subcutaneous fat will make inset difficult. This will reduce bulk and allow for better joint motion in the reconstructed thumb.
- During osteosynthesis, protect the neurovascular structures with an aperture made in a glove, or a moist gauze wrap. This retracts back the soft tissues and protects them from iatrogenic injury.
- Perform the microsurgical anastomosis proximally on reliable, large-calibre vessels at the wrist (for thumb reconstruction), particularly in cases where is there is aberrant anatomy or unreliable proximal flow. Our preference is to use a posterior wall anastomosis in end-to-end arterial and venous repair.
- Neuromas can help identify the proximal ends of digital nerves at the recipient site; these are resected under the microscope prior to neurroraphy.
- After traumatic thumb amputations it may be necessary to prepare for second toe transfer by initially optimizing the first web, for example, using a PIA flap or a free groin flap.

Pitfalls

- During second toe inset it is important not to close the skin tightly; if necessary apply split thickness skin grafts over areas (including the pedicle) if there is skin shortage.
- Ensure that as many cutaneous nerves are repaired with a tensionless nerve repair; nerve grafts may be used to bridge the segmental gaps.
- Avoid tight dressings and a so-called bloodcast, which can impair flap circulation.

- In congenital cases we wait till the age of 2–3 years, or later, as the vessels are larger calibre and microsurgical anastomoses are easier.
- Keep the patient warm and well hydrated and pain-free to avoid possible vasospasm. A sympathetic blockade provided by a supraclavicular or axillary block will help with peripheral vasodilation.

43.9 Selected Readings

- Tsai TY, Fries CA, Hsiao JC, et al. Patient-reported outcome measures for toe-to-hand transfer: a prospective longitudinal study. Plast Reconstr Surg. 2019;143(4):1122–32.
  Prospective patient-reported outcomes study including 23 patients. All the operated individuals reported an important increase in hand function, with no deterioration of foot function [6].
- Nikkhah D, Martin N, Pickford M. Paediatric toe-to-hand transfer: an assessment of outcomes from a single unit. J Hand Surg Eur Vol. 2016;41(3):281–94.
  Study demonstrating the technical aspects and outcomes of 31 second toe transfers in 19 children. The paper demonstrated excellent long-term motor and sensory outcomes (S2PD = 5 mm) and no failures [7].
- Sosin M, Lin CH, Steinberg J, et al. Functional donor site morbidity after vascularized toe transfer procedures: a review of the literature and biomechanical consideration for surgical site selection. Ann Plast Surg. 2016;76(6):735–42.
  Systematic review of donor site morbidity following toe transfer procedures [8].
- Zhao J, Tien HY, Abdullah S, Zhang Z. Aesthetic refinements in second toe-to-thumb transfer surgery. Plast Reconstr Surg. 2010;126(6):2052–9.
  This article presents modifications to the second toe transfer to improve its cosmetic appearance for thumb reconstruction [9].
- Kay SP, Wiberg M. Toe to hand transfer in children. Part 1: technical aspects. J Hand Surg Br. 1996;21(6):723–34.
- Kay SP, Wiberg M, Bellew M, Webb F. Toe to hand transfer in children. Part 2: functional and psychological aspects. J Hand Surg Br. 1996;21:735–45.
  This is a two-part article reviewing technical aspects of paediatric toe to thumb transfer and its functional and psychological benefits [10, 11].

References

1. Haeseker B. 1891-1991: the centenary of innovative reconstructive hand surgery by Carl Nicoladoni. Br J Plast Surg. 1991;44:306–9.
2. Buncke HJ Jr, Buncke CM, Schulz WP. Immediate Nicoladoni procedure in the Rhesus monkey, or hallux-to-hand transplantation, utilising microminiature vascular anastomoses. Br J Plast Surg. 1966;19:332–7.
3. Whitworthm IH, Pickford MA. The first toe-to-hand transfer: a thirty-year follow-up. J Hand Surg Br. 2000;25:608–10.
4. Henry SL, Wei F-C. Thumb reconstruction with toe transfer. J Hand Microsurg. 2010;2:72–8.
5. Spanio S, Wei F-C, Coskunfirat OK, Lin C-H, Lin Y-T. Symmetry of vascular pedicle anatomy in the first web space of the foot related to toe harvest: clinical observations in 85 simultaneous bilateral second-toe transfer patients. Plast Reconstr Surg. 2005;115:1325–7.
6. Tsai T-Y, Fries CA, Hsiao J-C, Hsu C-C, Lin Y-T, Chen S-H, Lin C-H, Wei F-C, Lin C-H. Patient-reported outcome measures for toe-to-hand transfer: a prospective longitudinal study. Plast Reconstr Surg. 2019;143:1122–32.
7. Nikkhah D, Martin N, Pickford M. Paediatric toe-to-hand transfer: an assessment of outcomes from a single unit. J Hand Surg Eur. 2016;41:281–94.
8. Sosin M, Lin C-H, Steinberg J, Hammond ER, Poysophon P, Iorio ML, Patel KM. Functional donor site morbidity after vascularized toe transfer procedures: a review of the literature and biomechanical consideration for surgical site selection. Ann Plast Surg. 2016;76:735–42.
9. Zhao J, Tien HY, Abdullah S, Zhang Z. Aesthetic refinements in second toe-to-thumb transfer surgery. Plast Reconstr Surg. 2010;126:2052–9.
10. Kay SP, Wiberg M. Toe to hand transfer in children. Part 1: technical aspects. J Hand Surg Br. 1996;21:723–34.
11. Kay SP, Wiberg M, Bellew M, Webb F. Toe to hand transfer in children. Part 2: functional and psychological aspects. J Hand Surg Br. 1996;21:735–45.

Great Toe Flaps

Dariush Nikkhah and Norbert Kang

44.1 Introduction

The great toe-to-thumb transplant was first reported in the Western literature by Cobbett; this case was followed up three decades later demonstrating an excellent outcome [1, 2]. 'Great toes make great thumbs' a term coined by Harry Buncke; however at the cost of donor morbidity [3]. Surgeons have over the years refined the great toe flap to improve on its appearance and also to reduce the donor site morbidity. Morrison described the 'Wrap-around flap' which involved transferring the soft tissue components and leaving behind the bony skeleton of the great toe minimising donor morbidity [4]. Fu Chan Wei refined the appearance of the great toe transfer by resecting the soft tissue and bony component of the tibial border of the great toe; the so-called trimmed toe flap [5]. The great toe pulp can also be transferred for volar oblique defects of the thumb, providing like for like reconstruction of the pulp with glabrous tissue.

The second toe-to-thumb transplant is more popular in Asian cultures owing to its reduced donor site morbidity. It is more commonly used in children with congenital differences; however, its small bulbous appearing pulp makes it hard to replicate a thumb. The ideal indication for a great toe transfer is traumatic loss of the thumb through the proximal phalanx with the toe-transplant reconstructing the interphalangeal joint of thumb. The more proximal the amputation the more challenging the reconstruction and if the amputation is proximal to the metacarpophalangeal joint; the metatarsophalangeal joint can be harvested in the great toe transplant but at the cost of donor site morbidity.

44.2 Anatomy

The great toe is supplied by the plantar and dorsal metatarsal arterial systems and drained by superficial veins which connect with the saphenous system [6]. The first dorsal metatarsal artery originates from the dorsalis pedis and courses either superficially or through the interosseous muscles. The vessel gives off branches to the metatarsals, muscles and joints. Between the great and second toe the dorsal metatarsal artery lies superficial to the deep transverse ligament. The first plantar metatarsal artery originates from the plantar arch and the deep plantar artery [6].

The dorsal system is the primary choice for the pedicle of the great toe owing to its superficial course and long pedicle. However in 10% of cases the dorsal system may be absent and the plantar system may need to be harvested as the primary pedicle, which has disadvantages of being significantly shorter and often needing lengthening with a vein graft. The anatomical variations of vasculature were described by Alain Gilbert in a study of 50 cadavers [7].

- **Types 1a and 1b** both metatarsal arteries arise independently—66% of cases: In type 1a the dorsal metatarsal artery passes superficially to the interosseous muscle, in Type 1b it passes through the first dorsal interosseous muscle.
- **Types 2a and 2b** 22% cases—In Type 2 cases the dorsal and plantar metatarsal arteries have a common trunk located under the first dorsal interosseous muscle (Inframuscular). In type 2a a slender superficial branch is present passing superficially to the muscle and uniting at the anterior part of the web space with the dorsal metatarsal artery. In contrast in type 2b the superficial arterial branch is not present.

Supplementary Information The online version contains supplementary material available at [https://doi.org/10.1007/978-3-031-07678-7_44].

D. Nikkhah (✉) · N. Kang
Royal Free Hospital, London, UK

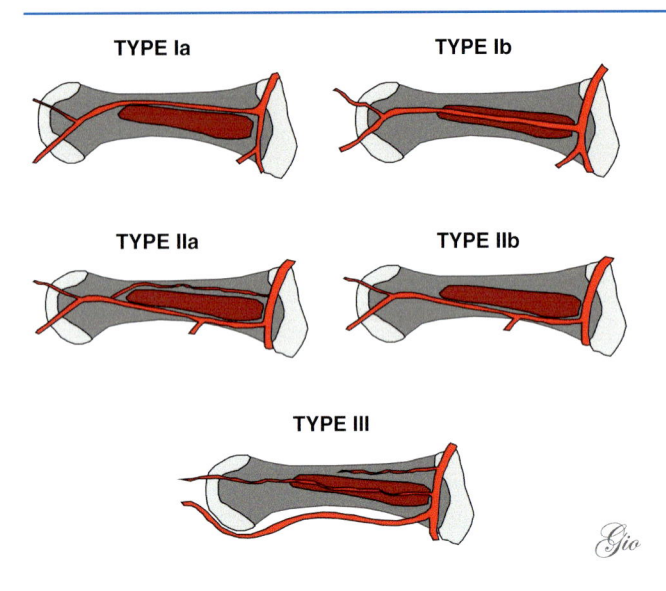

Fig. 44.1 Clinical illustration of the anatomical variations of great toe vasculature as described by Gilbert et al. Illustration courtesy of Dr Gio Pafitanis

- **Type 3** 12% cases: The first dorsal metatarsal artery (FDMA) is slender or absent. The first plantar metatarsal artery is well developed and the dominant circulation (Fig. 44.1).

44.3 Pre-operative Investigation

Pre-operative mapping with colour Doppler ultrasound can determine the course of the first dorsal metatarsal artery and whether it is absent. If this is not present, some groups use a hand-held Doppler to map out the course of the FDMA. A prominent signal would indicate a dorsal dominant system.

CT—angiogram has been described and would accurately indicate whether the great toe has a dorsal or plantar dominant circulation. Pre-operative investigations can help to determine if vein grafts will be needed in cases where there is a plantar dominant system.

44.4 Flap Design and Markings

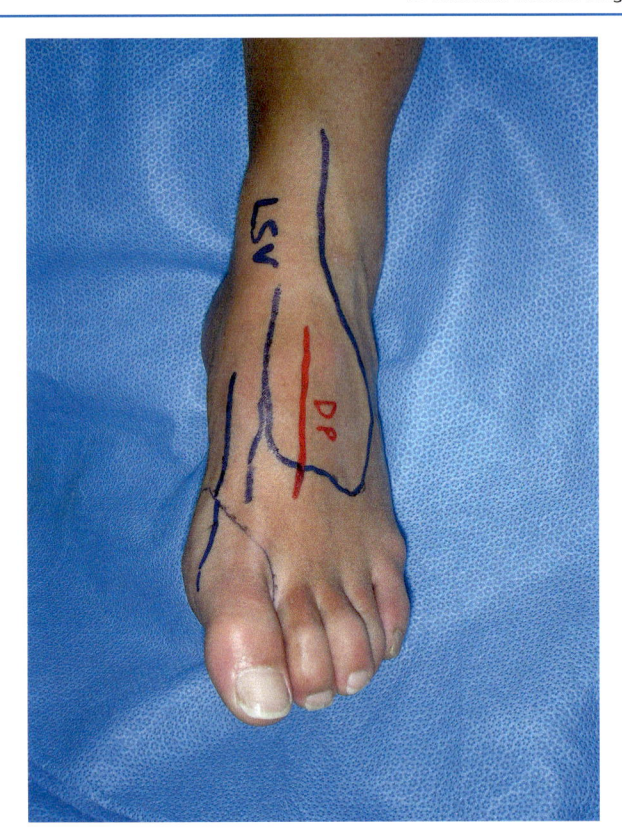

Great Toe Flap A racquet-shaped incision is made around the toe and a curvilinear incision is made proximally to the dorsalis pedis. Before tourniquet exsanguination the superficial veins are marked (Fig. 44.2).

Great Toe Pulp Transfer The lateral border of the great toe is marked, a curvilinear incision is marked proximally and an incision is marked on the plantar surface of the foot to harvest plantar vessels and nerves for transfer (Fig. 44.3).

We will illustrate the elevation and anatomy of the great toe flap using images from both case scenarios.

Fig. 44.2 A racquet-shaped incision is made around the toe and a curvilinear incision is made proximally to the dorsalis pedis. Before tourniquet exsanguination the superficial veins and long saphenous vein are marked

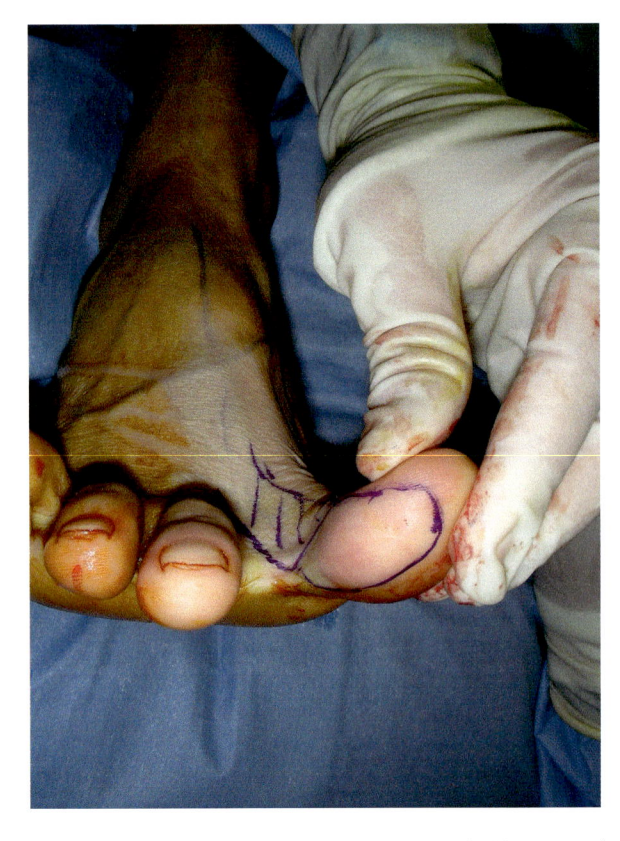

Fig. 44.3 The lateral border of the great toe is marked in preparation of a great toe pulp transfer

44.5 Flap Raise/Elevation: A Step-by-Step Guide

44.5.1 Great Toe Flap Elevation

- **Step 1 Incision and Approach:** The ipsilateral toe is used to reconstruct the thumb, the length of the toe is marked just proximal to the PIPJ (Fig. 44.4). Under tourniquet control the incision is started in the first webspace using a retrograde [8] or antegrade approach from the dorsalis pedis (Fig. 44.5).
- **Step 2 Venous Dissection:** The superficial veins over the dorsum of the foot that were marked are harvested, thin skin flaps should be raised. Multiple side branches from the superficial venous system should be ligaclipped (Figs. 44.6, 44.7, and 44.8). Fine microsurgical instruments should be used to dissect the vein to avoid damage.

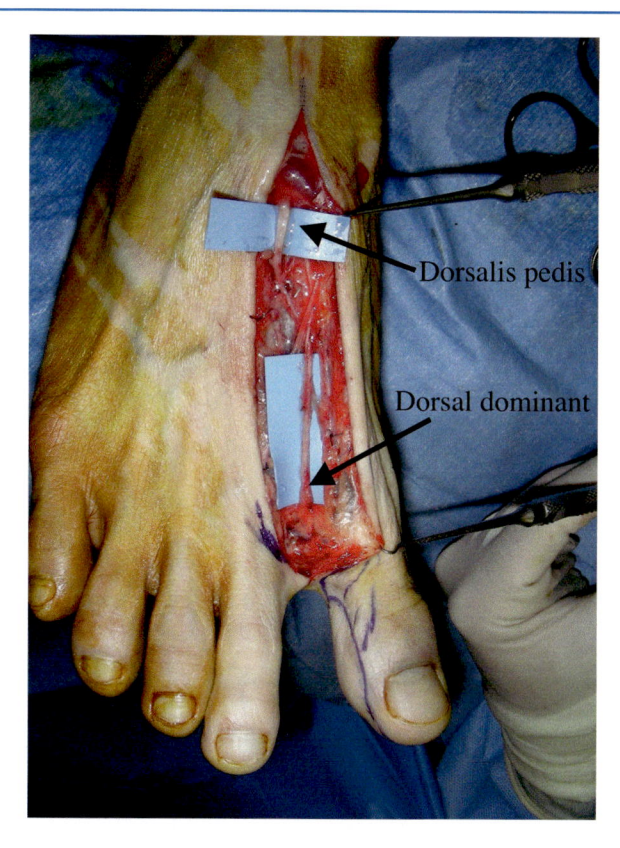

Fig. 44.5 Incision can be started retrograde in first webspace or antegrade from dorsalis pedis. The arrow demonstrates a dorsal dominant circulation emerging from the dorsalis pedis

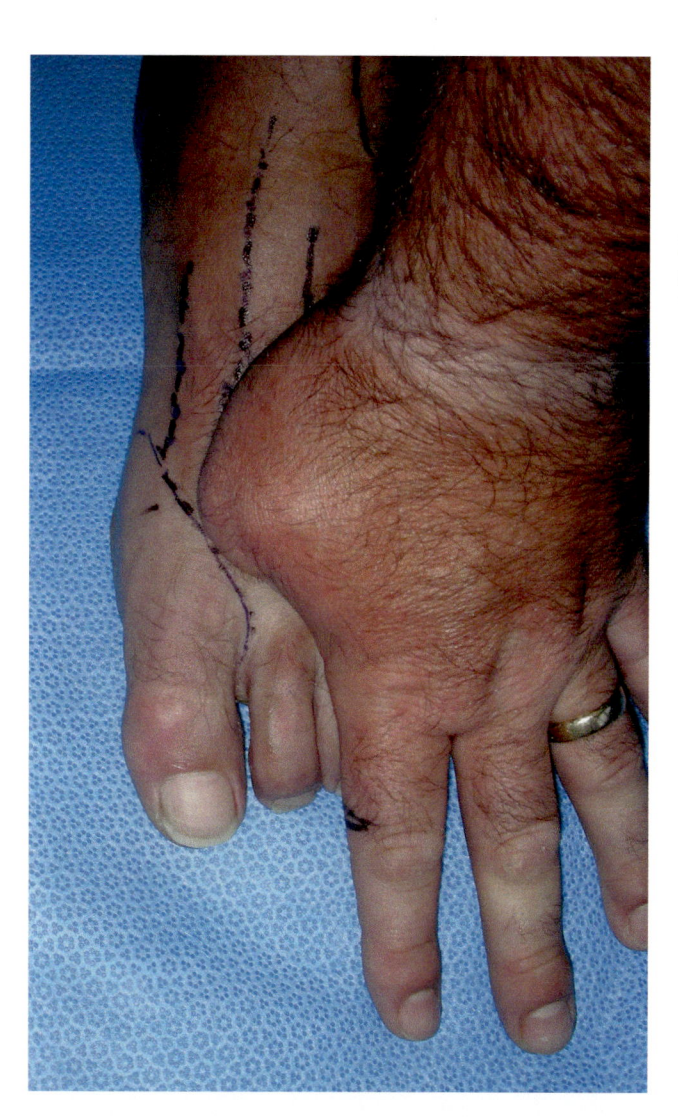

Fig. 44.4 The ipsilateral toe is used to reconstruct the thumb; the length of the toe is marked just proximal to the PIPJ

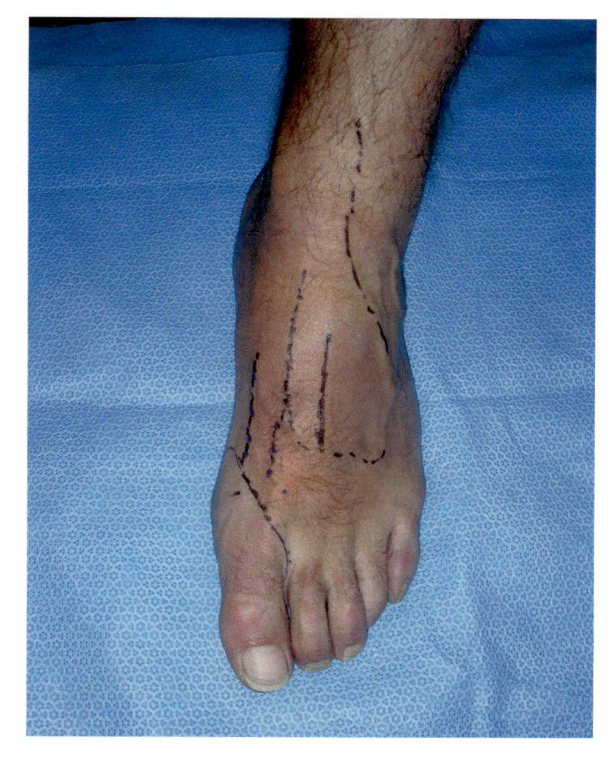

Fig. 44.6 Superficial veins are marked before exsanguination

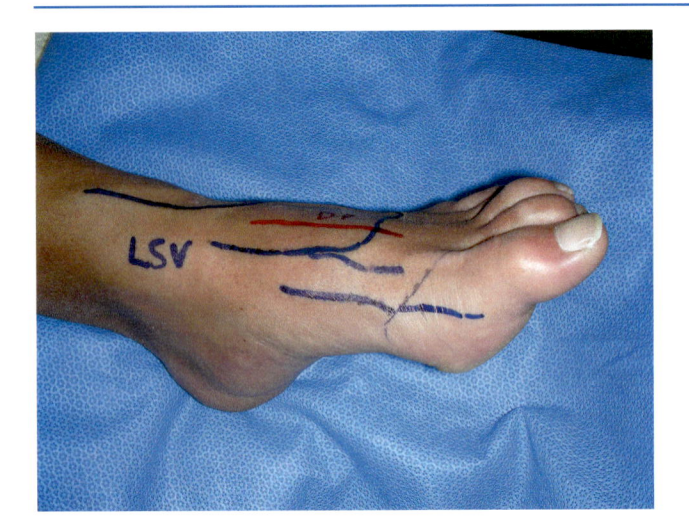

Fig. 44.7 Racquet-shaped incision over great toe with inclusion of long saphenous vein

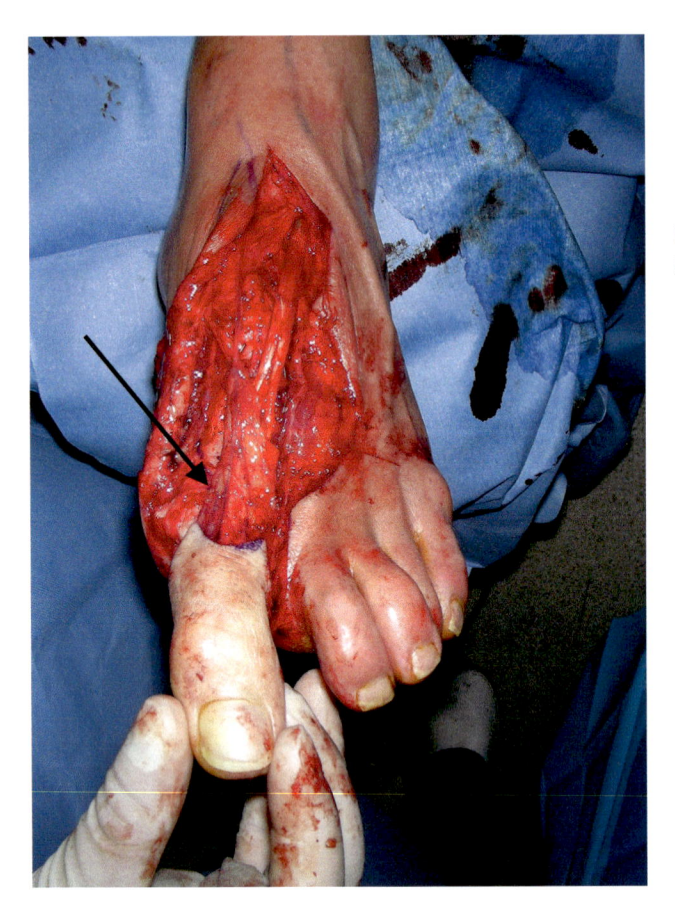

Fig. 44.8 Thin skin flaps are raised and all superficial veins (see arrows) are included, side branches are ligaclipped

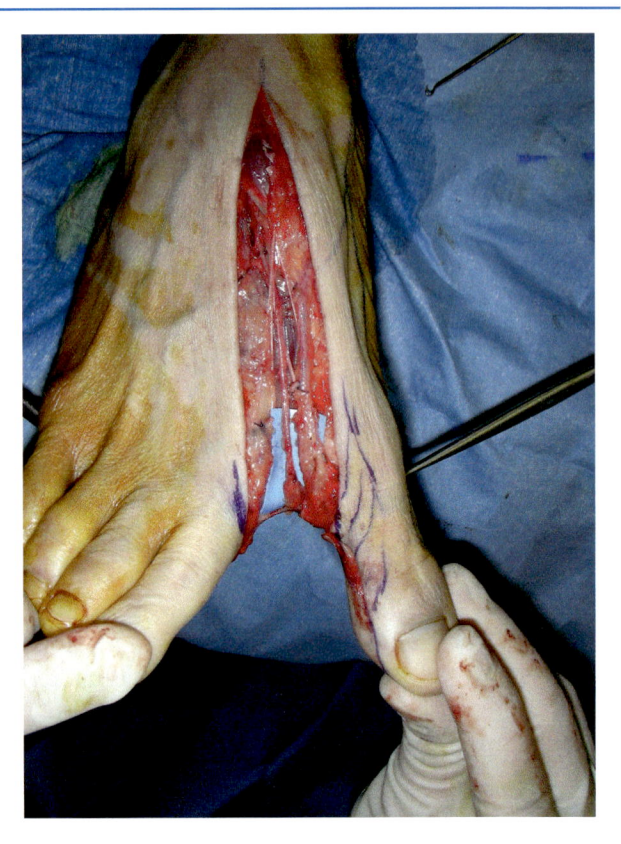

Fig. 44.9 If there is a dorsal system of adequate calibre, dissection proceeds along the first webspace

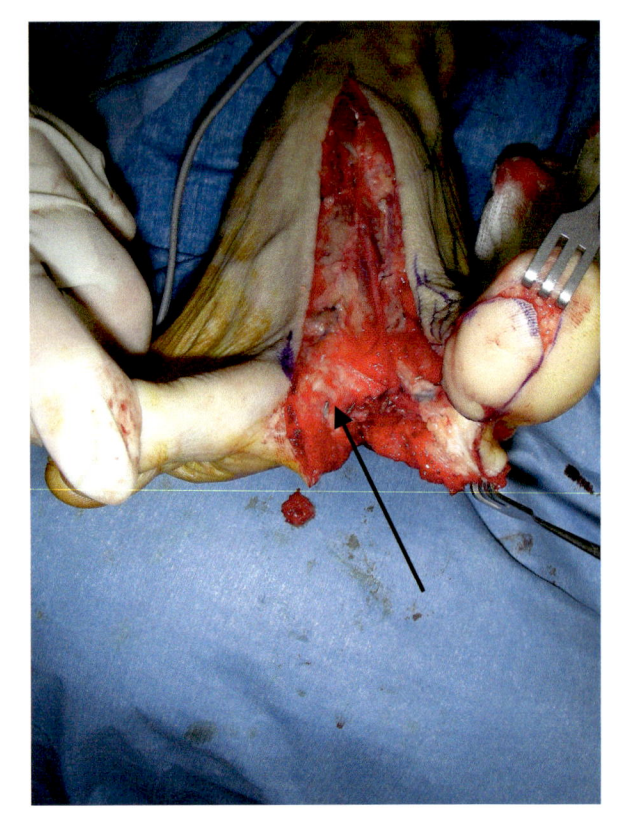

Fig. 44.10 The dorsal branch supplying the second toe is clipped off (arrow) and dissection continues to the dorsalis pedis

- **Step 3 Arterial Dissection:** If there is a dorsal system of adequate calibre, dissection proceeds along the first webspace, the dorsal branch supplying the second toe is clipped off and dissection continues to the dorsalis pedis (Figs. 44.9 and 44.10). Dissection is performed with bipolar cautery at a low setting. The dorsalis pedis is identified under the extensor hallucis brevis tendon which is divided. The dorsal peroneal nerve is identified. If there is no sufficient dorsal system the plantar arterial system is taken and a longitudinal incision is made over the plantar aspect of the foot. The medial and lateral plantar digital nerves are taken.

- **Step 4 Tendon Division and Disarticulation:** The extensor hallucis longus and flexor hallucis longus tendon are divided, taking sufficient length for tenoraphy at recipient site using Pulvertaft Weaves (Figs. 44.11 and 44.12). Once the arterial and venous drainage to the great toe is dissected free. The great toe is disarticulated at the metatarsophalangeal joint. Plantar digital nerves and the dorsal nerves are tagged with 6.0 nylon and divided—as many sensory nerves are taken for neurorraphy as possible. The tourniquet is then released assessing circulation to the toe.
- **Step 5 Recipient Vessels:** Preparing the recipient site for the great toe transfer should ideally be with a two-team approach. A second surgeon prepares the recipient artery and vein in the hand. In this case the radial artery in the snuff box or the wrist can be prepared (Figs. 44.13 and 44.14).
- **Step 6 Divide Pedicle:** After a sufficient length of pedicle is harvested, this is double checked at the recipient site with a ruler to see if it reaches and whether a vein graft is required. The veins and the arteries are clipped off and microsurgical clamps are placed in preparation for microsurgery. The nerves are also divided, and tagged with

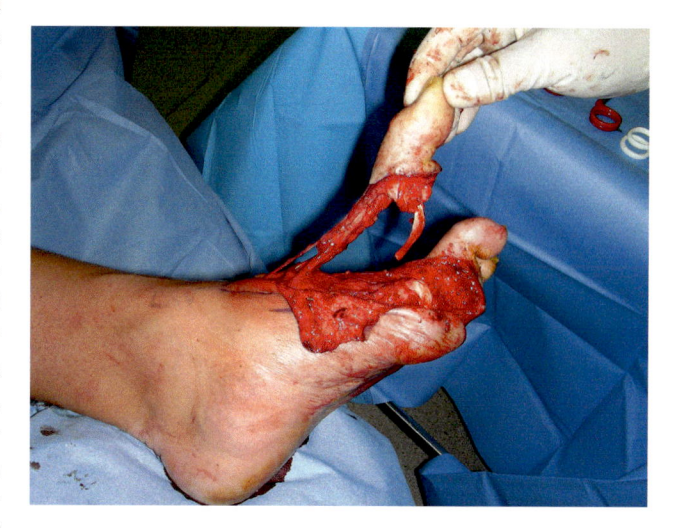

Fig. 44.12 The extensor hallucis longus and flexor hallucis longus tendon are divided—the toe remains attached by neurovascular structures

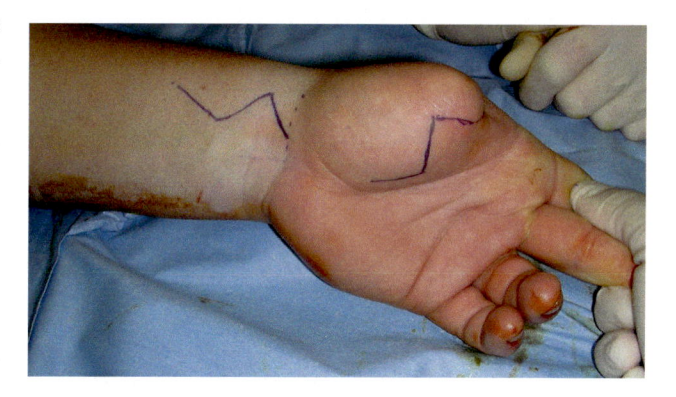

Fig. 44.13 Markings for preparing the recipient site for the great toe transfer; access incisions for the radial artery at the wrist are marked

Fig. 44.11 The great toe is disarticulated from the metatarsophalangeal joint

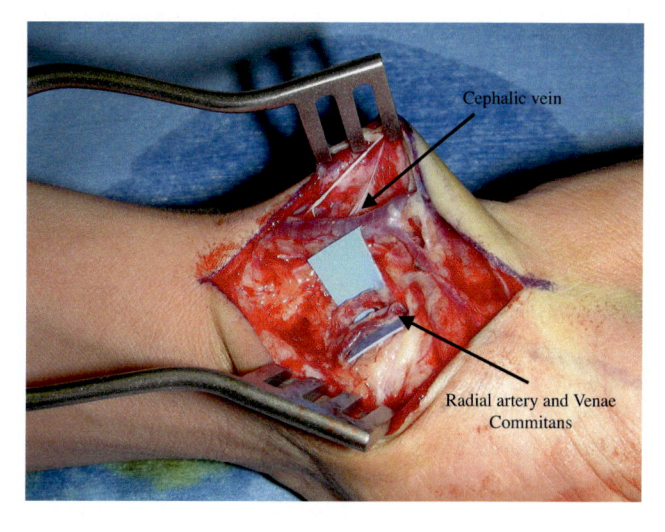

Fig. 44.14 The radial artery in snuff box with associated vena comitans (arrow). The cephalic vein is also prepared in the picture (arrow)

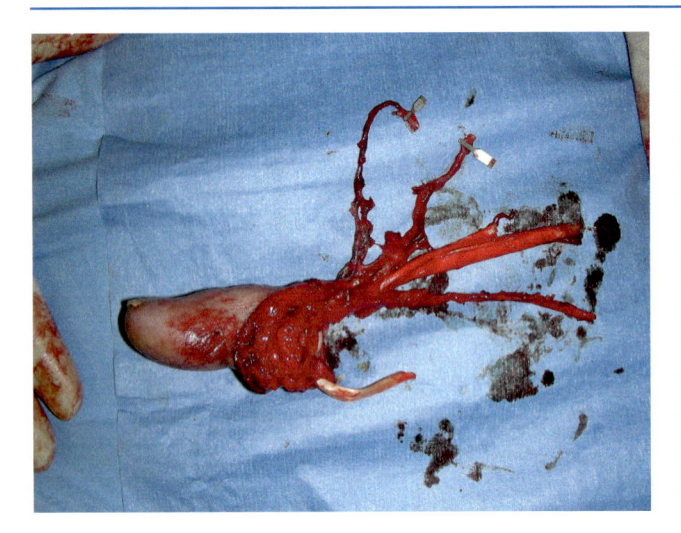

Fig. 44.15 Great toe divided and all structures marked for transfer. The vein and artery are clipped with microsurgical clamps in preparation for transfer

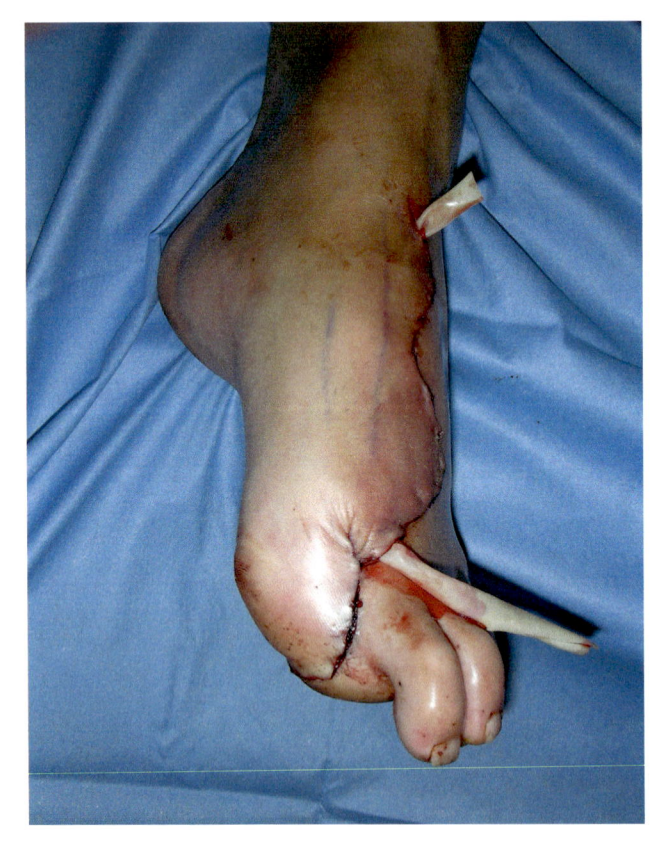

Fig. 44.16 Donor site closure ensuring padding over the metatarsophalangeal joint

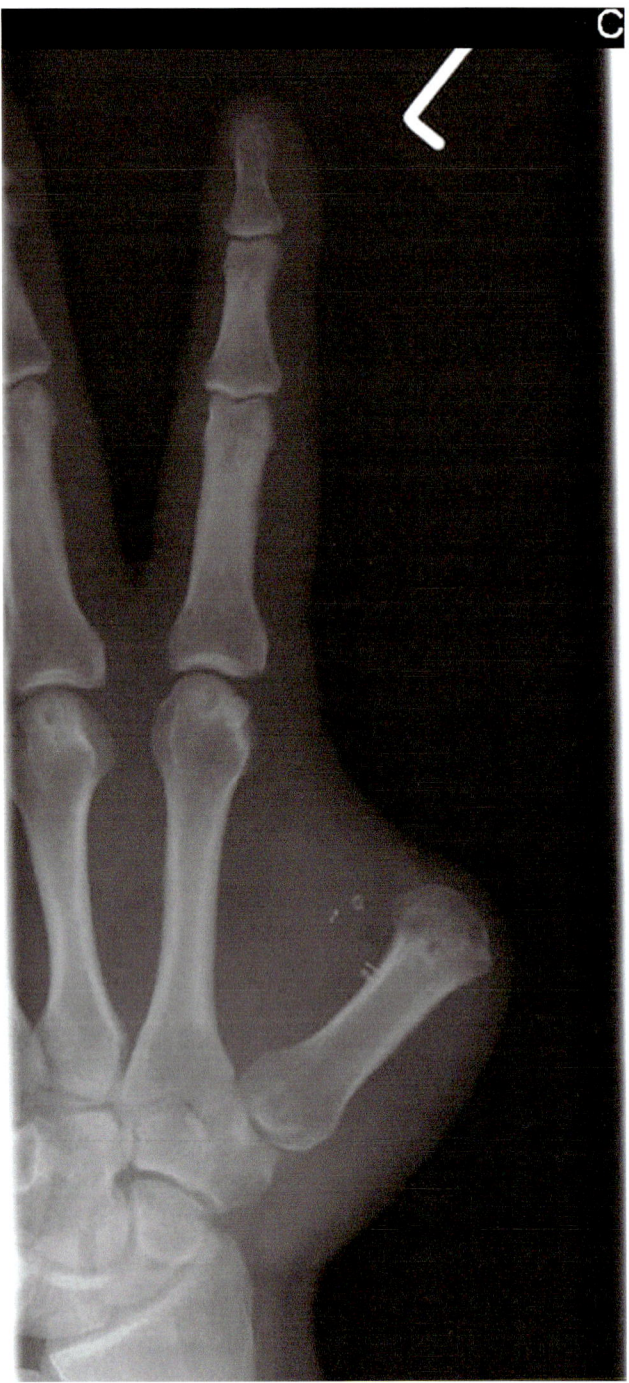

Fig. 44.17 Radiograph of recipient site, showing amputation through first metacarpal bone

either microsuture or blue dye for easy identification (Fig. 44.15).
- **Step 7 Donor Site Closure:** The donor site is closed in layers using 3.0 monocryl, ensuring there is enough padding over the metatarsal head which is preserved (Fig. 44.16).
- **Step 8 Osteosynthesis:** The recipient bone (Fig. 44.17) is prepared with an oscillating saw; the cartilaginous surface of the great toe is removed with an oscillating saw. Drill holes are made for interosseous wires, two can be used in parallel or at 90°. Another option is a lister loop with single Kirschner wire or a plate as illustrated in this case (Fig. 44.18).
- **Step 9 Tenorraphy and Neurorrhaphy**: After identification with a wide exposure at the recipient site (Fig. 44.19), both the extensor pollicus longus and flexor pollicus longus tendons are repaired with Pulvertaft weaves and 3.0

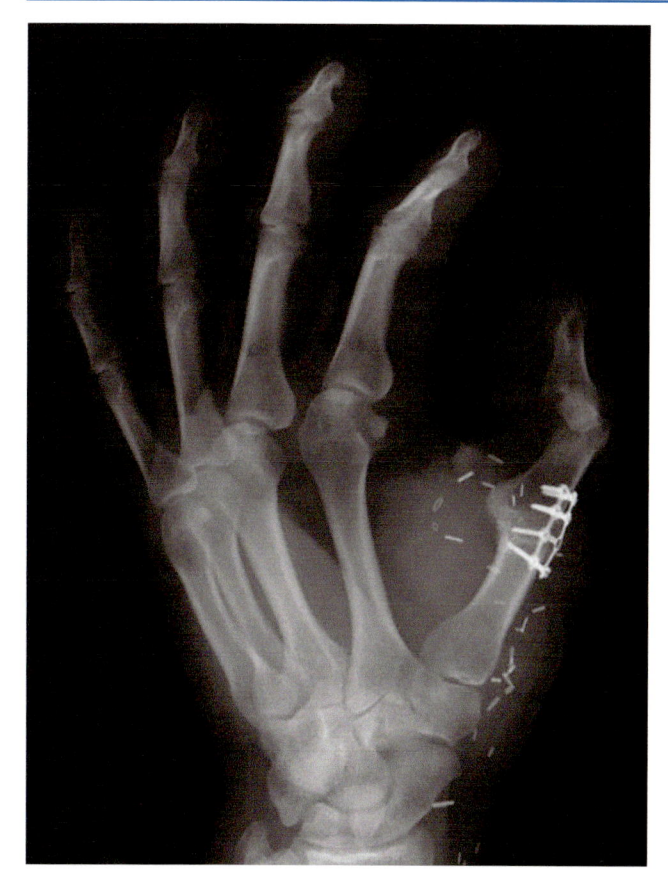

Fig. 44.18 Great toe osteosynthesis with plate fixation

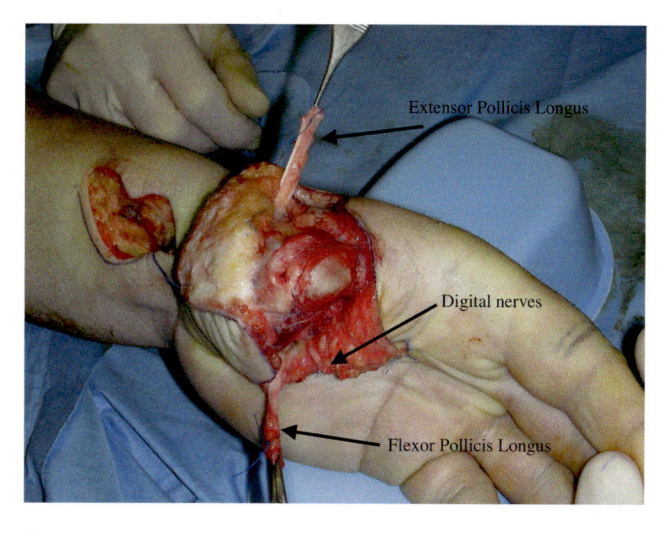

Fig. 44.19 The extensor pollicus longus and flexor pollicus longus are tagged and marked with 4.0 Prolene (arrows). The digital nerves are tagged with 8.0 nylon (arrow)

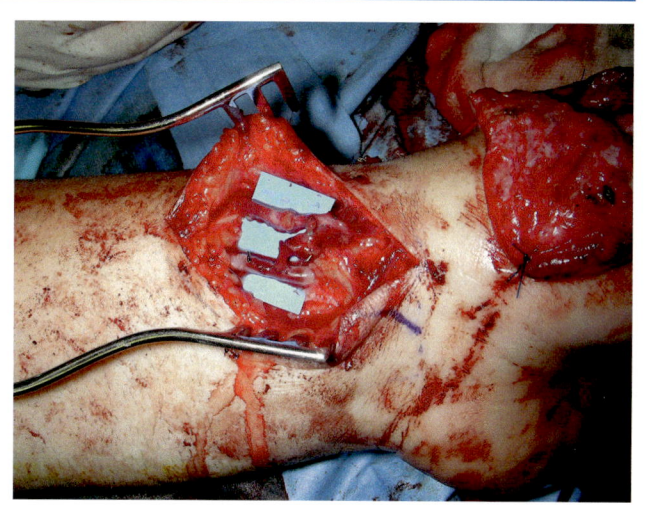

Fig. 44.20 The veins are anastomosed end to end. The arterial anastomosis is completed as an end to side anastomosis to the radial artery at the wrist

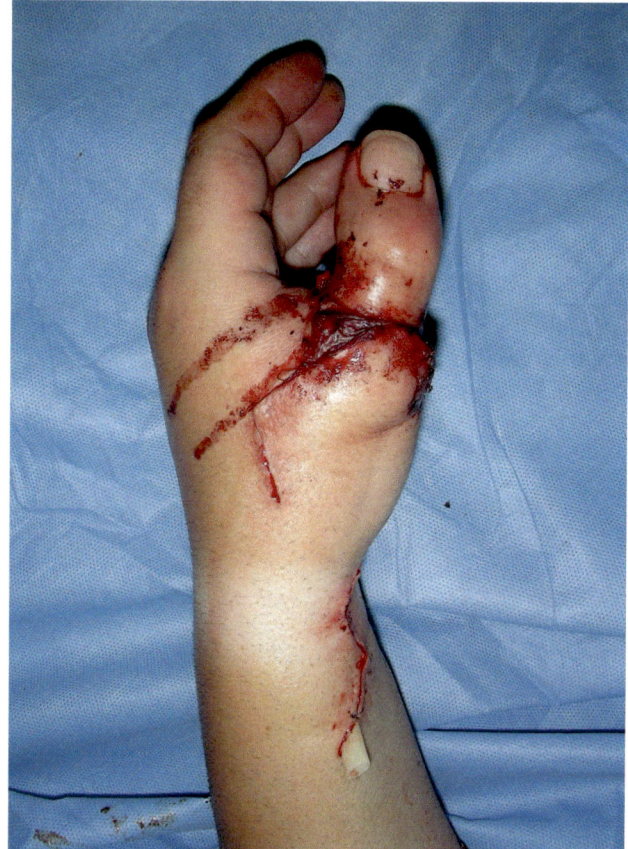

Fig. 44.21 Great toe is inset, skin grafts are applied over areas of tight closure

PDS suture. The plantar digital nerves and dorsal nerves are repaired under the microscope with 8.0 Nylon.

- **Step 10 Microsurgical Anastomosis and Inset**: The veins are repaired first using single clamps and a posterior wall technique using 9.0 Nylon (Fig. 44.20). The arterial anastomosis is completed in the same fashion after checking adequate inflow from the proximal artery, in this case an end to side anastomosis was performed to the radial artery at the wrist (Fig. 44.20). Skin closure is completed once circulation to the toe is sufficient. Skin grafts can cover areas where primary closure is not possible or tight closure would cause pedicle compression (Fig. 44.21).

44.6 Core Surgical Techniques in Flap Dissection

Arterial Anatomy Flap dissection during harvest of the great toe is best done with a retrograde approach unless there is certainty that there is a dorsal dominant circulation on pre-operative imaging. In 70% of cases, two sizeable vessels proceed in the first webspace in both the dorsal and plantar direction. The size of these vessels varies and dorsal vessel may traverse through the interosseous muscle. In 30% of cases, the plantar vessel is the more sizeable than the dorsal artery, which is either small or absent [9].

If both vessels (plantar and dorsal) have the same calibre, it is prudent to ligate the plantar system and take the dorsal system since dissection is easier and also it provides a longer pedicle (Fig. 44.22).

If the plantar dominance is identified and dissection proceeds, this can be destructive to the foot [9]. It is better to lengthen the pedicle in this scenario with a vein graft. The vein graft can be attached under the microscope to the plantar artery on a side table before toe inset. Some feel this technique obviates the need for CT angiogram or imaging; however, in our experience it is prudent to use all modalities to plan toe transfer.

Recipient Vessels Pedicle length is quickly judged after recipient vessel preparation, in traumatic cases it may be necessary to dissect out of the zone of trauma to the radial artery in the snuff box (Fig. 44.23).

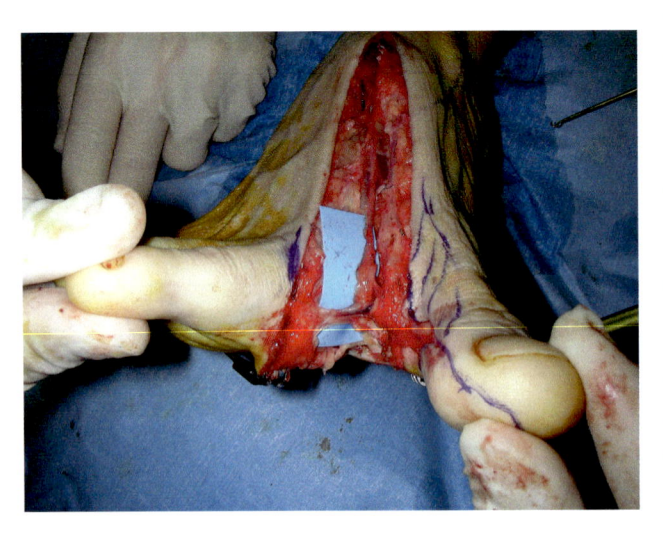

Fig. 44.22 Demonstration of a dorsal dominant system identified through dissection in the first webspace

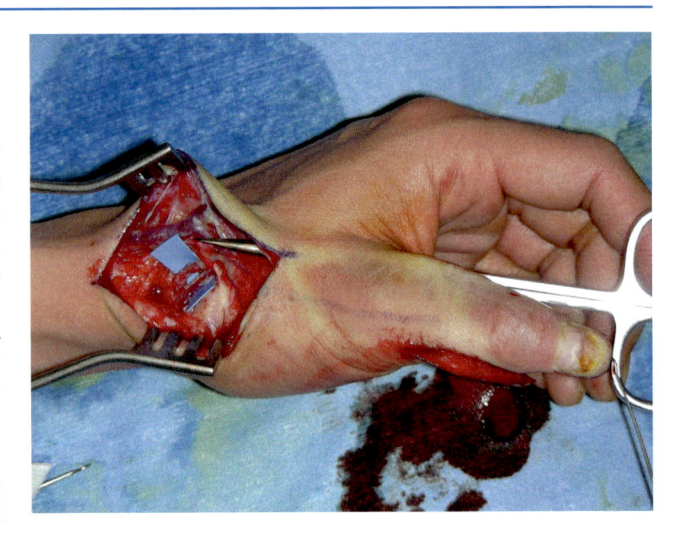

Fig. 44.23 As demonstrated here it is best to have large calibre recipient vessels in snuff box or wrist outside of the zone of injury or trauma

Instrumentation The vessels supplying the great toe are fragile and easily at risk of traction injury. Microsurgical instruments should be used to handle the veins and arteries and side branches should be ligaclipped to avoid thermal injury to pedicle. Bipolar cautery should be used carefully on a low setting and heat sink bipolar techniques should be utilised during side branch ligation.

Nerves If possible as many nerves should be harvested and repaired to improve sensory recovery. In children, toe transfer is associated with excellent static 2 point discrimination of 5 mm [10]. Adults are also expected to get acceptable sensory recovery of up to 10 mm static 2 point discrimination.

Veins Harvesting at least two veins reduces the chances of venous congestion, and the authors commonly perform a second venous anastomosis if there is a suitable calibre vein.

44.7 Clinical Scenario

44.7.1 Scenario A: Delayed Great Toe Flap Surgeon Norbert Kang

Patient A had oncological resection of his left thumb to the level of the MCPJ secondary to sarcoma (Fig. 44.24). A great toe transfer was performed to reconstruct the thumb, parts of the case are illustrated in the stepwise images for this chapter. His result at 4 years demonstrates excellent range of motion, sensibility and restoration of opposition (Fig. 44.25 and Videos 44.1 and 44.2) and an acceptable donor site morbidity (Fig. 44.26).

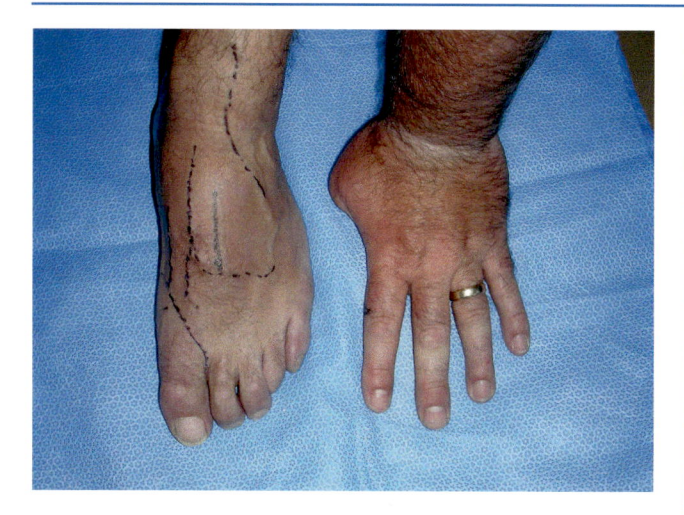

Fig. 44.24 This patient had oncological resection of his left thumb to the level of the MCPJ secondary to sarcoma. A great toe transfer was planned for reconstruction

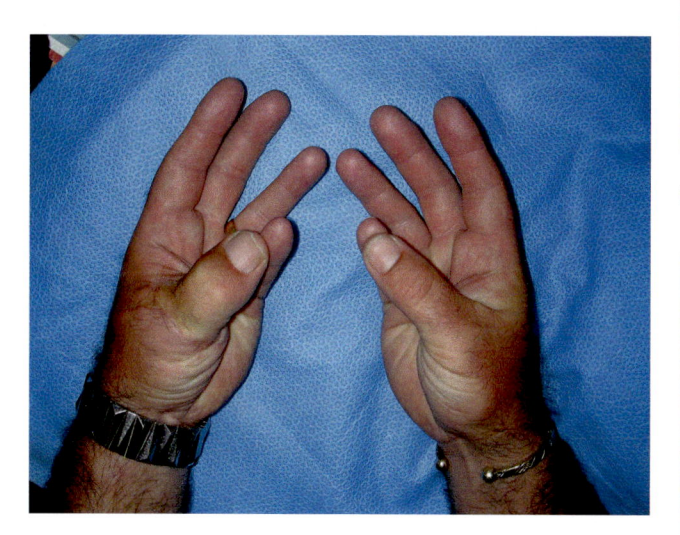

Fig. 44.25 4-year outcome after great toe transfer demonstrating excellent cosmesis and function

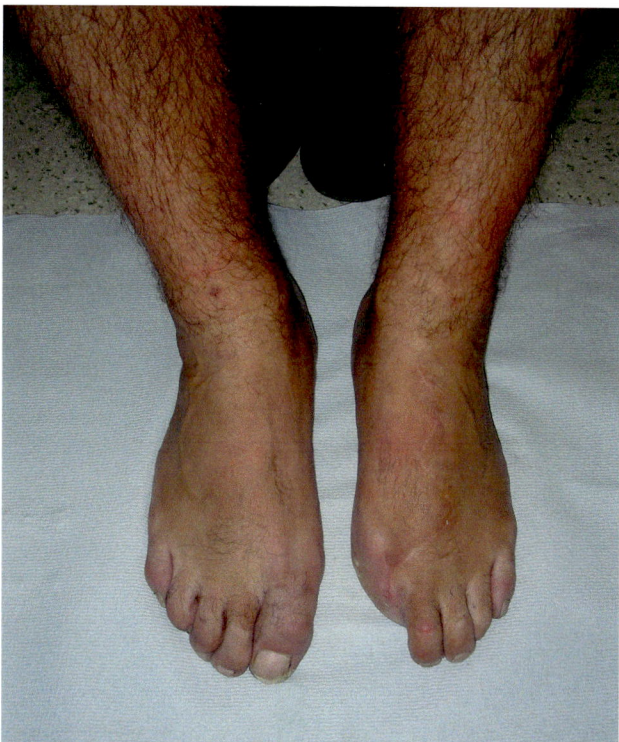

Fig. 44.26 Donor site outcome after great toe transfer

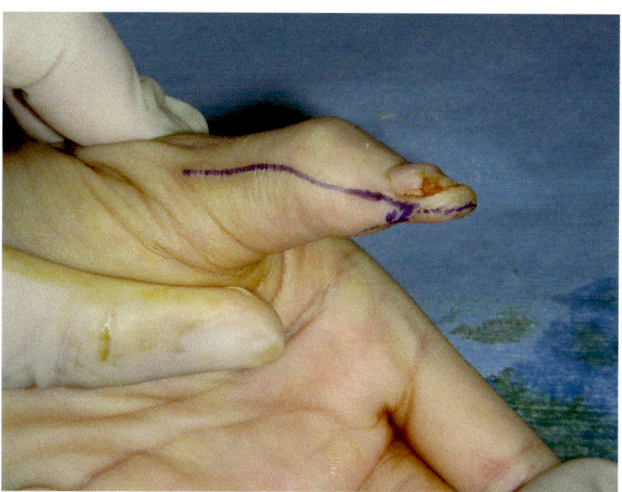

Fig. 44.27 Painful atrophic left thumb pulp

44.7.2 Scenario B: Delayed Great Toe Hemi-Pulp Transfer Surgeon Norbert Kang

Patient B developed a pulp space infection of his left thumb. The tissue was debrided and grafted with a split thickness skin graft. This left an atrophic and painful thumb tip (Fig. 44.27). The patient opted for a great toe pulp transfer to restore a well-padded and glabrous pulp (Fig. 44.28). The figure demonstrates an excellent outcome and restoration of the pulp with glabrous like for like tissue (Fig. 44.29). He had no donor site complaints apart from pigmentation from the full thickness graft inset over the lateral edge of the great toe (Fig. 44.30).

44.7.3 Scenario C: Immediate Great Toe to Hand Transplant Surgeon Dariush Nikkhah

Patient C had a traumatic amputation to his right dominant thumb at the level of the interphalangeal joint (IPJ). Revascularisation was unsuccessful and the pulp was necrotic and amputated (Fig. 44.31). An immediate great toe to hand

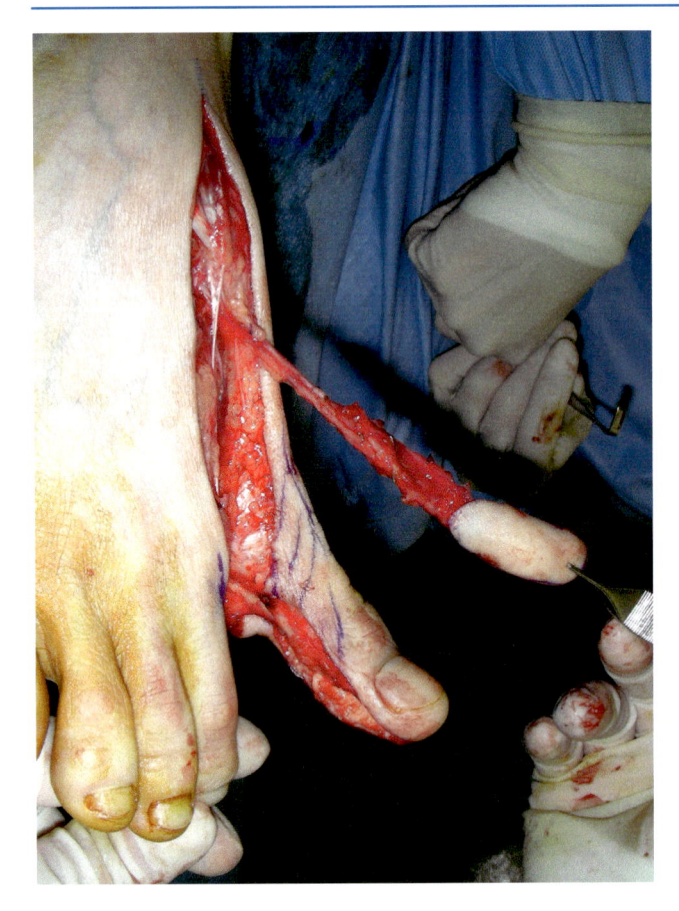

Fig. 44.28 Great toe pulp was taken from the lateral border of the great toe with associated neurovascular structures

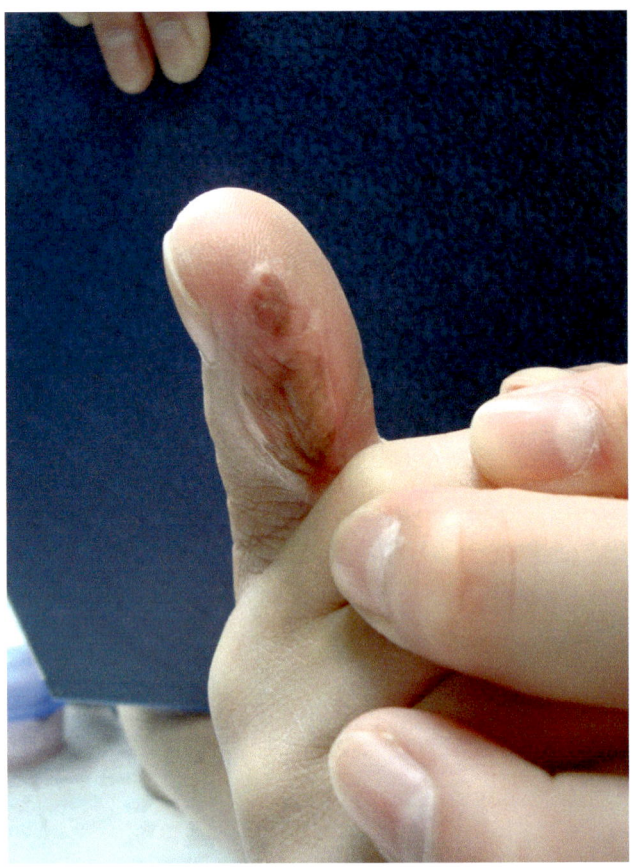

Fig. 44.30 Donor site from great toe pulp transfer demonstrates minor hyperpigmentation

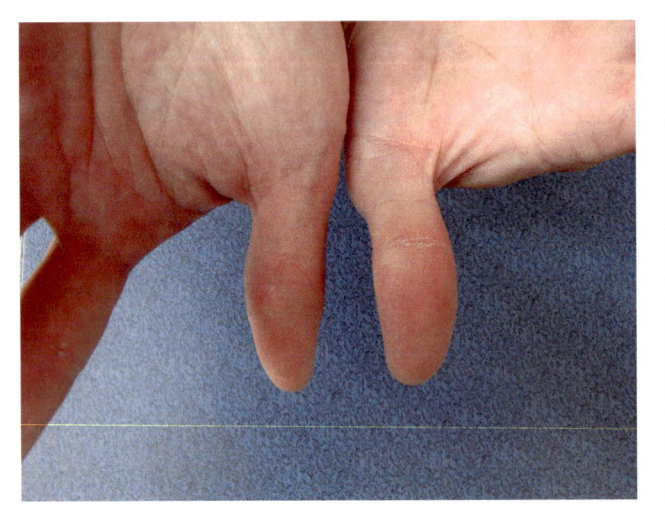

Fig. 44.29 2-year outcome of pulp transfer, it is indistinguishable from contralateral thumb

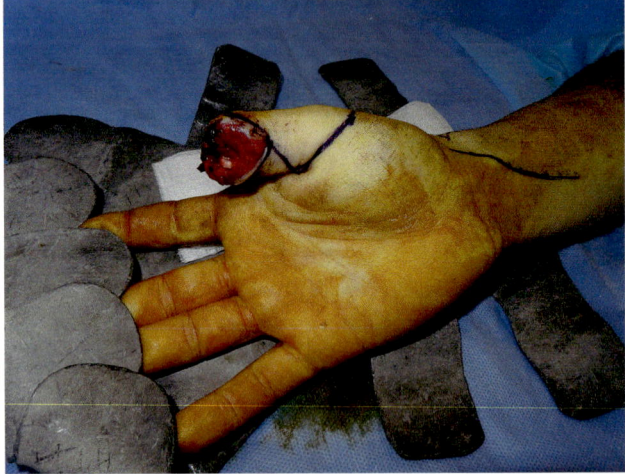

Fig. 44.31 Traumatic amputation of right thumb at level of IPJ

transplant was performed to preserve IPJ motion and restore thumb length (Fig. 44.32). A dorsal dominant circulation was identified and anastomosis was performed to the radial artery at the anatomical snuff box. The patient had a pulp plasty at 8 months to improve cosmesis. His result at 1 year demonstrates excellent range of motion, sensibility and restoration of opposition and an acceptable donor site morbidity (Figs. 44.33 and 44.34).

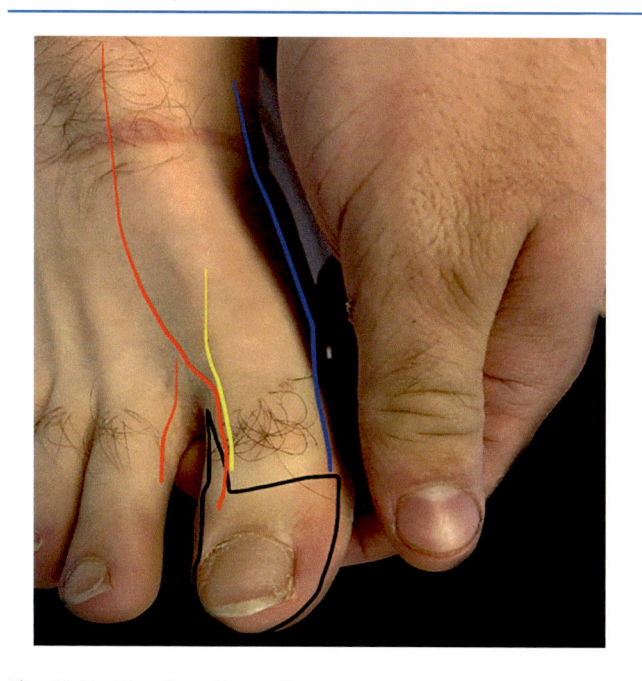

Fig. 44.32 Planning of immediate great toe to hand transfer

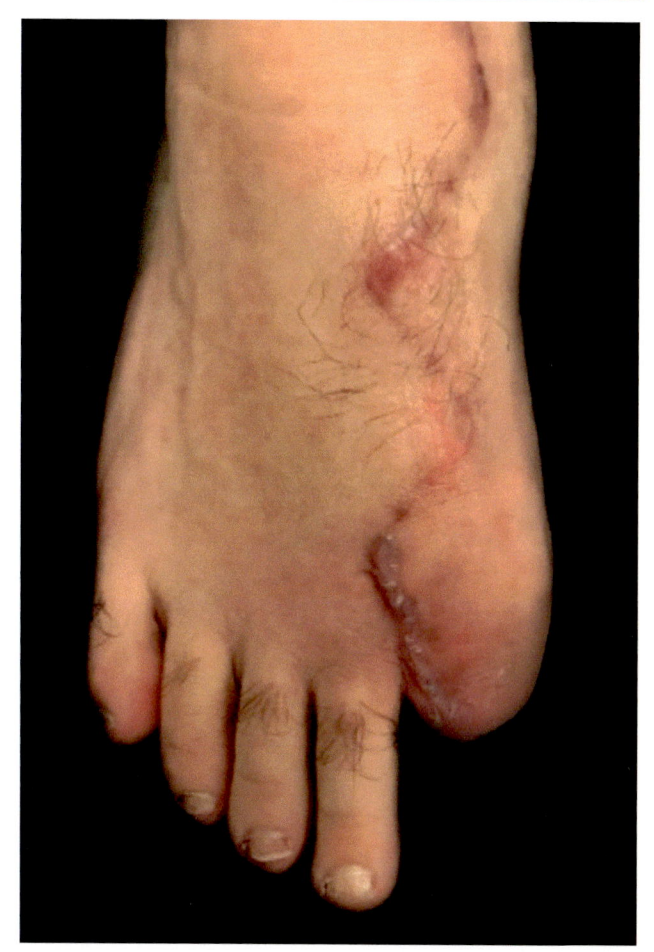

Fig. 44.34 Donor site outcome

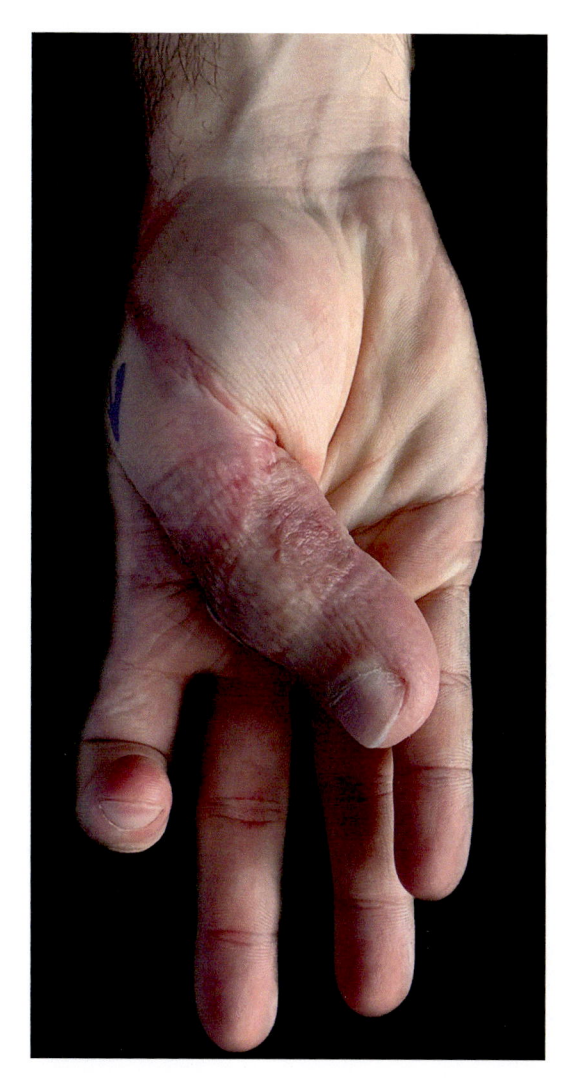

Fig. 44.33 Result of transfer at 1 year

44.8 Pearls and Pitfalls

Pearls
- Use a retrograde approach to determine the dominance of the circulation in toe transfer. The advantage of this method over the antegrade approach is that the surgeon can ascertain if there is a plantar or dorsal dominant circulation.
- The vessels should be dissected with microsurgical instruments and side branches ligaclipped with micro-ligaclips. To avoid thermal injury to the pedicle, a heat sink bipolar technique should be utilised.
- If the great toe is substantially larger than the thumb to be reconstructed, the tibial portion of skin, soft tissue and bone can be removed as a trimmed great toe. Secondary surgeries such as pulp plasty can also be performed to debulk the bulbous appearing pulp of the great toe transfer.
- Once the toe is raised, it is assessed for vascularity before transfer. In cases where there is vasospasm and the toe remains white, we recommend warm water and vasodilators such as lidocaine or papaverine.
- In an elective great toe transfer, the recipient site should be prepared with wide exposure to delineate dorsal veins, tendons, nerves and recipient arteries. This can be performed with a cruciate incision [9]. We prefer if feasible to do the microsurgery at the wrist or snuff box as vessels here are larger and the microsurgical anastomosis is less challenging.

Pitfalls
- Plantar dissection beyond the mid-metatarsal level can cause substantial morbidity to the foot. The incision if extended should be kept lateral to the weight bearing portion of the metatarsal head. We do extend by splitting the first web to achieve as much plantar vessel as possible, as this is an expensive operation, once started we feel we should do everything to make it work. It is far easier to reconstruct the first web in the donor foot than to save a failing toe transfer.
- The surgeon must ensure there is enough tissue to cover the donor site; it must be well padded and tension-free. We avoid resecting back the head of the metatarsal as this can affect gait. The great toe should not be taken proximal to the base of the proximal phalanx [9].
- Minimise periosteal stripping when performing osteosynthesis, and preserve up to 5 mm of bone for interosseous fixation or plate fixation [9].
- Use a light dressing; avoid circumferential dressing with Jelonet which can result in a blood cast and result in venous congestion.
- During the post-operative period, one must keep the patient warm and well hydrated. Use of brachial plexus block for the first 24 h can also induce vasodilation and reduce the chances of vasospasm in the early post-operative period.

44.9 Selected Readings

- Morrison WA, O'Brien BM, MacLeod AM. Thumb reconstruction with a free neurovascular wrap-around flap from the big toe. J Hand Surg Am. 1980;5(6):575–83.
- *This paper describes a method of thumb reconstruction with iliac crest bone graft and a neurovascular wrap-around flap from the great toe. The authors felt that this provided acceptable aesthetic outcome but minimising secondary morbidity at the donor site.*
- Wei FC, Chen HC, Chuang DC, Jeng SF, Lin CH. Aesthetic refinements in toe-to-hand transfer surgery. Plast Reconstr Surg. 1996;98(3):485–90.
- *The authors describe techniques to refine both the aesthetics and functional outcomes in toe transfers. They highlight how great toe transfer can be improved by the reduction of soft tissue, bone, interphalangeal joint, nail and by secondary pulp reduction and contouring procedures.*
- Gilbert A. Vascular anatomy of the first web space of the foot. In: Landi A, editor. Reconstruction of the thumb. London: Chapman and Hall; 1989. p. 1999.
- *Cadaveric study that examined the variation of the dorsal and plantar metatarsal arteries in 50 cadavers. The dorsal system is the primary choice for the pedicle of the great toe owing to its superficial course and long pedicle. However in 10% of cases the dorsal system may be absent and the plantar system may need to be harvested as the primary pedicle, which has disadvantages of being significantly shorter and often needing lengthening with a vein graft. Gilbert describes the anatomical subtypes seen in the dorsal and plantar metatarsal arteries.*

- Wei FC, Silverman RT, Hsu WM. Retrograde dissection of the vascular pedicle in toe harvest. Plast Reconstr Surg. 1995;96:1211–4.
- *Wei and colleagues describe the retrograde approach to second and great toe harvest, this enables swift identification of whether plantar or dorsal dominance is present in the toe. Furthermore the authors state it avoids the need for any pre operative imaging.*
- Henry SL, Wei FC. Thumb reconstruction with toe transfer. J Hand Microsurg. 2010;2(2):72–8.
- *A technical article from the Taiwanese group illustrating key techniques and steps in great toe, second toe and trimmed toe transfer. The authors describe common pitfalls and techniques to avoid difficulties.*
- Wei FC, Chen HC, Chuang CC, Noordhoff MS. Reconstruction of the thumb with a trimmed-toe transfer technique. Plast Reconstr Surg. 1988;82(3):506–15.
- *The article describes a new modification of the great toe transfer, the trimmed toe transfer. The technique involves reduction of bony and soft tissue elements along the medial aspect of the great toe in order to produce a normal-sized thumb. The first 20 transfers demonstrated excellent stability, grip strength and pinch strength but a modest reduction in range of motion at the interphalangeal joint.*
- Wei FC, Yim K. Pulp plasty after toe to hand transplantation. Plast Reconstr Surg. 1995;96(3):661–6.
- *This retrospective study looked at the effects of pulp plasty on the appearance and function in 82 digits on 51 patients. The procedure involves removal of a wedge of tissue from the centre of the pulp. In this series the procedure was considered effective in 87% of cases and it improved appearance and the function of the transplanted digit.*

References

1. Cobbett JR. Free digital transfer: report of a case of transfer of a great toe to replace an amputated thumb. J Bone Joint Surg. 1969;51B:677.
2. Whitworth IH, Pickford MA. The first toe-to-hand transfer: a thirty-year follow-up. J Hand Surg Br. 2000;25(6):608–10.
3. Valauri FA, Buncke HJ. Thumb reconstruction—great toe transfer. Clin Plast Surg. 1989;16(3):475–89.
4. Morrison WA, O'Brien BM, MacLeod AM. Thumb reconstruction with a free neurovascular wrap-around flap from the big toe. J Hand Surg Am. 1980;5(6):575–83.
5. Wei FC, Chen HC, Chuang DC, Jeng SF, Lin CH. Aesthetic refinements in toe-to-hand transfer surgery. Plast Reconstr Surg. 1996;98(3):485–90.
6. Strauch B, Yu H-L. Atlas of microvascular surgery. Anatomy and operative approaches. Stuttgart: Thieme; 1993.
7. Gilbert A. Vascular anatomy of the first web space of the foot. In: Landi A, editor. Reconstruction of the thumb. London: Chapman and Hall; 1989.
8. Wei FC, Silverman RT, Hsu WM. Retrograde dissection of the vascular pedicle in toe harvest. Plast Reconstr Surg. 1995;96:1211–4.
9. Henry SL, Wei FC. Thumb reconstruction with toe transfer. J Hand Microsurg. 2010;2(2):72–8.
10. Nikkhah D, Martin N, Pickford M. Paediatric toe-to-hand transfer: an assessment of outcomes from a single unit. J Hand Surg Eur. 2016;41(3):281–94.

The Medial Plantar Flap

Alexander E. J. Trevatt, Miguel A. Johnson, and Tiew C. Teo

45.1 Introduction

The medial plantar flap was first described by Shanahan and Gingrass in 1979 [1] who transposed the medial plantar flap based on an artery and nerve pedicle, to reconstruct heel defects. It was later described as an island fasciocutaneous flap by Harrison and Morgan in 1981 [2]. Morrison et al. subsequently described its use as a free flap [3]. It is a particularly versatile flap that can be used to provide 'like for like' reconstruction in the foot and ankle, with minimal donor site morbidity. It is ideally suited for defects in the foot and ankle region, where the stresses of ambulation require any reconstruction to provide durable sensate coverage. It is also an excellent option in the palmar region, where providing a sensate, durable reconstruction is particularly important. Duman et al. [4] demonstrated the versatility of the medial plantar flap in the palmar region by harvesting it with abductor hallucis muscle to simultaneously reconstruct defects of the thenar skin and muscle.

About 80% of standing body weight is supported by the heel, with the remainder supported by the metatarsals and distal sole [5]. Despite being essentially non-weight bearing, the medial plantar region retains the characteristics of the rest of the plantar region. The glabrous plantar skin is perfectly adapted for weight bearing and contains vertical fibrous septa, which extend from the fascia to the dermis, absorbing shock and resisting shear [6]. Medial plantar flaps can therefore provide durable coverage of defects in the foot and ankle, without affecting gait.

A. E. J. Trevatt (✉) · M. A. Johnson · T. C. Teo
Queen Victoria Hospital, East Grinstead, UK

45.2 Anatomy

Inferior to the medial malleolus, the posterior tibial artery enters the calcaneal canal and bifurcates at the level of the transverse septum between the abductor hallucis muscle and the flexor digitorum brevis muscle, into the medial and lateral plantar arteries. The mean length of the posterior tibial artery from the base of the medial malleolus to its bifurcation point is 2.7 cm [7].

On branching from the posterior tibial artery, the medial plantar artery (MPA) first passes superior to the abductor hallucis, before moving between it and the flexor digitorum brevis, where it supplies both muscles. It then runs inferiorly to the flexor hallucis longus tendon, before bifurcating into superficial and deep branch at the level of the talus-navicular joint. The mean length of the MPA from origin to bifurcation is 3 cm [8]. The superficial branch of the MPA usually has a larger calibre (average of 1.85 mm) than the deep branch (1.4 mm) [9]. The deep MPA is inconsistent and may be absent in up to 30–45% of cases [7].

Throughout its course, the MPA and superficial MPA provides 1–3 small perforators to the skin. These perforators have a mean diameter of 0.5 mm [10] and can be used as the basis of the MPA perforator flap [11].

The superficial MPA makes a number of variable anastomotic connections. There is usually a connection with the first plantar metatarsal artery (27–100%) [12, 13] which can be used to raise a reverse flow medial plantar flap [14]. There are often connections to the plantar arch via the first and second metatarsal arteries and there is a direct anastomosis with the deep plantar arch in up to 20% of cases [12].

The medial plantar nerve accompanies the medial plantar artery. It is a cutaneous sensory branch of the posterior tibial nerve, providing sensation to the medial plantar skin. It can be incorporated into the medial plantar flap to provide a sensate reconstruction. Concomitant veins also accompany the medial plantar artery, in addition to larger calibre subcutaneous tributaries of the great saphenous vein.

45.3 Pre-operative Investigation

Preoperative imaging is not routinely required, although CT angiography may be useful where there are concerns regarding the patency of the medial plantar artery, such as in peripheral vasculopathy or previous trauma.

In our experience, a handheld pencil Doppler is usually sufficient to localise the medial plantar artery and its perforators.

45.4 Flap Design and Markings

The medial plantar flap skin island should be centred around the strongest cutaneous perforator in the non-weight bearing aspect of the foot.

A large area can be raised including, if needed, part of the medial foot (Fig. 45.1). The posterior tibial artery is palpated just posterior to medial malleolus. Using the handheld Doppler, it is traced as it runs distally and branches into the medial plantar artery. A straight line is drawn connecting the posterior tibial artery at the medial malleolus to the plantar aspect of the first metatarsal space. This is divided into thirds with the main perforator generally being found at the junction of the middle and distal third (Fig. 45.2).

45.5 Flap Raise/Elevation: A Step-by-Step Guide

1. **Positioning.** The patient is placed in the lateral decubitus position (Fig. 45.3), or supine with the knee flexed, and the foot is elevated on a sandbag. A thigh tourniquet is applied. The medial malleolus along with the posterior tibial artery and skin paddle is marked preoperatively.
2. **Skin Flap Elevation.** The skin flap is raised from distal to proximal along the lateral plantar border down to plantar fascia (Fig. 45.4). If you have dopplered the pedicle

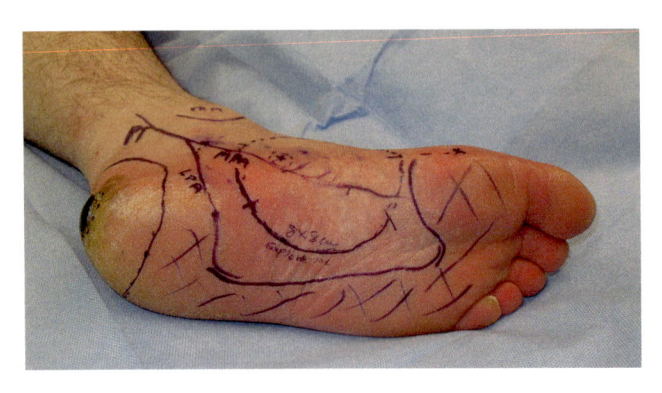

Fig. 45.1 Landmarks drawn before medial plantar flap transfer. Large flaps incorporating almost all of the non-weight bearing instep can be raised

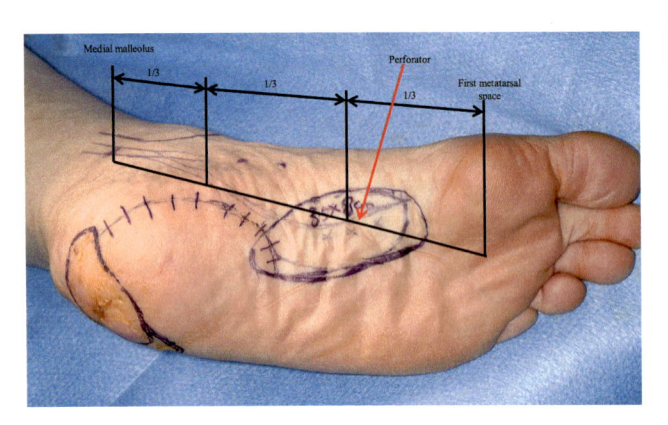

Fig. 45.2 A line is drawn from the posterior tibial artery at the level of the medial malleolus to the plantar aspect of the first metatarsal space. The main perforators are generally found two-thirds of the way along this line

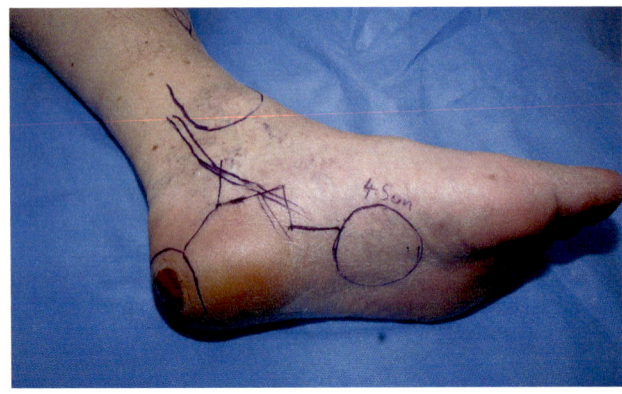

Fig. 45.3 The patient is placed in the lateral decubitus position and the flap is designed

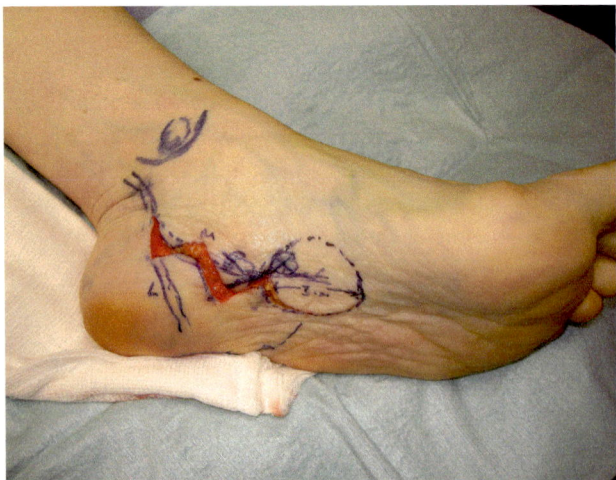

Fig. 45.4 The skin incision is made along the lateral border of the flap, down to the plantar fascia. In this case, the triangular skin incisions over the pedicle have also been made. The course pedicle was previously identified using doppler

and are happy with its course, you can also make the skin incisions over the pedicle at this point.

3. **Reflection of Plantar Fascia.** The plantar fascia is lifted to expose the medial plantar neurovascular bundle (Fig. 45.5) and the pedicle is appraised. The medial plantar neurovascular bundle can be found in the cleft between the abductor hallucis brevis and flexor digitorum brevis muscles. The distal end of the vessels are tied off and divided.

4. **Dissection of Medial Plantar Nerve.** Dissection of the medial plantar nerve should be performed at this stage. The nerve should be separated from the neurovascular bundle until the branch to the flap is identified (Fig. 45.6a). At this point, this branch is followed back to the trunk of the nerve and an intraneural dissection is performed to separate it from the trunk (Fig. 45.6b). Dissection is superficial to the muscles and just deep to the plantar fascia. The nerve is raised along with the pedicle of the flap.

5. **Pedicle Dissection** (Fig. 45.7). Following division of the distal end of the medial plantar vessels, the flap is raised from distal to proximal at the level between the plantar fascia and the flexor digitorum brevis. The length of pedicle needed will dictate how much we dissect the pedicle. Dissection often stops where the vessels emerge from the lateral border of abductor hallucis brevis. The pedicle may be further dissected proximally towards the posterior tibial artery to increase length where needed. At this point, if raising as a free tissue transfer, the pedicle can be clipped and divided at its origin. Following careful dissection, the medial plantar border of the skin is incised to island the skin flap on its pedicle.

6. **Flap Inset.** The flap is inset using 4–0 monocryl (Fig. 45.8). If performing free tissue transfer, anastomoses can be performed prior to this either as end-to-end or end-to-side, depending on the size of the recipient vessel. We routinely insert a passive corrugator drain.

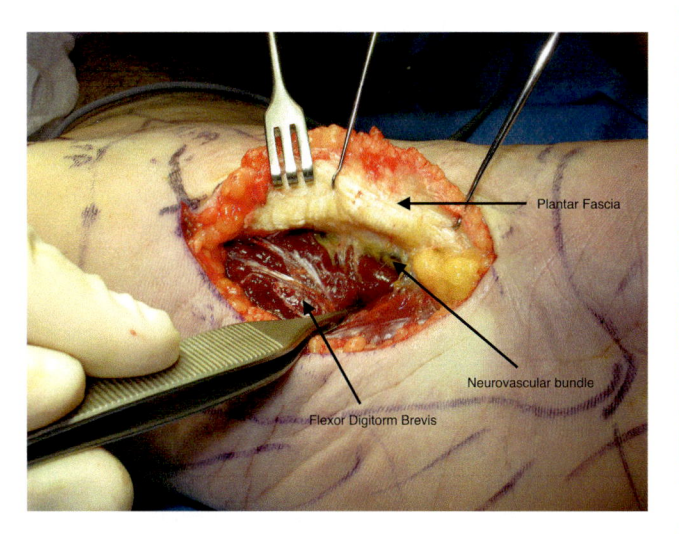

Fig. 45.5 The plantar fascia is reflected and a relatively avascular plain found

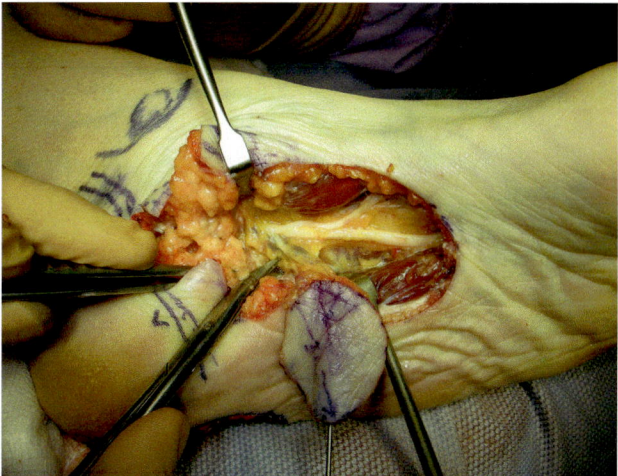

Fig. 45.7 The pedicle is carefully dissected until adequate length and mobility it achieved. Care is taken to remove all fascial attachments that would hinder mobility

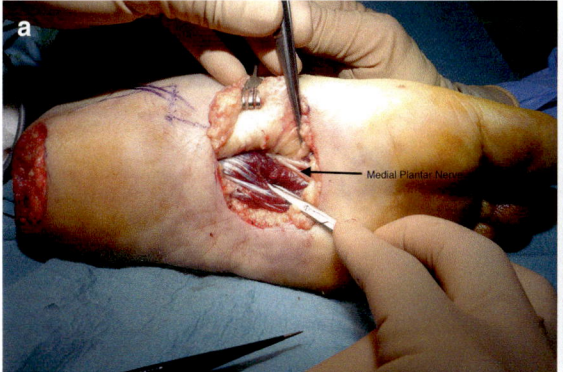

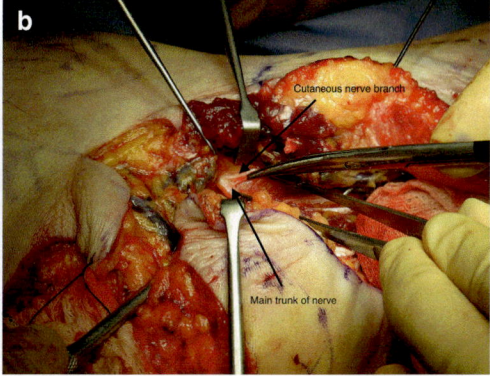

Fig. 45.6 (**a**) The medial plantar nerve is identified and carefully separated from the vessels. (**b**) The medial plantar nerve is traced back until cutaneous branches to the skin paddle are identified. At this point intraneural dissection is performed to separate it from the trunk

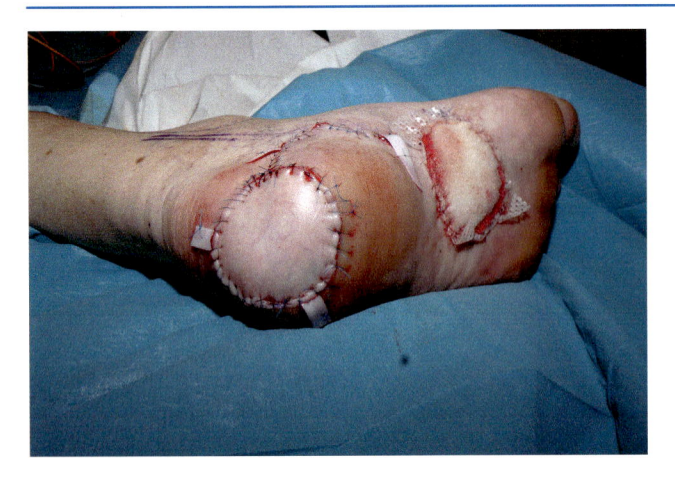

Fig. 45.8 The flap is inset and a passive corrugator drain is inserted

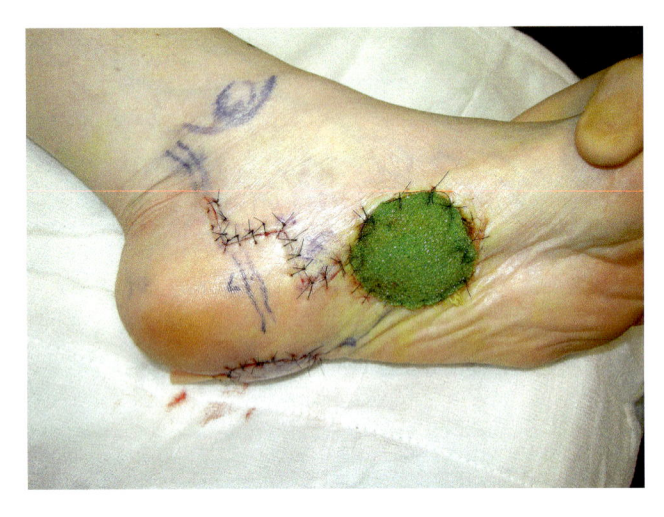

Fig. 45.9 The defect is reconstructed with a split skin graft and a bolster dressing is applied

7. **Donor Site Reconstruction.** The donor site defect is reconstructed with a split skin graft. This is bolstered with a dressing (Fig. 45.9) and the leg is elevated overnight. A window is made into the dressing to allow frequent monitoring of the flap.

45.6 Core Surgical Techniques in Flap Dissection

1. **Skin Flap Elevation.** This is done with a blade to incise the skin, followed by a finger switch diathermy. Care is taken to avoid avulsing the skin from the underlying fascia.
2. **Reflection of Plantar Fascia.** The fascia is incised with a ten blade and is held with either a Kilner retractor (catspaw) or skin hooks. Once you have incised the plantar fascia there is a relatively avascular plane which leads down to the vessels.
3. **Dissection of Medial Plantar Nerve.** The main trunk of the nerve is identified and is separated from the pedicle using Debakey forceps and Tenotomy scissors. A combination of sharp and blunt dissection continues until you see a cutaneous branch to the skin. This branch is then followed back to the main trunk of the nerve. Intraneural dissection is then performed to release the branch from the trunk. This is an important part of raising a sensate flap, otherwise the nerve would restrict movement of the flap. We usually continue the intraneural dissection until we have enough length to allow the flap to move the desired distance.
4. **Pedicle Dissection.** The MPA pedicle is dissected using both sharp and bipolar dissection. We prefer to tie off the pedicle distally, as ligaclips can be felt when weight bearing. Tenotomy scissors and Debakey forceps are used, along with bipolar diathermy where needed. We use vessel loops to retract vessels where necessary. The end point of dissection is where the lateral plantar artery branches, to avoid overly devascularising the foot. It has been reported however that if a longer pedicle is required, dissection can continue proximal to this, provided the dorsalis pedis is viable. However, in these cases we would opt for alternative solutions where there is less vascular disruption to the foot.
5. **Flap Inset.** We routinely insert a passive corrugator drain where using this flap to reconstruct foot and ankle defects. This is to minimise the risk of a haematoma putting pressure on the pedicle.

45.7 Clinical Scenario

Case Scenario 1 Surgeon TC Teo A 52-year-old man underwent excision of a malignant melanoma from his heel. A 5 × 5 cm defect was created and a medial plant flap was chosen for reconstruction to provide a durable, sensate, like for like reconstruction. The flap was raised as a pedicled flap and was able to comfortably reach the defect. A good long-term outcome was achieved, with the patient returning to normal ambulation (Figs. 45.10, 45.11, 45.12, 45.13, 45.14, and 45.15).

Case Scenario 2 Surgeon TC Teo A 41-year-old man underwent excision of a persistent verruca on the distal sole of his foot which had frequently recurred. A 3 × 4 cm defect was created that would have been too distal for a standard pedicled medial plantar flap. Instead a reverse flow pedicled medial plantar flap was raised and used to reconstruct the defect. The donor site was reconstructed with a split skin graft. This definitively treated the verruca with the patient suffering no further recurrences (Figs. 45.16, 45.17, 45.18, 45.19, 45.20, and 45.21).

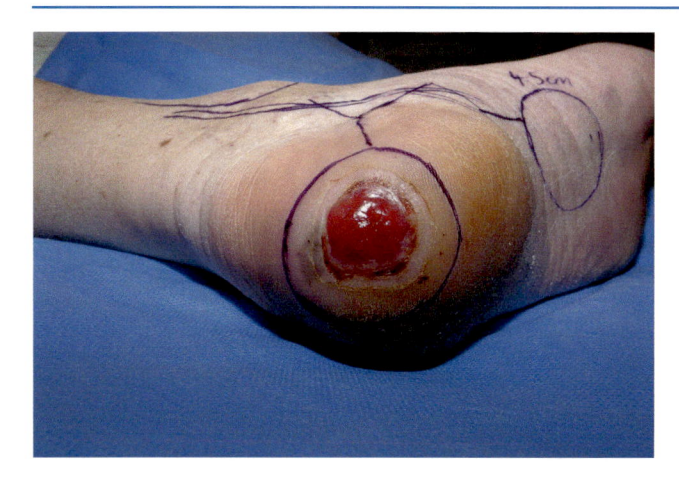

Fig. 45.10 A malignant melanoma requiring excision from the weight bearing aspect of the heel

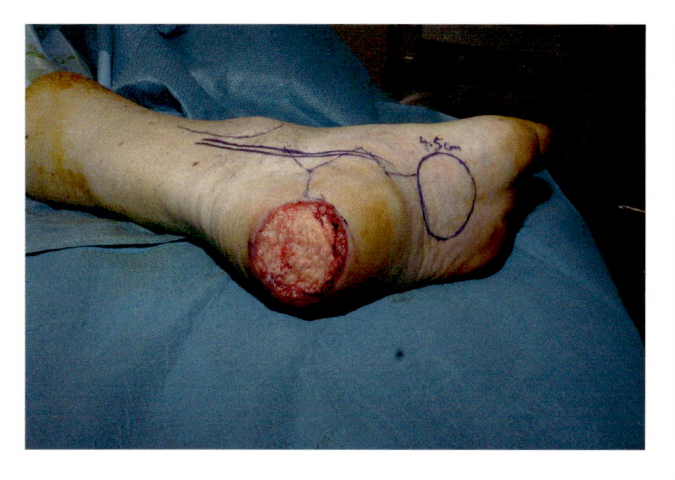

Fig. 45.11 Post-excision defect along with skin markings for pedicled medial plantar flap

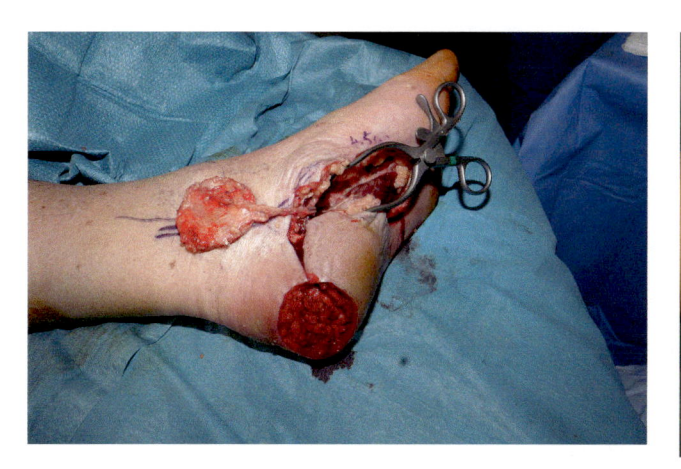

Fig. 45.12 Medial plantar flap raised on its pedicle, just before inset

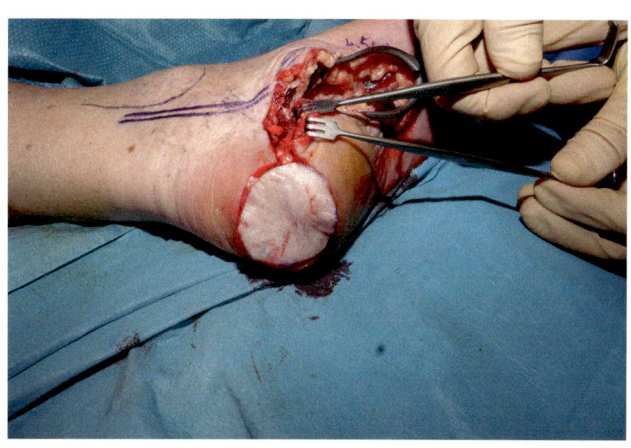

Fig. 45.13 Pedicled medial plantar flap easily reaching heel defect

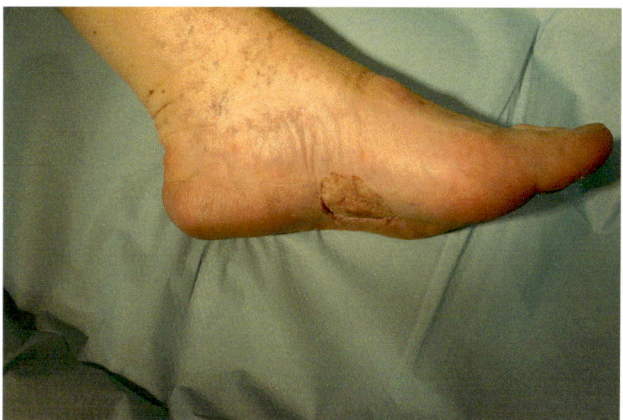

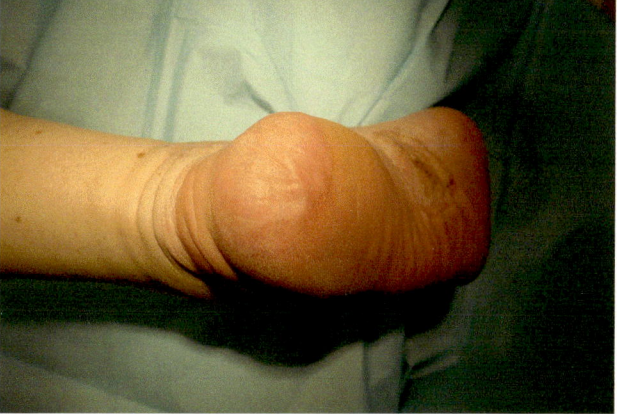

Fig. 45.14 Long-term outcome of pedicled medial plantar flap to heel

Fig. 45.15 Long-term outcome of pedicled medial plantar flap to heel

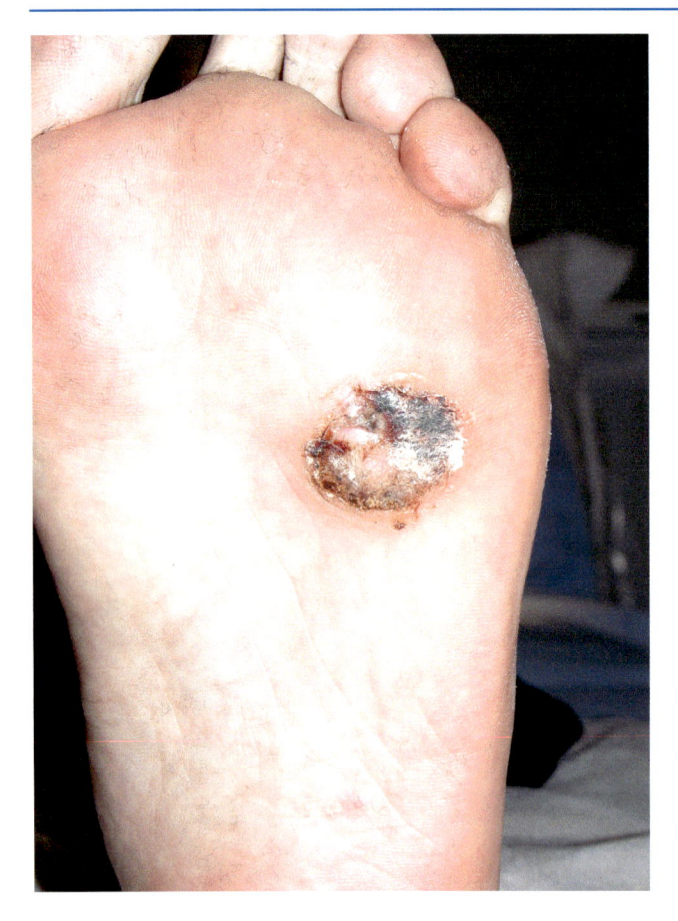

Fig. 45.16 Recurrent verruca on distal sole

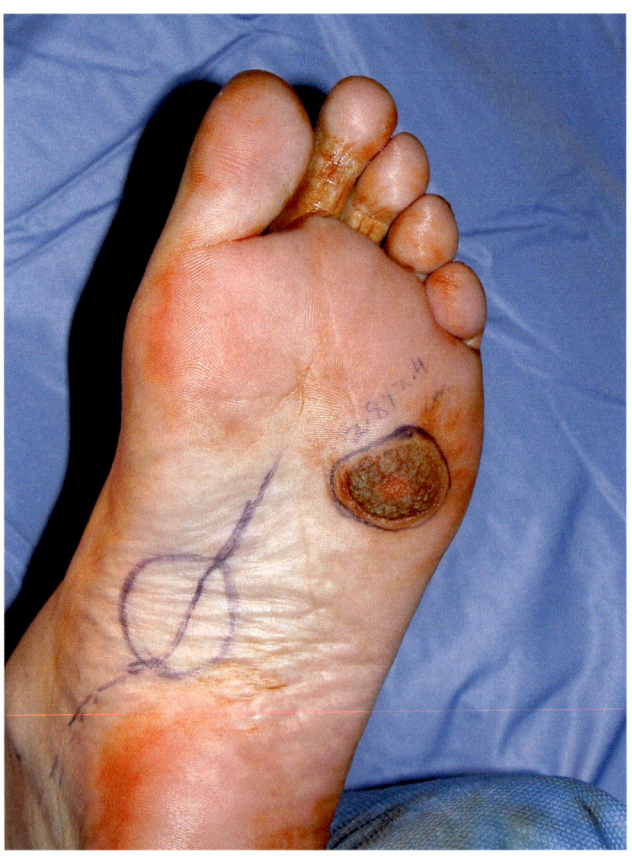

Fig. 45.17 Pre-operative skin markings for reverse flow medial plantar flap

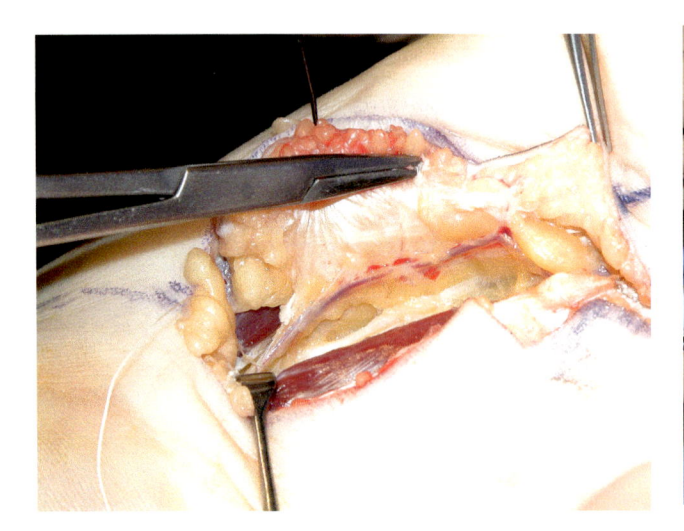

Fig. 45.18 Reverse flow medial plantar flap raised from proximal to distal

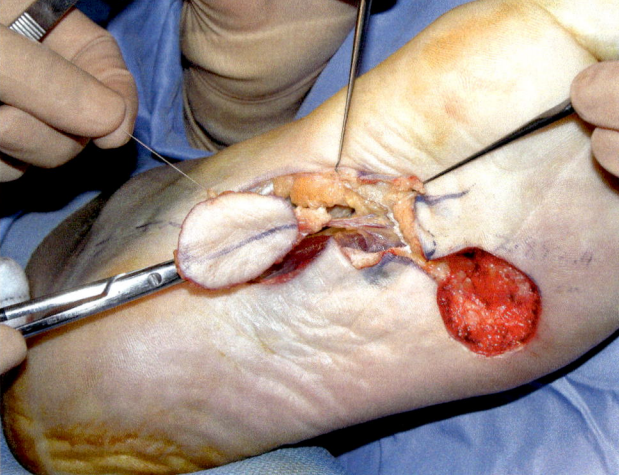

Fig. 45.19 Reverse flow medial plantar flap fully raised, just before inset

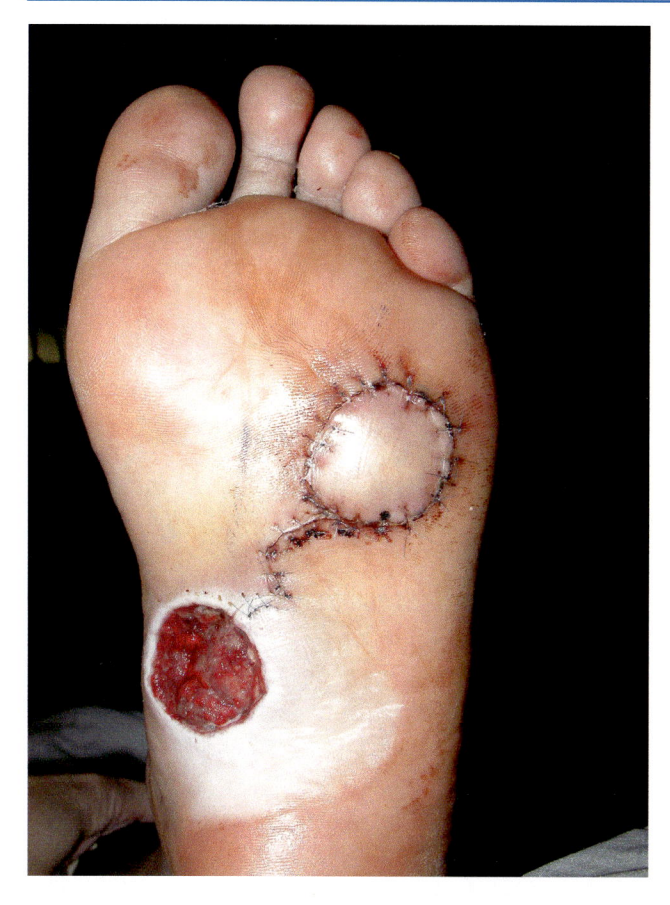

Fig. 45.20 Reverse flow medial plantar flap following inset. Donor defect was subsequently reconstructed with a split skin graft

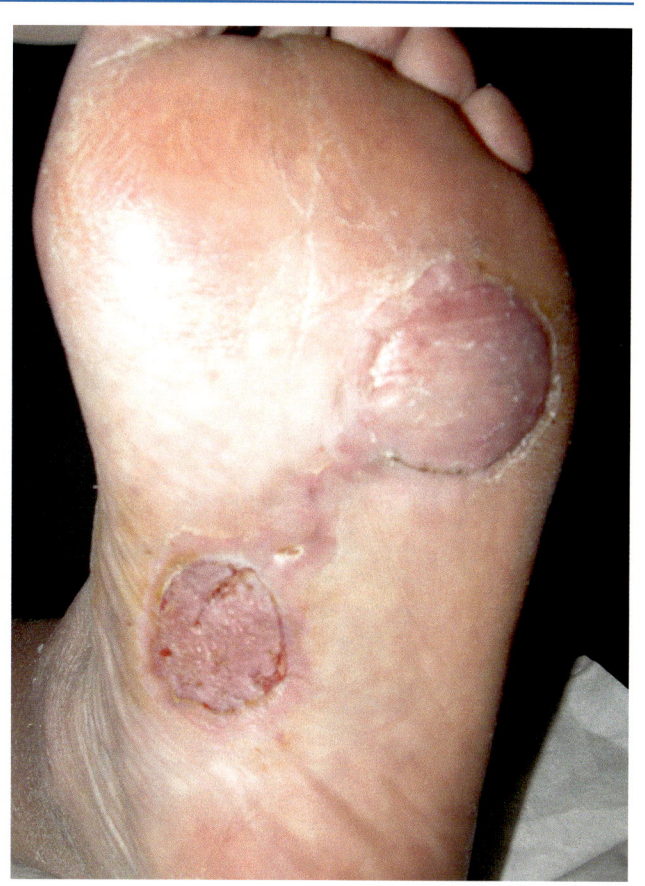

Fig. 45.21 Long-term outcome of reverse flow medial plantar flap to distal sole

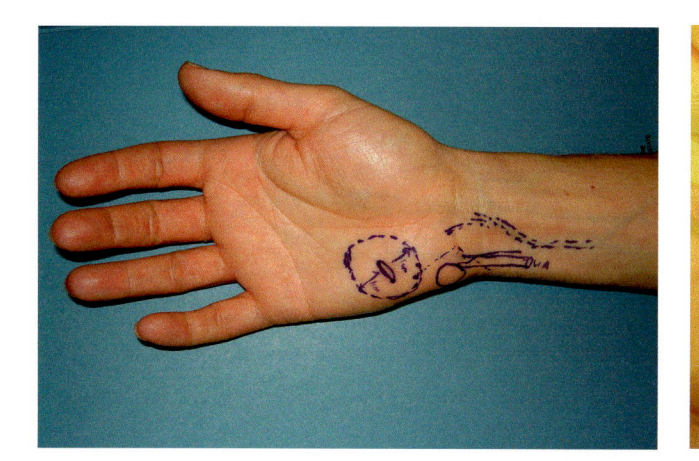

Fig. 45.22 Skin marking of malignant melanoma scar requiring wide local excision

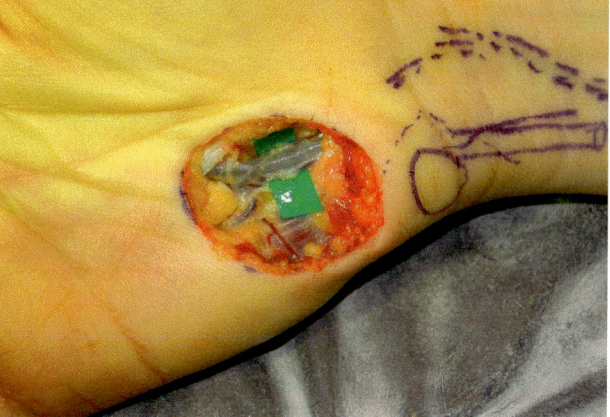

Fig. 45.23 2.5 × 2.5 cm defect on palm following wide local excision of malignant melanoma

Case Scenario 3 Surgeon TC Teo A 37-year-old man underwent wide local excision of a malignant melanoma scar from his palm. A 2.5 × 2.5 cm defect was created and a free medial plantar flap was chosen to provide a durable reconstruction that replicated the palmar skin. An end-to-end anastomosis was made to a branch of the ulnar artery (Figs. 45.22, 45.23, 45.24, 45.25, 45.26, 45.27a, b).

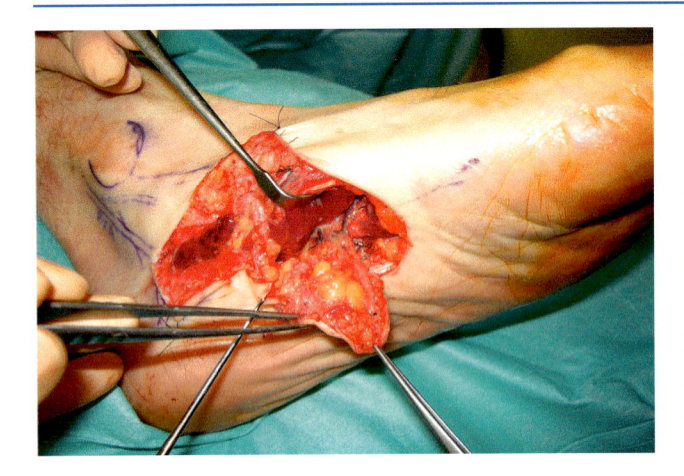

Fig. 45.24 A free medial plantar flap being raised

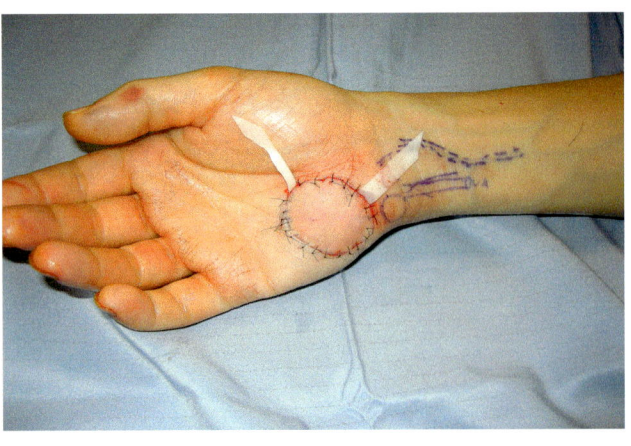

Fig. 45.26 A free medial plantar flap following inset into a branch of the ulnar artery on the palm

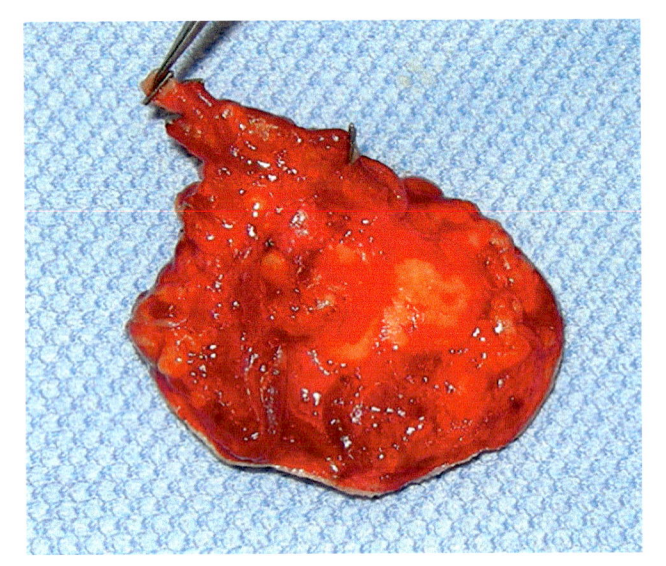

Fig. 45.25 A free medial plantar flap. In this case the flap has been raised without the fascia to keep it as thin as possible

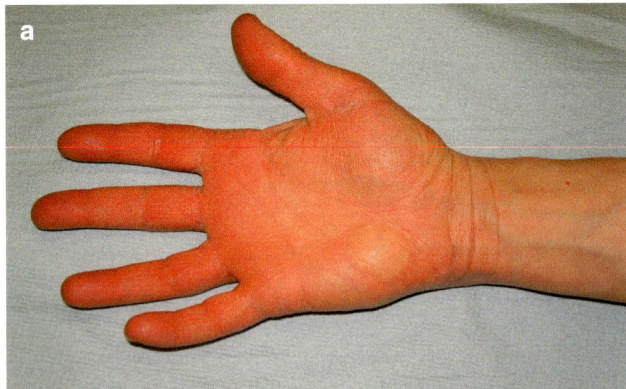

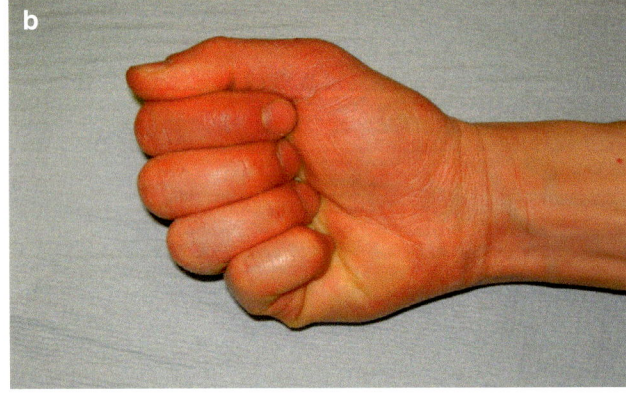

Fig. 45.27 (**a**) Long-term outcome of free medial plantar flap to palm. (**b**) Long-term outcome of free medial plantar flap to palm

45.8 Pearls and Pitfalls

Pearls
- If you require a longer pedicle, make your skin paddle as distal as possible within the non-weight bearing aspect of the foot.
- Where longer pedicle lengths are required, further mobilisation is possible by dividing or tunnelling under the abductor hallucis brevis muscle and the laciniate ligament, and tracing the medial plantar artery to its origin from the posterior tibial artery.
- If using the medial plantar flap to reconstruct distal foot defects, consider raising a reverse flow flap. In these cases, elevation should occur from proximal to distal and the medial plantar flap is tied off proximally.
- When dissecting the pedicle, ensure all the fascial attachments are released to allow for an uninhibited arc of rotation and to minimise the potential of kinking in pedicled flaps.
- If a thinner flap is required, the flap can be raised without the plantar fascia. This requires careful dissection of the perforator through the fascia.

Pitfalls
- At the level of the navicular tuberosity there is an extensive venous plexus. Since the branching pattern of the superficial and deep MPA are variable, caution must be taken to avoid isolation of the incorrect arterial supply.
- When raising a sensate flap, transecting the medial plantar nerve distally sacrifices sensation to the plantar medial distal foot and toes. This can be avoided by splitting the nerve through intraneural, extrafascicular dissection.
- During dissection, it is important to preserve the peritendinous structures overlying the abductor hallucis. If these are not maintained, the wound bed will not be suitably vascularised for skin grafting.
- Take care to ensure you apply only gentle traction when raising the skin paddle to avoid avulsion of the deep fascia from the skin.
- Rarely, the deep MPA can be the dominant vessel. It is therefore important to fully appraise the neurovascular bundle before committing to the dissection.

45.9 Selected Readings

- Guillier D, Cherubino M, Oranges CM, Giordano S, Raffoul W, di Summa PG. Systematic reappraisal of the reverse-flow medial plantar flap: from vascular anatomical concepts to surgical applications. J Plast Reconstr Aesthet Surg. 2020;73:421–33.
- *This recent review outlines the variations in MPA anatomy, along with their frequency.*
- Baker GL, Newton ED, Franklin JD. Fasciocutaneous island flap based on the medial plantar artery. Plast Reconstr Surg. 1990;85:47–58.
- *A selection of 12 clinical cases demonstrating the versatility of the medial plantar flap in the foot and ankle region.*
- Paget JT, Izadi D, Haj-Basheer M, Barnett S, Winson I, Khan U. Donor site morbidity of the medial plantar artery flap studied with gait and pressure analysis. Foot Ankle Surg. 2015;21:60–6.
- *A study demonstrating the minimal donor site morbidity of the medial plantar flap.*
- Scaglioni MF, Franchi A, Uyulmaz S, Giovanoli P. The bipedicled medial plantar flap: vascular enhancement of a reverse flow Y-V medial plantar flap by the inclusion of a metatarsal artery perforator for the reconstruction of a forefoot defect—a case report. Microsurgery. 2018;38:698–701.
- *A case report demonstrating how venous congestion can be reduced in reverse flow medial plantar flaps by raising a bipedicled flap.*

References

1. Shanahan RE, Gingrass RP. Medial plantar sensory flap for coverage of heel defects. Plast Reconstr Surg. 1979;64:295.
2. Harrison DH, Morgan BDH. The instep island flap to resurface plantar defects. Br J Plast Surg. 1981;34:315.
3. Morrison WA, Crabb DM, O'Brien BM, Jenkins A. The instep of the foot as a fasciocutaneous island and as a free flap for heel defects. Plast Reconstr Surg. 1983;72:56.
4. Duman H, Er E, Işík S, Türegün M, Deveci M, Nişancí M, Sengezer M. Versatility of the medial plantar flap: our clinical experience. Plast Reconstr Surg. 2002;109:1007–12.
5. Erdemir A, Sirimamilla PA, Halloran JP, van den Bogert AJ. An elaborated dataset characterizing the mechanical response of the foot. J Biomech Eng. 2009;131:094502.
6. Baker GL, Newton ED, Franklin JD. Fasciocutaneous island flap based on the medial plantar artery—clinical-applications for leg, ankle, and forefoot. Plast Reconstr Surg. 1990;85:47–58.
7. Macchi V, Tiengo C, Porzionato A, Stecco C, Parenti A, Mazzoleni F, et al. Correlation between the course of the medial plantar artery and the morphology of the abductor hallucis muscle. Clin Anat. 2005;18:580–8.
8. Rodriguez-Vegas M. Medialis Pedis flap in the reconstruction of palmar skin defects of the digits: clarifying the anatomy of the medial plantar artery. Ann Plast Surg. 2014;72:542–52.

9. Yoon E-S, Kim D-W, Chun D, Dhong E-S, Koo S-H, Park S-H, et al. An anatomic study and clinical application of medial pedis flap in Asians. Ann Plast Surg. 2007;58:517–22.
10. Zhang G-M, Syed SA, Tsai T-M. Anatomic study of a new axial skin flap based on the cutaneous branch of the medial plantar artery. Microsurgery. 1995;16:144–8.
11. Koshima I, Narushima M, Mihara M, Nakai I, Akazawa S, Fukuda N, et al. Island medial plantar artery perforator flap for reconstruction of plantar defects. Ann Plast Surg. 2007;59:558–62.
12. Masquelet AC, Penteado CV, Romana MC, Chevrel JP. The distal anastomoses of the medial plantar artery: surgical aspects. Surg Radiol Anat. 1988;10:247–9.
13. Song D, Yang X, Wu Z, Li L, Wang T, Zheng H, et al. Anatomic basis and clinical application of the distally based medialis pedis flaps. Surg Radiol Anat. 2016;38:213–21.
14. Bhandari PS, Sobti C. Reverse flow instep island flap. Plast Reconstr Surg. 1999;103:1986–9.

Part III
Common Recipient Vessels

Chest Wall Recipient Vessels Access

Pennylouise Hever, Dariush Nikkhah, Alexandra Molina, and Martin Jones

46.1 Indications

The internal mammary (IM) vessels have been used for microvascular reconstruction since 1947 in oesophageal reconstruction by Longmire, and later, in the 1970s and 1980s, for free superior gluteal myocutanoeous flap reconstruction post-mastectomy; first by Fujino and later by Shaw [1–3]. In 1980, Harashina described a case using the IM vessels as recipient vessels for a free groin flap reconstruction of the breast following radical excision of a large cavernous haemangioma [4]. Today the IM vessels remain the preferred recipient vessels for microvascular breast reconstruction for their constant anatomy, and ease of access.

The interest in the IMVs started with the popularisation of free abdominal tissue for autologous breast reconstruction—first with the TRAM flap and later the DIEP—, with the search for recipient vessels which would permit optimal flap positioning on the chest, with an adequate pedicle length. Four sets of possible recipient vessels in the chest were identified: the external carotid/jugular vein tributaries in the neck, branches of the subscapular artery and vein in the axilla, the thoracoacromial vessels on the superolateral anterior chest, and the IM vessels for the central anterior chest. The ones that are routinely used are the branches of the subscapular vessels (thoracodorsal, long thoracic, and the serratus branch of the circumflex scapular vessels) and the IM vessels. Advantages of the IM vessels include comparable vessel diameter match, more potent arterial flow, less demand for a long vascular pedicle, as compared to the vessels in the axilla, and the avoidance of lateral fullness of the breast. Disadvantages include the more complex, time-consuming dissection, vessel wall fragility following radiotherapy treatment, and anatomical variants which preclude their use. Furthermore, the dissection carries the additional risks of pneumothorax, intercostal neuralgia, and precludes the future use of the IMA for coronary artery bypass graft. Improved results have been demonstrated, however, with advances in microsurgery, including venous couplers, the rib-preserving approach, and IMA preserving end-to-side anastomosis.

46.2 Anatomy

Internal mammary vein anatomy has been widely studied, most notably by Arnez and Rohrich [5, 6]. Arnez et al. carried out the first anatomical study of the IMV in 1995 to assess the feasibility of anastomosis of the DIEP vessels with the IM recipient site. They proved the IM vessels to be present in all cadavers, and anastomosis to be safe and feasible. This finding was matched by Rohrich and other research groups in the years to follow. Only one notable study has reported the complete absence of the IMV. This rare finding was recorded by Pradas-Irun et al. in two patients; one who underwent immediate, and one delayed breast reconstruction following mastectomy and radiotherapy [7].

Four different patterns of IMV anatomy were described by Arnez et al., classifying the relationship of the IMV to the IMA [3]. The IMV was found medial to the IMA in 95% cases (types I and II), and lateral to the IMA in 5% (types III

P. Hever (✉) · D. Nikkhah
Royal Free NHS Foundation Trust, London, UK
e-mail: phever@nhs.net

A. Molina · M. Jones
Queen Victoria Hospital NHS Foundation Trust, East Grinstead, UK
e-mail: alexandramolina@doctors.org.uk

and IV). IMV division below the fifth rib was rare (1–2% cases). The type I pattern was most common (65%), in which the IMV ran medial to the IMA, dividing into two venae comitantes at the level of the third or fourth intercostal space. The type II pattern was the next most frequently observed (26%), consisting of a single IMV running medial to the IMA throughout its course, without division. Type III—the IMV running lateral to the IMA with division into two venae comitantes at the level of the third or fourth intercostal space—and type IV patterns, a single IMV running lateral to the IMA throughout its course without division, were rare. Tuinder et al. later reported an additional type V pattern, in which two IMVs were present, running parallel either side of the IMA, without further division [8] (Fig. 46.1a, b).

46.3 Pre-operative Investigation

In most cases, no pre-operative investigations are required due to the predictable anatomy of the IM vessels at the level of the third rib. Pre-operative mapping is therefore usually reserved for the abdominal wall perforators, to minimize exposure of the patient to unnecessary radiation. In exceptional cases (e.g. previous chest wall surgery), the diameter and flow of the IM vessels can be assessed pre-operatively by colour duplex scanning or CT/MR angiography.

There may be a role for pre-operative chest CT scanning to measure intercostal space width, to help plan for the rib-preserving vs. rib-sparing recipient vessel harvest technique. Most surgeons who favour the rib-preserving technique will, however, always attempt this approach at first, and only proceed to excise a small segment of rib cartilage if exposure is not deemed adequate. Routine chest CT is therefore not common practice.

46.4 Recipient Vessel Access (A Figure with Surface Markings)

Since the IMV never divides proximal to the third rib, it is best approached in the second or third intercostal space; preferentially in the second intercostal space due to much more predictable anatomy, with a wider space and single vein in 80% cases [9] (Fig. 46.2).

Traditionally the IMVs are accessed via the removal of a segment of costal cartilage (the rib-sacrificing approach). This approach provides excellent, reliable exposure of the vessels, with a wider space for vessel dissection and anastomosis. Several authors, however, have highlighted a number of disadvantages of this approach, including lon-

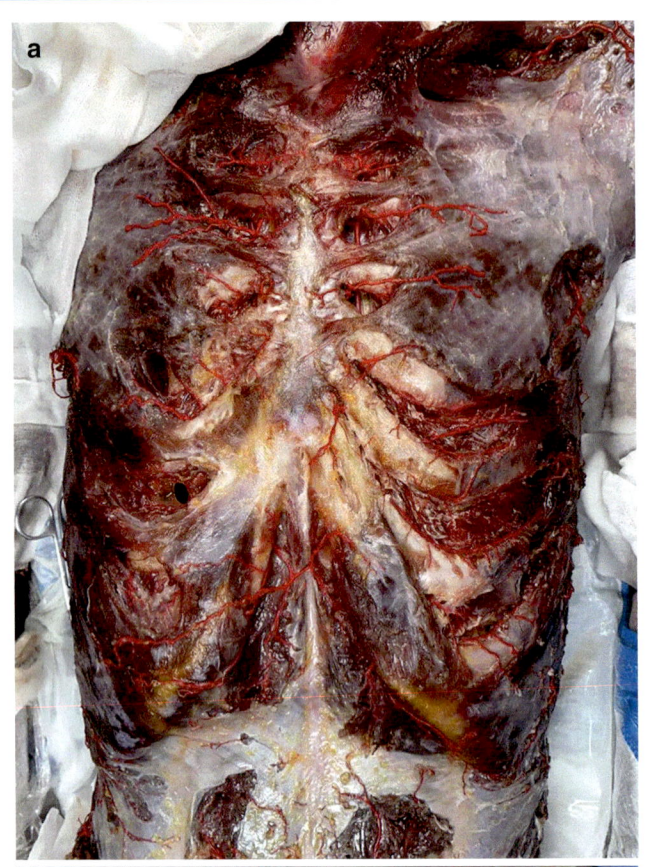

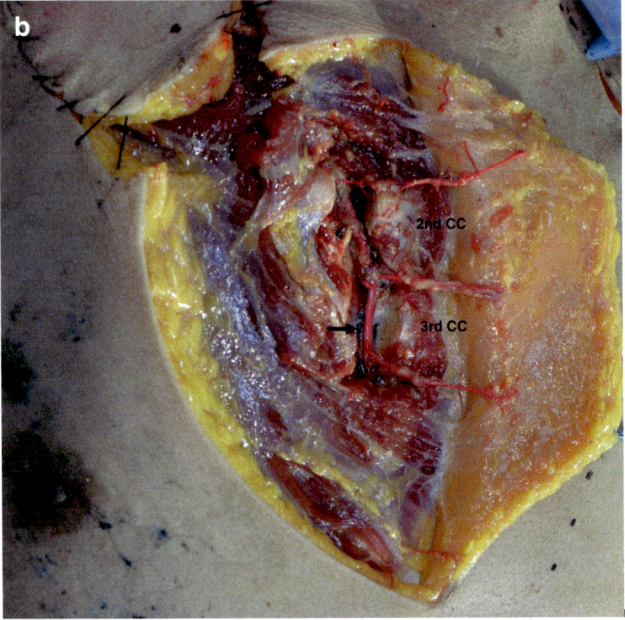

Fig. 46.1 (a) Latex injection dissection specimen demonstrating the anatomy of the IMA along its entire course. (b) Anatomy of the IMA perforators in relation to the second and third intercostal spaces. The IMV (arrow) has not yet divided, and therefore is best approached here (from Chap. 51 and provided by Dr Pafitanis and Dr Song)

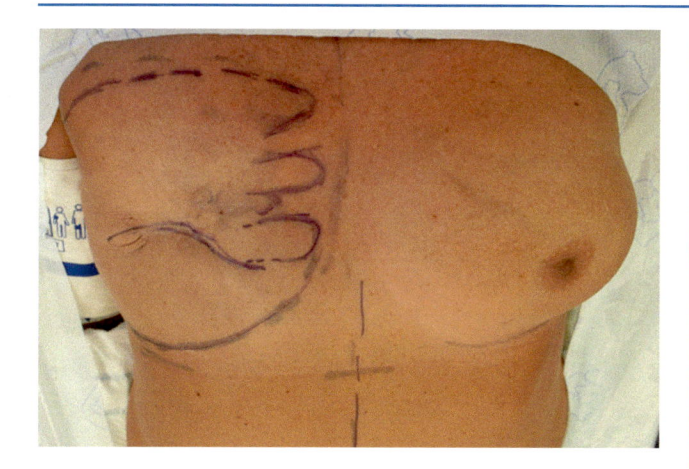

Fig. 46.2 Pre-op marking of the second–fourth ribs and corresponding intercostal spaces

ger post-operative pain and tenderness, and chest wall deformity [10]. With advances in microsurgery, the rib-preserving approach—first described by Parrett et al. in 2008—was developed, in which the IM vessels are accessed directly via the intercostal space, without the removal of the rib [11]. Significant advantages of this approach include reduced recipient site morbidity and post-operative pain relief requirements, and a potential radio-protective effect.

Though this approach provides an attractive alternative to the rib harvest technique, the narrower access to the recipient vessels can lead to increased flap ischaemic time and less available length, should revision anastomosis be required. A review of comparative studies has not provided a consensus as to which technique is superior [12]. The rib-preserving approach may therefore best be reserved for the experienced microsurgeon.

When alternative methods of autologous breast reconstruction are needed such as the TUG flap, the fourth rib is often removed due to the short length of its pedicle. This allows the flap to sit lower on the chest and match the inframammary fold of the other side. When two flaps are required for one breast reconstruction, by removing the fourth rib, the surgeon has a higher chance of utilizing anterograde anastomoses for the vein.

46.5 Recipient Vessel Dissection: A Step-by-Step Guide

- **Step 1** (Fig. 46.3)—In an immediate reconstruction, the second and third interspaces are marked before the mastectomy by palpating the ribs starting from the clavicle. In a delayed DIEP, the horizontal mastectomy scar is reopened down to the pectoralis major muscle.

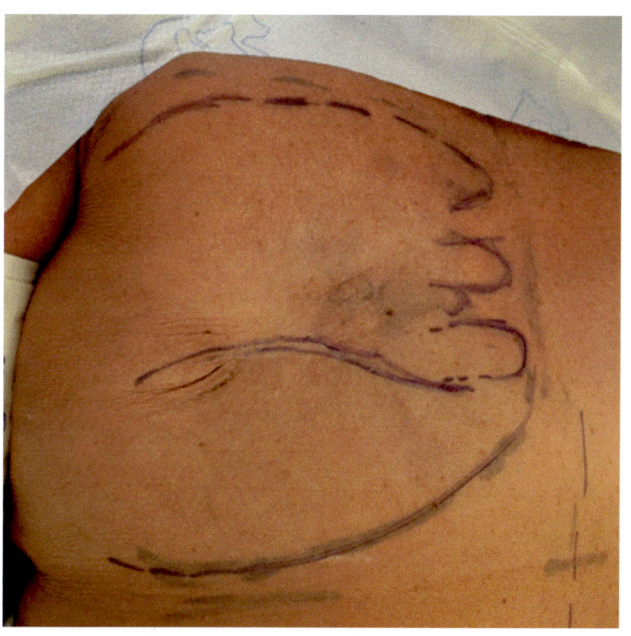

Fig. 46.3 Step 1—In an immediate reconstruction, the second and third interspaces are marked before the mastectomy by palpating the ribs starting from the clavicle. In a delayed DIEP, the horizontal mastectomy scar is reopened down to the pectoralis major muscle

- **Step 2** (Fig. 46.4a, b)—Pec major is split using monopolar diathermy from its insertion at the sternum along a length of 4–5 cm (Fig. 46.2a). Any chest wall perforators which are sizeable are protected for use of recipient vessels (Fig. 46.2b—depicted by arrow).
- **Step 3** (Fig. 46.5)—A self-retaining Traver's retractor is inserted to expose the second and third ribs, and fish hooks are used to retract the medial tissues. An alternative to fish hooks involves suturing 2.0 Vicryl sutures to the medial edge of the sternum and using these sutures as a retractor.
- **Step 4** (Fig. 46.6a, b)—The anterior perichondrium of the lower rib is marked and incised with diathermy.
- **Step 5** (Fig. 46.7a, b)—The anterior perichondrium is stripped from the cartilage using a periosteal elevator (Fig. 46.5a). In cases where there is significant scarring due to radiotherapy a Mitchells trimmer can be used (Fig. 46.5b). A cardiac Doyenne aids posterior dissection with gentle pushing medically once inserted into the correct plane between the posterior perichondrium below and the rib above.
- **Step 6** (Fig. 46.8)—Once the rib has been completely freed from the posterior perichondrium, it is protected laterally with a Howarth elevator or Cardiac Doyenne elevator before being cut with a knife.
- **Step 7** (Fig. 46.9a, b)—The rib is then disarticulated from the sternum, it can be removed as a single piece. If remnants of rib are still present medially; rongeurs can be

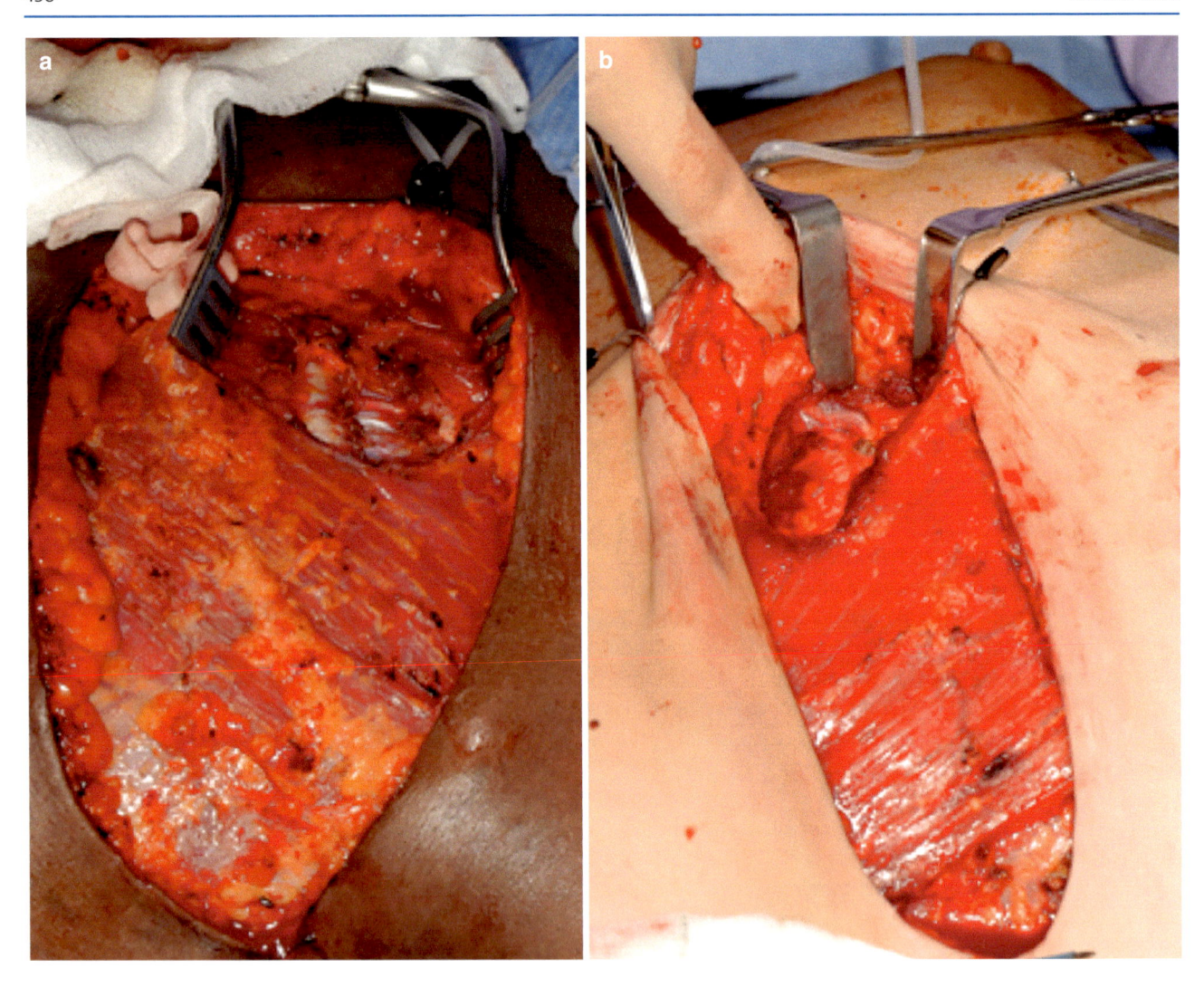

Fig. 46.4 (**a**) **Step 2**—Pec major is split using monopolar diathermy from its insertion at the sternum along a length of 4-5cm. (**b**) **Step 2**—Any chest wall perforators which are sizeable are protected for use of recipient vessels

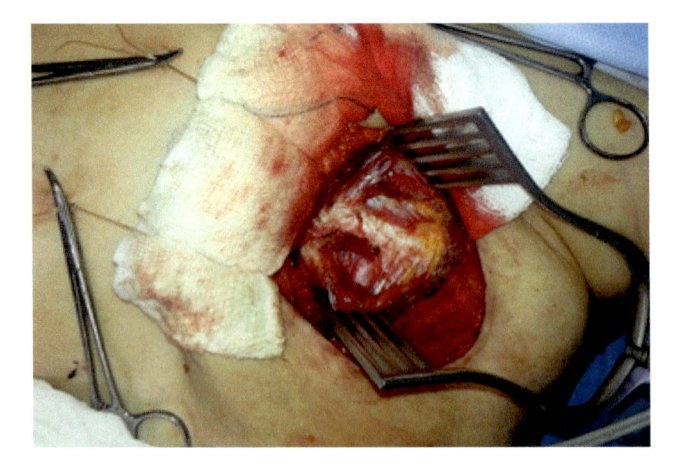

Fig. 46.5 **Step 3**—A self-retaining Traver's retractor is inserted to expose the second and third ribs, and fish hooks are used to retract the medial tissues. An alternative to fish hooks involves suturing 2.0 Vicryl sutures to the medial edge of the sternum and using these sutures as a retractor

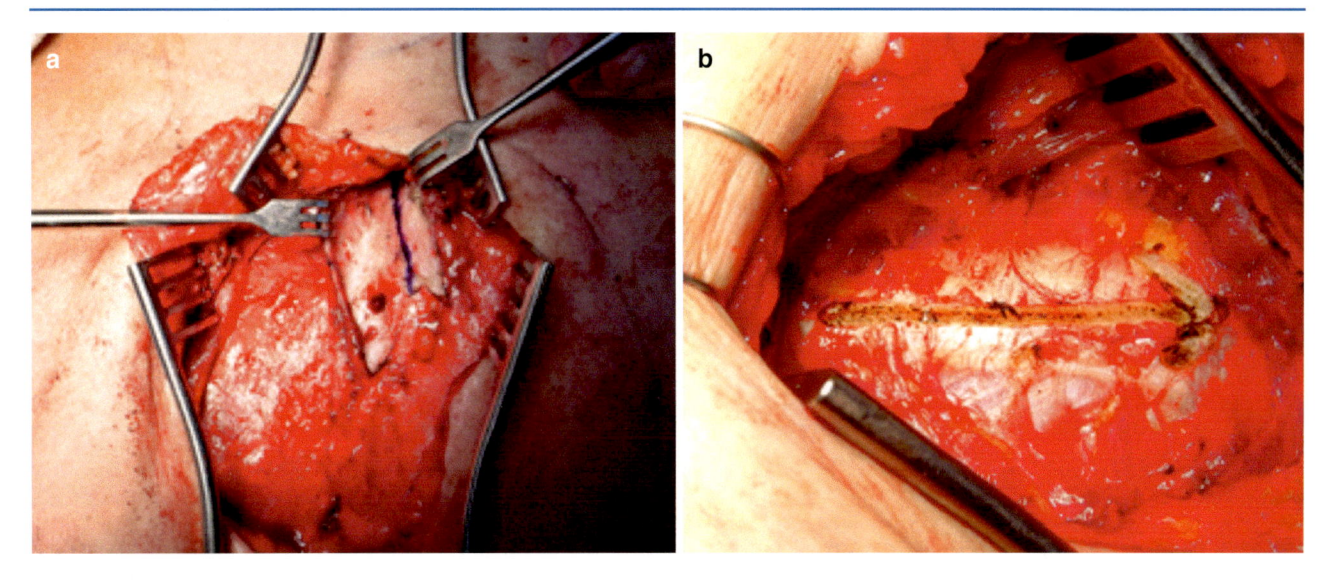

Fig. 46.6 (**a, b**) **Step 4** – The anterior perichondrium of the lower rib is marked (**a**) and incised with diathermy (**b**)

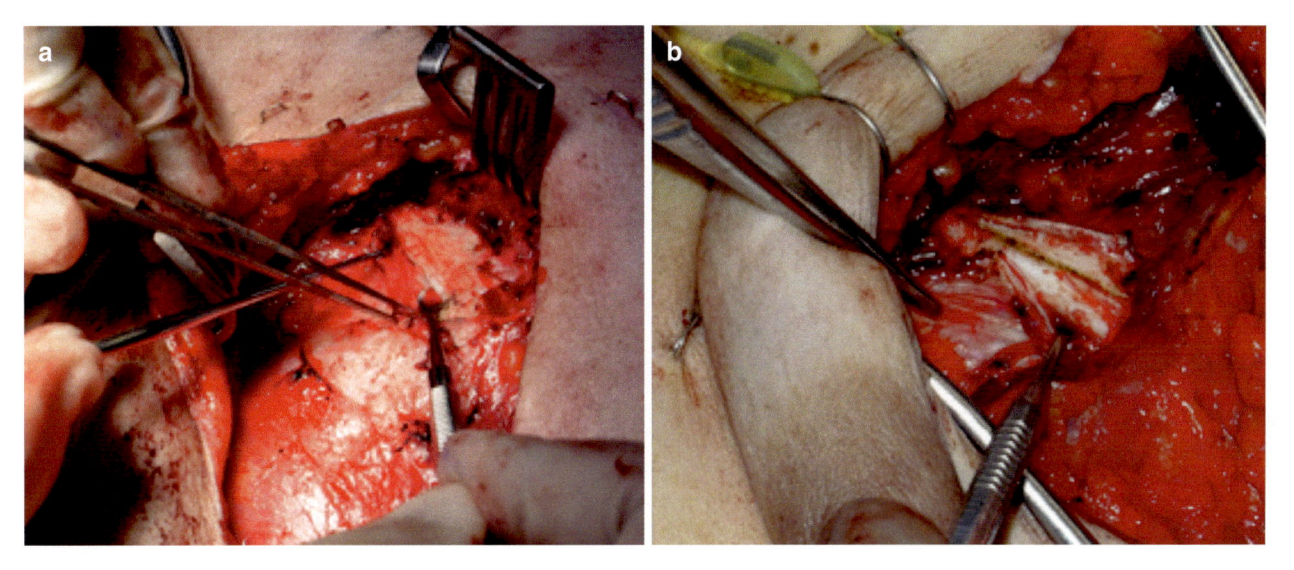

Fig. 46.7 (**a**) **Step 5**—The anterior perichondrium is stripped from the cartilage using a periosteal elevator. In cases where there is significant scarring due to radiotherapy a Mitchells trimmer can be used. (**b**) **Step 5**—A cardiac Doyenne aids posterior dissection with gentle pushing medially once inserted into the correct plane between the posterior perichondrium below and the rib above

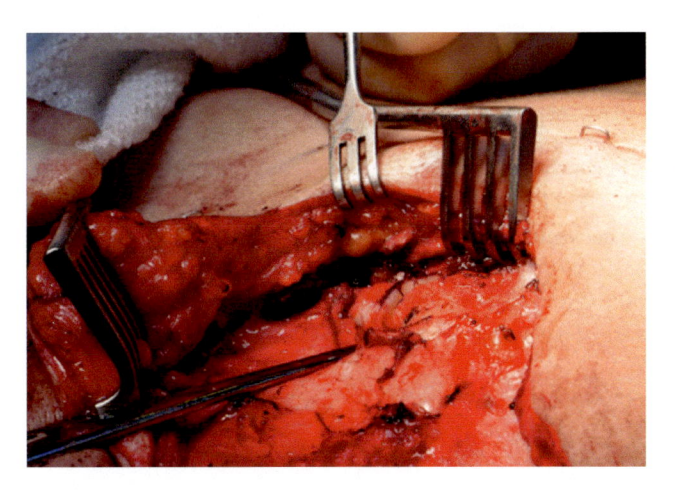

Fig. 46.8 **Step 6**—Once the rib has been completely freed from the posterior perichondrium, it is protected laterally with a Howarth elevator or Cardiac Doyenne elevator before being cut with a blade

used to remove rib medially until the sternum is reached. Care must be taken not to over-resect and iatrogenically remove sternum.

- **Step 8** (Fig. 46.10a, b)—The posterior perichondrium is dissected free using bipolar cautery from the underlying tissues. A damp swab can help to gently push and develop a plane between the overlying perichondrium and the vessels underneath. Care must be taken not to avulse or damage the underlying vessels particularly in cases where the chest is scarred due to radiotherapy—a nerve hook can help carefully dissect the perivascular tissues in these cases. To make the space wider, intercostal muscles are resected superiorly and inferiorly down to the second and fourth rib. The vessels are then dis-

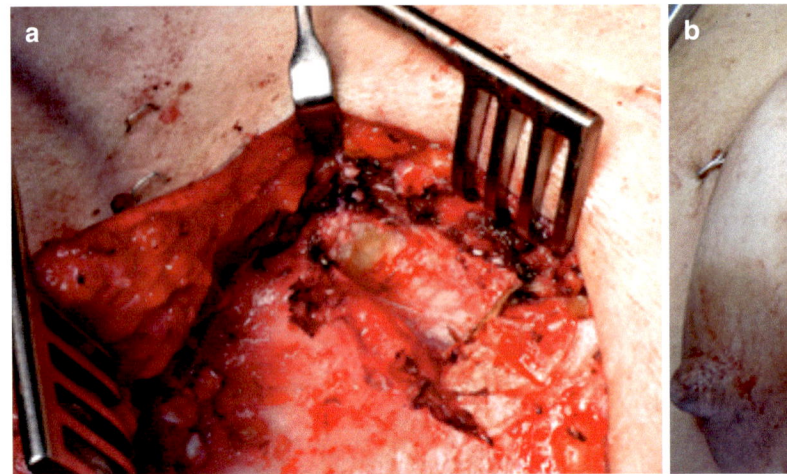

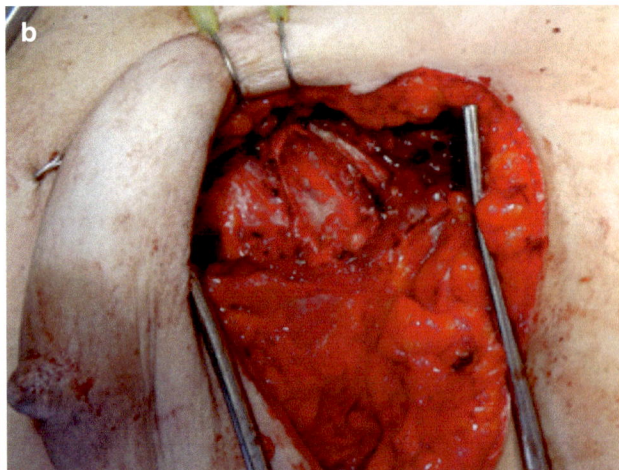

Fig. 46.9 (**a, b**) **Step 7**—The rib is then disarticulated from the sternum, it can be removed as a single piece. If remnants of rib are still present medially; rongeurs can be used to remove rib medially until the sternum is reached. Care must be taken not to over-resect and iatrogenically remove sternum

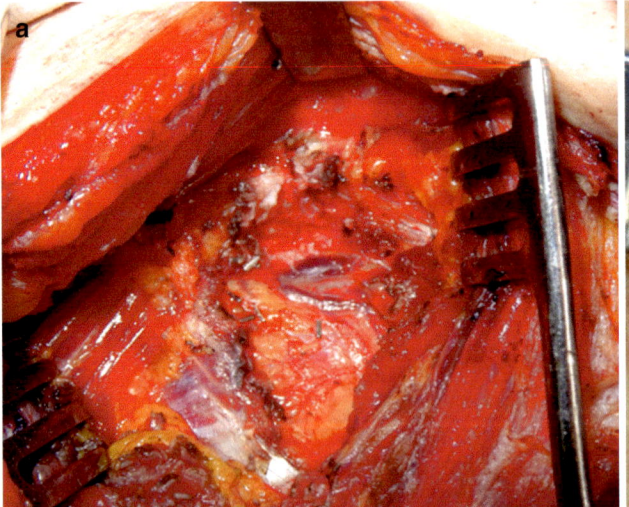

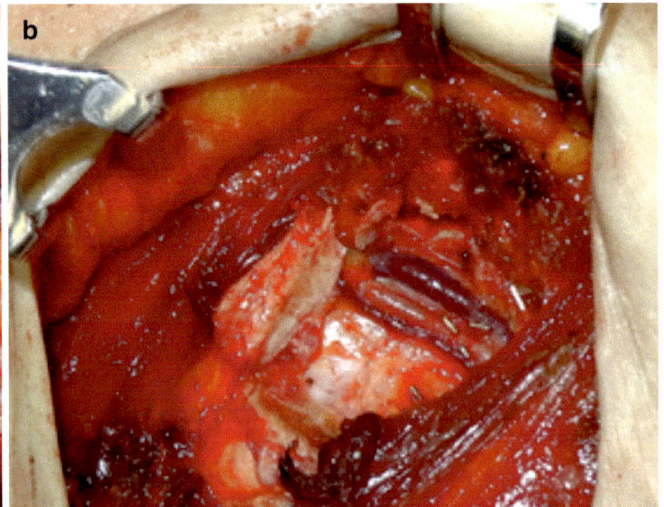

Fig. 46.10 (**a, b**) **Step 8**—The posterior perichondrium is dissected free using bipolar cautery from the underlying tissues. A damp swab can help to gently push and develop a plane between the overlying perichondrium and the vessels underneath. Care must be taken not to avulse or damage the underlying vessels particularly in cases where the chest is scarred due to radiotherapy – a nerve hook can help carefully dissect the perivascular tissues in these cases. To make the space wider, intercostal muscles are resected superiorly and inferiorly down to the second and fourth rib. The vessels are then dissected clean of perivascular fat and side branches – such as the anterior intercostal and sternal branches—cauterised or ligaclipped. Place ligaclips carefully, and angled appropriately, so they do not interfere with anastomosis

sected clean of perivascular fat and side branches—such as the anterior intercostal and sternal branches—cauterised or ligaclipped. Place ligaclips carefully and angled appropriately, so that they do not interfere with anastomosis.

Alternative Approach: The 'Rib-Preserving' Approach (Fig. 46.11) Another approach as is illustrated in this figure is to go between the ribs by raising an intercostal flap. The space for anastomosis can be narrow when using this approach, and is not favoured in cases of Bipedicled DIEP flaps, or without experience of the technique.

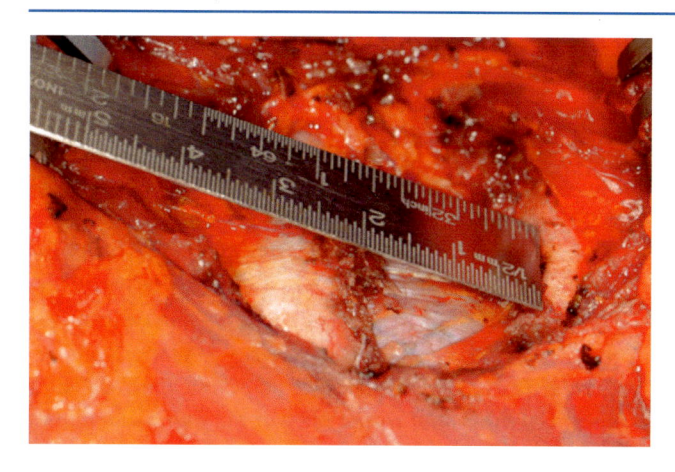

Fig. 46.11 Alternative approach: The rib preserving approach for internal mammary access—Another approach as is illustrated in this figure is to go between the ribs by raising an intercostal flap. The space for anastomosis can be narrow when using this approach, and is not favoured in cases of Bipedicled DIEP flaps, or without experience of the technique

46.6 Core Surgical Techniques in Recipient Vessel

We describe dissection of the internal mammary vessels in the second to third intercostal space following removal of the third rib, as this is the preferred point of access for the senior authors.

1. In an immediate reconstruction, the second and third interspaces are marked before the mastectomy by palpating the ribs starting from the clavicle (Fig. 46.3). In a delayed DIEP, the horizontal mastectomy scar is reopened down to the pectoralis major muscle, and the ribs palpated and marked.
2. Pec major is split using monopolar diathermy from its insertion at the sternum along a length of approximately 4–5 cm (Fig. 46.4a). Incision length is limited to 5 cm to permit suitable tension for retraction. Any sizeable perforator vessels are preserved for the anastomosis (Fig. 46.4b).
3. A self-retaining Traver's retractor is inserted to expose the second and third ribs, and fish hooks used to retract medial tissues. An alternative to fish hooks involves suturing 2.0 Vicryl sutures to the medial edge of the sternum and using these sutures as a retractor (Fig. 46.5).
4. A 3 cm line from the sternal edge is marked along the anterior perichondrium of the lower rib to the beginning of the bony rib, and incised with diathermy (Fig. 46.6a, b). {NB: The IM vessels are located within 2–2.5 cm of the sternal edge}.
5. A periosteal elevator is then used to strip the anterior perichondrium from the cartilage to its posterior surface (Fig. 46.7a). A Mitchells trimmer can be used in cases where there is significant irradiation of tissues, allowing for careful elevation of the anterior perichondrium (Fig. 46.7b). A cardiac Doyenne aids posterior dissection with gentle pushing medically once inserted into the correct plane between the posterior perichondrium below and the rib above.
6. The rib is then disarticulated from the sternum, with the aim to remove it as a single piece. If it is not removed as one piece, it can be removed piecemeal using rongeurs. Care must be taken here to avoid over resection, and iatrogenic disruption of the sternum.
7. The posterior perichondrium is dissected free using bipolar cautery from the underlying tissues. A damp swab cotton bud can help gently push and develop a plane between the overlying perichondrium and the vessels underneath. Sometimes perforators can guide the location of the internal mammary vessels. Care must be taken not to avulse or damage the underlying vessels particularly in cases where the chest is scarred due to radiotherapy. A nerve hook can help carefully dissect the perivascular tissues in these cases. To make the space wider, intercostal muscles are resected superiorly and inferiorly down to the second and fourth rib.
8. The perivascular fat of the IM vessels helps with identification once the posterior perichondrium has been dissected free (Fig. 46.10a). The vessels can then be cleaned of perivascular fat either with loupes or under the microscope, and side branches cauterised with bipolar diathermy on a low setting, or ligaclipped in preparation for the flap (Fig. 46.10b). Care must be taken to place ligaclips carefully and angled appropriately, so that they do not interfere with anastomosis. One can also preserve the intercostal nerve.
9. One should use the microscope early if there is significant scarring, or difficulty elevating posterior perichondrium off the vessels.
10. The vessels are then marked in their superior longitudinal axis with a series of dots. This helps twisting the pedicle which can compromise the anastomoses. This is especially important if using a venous coupler, as this can help propagate a twist superiorly and may go unnoticed beneath the superior rib.

46.7 Pearls and Pitfalls

Pearls

- The IM vessels, especially the vein, are typically smaller in caliber on the left than the right side [6, 13].
- When incising the pec major, it is important to avoid lateral extension of the incision beyond 4–5 cm to allow positioning of retractors with suitable tension. The medial extent of muscle split needs to be continued to the sternal edge to achieve sufficient exposure.
- In patients with previous chest radiotherapy, it may be easier to use a standard rib-sacrificing approach due to scarring and immobility of tissues. Often the segment of the IM vessels below the rib cartilage tend to be less friable than the segment within the interspace, suggesting a potential radio-protective effect of the rib.
- The fourth interspace usually has two venae comitantes, with the IMV most commonly branching at the level of the third or fourth rib (type I pattern). At this level, the vessels are of smaller diameter, are a better match for TUG flaps, and can allow double flap anterograde anastomoses to both venae comitantes.
- An internal mammary lymph node can frequently be encountered during dissection of the IM vessels. Although it may demonstrate inflammatory changes only, the identified node should be sent for histopathology in all patients with a cancer history, as this can alter stage and influence future treatment.

Pitfalls

- During perichondrial elevation, care must be taken in the irradiated chest to avoid puncturing of the perichondrium due to increased scarring. This manoeuvre should therefore always be performed laterally, away from the IM vessels.
- Likewise, extra care must be taken in the dissection of the IM vessels, as the planes between the vessels and the perichondrium and pleura are not so easily separated following radiotherapy.
- When removing the cartilage, it is important to ensure that the cartilage is removed right to the sternal edge to ensure adequate exposure of the IM vein—a common mistake is to not remove enough cartilage medially.

46.8 Selected Readings

- Arnez ZM, Valdatta L, Tyler MP, et al. Anatomy of the internal mammary veins and their use in free TRAM flap breast reconstruction. Br J Plast Surg. 1995;48(8):540–5.
- *A leading paper in the popularisation of the TRAM flap for breast reconstruction, this paper provides the first reported anatomical study of the IMV in human cadavers. Sixty-four internal mammary veins in 34 fresh human cadavers were studied, with 4 different patterns of venous anatomy identified. The type 1 pattern, in which the IMV runs medial and parallel to the IMA to the fourth intercostal space, where it divided into the medial and lateral IMV, was the most common pattern, observed in 69% of cases.*
- Clark CP, Rohrich RJ, Copit S, et al. An anatomic study of the internal mammary veins: clinical implications for free-tissue-transfer breast reconstruction. Plast Reconstr Surg. 1997;99(2):400–4.
- *Important anatomic study describing the anatomy of the internal mammary veins. The authors reported that there were veins of at least 3 mm diameter in the second ICS in 100% of cadavers. This was a landmark paper to support the use of the IM vessels as recipient vessels in free flap breast reconstruction.*
- Parrett B, Caterson SA, Tobias A, Lee BT. The rib-sparing technique for internal mammary vessel exposure in microsurgical breast reconstruction. Ann Plast Surg. 2008;60(3):241–3.
- *The first paper to describe the rib-sparing approach for IM vessel preparation. The authors reported a series of 74 flaps in which the rib-sparing technique was performed over a 3-year period, with no significant increase in complications, including revision of anastomosis (3%), fat necrosis (11%), or flap loss (1%), when compared with a group of 125 flaps undergoing rib resection. They demonstrated this approach to allow adequate exposure for safe and efficient microanastomosis, and to be reliable, bloodless, and reproducible.*
- Sasaki Y, Madada-Nyakauru RN, Samaras S. The ideal intercostal space for internal mammary vessel exposure during total rib-sparing microvascular breast reconstruction: a critical evaluation. J Plast Reconstr Aesthet Surg. 2019;72:1000–6.
- *In this paper, the authors present a series of 296 rib-preserving free flap breast reconstructions to support the safety and ease of the rib-preserving technique in microvascular breast reconstruction. They specifically looked at the ideal ICS, providing evidence for the preferential use of the second ICS. They analysed the vessel exposure times of different grades of surgeon, demonstrating exposure time to decrease with experience (resident to fellow to attending), with time taken plateauing off after seven*

cases. They argued the efficacy and safety of the technique, demonstrating a low intraoperative anastamotic revision rate and free flap failure rate.

- Hardwood N, Teotia S. Five steps to internal mammary vessel preparation in less than 15 minutes. Plast Reconstr Surg. 2017;140(5):884–6.
- *A useful paper describing five simple steps to efficient and safe internal mammary vessel preparation, with accompanying technical videos. Breast reconstruction was performed in 415 patients (715 breasts) using autologous tissue (850 flaps) from 2012 to 2016. In 97.6% of these breast reconstructions, the internal mammary vessels were used. The preparation of these vessels was routinely performed using the five-step technique described, within an average of approximately 15 min (range 7–45 min).*

Acknowledgements The authors give special thanks to Mr. Georgios Pafitanis of Barts Health NHS Trust and Dr. Yumao of Shanghai People's Hospital, China, for contributing Fig. 46.1a, b.

References

1. Longmire WP Jr, Ravitch MM. A new method for constructing an artificial oesophagus. Ann Surg. 1946;123:819–34.
2. Fujino T, Harashina T, Aoyagi F. Reconstruction for aplasia of the breast and pectoral region by microvascular transfer of a free flap from the buttock. Plast Reconstr Surg. 1975;56:335.
3. Shaw WW. Breast reconstruction by superior gluteal microvascular free flaps without silicone implants. J Plast Reconstr Aesthet Surg. 1983;72(4):490–501.
4. Harashina T, Imai T, Nakajima H, et al. Breast reconstruction with microsurgical free composite tissue transplantation. J Plast Reconstr Surg. 1980;33(1):30–7.
5. Arnez ZM, Valdatta L, Tyler MP, et al. Anatomy of the internal mammary veins and their use in free TRAM flap breast reconstruction. Br J Plast Surg. 1995;48(8):540–5.
6. Clark CP, Rohrich RJ, Copit S, et al. An anatomic study of the internal mammary veins: clinical implications for free-tissue-transfer breast reconstruction. Plast Reconstr Surg. 1997;99(2):400–4.
7. Pradas-Irun C, Azzawi K, Malata CM. A plea for recipient vascular pedicle versatility in microvascular breast reconstruction. Plast Reconstr Surg. 2012;129(2):383e–5e.
8. Tuinder S, Dikmans R, Schipper R, et al. Anatomical evaluation of the internal mammary vessels based on magnetic resonance imaging (MRI). J Plast Reconstr Aesthet Surg. 2012;65:1363–7.
9. Sasaki Y, Madada-Nyakauru RN, Samaras S. The ideal intercostal space for internal mammary vessel exposure during total rib-sparing microvascular breast reconstruction: a critical evaluation. J Plast Reconstr Aesthet Surg. 2019;72:1000–6.
10. Rosich-Medina A, Bouloumpasis S, Di Candia M. Total 'rib'-preserving technique of internal mammary vessel exposure for free flap breast reconstruction: a 5-year prospective cohort study and instructional video. Ann Med Surg. 2015;4:293–300.
11. Parrett B, Caterson SA, Tobias A, Lee BT. The rib-sparing technique for internal mammary vessel exposure in microsurgical breast reconstruction. Ann Plast Surg. 2008;60(3):241–3.
12. Jeevaratnam J, Nikkhah D, Dheansa B. The evolution of internal mammary vessel preparation in microsurgical breast reconstruction: what is the current evidence? J Plast Reconstr Aesthet Surg. 2014;67(9):e226–7.
13. Dupin CL, Allen RJ, Glass CA, Bunch R. The internal mammary artery and vein as a recipient site for free-flap breast reconstruction: a report of 110 consecutive cases. Plast Reconstr Surg. 1996;98(4):685–9.

Head and Neck Recipient Vessels Access

Alexandra O'Neill, Juan Enrique Berner, and Georgios Pafitanis

47.1 Indications

Head and neck reconstruction poses unique challenges due to the highly specialised anatomy, and cosmetic importance of the region. Microvascular free tissue transfer reconstruction has become the mainstay for large or composite defects and the guiding principles are to restore integrity, form, and function while aiming for an acceptable aesthetic outcome. Most reconstructions are performed following oncological surgery, which for intraoral and aerodigestive malignancies is frequently associated with concurrent neck dissection. However, secondary management of complications such as fistulae or osteoradionecrosis is also common in specialist services. Recipient vessel selection is influenced by defect site, indication for concurrent neck dissection, free flap pedicle length and caliber, and patient factors including prior surgery or radiotherapy.

47.2 Anatomy

47.2.1 Arterial Anatomy

At the level of the hyoid bone the common carotid artery (CCA) bifurcates into an internal and external carotid artery (ICA and ECA). The ICA slopes up in the carotid sheath beside the pharynx entering the base of skull via the carotid canal without giving off any branches throughout its course. The ECA continues anterior to the ICA passing deep to the posterior belly of digastric and stylohyoid before piercing the deep lamina of the parotid fascia and dividing into its terminal branches the maxillary artery and superficial temporal artery.

A. O'Neill (✉)
Department Plastic and Reconstructive Surgery, Royal Perth Hospital, Perth, WA, Australia

J. E. Berner · G. Pafitanis
London Reconstructive Microsurgery Unit (LRMU), Department of Plastic Surgery, Emergency Care and Trauma Division, The Royal London Hospital, Barts Health NHS Trust, London, UK

The non-terminal branches of the ECA include three anterior branches (superior thyroid, lingual and facial), one medial branch (ascending pharyngeal), and two posterior branches (occipital and posterior auricular). The anterior branches of the ECA are commonly utilised recipient vessels for neck and lower facial reconstruction due to their favourable orientation. The arterial anatomy is fairly constant, except for the facial and lingual arteries that can occasionally arise from a common trunk, the fascio-lingual trunk. The superficial temporal artery courses behind the temporomandibular joint anterior to the mastoid and external ear and crosses the posterior aspect of the zygomatic arch where it can be palpated in the pre-auricular region. The superficial temporal vessels are easily accessible for upper face, temple, and scalp reconstructions.

The transverse cervical artery (TCA), a branch of the thyrocervical trunk, is usually spared in most neck dissections and radiotherapy field for intraoral and aerodigestive tract malignancies. It passes across the lower aspect of the posterior triangle just superior to the clavicle and anterior to scalenus anterior. It is usually the vessel of choice in hostile and vessel-depleted necks (Fig. 47.1).

47.2.2 Venous Anatomy

The external jugular vein (EJV), formed by the posterior branch of the retromandibular vein and the posterior auricular vein, courses down in the subcutaneous tissue over sternocleidomastoid, piercing the investing layer of the deep cervical fascia approximately 1 cm above the midpoint of the clavicle to empty into the subclavian vein. The anterior branch of the retromandibular vein joins the facial vein emptying into the continuation of the sigmoid sinus to form the internal jugular vein (IJV) which typically receives the superior thyroid vein and the vena commitantes of the hypoglossal nerve. The IJV lies posterior to the ICA within the loose lateral aspect of the carotid sheath receiving numerous tributaries along its course.

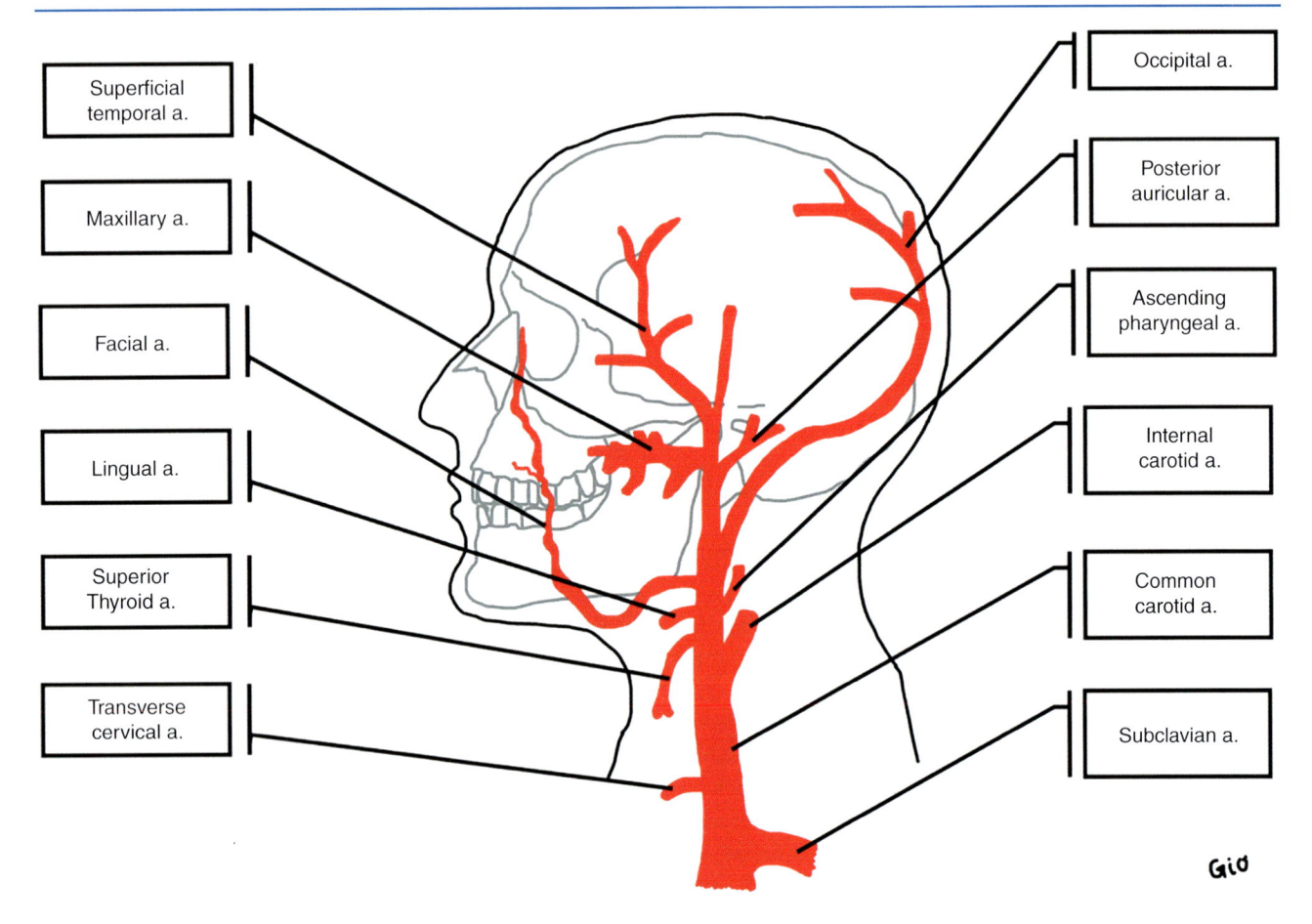

Fig. 47.1 Commonly used vessels in head and neck reconstruction

47.3 Pre-operative Investigation

Head and neck cancer patients tend to be older, smokers, and with comorbidities and require thorough pre-operative work up, including nutritional arrangements for the peri-operative period. Patients undergoing immediate reconstruction following tumour excision typically undergo pre-operative staging scans to assess the primary tumour, the nodal basin and investigate for metastatic disease with a combination of computed topography (CT) of the head and neck, magnetic resonance imaging (MRI), and positron emission tomography (PET) for selected cases. Specific imaging to assess recipient vessels is not routinely performed in head and neck reconstruction; however, CT-angiography can be considered for high-risk patients that have undergone prior surgery or radiotherapy.

47.4 Recipient Vessel Access

A variety of skin incisions have been described for performing neck dissections. The aim of these is to allow generous exposure to sub-platysma neck structures while raising robust skin flaps. Incision selection may change depending on which lymphatic levels and adjacent structures need to be addressed (for example: Conley, Schobinger, Macfee, Ariyan skin incisions). If no oncological neck dissection is indicated, an access neck dissection can be performed to prepare recipient vessels. This incision is placed preferably on skin crease 3 cm inferior to the border of the mandible. The incision continues through subcutaneous tissues and the platysma muscle. This approach allows identification and protection of the marginal mandibular nerve while exposing the investing layer of the deep cervical fascia (Fig. 47.2).

Fig. 47.2 Examples of described incisions for performing a neck dissection

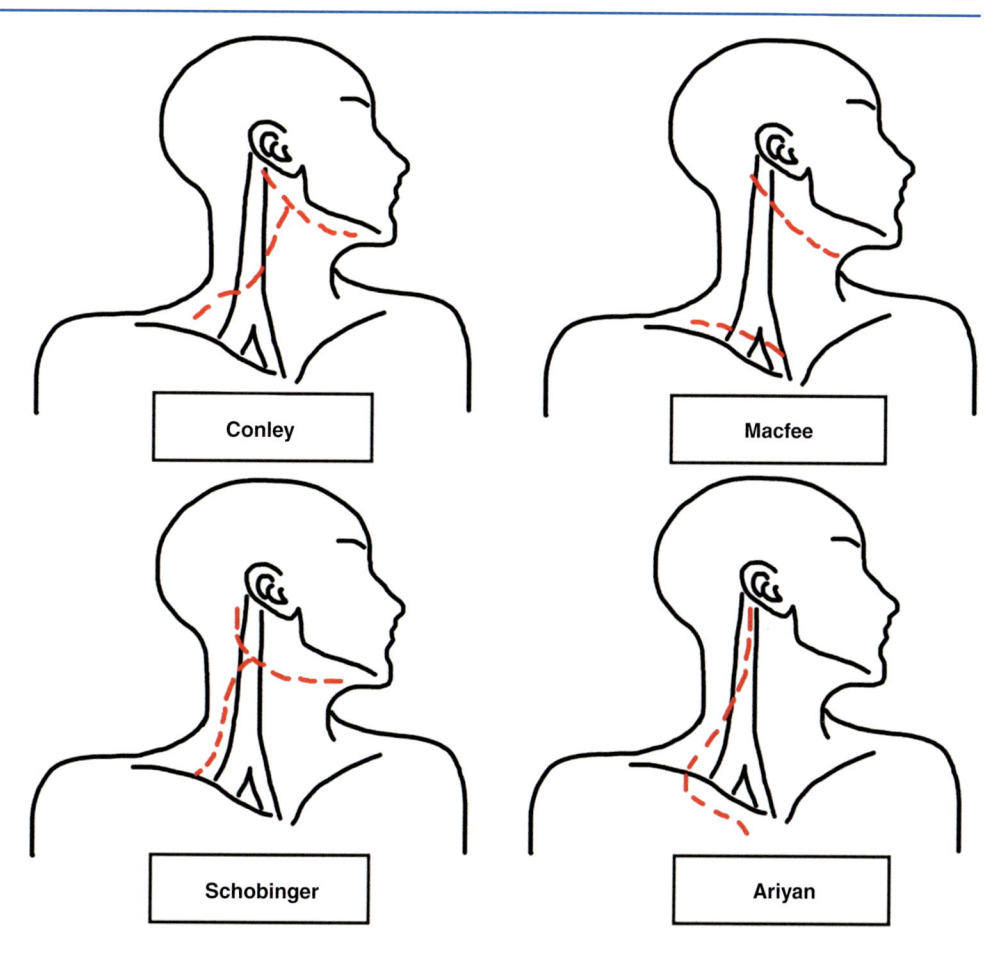

47.5 Recipient Vessel Dissection: A Step-by-Step Guide

Recipient vessel selection is of paramount importance in head and neck microsurgical reconstruction. The decision will be influenced by the location of the reconstruction, the pedicle length of the chosen free flap, and the availability of vessels in the region. For defects in the upper third of the face and scalp, the superficial temporal vessels tend to be ideally positioned, however, for defects of the lower two-thirds the facial artery offers easier access. For aerodigestive tract or neck resurfacing, the superior thyroid vessels are usually preferred. The transverse cervical vessels offer a lifeboat alternative in vessel-depleted necks, as it is spared in selective anterolateral neck dissections and radiotherapy fields. This algorithm should only be a guide, the ideal vessels for a given location may not be available, necessitating exploration of nearby alternatives. In this scenario having a long flap pedicle is preferred, with vein grafts being a last resort.

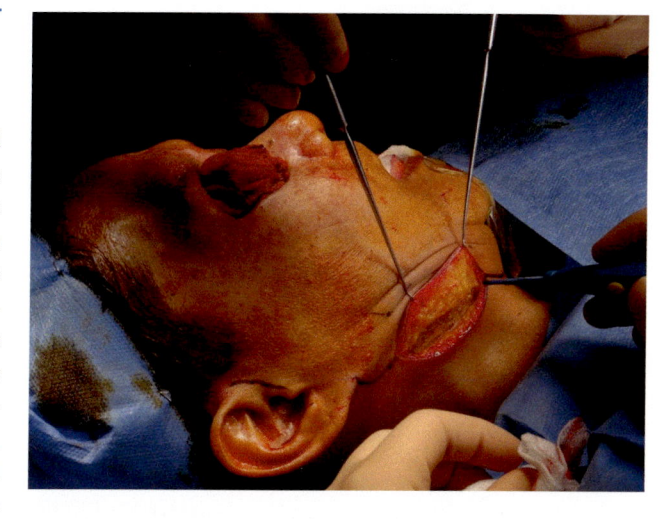

Fig. 47.3 Incision for accessing facial vessels

47.5.1 Facial Artery (FA)

- **Step 1:** The facial artery is palpated against the mandible and marked (Fig. 47.3).
- **Step 2:** Skin and subcutaneous tissues are incised; platysma is then divided. Flaps are raised on the sub-platysma plane, allowing identification of the marginal mandibular nerve (Fig. 47.4).
- **Step 3:** Protecting the nerve, the deep investing fascial layer of the neck can be incised and reflected superiorly. This exposes the facial artery (Fig. 47.5), which can be dissected proximally and distally.
- **Step 4:** Removal of the submandibular gland and transposing the facial artery stump below the posterior body of digastric allows mobilisation of this recipient vessel (Fig. 47.6).

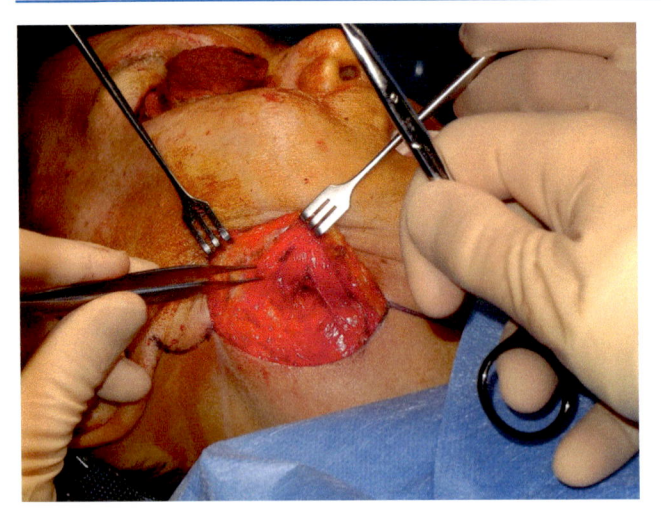

Fig. 47.4 Subplatysmal dissection

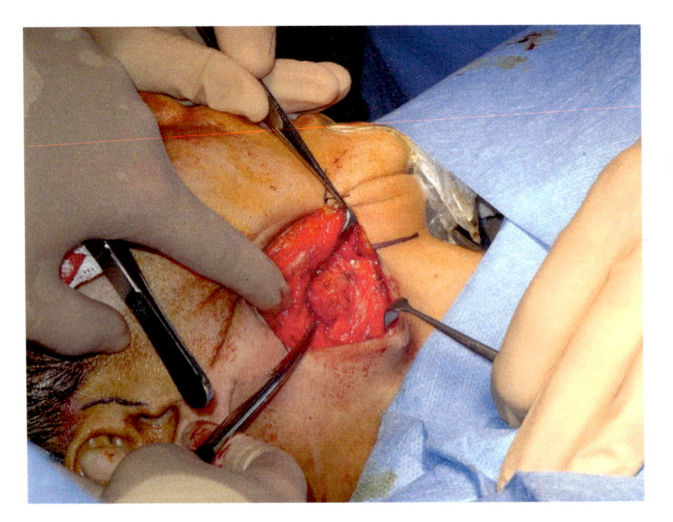

Fig. 47.5 Facial vessels are identified, while protecting marginal mandibular branch of facial nerve

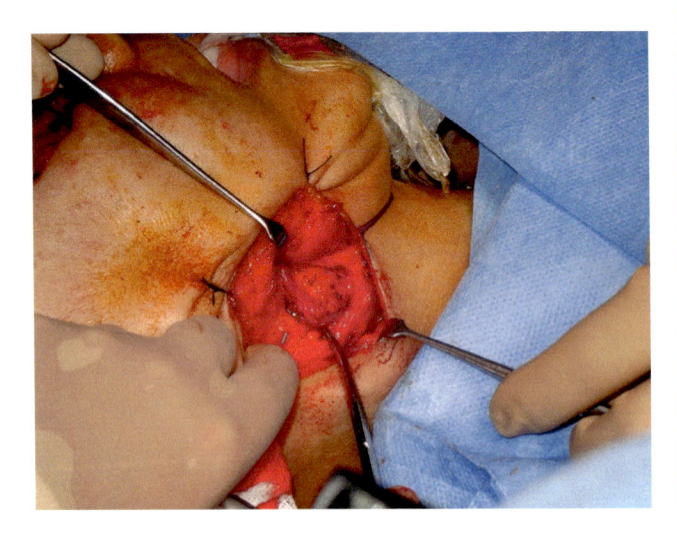

Fig. 47.6 Facial artery can be traced superiorly to augment the length of recipient vessels

47.5.2 Superior Thyroid Artery (STA)

- **Step 1:** The superior thyroid artery is usually accessed in the context of an anterolateral neck dissection.
- **Step 2:** The artery is identified as it arises from the external carotid artery and travels caudally to the thyroid gland within the carotid sheath.
- **Step 3:** The vessels are prepared carefully as they have a smaller calibre than the facial artery, providing a good match for SCIP or lateral arm flaps (Fig. 47.7).
- **Step 4:** The artery can be mobilised cranially to facilitate anastomosis.

47.5.3 Superficial Temporal Artery (SuTA)

- **Step 1:** A pre-auricular incision can be continued superiorly, or a hemi-coronal incision can be utilised to access the superficial temporal fascia in the temple region.

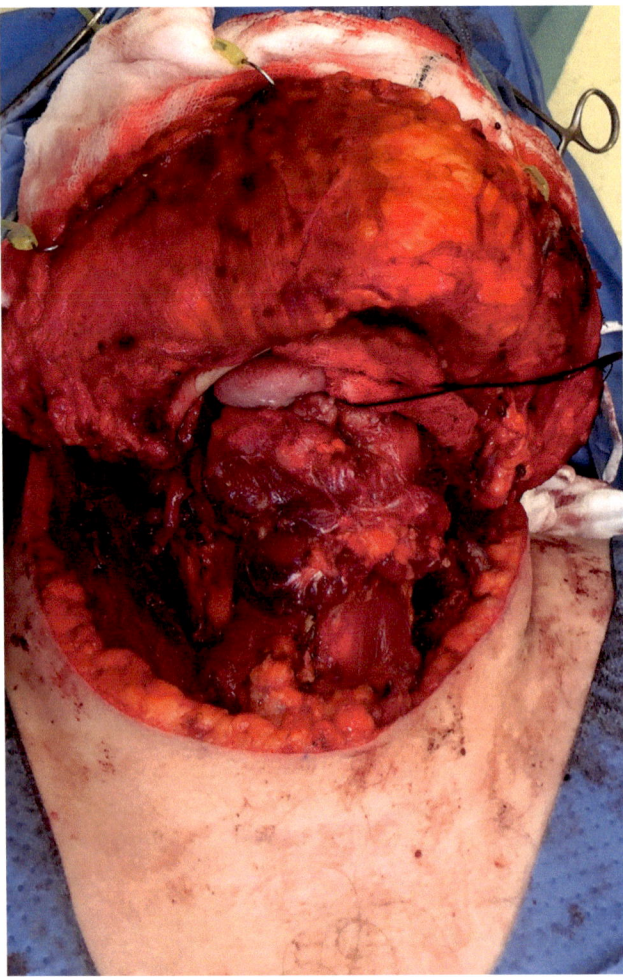

Fig. 47.7 Superior thyroid vessels are ideally positioned for microsurgical pharyngeal reconstruction

- **Step 2:** The superficial temporal vessels are identified under the superficial temporal fascia. Approximately 2–4 cm superior to the zygomatic arch the SuTA divides into its terminal branches.
- **Step 3:** The superficial temporal vessels are dissected and prepared. If small, they can be dissected inferiorly into the parotid gland, where their calibre increases.

47.5.4 Transverse Cervical Artery (TCA)

- **Step 1:** The transverse cervical vessels are located at the base of the posterior triangle of the neck, and are usually accessed in the context of a neck dissection.
- **Step 2:** The vessels can be identified as they pass laterally from their origin, the thyrocervical artery, across the posterior triangle on scalenus anterior, just above the clavicle.
- **Step 3:** The vessels are ligated just prior to their division into superficial and deep branches, facilitating superior transposition of the vessel to make it reach the level of the hyoid. Vessel length ranges from 4 to 7 cm and has mean diameter of 2.65 mm [1] (Fig. 47.8).

47.5.5 Venous Recipients

The EJV can be marked pre-operatively in slim patients; however, this is rarely required. Commonly, the EJV is divided during the neck dissection, where it is ligated as high as feasible and dissected a few centimetres proximally in its subcutaneous course to facilitate unrestricted mobility. Good communication between the reconstructive team and resecting teams is imperative to optimise EJV preservation during the nodal dissection. The EJV provides a reliable, easily accessible choice for end-to-end venous anastomosis (Fig. 47.9).

The IJV is exposed through its entire cervical course during a neck dissection and its many tributaries ligated, thereby providing multiple viable recipient vessels (Fig. 47.10).

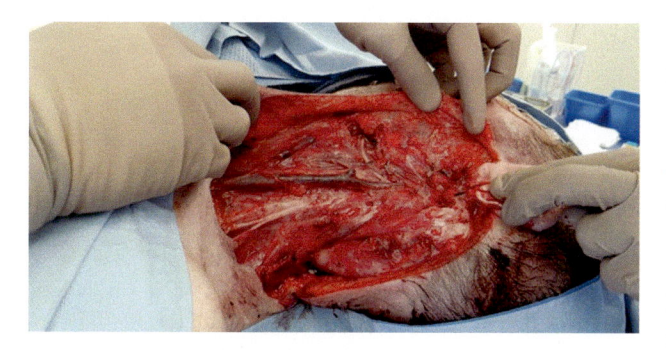

Fig. 47.8 Transverse cervical vessels can be found in the posterior triangle of the neck during a comprehensive or radical neck dissection

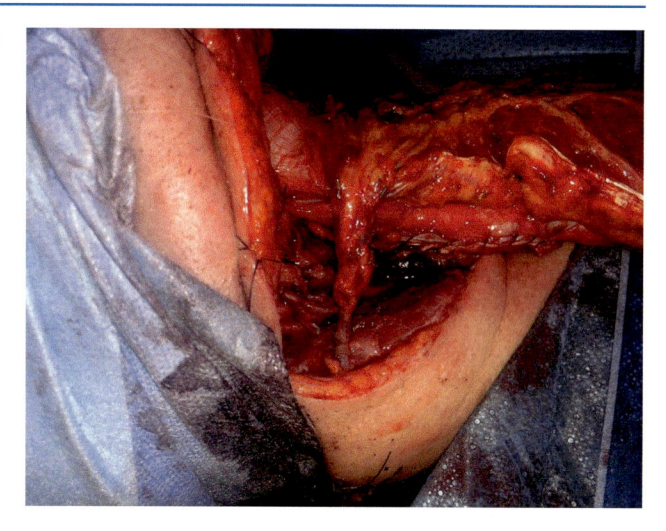

Fig. 47.9 The EJV can be mobilised to achieve an end-to-end anastomosis, using a coupler device for this case

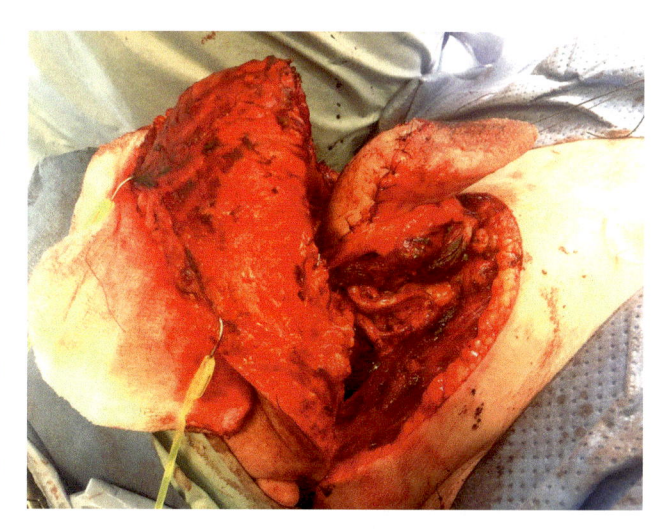

Fig. 47.10 End-to-side anastomosis to IJV

Anastomoses can be performed end to end onto one of its tributaries or end to side on to the IJV itself. If a side branch is to be used, standard microvascular clamps can be applied to the vessel base. For end-to-side anastomoses a paediatric Satinsky clamp can be applied to the IJV to facilitate anastomosis, this should be applied after the venotomy site is marked, as the vessel collapse can obscure the ideal site and size required.

47.6 Core Surgical Techniques in Recipient Vessel Harvesting

Recipient vessel selection and preparation is largely determined by whether a neck dissection is indicated at the time of reconstruction and the type of dissection planned including what structures are anticipated to be sacrificed [2].

Subplatysmal flaps are raised via the surgeon's preferred neck dissection incision and the EJV is dissected and ligated as a potential recipient vein. The sternocleidomastoid muscle is retracted laterally with a conventional or self-retaining retractor or, alternatively, a nylon tape, to expose the underlying carotid sheath and its contents. The IJV is dissected cranial with preservation of tributary stumps, provided its sacrifice is not planned with the oncologic resection. The external carotid artery is dissected, and particular attention paid to the anterior branches, notably the facial and superior thyroid arteries which are conveniently positioned to facilitate microvascular anastomosis. Recipient vessels should be mobilised 1–2 cm where possible to provide adequate length and reduce the risk of kinking. Patency and pulsatile flow are confirmed, and a microvascular clamp is applied in anticipation for flap transfer (Table 47.1).

Table 47.1 Proposed algorithm for recipient vein selection in head and neck reconstruction

Algorithm for recipient vein selection in Head and Neck free tissue transfer
1°: Venous comitant vein of the selected recipient artery
2°: Branches of the Internal Jugular Vein (IJV) in proximity to the selected recipient artery
3°: External Jugular Vein (EJV)
4°: Internal Jugular Vein (IJV) in an end-to-side configuration
5°: Long Vein grafting to the contralateral neck veins (IJV branches or contralateral EJV)
6°: Cephalic vein transposition

47.6.1 Microvascular Anastomosis

Once the flap is transferred to the recipient site, the pedicle is checked to ensure no twist has occurred during transfer (Fig. 47.10). The decision in terms of sequence for venous and arterial anastomoses should consider the position of the recipient vessels and the difficulty of access. Reconstruction of head and neck defects often requires partial flap inset prior to microvascular anastomoses, and this should be factored into the surgical planning. An algorithm for recipient arteries is displayed in Table 47.2.

47.7 Pearls and Pitfalls

Pearls
- The decision to perform end-to-end or end-to-side arterial and venous anastomoses is best decided on a case by case basis with consideration of the configuration of recipient and pedicle vessels, vessel calibre, and potential size mismatch rather than a dogmatic approach that has been traditionally taught [3–5].
- Consider the transverse cervical vessels or the contralateral neck in irradiated fields and patients with prior neck dissections. The TCA is less affected by atherosclerosis than the carotid system [1, 6, 7].
- Two venous anastomoses are better than one where possible [8]. Studies have demonstrated IJV thrombosis rated between 0 and 26% at 1 week post free flap reconstruction [9, 10].

Pitfalls
- Where two free flaps are required to reconstruct large or composite defects and recipient vessels are limited, the first flap can be used as a recipient vessel to the second flap. In this situation, the second flap can be vascularised by either a proximal muscle branch off the flap pedicle (a pseudo-chimeric flap) or by distal run off from the first flap (flow-through style flap [11]). This technique does carry a high rate of partial and total flap failure but can provide a bailout in the vessel-deplete neck.
- The contralateral neck, internal mammary vessels and the cephalic vein are alternatives for vessel-depleted necks for which the transverse cervical vessels are not available. The pectoralis major is still a robust regional flap option when no recipient vessels are available for soft tissue transfer.

Table 47.2 Proposed algorithm for vessel selection in head and neck reconstruction

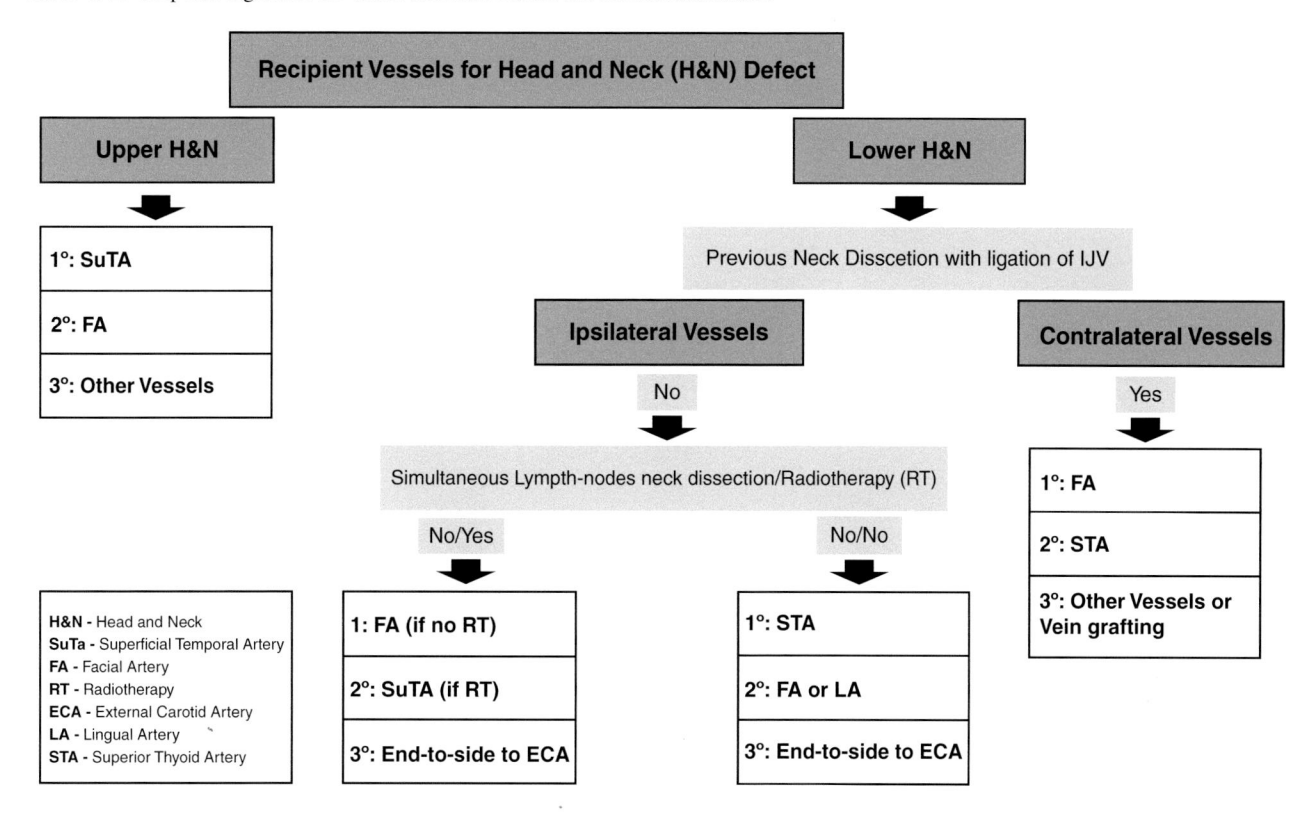

```
                    Recipient Vessels for Head and Neck (H&N) Defect
                              │                              │
                    ┌─────────┘                              └─────────┐
                    ▼                                                  ▼
                Upper H&N                                          Lower H&N
                    │                                                  │
                    ▼                                                  ▼
               1°: SuTA                         Previous Neck Dissection with ligation of IJV
                                                           │
               2°: FA                          ┌───────────┴───────────┐
                                               ▼                       ▼
               3°: Other Vessels         Ipsilateral Vessels     Contralateral Vessels
                                               │                       │
                                              No                      Yes
                                               ▼                       ▼
                              Simultaneous Lymph-nodes neck        1°: FA
                              dissection/Radiotherapy (RT)
                                  │              │                2°: STA
                               No/Yes         No/No
                                  ▼              ▼                3°: Other Vessels or
                          1: FA (if no RT)    1°: STA                  Vein grafting

                          2°: SuTA (if RT)    2°: FA or LA

                          3°: End-to-side     3°: End-to-side
                              to ECA              to ECA
```

H&N - Head and Neck
SuTa - Superficial Temporal Artery
FA - Facial Artery
RT - Radiotherapy
ECA - External Carotid Artery
LA - Lingual Artery
STA - Superior Thyoid Artery

47.8 Selected Readings

- Chummun S, McLean NR, Ragbir M. Surgical education: neck dissection. Br J Plast Surg. 2004;57(7):610–23. https://doi.org/10.1016/j.bjps.2004.05.011. PMID: 15380694.
- Kushida-Contreras BH, Manrique OJ, Gaxiola-García MA. Head and neck reconstruction of the vessel-depleted neck: a systematic review of the literature. Ann Surg Oncol. 2021;28(5):2882–95. https://doi.org/10.1245/s10434-021-09590-y. Epub 2021 Feb 6. PMID: 33550502.
- Chia HL, Wong CH, Tan BK, Tan KC, Ong YS. An algorithm for recipient vessel selection in microsurgical head and neck reconstruction. J Reconstr Microsurg. 2011;27(1):47–56. https://doi.org/10.1055/s-0030-1267829. Epub 2010 Oct 25. PMID: 20976669.
- Tessler O, Gilardino MS, Bartow MJ, St Hilaire H, Womac D, Dionisopoulos T, Lessard L. Transverse cervical artery: consistent anatomical landmarks and clinical experience with its use as a recipient artery in complex head and neck reconstruction. Plast Reconstr Surg. 2017;139(3):745e–51e. https://doi.org/10.1097/PRS.0000000000003085. PMID: 28234854.

References

1. Tessler O, et al. Transverse cervical artery: consistent anatomical landmarks and clinical experience with its use as a recipient artery in complex head and neck reconstruction. Plast Reconstr Surg. 2017;139(3):745e–51e.
2. Yagi S, et al. Recipient vessel selection in head and neck reconstruction based on the type of neck dissection. Yonago Acta Med. 2016;59(2):159–62.
3. Nahabedian MY, et al. Recipient vessel analysis for microvascular reconstruction of the head and neck. Ann Plast Surg. 2004;52(2):148–55; discussion 156–7.
4. Chia HL, et al. An algorithm for recipient vessel selection in microsurgical head and neck reconstruction. J Reconstr Microsurg. 2011;27(1):47–56.
5. Ahmadi I, et al. End-to-end versus end-to-side microvascular anastomosis: a meta-analysis of free flap outcomes. J Reconstr Microsurg. 2017;33(6):402–11.
6. Yu P. The transverse cervical vessels as recipient vessels for previously treated head and neck cancer patients. Plast Reconstr Surg. 2005;115(5):1253–8.
7. Yazar S. Selection of recipient vessels in microsurgical free tissue reconstruction of head and neck defects. Microsurgery. 2007;27(7):588–94.
8. Christianto S, et al. One versus two venous anastomoses in microsurgical head and neck reconstruction: a cumulative meta-analysis. Int J Oral Maxillofac Surg. 2018;47(5):585–94.
9. Prim MP, et al. Patency and flow of the internal jugular vein after functional neck dissection. Laryngoscope. 2000;110(1):47–50.
10. Wax MK, et al. Internal jugular vein patency in patients undergoing microvascular reconstruction. Laryngoscope. 1997;107(9):1245–8.
11. Dancey A, Blondeel PN. Technical tips for safe perforator vessel dissection applicable to all perforator flaps. Clin Plast Surg. 2010;37(4):593–606, xi-vi.

Upper Limb Recipient Vessels Access

Zhi Yang Ng, Calum Honeyman, Amir Sadr, and Dariush Nikkhah

48.1 Indications

The requirement for upper limb microsurgery is varied and includes reconstruction following trauma, burns, infection, neoplasia and congenital differences for both elective free tissue transfers, and emergency cases such as replantation, revascularisation, fasciotomies and amputations. Selection of the most appropriate recipient vessels depends on the size and composition of the defect to be addressed, osteosynthesis required (e.g. external fixator), quality of vessels (particularly veins) and the pedicle length available; vein and nerve grafts may also be needed and should be marked out at the start of the case on the same limb.

It is also important to consider the long-term reconstructive plan for patients from the outset. In the upper extremity, staged reconstruction to optimise function is commonly required. The addition of future free functioning muscle or toe transfers should be carefully planned when choosing recipient vessels to prevent burning future bridges.

This chapter details the relevant clinical anatomy of the most commonly used recipient vessels in upper limb free tissue transfer, up to and including the antecubital fossa proximally. In addition, the pre-operative work up, surgical approach and technical pearls and pitfalls are discussed, with the aim of maximising functional and aesthetic outcomes for this highly challenging group of patients.

48.2 Anatomy

48.2.1 Antecubital Fossa

The boundaries of the antecubital fossa are the brachioradialis (BR) muscle laterally, the pronator teres muscle medially and a theoretical line between the medial and lateral epicondyles proximally. The floor is made up of the brachialis and supinator muscles, and the roof by skin, fat, fascia, the median cubital vein and the bicipital aponeurosis (lacertus fibrosus). The brachial artery, a continuation of the axillary artery, originates at the distal edge of the teres major muscle, where it is generally accompanied by two sizeable venae comitantes. Numerous subcutaneous veins are encountered when accessing the antecubital fossa from the medial side, including the large basilic vein, which runs superficial and medial to the brachial artery, accompanied by the medial antebrachial cutaneous nerve (MABCN) in the subcutaneous plane. Ultimately, the brachial artery divides into the radial and ulnar arteries approximately 2 cm distal to the flexion crease of the elbow (Fig. 48.1). This bifurcation occurs medial to the insertion of the biceps tendon, and lateral to the median nerve (Fig. 48.2). While anatomical variations of the brachial artery have been described that include an accessory brachial artery, trifurcation and even complete absence [1], this is usually not of clinical significance.

48.2.2 Forearm/Wrist

In the proximal third of the forearm, the radial artery is usually located in a plane deep to the BR (but can be superficial to BR [2]) and flexor carpi radialis (FCR) muscle bellies. At this level, the ulnar artery lies in a plane on top of the brachialis and flexor digitorum profundus muscles (FDP) and beneath the muscle bellies of pronator teres (PT), FCR and flexor digitorum superficialis (FDS) arising from the common flexor origin. In the distal third of the forearm, the

Z. Y. Ng
Oxford Deanery, Oxford, UK

C. Honeyman
Canniesburn Plastic Surgery and Burns Unit, Glasgow Royal Infirmary, Glasgow, UK

A. Sadr · D. Nikkhah (✉)
The Royal Free Hospital NHS Foundation Trust, London, UK
e-mail: d.nikkhah@nhs.net

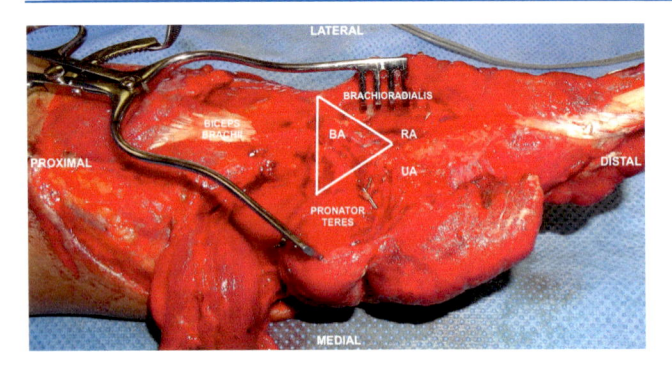

Fig. 48.1 Bifurcation of the brachial artery (BA) into the radial (RA) and ulnar (UA) arteries approximately 2 cm distal to the flexion crease of the elbow. Triangle represents the boundaries of the antecubital fossa

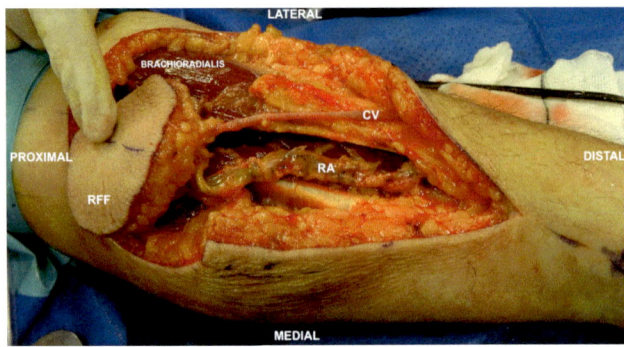

Fig. 48.3 Reverse radial forearm flap (RFF) based on retrograde flow through the radial artery (RA) (note accompanying pair of venae comitantes) and cephalic vein (CV)

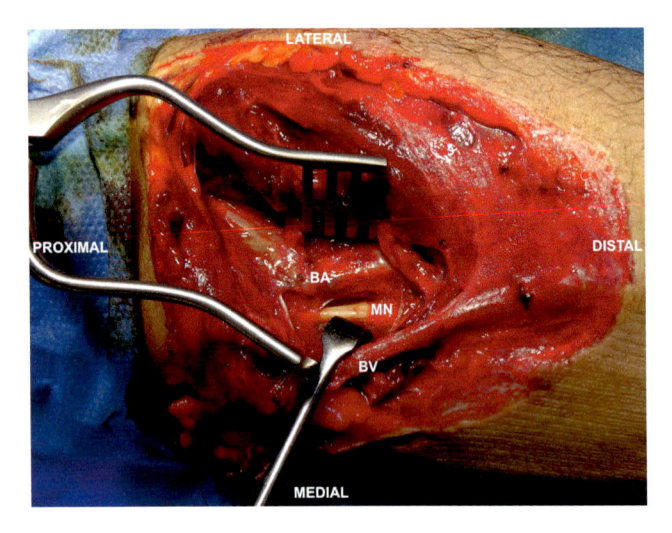

Fig. 48.2 Median nerve (MN) lies medial to the brachial artery (BA) at the antecubital fossa; basilic vein (BV) retracted

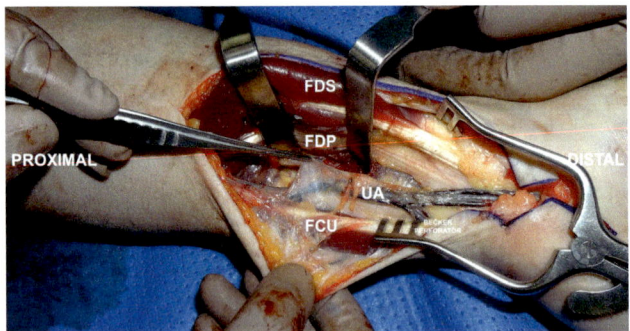

Fig. 48.4 Ulnar artery with accompanying venae comitantes; The FDS and FDP are retracted radially while FCU is retracted ulnarly. Note dorsal branch of ulnar artery i.e. perforator used for Becker flap arborising into the skin

radial artery continues in the lateral intermuscular septum, easily accessed between the tendons of the FCR muscle ulnarly and brachioradialis radially. The ulnar artery courses on the medial side of the ulnar nerve, in a plane between the FCU tendon ulnarly and FDS radially, sitting on top of the FDP tendons before entering Guyon's canal at the wrist.

The cephalic vein (3 mm or more) has a suprafascial course along the radial aspect of the forearm (Fig. 48.3) and crosses the anatomical snuffbox distally in the wrist. Correspondingly, the basilic vein can be found on the medial aspect of the arm before joining the median cubital vein in the antecubital fossa and extends distally along the ulnar aspect of the forearm. Both radial and ulnar arteries are commonly accompanied by a pair of venae comitantes (around 1.5 mm each) (Fig. 48.4).

48.2.3 Hand

The ulnar artery exits the wrist on the radial side of the pisiform and distal FCU tendon, entering Guyon's canal with the ulnar nerve located ulnarly. Guyon's canal is approximately 4 cm in length and sits on top of the transverse carpal ligament bounded by the pisiform and pisohamate ligament ulnarly and the hamate radially. Ultimately, the ulnar artery becomes the superficial palmar arch in 39% of cases, or anastomoses with the superficial palmar branch of the radial artery in 35% of cases to form the superficial palmar arch [2] at the level of Kaplan's line, with other anatomical variations comprising the rest. Correspondingly, the radial artery leaves the distal wrist and enters the anatomical snuff box between the tendons of abductor pollicis longus (APL), extensor pollicis brevis (EPB) and extensor pollicis longus (EPL); deep to the fascia of the snuff box, the radial artery and its two venae comitantes are found coursing obliquely in the space on top of the first and second metacarpals. The superficial palmar branch of the radial artery is also superficial to the flexor tendons and common digital nerves from the median nerve but deep to the superficial palmar fascia.

Three common digital arteries then arise from the superficial palmar arch and subsequently bifurcate into proper palmar digital arteries around 1 cm proximal to the webspaces. The proper digital arteries continue into the digits deep to the digital nerves (Fig. 48.5), and are covered by Grayson's ligaments volarly, and Cleland's ligaments dorsally [3]. Ultimately, these form an arch at the level of the pulp, which is distal to the distal interphalangeal joint before terminating in the central artery of the pulp. Of note, the thumb is unique in that it has a palmar (proper digital arteries) and dorsal blood supply (variable origins from first dorsal metacarpal artery to the dorsal branch of radial artery) [4].

An abundant network of highly variable veins is present on the dorsum of the hand and fingers which ultimately drain into the basilic and cephalic veins. Superficially, the cephalic vein and superficial radial nerve branches are encountered in the snuffbox. Small volar veins are also present in the digits and can be used as recipient outflow for distal replants and in bespoke super microsurgical finger free flaps.

48.3 Pre-operative Investigation

Careful pre-operative clinical examination of the upper extremities prior to microsurgical intervention is essential to ascertain signs of neurovascular compromise, associated functional deficits, size and composition of potential defects and the true extent of the zone of injury, if applicable. Observation for signs of intravenous drug use or in situ or previous venous and arterial lines is also important.

Physical examination typically requires documentation of the results from Allen's test, especially when raising flaps based on the radial or ulnar artery, to avoid subsequent hand ischaemia. This occurs when colour (i.e. perfusion) fails to return during an Allen's test, suggesting that the blood sup-

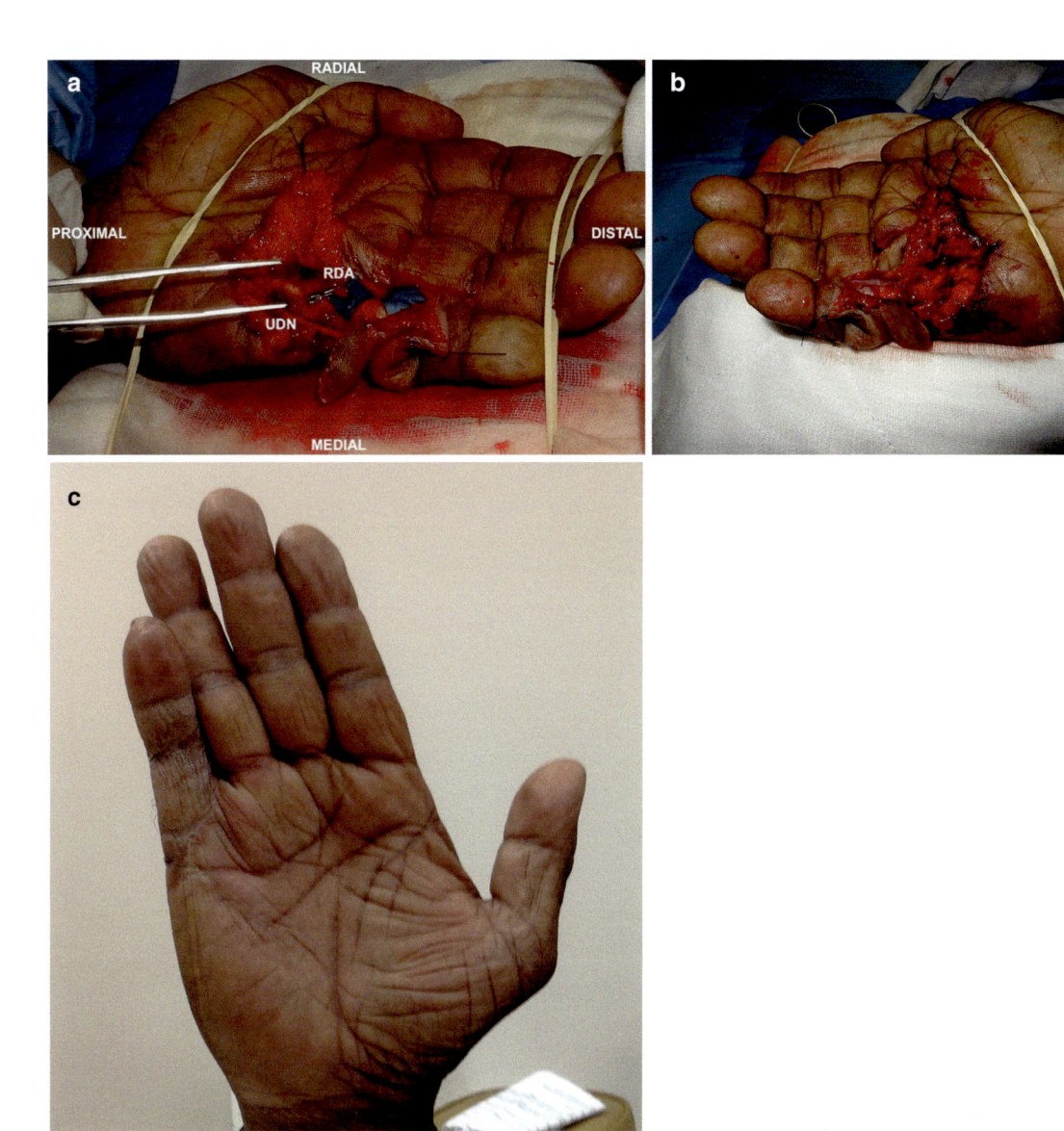

Fig. 48.5 (**a**) Ring avulsion injury (Urbaniak Class II) of the little finger, demonstrating an intact ulnar digital nerve (UDN) and microsurgical repair (with vein graft, not shown) of the radial digital artery (RDA). (**b**) Reperfused digit after reversed interpositional vein graft taken from distal forearm. (**c**) Outcome after salvage

ply to the palmar arch is incomplete (e.g. blood flow from the ulnar artery is compromised if the radial artery is compressed and pallor persists, and vice versa). Interestingly, head and neck reconstruction studies based on the radial forearm free flap have suggested an incidence of a variant, superficial ulnar artery in 0.43% of cases, which suggests radial dominance based on Allen's test although true figures are believed to be much higher [5].

Of note, the superficial location of the cephalic and basilic veins is such that both can be lost as a result of trauma. Therefore, there has been increasing argument for CT angiography to assess both the arterial and venous systems, especially in paediatric patients where clinical findings may be equivocal, or in mutilating injuries, as the surgical plan may change. Finally, colour Doppler ultrasound is increasingly being used to map out perforators arising from both the radial [6] and ulnar [7] arteries.

48.4 Recipient Vessel Access (A Figure with Surface Markings)

Typical incisions for access to the (a) brachial artery and bifurcation into radial and ulnar arteries; (b) radial artery along the proximal, middle or distal forearm; within the anatomical snuffbox (c); and (d) ulnar artery along the middle or distal forearm, and (e) wrist (Fig. 48.6).

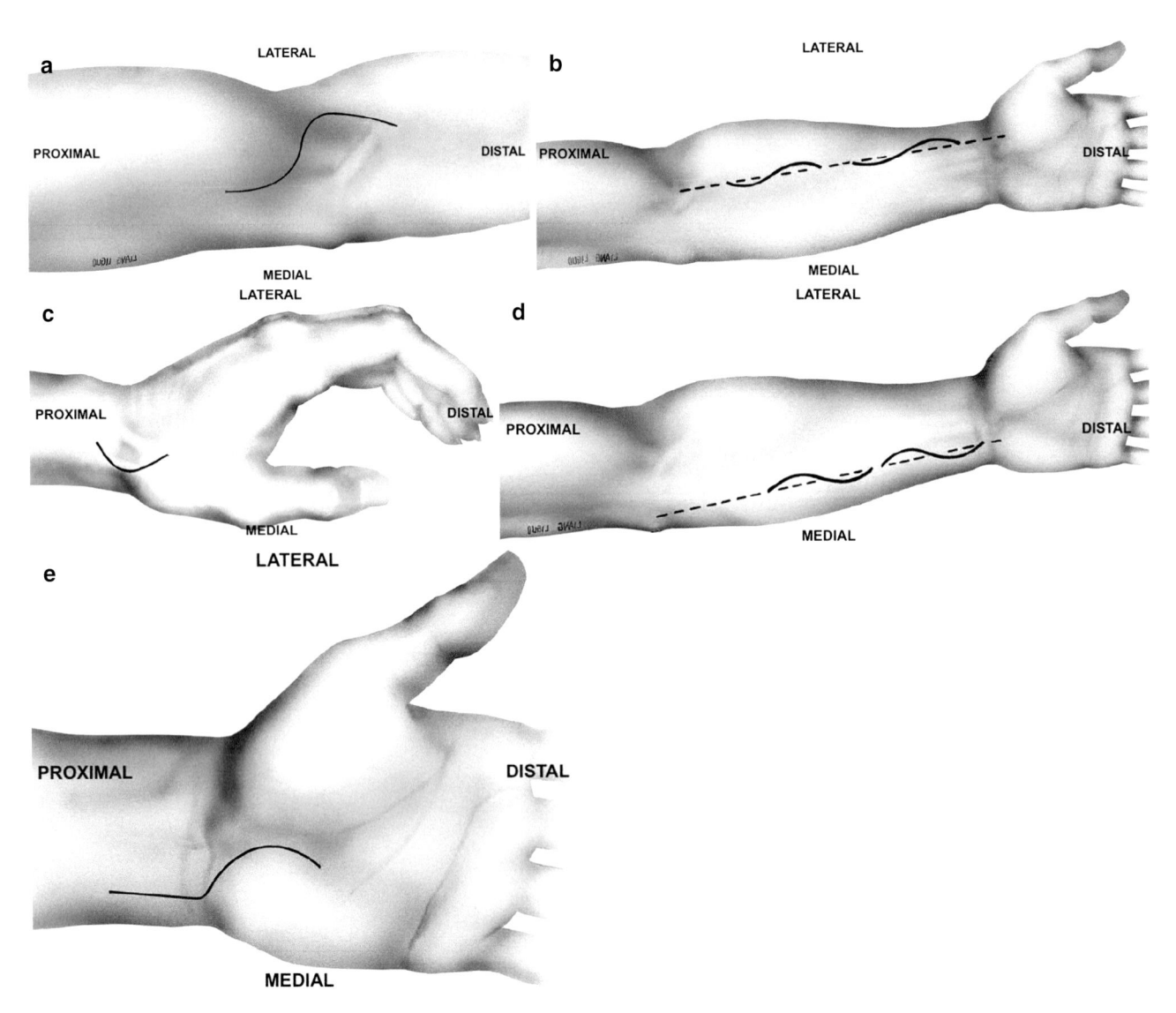

Fig. 48.6 Typical incisions for exposure of the (**a**) brachial artery and bifurcation, radial artery along the forearm (**b**) and within the anatomical snuffbox (**c**), and the ulnar artery along the forearm (**d**) and in the hand/wrist (**e**). (Modified from Strauch, B. and Yu, H., 2006. Atlas of Microvascular Surgery. New York: Thieme)

48.5 Recipient Vessel Dissection: A Step-by-Step Guide

Following general or regional anaesthesia, patients are typically positioned supine with their arm outstretched on a hand table and an upper arm tourniquet applied. Figure 48.6 shows classical placement of skin incisions for access to the main recipient vessels of the upper limb; the accompanying venae comitantes are usually sufficient for microsurgery. However, in trauma, infection and oncology, the final soft tissue defect may be far more extensive following debridement or R0 resection and may incorporate or even be "joined up" with these incisions.

48.5.1 Brachial Artery: Antecubital Fossa
(Fig. 48.6a)

NB: To access the brachial artery in the arm, a removable sterile tourniquet or pre-operative subcutaneous administration of local anaesthetic with adrenaline can be useful.

1. Palpate the brachial artery (BA) in the distal arm by rolling your fingers medially and deep to the biceps tendon.
2. Place the skin incision slightly medial to the artery beginning 4–5 cm proximal to the elbow crease. Extend the incision distally, crossing the flexion crease of the elbow at 90° before terminating the incision into the forearm to permit access to the bifurcation of the BA into the radial and ulnar arteries as required.
3. When approaching the BA from medial to lateral, the following structures will be encountered and should be preserved: the MABCN, the median nerve (larger than the MABCN and just medial to the BA), the basilic vein, the median cubital vein and, finally, the BA.
4. Incise the deep fascia overlying the BA.
5. Further exposure of the bifurcation, if required, can be achieved by incising the bicipital aponeurosis (lacertus fibrosus) and retracting the pronator teres and brachioradialis.

48.5.2 Radial Artery; Distal Forearm
(Fig. 48.6b)

1. Palpate and identify the radial artery (RA) in the distal forearm between the tendons of FCR and BR (radially).
2. A curvilinear skin incision is made directly over the RA.
3. Incise the deep fascia over the RA and insert a West self-retaining retractor to optimise exposure.

48.5.3 Radial Artery: Anatomical Snuffbox
(Fig. 48.6c)

1. A curvilinear incision is placed over the radial side of the snuffbox to expose the EPL and APL/EPB; the superficial branch of the radial nerve and the cephalic vein run superficial to the fascia and should be identified and preserved.
2. Incision of the deep fascia between EPL and APL/EPB followed by blunt dissection exposes the radial artery (Fig. 48.7).

48.5.4 Ulnar Artery: Distal Forearm
(Fig. 48.6d, e)

1. Place skin incision radial to the FCU to expose the antebrachial fascia medially and the FCU ulnarly.
2. Incision of the fascia exposes the ulnar artery which lies deep to the FCU. If necessary, further distal exposure can be achieved with a curvilinear incision across the wrist crease placed between the pisiform and hook of hamate.
3. The volar carpal ligament (which forms the roof of Guyon's canal) and palmaris brevis are then divided with bipolar cautery with further extension into the proximal palm (Fig. 48.8). At this level the ulnar nerve continues to lie laterally so due care must be taken to avoid the deep branch of the ulnar nerve when accessing this area.

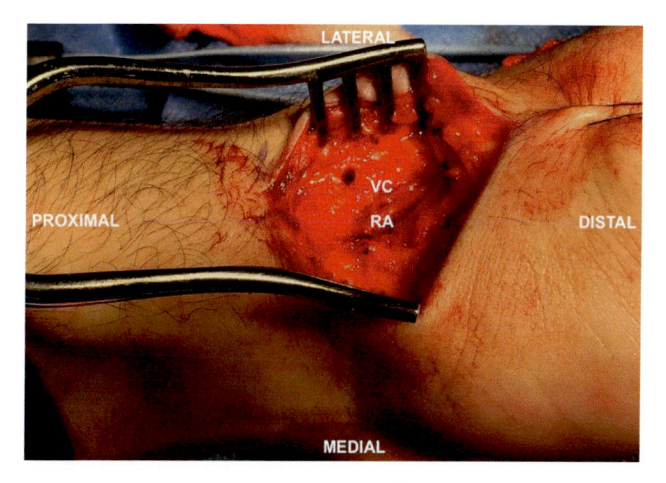

Fig. 48.7 Exposure of the radial artery (RA) and accompanying venae comitantes (VC) within the anatomical snuff box

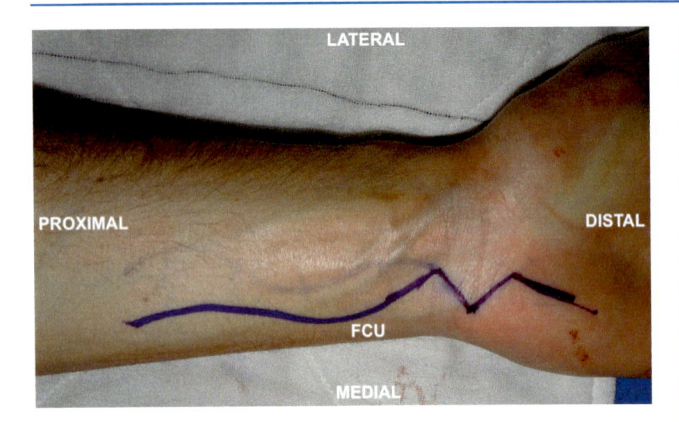

Fig. 48.8 Skin incision radial to the FCU for exposure of the ulnar artery and accompanying venae comitantes, with distal, zig-zag extension across the wrist crease into the proximal palm

48.6 Core Surgical Techniques in Recipient Vessel Harvest

Generally, using one or two West self-retaining retractors helps to maximise recipient vessel exposure and frees up the assistant(s) to help with preparing for microsurgical anastomosis. Identify and preserve the important and relevant neurovascular structures encountered with vessel loops; vessel side branches can be ligated with electrocautery alone, clips alone, or a combination of both (with heatsink technique) so that adequate recipient vessel length can be achieved. Dissect and clip superficial veins encountered during access incisions in the upper limb as potential venous outflow options.

48.6.1 Brachial Artery

1. Use tenotomy scissors or knife to progress through subcutaneous tissue proximal to the antecubital fossa (Step #2 above).
2. Distal to the elbow flexion crease, following dissection and preservation of key neurovascular structures (Steps #3 and #4 above), preserve any sizeable cutaneous nerves (potential nerve graft donor) that run along with the basilic vein.
3. Use microsurgical Acland clamps for proximal and distal control and microsurgical scissors for cutting back trimmed ends and/or making an arteriotomy for ETS anastomosis.

48.6.2 Radial Artery

1. This is usually of sufficient calibre at the distal forearm to permit ETS anastomosis to preserve distal perfusion to the hand (Step #2 above) to avoid potential sequelae including cold intolerance and pain.
2. When the dissection is extended more distally (but proximal to the wrist crease), the superficial palmar branch (variable calibre, 0.8–3.0 mm) of the radial artery may be identified and can be used for ETE anastomosis (Step #3); distal to the wrist crease, careful blunt dissection in the first dorsal compartment will expose the radial artery at the base of the snuffbox (Step #4) (Fig. 48.9).

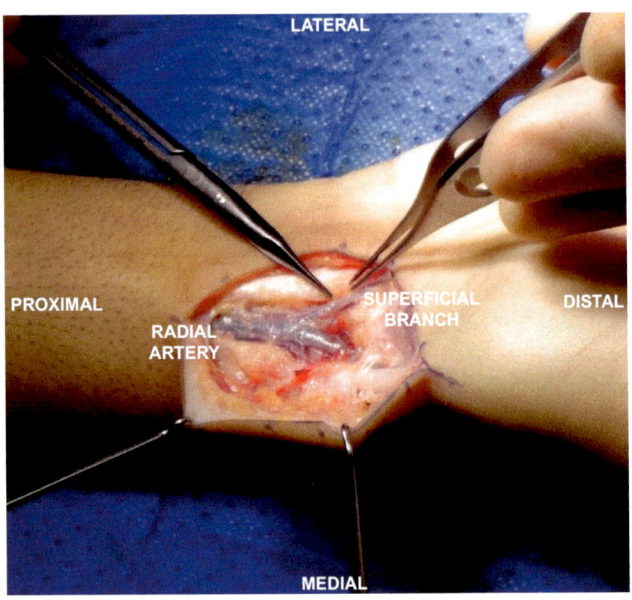

Fig. 48.9 Superficial palmar branch of radial artery seen entering thenar eminence (Demonstrated by tenotomy forceps). This serves as the basis for the free thenar flap, it can also be used as a recipient vessel

48.6.3 Ulnar Artery

1. It is usually radial and superficial to the ulnar nerve at the wrist although in a small number of cases, it can be suprafascial and at risk of inadvertent injury.
2. Further dissection under palmaris brevis into the palm for distal exposure can be performed (Step #4).
3. After Guyon's canal is opened, the hook of the hamate is identified by palpation, the ulnar neurovascular bundle retracted medially, and the deep motor branch of the ulnar nerve is identified and preserved after dissection of the proximal edge of the hypothenar muscles with tenotomy scissors.

48.7 Pearls and Pitfalls

Pearls
- Consider preservation of perforators from the brachial artery around the elbow to permit end-to-end (ETE) anastomosis (e.g. perforator to perforator) instead of end-to-side (ETS) to the brachial artery.
- Following the radial artery distally after exposure of the bifurcation leads to several branches including the recurrent radial artery, and also the superficial palmar branch of the radial artery both of which can also be used for ETE anastomosis.
- Release of the brachioradialis from the distal radius may occasionally be necessary for adequate vessel exposure.
- The main blood supply to the hand is usually from the ulnar artery. ETS anastomosis to the ulnar artery is preferable or perforator to perforator ETE anastomosis.
- CT angiogram can be helpful in planning microsurgical anastomosis in free tissue transfer to the upper extremity, with identification of perforators and suitable recipient vessels.

Pitfalls
- Under the operating microscope, assess for intimal damage, particularly in the case of digital revascularisation for avulsion injuries.
- In extremity replantation dissect back outside the zone of injury under the operating microscope.
- Check for good proximal flow before microsurgical anastomosis (Fig. 48.10a).
- Prepare extra donor sites in the lower limb (e.g. saphenous vein, which will need to be reversed in direction, and sural nerve for cable grafting) and/or the volar forearm for potential vein or nerve grafts for digital revascularisation (posterior interosseous nerve, MABC nerve) (Fig. 48.10b).
- Wherever possible do not sacrifice the main vessels (radial artery and ulnar artery) in the upper extremity when performing free tissue transfer, ETS anastomosis or ETE perforator to perforator anastomosis should be considered first.

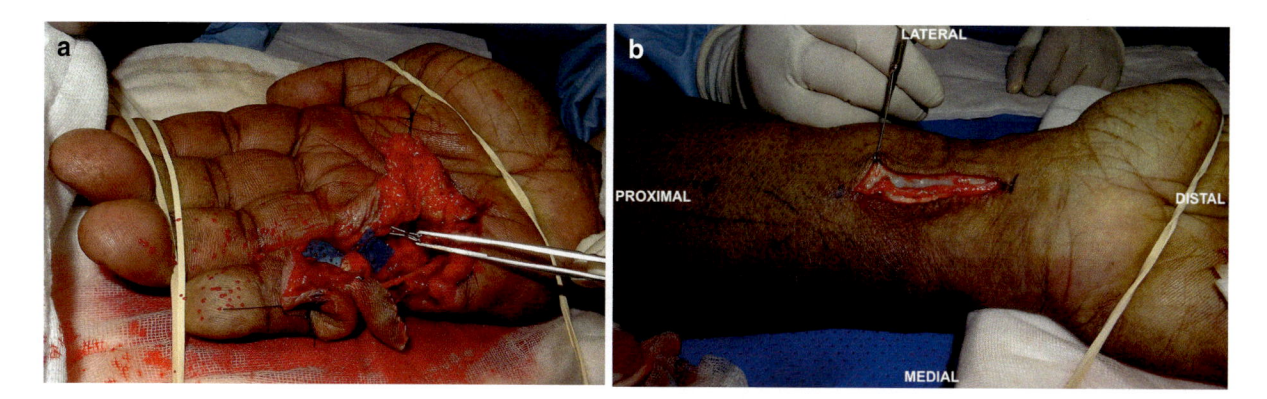

Fig. 48.10 (a) Acland clamp released demonstrating good proximal flow from digital. (b) Harvest of a superficial cutaneous vein from the volar forearm for interpositional vein grafting in a case of a ring avulsion injury as demonstrated in figure 48.5

48.8 Selected Readings

- Bogdan MA, Klein MB, Rubin GD, McAdams TR, Chang J. CT angiography in complex upper extremity reconstruction. J Hand Surg Br. 2004;29:465–9.
- *Over 20 months, 17 outpatient contrast-enhanced CT angiograms were performed in 14 patients. While intraoperative findings corroborated CT findings, two patients required a change in surgical plan due to pre-operative imaging results.*
- Hsu CS, Hellinger JC, Rubin GD, Chang J. CT angiography in pediatric extremity trauma: preoperative evaluation prior to reconstructive surgery. Hand (N Y). 2008;3:139–45.
- *In paediatric patients with suspected, traumatic extremity vascular injuries (n = 5 each for upper and lower limb) requiring reconstruction, findings from CT angiography were confirmed intra-operatively with no complications at up to a mean of 28 months' follow-up post-operatively.*
- Unal C, Yasar EK, Sarisoy TH. The role of preoperative radiological assessment of vascular injury on surgical decision making in mutilating injuries of the upper extremity. Ann Plast Surg. 2013;70:289–95.
- *Pre-operative digital subtraction angiography (DSA) and CT angiography were performed in seven adult patients with upper extremity injuries. This led to the change in flap type that was planned for in five patients, and the anastomosis plan had to be revised in seven.*
- Nasr AY. The radial artery and its variations: anatomical study and clinical implications. Folia Morphol (Warsz). 2012;71:252–62.
- *Cadaveric dissection of 100 upper limbs (30 men) showed different branching patterns and 3 modes of termination. Most importantly, the diameters at 1 cm distal to its origin, and at 2 cm proximal to the styloid process, ranged between 3.1 and 3.3 mm in both males and females, confirming adequacy for microsurgical anastomoses.*
- Ozkus K, Peştelmaci T, Soyluoğlu AI, Akkin SM, Ozkus HI. Variations of the superficial palmar arch. Folia Morphol (Warsz). 1998;57:251–5.
- *Cadaveric dissection of 80 hands demonstrated variation in radial and ulnar artery contribution to the superficial palmar arch; 17.5% was formed by the ulnar artery alone. This supports the importance of pre-operative Allen's test prior to flap design based on the radial or ulnar artery.*

References

1. Funk GF, Valentino J, McCulloch TM, Graham SM, Hoffman HT. Anomalies of forearm vascular anatomy encountered during elevation of the radial forearm flap. Head Neck. 1995;17:284–92.
2. Strauch B, Yu HL. Forearm region. In: Atlas of microvascular surgery anatomy and operative techniques. 2nd ed. New York: Thieme; 2006. p. 40–108.
3. de-Ary-Pires B, Valdez CF, Shecaira AP, de Ary-Pires R, Ary Pires-Neto M. Cleland's and Grayson's ligaments of the hand: a morphometrical investigation. Clin Anat. 2007;20:68–76.
4. Earley MJ. The arterial supply of the thumb, first web and index finger and its surgical application. J Hand Surg Br. 1986;11:163–74.
5. Bell RA, Schneider DS, Wax MK. Superficial ulnar artery: a contraindication to radial forearm free tissue transfer. Laryngoscope. 2011;121:933–6.
6. Onode E, Takamatsu K, Shintani K, et al. Anatomical origins of radial artery perforators evaluated using color Doppler ultrasonography. J Reconstr Microsurg. 2016;32:594–8.
7. Ishiko M, Yano K, Onode E, Takamatsu K. Identification of ulnar artery perforators using color Doppler ultrasonography. J Reconstr Microsurg. 2020;36:667. https://doi.org/10.1055/s-0040-1713601.

Lower Limb Recipient Vessels Access

Yezen Sheena, Georgios Pafitanis, Dariush Nikkhah, Edmund Fitzgerald O'Connor, and Jeremy Rawlins

49.1 Indications

Lower limb reconstruction by free tissue transfer is required in a variety of settings and not uncommonly after trauma, infection, or oncological resections. In general, limb-salvage is the aim, and the only absolute contraindication is when the patient's life is threatened by achieving this. The defect location, size, composition and availability of donor sites are important when considering the best flap and recipient vessels. It is useful, particularly in trauma, to obtain angiographic imaging to confirm the anatomy and condition of leg vessels. By communication with the patient and colleagues, the microsurgeon must anticipate the whole reconstructive and rehabilitation journey tailoring a dynamic approach to staged orthopaedic treatment, integrating complication management (keeping 'lifeboats' without 'burning bridges') towards returning the patient to normal ambulatory function.

49.2 Anatomy

Reviewing lower limb vascular anatomy is relevant and a summary is provided here with brief details on the approach, to access common recipient vessels for microsurgery to fol-

Supplementary Information The online version contains supplementary material available at [https://doi.org/10.1007/978-3-031-07678-7_49].

Y. Sheena (✉)
Royal Perth Hospital, Perth, WA, Australia

G. Pafitanis · E. F. O'Connor
Guys & Thomas' and Kings College Hospital NHS Foundation Trusts, London, UK

D. Nikkhah
The Royal Free Hospital NHS Foundation Trust, London, UK

J. Rawlins
Department of Plastic and Reconstructive Surgery, Royal Perth Hospital, Perth, WA, Australia

low. The femoral artery, a continuation of the external iliac artery distal to the inguinal ligament, provides the main blood supply to the lower limb. At its origin within the femoral triangle it gives off the profunda femoris artery. This courses posteriorly and distally giving off three main branches: (1) Lateral femoral circumflex—crosses anterior femur supplying lateral thigh muscles and skin; (2) Medial femoral circumflex—wraps round posterior femur supplying the bone's head and neck; (3) Perforators supplying adductor magnus. The Superficial Femoral Artery (SFA) descends from the femoral triangle, entering the adductor canal supplying the anterior thigh muscles, and becomes the Popliteal Artery (PA) as it leaves this canal via the adductor (magnus) hiatus. The PA gives off genicular branches supplying the knee joint, then descends through and exits the popliteal fossa between gastrocnemius and popliteus muscles where it terminates by dividing into the Anterior Tibial Artery (ATA) and Tibio-Peroneal Trunk. The latter bifurcates into the Posterior Tibial Artery (PTA) and Peroneal or Fibular Artery (FA). The FA descends posterior to the fibula in the posterior leg giving off perforators supplying the lateral leg muscles. The PTA descends in the deep posterior leg compartment entering the foot via the tarsal tunnel where it bifurcates into medial and lateral plantar arteries (contributing to the sole of the foot and toes via the deep plantar arch). The ATA is conducted anteriorly through a gap in the interosseous membrane between tibia and fibula and descends the anterior compartment of the leg becoming the Dorsalis Pedis Artery (DPA) beyond the ankle to supply the dorsal foot and joins the lateral plantar artery forming the deep plantar arch.

49.3 Pre-operative Investigation

Beyond a thorough pre-operative clinical examination of the lower limb's injury and neurovascular status, the majority of microsurgeons utilise some form of imaging to define the recipient lower limb vascular anatomy. Anatomical land-

© Springer Nature Switzerland AG 2023
D. Nikkhah et al. (eds.), *Core Techniques in Flap Reconstructive Microsurgery*, https://doi.org/10.1007/978-3-031-07678-7_49

marks guide the approach and thigh vasculature is less prone to variation, but it is worth being aware of differences (even within the same individual on the contralateral side) in the origin, calibre and course of leg vessels. One important variant being the Peronea Arteria Magna, where one or both of the Anterior and Posterior Tibial arteries are congenitally small or absent, making the Fibular artery the dominant blood supply to the distal leg in 5–9% of patients [1, 2]. It is wise to note the risks of atherosclerotic occlusive or deep venous thrombotic disease, and some would argue colour Doppler ultrasound performed by radiologically trained surgeons gives the most useful dynamic information on the condition of the vessels for microsurgery [3, 4]. In elective oncological or chronic infection cases, vessels involvement is worth investigating and in trauma—fractures, penetrating injuries and external forces may have caused vessel damage precluding their use or mandating vascular reconstruction during microsurgery. It is our common practice to utilise thermal imaging and hand-held Doppler for skin perforator mapping/flap design, and all our trauma patients have routine pre-operative CT angiography, which many use as the 'gold standard' investigation [5, 6] to define the pre-operative vascular state, relationship to orthopaedic injuries and to plan microsurgical reconstruction (see Fig. 49.1).

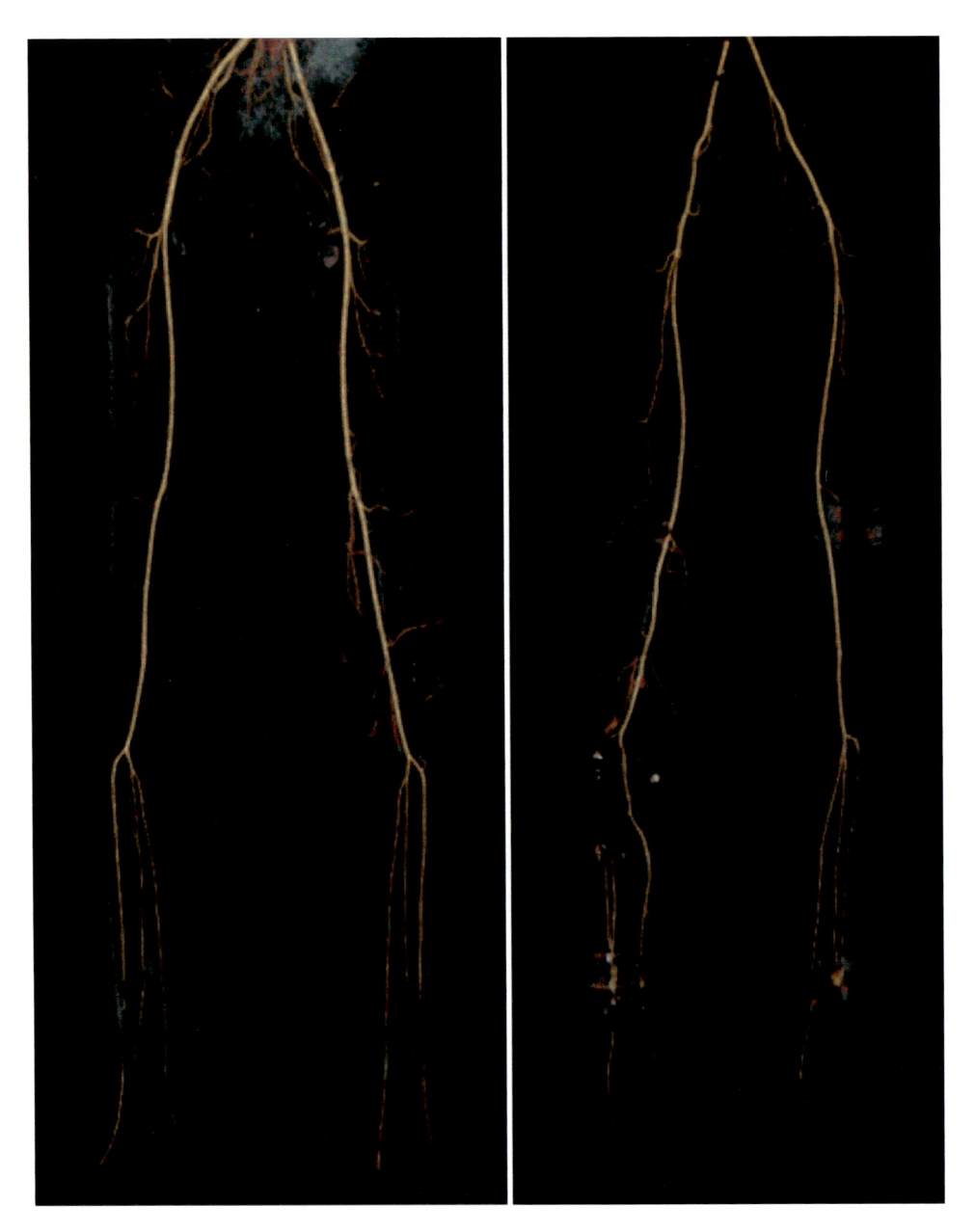

Fig. 49.1 CT angiograms on the left showing normal bilateral 3-vessel run off; and on the right in an open left tibia and fibula fracture with arterial injury signified by no flow in the proximal 10 cm of the anterior tibial and peroneal arteries

49.4 Recipient Vessel Access [See Fig. 49.2 for Leg Surface Markings]

If appropriate recipient vessels are not available within the defect to be reconstructed, the principle of access is to connect the defect to the safe fasciotomy lines [7] via the shortest necessary incisions (see Fig. 49.2). The incisions go through skin, subcutaneous fat, fascia and into the relevant plane retracting tendons/muscles/nerves to isolate the selected recipient vessels with the final preparation performed under the microscope. The most commonly used recipient vessels are the anterior or posterior tibials. There are pros/cons of each and we are aware of past schools of thought preferring the PTA [8], with Godina describing a mid-axial approach splitting the medial and lateral gastrocnemius muscle [9]. More recent experience shows the ATA to be just as reliable, even when the vessels are damaged in the zone of trauma, they have equivalent flap success rates when dissected proximal to injury [10]. Other not infrequently utilised recipient vessels include the dorsalis pedis, superficial femoral and its descending genicular branches. Less commonly utilised 'get out of jail' vessels include the fibular, popliteal and vein grafts or AV loops to more proximal thigh vessels. The PTA is commonly dominant in supplying blood distally, so we rarely perform end-to-end anastomosis on this artery. It has predictable perforators to surrounding muscles and medial leg skin (described at 5, 10 and 15 cm above the medial malleolus) and these are ideal recipients for free flap microsurgery. We prefer to perform end-to-side arterial anastomoses to maintain axial limb blood flow, especially when less than three healthy vessels perfuse the distal leg or in patients with peripheral vascular disease [11]. In a 'one vessel' leg our preference is to use a 'flow-through' free flap to reconstruct the damaged vessels, and some surgeons believe these may be associated with improved flap survival [12]. Some cases with figures to illustrate vessel access follow.

1. *Dorsalis Pedis Vessels* [Figs. 49.3 and 49.4]:
   Useful for dorsal foot wounds when the vessels are available. DPA is the continuation of the ATA distal to the ankle joint and terminates as the First Dorsal Metatarsal Artery and the Deep Plantar Artery. Its course can be surface landmarked by the line joining the mid-point of the malleoli and the proximal first metatarsal interval. Find the pulse just lateral to Extensor Hallucis Longus (EHL) and medial to Extensor Digitorum Longus (EDL) most readily palpable at the distal navicular bony prominence. During dissection, identify and protect the adjacent deep peroneal nerve.
2. *Anterior Tibial Vessels* [Figs. 49.5, 49.6, 49.7, 49.8, 49.9, and 49.10]:

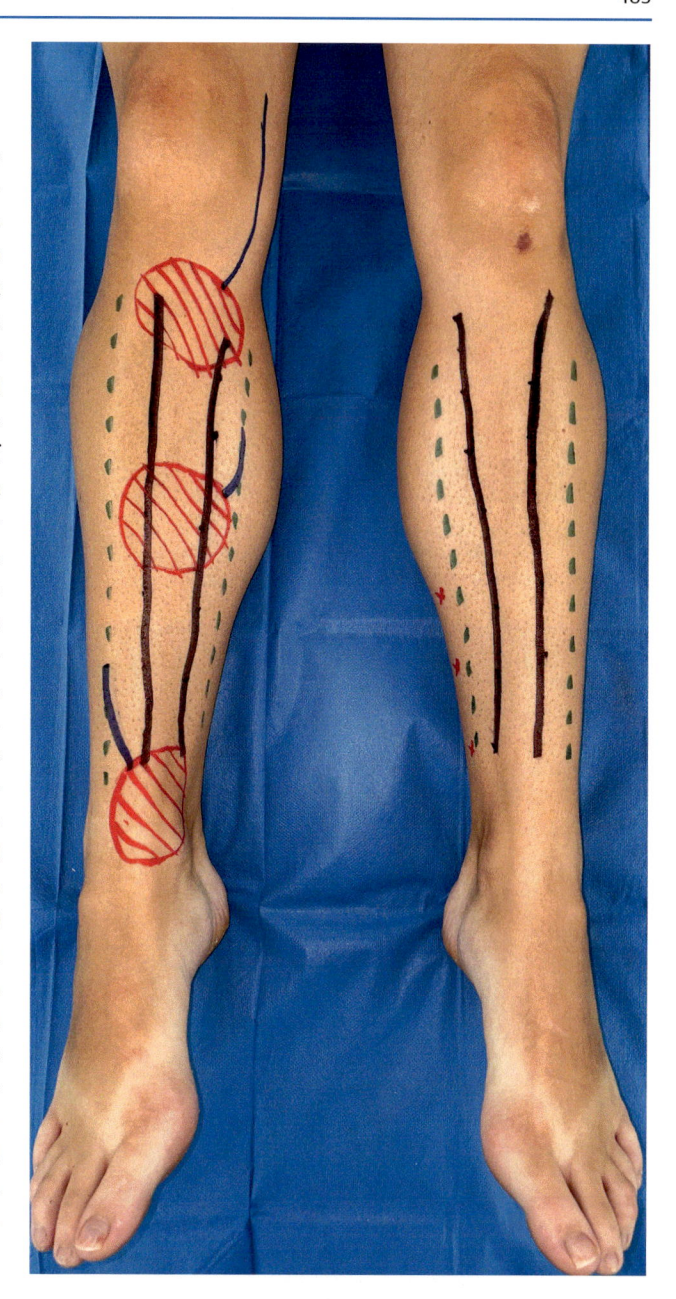

Fig. 49.2 Image of left leg with subcutaneous Tibial borders (Black solid lines), fasciotomy election lines (Green dashed) and PTA perforators medially (Red crosses); and Right leg illustrating three potential open fracture soft tissue defects (Red hatched) with access incisions (Blue curved lines) in relation to fasciotomy lines. The inferior defect to ATA, middle 1/3 defect to PTA and proximal defect to DGA or SFA

The surface landmark line of the ATA is described by a line joining the medial fibula head to the dorsal mid-malleolar point. Find these vessels distally between the Tibialis Anterior (TA) and EHL tendons. More proximally these vessels become deeper between the muscles of TA medially and EDL laterally. Protect the adjacent deep peroneal nerve during vessel dissection. The images show a lateral ankle open fracture (fixed by diastasis

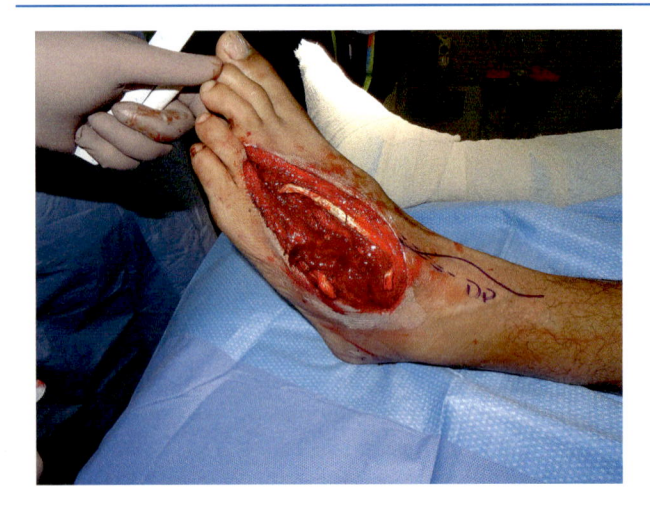

Fig. 49.3 Left dorsal foot defect with skin surface markings for access to the dorsalis pedis vessels

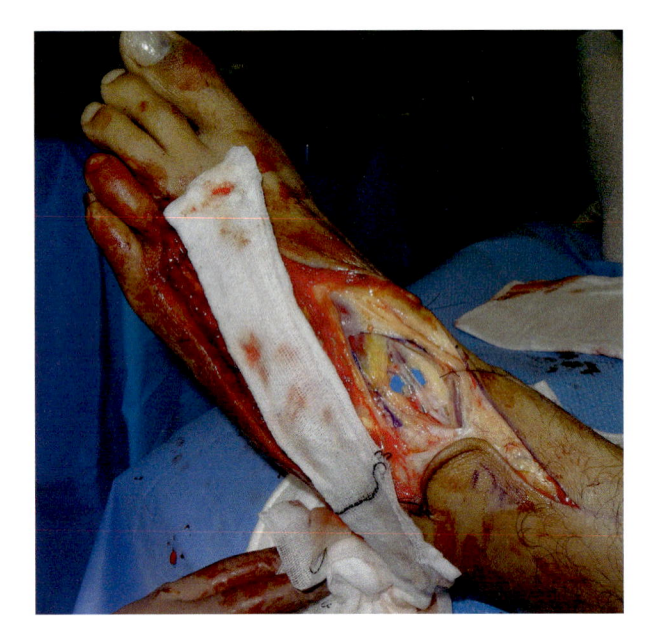

Fig. 49.4 DPA with its two VCs dissected and clear for microsurgery at site with blue background

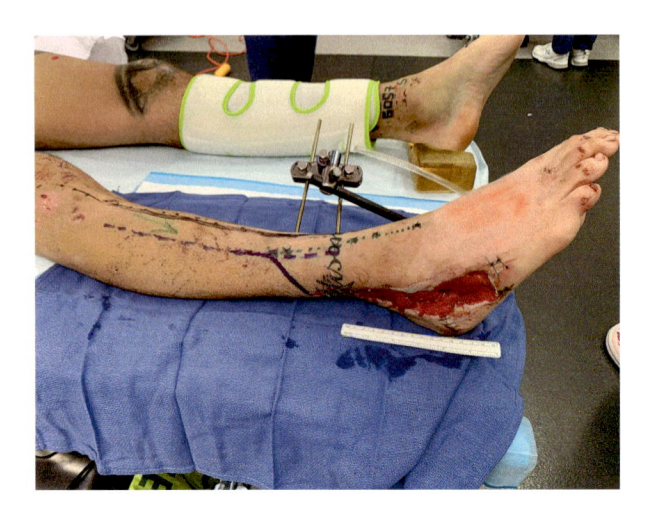

Fig. 49.5 Right lateral ankle defect with surface markings for access to anterior tibial vessels

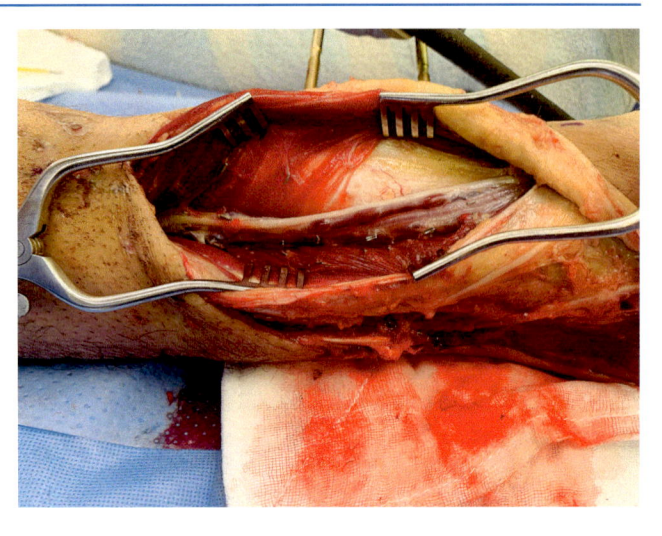

Fig. 49.6 Right ATA prepared for microsurgery with its two flanking VCs between tibialis anterior (retracted medially/above) and the EHL/EDL muscles (retracted laterally/below, along with the deep peroneal nerve seen distally on right side of wound in image)

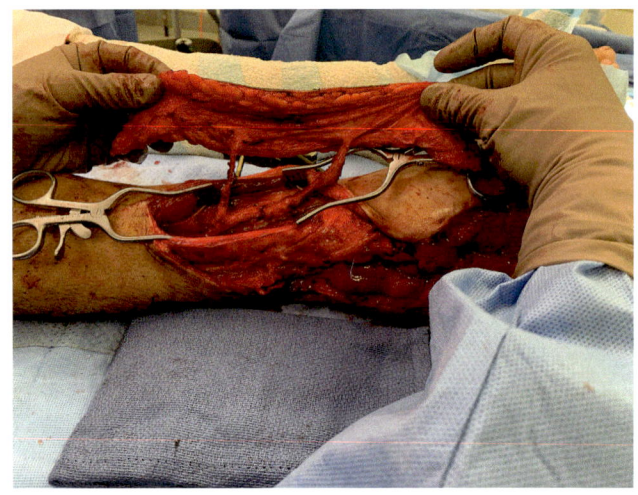

Fig. 49.7 Two-perforator ALT flap connected end-to-end on to the right ATA seen from lateral side

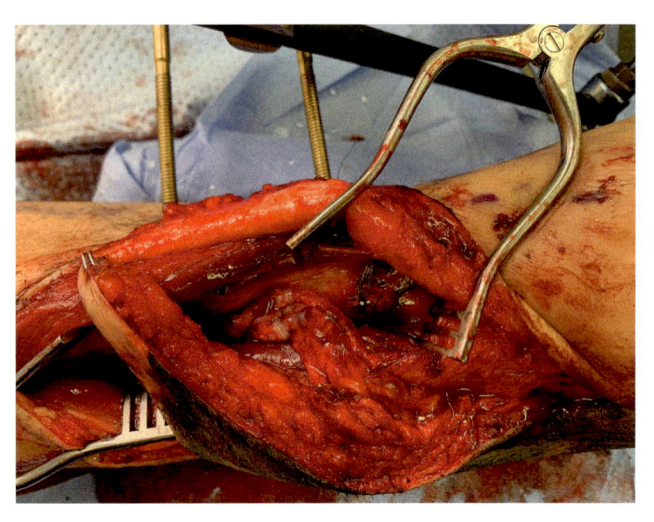

Fig. 49.8 ALT flap anastomoses showing two venous couplers end-to-end on to ATA VCs

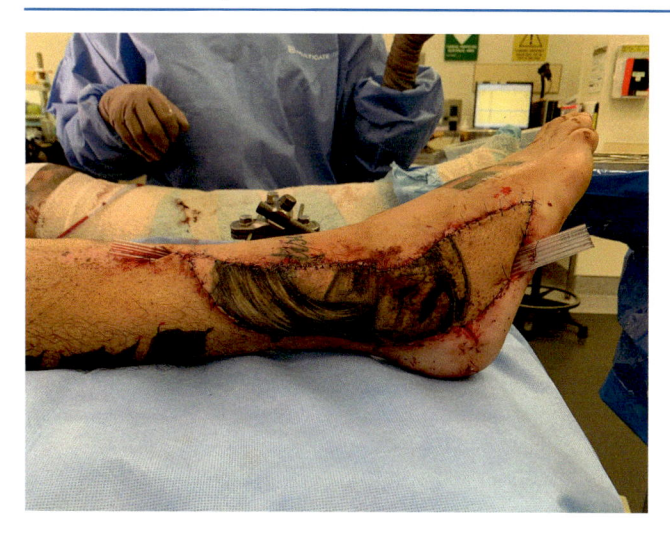

Fig. 49.9 ALT flap inset to cover the defect distally and the vessel access incision/wound proximally

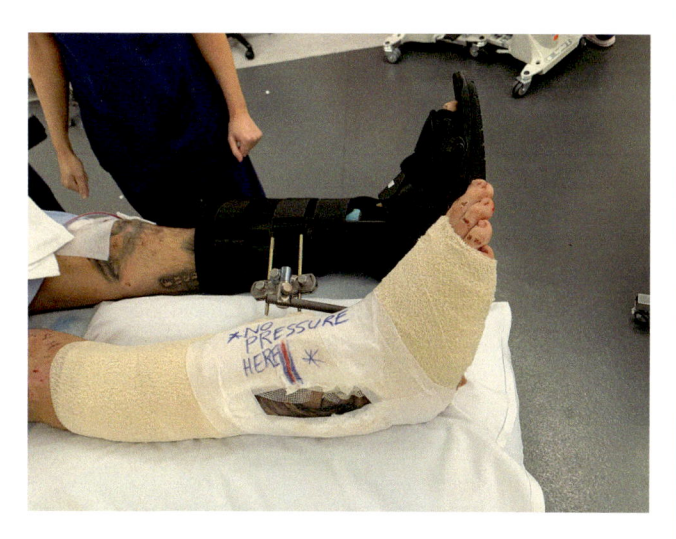

Fig. 49.10 ALT flap dressings at end of procedure demonstrating monitoring window and pressure care instructions around anastomosis site

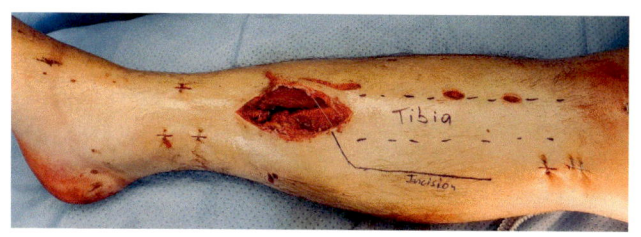

Fig. 49.11 Right distal tibial open fracture with IM nail in situ showing access incision to PTA

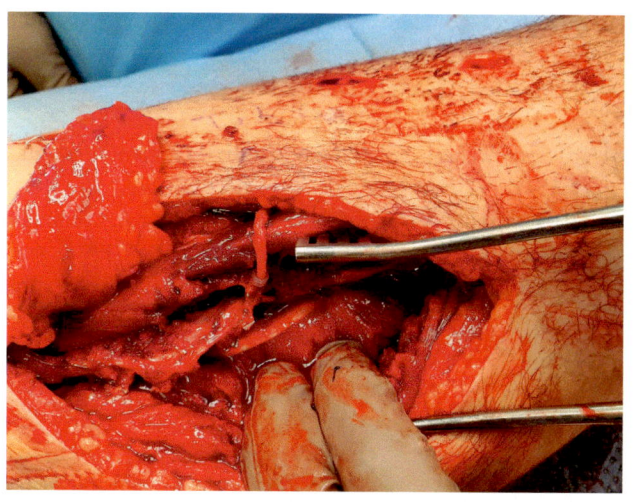

Fig. 49.12 MSAP flap over tibial defect with end-to-side anastomosis to PTA and one flap vein coupled to its VC and the second to a superficial system vein

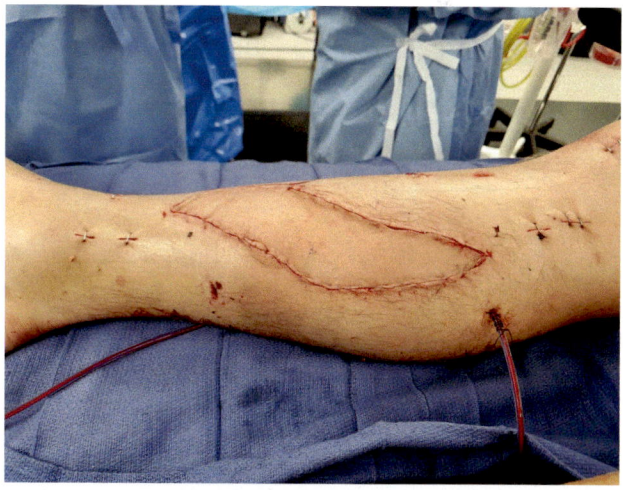

Fig. 49.13 MSAP flap inset resurfacing defect. Note proximal half of flap utilised to cover vessels

screw) with a soft tissue defect in a leg with three-vessel run-off with an access incision towards the distal anterior tibial vessels allowing an end-to-end arterial hand-sewn and two venous coupled ALT (double perforator) flap anastomoses.

3. *Posterior Tibial Vessels* [Figs. 49.11, 49.12, and 49.13]:
   The PTA runs from the end of the PA (2.5 cm below the mid-Popliteal fossa) to a point between the medial malleolus and the heel where the pulse should be easily palpable. Passing under the ankle flexor retinaculum the mneumonic 'Tom, Dick and Nervous Harry' serves to remind of the anterior to posterior relationships of Tibialis Posterior, Flexor Digitorum Longus, the Tibial Artery, Tibial Nerve and Flexor Hallucis Longus. In the leg, the PTA travels with its Venae and the Tibial nerve in the deep posterior compartment (deep to the transverse intermuscular septum superficial to the Tibialis Posterior muscle) between the FDL and FHL muscles. It is usually

approached medially, taking care not to injure the Great Saphenous Vein (GSV) and Saphenous Nerve, by releasing and retracting the crural fascia and Soleus off the posterior-medial Tibial border. Care must be taken not to injure the Tibial nerve. This open Tibial fracture had IM nail fixation and immediate contralateral MSAP free flap reconstruction. The incision allowed access to the PTA, its VCs and a superficial vein were also identified, dissected and utilised. An end-to-side arterial and two coupled venous anastomoses (one to deep VC and one to the superficial recipient). Note that swelling in the acute trauma setting often requires larger flaps be harvested in anticipation of failure to close the vessel access incision and to cover the pedicle.

4. *Superficial Femoral and Descending Genicular Vessels* [49.14].

These vessels are useful in cases of higher leg, knee or thigh defects that require reconstruction. The SFA is surface marked by the upper two-thirds of a line from the mid-inguinal point (midpoint between Pubic Symphasis Pubis and Anterior Superior Iliac Spine) and the Adductor Tubercle. As aforementioned, it travels under Sartorius and can be accessed between Adductor Longus (easily palpable with the relaxed thigh abducted and externally rotated). The SFA usually gives off a branch medially called the Descending Genicular Artery (DGA) approximately 13 cm above the knee joint, which travels between Sartorius and Vastus Medialis in close proximity to the Saphenous nerve. This nerve and the GSV should be identified and protected when preparing these vessels. See Fig. 49.14 for an image showing DGA vessel preparation to receive an LD free flap to reconstruct a proximal tibial Gustillo 3B fracture with single vessel distal run off and poor Popliteal branches on CTA.

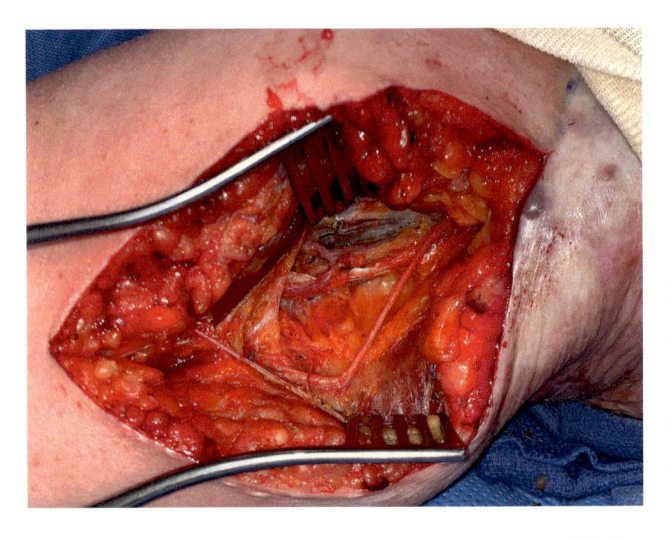

Fig. 49.14 Medial thigh access incision showing the DGA utilised as recipient vessel for proximal tibial reconstruction

49.5 Core Surgical Techniques in Recipient Vessel Harvest

To summarise:

1. Recipient vessel selection is based on defect location and the condition of local vessels on CTA.
2. Surface landmarks and hand-held Doppler confirm access incision placement. Utilise shortest line from defect to safe fasciotomy lines (see Fig. 49.2).
3. Tourniquet control dissection for bloodless field and Loupe magnification allow accurate identification of nerves, superficial veins (that may be utilised during primary or rescue anastomoses).
4. Adequate assistance and good retraction allows safe identification and control of selected vessels.
5. Final preparation under microscope to confirm satisfactory vessel walls, an arterial 'squirt test' and low pressure venous 'flush test' are key requirements.
6. Aim for perforator-to-perforator (when available) end-to-end anastomosis or an end-to-side anastomosis with more major recipient vessels. End-to-side anastomosis has comparable patency and flap outcomes, addresses vessel size mismatch and preserves distal limb perfusion and preserves recipient vessel options if subsequent reconstruction or further free flap surgery is ever required.
7. Check for venous backflow and low resistance heparinised saline flushing. Anastomosis proximity to valves is not usually an issue. There must be a low threshold in connecting an extra vein to the flap, if possible, especially if turgid second flap vein with first vein flowing, or if high pressure recipients (we mitigate DVT risk by utilising a superficial second vein recipient if available).
8. Assess immediate flow with Acland test, note darker blood return to vein on clamps down and usual flap observations noting colour of bleeding from dermal edges with low threshold to revision/additional vein anastomoses or Vein Grafts if required.

49.6 Pearls and Pitfalls

Pearls
- Utilise pre-operative imaging—Angiography or Colour Doppler Ultrasound (CDU).
- Identify/protect any superficial veins around defect for reconstruction. We aim to anastomose two veins if the flap pedicle has two VCs. Utilising a recipient site VC and a superficial vein mitigates the risks of relying on just the deep or superficial venous systems.

- Assess vein wall condition, blood backflow on cutting and ease of flushing with heparinised saline.
- Careful flap templating taking extra skin to account for and cover the vessels and access incision.
- Arterial assessment considers non-contused appearance, visible/palpable pulsatility (we use intraoperative pencil Doppler) and most importantly the 'squirt test' to confirm adequate flow pressure. After microsurgery confirm vessels not twisted, kinked, or under tension/pressure. We sometimes utilise a small piece of fat to help cushion the pedicle around the anastomosis site.

increase flap salvage rates. Pedicle positioning to avoid any tension, twisting/kinking or external compression is crucial (this may require vein grafts). Sometimes the flap may require inset adjustments necessitating skin grafts to less crucial wound areas. We recognise the lack of evidence base, but when anticoagulation is not contraindicated, we favour Heparin IV bolus on releasing microvascular clamps and a low dose post-operative infusion for 3 days in the revision setting.

Pitfalls
- Regardless of microsurgical planning and execution, the adequacy of excision margins **will** determine outcome. It is complete oncological clearance or radical wound excision to healthy tissues in the infective or trauma setting that will minimise cancer recurrence, infection and non-union. It is crucial for the microsurgeon to perform this well or work closely with the ablative surgeon to do so.
- Any factor from the pre- to the post-operative course can compromise the vessels, flap and entire reconstruction. The adequacy of your local preoperative clinical and radiological assessment helps guide the operative vessel selection and it is well worth learning to correlate your local angiography procedure (for DSA, CTA, MRA, etc.) with operative findings.
- Adequate arteries are necessary, but not sufficient for flap success. Venous congestion is the greater risk so identifying injuries or deep vein thrombosis preoperatively can help plan to mitigate flap venous compromise. Colour Doppler ultrasound may have an imaging advantage in dynamically assessing flow velocities.
- To mitigate venous compromise, we utilise couplers as they are efficient and effective for anastomosis patency and assess blood flow and colour on taking clamps off (dark blood initially after ischaemia time). Turgor within other available flap veins is a sign another venous anastomosis might be of benefit and is considered along with flap colour, capillary refill time and dermal bleeding assessment.
- Effective flap observations by experienced clinical staff and prompt re-exploration in theatre if any signs of compromise are recognised measures to

49.7 Selected Readings

- Duymaz A, Karabekmez FE, Vrtiska TJ, Mardini S, Moran SL. Free tissue transfer for lower extremity reconstruction: a study of the role of computed angiography in the planning of free tissue transfer in the post-traumatic setting. Plast Reconstr Surg. 2009;124(2): 523–9.

  In 76 lower extremity trauma patients who underwent preoperative CTA for free flap reconstruction of the lower limb the incidence of traumatic occlusion was recorded. The authors concluded that the incidence of single-vessel traumatic arterial occlusion within traumatized lower limbs undergoing free tissue transfer may be as high as 29%. Computed tomographic angiography provided excellent visualization of lower extremity vasculature, and its routine use for trauma patients is safe. Flap failure rates were low when using this technique for preoperative planning. Flap failure occurred only in patients with evidence of arterial injury. Evidence of arterial occlusion on computed tomographic angiography may be a risk factor for limb loss.

- Eccles S, Handley B, Khan U, Nanchahal J, Nayagam S, McFadyen I, editors. Standards for the management of open fractures. Published: August 2020.

  Standards for the Management of Open Fractures provides an evidence-based approach for the management of open fractures, focusing on lower limb injuries. It builds on and expands the National Institute for Health and Care Excellence (NICE) Guidelines to provide a practical approach with supporting evidence. The new edition has been extensively updated and expanded to include key aspects of management, ranging from setting up an orthoplastic service, through to dealing with bone and soft tissue injuries, including in young and older people, patient rehabilitation and psychological care, blast injuries, as well as complications such as infection.

- Chen HC, Chuang CC, Chen S, Hsu WM, Wei FC. Selection of recipient vessels for free flaps to the distal leg and foot following trauma. Microsurgery. 1994;15(5):358–63.

  This classic paper by the Chen and colleagues examined 126 patients with Gustillo Type III open fractures that required free tissue transfer. They found the anterior tibial artery had a much higher incidence of injury compared to the posterior tibial artery. This should be borne in mind when the anterior tibial artery is selected as the recipient artery in order to prevent reexploration and failure of the flaps. However, the posterior tibial artery is much less vulnerable to damage in most injuries and is more reliable as the recipient artery.

- Godina M. Preferential use of the posterior approach to blood vessels of the lower leg in microvascular surgery. Plast Reconstr Surg. 1991;88:287–91.

  This classic paper by Marco Godina describes a mild muscle splitting approach that provides a wide exposure to the posterior tibial artery. End to side anastomosis can be performed in the lateral decubitus position.

References

1. Rosson GD, Singh NK. Devascularising complications of free fibula harvest: peronea arteria magna. J Reconstr Microsurg. 2005;21(8):533–8.
2. Abou-Foul AK, Borumandi F. Anatomical variants of lower limb vasculature and implications for free fibula flap: systematic review and critical analysis. Microsurgery. 2016;36(2):165–72.
3. Cho MJ, Kwon JG, Pak CJ, Suh HP, Hong JP. The role of duplex ultrasound in microsurgical reconstruction: review and technical considerations. J Reconstr Microsurg. 2020;36(7):514–21.
4. Oni G, Chow W, Ramakrishnan V, Griffiths M. Plastic surgeon led ultrasound. Plast Reconstr Surg. 2018;141(2):300e–9e.
5. Lee GK, Fox PM, Riboh J, Hsu C, Saber S, Rubin GD, Chang J. Computed tomography angiography in microsurgery: indications, clinical utility, and pitfalls. Eplasty. 2013;13:e42.
6. Gakhal MS, Sartip KA. CT angiography signs of lower extremity vascular trauma. AJR Am J Roentgenol. 2009;193:W49–57.
7. https://oxfordmedicine.com/view/10.1093/med/9780198849360.001.0001/med-9780198849360.
8. Chen HC, Chuang CC, Chen S, Hsu WM, Wei FC. Selection of recipient vessels for free flaps to the distal leg and foot following trauma. Microsurgery. 1994;15(5):358–63.
9. Godina M, Arnez ZM, Lister GD. Preferential use of the posterior approach to blood vessels of the lower leg in microvascular surgery. Plast Reconstr Surg. 1991;88(2):287–91.
10. Yazar S, Lin CH. Selection of recipient vessel in traumatic lower extremity. J Reconstr Microsurg. 2012;28(3):199–204.
11. Broer PN, Moellhoff N, Mayer JM, Heidekruger PI, Ninkovic M, Ehrl D. Comparison of outcomes of end-to-end versus end-to-side anastomoses in lower extremity free flap reconstructions. J Reconstr Microsurg. 2020;36(6):432–7.
12. Fujiki M, Miyamoto S, Sakuraba M. Flow-through anastomosis for both the artery and vein in leg free flap transfer. Microsurgery. 2015;35:536–40.

Lymphatic Supermicrosurgery

Takumi Yamamoto and Nana Yamamoto

50.1 Indications of Lymphatic Supermicrosurgery

Lymphatic supermicrosurgery includes supermicrosurgical dissection and anastomosis of the collecting lymph vessels. Since the collecting lymph vessels are usually smaller than 0.5 mm in diameter, supermicrosurgical techniques are required to anastomose them. There are two indications of lymphatic supermicrosurgery; obstructive disease (lymphedema) and diseases of leakage (lymphorrhea and lymphocyst).

Lymphedema is a progressive edematous disease caused by lymph flow obstruction. Lymphatic bypass is effective to improve lymph flows. As lymph originally flows into venous circulation at the venous angle, lymph-to-venous shunt addresses pathophysiology of obstructive lymphedema. Supermicrosurgical **lymphaticovenular anastomosis (LVA)**, in which a lymph vessel is anastomosed to a nearby venule or a small vein in an intima-to-intima coaptation, diverts congested lymph flows into venous circulation.

Lymphorrhea and lymphocyst occur after trauma or surgery to lymph-rich regions, i.e., lymphadenectomy. Surgical treatment is considered when refractory to conservative therapy. Precise identification of the ruptured lymph vessels is a key to successful management. The lymph vessels should be reconstructed, if possible, with supermicrosurgical **lymphaticolymphatic anastomosis (LLA)** or LVA. If there is no suitable recipient vessel, the lymph vessel is supermicrosurgically ligated, but secondary lymphedema may occur because the major lymph flow is obstructed by the ligation.

T. Yamamoto (✉) · N. Yamamoto
Department of Plastic and Reconstructive Surgery, National Center for Global Health and Medicine, Tokyo, Japan
e-mail: tyamamoto-tky@umin.ac.jp

50.2 Anatomy and Preoperative Imaging of Lymphatic System

Major lymph pathways run along the major subcutaneous veins such as the saphenous vein, the cephalic vein, and the basilic vein. However, precise anatomy is slightly different from venous anatomy, and lymphatic imaging studies play a crucial role in lymphatic supermicrosurgery. The gold standard of lymph flow imaging is lymphoscintigraphy, but its images are too obscure as preoperative mapping for lymphatic supermicrosurgery. MR lymphography and SPECT/CT allow three-dimensional localization of lymphatics, but it is not easy to accurately localize the found lymphatics onto the skin surface for incision site design. Currently, indocyanine green (ICG) lymphography is the most useful imaging method for diagnosis and preoperative evaluation.

ICG lymphography is performed as follows; 0.1–0.2 mL of 0.25% ICG is intradermally injected at the distal limb (usually at second web space of the hand/foot, and several points), and fluorescent images are obtained using a near-infrared camera system. **Dynamic ICG lymphography**, dual-phase observation ICG lymphography, is important for thorough examination of lymphatic system; observed immediately after ICG injection (early transient phase), and 2–72 h after injection (late plateau phase) [Fig. 50.1]. Typical ICG lymphography findings include normal linear pattern and abnormal dermal backflow (DB) patterns (Splash, Stardust, and Diffuse pattern) [Fig. 50.2]. At an early phase, Linear pattern is marked to localize lymph vessels. At a late phase, extension of DB pattern is marked for severity evaluation of lymphedema.

ICG lymphography stage is useful for pathophysiological severity staging of secondary lymphedema and to consider indication of LVA [Table 50.1]. LVA is best indicated for ICG stage II-IV. Prophylactic LVA may be considered for ICG stage I, and lymph node transfer is better indicated for ICG stage V.

Fig. 50.1 Dynamic ICG lymphography; dual-phase observation at an early transient phase, and at a late plateau phase

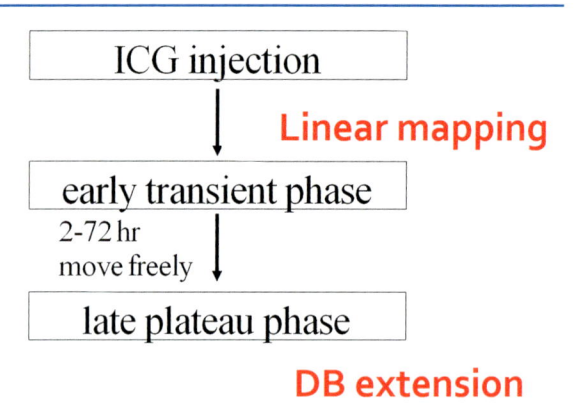

Fig. 50.2 Characteristic ICG lymphography findings

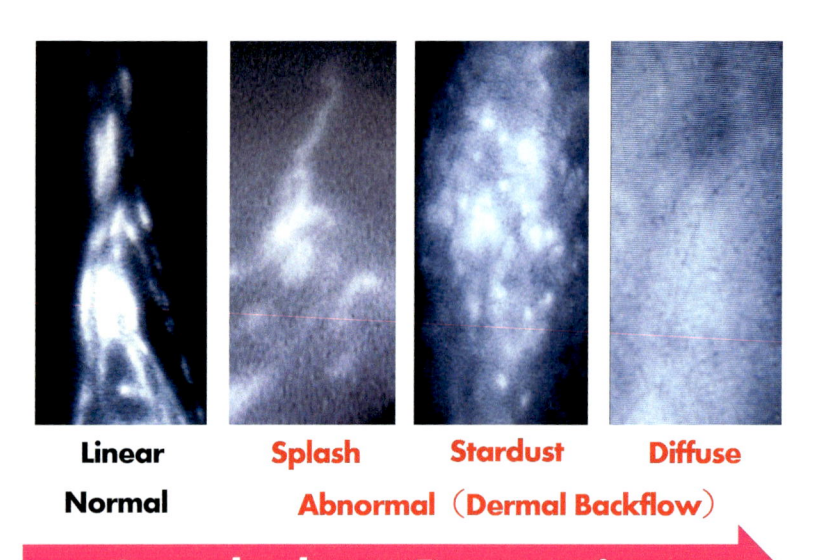

Table 50.1 ICG lymphography stage

ICG stage	Lymphographic findings
Stage 0	Linear pattern only (no DB pattern)
Stage I	Linear pattern + splash pattern[a]
Stage II	Linear pattern + DB pattern (1 region)[b]
Stage III	Linear pattern + DB pattern (2 regions)[b]
Stage IV	Linear pattern + DB pattern (3 regions)[b]
Stage V	DB pattern only (no linear pattern)

ICG indocyanine green, *DB* dermal backflow
[a] Splash pattern is usually seen around the axilla/groin
[b] Upper/lower extremity is divided into three regions; the upper-arm/thigh, the forearm/lower-leg, and the hand/foot. Stardust pattern is usually seen in DB pattern; diffuse pattern may be seen

Table 50.2 Lymphosclerosis severity classification

	Lymph vessel characteristics			
Severity	Appearance	Expandability	Lumen	Wall thickness
s0	Translucent	Expandable	Identifiable	Very thin
s1	White	Expandable	Identifiable	Thin
s2	White	Not expandable	Identifiable	Thick
s3	White	Not expandable	Not identifiable	Very thick

50.3 Recommended Surgical Sites for Lymphedema and Lympho-rrhea/-cyst (A Figure with Surface Markings)

In LVA for lymphedema treatment, slightly sclerotic lymph vessels are recommended for anastomosis. With lymphedema progression, lymph vessels become sclerotic with less lymph flows inside; lymphosclerosis. **Lymphosclerosis** grades are divided into "s0," "s1," "s2," and "s3" [Table 50.2]. A slightly sclerotic "s1" lymph vessel usually has high lymph flow, and is best indicated for LVA. "s1" lymph vessels can be most frequently found in the "overlapping region." The **"overlapping region"** is identified by dynamic ICG lymphography, where Linear pattern is seen at an early phase and DB pattern at a late phase [Fig. 50.3]. Incision sites for LVA should be designed in the overlapping regions revealed by dynamic ICG lymphography.

Fig. 50.3 Skin incision sites in LVA surgery for lymphedema. Overlapping region revealed by dynamic ICG lymphography

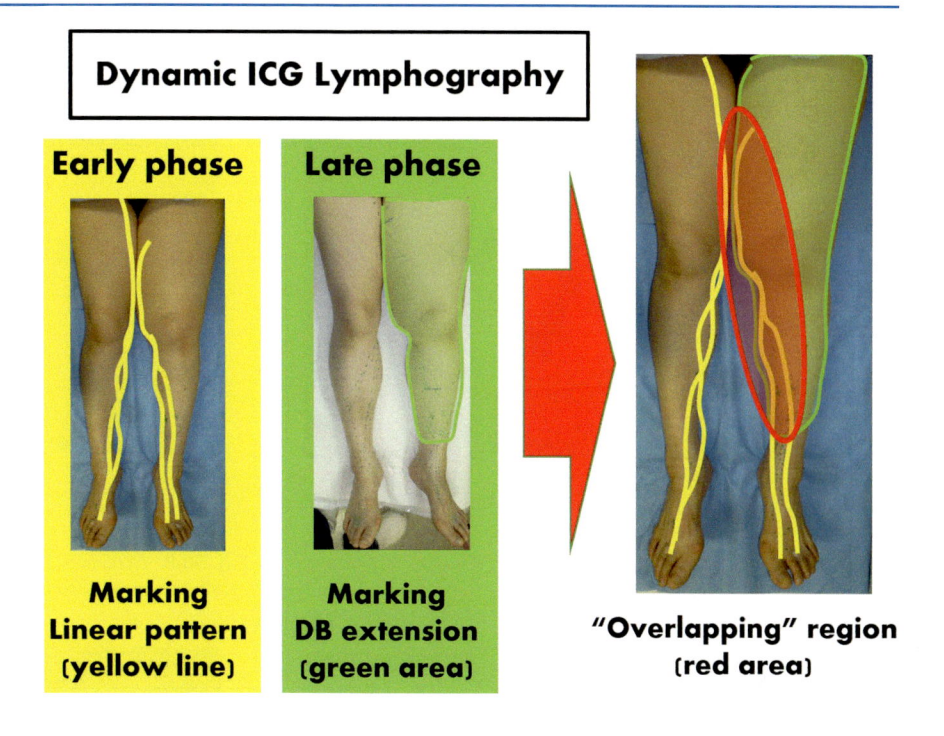

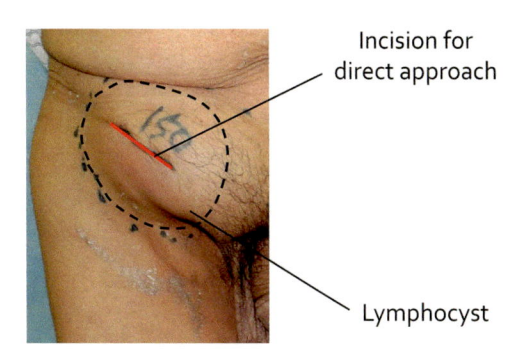

Fig. 50.4 "Direct approach" skin incision site (red line) for lympho-rrhea/-cyst

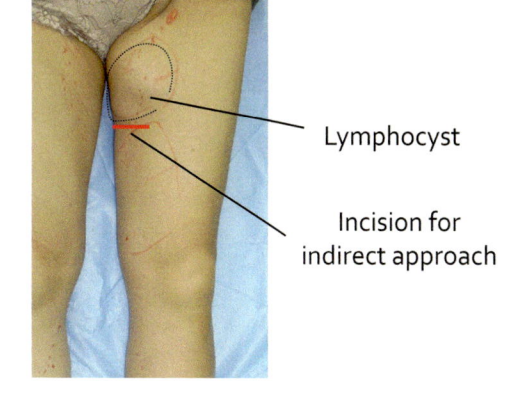

Fig. 50.5 "Indirect approach" skin incision site (red line) for lympho-rrhea/-cyst

For lympho-rrhea/-cyst treatment, skin incision should be designed on the lesion, if possible [50.4]. Direct approach allows secure identification and reconstruction of causative ruptured lymph vessels, and capsulectomy for lymphocyst if needed. When the direct approach is difficult, for example, as wound problem risk is considered high due to radiation or exposed artificial materials, indirect approach is applied; skin incision should be designed distally to the lesion as close as possible, according to preoperative ICG lymphography findings [Fig. 50.5].

50.4 Supermicrosurgical LVA for Lymphedema: A Step-by-Step Guide

- **Step 1. Careful Skin Incision** [Fig. 50.6]. After local infiltration anesthesia with 1% lidocaine with 1:100,000 epinephrine, skin incision is made on a designed line. Attention is paid not to injure the subdermal veins. Whole procedures, from skin incision to skin closure, should be performed under an operating microscope.

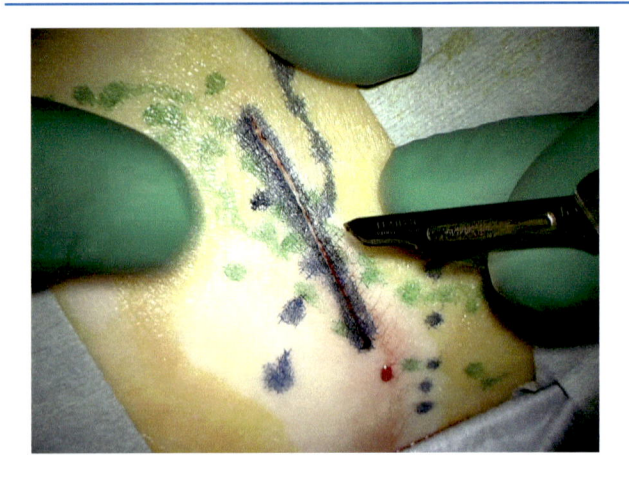

Fig. 50.6 LVA step 1. Skin is incised carefully with a surgical scalpel

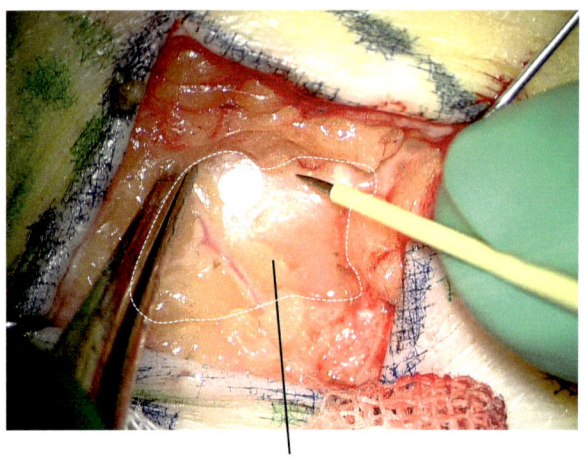

Fig. 50.8 LVA step 3. The superficial fascia is widely exposed, and carefully incised with a needle-tip electric cautery

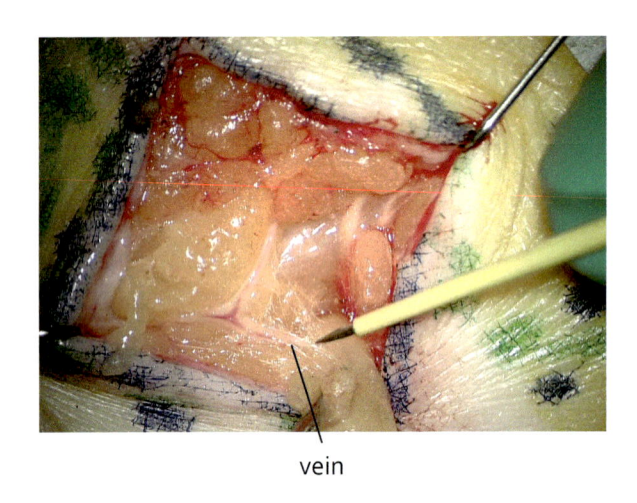

Fig. 50.7 LVA step 2. A vein is dissected with inter-lobular dissection method in the superficial fat layer above the superficial fascia

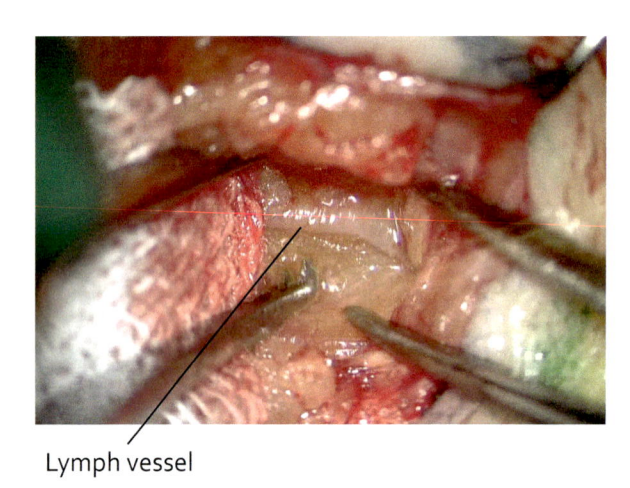

Fig. 50.9 LVA step 4. A lymph vessel is dissected with inter-lobular dissection method in the deep fat layer below the superficial fascia

- **Step 2. Dissection of Recipient Vein** [Fig. 50.7]. Using a needle-tip electric cautery with power level set at 5–7, the superficial fat layer is dissected to seek for a recipient vein. Dissection should go between the fat lobules; **inter-lobular dissection**. A vein is dissected and cut as distally as possible to include many valves inside; important to prevent venous reflux which is a major risk factor of LVA site thrombosis.
- **Step 3. Exposure and Careful Incision of the Superficial Fascia** [Fig. 50.8]. Inter-lobular dissection continues deeply to the superficial fascia. The superficial fascia should be explored as widely as possible in a surgical field. The superficial fascia is very carefully incised with a needle-tip electric cautery; lymph vessels, if present, lie just below the superficial fascia.
- **Step 4. Dissection of Lymph Vessel** [Fig. 50.9]. Deep fat layer is dissected inter-lobularly with a dissector or a fine-tip mosquito to seek for lymph vessels. Every inter-lobular space should be explored throughout the field. A lymph vessel, when found, is marked with 3–0 nylon thread not to lose it.
- **Step 5. Supermicrosurgical Anastomosis in an Intima-to-Intima Coaptation** [Fig. 50.10]. A lymph vessel is anastomosed to a vein in an intima-to-intima coaptation manner using 11–0 (65 μm needle), 12–0 (50 μm needle), or 12–0 s (30 μm needle) supermicrosutures; 11–0 for 0.4–1.0 mm vessel, 12–0 for 0.2–0.6 mm vessel, and 12–0 s for 0.1–0.3 mm vessel. Usually, six stiches are put for one end-to-end anastomosis.

- **Step 6. Evaluation of Anastomosis Patency** [Fig. 50.11]. Patency is evaluated with venous expansion filled with translucent lymph. Intraoperative ICG lymphography is useful to rule out minor leakage.
- **Step 7. Protection of the Anastomosis Site and Vessels** [Fig. 50.12]. The anastomosis site and vessels are covered with the surrounding fat tissue to place them as deep as possible.
- **Step 8. Careful Skin Closure** [Fig. 50.13]. Skin is closed carefully under an operating microscope, not to affect the anastomosis site and vessels.

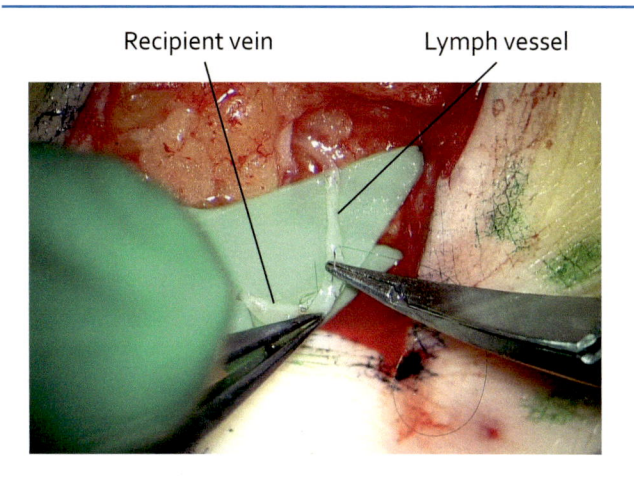

Fig. 50.10 LVA step 5. Supermicrosurgical anastomosis is done in an intima-to-intima coaptation manner

Fig. 50.11 LVA step 6. Anastomosis is evaluated regarding patency and leakage. Intraoperative ICG lymphography (right)

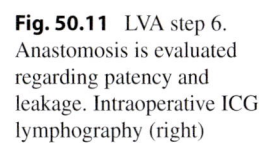

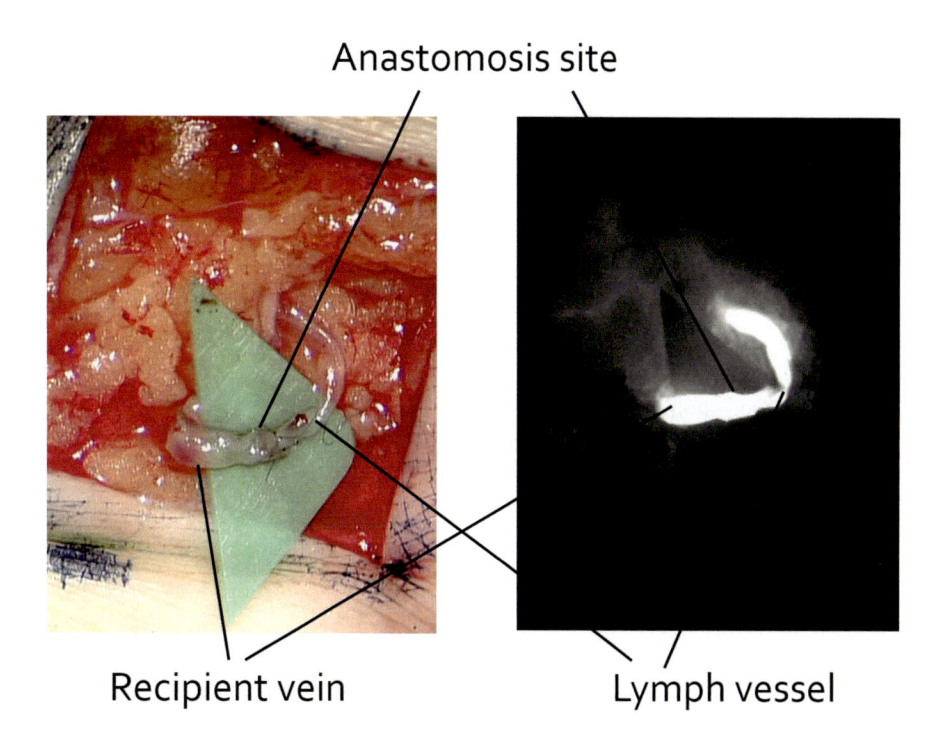

Fig. 50.12 LVA step 7. The anastomosis site and vessels are covered with the surrounding fat tissue

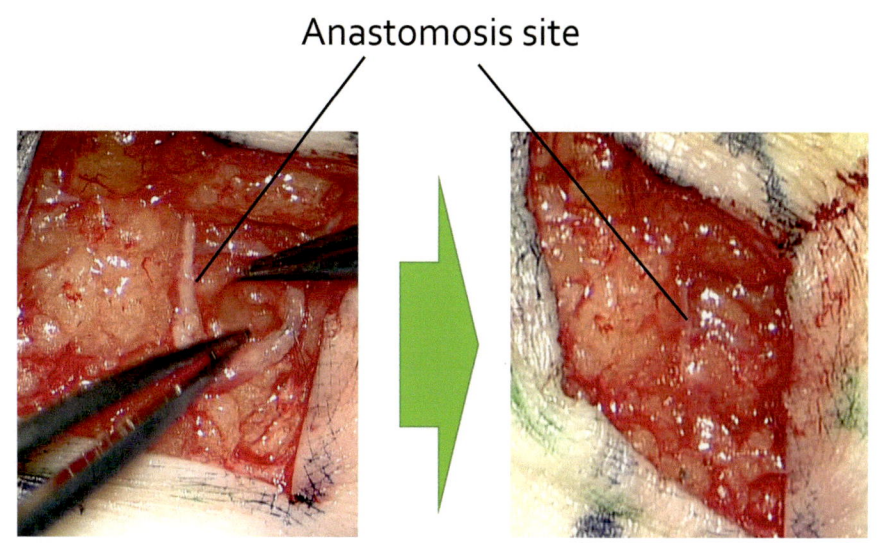

Fig. 50.13 LVA step 8. Skin is closed carefully not to affect the anastomosis site and vessels

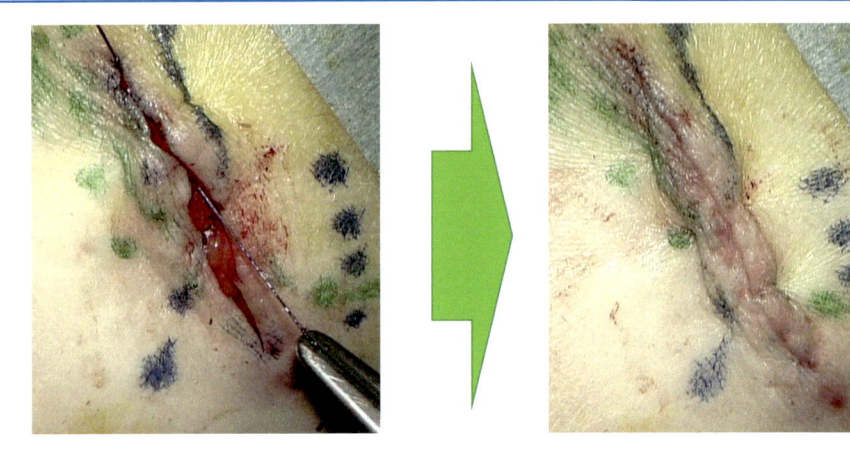

50.5 Supermicrosurgical LLA for Lymphorrhea/-cyst: A Step-by-Step Guide

- **Step 1. Exploration Inside a Cyst** [Fig. 50.14]. Usually, there is a cyst formation in the lesion, which is opened up to explore inside. If the history is long, capsulectomy should be done. As in LVA, whole procedures are done under an operating microscope.
- **Step 2. Identification of Ruptured Lymph Vessel** [Fig. 50.15]. Careful observation is conducted to seek for ruptured lymph vessels under intraoperative ICG lymphography navigation; if ICG is not available, dye injection is helpful. The ruptured lymph vessel, when found, is dissected distally for subsequent anastomosis.
- **Step 3. Dissection of Recipient Vessel** [Fig. 50.16]. Nearby intact lymph vessel is searched under intraoperative ICG lymphography. When found close enough to the ruptured lymph vessel, the recipient lymph vessel is dissected proximally and distally for subsequent end-to-side LLA. If there is no recipient lymph vessel suitable for LLA, a vein is searched for LVA. If there is no recipient lymph or vein, the ruptured lymph vessel is just supermicrosurgically ligated for secure closure.
- **Step 4. Supermicrosurgical Anastomosis in an Intima-to-Intima Coaptation** [Fig. 50.17]. Lymphotomy is performed on the recipient lymph vessel, and end-to-side LLA is performed; the ruptured lymph vessel stump is anastomosed to a side of the recipient lymph vessel to preserve native lymph flow in the recipient.
- **Step 5. Evaluation of Patency and Leakage** [Fig. 50.18]. Anastomosis site is evaluated under intraoperative ICG lymphography navigation; there should be good flow and no leakage.
- **Step 6. Placement of Drain and Skin Closure**. Wound is closed layer by layer, after placement of a drain.

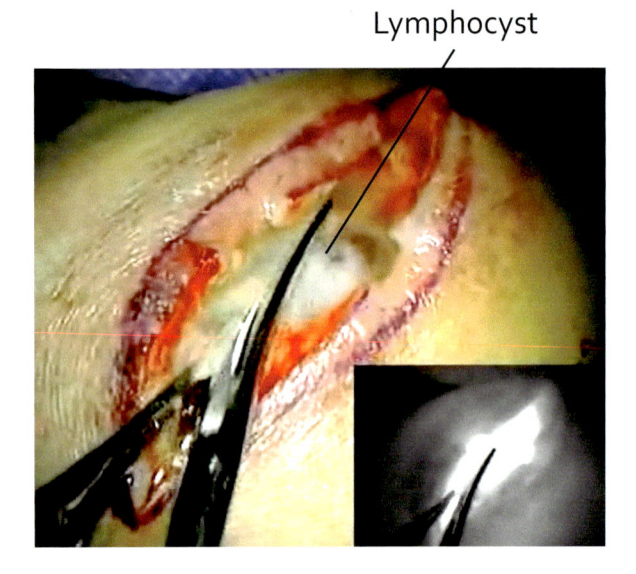

Fig. 50.14 LLA step 1. A lymphocyst is opened to seek for ruptured lymph vessels. Intraoperative ICG lymphography navigation (lower right)

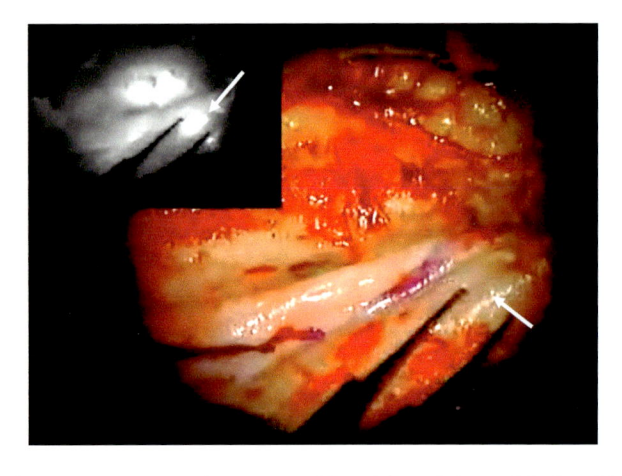

Fig. 50.15 LLA step 2. A ruptured lymph vessel (arrows) is found in the lesion. Intraoperative ICG lymphography navigation (upper left)

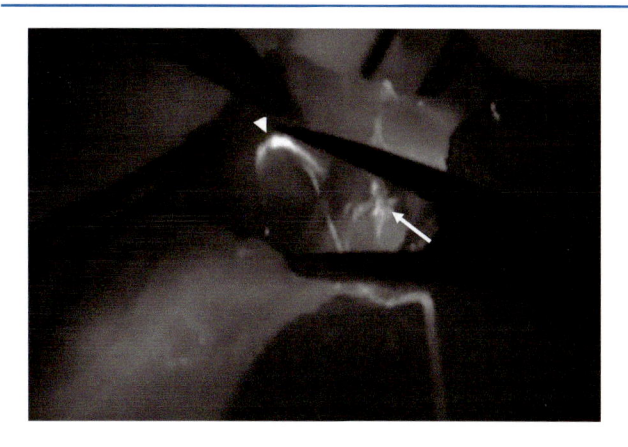

Fig. 50.16 LLA step 3. An intact lymph vessel (arrowhead), located close to the ruptured lymph vessel (arrow), is dissected under intraoperative ICG lymphography navigation

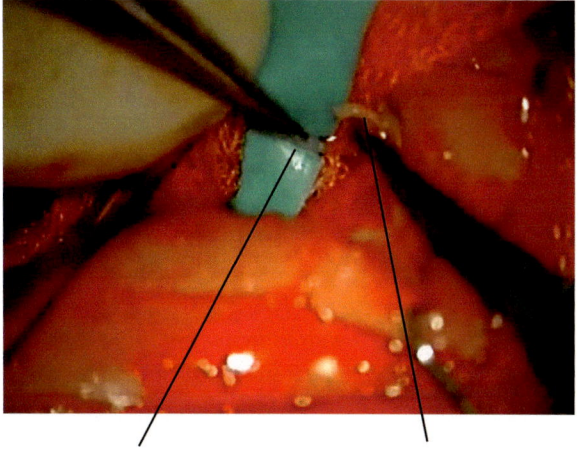

Fig. 50.17 LLA step 4. End-to-side LLA is performed using 12–0 supermicro-suture

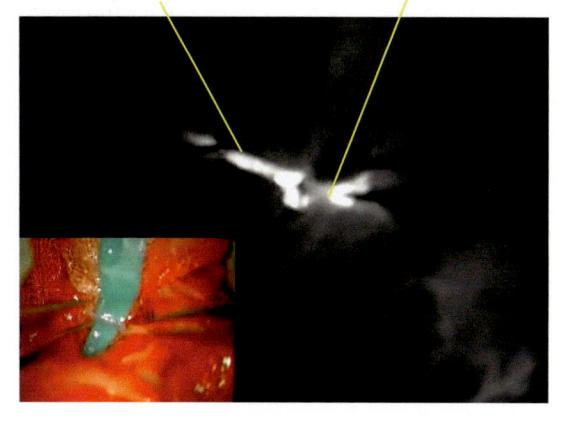

Fig. 50.18 LLA step 5. Anastomosis site is evaluated regarding patency and leakage under intraoperative ICG lymphography navigation. Conventional microsurgical view (lower left)

50.6 Pearls and Pitfalls

Dynamic ICG lymphography is important for evaluation of lymphatic disease before lymphatic supermicrosurgery. LVA is best indicated for ICG stage II–IV cases.

Slightly sclerotic "s1" lymph vessel should be used for LVA. "Overlapping region," revealed by dynamic ICG lymphography, is best for LVA.

Intact lymph vessel should be preserved; LVA should not be performed in a non-edematous region where ICG lymphography shows linear pattern only.

Bloodless inter-lobular dissection is a key to successful supermicrosurgery; all important structures, blood vessel, nerve, and lymph vessel exist between the fat lobules. Once a field is stained or contaminated with blood, it is impossible to securely dissect translucent lymph vessels from the surrounding yellow fat tissues.

Intima-to-intima coaptation anastomosis is a basis of supermicrosurgery; a supermicrosurgeon has to be used to 11–0, 12–0, and 12–0 s supermicro-sutures.

50.7 Selected Readings

- Yamamoto T, Narushima M, Doi K, Oshima A, Ogata F, Mihara M, Koshima I, Mundinger GS. Characteristic indocyanine green lymphography findings in lower extremity lymphedema: the generation of a novel lymphedema severity staging system using dermal backflow patterns. Plast Reconstr Surg. 2011;127(5):1979–86.
- *The first description of characteristic ICG lymphography findings and pathophysiological severity staging system for lower extremity lymphedema based on ICG lymphography findings. Linear, Splash, Stardust, and Diffuse patterns are introduced.*
- Yamamoto T, Yamamoto N, Yoshimatsu H, Narushima M, Koshima I. Factors associated with lymphosclerosis: an analysis on 962 lymphatic vessels. Plast Reconstr Surg 2017;140(4):734–41.
- *Severity grade for lymphosclerosis, consisting of "s0," "s1," "s2," and "s3", is described. Comprehensive analysis with multivariate analysis reveals independent factors associated with lymphosclerosis.*
- Yamamoto T, Narushima M, Yoshimatsu H, Yamamoto N, Kikuchi K, Todokoro T, Iida T, Koshima I. Dynamic indo-

cyanine green lymphography for breast cancer-related arm lymphedema. Ann Plast Surg. 2014;73(6):706–9.
- *The first description of dynamic ICG lymphography. Protocol of dynamic ICG lymphography is reported, and lymph pump function, measured with ICG velocity, is evaluated according to ICG lymphography stage.*
- Yamamoto T, Narushima M, Doi K, Oshima A, Ogata F, Mihara M, Koshima I, Mundinger GS. Characteristic indocyanine green lymphography findings in lower extremity lymphedema: the generation of a novel lymphedema severity staging system using dermal backflow patterns. Plast Reconstr Surg. 2011;127(5):1979–86.
- *The first description of ICG lymphography-based pathophysiological severity staging system for upper extremity lymphedema. Characteristic ICG lymphography findings in upper extremity lymphedema are introduced, and evaluated according to clinical stage.*
- Yamamoto T, Narushima M, Yoshimatsu H, Seki Y, Yamamoto N, Oka A, Hara H, Koshima I. Minimally invasive lymphatic supermicrosurgery (MILS): indocyanine green lymphography-guided simultaneous multi-site lymphaticovenular anastomoses via millimeter skin incisions. Ann Plast Surg. 2014;72(1):67–70.
- *Application of intraoperative ICG lymphography to further minimize invasiveness of LVA surgery. LVA can be performed via a millimeter skin incision with appropriate ICG lymphography mapping.*
- Yamamoto T, Yamamoto N, Azuma S, Yoshimatsu H, Seki Y, Narushima M, Koshima I. Near-infrared illumination system-integrated microscope for supermicrosurgical lymphaticovenular anastomosis. Microsurgery 2014;34(1):23–7.
- *Application of intraoperative ICG lymphography to navigate LVA surgery. Lymph vessels can be easily found even in DB region under intraoperative ICG lymphography navigation.*
- Yamamoto T, Yoshimatsu H, Koshima I. Navigation lymphatic supermicrosurgery for iatrogenic lymphorrhea: supermicrosurgical lymphaticolymphatic anastomosis and lymphaticovenular anastomosis under indocyanine green lymphography navigation. J Plast Reconstr Aesthet Surg. 2014;67(11):1573–9.
- *First description of LLA for intractable lymphorrhea cases. Surgical strategy for intractable lymphorrhea cases are described, including end-to-side LLA and conventional LVA under intraoperative ICG lymphography navigation.*
- Yamamoto T, Yamamoto N, Yamashita M, Furuya M, Hayashi A, Koshima I. Efferent lymphatic vessel anastomosis (ELVA): supermicrosurgical efferent lymphatic vessel-to-venous anastomosis for the prophylactic treatment of subclinical lymphedema. Ann Plast Surg. 2016;76(4):424–7.
- *First description of efferent lymphatic vessel anastomosis for prophylactic treatment of subclinical lymphedema. Ideal way of secondary prophylaxis is described.*
- Yamamoto T, Yoshimatsu H, Yamamoto N. Complete lymph flow reconstruction: a free vascularized lymph node true perforator flap transfer with efferent lymphaticolymphatic anastomosis. J Plast Reconstr Aesthet Surg. 2016;69(9):1227–33.
- *A special case of LLA combined with lymph node transfer, showing the first evidence of lymph drainage after lymph node transfer. The efferent lymph vessel of the transferred lymph node is anastomosed to contralateral iliac lymph vessel, to achieve complete lymph flow reconstruction.*
- Yamamoto T, Narushima M, Kikuchi K, Yoshimatsu H, Todokoro T, Mihara M, Koshima I. Lambda-shaped anastomosis with intravascular stenting method for safe and effective lymphaticovenular anastomosis. Plast Reconstr Surg. 2011;127(5):1987–92.
- *Introduction of int ravascular stenting method for lambda-shaped LVA. Bidirectional bypass LVA can be safely performed even by a beginner supermicrosurgeon with modified intravascular stenting method.*

Part IV
Appendix

Cadaveric Anatomy: Microvascular Flaps Dissection

51

Georgios Pafitanis, Dajiang Song, and Youmao Zheng

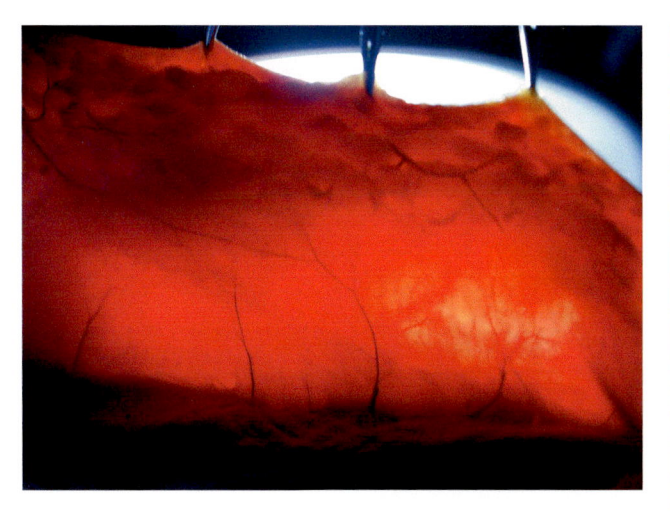

Fig. 51.1 Fasciocutaneous flap perforators dissection

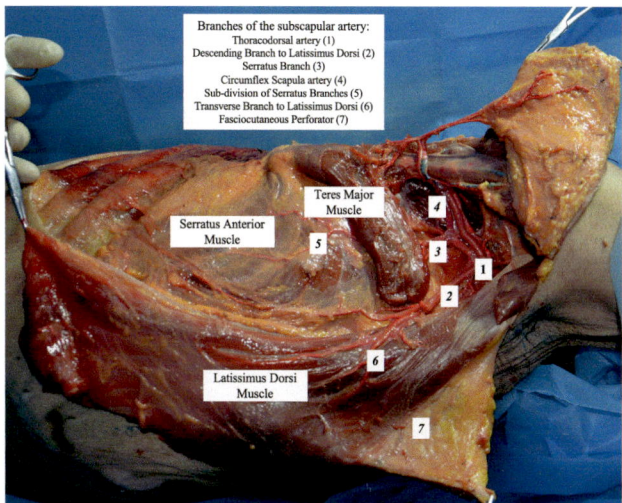

Fig. 51.2 Chapter 14: LD muscle flap

G. Pafitanis (✉)
Department of Plastic Surgery, Emergency Care and Trauma Division (ECAT), The Royal London Hospital, Barts Health NHS Trust & University College Hospital London (UCLH), London, UK
e-mail: georgios.pafitanis@nhs.net

D. Song
Department of Oncology Plastic Surgery, Hunan Cancer Hospital and The Affiliated Cancer Hospital of Xiangya School of Medicine, Central South University, Changsha, Hunan, China

Y. Zheng
Department of Hand and Foot Surgery, Taizhou Hospital, Wenzhou Medical University and The Third Affiliated Hospital of Southern Medical University, Taizhou, Zhejiang Province, China

© Springer Nature Switzerland AG 2023
D. Nikkhah et al. (eds.), *Core Techniques in Flap Reconstructive Microsurgery*, https://doi.org/10.1007/978-3-031-07678-7_51

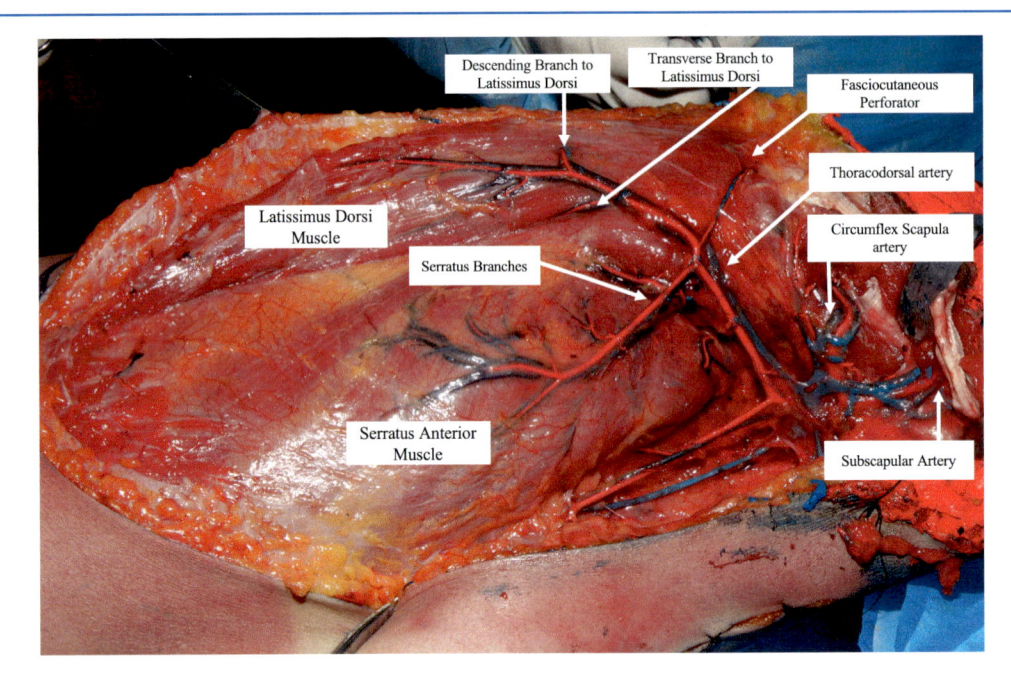

Fig. 51.3 Chapter 15: TDAP fc flap

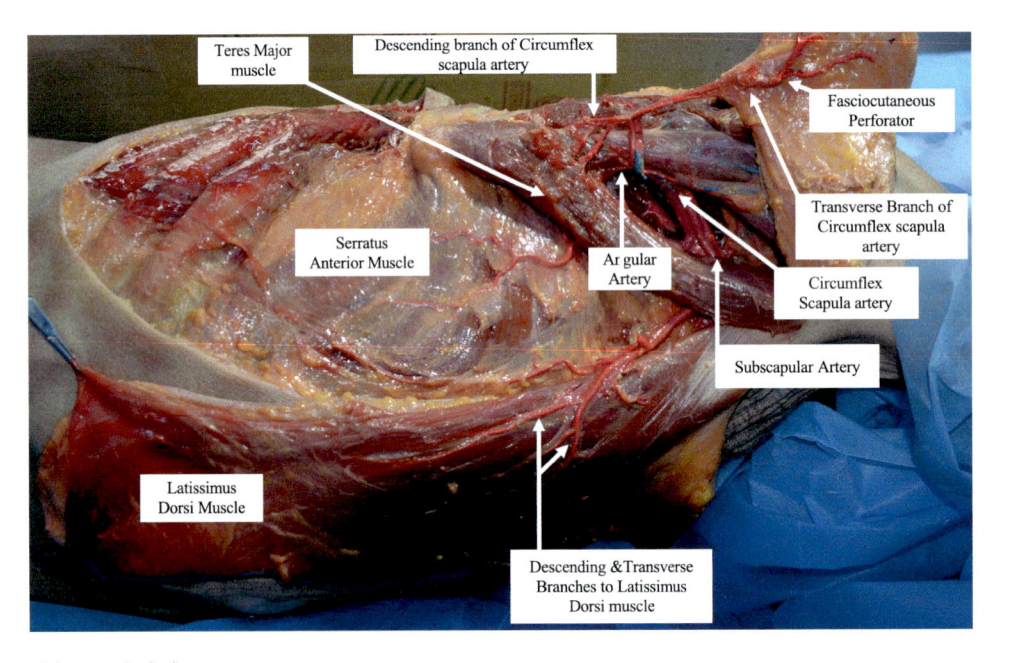

Fig. 51.4 Chapter 16: scapula fc flap

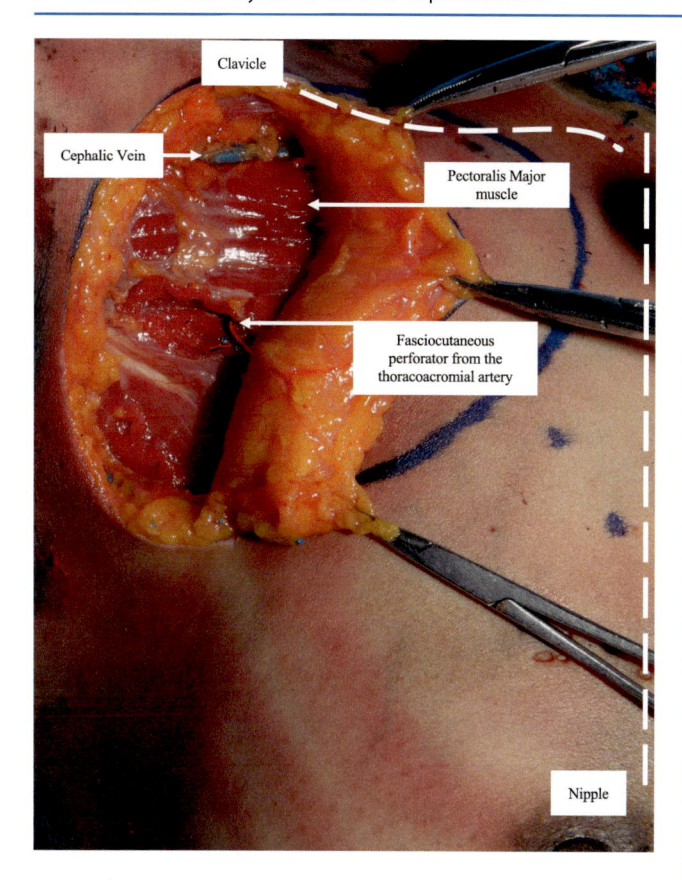

Fig. 51.5 Chapter 17: TAAP fc clap

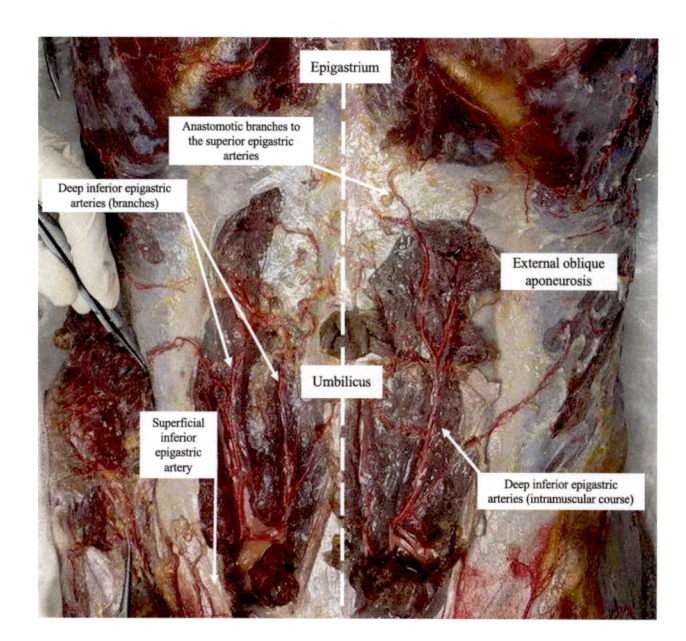

Fig. 51.6 Chapter 19: DIEAP flap

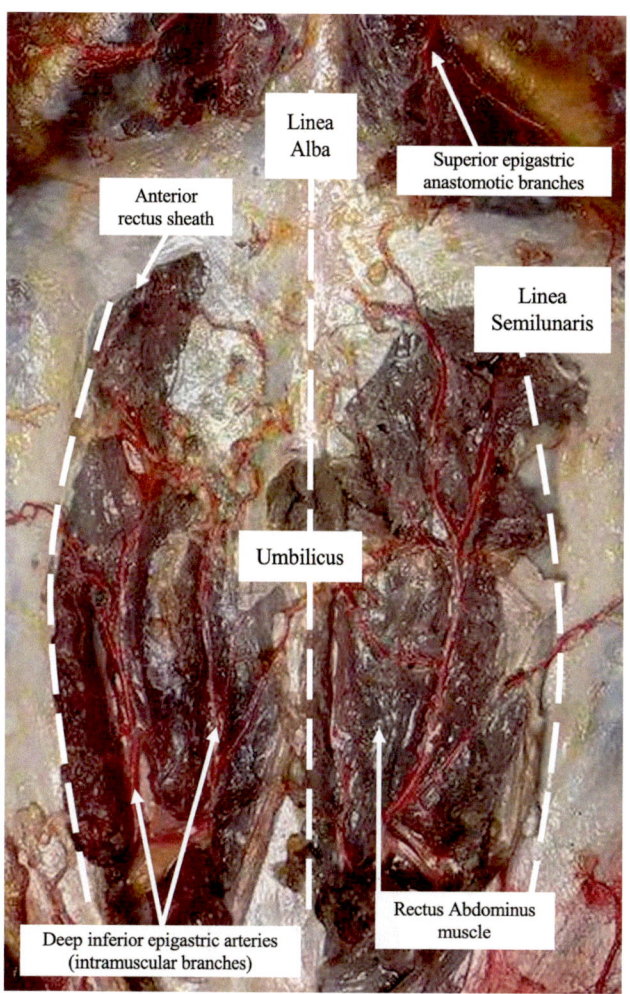

Fig. 51.7 Chapter 20: rectus mc flap

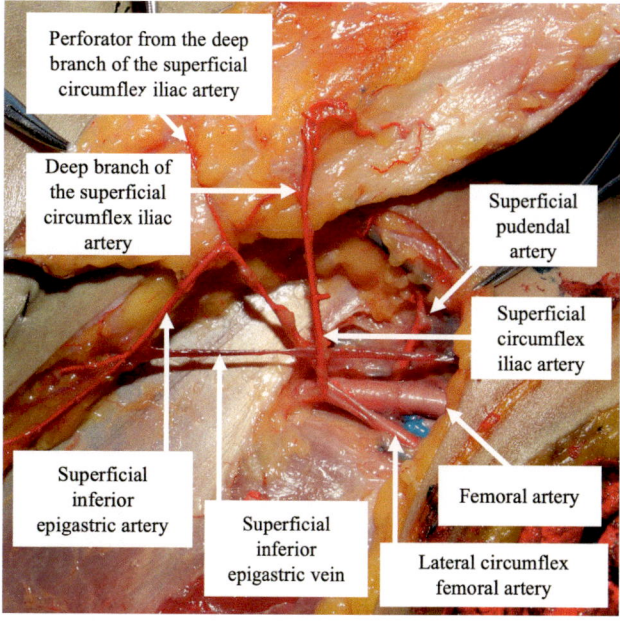

Fig. 51.8 Chapter 21: SCIA SIAE flaps

Fig. 51.9 Chapter 22: SGA flaps

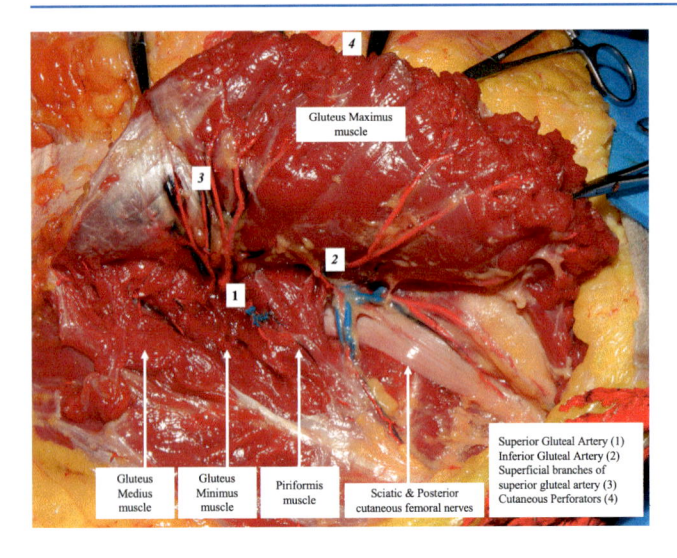

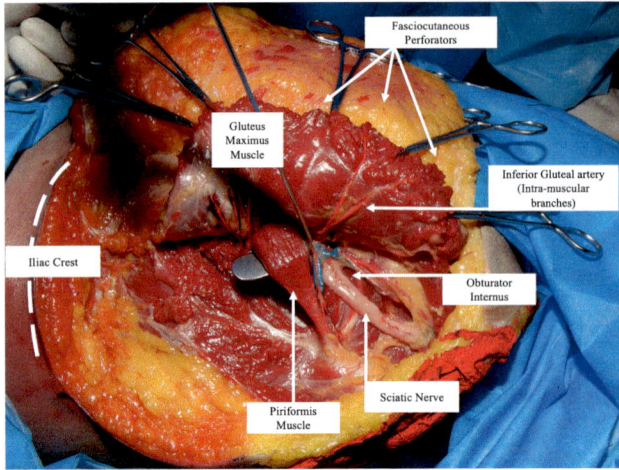

Fig. 51.10 Chapter 23: IGA flaps

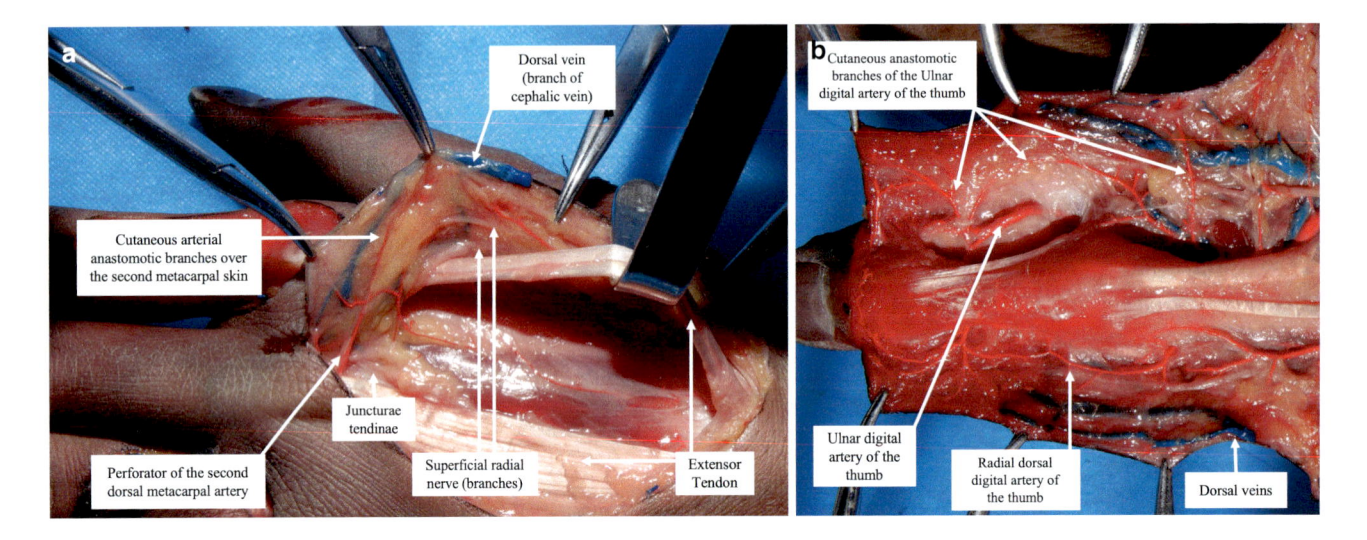

Fig. 51.11 Chapter 26: dorsal metacarpal flaps

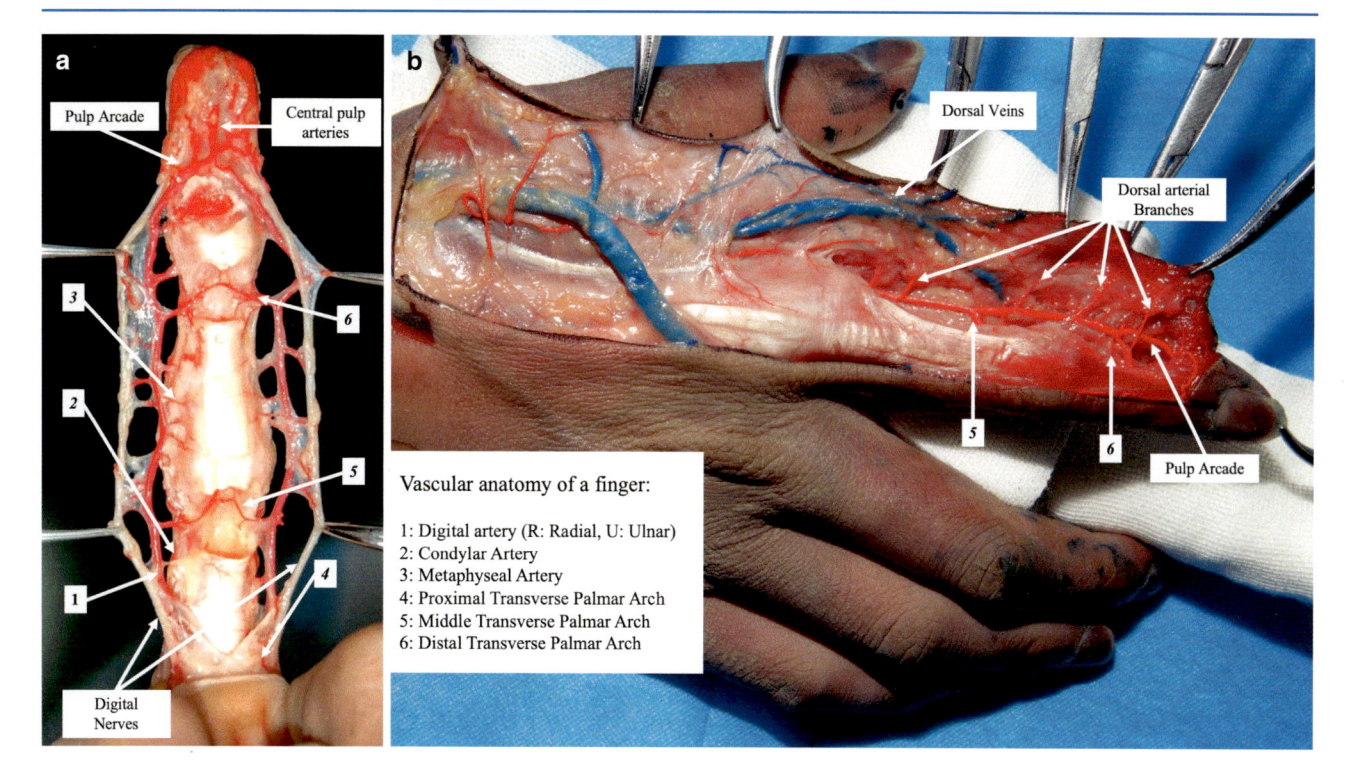

51 Cadaveric Anatomy: Microvascular Flaps Dissection

Fig. 51.12 Chapter 27: digital artery flaps

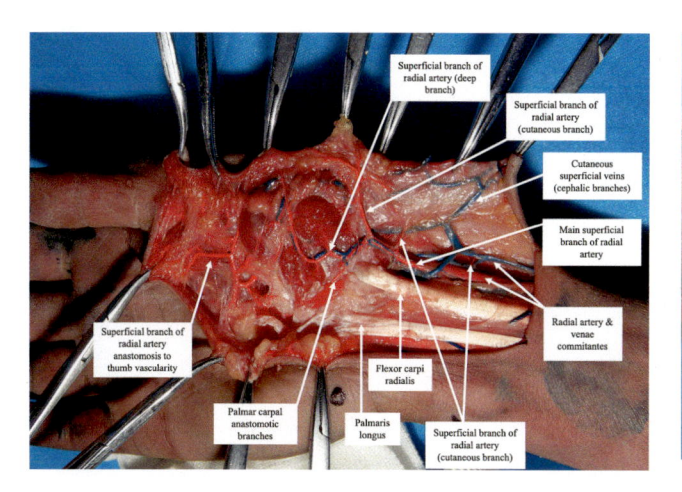

Fig. 51.13 Chapter 28: radial artery flaps

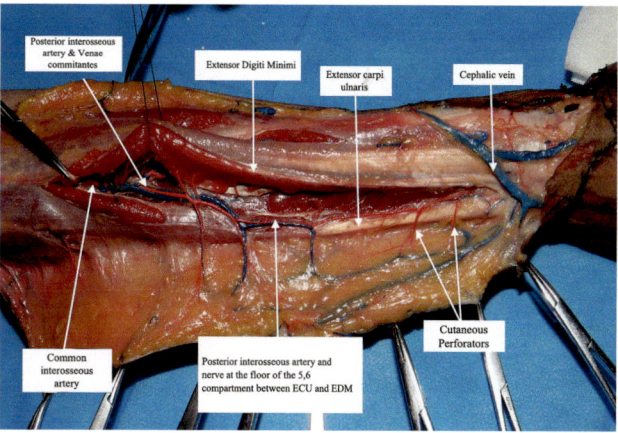

Fig. 51.14 Chapter 29: posterior interosseous flap

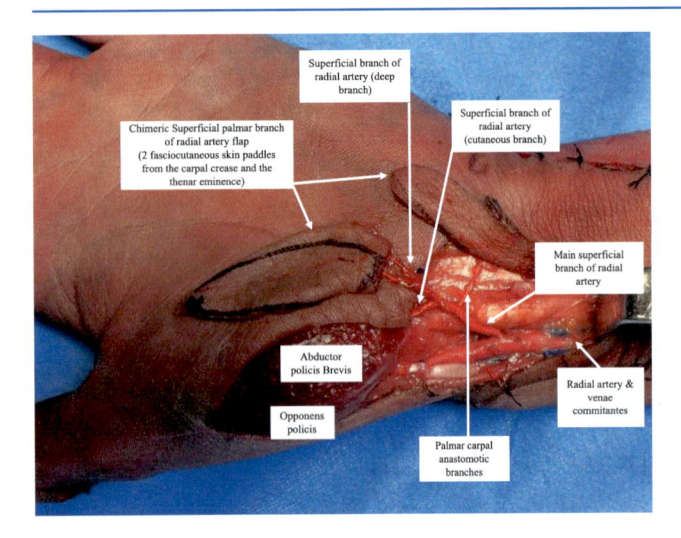

Fig. 51.15 Chapter 31: superficial radial artery flap

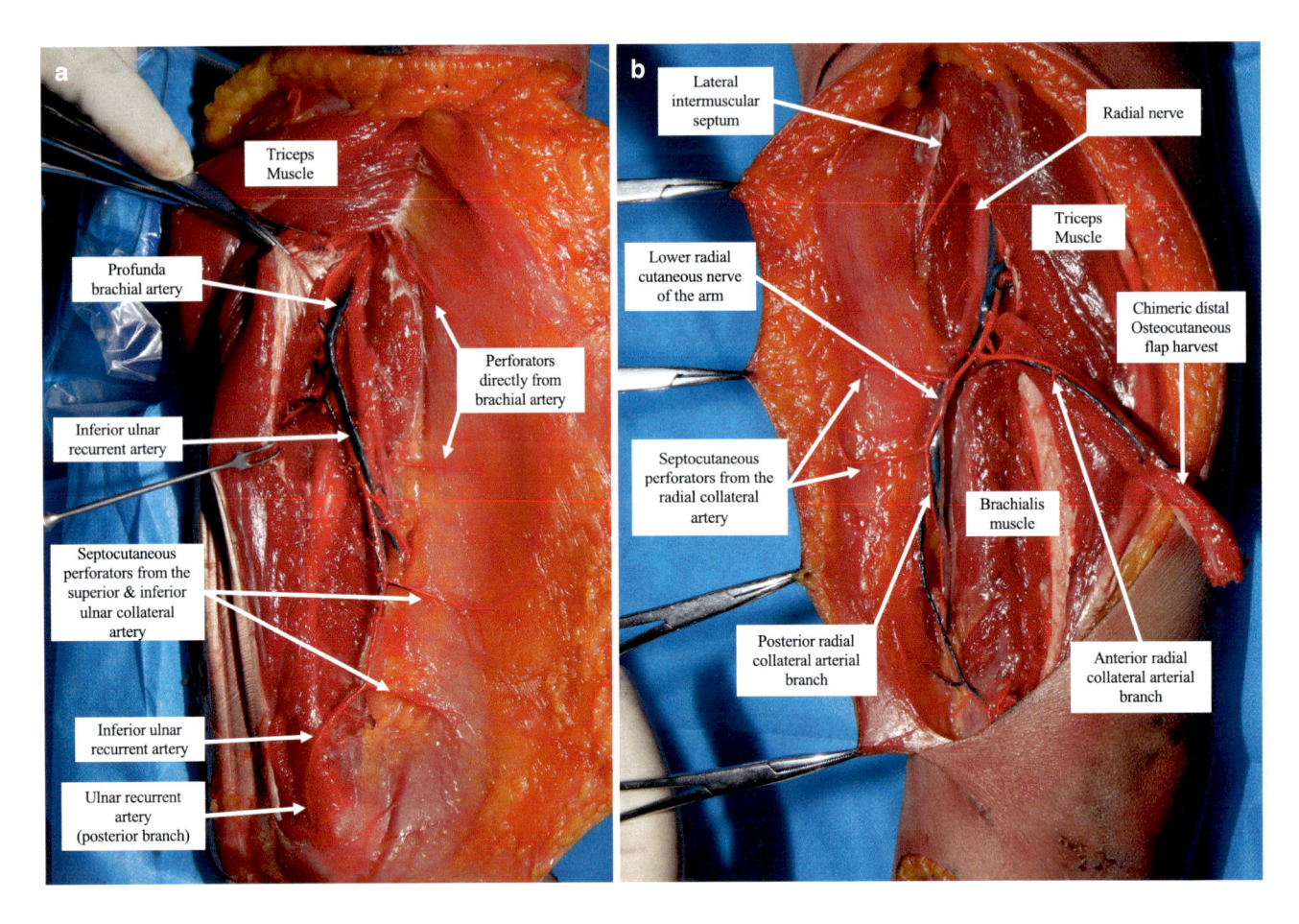

Fig. 51.16 Chapter 32: medial and lateral arm flaps

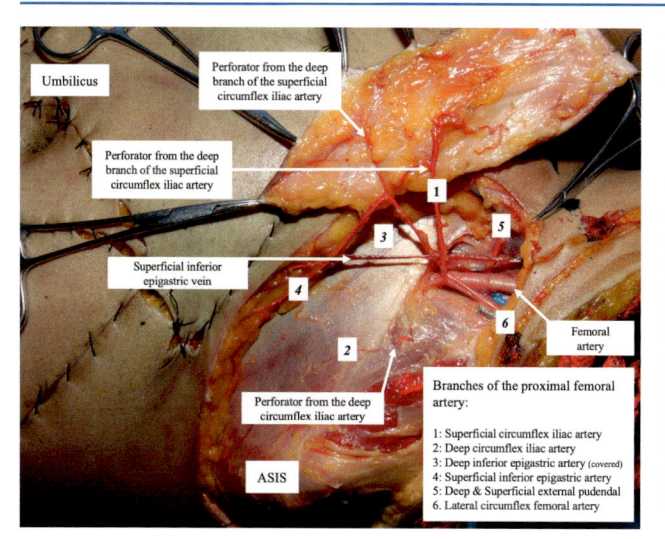

51 Cadaveric Anatomy: Microvascular Flaps Dissection

Fig. 51.17 Chapter 34: SCIP flaps

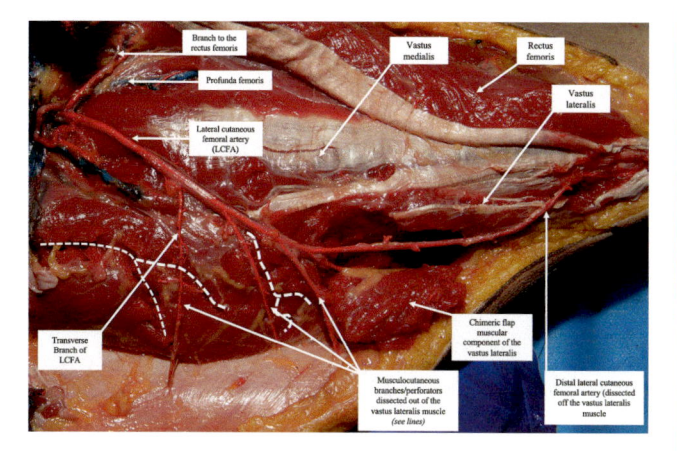

Fig. 51.18 Chapter 35: LCFA flaps

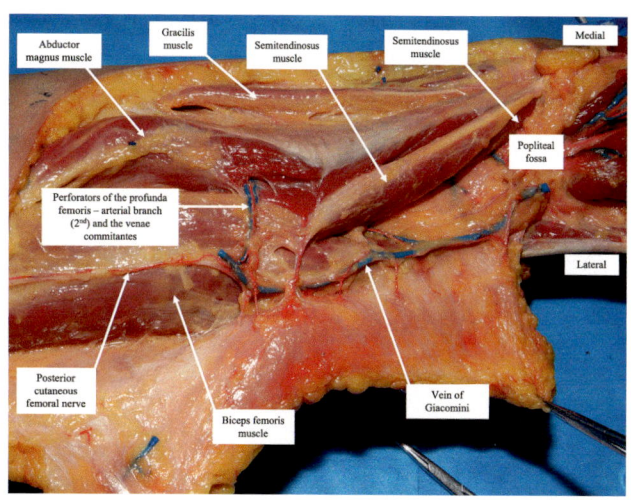

Fig. 51.19 Chapter 38: PAP flap

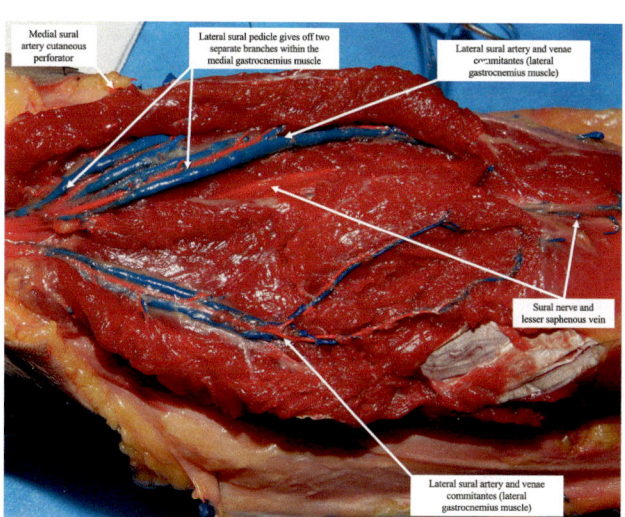

Fig. 51.20 Chapter 40: MSAP—gastrocnemius flap

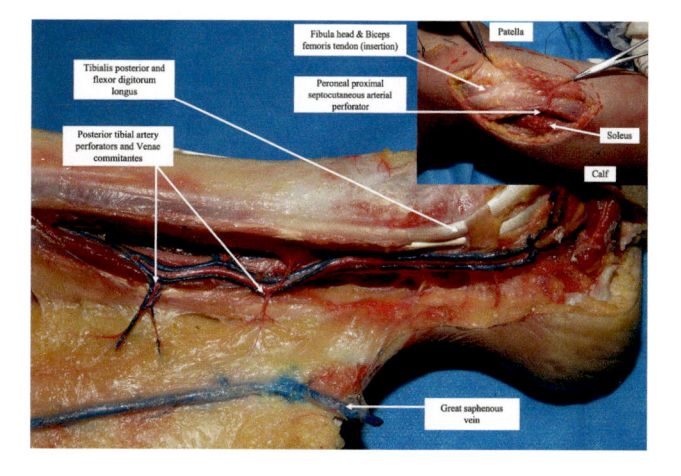

Fig. 51.21 Chapter 42: PTA—peroneal perforators

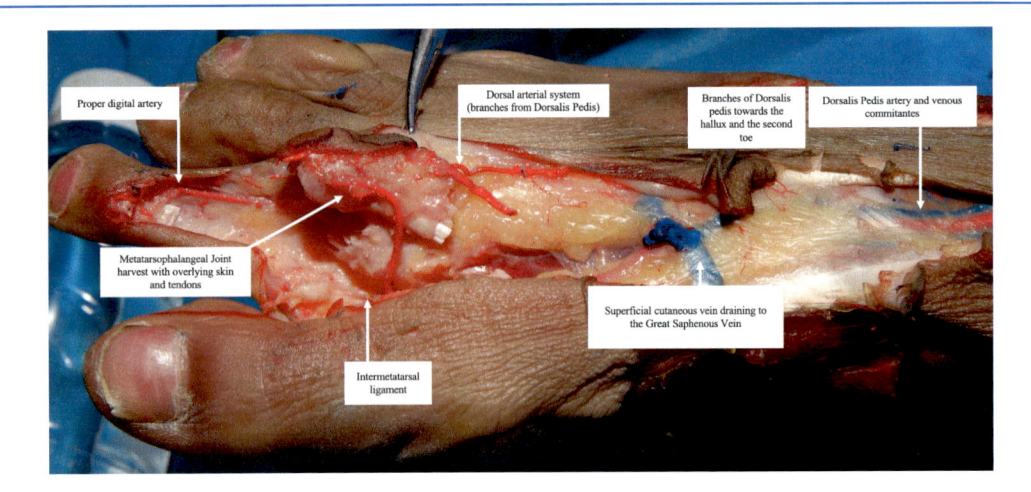

Fig. 51.22 Chapter 43: second toe flap

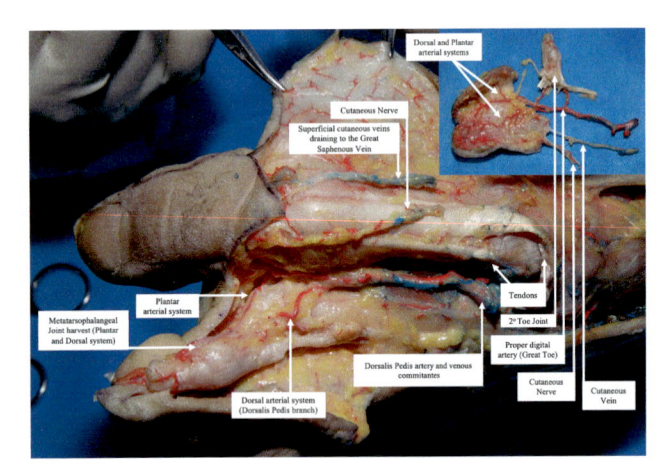

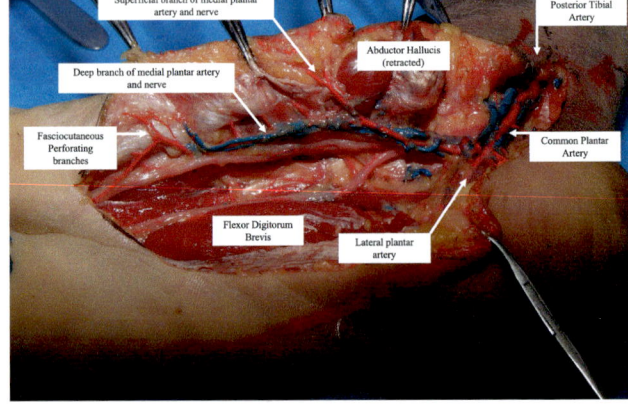

Fig. 51.23 Chapter 44: great toe flap

Fig. 51.24 Chapter 45: medial plantar flap

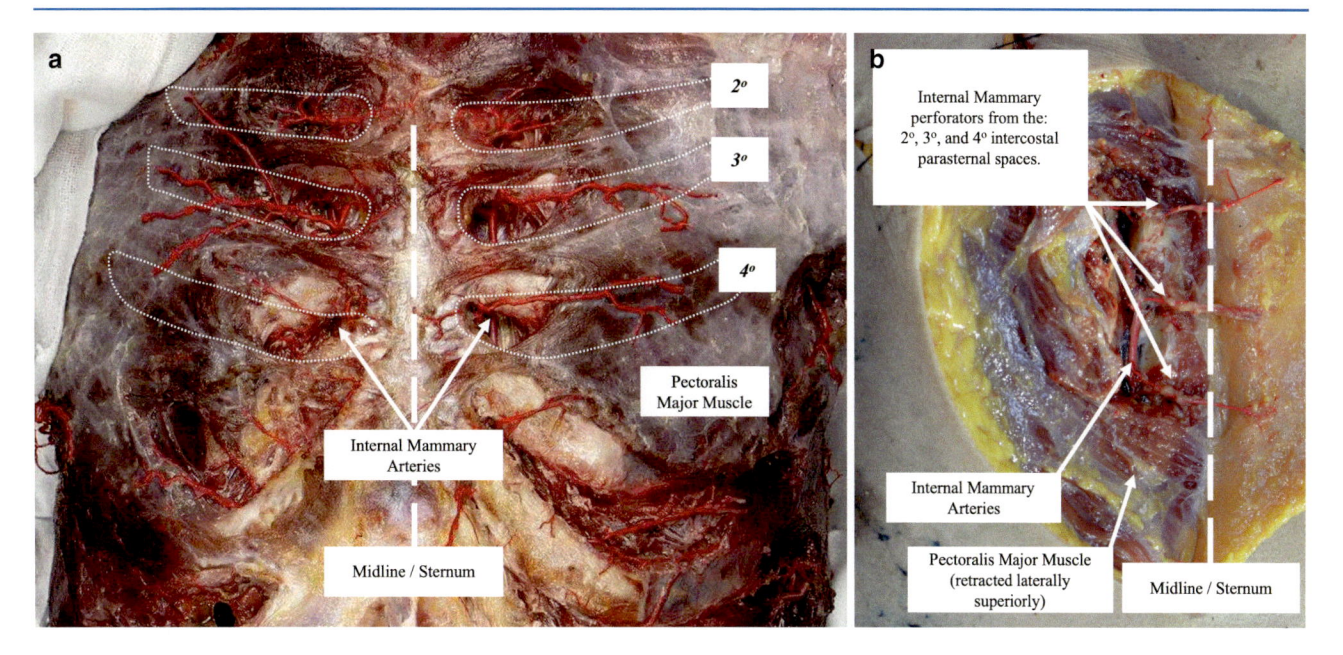

51   Cadaveric Anatomy: Microvascular Flaps Dissection   507

Fig. 51.25 Chapter 46: Internal mammary artery perforators

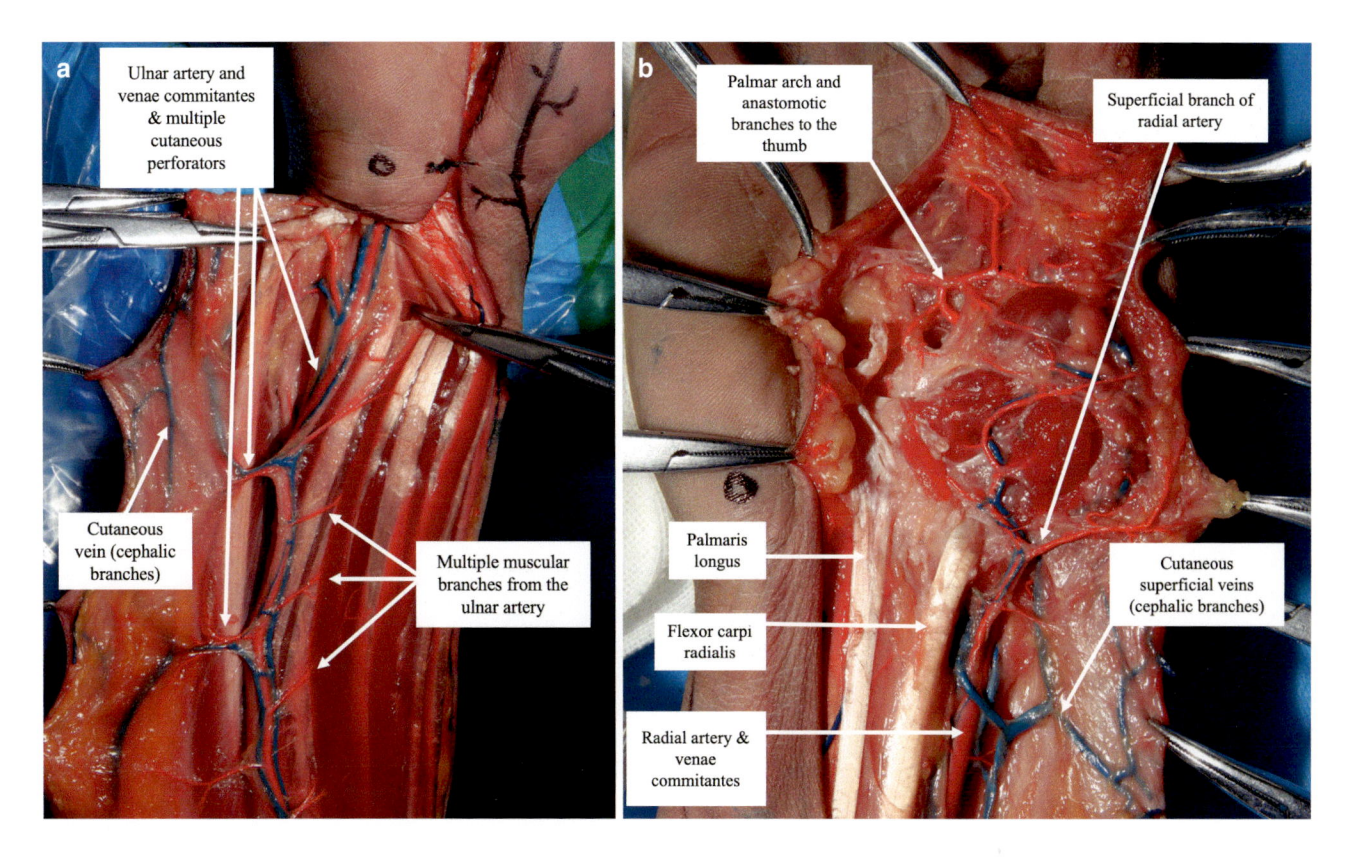

Fig. 51.26 Chapter 48: Upper Limb Vessels

Fig. 51.27 Chapter 49: Posterior Tibial Artery Perforators

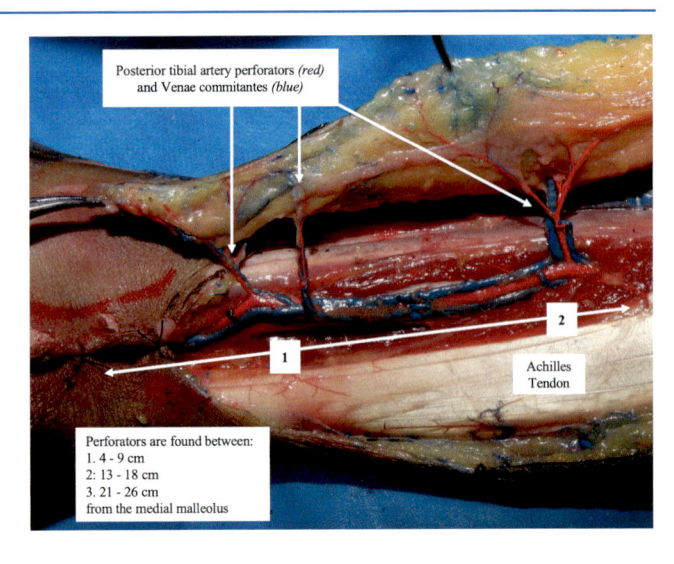